J. Rello · M. Kollef · E. Díaz · A. Rodríguez (Eds.) Infect

J. Rello · M. Kollef · E. Díaz · A. Rodríguez (Eds.)

Infectious Diseases in Critical Care

With 57 Figures and 137 Tables

Springer

Jordi Rello, MD, PhD
Critical Care Department, Joan XXIII University Hospital
Carrer Mallafré Guasch, 4
E-43007 Tarragona, Spain

Marin Kollef, MD
Professor of Medicine
Director, Medical Intensive Care Unit
Washington University School of Medicine
Barnes-Jewish Hospital
660 South Euclid Avenue
Campus Box 8052
St. Louis, MO 63110-1093, USA

Emili Díaz, MD
Intensive Care Department, Joan XXIII University Hospital
Carrer Mallafré Guasch, 4
E-43007 Tarragona, Spain

Alejandro Rodríguez, MD, PhD
Critical Care Department, Joan XXIII University Hospital
Carrer Mallafré Guasch, 4
E-43007 Tarragona, Spain

ISBN 978-3-540-34405-6 Springer-Verlag Berlin Heidelberg New York

Library of Congress Control Number: 2006933721

Springer is a part of Springer Science+Business Media
http://www.springer.com

Printed in Germany

Editor: Dr. Ute Heilmann
Desk Editor: Dörthe Mennecke-Bühler
Production Editor: Joachim W. Schmidt

Cover design: eStudio Calamar, Spain

Typesetting: FotoSatz Pfeifer GmbH, D-82166 Gräfelfing
Printed on acid-free paper – 24/3150 – 5 4 3 2 1 0

Preface

Infections and their complications are a very important clinical area in the intensive care unit setting. Community-acquired infections and nosocomial infections both contribute to the high level of disease acquisition common among critically ill patients. The accurate diagnosis of nosocomial infections and the provision of appropriate therapies, including antimicrobial therapy effective against the identified agents of infection, have been shown to be important determinants of patient outcome. Critical care practitioners are in a unique position in dealing with infectious diseases. They are often the initial providers of care to seriously ill patients with infections.

Additionally, they have a responsibility to ensure that nosocomial infections are prevented and that antimicrobial resistance is minimized by prudently employing antibiotic agents. It is the editors' hope that this book will provide clinicians practicing in the intensive care unit with a reference to help guide their care of infected patients. To that end they have brought together a group of international authors to address important topics related to infectious diseases for the critical care practitioner.

February 2007

Jordi Rello
Marin H. Kollef
Emili Díaz
Alejandro Rodríguez

Contents

VI Infections with Surgical Implications

List of Contributors

Antonio Anzueto, MD
VERDICT (11C6), South Texas Veterans Health Care System, Audie L. Murphy Division, San Antonio
7400 Merton Minter Boulevard
San Antonio, TX 78284, USA

Abhijit M. Bal, MD
Department of Medical Microbiology, Aberdeen Royal Infirmary, Foresterhill
Aberdeen, AB25 2ZN, UK

Josep-E. Baños, MD, PhD
Department of Experimental and Health Sciences
Universitat Pompeu Fabra, Dr. Aiguader 80
08003 Barcelona, Spain

Philip S. Barie, MD
Department of Surgery, Anne and Max A. Cohen Surgical Intensive Care Unit, P713A, New York-Presbyterian Hospital, Weill Cornell Medical Center
525 East 68th Street
New York, NY 10021, USA
Division of Critical Care and Trauma, Weill Medical College of Cornell University, New York, USA

Rosemary A. Barnes, MD, MSc
Department of Medical Microbiology, School of Medicine, Cardiff University, Heath Park
Cardiff CF14 4XN, UK

Nicolau Barquet, MD, PhD
CAP Bordeta-Magòria, Institut Català de la Salut
Calvet 47 – 49 entresòl A
08021 Barcelona, Spain

Torsten T. Bauer, MD
Abteilung für Pneumologie, Allergologie und Schlafmedizin, Medizinische Klinik und Poliklinik
Bochum, Germany

Susan J. Bersoff-Matcha, MD
Kaiser-Permanente West End Medical Center
2100 Pennsylvania Avenue, NW
Washington, DC 20037, USA

Kavita P. Bhavan
Division of Infectious Diseases, Washington University School of Medicine, 660 South Euclid Avenue
Saint Louis, MO 63132, USA

Stijn Blot, PhD
Department of Intensive Care, Ghent University Hospital, De Pintelaan 185
9000 Ghent, Belgium

María Bodí, MD, PhD
Critical Care Department, Hospital Universitari Joan XXIII de Tarragona, Mallafré Guasch, 4
43007 Tarragona, Spain

Emilio Bouza, MD, PhD
Department of Clinical Microbiology and Infectious Diseases, Hospital General Universitario Gregorio Marañón, University of Madrid, Dr. Esquerdo 46
28007 Madrid, Spain

Peter R. Brookmeyer, MD
Washington University School of Medicine
St. Louis MO 63110, USA
316 N Meade Ave., Colorado Springs
CO 80909, USA

Erwin M. Brown, MD
Department of Medical Microbiology, Frenchay Hospital, Frenchay Park Road
Bristol, BS16 1LE, UK

Culley Carson, MD
Division of Urologic Surgery, University of North Carolina at Chapel Hill
Chapel Hill, NC 27599, USA

Xavier Castella, MD
Intensive Care Unit, Hospital Nostra Senyora de Meritxell
Escaldes, Andorra

Pedro Castro Rebollo, MD
Critical Care Department, Hospital Clinic, IDIBAPS School of Medicine, University of Barcelona, Villarroel 170
08030 Barcelona, Spain

José M. Cisneros, MD, PhD
Servicio de Enfermedades Infecciosas, Hospital Universitario Virgen del Rocío
Avda. Manuel Siurot s/n
41013 Seville, Spain

Jeremy Cohen, BSc, MRCP
Department of Intensive Care Medicine, Ned Hanlon Building, Royal Brisbane and Women's Hospital
Butterfield Street, Herston
Brisbane 4029 Queensland, Australia

Jon Cohen, MB, FRCP
Department of Infectious Diseases, Faculty of Medicine, Imperial College
London, W12 0NN, UK

Elisa Cordero, MD
Servicio de Enfermedades Infecciosas, Hospital Universitario Virgen del Rocío
Avda. Manuel Siurot s/n
41013 Seville, Spain

Humberto Correa, MD
Joan XXIII University Hospital, Carrer Dr. Mallafré Guasch 4, 43007 Tarragona, Spain

Stephen W. Crawford, MD, CPHRM
CIGNA Healthcare, LIFESOURCE Transplant Network
3200 Park Lane Office Center
Pittsburgh, Pennsylvania, 15275, USA

Núria Cruz, MD
Servei de Farmacologia Clínica, Unitat d'Avaluació Suport i Prevenció (UASP), Institut d'Investigacions Biomèdiques August Pi i Sunyer (IDIBAPS), Hospital Clínic, Villarroel 170
08036 Barcelona, Spain

H. Dele Davies, MD, MSc
Departments of Pediatrics and Human Development Michigan State University, College of Human Medicine, B240 Life Sciences Building
East Lansing, MI 48824, USA

Pieter Depuydt, MD
Department of Intensive Care, Ghent University Hospital, De Pintelaan 185
9000 Ghent, Belgium

Emili Díaz, MD, PhD
Critical Care Department, University Rovira & Virgili Medical School, Institut Pere Virgili, Joan XXIII University Hospital, Carrer Mallafré Guasch, 4
43007 Tarragona, Spain

George Dimopoulos, MD, PhD
Department of Intensive Care, ATTIKO University Hospital, Medical School, University of Athens
7 Kiprou Av., 14569, Anixi, Attiki, Athens, Greece

Pere Domingo, MD, PhD
Department of Internal Medicine, Hospital de la Santa Creu i Sant Pau, Terol 2–4 2nd
08012 Barcelona, Spain

Soumitra R. Eachempati, MD
Division of Critical Care and Trauma, Weill Medical College of Cornell University, New York, USA

Charles E. Edmiston, Jr, PhD, CIC
Department of Surgery, Medical College of Wisconsin & Froedtert Hospital, 9200 West Wisconsin Avenue
Milwaukee, WI 53226, USA

Magí Farré, MD, PhD
Department of Pharmacology, Institut Municipal d'Investigació Mèdica, Dr Aiguader, 80
08003 Barcelona, Spain
Department of Pharmacology, Therapeutics and Toxicology, School of Medicine, Universitat Autònoma de Barcelona 08193 Bellaterra, Spain

Charles Feldman, MB, PhD
Department of Medicine, Johannesburg Hospital and University of the Witwatersrand
7 York Road, Parktown
2193, Johannesburg, South Africa

Ross Freebairn, MB, ChB
Intensive Care Services, Hawke's Bay Hospital
Hastings, New Zealand

José Garnacho-Montero, MD
Critical Care Department, Vírgen del Rocío University Hospital, Avda. Manuel Siurot, s/n
41013 Seville, Spain

Josep Maria Gatell, MD
Department of Infectious Diseases, Hospital Clinic IDIBAPS, School of Medicine, University of Barcelona
Villarroel 170, 08030 Barcelona, Spain

Joan Gavaldà, MD, PhD
Infectious Diseases Department, Hospital Vall d'Hebron, P. Vall d'Hebron 119–129
08035 Barcelona Spain

Clare N. Gentry, MD
Division of Infectious Diseases, Washington University School of Medicine, 660 S. Euclid Ave.
Campus Box 8051, St. Louis, MO 63110, USA

Ian M. Gould, MD
Department of Medical Microbiology, Aberdeen Royal Infirmary, Foresterhill, Aberdeen, AB25 2ZN, UK

Bonnie F. Grahn, BSN, CIC
Infection Control Section, Froedtert Hospital
9200 West Wisconsin Avenue
Milwaukee, WI 53226 USA

Maritza L. Groth, MD
Medical Intensive Care Unit, Winthrop University Hospital, Mineola, NY, USA

Juan J. Guardiola, MD
Department of Pulmonary, Critical Care and Sleep Medicine, University of Louisville, 550 S. Jackson Street, ACB-3, Louisville, KY 40202, USA

Laure Hammer, MD
Department of Cardiology and Hypertension, University Hospital Albert Michallon, BP 217
38043 Grenoble Cedex 9, France

Ravishankar Hasanadka, MD
Division of Vascular Surgery, Medical College of Wisconsin, 9200 West Wisconsin Avenue
Milwaukee WI 53226, USA

Thomas L. Husted, MD
Department of Surgery, University of Cincinnati College of Medicine, 231 Albert Sabin Way
Cincinnati OH 45267-0558, USA

Mubeen A. Jafri, MD
Department of Surgery, University of Cincinnati College of Medicine, 231 Albert Sabin Way
Cincinnati OH 45267-0558, USA

Christopher P. Johnson, MD
Division of Transplant Surgery, Froedtert and Medical College Transplant Center, 9200 West Wisconsin Avenue, Milwaukee, WI 53226, USA

Marin H. Kollef, MD
Department of Pulmonary and Critical Care Medicine, Washington University School of Medicine
Barnes-Jewish Hospital, 660 South Euclid Ave.
Campus Box 8052, St. Louis, MO 63110-1093, USA

Despoina Koulenti, MD
Joan XXIII University Hospital, Carrer Dr. Mallafré Guasch 4, 43007 Tarragona, Spain

Tiffany M. Lasky, DO
Department of Surgery, University of Cincinnati College of Medicine, 231 Albert Sabin Way
Cincinnati, OH 45269-0558, USA

Kevin B. Laupland, MD, MSc
Departments of Medicine and Critical Care Medicine
University of Calgary, Room 1W-415, #9
3535 Research Road NW, Calgary, Alberta, Canada
T2L 2K8

Oscar Len, MD, PhD
Infectious Diseases Department, Hospital Vall d'Hebron, P. Vall d'Hebron 119–129
08035 Barcelona Spain

Carlos Ortiz Leyba, MD
Intensive Care Unit, Vírgen del Rocío University Hospital, Avda. Manuel Siurot, s/n
41013 Seville, Spain

Jeffrey Lipman, MD
Department of Intensive Care Medicine, 3rd Floor Ned Hanlon Building, Royal Brisbane and Women's Hospital, Butterfield Street, Herston
Brisbane 4029, Queensland, Australia

Martin Llewelyn, MB, MRCP, PhD
Infectious Diseases & Therapeutics, Brighton and Sussex Medical School, Medical Research Building
University of Sussex
Falmer, BN1 9PS, UK

Raúl Lombardi, MD
Department of Critical Care Medicine, IMPASA, L.A. de Herrera 2275, CP 11600, Montevideo, Uruguay
Dialysis Unit, Instituto de Nefrología y Urología
Montevideo, Uruguay

Diego López Mendoza, MD
Fundación Jiménez Díaz-Capio University Hospital, Madrid, Spain

Jay R. McDonald, MD
Washington University School of Medicine, Division of Infectious Diseases, St. Louis VA Medical Center
915 N. Grand Blvd. (151/JC), St. Louis, MO 63106
USA

Daniel McRackan, MD
Division of Urologic Surgery, University of North Carolina at Chapel Hill, Chapel Hill, NC 27599, USA

Francesc Marco, MD
Department of Microbiology, Hospital Clinic, IDIBAPS, School of Medicine, University of Barcelona
Villarroel 170, 08030 Barcelona, Spain

Javier Aznar Martín, MD, PhD
Microbiology Service, Virgen del Rocío University Hospital, 41013 Seville, Spain

José Antonio Martínez, MD, PhD
Department of Infectious Diseases, IDIBAPS, School of Medicine, University of Barcelona, Villarroel 170
08030 Barcelona, Spain

Scott T. Micek, PharmD
Department of Pharmacy, Barnes-Jewish Hospital, Washington University School of Medicine
St. Louis, Missouri, USA

Lee Morrow, MD, MSc
Pulmonary and Critical Care Division, Creighton University Medical Center, Suite #3820, 601 North 30th Street, Omaha, NE 68131, USA

Eric W. Mueller, MD
Department of Surgery, University of Cincinnati College of Medicine, 231 Albert Sabin Way
Cincinnati OH 45267-0558, USA

Linda M. Mundy, MD
School of Public Health, Saint Louis University
3545 Lafayette Avenue, St. Louis, MO 63104, USA

Patricia Muñoz, MD, PhD
Department of Clinical Microbiology and Infectious Diseases, Hospital General Universitario Gregorio Marañón, University of Madrid, Dr. Esquerdo 46
28007 Madrid, Spain

Josep Maria Nicolás, MD
Critical Care Department, Hospital Clinic, IDIBAPS School of Medicine, University of Barcelona Villarroel 170, 08030 Barcelona, Spain

Michael S. Niederman, MD
Department of Medicine, Winthrop-University Hospital, 222 Station Plaza N., Suite 509
Mineola, NY 11501, USA

Jerónimo Pachón, MD
Servicio de Enfermedades Infecciosas, Hospital Universitario Virgen del Rocío
Avda. Manuel Siurot s/n
41013 Seville, Spain

Albert Pahissa, MD, PhD
Infectious Diseases Department, Hospital Vall d'Hebron, P. Vall d'Hebron 119–129
08035 Barcelona, Spain

José Artur Paiva, MD, PhD
Serviço de Cuidados Intensivos, Hospital de S. João
Porto, Portugal

José Manuel Pereira, MD
Serviço de Cuidados Intensivos, Hospital de S. João
Porto, Portugal

Omar J. Pérez-Jimenez, MD
Bella Vista Hospital
351 Hostos Ave., Suite 202
Mayaguez, Puerto Rico 00680-1503

Fredric M. Pieracci, MD
Departments of Surgery and Public Health, New York-Presbyterian Hospital, Weill Cornell Medical Center
525 East 68th Street, New York, NY 10021, USA

Alejandro Ramírez, MD
Intensive Care Unit, University Hospital Puerta del Mar, University of Cádiz, Av. Ana de Viya 21
11009 Cádiz, Spain

Jordi Rello, MD, PhD (jrello.hj23.ics@gencat.net)
Critical Care Department, University Rovira & Virgili Medical School, Institut Pere Virgili, Joan XXIII University Hospital, Carrer Mallafré Guasch 4
43007 Tarragona, Spain

Marcos I. Restrepo, MD, MSc
VERDICT (11C6), South Texas Veterans Health Care System, Audie L. Murphy Division, San Antonio
7400 Merton Minter Boulevard
San Antonio, TX 78284, USA

Guy A. Richards, MB, PhD
Department of Medicine, Johannesburg Hospital and University of the Witwatersrand, 7 York Road Parktown, 2193, Johannesburg, South Africa

Jason A. Roberts, BAppSc, BPh
Department of Intensive Care Medicine, 3rd Floor, Ned Hanlon Building, Royal Brisbane and Women's Hospital, Butterfield Street, Herston
Brisbane 4029, Queensland, Australia

Alejandro Rodríguez, MD, PhD
Critical Care Department, University Rovira & Virgili Medical School, Institut Pere Virgili, Joan XXIII University Hospital, Carrer Mallafré Guasch 4
43007 Tarragona, Spain

Jorge Roig, MD, PhD
Pulmonary Division, Hospital Nostra Senyora de Meritxell, 1–13 Fiter Rosell, Escaldes, Andorra AD700

Mohamed Saad, MD
Department of Pulmonary, Critical Care and Sleep Medicine, University of Louisville, 550 S. Jackson Street, ACB-3, Louisville, KY 40202, USA

Miquel Sabria, MD, PhD
Infectious Diseases Department, Hospital Universitari Germans Trias i Pujol, Badalona, Barcelona, Spain

Alberto Sandiumenge Camps, MD
Critical Care Department, University Hospital Joan XXIII, 43007 Tarragona, Spain

Dan Schuller, MD
Pulmonary and Critical Care Division, Creighton University Medical Center, 601 North 30th Street
Suite #3820, Omaha, NE 68131, USA

Gary R. Seabrook, MD
Division of Vascular Surgery, Medical College of Wisconsin, 9200 West Wisconsin Avenue
Milwaukee, WI 53226, USA

Rafael Sierra, MD, PhD
Intensive Care Unit, University Hospital Puerta del Mar, University of Cádiz, Av. Ana de Viya 21
11009 Cádiz, Spain

Jaisi Sinha, MRCPath
National Public Health Service Cardiff, University Hospital of Wales, Heath Park, Cardiff, CF14 4XW, UK

Antonio Sitges-Serra, MD
Department of Surgery, Hospital Universitari del Mar, P. Marítim 25–29, 08003 Barcelona, Spain

Joseph S. Solomkin, MD, PhD
Department of Surgery, University of Cincinnati College of Medicine, 231 Albert Sabin Way
Cincinnati, OH 45267-0558, USA

Jean-François Timsit, MD, PhD
Medical Intensive Care Unit, University Hospital Albert Michallon, 38043 Grenoble, & INSERM U578 Grenoble, France

Antoni Torres, MD, PhD
Respiratory Intensive Care Unit (UVIR), Pulmonology Department, Hospital Clínic, C/ Villarroel 170
08036 Barcelona, Spain

Mauricio Valencia, MD
Respiratory Intensive Care Unit (UVIR), Pulmonology Department, Hospital Clínic, C/Villarroel 170
08036 Barcelona, Spain

Jordi Valles, MD, PhD
Critical Care Department, Institut Universitari Parc Tauli, Hospital Sabadell, Parc Taulí, s/n
08208 Sabadell, Spain

Koenraad Vandewoude, MD
Department of Intensive Care, Ghent University Hospital, De Pintelaan 185, 9000 Ghent, Belgium

Loreto Vidaur, MD
Critical Care Department, University Rovira & Virgili Medical School, Institut Pere Virgili, Joan XXIII University Hospital, Carrer Mallafré Guasch, 4
43007 Tarragona, Spain

Jordi Vila, MD, PhD
Department of Microbiology, Hospital Clinic IDIBAPS, School of Medicine, University of Barcelona Villarroel 170, 08030 Barcelona, Spain

David K. Warren, MD
Division of Infectious Diseases, Washington University School of Medicine, Campus Box 8051
660 South Euclid Avenue, Saint Louis, MO 63110, USA

Grant W. Waterer, MBBS, PhD
School of Medicine and Pharmacology, University of Western Australia, 4th Floor MRF Building, Royal Perth Hospital, GPO Box X2213, Perth, 6847, Australia

Patti J. Wilson, BSN, CIC
Infection Control Section, Froedtert Hospital, 9200 West Wisconsin Avenue, Milwaukee, WI 53226, USA

Keith F. Woeltje, MD, PhD
Division of Infectious Diseases, Washington University School of Medicine, Campus Box 8051
660 South Euclid Avenue, St. Louis, MO 63110, USA

Richard G. Wunderink, MD
Northwestern University Feinberg School of Medicine, 240 E. Huron St., McGaw M300
Chicago, IL 60611 USA

Jerry Yu, PhD
Department of Pulmonary, Critical Care and Sleep Medicine, University of Louisville, 550 S. Jackson Street, ACB-3, Louisville, KY 40202, USA

Jean-Ralph Zahar, MD
Infection Control, Hygiene and Antibiotic Consulting Unit, CHU Necker-Enfants Malades, Paris; INSERM U570, Paris 5 University, Paris, France

Section I

General Aspects

I

Approach to the Febrile Patient in the Intensive Care Unit

G.T. Dimopoulos

1.1 Introduction

Fever occurs in approximately one-third of all medical patients during their hospital stay and in more than 90% of critically ill patients with severe sepsis [1]. According to the Society of Critical Care Medicine (SCCM) and the Infectious Diseases Society of America (IDSA), a temperature above 38.3 °C (101 °F) should be considered as fever necessitating a clinical assessment. The mean body temperature in healthy individuals is 36.8 °C (98.2 °F), with a range of 35.6 °C (96 °F) to 38.2 °C (100.8 °F) and a slight diurnal/circadian variation of between 0.5 and 1.0 °C [2, 3]. Patients with elevated temperature in the ICU are in a closed monitoring system undergoing accurate and reproducible measurements using a variety of methods (instruments and techniques) at different body sites (Table 1.1) [4].

The febrile response (fever is one of the components) is a complex physiological reaction to disease involving a cytokine-mediated rise in core body temperature, generation of acute-phase reactants and activation of numerous physiological, endocrinologic and immunologic systems. Fever, with its beneficial and deleterious effects, occurs as a response to infection, increasing several parameters of immune function (cytokine production, T-cell activation, neutrophil and macrophage function).

However, the management of the critically ill febrile patient can be characterized as a diagnostic dilemma *(infectious or non-infectious cause)* and a response from the physician and staff *(to treat or not to treat)* which varies institutionally. Frequently in the same ICU fevers of mixed causes are seen on evaluation of the patient, and before the cause of fever is confirmed pharmacologic and/or mechanical antipyretic therapy is administered. This traditional point of view shows the misconceptions about the detrimental effects of fever (seizures, brain damage, etc.) and the response from the physician to psychosocial pressure, which however leads to increased medical costs (use of paracetamol, icepacks, cooling blankets) and organ dysfunction (in volume depleted patients or in those with renal and kidney diseases) despite the evidence that fever is a beneficial response to infection [5, 6].

1.2 Physiology and Pathogenesis of Fever

After the action of exogenous stimuli (endotoxin, viruses, etc.), different endogenous pyrogens [interleukin (IL)-1, tumor necrosis factor (TNF), IL-6 and interferons] released by monocytic cells bind to specific receptors located to the preoptic region of the anterior hypothalamus [7]. The subsequent manifestation of fe-

Table 1.1. Measurement of fever

Site	Method	Comment
Pulmonary artery	Mixed venous blood	Pulmonary artery catheter
Infrared ear	Thermometer	Values a few tenths below values in the pulmonary artery catheter and brain
Rectal temperature	Mercury thermometer or electronic probe	A few tenths higher than core temperature
		Unpleasant and intrusive for patients
Oral measurement	Thermometer	Influenced by warmed gases delivered by respiratory devices, by eating and drinking
Axillary measurement	Thermometer	Underestimates core temperature, lacks reproducibility

ver appears to be an upregulation of the thermostatic set point for body temperature in this preoptic area. The brain is protected from large proteins, such as pyrogens (15,000 – 30,000 daltons), entering in a sufficient quantity by a blood-brain barrier recognizing them at certain sites known as circumventricular organs, which represent small neuronal cell groups with fenestrated capillaries allowing neurons to come into contact with different circulating substances directly from the bloodstream. This leakage allows the central nervous system to sense the presence of endogenous pyrogens, which lead to the production of fever from the organum vasculosum of the lamina terminalis (direct response of the neurons within the organum vasculosum to cytokines or response of astrocytes or microglia to cytokines by producing prostaglandins) [8]. The interaction of the cytokine receptors leads to phospholipase A_2 production, arachidonic acid liberation as substrate for the cyclo-oxygenase-2 (COX-2) pathway and elevation of prostaglandin E_2 levels, decreasing the rate of firing of sensitive neurons and leading to decreased heat loss and increased heat production [9, 10]. The role of COX-2 is important because these components induce fever development while its activity is inhibited by selective inhibitors including NSAIDS (non-steroidal anti-inflammatory drugs) and acetaminophen [11].

The febrile response is characterized by endocrine/metabolic, autonomic and behavioral components (Fig. 1.1) [8]. A slight elevation of body temperature improves the efficiency of macrophages in killing invading bacteria, impairs the replication of many microorganisms, minimizes the availability of glucose (substrate for bacterial growth), reduces the demands of muscles for energy expenditure, produces acute-phase reactants which bind divalent cations necessary for the proliferation of microorganisms and increases cortisol and corticotropin secretion, aiding the organism to cope with the stress. The beneficial effects of fever have been shown (a) in mammalian models where the increased body temperature led to enhanced resistance to infection and (b) in clinical trials in adults with a positive correlation between maximum temperature on the bacteremia day and survival or between a temperature >38 °C and survival in spontaneous bacterial peritonitis [12, 13]. The deleterious effects of fever affect mainly patients with cardiorespiratory symptoms (poorly tolerated due to the increased cardiac output, elevated oxygen consumption, increased carbon dioxide production and elevated energy expenditure) and neurosurgical patients with head injuries or cerebrovascular accidents (moderate elevations of brain temperature exacerbate the resulting injury) [14, 15].

1.3 Causes of Fever in the ICU

Fever in the ICU arises from non-infectious and infectious causes. The non-infectious causes (Table 1.2) account for half of fevers in the ICU not usually exceeding 38.3 °C (101 °F) [16]. These diseases are often obvious without additional diagnostic procedures being necessary. The medical history (recent medical interventions, transfusions, recent antibiotics, other medications) along with the physical examination aids the clinician in narrowing down the differential diagnosis.

In Cardiac Care Units the non-infectious causes of fever [which rarely exceeds 38.3 °C (101 °F)] include myocardial infarction, Dressler's syndrome with pericarditis, thromboembolism (complications >10% of

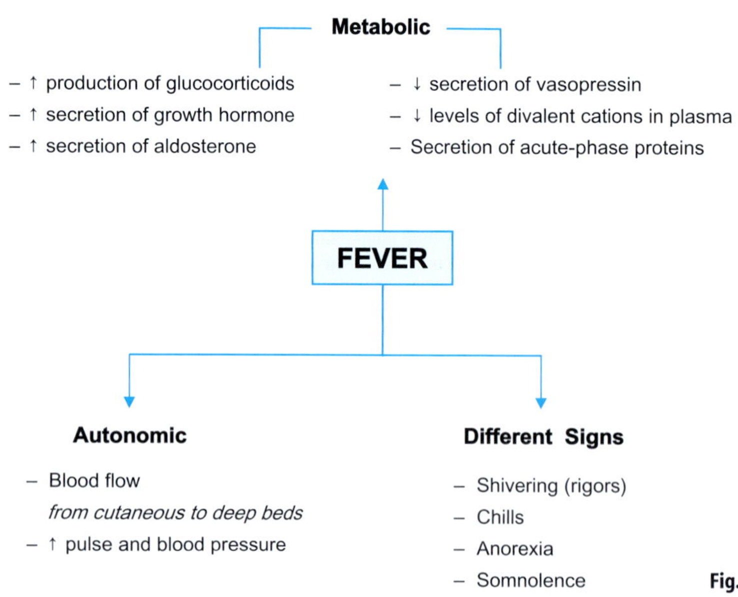

Fig. 1.1. Fever and responses from different organs

Table 1.2. Causes of fever in the ICU

System	Infectious causes	Non-infectious causes
CNS	Meningitis, encephalitis	Posterior fossa syndrome, central fever, seizures, cerebral infarction, hemorrhage, cerebrovascular accident
Cardiovascular	Central line, infected pacemaker, endocarditis sternal osteomyelitis, viral pericarditis	Myocardial infarction, myocardial/perivalvular abscess, balloon pump syndrome, postpericardiotomy syndrome
Pulmonary	VAP, mediastinitis, tracheobronchitis, empyema	Pulmonary emboli, ARDS, atelectasis (without pneumonia), BOOP, bronchogenic carcinoma without postobstructive pneumonia, systemic lupus erythematosus pneumonitis
Gastrointestinal	Intra-abdominal abscess, cholangitis, cholecystitis, viral hepatitis, peritonitis, diarrhea (*Clostridium difficile*)	Pancreatitis, acalculous cholecystitis, ischemia of the bowel, bleeding, cirrhosis, ischemic colitis, irritable bowel syndrome
Urinary tract	Catheter-associated bacteremia, urosepsis, pyelonephritis, cystitis	
Skin/soft tissue	Decubitus ulcers, cellulitis, wound infection	
Bone/joint	Chronic osteomyelitis, septic arthritis	Acute gout
Other	Transient bacteremias, sinusitis	Adrenal insufficiency, phlebitis/thrombophlebitis, neoplastic fever, alcohol/drug withdrawal, delirium tremens, drug fever, fat emboli, deep venous thrombosis, postoperative fever (48 h), fever after transfusions

ARDS acute respiratory distress syndrome, *CNS* central nervous system, *VAP* ventilator associated pneumonia, *BOOP* bronchiolitis obliterans organizing pnuemonia

myocardial infarctions), thrombolytic therapy with hemorrhagic complications and administration of antiarrhythmic medication (procainamide, quinidine) [17]. Fever also occurs in deep venous thrombosis without, however, the necessity for routine venography as the initial diagnostic procedure of pyrexia [1].

In neurosurgical ICU patients, the commonest causes of fever include posterior fossa syndrome, drug fever, central causes, IV-line sepsis, meningitis, wound infections and nosocomial pneumonia [18]. Wound infections are caused mainly by the skin flora of the head (group A streptococci, *Staphylococcus aureus*) or by gram-negative pathogens after open-head trauma resulting in low-grade fevers where the diagnosis is simple with the aid of culture materials. Postoperative meningitis is common after open-head trauma procedures characterized by a persistent fever after the initial postoperative period. The diagnosis is made by Gram's stain and cerebrospinal fluid (CSF) culture. Posterior fossa syndrome mimics meningitis, presenting stiff neck, low level of glucose/increased level of protein and predominance of polymorphonuclear leukocytes in CSF. These findings are consequences of blood insertion in CSF, and the differential diagnosis from bacterial meningitis is based on the negative cultures and the gradual lessening of meningeal symptoms as the number of red blood cells decreases in the CSF with time [18]. Other causes include central fever resistant to antipyretics (intracranial lesion, trauma affecting the brain or hypothalamus) which exceeds 39°C (106°F) and which is characterized by absence of perspiration, anticonvulsive medications and deep venous thrombosis including fat embolism in trauma patients [18]. Pyrexia in the acute phase after head injury is extremely frequent and deleterious for cerebral perfusion pressure (CCP) affecting intracranial pressure (ICP) [19]. In tense patients antipyretic therapy is poorly effective for controlling body temperature and is correlated with a longer ICU stay [19].

Acalculous cholecystitis is the result of gallbladder ischemia and bile stasis, and is frequently unrecognized as a cause of fever in critically ill patients (estimated incidence of 1.5%) [20]. The diagnosis remains difficult especially in septic patients or in patients recovering from abdominal sepsis because of the non-specific clinical signs (pain in the right upper quadrant, nausea, vomiting, fever) and laboratory workup. The radiologic investigation is performed with (a) ultrasound indicating a wall thickness >3 mm, intramural lucencies, gallbladder distension, pericholecystic fluid and intramural sludge; (b) CT scanning presenting high sensitivity and specificity; and (c) hepatobiliary scintigraphy which is associated with a high false-positive rate (>50%) [20]. Acalculous cholecystitis is related to a delayed diagnosis which often progresses to ischemia, gangrene and perforation, indicating the necessity for a high index of suspicion. Percutaneous cholecystostomy is the procedure of choice for the definitive therapy but if the abdominal signs, fever and leukocytosis have not ameliorated open cholecystectomy is recommended [21].

Fever due to drug hypersensitivity reaction or so-called "drug fever" is a non-infectious cause of fever characterized by unknown incidence (3–7% of febrile episodes are attributed to drug reactions but many more cases remain undiagnosed), a temperature range of 38.8°C (102°F) to 40°C (104°F), difficult diagnosis (usually established by exclusion because of the non-specific signs and laboratory tests), shaking chills and spiking temperatures [1, 22]. The usual scenario in the ICU includes a critically ill patient in whom the infection is resolved and after an initial defervescence in temperature a recurrence of fever is noticed. In this patient if the infection has resolved or has not been detected at other sites, the antibiotics should be stopped. If the patient is clinically stable but the infection has not been resolved the antibiotics should be changed to a combination with the same spectrum of pathogens but without sensitizing potential. The presumed offending agent in suspected drug fever should be withdrawn. Taking into account the difficult diagnosis of drug fever, the clinician has to evaluate non-specific signs or symptoms, to avoid needless therapy and to discontinue with safety the offending medication. A concomitant maculopapular rash makes the diagnosis simple but accompanies the fever in only 5–10% of cases. Rarely present are an increased WBC count with a left shift, a moderate elevation of serum transaminases, peripheral eosinophilia and a markedly elevated erythrocyte sedimentation rate (> 100 mm/h). Drug fever is associated with a lack of appropriate pulse rate response and a relative bradycardia (in the absence of intrinsic conduction defects or beta-blockade) [23]. The medications considered as high risk for drug-fever development are all antibiotics (especially α-lactams), diuretics, α-methyldopa, quinidine, hydralazine, procainamide, diphenylhydantoin, antiseizures and stool softeners. Antibiotics with minimal risk for drug-fever development include clindamycin, vancomycin, chloramphenicol, aztreonam, doxycycline erythromycin, imipenem, quinolones and aminoglycosides [1, 23]. After the discontinuation of the offending medication, the fever resolves usually within 72 h but when a rash is present it persists for days or weeks.

Atelectasis is listed as a usual cause of fever in the ICU leading to significantly increased levels of IL-1 and TNF-α of macrophages in the atelectatic lung [24]. Blood transfusions (especially platelet transfusion) indicating an incidence of 0.5% are associated with a febrile response within 30 min to 2 h after the transfusion is begun and last 2–24 h preceded by chills (usually an acute leukocytosis for up to 12 h has been present) [25]. Acute respiratory distress syndrome (ARDS) patients in the late stage of the disease present with pulmonary fibroproliferation, fever and leukocytosis in the absence of infection as a result of the inflammatory-fibrotic process in the airspace of the lungs [26].

In the initial postoperative period the majority of fevers in the ICU are non-infectious (72% of fevers occur in the first 48 h of surgery) caused by the release of endogenous pyrogens into the bloodstream [2]. Postoperative fever warrants a careful evaluation to rule out infection, which is increasingly likely with time. In these patients specific predisposing factors (specific type and site of surgery) and underlying comorbidities leading to certain postoperative infections (pneumonia is most common in patients undergoing upper abdominal or thoracic surgeries, wound infections usually occur in upper abdominal surgery, urinary tract infections are usually associated with lower abdominal procedures) must be taken into account.

Malignant hyperthermia occurs after general anesthesia with depolarizing paralytic agents inducing mutation in the calcium channel of muscle sarcoplasmic reticulum. Malignant neuroleptic syndrome is considered a consequence of blockade of dopamine receptors from antipsychotic drugs inducing muscular rigidity and inhibiting hypothalamic heat-conserving mechanisms and malignant neuroleptic syndrome. Heatstroke is seen more often in patients under psychotropic medication or anticholinergic drugs which inhibit normal heat loss through sweating characterized by a temperature exceeding 41°C [8]. Malignant hyperthermia and malignant neuroleptic syndrome respond to administration of dantrolene and dopamine agonists (bromocriptine) to prevent tissue damage although a diligent and simultaneous search is indicated for an underlying cause of fever. The management of heatstroke includes discontinuation of anticholinergic drugs and external cooling of the body (first with ice baths and later with cooling blankets).

The ICU-acquired infections show a prevalence of between 10% (NNIS) and 20.6% (EPIC study), with ventilator associated pneumonia (VAP) being the most common followed by sinusitis, bloodstream and catheter-related infection, nosocomial diarrhea and wound infections [27, 28]. Almost all cases of nosocomial pneumonia developing in the ICU occur in patients under mechanical ventilation. VAP occurs in 25% of mechanically ventilated patients presenting with leukocytosis, purulent tracheal secretions and new or worsening infiltrates on the chest roentgenogram, but it is difficult to differentiate from other conditions characterized by the same symptoms and signs [29]. The most aggressive diagnostic approach for VAP includes bronchoscopy, bronchoalveolar lavage (BAL), semiquantitative mini-BAL and protected specimen brush performance. However, with prior antibiotic therapy these techniques are considered of limited diagnostic value [30]. The intensivist frequently has to differentiate pneumonia from ARDS (acute respiratory distress syndrome) and LVF (left ventricular failure) because of the same pattern of pulmonary infiltrates. ARDS is characterized in the chest X-ray by the low lung volume and LVF from the immediate and permanent improvement of pulmonary infiltrates after the administration of aggressive therapy.

Gram-negative microorganisms account mainly for nosocomial sinusitis while in 50% of cases isolates are polymicrobial, indicating the pathogens commonly colonize ICU patients. Sinusitis occurs with an incidence of 5% of all nosocomial infections in the ICU characterized by fever and leukocytosis (purulent nasal discharge is often lacking) commonly affecting neurosurgical or trauma patients [22]. The diagnosis is made by CT scan of the sinus, and predisposing factors are considered to be nasotracheal and nasogastric tube placement, nasal packing, facial fractures and steroid administration. Fever is present in a few cases of nosocomial sinusitis and when a CT scan is performed the fever may be attributed to a concomitant infection.

Bloodstream infections (bacteremias) in the absence of an IV-line or catheters in the ICU patient originate from gastrointestinal and genitourinary systems. Catheter related infection/sepsis (a bloodstream infection due to a pathogen that has colonized a vascular device) occurs with an incidence of 10 infections/1,000 catheter days, which increases with the length of time (the catheter in situ), the number of ports and the number of manipulations. The pathogens which commonly colonize/infect the catheters are *Staphylococcus aureus*, coagulase-negative *Staphylococci* followed by enterococci, Gram-negative bacteria and *Candida* species. The management of catheter colonization remains controversial including topical antibiotics and antimicrobial solution administration, subcutaneous tunnelling of catheters and silver-impregnated subcutaneous cuffs. The most effective method to reduce colonization seems to be the antimicrobial bonding of central venous catheters using chlorhexidine gluconate, silver sulfadiazine, minocycline and rifampin [31]. In the case of catheter sepsis the catheter should be changed to a new site and the tip must be cultured (quantitative or semiquantitative). The replacement of the colonized catheter should not be performed by guidewire because of the rapid recolonization.

Intensive care unit patients frequently present with diarrhea of infectious or non-infectious causes. Diarrheas of infectious origin are antibiotic associated and present fever of low grade. The principal pathogen is *Clostridium difficile*. A negative stool culture for *C. difficile* excludes the infectious origin of diarrheas and enteral feeding must be reconsidered because of the high osmolality/flow rate of the enteral solution. In these patients the decreased volume (by one half) of enteral nutrition allows the cessation of diarrheas within 12–24 h [32].

Intra-abdominal infections could be the main cause of ICU admission or a secondary cause after abdominal surgery. Abscess formation is the most common infection and is frequently complicated by acalculous cholecystitis, biliary sepsis and diarrhea due to *C. difficile* [22]. Detection of the infection site is performed by CT scan of the abdomen, ultrasound and nuclear medicine techniques (gallium-67, indium-111 white blood cell scintigraphy). Nuclear medicine techniques are used to detect infections with non-localizing signs. CT scans and ultrasound are used to evaluate focal findings (CT scan is used mainly to detect infections sited in the mid-lower abdomen/peritoneal cavity and ultrasound for evaluation of infections in the pelvis and right upper quadrant of the abdomen) [33].

Fungi (mainly *Candida* spp.) are important opportunistic pathogens in the ICU associated with certain predisposing factors characterized by the difficult diagnosis because of the lack of a laboratory method able to distinguish colonization from infection. The diagnosis of these infections is made by the identification of the fungi from sterile or histologic specimens [34]. During recent years cytomegalovirus (CMV) antigenemia has been proposed as a cause of unexplained prolonged fever in severely ill immunocompetent ICU patients [35]. The significance of CMV detection is unknown because the differentiation between CMV detection and CMV disease represents a diagnostic dilemma, although patients with detectable CMV tend to have a higher morbidity and mortality compared with patients in whom the virus remains undetectable [35].

Intensive care unit-acquired urinary tract infections (UTIs) have an incidence of 9.6/1,000 ICU days, commonly affect women/medical patients and despite the increased morbidity associated with critical illness are not a significant attributable cause of mortality in the ICU [36]. The main pathogens associated with ICU-acquired UTI development are *Escherichia coli* (23%), *Candida albicans* (20%), and *Enterococcus* species (15%) [37]. The management of UTIs includes antibiotic administration after urine culture performance and specific preventive measures (use of a catheter valve instead of a standard drainage system, use of a silver-alloy, hydrogel-coated latex urinary catheter instead of uncoated catheters). The term "asymptomatic bacteriuria" is frequently used to define the colonization of the urinary tract without bacterial invasion and acute inflammatory response. Bacteriuria should be treated with antibiotics only after urinary tract manipulations/surgery, in patients with kidney stones and in patients with obstruction.

1.4 Approach to the Febrile Critically Ill Patient and Treatment

The approach to the febrile patient in the ICU includes (a) an overview of the medical record (comorbidities, recent procedures, current medications, indwelling devices), (b) physical examination/review of the chest X-ray and (c) evaluation of fever characteristics (magnitude, duration, relationship to the patient's pulse rate, temporal relationship to both diagnostic and therapeutic interventions). In the ICU, fever could arise as remittent or intermittent, sustained or appearing at different point times in the course of the patient's illness, after 48 h from mechanical ventilation initiation (VAP), 5–7 days postoperatively (abscess formation) or at the 10–14th ICU day (fungal infections). The cause of fever varies according to the types of ICU and patient population. In medical ICUs the commonest causes of fever are secondary to myocardial infarction, pulmonary emboli, acute pancreatitis, adrenal insufficiency, gastrointestinal bleeding, central catheter related infections, ventilator associated pneumonia (VAP) or drug reactions. In surgical ICUs are additionally seen wound infections, peritonitis or abscesses. In cases of unknown origin where fever may fluctuate widely within a 24-h period a graph of temperature and pulse rate is used in relation to procedural intervention timing and transfusions.

Critically ill patients often show single spikes of temperature which return to normal without treatment (are considered to have no clinical significance) related to intervention inducing bacteremia, endotracheal suctioning, urinary catheter placement and transfusion of blood products. The fever related to an invasive procedure or manipulation of an indwelling device with or without transient bacteremia frequently resolves spontaneously, while fever due to underlying chronic diseases, current medical illness or its complications or reactions following drug therapy may be persistent.

In all febrile ICU patients (Fig. 1.2) and before the initiation of any treatment (empiric antibiotic therapy, antipyretic treatment), blood cultures (at least two and no more than three sets obtained by separate needles from different sites) as well as other appropriate cultures must be performed. Bacteremia is an important cause of morbidity and mortality in the ICU leading to fever and chills 1–2 h after the presence of microorganisms in the blood (the initiating event), therefore explaining the frequently negative blood cultures at the time of the temperature spike [38].

In the case of unexplained fever or fever of unknown origin with unexplained leukocytosis, anion gap acidosis, hypotension or persistent tachycardia and tachypnea, the initial evaluation of the patient must focus on ruling out a possible infection (most commonly in the ICU urinary tract infections, pneumonia, phlebitis, wound infection and bacteremia) with the aid of certain laboratory tests including a complete blood count (CBC), urine examination with culture, blood cultures and a chest roentgenogram (especially in patients on mechanical ventilation). In patients with progressive

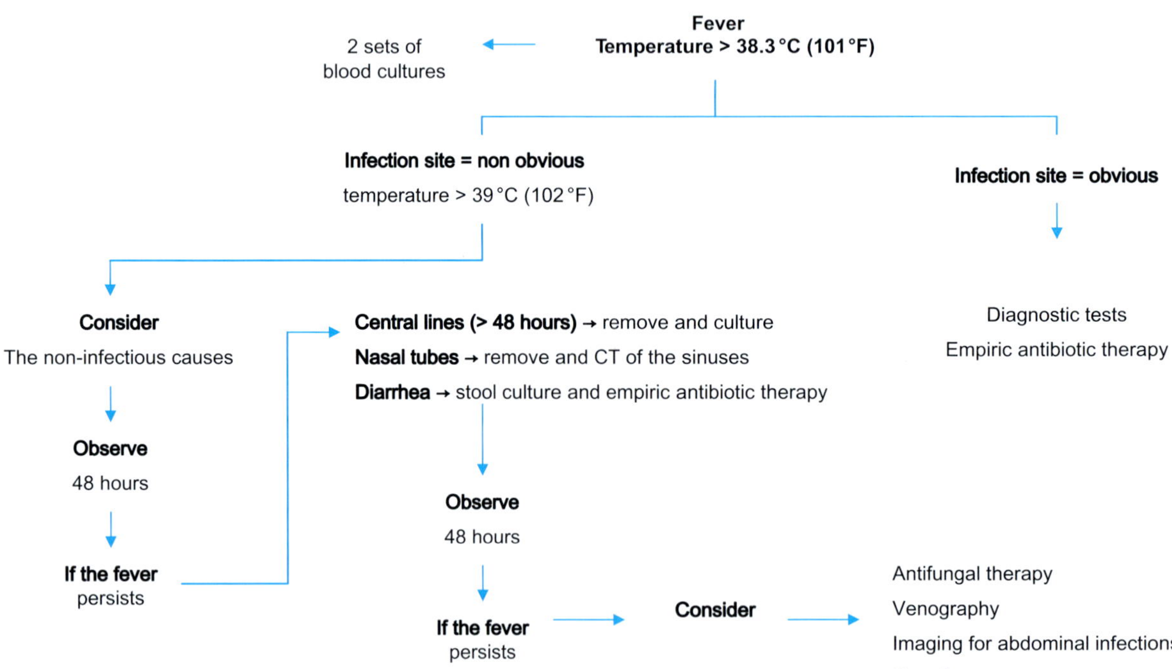

Fig. 1.2. Approach to the febrile critically ill patient

signs of severe sepsis and in all neutropenic patients with fever, broad-spectrum antimicrobial therapy should be started immediately after cultures have been obtained. In patients with no clinically obvious signs of infection all the central lines (placed > 48 h) and the nasal tubes should be removed and cultured (with semiquantitative or quantitative cultures), while in the case of diarrhea, stool cultures for WBC count and toxin against *C. difficile* should be performed. CT scanning of the abdomen is indicated in patients with abdominal sepsis or with signs of abdominal infection (tenderness, distension, etc.). If fever persists after 48 h despite empiric antibiotic treatment and without the cause or the source of the infection being identified, the patient must be reevaluated for risk factors associated with fungal infections (antifungal treatment is indicated) and with additional diagnostic tests being performed including venography, blood cultures for eosinophils (drug fever) and abdominal imaging.

For the suppression of fever in the ICU, antipyretic agents (acetaminophen, cyclooxygenase 2, non-steroidal, metamizol, propacetamol) and external cooling methods are used. Antipyretics include agents capable of blocking or reversing the fever's cytokine-mediated rise in core temperature without affecting body temperature in the afebrile state and must be distinguished from hypothermia agents which are able of lowering core temperature even in the absence of fever [39]. External cooling methods include hypothermia blanket placement, the use of which, however, is characterized by certain side effects including large temperature fluctuations, rebound hyperthermia, increased hypermetabolism and elevated oxygen consumption leading to increased epinephrine and norepinephrine levels [40].

Fever is a normal adaptive brain response to circulating cytokines during systemic inflammation and no harm is done by letting it take its natural course [41]. In the ICU fever should be treated in cardiorespiratory patients and neurosurgical individuals and in those patients in whom the temperature exceeds 40 °C (104 °F). Antipyretic therapy must be justified regardless of the metabolic cost (if the fever exceeds its physiological benefit), the result (if the symptomatic relief adversely affects the course of the febrile illness) and the side effects of the antipyretic regimens (in patients with reduced glutathione reserves such as alcoholics, malnourished patients, etc., regular doses of acetaminophen are associated with acute hepatitis).

References

1. Cunha BA, Shea KW (1996) Fever in the intensive care unit. Infect Dis Clin North Am 10:185 – 209
2. O'Grady NP, Barie PS, Bartlett J, Bleck T, Garvey G, Jacobi J, Linden P, Maki DG, Nam M, Pasculle MD, Triblett DL, Masur H (1998) Practice parameters for evaluating new fever in critically ill adult patients. Task Force of the American College of Critical Care Medicine of the Society of Critical Care Medicine in collaboration with the Infectious Disease Society of America. Crit Care Med 26:392 – 408
3. Mackoviak PA, Wassermann SS, Levine MM (1992) A critical appraisal of 98.6 degrees F, the upper limit of the normal body temperature and other legacies of Carl Reinhold August Wunderlich. JAMA 268:1576 – 1580
4. Erikson RS, Kirklin SK (1993) Comparison of ear-based, bladder, oral and axillary methods for core temperature measurement. Crit Care Med 1:1528 – 1534
5. Ipp M, Jaffre D (1993) Physicians' attitudes toward the diagnosis and management of fever in children 3 months to 2 years of age. Clin Pediatr (Phila) 32:66 – 70
6. Gozzoli V, Schottker P, Suter PM, Ricou B (2001) Is it worth treating fever in intensive care unit patients? Preliminary results from a randomized trial of the effect of external cooling. Arch Intern Med 161:121 – 123
7. Leon L (2002) Cytokine regulation of fever: studies using gene knockout mice. J Appl Physiol 92:2648 – 2655
8. Saper CB, Breder CD (1994) The neurologic basis of fever. N Engl J Med 330:1880 – 1886
9. Ryan M, Levy MM (2003) Clinical review: fever in intensive care unit patients. Crit Care 7:221 – 225
10. Luheshi GN (1998) Cytokines and fever. Mechanisms and sites of action. Ann NY Acad Sci 856:83 – 89
11. Simmons DL, Wagner D, Westover K (2000) Nonsteroidal anti-inflammatory drugs, acetaminophen, cyclooxygenase 2 and fever. Clin Infect Dis 31(Suppl 5):S211–S218
12. Anderson KJ, Kuhn RE (1989) Elevated environmental temperature enhances immunity in experimental Chagas' disease. Infect Immunol 57:13 – 17
13. Weinstein MP, Iannini PB, Stratton CW, Eickhoff TC (1978) Spontaneous bacterial peritonitis. A review of 28 cases with emphasis on improved survival and factors influencing prognosis. Am J Med 64(4):592 – 598
14. Manthous CA, Hall JB, Olson D, Singh M, Chatila W, Pohlman A, Kushner R, Schmidt GA, Wood LD (1995) Effect of cooling on oxygen consumption in febrile critically ill patients. Am J Respir Crit Care Med 151(1):10 – 14
15. Ginsberg MD, Busto R (1998) Combating hyperthermia in acute stroke: a significant clinical concern. Stroke 29: 529 – 534
16. Cunha BA (1994) Intensive care, not intensive antibiotics. Heart Lung 23:361 – 362
17. Cunha BA (1996) The clinical significance of fever patterns. Infect Dis Clin North Am 10:33 – 44
18. Cunha BA, Tu RP (1988) Fever in the neurosurgical patient. Heart Lung 17:608 – 615
19. Stocchetti N, Rossi S, Roncati Zanier E, Colombo A, Beretta L, Citerio G (2002) Pyrexia in head-injured patients admitted to intensive care. Intens Care Med 28:1555 – 1562
20. Barie PS, Fischer E (1995) Acute acalculous cholecystitis. J Am Coll Surg 180:232 – 234
21. Kiviniemi H, Makela JT, Autio R, Tikkakoski T, Leinonen S, Siniluoto T, Perala J, Paivansalo M, Merikanto J (1998) Percutaneous cholecystostomy in acute cholecystitis in high-risk patients: an analysis of 69 patients. Int Surg 83:299 – 302
22. Marik PE (2000) Fever in the ICU. Chest 117(3):855 – 869
23. Wood AJJ (1998) Adverse drug reactions. In: Fauci AS, Braunwald E, Isselbacher KJ, et al. (eds) Harrison's principles of internal medicine. McGraw-Hill, New York, NY, pp 422 – 430
24. Engoren M (1995) Lack of association between atelectasis and fever. Chest 107:81 – 84
25. Fenwick JC, Cameron M, Naiman SC, Haley LP, Ronco JJ, Wiggs BR, Tweeddale MG (1994) Blood transfusion as a

cause of leucocytosis in critically ill patients. Lancet 344 (8926):855–856
26. Meduri GU, Headley AS, Golden E, Carson SJ, Umberger RA, Kelso T, Tolley EA (1999) Effect of prolonged methylprednisolone therapy in unresolving acute respiratory distress syndrome: a randomized controlled trial. JAMA 280:159–165
27. Jarvis WR, Edwards JR, Culver DH, Hughes JM, Horan T, Emori TG, Banerjee S, Tolson J, Henderson T, Gaynes RP, et al. (1991) Nosocomial infection rates in adult and pediatric intensive care units in the United States. National Nosocomial Infections Surveillance System. Am J Med 91(3B): 185S–191S
28. Vincent JL, Bihari DJ, Suter PM, Bruining HA, White J, Nicolas-Chanoin MH, Wolff M, Spencer RC, Hemmer M (1995) The prevalence of nosocomial infection in intensive care units in Europe. Results of the European Prevalence of Infection in Intensive Care (EPIC) Study. EPIC International Advisory Committee. JAMA 274(8):639–644
29. Rello J, Diaz E, Rodriguez A (2005) Advances in the management of pneumonia in the intensive care unit: review of current thinking. Clin Microbiol Infect Suppl 5:30–38
30. Rello J, Gallego M, Mariscal D, Sonora R, Valles J (1997) The value of routine microbial investigation in ventilator-associated pneumonia. Am J Respir Crit Care Med 156: 196–200
31. McConnell SA, Gubbins PO, Anaissie EJ (2004) Are antimicrobial-impregnated catheters effective? Replace the water and grab your washcloth, because we have a baby to wash. Clin Infect Dis 39 (12):1829–1833
32. Caines C, Gill MV, Cunha BA (1997) Non-*Clostridium difficile* nosocomial diarrhea in the intensive care unit. Heart Lung 26(1):83–84
33. Meduri GU, Belenchia JM, Massie JD, Eltorky M, Tolley EA (1996) The role of gallium-67 scintigraphy in diagnosing sources of fever in ventilated patients. Intens Care Med 22:395–403
34. Peres-Bota D, Rodriguez-Villalobos H, Dimopoulos G, Melot C, Vincent JL (2004) Potential risk factors for infection with *Candida* spp. in critically ill patients. Clin Microbiol Infect 10(6):550–555
35. Jaber S, Chanques G, Borry J, Souche B, Verdier R, Perrigault PF, Eledjam JJ (2005) Cytomegalovirus infection in critically ill patients: associated factors and consequences. Chest 127:233–241
36. Laupland KB, Bagshaw SM, Gregson DB, Kirkpatrick AW, Ross T, Church DL (2005) Intensive care unit-acquired urinary tract infections in a regional critical care system. Crit Care 9(2):R60–65
37. Gaynes R, Edwards JR (2005) National Nosocomial Infections Surveillance System Overview of nosocomial infections caused by gram-negative bacilli. Clin Infect Dis 41(6):848–854
38. Pronovost PJ, Holzmueller CG (2004) Partnering for quality. J Crit Care 19(3):121–129
39. Mackowiak PA (2000) Physiological rationale for suppression of fever. Clin Infect Dis 31 (Suppl 5):S185–189
40. Gozzoli V, Treggiari MM, Kleger GR, Roux LP, Fathi M, Pichard C, Romand JA (2004) Randomized trial of the effect of antipyresis by metamizol, propacetamol or external cooling on metabolism, hemodynamics and inflammatory response. Intens Care Med 30(3):401–407
41. Mackowiak PA, Boulant JA (1996) Fever's glass ceiling. Clin Infect Dis 22:525–536

Chapter 2

Cardiovascular Monitoring in Severe Sepsis or Septic Shock

2

J.J. Guardiola, M. Saad, J. Yu

2.1 Introduction

The American College of Chest Physicians & Society of Critical Care Medicine Consensus [1] defines sepsis as the systemic inflammatory response syndrome (SIRS) as a result of infection. Septic shock is defined as sepsis-induced hypotension despite adequate fluid resuscitation along with the presence of perfusion abnormalities. These abnormalities may include, but are not limited to, lactic acidosis, oliguria or an acute alteration in mental status. Patients who are receiving inotropic or vasopressor agents may not be hypotensive at the time that perfusion abnormalities are measured. During the years 1950–1991 mortality soared 13-fold [2]. Alone sepsis carries a 30–40% lethality [2], but when aggravated by shock it has a 40–60% mortality [3]. Recently the effectiveness of invasive hemodynamic monitoring in septic shock has undergone intense scrutiny. A lack of well designed prospective studies assessing this problem has cast a shadow of doubt over the lowering of morbidity or mortality (attributable to the right heart catheterization). A moratorium on their placement was suggested in the literature, which prompted a consensus conference in 1997 to help clarify the role of the pulmonary artery catheter in the critically ill [4]. Minimally invasive and non-invasive cardiovascular monitoring devices are being examined and are increasingly being researched.

2.2 Shock States and Differential Diagnosis

Shock is the state in which the circulatory system fails to maintain adequate tissue perfusion. As a consequence of inadequate tissue perfusion, cellular and organ dysfunction ensues, which becomes irreversible unless corrected promptly. Clinical features of shock are arterial hypotension, tachycardia, tachypnea, decreased mentation, oliguria and metabolic acidosis. Blood pressure (BP) is equal to cardiac output (CO) times systemic vascular resistance (SVR). Because hypotension can result from a reduction in either CO or SVR, shock may be categorized as distributive, cardiogenic, extracardiac obstructive or hypovolemic. Distributive shock is caused by a maldistribution of blood flow in the microcirculation with a decreased SVR (e.g., sepsis, anaphylaxis, spinal cord injury, barbiturate overdose, etc.). Cardiogenic shock's most common cause is acute myocardial infarction, while extracardiac obstructive shock may be caused by cardiac tamponade, massive pulmonary embolus or tension pneumothorax. Hypovolemic shock causes include massive losses of gastrointestinal fluids or frank hemorrhage.

Bedside clinical assessment provides a good indication of cardiac output and filling pressures of the heart. Based on this clinical assessment, an early diagnosis of the type of shock can be made (Tables 2.1, 2.2).

Table 2.1. Bedside diagnosis of the type of shock [5] based on cardiac output

Signs	High cardiac output	Low cardiac output
Pulse pressure	Increased	Decreased (pulsus paradoxus in cardiac tamponade)
Skin and digits	Warm and pink	Cool, cyanotic mottling
Capillary refill (nailbed)	Rapid	Slow
Heart sounds	Loud and clear	Soft and muffled
Temperature	Fever or hypothermia	Normal temperature
White blood cell count	Leukocytosis or leukopenia (shift to immature forms)	Normal to mild leukocytosis
Source of infection	E.g., pneumonia or pyelonephritis	No source of infection
Possible diagnosis	*Septic shock*	*Cardiogenic shock* *Obstructive shock* *Hypovolemic shock*

Table 2.2. Bedside diagnosis of the type of shock [5] based on filling pressures of the heart

Filling pressures	Increased filling pressure	Decreased filling pressure
Clinical setting	Chest pain	Bleeding, vomiting or diarrhea
Jugular venous pressure	Jugular venous distension	Jugular veins collapse when supine
Cardiac auscultation	Gallop rhythm	Absent gallop
Pulmonary crepitant rales	Present	Clear lungs
Chest roentgenogram	Cardiomegaly – Pulmonary venous congestion – Pulmonary edema – Clear in pulmonary embolus and cardiac tamponade	Normal (except when shock is due to pneumonia)
Electrocardiogram	MI-ST segment elevation PE – $S_I\ Q_3\ T_3$ Tamponade – decreased voltage	Normal
Cardiac enzymes	Increase in MI	Normal
Possible diagnosis	*Cardiogenic shock* *Obstructive shock*	*Hypovolemic shock*

Table 2.3. Hemodynamic profiles in shock

Type of shock	CO	SVR	SvO_2	CVP	PAP	PCWP
Cardiogenic (e.g., MI[a])	↓	↑	↓	↑	↑	↑
Hypovolemic (e.g., hemorrhage)	↓	↑	↓	↓	↓	↓
Distributive (e.g., sepsis[b])	↑	↓	N – ↑	N – ↓	N – ↓	N – ↓
Obstructive (massive PE[c])	↓	↑ – N	↓	↑	↑	N – ↓
Obstructive (cardiac tamponade[c,d])	↓	↑	↓	↑	↑	↑

CO cardiac output, *CVP* central venous pressure (right atrial pressure), *PCWP* pulmonary capillary wedge pressure, *SVR* systemic vascular resistance, SvO_2 mixed venous oxygen saturation, *PAP* pulmonary artery pressure, *N* normal

[a] In the presence of a right ventricular infarct, PCWP may not increase in cardiogenic shock

[b] In the late stages of septic shock, CO falls and SVR rises due to myocardial depression

[c] PCWP is decreased in massive pulmonary embolus, but increased in cardiac tamponade

[d] Equalization of mean CVP, mean PCWP, right ventricular diastolic pressure and diastolic PAP establishes the diagnosis cardiac tamponade

Invasive hemodynamic monitoring with a pulmonary artery catheter (PAC) allows the classification of a patient with shock into one of four types: cardiogenic, hypovolemic, distributive or obstructive (Table 2.3).

2.3 Hemodynamics in Septic Shock [6–9]

Septic shock has a characteristic hemodynamic profile consisting of tachycardia, systemic arterial hypotension, low SVR, high CO, low to normal pulmonary capillary wedge pressure (PCWP) and normal or elevated mixed venous oxygen saturation (SvO_2). This "high output-low resistance" state (or hyperdynamic circulation) is seen in more than 90% of patients with septic shock who have been aggressively fluid resuscitated to correct hypovolemia. In a minority of patients, left ventricular dysfunction with a low cardiac output may occur. The responses to sepsis include vascular changes and myocardial dysfunction.

2.3.1 Systemic Vascular Resistance

Severe sepsis is commonly associated with a decrease in SVR which results in hypotension despite a normal or increased cardiac index (CI). Most non-survivors of septic shock demonstrate a persistent vasodilatation and hence refractory hypotension.

2.3.2 Generalized Blood Flow Redistribution

Although the CO is increased in sepsis, this flow is not uniformly distributed. There is a reduction in the splanchnic blood flow resulting in mucosal ischemia of the gastrointestinal tract, while blood flow to the other vital organs (e.g., brain and heart) is preserved. Intestinal ischemia has been considered to play a central role in the development of irreversible shock and the multiple organ dysfunction syndrome (MODS).

2.3.3 Microcirculatory Blood Flow Maldistribution

Many vascular beds are dilated but some are constricted while arteriovenous shunts may open and bypass the capillary bed resulting in impaired organ perfusion.

2.3.4 Venous Capacitance

Venous tone decreases in the large capacity vessels and venous pooling occurs resulting in relative hypovolemia.

2.3.5 Capillary Permeability

A generalized increase in endothelial permeability ("capillary leak") leads to "third-spacing" and intravascular volume depletion; thus the effective intravascular volume is reduced in sepsis due to the multiple factors including an increase in venous capacitance with venous pooling and decreased intravascular volume secondary to a capillary leak.

2.3.6 Myocardial Depression

Depressed myocardial contractile function is a common consequence of severe sepsis. This reversible cardiac dysfunction is manifested by a decrease in left and right ventricular ejection fraction with biventricular dilatation. Since ejection fraction declines, ventricular dilation can be a compensatory mechanism to maintain stroke volume at a constant level by the Frank Starling mechanism. Early septic shock is characterized by an increased cardiac output owing to an increased heart rate and a constant stroke volume. With recovery, CO falls as heart rate decreases and the stroke volume remains constant but there is a reduction in ventricular size and an increase in ejection fraction. Myocardial depression may be the effect of the cytokine – tumor necrosis factor. Myocardial ischemia does not play a significant role since coronary flow is preserved in septic shock [10].

In a minority of patients with septic shock, left ventricular dysfunction is not compensated and these patients die of myocardial pump failure with a low CI. However, most patients who die of septic shock either succumb in the early stage owing to persistently low SVR with refractory hypotension or die at a later stage as a result of sepsis induced MODS.

2.4 Cellular Metabolism in Septic Shock

Distributive abnormalities of systemic blood flow (intestinal ischemia) and maldistribution of blood flow in the microcirculation (arterial-venous shunting) limit effective oxygen extraction during septic shock. In addition to blood flow maldistribution, in some septic patients, a "metabolic block" exists at the cellular level preventing adequate oxygen utilization [11]. As a consequence of the inability of systemic tissues to maximally extract oxygen from the blood, anaerobic metabolism occurs with increased blood lactate concentrations despite near normal mixed venous oxygen saturation and a narrow difference in the arterial-venous oxygen content.

2.5 Monitoring the Septic Patient

2.5.1 Basic Monitoring

2.5.1.1 Electrocardiogram (ECG)

Continuous ECG monitoring is used in almost all patients in the intensive care unit (ICU). ECG monitoring will measure heart rate, and detect arrhythmias and myocardial ischemia.

2.5.1.2 Non-invasive Blood Pressure Monitoring (NIBP)

Automated NIBP is widely available in the ICU, usually as a part of a multicomponent monitor along with continuous ECG and pulse oximetry monitoring. It is frequently used on admission to the ICU before insertion of an arterial cannula. Measurements are unreliable in obesity, in low cardiac output states and in the presence of many arrhythmias.

2.5.1.3 Arterial Line

Intra-arterial monitoring is accurate, allowing immediate beat-to-beat analysis and frequent arterial blood gas sampling. In hypotensive septic patients receiving high-dose vasopressor therapy, radial artery pressure underestimates central pressure. Clinical management based upon radial pressure may lead to excessive vasopressor administration. Awareness of this phenomenon may help to minimize the adverse effects of these potent agents by enabling dosage reduction [12].

2.5.1.4 Pulse Oximetry

A pulse oximeter attached to a finger or earlobe allows for transcutaneous estimates of hemoglobin oxygen saturation. Accuracy depends on satisfactory arterial perfusion of the skin. Inaccurate readings are seen with low cardiac output states, vasoconstriction and in hypothermia.

2.5.1.5 Arterial Blood Gases

Arterial blood gases are useful for monitoring pulmonary function and acid-base status in septic patients.

2.5.1.6 Urinary Output

A Foley catheter is inserted and connected to a graduated collecting device (urimeter) so that urinary output can be measured hourly. Urine output is a reliable guide to tissue perfusion. A significant fall in renal perfusion is associated with oliguria, which if allowed to persist, may progress to acute tubular necrosis.

2.5.1.7 Central Venous Catheter (CVC)

Central venous pressure (CVP) is measured by inserting a catheter into the central venous circulation, usually in the internal jugular or subclavian vein. CVP reflects the right atrial pressure and therefore the filling pressure of the right ventricle. The pulmonary artery wedge pressure on the other hand reflects the left atrial pressure, and therefore the filling pressure of the left ventricle. CVC allows monitoring of central venous oxygen saturation ($ScvO_2$), either continuously via fiberoptic oxymetry or intermittently by obtaining venous blood gases. Central lines are also used for administration of fluids and medications.

2.5.1.8 Pulmonary Artery Catheter (PAC)

The PAC, balloon flotation catheter or Swan-Ganz catheter was described by Jeremy Swan and William Ganz in 1970. The PAC enables the acquisition of three types of data:

1. Cardiac output (CO) using the thermodilution method
2. Central venous pressure (CVP), pulmonary artery pressure (PAP) and pulmonary capillary wedge pressure (PCWP) (Fig. 2.1)
3. Mixed venous blood for oxygen saturation (SvO_2)

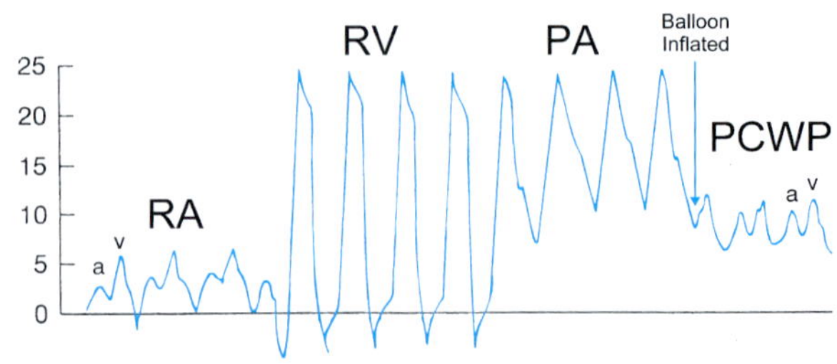

Fig. 2.1. Waveforms and pressures seen during insertion of PAC. *RA* right atrium, *RV* right ventricle, *PA* pulmonary artery, *PCWP* pulmonary capillary wedge pressure

Cardiac output is equal to heart rate times stroke volume. Stroke volume depends on preload, afterload and contractility. Preload physiologically is the muscle fiber length at end diastole. Frank Starling's law of the heart is a fundamental property of heart muscle in which the force of contraction at any given tension depends on the end-diastolic fiber length. Afterload represents the force opposing muscle fiber shortening. This is dictated by the wall tension in the left ventricle (LV) during systole. Tension (T) is directly related to pressure (P) and radius (r) while being inversely related to the thickness (h) of the chamber ($T=Pr/2\,h$). Systemic vascular resistance will affect the afterload by virtue of its direct effect on intraventricular pressure. Contractility or inotropic state is the ability of the heart at any given length to generate tension.

PAC is used to measure pressures (Fig. 2.1), but what pressures are we really measuring? Any indwelling catheter that measures pressures encompasses intravascular pressure, driving pressure and transmural pressure. Intravascular pressure is the pressure inside vessels relative to ambient room pressure at the same level. Driving pressure, in the case of the pulmonary circulation, is the pressure difference between the pulmonary artery and left atrium. Transmural pressure is the pressure differential between the inside and outside of the blood vessel. When we measure the pulmonary capillary wedge pressure (PCWP), we are measuring *estimates* of the left ventricular end diastolic volume (preload). PCWP measures the left atrial pressure, which is an indirect measurement of the left ventricular pressure at end diastole. This in turn is an estimate of the left ventricular end diastolic volume. There is a linear relationship between volume and pressure. This relationship does not always hold true and supposes there is normal left ventricular compliance and juxtacardiac pressure. As we know, this is not always the case with our patients. Left ventricular (LV) compliance is the change in volume per unit of pressure as the LV fills with blood from the left atrium. LV compliance may be compromised (left ventricular hypertrophy, hypertrophic cardiomyopathy, restrictive cardiomyopathy, myocardial ischemia RV overload with septal shift and pulmonary hypertension), leading to a greater elevation in pressure for any given volume. Mitral valve disease may negate this relationship.

Transmural pressure (P_{tm}) is the gradient between the intracavitary pressure (PCWP) and the juxtacardiac pressure (P_{jc}), which represents intrathoracic pressure (intrapleural pressure). Juxtacardiac pressures may be elevated by elevated intrathoracic pressures [e.g. – mechanical ventilation with positive end-expiratory pressure (PEEP), auto-PEEP, and pneumothorax] or lowered by negative intrathoracic pressure (as in normal or labored breathing). Measurements should be made at end expiration. P_{jc} may be assessed directly by esophageal manometry (a measure of intrapleural pressure).

Proper location of the PAC is important. Measurement should be made in a Zone III condition (where alveolar pressure is less than that of the pulmonary artery or vein). Zone III may be reduced in size with increasing alveolar distension (obstructive lung physiology, auto- or excessive PEEP) or diminished pulmonary vascular pressures (severe hypovolemia). Anteroposterior and lateral films may confirm the good position of the catheter. When the patient lies supine, Zone III is in the dependent part of the lung; therefore the tip of the catheter has to be in this area to produce reliable results. The position of the tip should be below the posterior border of the left atrium on a supine lateral chest X-ray. The nasogastric tube is a useful landmark since the esophagus traverses posterior to the left atrium.

The PAC allows for true mixed venous oxygen sampling, whereas central lines do not. The blood returning from the superior vena cava usually has a lower saturation due to a high oxygen extraction. The inferior vena cava usually has a higher saturation owing to shunts such as the renal circulation.

Table 2.4. Complications of pulmonary artery catheterization [15]

Complication	Incidence	Citation
Arterial sticks	10 %	
Pneumothorax	0.5–6 %	
Venous air embolism	0.5 %	
Thoracic duct injury	1 % of left-sided attempts	
Premature ventricular beats	68 %	
Transient ventricular tachycardia	33 %	
Persistent ventricular tachycardia	3 %	
Right bundle branch block	6–12 % (resolved in 24 h)	
Right bundle branch block with existing left bundle branch block	23 %	
Misplacement of catheter	19 % internal jugular	
Misplacement of catheter	16 % subclavian	
Pulmonary artery rupture	0.034–0.125 %	
Pulmonary artery ruptures that result in death	70 %	
Thrombosis	1–11 %	
Valvular lesions	Up to 31 %	
Infection of catheter or sheath	5.9–29.1 %	
Catheter associated bacteremia	0–4.6 %	
Inaccurate PCWP	15 %	
Inaccurate interpretation by doctors	54 %	17
Inaccurate interpretation by nurses	42 %	16

1. *Complications:* Cardiac output measurements may also be riddled with inaccuracy. Thermodilution is used but can be inaccurate owing to slow injection of fluid, measurements taken at different times of the respiratory cycle, tricuspid regurgitation, intracardiac shunts or distal location of the PAC. Placement of the PAC with its introducer has associated morbidity as noted in Table 2.4 [15]. This is not an all-inclusive list. The most concerning findings are the last two. If we chose to use the PAC it is incumbent upon the critical care team to resolutely endeavor for correct capture and interpretation of data. For if the data is interpreted wrongly, then inappropriate therapy will likely be prescribed.
2. *Controversy and consensus:* Of late, significant controversy has surrounded the PAC. Connors et al. suggest that careful consideration should be given as to whether or not one should be placed. Findings that lead to their conclusions were an increased 30-day mortality (4.5 % higher), higher cost and protracted intensive care requirement. Proponents of the right heart catheter criticize that this was not a randomized prospective trial. Since it allows for earlier intervention and often leads to a change in therapy, then it must logically improve outcome. However, we are reminded of the CAST trial that clearly showed postmyocardial infarction antiarrhythmics are detrimental, counterintuitive to the rationale of the time. The risks and its indiscriminate use in the low benefit patient may negate the benefits of the catheter. Compounding this is a high degree of misinterpretation by trained intensive care physicians [17] and nurses [16]. Pulmonary artery occlusion pressure is inaccurate 15 % of the time and in the critically ill does not always correlate with left ventricular end diastolic volume [32]. This controversy prompted a consensus statement [4] endorsed by the American Association of Criti-

Table 2.5. Summary of consensus statement – based upon clinical situation [4]

Situation	Findings
Improve outcome in MI with cardiogenic shock	Yes
Improve outcome in MI with mechanical complications	Yes
Improve outcome in MI with right ventricular infarction	Yes
Improve outcome in refractory congestive heart failure	Uncertain
Improve outcome in pulmonary hypertension	Uncertain
Improve outcome in shock or hemodynamic instability	Uncertain
Reduce complications and mortality in cardiac surgery – low risk patients	No
Reduce complications and mortality in cardiac surgery – high risk patients	Uncertain
Reduce perioperative complications in peripheral vascular surgery	Yes
Reduce mortality in peripheral vascular surgery	Uncertain
Reduce perioperative complications and mortality in aortic surgery – low risk patients	Uncertain
Reduce perioperative complications and mortality in aortic surgery – high risk patients	Yes
Reduce perioperative complications and mortality in geriatric patients	No
Reduce perioperative complications and mortality in neurosurgical patients	Uncertain
Reduce complications and mortality in patients with preeclampsia	No
Alter diagnosis and improve functional outcome in traumatically injured patients	Yes
Alter mortality in traumatically injured patients	Uncertain
Improve outcomes in patients with sepsis or septic shock	Uncertain
Alter diagnosis and treatment in patients with respiratory failure	Yes
Alter outcomes in patients with respiratory failure	Uncertain
Clarify cardiopulmonary physiology in critically ill infants and children	Yes
Improve organ function or survival when PAC used to achieve supranormal oxygen delivery after onset of SIRS from sepsis, trauma or postoperative complication	Uncertain
Improve organ function or survival when PAC used to achieve supranormal oxygen delivery after onset of SIRS from sepsis, trauma or postoperative complication	Uncertain
Are continuous venous oximetry, right ventricular ejection fraction and continuous cardiac output pulmonary artery catheter devices accurate	Yes

MI myocardial infarction, *PAC* pulmonary artery catheter, *SIRS* systemic inflammatory response syndrome

cal Care Nurses, American College of Chest Physicians, American Thoracic Society and Society of Critical Care Medicine. It called for an improved knowledge of interpretation of the data obtained from the pulmonary artery catheter and the complications of the placement. Furthermore, no moratorium should be invoked and the clinician shall carefully weigh the benefits and risks of the catheter before placing it with informed consent. It was agreed that there should be a controlled randomized study to determine indications for placement. Outlined in Table 2.5 is a portion of their findings based upon the clinical situation.

The Pulmonary Artery Catheter Consensus Conference (PACCC) [4] stated that it is *uncertain* whether pulmonary artery catheter-guided management improves outcomes in patients with sepsis or septic shock. This statement was based upon non-randomized studies with contemporaneous controls. These studies do not answer whether the changes in therapy that are made, based on hemodynamic measurements, alter the outcome of the patient.

The PACCC recommended:

1. The PAC may be useful in patients with septic shock who have not responded to initial aggressive fluid resuscitation and low dose inotropic/vasoconstrictor therapy.
2. Various management strategies for sepsis and septic shock (IV fluids, vasoactive and inotropic drugs, etc.) should be evaluated in prospective, randomized, controlled trials. Investigations should be designed to determine both the effectiveness of the PAC in accurate diagnosis and in monitoring patient response to therapeutic intervention. Management protocols need to be defined for both the PAC-guided and non-PAC-guided groups.

Since the consensus statement was published in 1997, the results of several trials have been presented. The trial by Richard and colleagues [18] for the French Pulmonary Artery Catheter Study Group was conducted in 36 intensive care units in France. A total of 681 patients were randomized to receive PAC or none. The treatment based on data obtained from the PAC was at the discretion of the treating physicians. The main conclusion of the study was that clinical management involving the early use of PAC in patients with shock, ARDS or both did not significantly affect mortality at 28 days (mortality with PAC was 59.4% vs. 61.0% without PAC).

The PAC-Man trial by Harvey and colleagues [19] was also to answer the question about whether the use of PAC in the ICU affects mortality. This was a randomized trial involving over 1,000 patients from 65 ICUs in the UK; 519 patients were managed with a PAC, 522 without. The ICU doctors had the option of using an alternative cardiac output monitoring device in the control group (such as esophageal Doppler and arterial pulse contour analysis, presumably the most common alternatives to PAC). The timing of insertion and subsequent clinical management were at the discretion of the treating physician. No difference was noted in hospital all cause mortality between patients managed with or without a PAC (68% vs. 66%, respectively).

These findings indicate no clear evidence of benefit or harm by managing critically ill patients with a PAC.

The results of the Fluid and Catheters Treatment Trial (FACTT) [20] of the ARDS Net sponsored by the National Heart, Lung, and Blood Institute of the USA have recently been published [20 bis]. This trial compares treatment of ARDS patients with and without PAC and for each group compares "fluid conservative" versus "fluid liberal" approach. Of all PAC trials, this is the only one simultaneously assessing the benefits or harms of both methods of monitoring (comparing PAC to CVC) and the treatment strategy guided by the monitoring. PAC-guided therapy did not improve survival or organ function, but was associated with more complications than CVC-guided therapy. In conclusion, we now have solid evidence based on randomized control trials in specific conditions to be able to say, that for these disease states, routine use of the PAC does not improve outcomes.

2.5.2 Indices of Global Perfusion

2.5.2.1 Physical Examination

Physical signs of decreased perfusion are acutely diminished mental status, cool skin, mottled skin, delayed capillary refill and oliguria.

2.5.2.2 Blood Lactate Concentration

In most forms of shock (hypovolemic, cardiogenic, obstructive), elevated blood lactate concentration reflects anaerobic tissue metabolism due to hypoperfusion resulting from a decrease in cardiac output. In severe sepsis and septic shock several studies have suggested that elevated lactate may result from a "metabolic block" at the mitochondrial level rather than from global hypoperfusion. The prognostic value of elevated blood lactate concentration is well established in septic shock [12]. The trend of lactate concentration is a better prognostic indicator than a single value [13]. Early lactate clearance is associated with improved outcome in severe sepsis and septic shock [21]; in other words a decrease of an elevated lactate during early resuscitation means a favorable outcome.

2.5.2.3 Venous Oxygen Saturation (SvO_2, $ScvO_2$)

Venous oxygen saturation assesses the relation between oxygen delivery and oxygen consumption. The amount of oxygen delivered to the tissues for use in aerobic metabolism is determined by three variables: hemoglobin concentration, oxygen saturation of hemoglobin and cardiac output. These three variables represent the three organ systems that constitute the three pillars of aerobic metabolism: blood, lungs and cardiovascular systems (Fig. 2.2).

$$O_2 \text{ delivery } (DO_2) = \text{Hb (g/dl)} \times 1.36 \times O_2 \text{ saturation} \times \text{cardiac output (ml/minute)}$$

This equation determines oxygen delivery only for oxygen combined with hemoglobin. The dissolved portion is very small and is ignored. Oxygen consumption (VO_2) is the percentage of the delivered oxygen the tissues extract for cellular respiration. Oxygen consumption is increased with fever, shivering, stress, pain, agitation and work of breathing and is decreased with hypothermia, sedation and paralysis.

After the tissues extract oxygen from the blood, the remaining oxygenation of the venous blood can be measured from the pulmonary artery (mixed venous oxygen saturation, SvO_2) or from the central venous circulation (central venous oxygen saturation, $ScvO_2$). Under normal conditions the $SaO_2 - SvO_2$ difference is 20–25%, yielding a SvO_2 of 65–75%. Normally the O_2 saturation is lower in the superior vena cava, but the reverse is true in shock, where the $ScvO_2$ values are approximately 5–15% greater than SvO_2 values. Redistribution of blood flow away from the hepatosplanchnic region (non-vital organs) toward the cerebral and coronary circulation (vital organs) causes increased oxygen extraction in the hepatosplanchnic region, resulting in reduced oxygen saturation in the inferior vena cava.

Global tissue hypoxia develops when systemic oxygen delivery is inadequate to meet tissue oxygen consumption, resulting in low venous oxygen saturation and an increased serum lactate concentration. On the other hand, normal venous saturation and serum lactate level suggest that oxygen delivery is adequate to meet

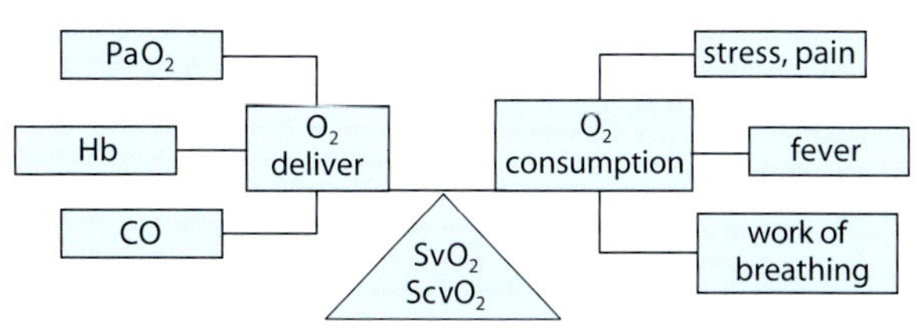

Fig. 2.2. The oxygen delivery to consumption ratio. *PaO_2* arterial partial pressure of oxygen, *Hb* hemoglobin, *CO* cardiac output, *SvO_2* mixed venous oxygen saturation, *$ScvO_2$* central venous oxygen saturation

tissue oxygen demands. A normal or high oxygen venous saturation with increased serum lactate concentration in a patient with sepsis indicates that despite adequate global systemic oxygen delivery the tissues are unable to extract the oxygen either due to microvascular shunting or mitochondrial dysfunction, "metabolic block."

In the resuscitation of severe sepsis and septic shock, $ScvO_2$ has been shown to be a better indicator of tissue oxygenation than vital signs (blood pressure, heart rate, urinary output and central venous pressure) when used to guide the early treatment of sepsis and septic shock. A recent prospective randomized study [22] comparing two strategies for early goal-directed therapy (EGDT) in patients with severe sepsis and septic shock showed that maintenance of continuously measured $ScvO_2$ above 70% in addition to maintaining central venous pressure above 8 – 12 mmHg, mean arterial pressure above 65 mmHg, and urinary output above 0.5 ml/kg per hour resulted in a 15% absolute reduction in mortality compared to the same treatment without $ScvO_2$ monitoring. In conclusion, EGDT that aims to restore the balance between oxygen supply and demand in the early management of severe sepsis and septic shock improves mortality.

2.5.3 Indices of Regional Perfusion

2.5.3.1 Gastric Tonometry

Gastric tonometry is a method to assess regional perfusion in the gut. The splanchnic bed has a countercurrent circulation at the mucosal level, rendering it especially vulnerable to ischemia. Global oxygen assessment may underestimate intestinal perfusion. This may lead to endotoxin or bacterial translocation across the gut wall to further compound problems. Intramucosal CO_2 (P_ICO_2) may be used to derive intramucosal pH_I using the Henderson-Hasselbach equation. A gastric probe is placed with a balloon and inflated with gas or a buffered solution for 90 min. After this time, the fluid is removed and analyzed. Low pH_I correlates with a poor outcome. Its utility in guiding therapy is still unclear.

2.5.3.2 Sublingual Capnography ($PslCO_2$)

Sublingual capnography is less invasive and more simple to use than gastric tonometry. In Marik's study [23], sublingual PCO_2 correlated well with gastric PCO_2. Elevated CO_2 in the gastrointestinal tract, either the gastric mucosa or the sublingual mucosa, indicates tissue dysoxia. The source of increased tissue CO_2 is intracellular buffering of excess hydrogen ions by bicarbonate. The excess of hydrogen ions is caused by excessive production of lactic acid during anaerobic metabolism either due to decreased oxygen supply (e.g., tissue hypoperfusion) or diminished ability to utilize oxygen.

2.5.3.3 Orthogonal Polarization Spectral Imaging (OPS)

Recently, investigations have used OPS to assess the microcirculation blood flow. De Baker and coworkers [24] used this technique to visualize the sublingual circulation. They observed a reduction of approximately half in the density of small vessels in patients with severe sepsis. Sakr et al. [25] from the same group found that microcirculatory alterations improved rapidly in septic shock survivors but not in non-survivors dying with multiple organ failure, regardless of whether shock was resolved. Hence microvascular recruitment (opening the microcirculation) can be a new goal for resuscitation in patients with septic shock.

2.5.4 Minimally and Non-invasive Devices

Recent approaches have sought minimally and non-invasive devices. Pulse contour analysis, transesophageal Doppler stroke volume, and transesophageal and transthoracic echocardiograms are the most commonly used methods.

2.5.4.1 Pulse Contour Analysis

Pulse contour analysis is based on the concept that the contour of the arterial pressure waveform is proportional to stroke volume (SV). According to Wesseling's formula, stroke volume is directly proportional to the systolic area of the aortic pressure (As) and inversely proportional to the vascular impedance (Z):

$$SV = As/Z$$

Edwards Lifesciences has recently introduced the Flotrac sensor and Vigileo monitor system for monitoring cardiac output continuously from the arterial line.

Calculation of the stroke volume from the arterial pressure wave according to the Flotrac/Vigileo system is as follows:

1. Pulse pressure: the difference between systolic and diastolic pressure is proportional to stroke volume. The algorithm calculates the pulsatility from the systolic and diastolic pressures over time and calculates the standard deviation of the arterial pressure over a 20-s window.
2. Software takes into account two additional key factors affecting the arterial pulse:

a) Large vessel compliance influenced by age, body surface area and gender.
b) Real time changes in peripheral resistance calculated by analysis of key waveform characteristics (e.g., change in MAP, time from start to end of a pulse, distribution of pressure over a pulse wave, angle and shape of waveform).

SV = $K \times$ SD(BP) where K is a constant quantifying arterial compliance and vascular resistance and SD(BP) is the standard deviation of the arterial pressure wave over a 20-s interval.

Cardiac output (CO) is then calculated by multiplying the SV by the heart rate. If a central venous pressure catheter has been placed, its signal can be interfaced with the Vigileo monitor, allowing for the calculation of the systemic vascular resistance (SVR). When used with a central venous oximetry catheter, the Vigileo monitor also provides continuous central venous oxygen saturation ($ScvO_2$). Small validation studies have shown good correlation of arterial pressure waveform based CO with CO obtained by thermodilution using the pulmonary artery catheter.

2.5.4.2 Esophageal Doppler Monitor [26]

The esophageal Doppler is a flexible ultrasound probe about the size of a nasogastric tube that can obtain a continuous cardiac output by measuring blood flow velocity in the descending thoracic aorta. Stroke volume is calculated as the product of mean velocity and cross-sectional area of the descending aorta. Area of the aorta is estimated using a nomogram based on the patient's age, height and weight. In adults, the measures of cardiac output made simultaneously with the esophageal Doppler monitor and standard thermodilution show good correlation. An attribute of this technique is easy probe insertion since it can be placed within minutes without major complications and requires minimal technical skill. The probe may be left in place for over 2 weeks. Disadvantages are difficulty in maintaining an optimal probe position and the fact that it cannot provide direct measurements of pulmonary artery and wedge pressures.

2.5.4.3 Echocardiogram

Using echocardiography, the same principles may be applied to determine cardiac output. Measuring the left ventricular outflow tract (LVOT) diameter (d) and time velocity integral (TVI) as determined by Doppler signal, a cardiac output (CO) may be calculated. CO in liters per minute = TVI × (d^2 × 0.785) × heart rate [26–30]. There is agreement over a wide range of values, when referenced to the PAC [31]. Sinus rhythm is required for factual results. In the unstable patient it may still be used safely but will not allow for ongoing monitoring to aid in titration of therapy [32]. Transesophageal echocardiogram (TEE), in certain instances, may be more revealing than the transthoracic approach [33]. TEE [34] assumes an increasingly important role in the non-invasive evaluation of the hemodynamically unstable patient [32]. With experienced personnel, TEE can be performed safely in critically ill patients with a high success rate. TEE facilitates prompt definitive diagnosis of major cardiac disorders that can be surgically correctable (endocarditis, cardiac tamponade, aortic dissection, mechanical complications of myocardial infarction). TEE can also help to determine the non-surgical cardiac contribution to hemodynamic instability. The patient with hypovolemic hypotension shows a small left ventricular cavity and hyperdynamic function. Intracavitary gradients due to mid-ventricular obstruction or systolic anterior motion of the mitral valve are often identified by Doppler echocardiography in such situations. Administration of fluids and withdrawal of inotropic agents results in paradoxical increases in blood pressure and lessening of pulmonary congestion as the intracavitary gradient decreases [34].

2.6 Clinical and Hemodynamic Goals in Patients with Septic Shock

Based upon recent studies [22, 35–37], it seems most reasonable to attempt to achieve a normal oxygen delivery and perfusion pressure that is associated with evidence of adequate organ oxygenation and perfusion. Oxygen delivery is determined by the product of cardiac output and oxygen content while perfusion pressure

Table 2.6. Goals of hemodynamic management

Hemodynamic goals	Oxygen delivery goals	Organ perfusion goals
MAP ≥65 mmHg	Cardiac index ≥2.5 l/m²/min Hct ≥30%	CNS – normal sensorium
CVP = 8–12 mmHg PCWP = 12–15 mmHg	SaO_2 >92%	Skin – pink, warm and dry
Cardiac index ≥2.5 l/m²/min	Serum lactate <2 mM/l SvO_2 ≥70%	Renal – urine output ≥0.5 ml/kg/h

is best reflected by mean arterial pressure. Interventions designed to achieve supranormal oxygen delivery in septic shock (with fluids and inotropes) have not demonstrated a benefit and such therapy may actually be associated with a reduced survival rate. The ideal goals are listed in Table 2.6.

2.7 Early Goal Directed Therapy (EGDT) [22]

Early goal directed therapy can significantly decrease in-hospital mortality in patients with severe sepsis or sepsis induced tissue hypoperfusion (hypotension with systolic BP 90 mmHg after a crystalloid fluid challenge of 20–30 ml/kg of body weight over 30 min or lactic acid level ≥4 mmol/l) as shown in the study of Rivers et al. During the first 6 h resuscitation of sepsis, induced hypoperfusion should include all of the following (Fig. 2.3.):

1. Central venous pressure 8–12 mmHg. In mechanically ventilated patients a CVP of 12–15 mmHg is considered to account for the increased intrathoracic pressure. If a PAC is inserted, a PCWP target of 12–15 mmHg replaces the CVP target.
2. Mean arterial pressure ≥65 mmHg, and ≤90 mmHg
3. Urine output ≥0.5 ml/kg/h
4. $ScvO_2$ or SvO_2 ≥70%

Although the cause of the tachycardia in septic patients may be multifactorial, a decrease in elevated heart rate with fluid resuscitation is often a useful marker for improving intravascular filling.

The protocol used in this study targeted an increase in venous oxygen saturation to ≥70%. This was achieved by sequential institution of initial fluid resuscitation, then packed RBC and then dobutamine.

This protocol was associated with a significant improvement in survival.

A point not addressed but of equal importance for rapid resuscitation is the need to start appropriate antibiotics within 60 min of diagnosing severe sepsis.

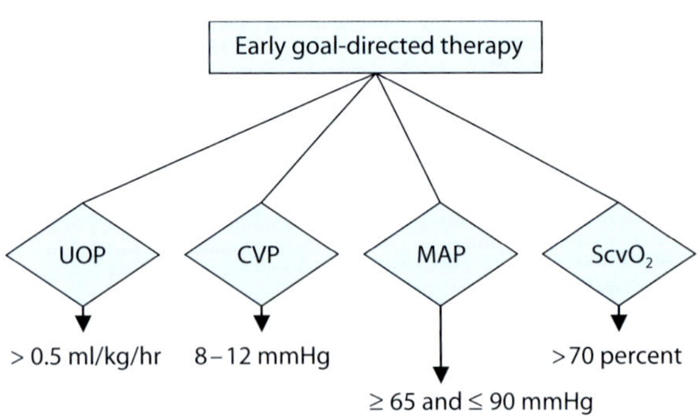

Fig. 2.3. Early goal-directed therapy

Appendix

Pulmonary Artery Catheter Measurements: Normal

Parameter	Symbols	"Normal" range
Right atrial pressure (central venous pressure)	RAP or CVP	2–7 mmHg
Right ventricular systolic pressure	RVSP	15–25 mmHg
Right ventricular diastolic pressure	RVDP	0–8 mmHg
Pulmonary artery systolic pressure	PASP	15–25 mmHg
Pulmonary artery diastolic pressure	PADP	8–15 mmHg
Pulmonary artery mean pressure	PA mean	10–20 mmHg
Pulmonary capillary wedge pressure	PCWP	6–12 mmHg
Cardiac output	CO	3.5–5.5 l/min
Cardiac index	CI	2.8–3.2 $l/min/m^2$
Pulmonary vascular resistance	PVR	150–250 dyne s/cm^5
Systemic vascular resistance	SVR	800–1200 dyne s/cm^5
Right ventricular stroke work index	RVSWI	7–12 $g\,m/m^2$
Left ventricular stroke work index	LVSWI	43–61 $g\,m/m^2$
Arterial oxygen content	CaO_2	20 vol%
Mixed venous oxygen saturation	SvO_2	75%
Mixed venous oxygen content	CvO_2	15 vol%
Oxygen delivery	DO_2	800–1,200 ml/min
Oxygen consumption	VO_2	225–275 ml/min
Oxygen extraction	O_2 extraction	25%

Formulas

Pulse Pressure = SBP – DBP

$$\text{Mean Arterial Pressure} = \frac{SBP + 2\,(DBP)}{3}$$

CO = SV × HR

CI = CO/BSA

SV Index = SV/BSA

$$PVR = \frac{(PAP - PCWP)\,80}{CO}$$

$$SVR = \frac{(MAP - CVP)\,80}{CO}$$

$CaO_2 = 1.36\,(Hgb)\,(SaO_2) + 0.003\,(PaO_2)$

$CvO_2 = 1.36\,(Hgb)\,(SvO_2) + 0.003\,(PvO_2)$

$Cc'_{O_2} = 1.36\,(Hgb)\,(100\%) + 0.003\,(PAO_2)$

(PAO_2 is the calculated alveolar pressur of O_2)

Arterio-venous O_2 content difference = $CaO_2 - CvO_2$

$Do_2 = CO \times CaO_2$

$\dot{V}o_2 = CO\ (CaO_2 - CvO_2)$

Fick equation: $CO = \dot{V}O_2 / (CaO_2 - CvO_2)$

O_2 Extraction fraction: $(CaO_2 - CvO_2) / CaO_2$

Shunt Fraction: $Q_s/Q_t = \dfrac{Cc'O_2 - CaO_2}{Cc'O_2 - CvO_2}$

References

1. American College of Chest Physicians & Society of Critical Care Medicine Consensus Conference (1992) Definitions for sepsis and multiple organ failure and guidelines for the use of innovative therapies in sepsis. Crit Care Med 20:864–874
2. Marik PE, Varon J (1998) The hemodynamic derangements in sepsis. Chest 114(3):854–860
3. Connors AF (1997) Right heart catheterization: Is it effective? New Horizons 5(3):195–200
4. Pulmonary Artery Catheter Consensus Conference Participants (1997) Consensus statement. Crit Care Med 25 (6):910–924
5. Wood LDH (1998) The pathophysiology of the circulation in critical illness. In: Hall JB, Schmidt GA, Wood LDH (eds) Principles of critical care, 2nd edn. McGraw-Hill, New York, p 268
6. Parillo JE (1993) Pathogenic mechanisms of septic shock. N Engl J Med 328:1471–1477
7. Parker MM (1998) Pathophysiology of cardiovascular dysfunction in septic shock. New Horizons 6:130–138
8. Marik PE, Varon J (1998) The hemodynamic derangements in sepsis: Implications for treatment strategies. Chest 114:854–860
9. Astiz ME, Rackow EC (1998) Septic shock. Lancet 351: 1501–1505
10. Cunnion RE, Schaer GL, Parker MM, et al. (1986) The coronary circulation in human septic shock. Circulation 73: 637–644
11. Rackow EC, Astiz ME, Weil MH (1988) Cellular oxygen metabolism during sepsis and shock. JAMA 259:1989–1993
12. Weil MH, Afifi AA (1970) Experimental and clinical studies in lactate and pyruvate as indicators of the severity of acute circulatory failure (Shock). Circulation 41:989
13. Vincent JL, Dufaye P, Berk J (1983) Serial lactate determination during circulatory shock. Crit Care Med 11:449
14. Dorman T, Breslow MJ, Lipsett PA, et al. (1998) Radial artery pressure monitoring underestimates central arterial pressure during vasopressor therapy in critically ill surgical patients. Crit Care Med 26:1646–1649
15. Coulter TD, Wiedemann HD (1999) Complications of hemodynamic monitoring. Clinics Chest Med 2:249–267
16. Iberti TJ, Daily EK, Leibowitz AB, Schecter CB, Fischer EP, Silverstein JH (1994) Assessment of critical care nurses' knowledge of the pulmonary artery catheter. Crit Care Med 22:1674–1678
17. Iberti TJ, Fischer EP, Leibowitz AB (1990) A multicenter study of physicians' knowledge of the pulmonary artery catheter. JAMA 264(22):2928–2932
18. Richard C, Warszawski J, Anguel N, et al., for the French Pulmonary Catheter Study Group (2003) Early use of pulmonary artery catheter and outcomes in patients with shock and acute respiratory distress syndrome: a randomized controlled trial. JAMA 290:2713–2720
19. Harvey S, Harrison DA, Singer M, et al. (2005) Assessment of the clinical effectiveness of pulmonary artery catheter in management of patients in intensive care (PAC-MAN): a randomized controlled trial. Lancet 366:472–7
20. ARDSnet. Prospective, randomized multicenter trial of pulmonary artery catheter (PAC) vs central venous catheter (CVC) for management of acute lung injury (ALI) and acute respiratory syndrome (ARDS). Prospective, randomized multi-center trial of "fluid conservative" vs "fluid libral" management of acute lung injury (ALI) and acute respiratory distress syndrome (ARDS). Available at: http://www.ards.org/fact.php

20 bis. The National Heart, Lung, and Blood Institute (2006) Acute Respiratory Distress Syndrome (ARDS) Clinical Trials Network. Pulmonary-artery versus central venous catheter to guide treatment of acute lung injury. N Engl J Med 354:2213–2224

21. Nguyen HB, Rivers EP (2004) Early lactate clearance is associated with improved outcome in severe sepsis and septic shock. CCM 32:1637–1643
22. Rivers EP, Nguyen HB, Havstad S, Ressler J, Muzzin A, Knoblich B, Peterson E, Tomlanovich M, for the Early Goal-Directed Therapy Collaborative Group (2001) Early goal-directed therapy in the treatment of severe sepsis and septic shock. N Engl J Med 345:1368–1377
23. Marik PE (2001) Sublingual capnography. A clinical validation study. Chest 120:923–927
24. De Backer D, Creteur J, Preiser J-C, Dubois M-J, Vincent J-L (2002) Microvascular blood flow is altered in patients with sepsis. Am J Respir Crit Care Med 166:98–104
25. Sakr Y, Dubois MJ, De Baker D, et al. (2004) Persistent microcirculatory alterations are associated with organ failure and death in patients with septic shock. Crit Care Med 32:1825–1831
26. Gan TJ, Arrowsmith JE (1997) The esophageal Doppler monitor. A safe means of monitoring circulation. BMJ 315:893–894
27. Nishimura RA, et al. (1984) Non-invasive measurement of cardiac output by continuous wave Doppler echocardiography: Initial experience and review of the literature. Mayo Clin Proc 59(7):484–489
28. Hattle L, Angelsen B (1985) Doppler ultrasound in cardiology, 2nd edn. Lea and Febiger, Philadelphia
29. Baker DW (1980) Applications of pulsed Doppler. Rad Clin North Am 18:79–103
30. Nishimura RA, et al. (1985) Doppler echocardiography: Theory, instrumentation, technique and application. Mayo Clin Proc 60(5):321–343
31. Dabaghi SF, Rokey R, et al. (1995) Comparison of echocardiographic assessment of cardiac hemodynamics in the intensive care unit with right-sided cardiac catheterization. Am J Cardiol 76:392
32. Sohn D-W, Shin G-J, Oh JK, Tajik AJ, Click RL, Miller FA, Seward JB (1995) Role of transesophageal echocardiography in hemodynamically unstable patients. Mayo Clin Proc 70:925–931
33. Heidenreich J, Raymond F, et al. (1995) Transesophageal echocardiography predicts mortality in critically ill patients with unexplained hypotension. Am Coll Cardiol 26:152–158
34. Pearson AC (1995) Noninvasive evaluation of the hemodynamically unstable patient: the advantage of seeing clearly. Mayo Clin Proc 70:1012–1014
35. Hayes MA, Timmins AC, Yau H, Palazzo M, et al. (1994) Elevation of systemic oxygen delivery in the treatment of critically ill patients. N Engl J Med 330:1717–22
36. Gattinoni L, Brazzi L, Pelosi P, Latini R, Tognoni G, Pesenti A, Fumagalli R, for The SvO_2 Collaborative Group (1995) A trial of goal-oriented hemodynamic therapy in critically ill patients. N Engl J Med 333:1025–32
37. Heyland DK, Cook DJ, et al. (1996) Maximizing oxygen delivery in critically ill patients. A methodologic appraisal of the evidence. Crit Care Med 24:517

3 Cardiopulmonary Resuscitation and Infection

L. Hammer, J.-F. Timsit

3.1 Introduction

The survival to hospital discharge after an out-of-hospital cardiac arrest due to cardiac disease is only 7% [1]. The continuous provision of information to the public and healthcare workers about cardiopulmonary resuscitation (CPR) in the 1970s has led to a dramatic improvement in immediate survival from cardiac arrest. Survival to discharge after in-hospital cardiac arrest is 17–37% [2, 3].

But, the AIDS epidemic as well as the rapid progression of hepatitis C have changed this situation. Even if CPR with mouth-to-mouth ventilation (MTMV) is associated with a 5- to 30-fold increase in survival, due to fear of transmitted infectious diseases, persons willing to perform this procedure are rare. In addition, after initial CPR, survivors are at risk of nosocomial pneumonia, especially aspiration pneumonia and bacteremia, which must be recognized and treated promptly.

These two sides of the relationship between CPR and infection are discussed in this chapter. We review the risk of acquisition of infection in patients surviving from initial CPR and the risk of transmission of infection between the patient and the caregivers, and the way to prevent it.

3.2 Infection Acquired During CPR: Estimating the Risk for the Caregiver

3.2.1 Reluctance of Caregivers To Perform Cardiopulmonary Resuscitation and Mouth-to-Mouth Ventilation (MTMV)

The only interventions that have been shown unequivocally to improve long-term survival after cardiac arrest are basic life support and defibrillation [4].

The value of MTMV is currently under discussion because of a widespread fear of transmission of infectious diseases. Healthcare professionals have stated in several studies that they may hold back from providing MTMV when confronted with a cardiac arrest in a stranger. Although infection by *Mycobacterium tuberculosis* is more likely than one by human immunodeficiency virus (HIV) via MTMV, people's fear is understandable. For example, a reluctance of lay and medical personnel to perform MTMV in hospital and community settings has been documented, with 45% of respondents declining to perform MTMV on a stranger [5].

An expert committee of the American Heart Association stated that MTMV may be omitted in the initial phase of cardiac arrest, and considered recommending chest compressions only if the emergency medical support was going to arrive rapidly. However, in anesthetized volunteers, ventilation was not capable of providing sufficient gas exchange, especially when the airway was not protected.

Hew et al. examined whether the perceived risk and fear of contracting infectious diseases diminishes the willingness of paramedics and emergency medical technicians (EMTs) to perform mouth-to-mouth resuscitation (MMR) [6]. Seventy-seven EMTs and 27 paramedics responded to a questionnaire, administered by one of two physicians, containing mock cardiac arrest scenarios that were designed to assess willingness to perform MTMV as a citizen responder. Faced with a situation in which an adult stranger required MTMV, 57% of the participating EMTs and all of the paramedics stated that they would refuse to perform MTMV. Moreover, none of the paramedics and only 32.5% of the EMTs stated that they would perform MTMV on a man in a gay neighborhood. In addition, 23% of the EMTs and 37% of the paramedics indicated that they would refuse to perform MTMV on a child. Twenty-nine percent of the prehospital-care providers had been in situations requiring MTMV in the community, and 40% either had walked away or only did external compression. Of those participating paramedics and EMTs who had performed MTMV in emergency situations, only 45% indicated that they would do so again. The respondents indicated that they would not be willing to administer MTMV because of the fear of contracting infectious agents, especially HIV. Despite the proven effectiveness of MMR in saving lives, paramedics and EMTs are highly reluctant to perform MMR as citizen responders. Their perceived risks of contracting infectious agents during MMR are high, despite the low actual risks.

3.2.2 Risks of Infection for Caregivers

The possibility of transmission of infection between a victim and a rescuer has caused much concern, especially more recently with the heightened anxiety over viral hepatitis and AIDS. Even if cases are probably underreported, the number of infections convincingly related to resuscitation is estimated to be less than 1/200,000 [7].

There are two main ways of acquiring infectious diseases while performing CPR: MTMV and needlestick transmission.

3.2.2.1 Mouth-to-Mouth Transmission

***Neisseria* Meningitidis.** The risk of salivary transmission of *N. meningitidis* is high especially in the case of systemic infection [8] and may explain why four cases of meningococcal infections have been linked to MTMV performed by healthcare workers. One case of meningococcal meningitis after tracheal intubation of a child suspected of having meningoencephalitis has also been described [9]. Providers who have experienced such an exposure should be offered chemoprophylaxis.

***Mycobacterium* Tuberculosis.** Although the risk of acquiring tuberculosis after performing MTMV on a patient with active tuberculosis should likely be very high, a unique case of tuberculosis in a healthcare worker has been described. However, a rescuer who has given MTMV should be followed up for conversion and/or active tuberculosis. It seems logical to recommend serial tuberculin tests and/or a chest radiograph in this case [10].

3.2.2.2 Enteric Pathogens

Mouth-to-mouth transmission of enteric pathogens has been described for *Shigella sonnei*, *Salmonella infantis* and possibly for *Helicobacter pylori.*

3.2.2.3 Risk of Transmission of Viruses Through MTMV

HIV is rarely isolated from the saliva of HIV infected patients and then in very low concentrations. This finding might explain the low risk of salivary transmission. For example, 1,309 dental professionals who had no behavioral risk factors for HIV infection but have cared for multiple patients known to have AIDS were screened. Only one dentist was seropositive for HIV [11].

On the other hand, hepatitis B virus (HBV) poses substantial risks to caregivers. Although no case of HBV transmission has ever been reported, salivary exchange is considered to be one of the mechanisms of non-parenteral transmission of HBV within families [12], and human bites are responsible for the acquisition of HBV [13].

Little is known about the risk of hepatitis C (HCV) transmission during MTMV. The prevalence of HCV positivity in saliva ranged between 20% and 62% of HCV infected patients [7]. However, only a single case of saliva transmission after a human bite has been reported.

3.2.2.4 Needlestick Transmission

Although the risk of acquiring infection should be considered as being very low, the risk of acquiring infection during emergency cardiopulmonary resuscitation exists especially because the scene of resuscitation is often chaotic, resulting in a high risk of needlestick or other sharp injuries.

Usually, the risk resulting for parenteral exposure is greatest with HBV (13.1%), intermediate with HCV (5.8%) and lowest with HIV (0.32%) [14–16]. A particular effort in preventing sharp injuries in this situation is the main and essential way to prevent infection acquisition for caregivers (see Appendix).

3.3 Nosocomial Infections After CPR

3.3.1 Pathophysiology of Infection After CPR

Postresuscitation abnormalities after cardiac arrest mimic the immunologic and coagulation disorders observed in severe sepsis and multiple organ dysfunction syndrome [17]. Postresuscitation disease is characterized by high levels of circulating cytokines and adhesion molecules, the presence of plasma endotoxin in ≈ 50% of patients, and dysregulated leukocyte production of cytokines [18]. This could be due to the intensity of the ischemia and reperfusion which is known to activate nuclear factor kB [19] or other signaling pathways and then induce the production of cytokines such as TNF-α, IL-1 or IL-8 [20] as well as oxygen radicals. Ischemia reperfusion also promotes the adhesion of leukocytes to the endothelium. Consequently plasma protein C and S levels after successful resuscitation are lower in non-survivors than in survivors [21]. Low baseline cortisol levels may be associated with an increased risk of fatal dysfunction in these patients [18, 22].

After the initial phase of injury, negative feedback downregulates early systemic inflammatory response syndrome (SIRS) to limit potential autodestructive inflammation. The early hypoinflammatory response consists of a release of anti-inflammatory cytokines (IL-4, IL-10) and is followed by a long-lasting hypoinflammatory state called "compensatory anti-inflammatory response syndrome" (CARS) [23]. This could lead to a delayed immunosuppression [24], which could be associated with major infectious complications. This potential mechanism has not been yet demonstrated clinically.

3.3.2 Problems in Diagnosing Nosocomial Infections After CPR

The proinflammatory cascade might explain fever occurring after CPR [25]. Fever is also a poor marker of infection. It is frequently encountered, as well as sepsis syndrome, after successful CPR and is frequently considered as a marker of poor neurologic outcome [26]. Hyperthermia is responsible for an increase of the volume of the cerebral infarction after occlusion of the cerebral blood flow in animal models [27]. Fever, even moderate fever during the day following brain ischemia, may markedly exacerbate brain injury. It is probably due to ischemia related factors, thermodysregulation of central nervous system origin and/or decreased heat loss or altered distribution of body heat due to vasoconstriction [28]. For example, Takino and Okada [25] found 18 patients with restoration of spontaneous circulation and who were not considered brain-dead within the first 48 h. Fourteen had hyperthermia (temperature >38 °C) occurring in the initial 48 h after resuscitation. Eight patients with later brain death showed significant hyperthermia and a high peak temperature (median 39.8 °C), and six out of the seven patients with prolonged coma had a peak body temperature of greater than 38 °C (median 38.3 °C). None of these patients had evidence of infection. On the contrary, in another study, only six out of 13 patients with bacteremia after cardiac arrest had hypothermia (<36 °C, $n=3$) or hyperthermia (>38.5 °C, $n=3$) [29].

On the other hand, hypothermia is often used by intensivists to prevent brain injury. The efficacy of hypothermia in preserving neurologic function when instituted before and during the no flow cardiovascular state has been well documented both clinically and experimentally since the 1950s. Recent experimental and clinical (for cardiac arrest due to ventricular fibrillation) evidence has shown that hypothermia induced after cardiac arrest does indeed mitigate the effects of postresuscitation syndrome, improves neurologic function and reduces histologic brain damage [28]. Such benefit can be demonstrated with mild (34–36 °C) hypothermia [30], thus minimizing complication and requiring less time for induction of hypothermia. Mild hypothermia is considered as an important and secure component for cerebral preservation and resuscitation during, and after, global ischemia and it is often considered as a useful method of cerebral resuscitation after global ischemic states, thereby promoting the prevention of neuromental diseases [31].

Evidence from clinical and in vitro studies shows that hypothermia can impair immune function. Indeed, inhibition of inflammatory responses may be one of the mechanisms through which hypothermia exerts neuroprotective effects [32]. A number of studies, mostly in patients with stroke or traumatic brain injury, have indeed reported higher risks of pneumonia when therapeutic hypothermia is used over longer periods of time (≥48–72 h) [33, 34]. Short-term cooling (≤24 h) does not appear to increase the risk of infection [31, 35, 36].

3.3.3 Role of the Digestive Tract

The importance of intestinal injury is directly related to the duration of ischemia and to the reperfusion injury via the O_2 free production [37].

Infection is considered to be partly due to digestive ischemia and bacterial translocation occurring during CPR. After CPR, early onset nosocomial infections are frequent. In 67 patients who survived from CPR at least 72 h, 51 developed early onset nosocomial infections (76% pneumonia and 9% bacteremia) [38]. Microorganisms responsible for these infections were Enterobacteriaceae (32%), *Enterococcus* (9%), *Staphylococcus* spp. (12%) and *S. pneumoniae* (9%) [38], which correspond mainly to endogenous flora. These patients present digestive symptoms in two-thirds of cases (vomiting or hiccoughing 52%, diarrhea or ileus 16%, digestive hemorrhage 32%). In another study [29], Gaussorgues et al. found that 12 out of 13 patients with early onset bacteremia after CPR had fetid diarrhea a few hours after their ICU admission. Moreover, the same microorganisms were found in blood and feces. In addition, 13 out of 19 patients underwent digestive endoscopy showing esophageal, stomach or colonic ischemia, profound ulceration or necrosis. Non-occlusive mesenteric infarction could also be involved in the genesis of these bacteremia [39]. In another study [40], ten out of 56 patients had documented episodes of diarrhea or gastrointestinal bleeding during the first 48 h after CPR but none of them developed bloodstream infection.

The digestive lesions together with the microorganisms recovered are strong arguments for the predominant role of the digestive tract in the genesis of infection.

3.3.4
Lower Respiratory Tract Infections Following Cardiac Arrest and Successful CPR

Patients surviving CPR are at high risk of lower respiratory tract infections. They accumulate major risk factors such as emergency tracheal intubation, a decreased level of consciousness and bronchoaspiration. Animal models indicate that lower esophageal sphincter pressure may decrease rapidly to 5 cmH_2O during cardiac arrest, which may further increase the risk of gastric inflation and subsequent regurgitation, aspiration and pneumonia during ventilation with an unprotected airway [5]. Gastric regurgitation was recorded to have occurred in 180 out of 797 (22.6%) patients with cardiac arrest [41].

Complications of tracheal intubation performed on emergency have been prospectively evaluated: among 297 tracheal intubations, radiological pictures of pulmonary aspiration have been found in 4% of cases and might partly explain the high rate of early onset pneumonia after CPR [42].

The incidence of lower respiratory tract infection in CPR survivors was as high as 28.1% using protected specimen brush and bronchoalveolar lavage culture techniques [43] and was higher than that observed in the other general ICU ventilated population.

Rello et al. [44] have shown that cardiopulmonary resuscitation is independently associated with development of very early-onset pneumonia (within the first 48 h of intubation). CPR [odds ratio: 5.13 (2.14–12.26)] and continuous sedation [odds ratio: 4.4 (1.8–10.6)] were significant risk factors of pneumonia, while antibiotic use [odds ratio: 0.29 (0.12–0.69)] showed a protective effect. Gajic et al. reported that 30% of cardiac arrest patients developed new pneumonia after resuscitation [40]. *S. aureus* is the most frequently isolated organism of pneumonia in their study. The occurrence of pneumonia was also reported in 29% of survivors of ventricular fibrillation [31]. Tsai et al. reported pneumonia in 61% out-of-hospital cardiac arrest survivors in the first 7 days. However, in contrast to findings in the other studies, gram-negative bacteria accounted for 78.9% of cases of pneumonia (the most common organisms of pneumonia were *Klebsiella pneumoniae* and *Acinetobacter baumanii*) [45].

3.3.5
Catheter-Related Infections and Bacteremia

After 7.5 min experimental cardiac arrest in dogs, bacteremia was present in all animals [46]. Bacteremia was demonstrated in patients admitted to the ICU after successful CPR. Gaussorgues and colleagues [29] found that 13 out of 33 patients had at least two positive peripheral blood cultures in the first 12 h after admission. Bacteremia was considered as being due to mesenteric ischemia as 12 patients had fetid diarrhea during 3–5 h following cardiac arrest. The microorganisms isolated were found in both blood and feces in 12 cases. One *S. aureus* catheter-related septicemia occurred after emergency insertion of a central line. Tsai et al. found 13% bacteremia. The most commonly isolated organisms of bacteremia were *Staphylococcus* spp. (*S. aureus* and *S. epidermidis*) and *Burkholderia cepacia* [45]. In the Gajic et al. study, 5 patients out of 79 had positive blood cultures: *S.aureus* in three, *Streptococcus pneumoniae* in one, and combined *S. epidermidis* and *Candida* spp. in one [40]. In most cases, during CPR, maximal sterile barriers are not used during insertion of central venous catheters. Moreover, the femoral route is frequently chosen. This could explain the high risk of catheter-related infection in this situation [47, 49]. In a study involving prospectively 300 catheters inserted into 204 patients, Goetz and coworkers [48] found that emergent insertion was associated with a sixfold increase in the risk of catheter contamination (clinical infection or colonization with >15 colonies on semi-quantitative culture) [odds ratio 6.2; 95% confidence interval (CI95) 1.1–36.7; $P = 0.04$].

Even if reasonable, there is currently no recommendation for the removal of central catheters inserted under emergency conditions, where breaks in aseptic technique are likely to have occurred [49].

3.3.6
Other Infections

Other anecdotal infectious complications have been described such as acute *S. aureus* mediastinitis complicating sternal fracture during chest compressions and a resulting retrosternal hematoma [50–52].

3.3.7
Consequences of Infections on the Prognosis of CPR Patients

The impact of infections on the prognosis of CPR patients is still under debate. Although old studies reported an increased risk of death associated with infection [29, 53], more recent studies did not [40, 45].

3.4
Prevention of Infection

3.4.1
For the Patient

During ventilation of unprotected airways, tidal volumes of 0.5 l instead of 0.8–1 l may have an advantage as they decrease the risk of gastric inflation and subsequent aspiration and pneumonia [5]. The use of the laryngeal mask airway alone or after bag valve mask ventilation has been shown to reduce the risk of regurgitation [41].

In the study of Rello et al. [44], exposure to antibiotic independently prevented development of pneumonia during the first 2 days of ventilation but has no effect on late onset pneumonia frequently related to multiresistant strains. Indeed, other studies have reported the protective effect of antibiotics specifically on episodes caused by primary endogenous flora [54]. However, the protective effect of antibiotics has been shown to attenuate when the time in the ICU increases [55]. Moreover, antibiotic use increases the risk of antimicrobial resistance. Antimicrobial intravenous prophylaxis cannot be recommended. However, in the case of fever, after microbiological samples have been taken, the threshold for instituting antimicrobial therapy, if there is any suspicion of pneumonia or sepsis developing, should be lowered.

3.4.2 Precautions To Reduce the Risk for the Caregivers During CPR

Healthcare workers know the "universal precautions" for the prevention of cross-transmission of infectious diseases. Guidelines for prevention and management of biohazardous exposures during CPR are summarized in the Appendix. However, in urgent situations, such as cardiac arrest, it is often difficult to take the time to follow these precautions. So, to decrease the risk for caregivers, it is important to facilitate the use of new devices such as needleless systems. One-way valve mouth-to-mask systems or bag-valve masks [56] are of interest in preventing direct mouth-to-mouth contact between rescuer and patient. They seem to prevent transmission from the oral flora to the rescuer's side of the device.

Adequate training in CPR is one of the determinants of the efficacy of CPR [57]. This training must address protection from infection during CPR, with a great focus on measures for avoiding sharp injuries.

3.5 Conclusion

The benefit of initiating lifesaving resuscitation in a patient in cardiac arrest greatly outweighs the risk of secondary infection in the rescuers or the patient. Nevertheless, use of simple infection-control measures during CPR can reduce a very low level of risk even further.

Instruction in CPR for providers of pre-hospital care, the medical community, and the general public should emphasize the benefits of providing MTMV, the actual low risks of contracting infectious diseases during administration of MTMV, and the use of widely available and effective barrier masks to minimize any risks due to administration of MTMV. The strategy to compress the thorax first and then maintain the airway and perform ventilation may only be advantageous for the first 30 s of CPR.

After successful initial CPR, hyperthermia is frequent and might be due to early onset nosocomial infection, which requires immediate diagnosis and treatment.

Appendix

Guidelines for Prevention and Management of Biohazardous Exposures During Cardiopulmonary Resuscitation (Adapted from Mejicano and Maki [7])

1. Healthcare workers and public protection personnel likely to be called on to give CPR must be aware of the potential catastrophic sequelae of biohazardous exposure, especially needlestick injuries, and of guidelines for prevention. This can be effected through inclusion in all CPR training programs.
   - Recapping or resheathing used needles must be strongly discouraged. Effective and safe needle-disposal units should be made widely and conveniently available throughout the hospital, especially in locations that facilitate their immediate use.
   - Receptacles in metal or other impervious material should be available and emptied according to an established routine.
   - Needleless systems now available should be encouraged and made available in various sites, including resuscitation carts and emergency transport vehicles.
   - Healthcare workers and public protection professionals must be apprised of the importance of obtaining adequate assistance when administering injections or infusion therapy to patients.
   - Personnel must be apprised of the need to use extreme care in cleaning up after CPR and other procedures that involve needles, such as insertion of central lines.
2. Oral barrier devices should be widely and conveniently available throughout hospitals and clinics and in emergency transport vehicles where CPR is likely to be performed.
   - After every CPR procedure, especially if mouth-to-mouth ventilation was done, an effort should be made to determine whether the patient may have had a dangerous, contagious infection, such as pulmonary tuberculosis, meningococcal or streptococcal sepsis, or overwhelming pneumonia. If the patient does not survive, cultures and blood specimens should be obtained. If an autopsy is carried out, evidence of undiagnosed infection should specifically be sought.

3. If a clear-cut biohazardous exposure to a patient's blood occurred through a needlestick, a blood splash into the mouth or eyes, or broken skin, or if blood or open sores were seen in the patient's mouth and mouth-to-mouth ventilation was given, the patient must be tested for evidence of infection with HIV, HBV, and HCV to determine the need for postexposure prophylaxis.
   - With biohazardous exposures, especially needlestick injuries, the exposure should be immediately reported to the employee health service, where the exposed person can be evaluated and managed most consistently and inexpensively and surveillance of all work related injuries can be facilitated.
   - Management of biohazardous injuries must be possible 24 h a day, 7 days a week, by emergency department personnel trained in the institutional biohazardous injury protocol.
   - Particular attention should be given to persons who have sustained repeated injuries to identify accident-prone activities or persons.

4. Institutions should maintain continuous surveillance of all biohazardous injuries. This can form the basis for preventive programs and for assessment of their effectiveness.

5. It is imperative that every hospital has a protocol that provides unambiguous management guidelines specifically focussing on the following:
   - Clear definitions of biohazardous exposures
   - Procedures for immediate care of the injury at the time of occurrence, such as squeezing the puncture wound to induce bleeding and using immediate cutaneous disinfection with a virucidal agent, such as an iodophor
   - Procedures to expeditiously determine the magnitude of risk (for example, screening the resuscitated patient for evidence of active with HBV, HCV, and HIV)
   - Guidelines for postexposure evaluation and treatment, where indicated, especially for exposures to hepatitis A virus, HBV, HCV, HIV, *Mycobacterium tuberculosis* and *Neisseria meningitidis*
   - Provisions for long-term follow-up of the exposed rescuer, especially after exposures to HBV, HCV and HIV
   - Provisions for administrative follow-up of all injuries (to minimize recurrences)
   - Review and revision of the protocol at least annually
   - Public protection professionals who are likely to provide CPR in the community must also have access to an educational program and postexposure protocol, which will be most efficiently and consistently effected through a local hospital.

References

1. Pell JP, Sirel JM, et al. (2003) Presentation, management and outcome of out of hospital cardiopulmonary arrest: comparison by underlying aetiology. Heart 89:839–842
2. Gwinnutt CL, Columb M, et al. (2000) Outcome after cardiac arrest in adults in UK hospitals: effect of the 1997 guidelines. Resuscitation 47:125–135
3. Herlitz J, Bang A, et al. (2001) Characteristics and outcome among patients suffering in-hospital cardiac arrest in monitored and non-monitored areas. Resuscitation 48: 125–135
4. Advanced Life Support Working Group of the European Resuscitation Council (1998) The 1998 European resuscitation council guidelines for adult advanced life support. BMJ 37:81–90
5. Wenzel V, et al. (1997) Ventilation during cardiopulmonary resuscitation. A literature study and analysis of ventilation strategies. Anaesthesist 46:133–141
6. Hew P, et al. (1997) Reluctance of paramedics and emergency medical technicians to perform mouth-to-mouth resuscitation. J Emerg Med 15(3):279–284
7. Mejicano GC, Maki DG (1998) Infections acquired during cardiopulmonary resuscitation: estimating the risk and defining strategies for prevention. Ann Intern Med 129: 813–828
8. Jacobson JA, Fraser DW (1976) A simplified approach to meningococcal disease prophylaxis. JAMA 236:1053–1054
9. Gehanno JF, Kohen-Couderc L, et al. (1999) Nosocomial meningococcemia in a physician. Infect Control Hosp Epidemiol 20:564–565
10. Bass JB Jr, Farer LS, et al. (1994) Treatment of tuberculosis and tuberculosis infection in adults and children. American Thoracic Society and the Center for Disease Control and Prevention. Am J Respir Crit Care Med 149:1359–1374
11. Klein RS, Phelan JA, et al. (1988) Low occupational risk of human immunodeficiency virus infection among dental professionals. N Engl J Med 318:86–90
12. Powell E, Duke M, et al. (1985) Hepatitis B virus infection within families: potential importance of saliva as a vehicle of spread. Aust N Z J Med 15:717–720
13. MacQuarrie MB, Forghani B, et al. (1974) Hepatitis B transmitted by a human bite. JAMA 230:723–724
14. Gerberding JL (1996) Prophylaxis of occupational exposure to HIV. Ann Intern Med 125:497–501
15. Seef LB, Wright HL, et al. (1978) Type B hepatitis after needle-stick exposure: prevention with hepatitis B immune globulin. Final report of the veteran administration cooperative study. Ann Intern Med 88:285–293
16. Kiyosawa K, Sodeyama T, et al. (1991) Hepatitis C in hospital employees with needlestick injuries. Ann Intern Med 115:367–369
17. Adrie C, Adib-Conquy M, et al. (2002) Successful cardiopulmonary resuscitation after cardiac arrest as a "sepsis-like" syndrome. Circulation 106:562–568
18. Adrie C, Laurent I, et al. (2004) Postresuscitation disease after cardiac arrest: a sepsis-like syndrome? Curr Opin Crit Care 10:208–212
19. Moine P, Shenkar R, et al. (1997) Systemic blood loss affects NF kappa B regulatory mechanisms in the lung. Am J Physiol 273:L185–L192
20. Wan S, Leclerc JL, et al. (1997) Inflammatory response to cardiopulmonary bypass: mechanisms involved and possible therapeutic strategies. Chest 112:676–692
21. Adrie C, Monchi M, et al. (2005) Coagulopathy after successful cardiopulmonary resuscitation following cardiac arrest. JACC 46:21–28

22. Hekimian G, Baugnon T, et al. (2004) Cortisol levels and adrenal reserve after successful cardiac arrest resuscitation. Shock 22:116–119
23. Bone RC (1996) Sir Isaac Newton, sepsis, SIRS and CARS. Crit Care Med 24:1125–1128
24. Soppi E, Lindroos M, et al. (1984) Effect of cardiopulmonary resuscitation-induced stress on cell-mediated immunity. Intensive Care Med 10:287–292
25. Takino M, Okada Y (1991) Hyperthermia following cardiopulmonary resuscitation. Intensive Care Med 17:419–420
26. Torres A, Pickert CB, et al. (1997) Long term functional outcome of inpatient pediatric cardiopulmonary resuscitation. Pediatr Emerg Care 13:369–373
27. Kim Y, Busto R, et al. (1996) Delayed postischemic hyperthermia in awake rats worsens the histopathological outcome of transient focal cerebral ischemia. Stroke 27:2274–2280
28. Safar P (1988) Resuscitation from clinical death: pathophysiologic limits and therapeutic potentials. Crit Care Med 16:923–941
29. Gaussorgues P, Gueugniaud PY, et al. (1988) Bacteremia following cardiac arrest and cardiopulmonary resuscitation. Intensive Care Med 14:575–577
30. Sterz F, Zeiner A, et al. (1996) Mild resuscitative hypothermia and outcome after cardiopulmonary resuscitation. J Neurosurg Anesthesiol 8:88–96
31. Hypothermia After Cardiac Arrest Study Group (2002) Mild therapeutic hypothermia to improve the neurologic outcome after cardiac arrest. N Engl J Med 346:549–556
32. Polderman K (2004) Application of therapeutic hypothermia in the intensive care unit. Intensive Care Med 30: 757–769
33. Shiozaki T, Hayakata T, et al. (2001) A multicenter prospective randomized controlled trial of the efficacy of mild hypothermia for severely head injured patients with low intracranial pressure. J Neurosurg 94:50–54
34. Schwab S, Georgiadis D, et al. (2001) Feasibility and safety of moderate hypothermia after massive hemispheric infarction. Stroke 32:2033–2035
35. Marion DW, Penrod LE, et al. (1997) Treatment of traumatic brain injury with moderate hypothermia. N Engl J Med 336:540–546
36. Bernard SA, Gray TW, et al. (2002) Treatment of comatose survivors of out-of-hospital cardiac arrest with induced hypothermia. N Engl J Med 346:557–563
37. Haglund U, Hulten L, et al. (1975) Mucosal lesions in the human small intestine in shock. Gut 16:979–984
38. Fourel D, L'Her E, et al. (1999) Infections nosocomiales après arret cardiocirculatoire extra-hospitalier: rôle du tube digestif. Ann Fr Anesth Reanim 18:292S
39. Morgan RJ, White PW, et al. (1985) Treatment of non-occlusive mesenteric infarction after cardiopulmonary resuscitation. Crit Care Med 13:53–54
40. Gajic O, Festic E, et al. (2004) Infectious complications in survivors of cardiac arrest admitted to the medical intensive care unit. Resuscitation 60:65–69
41. Stone BJ, Chantler PJ, et al. (1998) The incidence of regurgitation during cardiopulmonary resuscitation: a comparison between the bag valve mask and laryngeal mask airway. Resuscitation 38:3–6
42. Schwartz DE, Matthay MA, et al. (1995) Death and other complications of emergency airway management in critically ill adults: a prospective investigation of 297 tracheal intubations. Anesthesiology 82:367–376
43. Rello J, Valles J, et al. (1995) Lower respiratory tract infections following cardiac arrest and cardiopulmonary resuscitation. Clin Infect Dis 21:310–314
44. Rello J, Diaz E, et al. (1999) Risk factors for developing pneumonia within 48 hours of intubation. Am J Respir Crit Care Med 159:1742–1746
45. Tsai MS, Chiang WC, et al. (2005) Infections in the survivors of out-of-hospital cardiac arrest in the first 7 days. Intensive Care Med 31:621–626
46. Cerchiari EL, Safar P, et al. (1993) Visceral, hematologic and bacteriologic changes and neurological outcome after cardiac arrest in dogs. The visceral post-resuscitation syndrome. Resusciation 25:119–136
47. Richet H, Hubert B, et al. (1990) Prospective multicenter study of vascular catheter-related complications and risk factors for positive central catheter cultures in intensive care unit patients. J Clin Microbiol 28:2520–2525
48. Goetz AM, Wagener MM, et al. (1998) Risk of infection due to central venous catheters: effect of site of placement and catheter type. Infect Control Hosp Epidemiol 11:842–845
49. Pearson ML (1996) Guidelines for prevention of intravascular-device-related infections. Infect Control Hosp Epidemiol 17:438–473
50. Mensah GA, Gold JP, et al. (1988) Acute purulent mediastinitis and osteomyelitis after closed chest cardiopulmonary resuscitation: a case report and review of the literature. Ann Thorac Surg 46:353–355
51. Werhens XH, Doevendans PA, et al. (1996) Infected sternal fracture hematoma after cardiopulmonary resuscitation initially seen as pericarditis. Am Heart J 132:685–686
52. Mallinson RH, Tremlett CH, et al. (1999) Sternal osteomyelitis after cardiopulmonary resuscitation. J R Soc Med 92:87
53. Bjork RJ, Snyder BD, et al. (1982) Medical complications of cardiopulmonary arrest. Arch Intern Med 142:500–503
54. Sirvent JM, Torres A, et al. (1997) Protective effect of intravenously administered cefuroxime against nosocomial pneumonia in patients with structural coma. Am J Respir Crit Care Med 155:1729–1734
55. Cook DJ, Walter SD, et al. (1998) For the Canadian Critical Care Trials Group (1998) Incidence and risk factors for ventilator associated pneumonia in critically ill patients. Ann Intern Med 129:433–440
56. Cydulka RK, Connor PJ, et al. (1991) Prevention of oral bacterial flora transmission by using mouth to mask ventilation during CPR. J Emerg Med 9:317–321
57. Cobb LA, Fahrenbruch CE, et al. (1999) Influence of cardiopulmonary resuscitation prior to defibrillation in patients with out-of-hospital ventricular fibrillation. JAMA 281:1182–1188

Chapter 4

Opportunistic Infections in the Intensive Care Unit: A Microbiologic Overview

4

J. Vila, J.A. Martínez

4.1 Introduction

The word "opportunistic" refers to those microorganisms which do not usually cause disease in people with intact host defence systems; yet they can clearly cause devastating disease in many hospitalised and immunocompromised patients. Therefore, it is probable that virtually any microorganism with a capacity for sustained multiplication in humans can cause disease more readily in individuals with underlying chronic diseases or in those who are otherwise compromised. This concept of "opportunistic" pathogen should be distinguished from "principal" pathogen, which refers to microorganisms causing diseases in a proportion of susceptible individuals with apparently intact specific and non-specific defence systems. Normal human flora is defined as microorganisms that are frequently found on or within the body of a person, normally colonising the epithelia or the skin, and such microorganisms may be permanent or transient and they can be a source of many opportunistic infections. Moreover, opportunistic infections can also by caused by microorganisms found in the inanimate environment.

It is currently recognised that patients in the ICU have a five- to tenfold higher risk of acquiring nosocomial infections than patients elsewhere in the hospital. Overall, two types of infections may be considered in patients in the ICU. The first type is when the infection is the cause of admission to the ICU and the second is the infection acquired during hospitalisation in the ICU. We will refer to the microorganisms associated with the latter in this chapter. According to the presence of the pathogen at the time of admission of the patient in the ICU, the infection can be classified as endogenous primary infection, endogenous secondary infection or exogenous infection. In the first case, the pathogen is present in the nose, pharynx or intestinal tract at the time of admission and the second is mainly caused by nosocomial pathogens, which are not present in the patient at the time of admission but rather, the patient becomes colonised during the stay in the ICU. Exogenous infections refer to those caused by pathogens which do not have a previous step of transient colonisation.

4.2 Factors Predisposing Opportunistic Infections

Several factors contribute to the acquisition of opportunistic infections in the ICU: (1) use of invasive tools, which alter the natural defensive barriers favouring the colonisation of deep tissue; (2) use of devices, such as humidifiers, that can be reservoirs for microorganisms [1]; (3) use of lines and tubes for invasive monitoring and therapy, which can bypass natural defence mechanisms; (4) underlying diseases or impaired immune function resulting from critical illness; (5) patient care in the ICU involves close contact with hospital staff, leading to possible cross-contamination from other patients or the environment [2, 3]. The consequent colonisation of patients is generally accepted as a prerequisite for developing most nosocomial infections. The incidence of colonisation increases significantly after admission to hospital.

4.3 Bacterial Opportunistic Infections

Overall, Gram-negative bacilli belonging to the Enterobacteriaceae family are the most frequently encountered bacterial isolates recovered from clinical specimens. Thus, members of this family may be incriminated in virtually any type of infectious diseases and recovered from any specimen received in the laboratory. These microorganisms are ubiquitous in nature, found both in the general environment and on mucosal surfaces of mammals. Among the species belonging to this family, *Escherichia coli*, *Enterobacter* spp., and *Klebsiella* spp. are the most frequently related to infections in the ICU (Table 4.1). Urinary tract infections are responsible for 20–30 % of nosocomial infections in this setting [4, 5], and *E. coli* is, by far, the most frequently found etiological agent. Moreover, this species, as well as *Klebsiella* spp., is involved in peritonitis, cholangitis and intra-abdominal infections. *Enterobacter aerogenes* and *Enterobacter cloacae*, the most commonly isolated species of the genus *Enterobacter*, cause a variety of infections including bacteraemia, urinary tract

Table 4.1. Main aetiological agents of opportunistic infections in the ICU

Wound infections	
Clean	Streptococci, staphylococci
Clean-contaminated	Polymicrobial aerobic and anaerobic (streptococci, staphylococci, Enterobacteriaceae, *Pseudomonas*, enterococci, anaerobes)
Contaminated	Polymicrobial aerobic and anaerobic (streptococci, staphylococci, Enterobacteriaceae, *Pseudomonas*, enterococci, anaerobes)
Prosthetic devices	
Cerebrospinal fluid (shunt-associated infections)	Coagulase-negative staphylococci (50%) *Staphylococcus aureus* (20%) Streptococci (10%) Gram-negative bacilli (5–15%) *Corynebacterium* spp. plus *Propionibacterium acnes* (5–10%)
Orthopaedic devices	Coagulase-negative staphylococci plus *Staphylococcus aureus* (50%) Enterobacteriaceae and streptococci
Catheter-related bacteraemia	Coagulase-negative staphylococci (37%) *Staphylococcus aureus* (26%) *Pseudomonas aeruginosa* (5%) Other Gram-negative bacilli (11%) *Streptococcus* and *Enterococcus* spp. (5%) *Candida* spp. (16%)
Catheter-associated urinary tract infections	*Escherichia coli* (24%) *Candida* spp. *Enterococcus* spp. *Pseudomonas aeruginosa* (9%)
Ventilated-associated pneumonia	*Pseudomonas aeruginosa* (15.9–33.9%) *Streptococcus* spp. (3.3–13.5%) MRSA (3.3–19.3%) MSSA (12.6–14.7%) *Acinetobacter baumannii* (3.8–12.6%) Enterobacteriaceae (3.7–9%)

MRSA methicillin-resistant *Staphylococcus aureus*, *MSSA* methicillin-susceptible *Staphylococcus aureus*

and surgical wound infections [6]. Although the causative organisms of ventilator-associated pneumonia vary widely from ICU to ICU, these three genera of Enterobacteriaceae account for around 9% of the total number of bacteria causing this type of pneumonia [7].

Enterobacteria grow well in the usual culture media and are easy to identify with biochemical tests. Special attention should be given to the antimicrobial susceptibility testing of these bacteria due to the increased problem of the extended-spectrum β-lactamase-producing Enterobacteria, mainly *Klebsiella* spp. and *E. coli*. Twenty-five percent of *Klebsiella* isolates from European ICUs produce extended-spectrum β-lactamases [8].

Pseudomonas aeruginosa and *Acinetobacter baumannii* are the two most relevant non-fermentative Gram-negative bacilli associated with infections in the ICU. These microorganisms usually present multiresistance. They have minimal requirements for growth and tolerate a wide range of physical conditions, favouring the acquisition of multiresistance [9]. *P. aeruginosa* is a common cause of bacteraemia and urinary tract infections, often as a result of catheter use. In addition, it has been identified as one of the commonest causes of ventilator-associated pneumonia [10] (Table 4.1). In the last decade, *A. baumannii* has emerged worldwide as an important pathogen in hospitalised patients, causing high mortality rates. This microorganism can cause many infections including pneumonia, bacteraemia, meningitis, urinary tract infections, and skin and soft-tissue infections. However, differentiating genuine infection from colonisation is sometimes difficult and the diagnosis is often based on clinical judgement.

These two microorganisms grow well in MacConkey agar, and identification of *P. aeruginosa* includes pigment (pyocyanin – blue-green and pyoverdin – green-yellow) production and biochemical reactions. *P. aeruginosa* is oxidase positive, in contrast to *A. baumannii* and Enterobacteriaceae, which are oxidase negative. Differentiation of *A. baumannii* from the remaining species of the genus *Acinetobacter* should be made by genotypic methods, since phenotypic methods are not able to separate *A. baumannii* from *Acinetobacter calcoaceticus, Acinetobacter* genospecies 3 and *Acinetobacter* genospecies 13.

Obligate anaerobes are bacteria that cannot survive in the presence of a high oxygen content. Strict anaerobes cannot grow in healthy tissues because of the oxygen content, while tissue injury with limitation of the blood (and oxygen) supply creates conditions for opportunistic growth of obligate anaerobes. Simultaneous infection with a facultative anaerobe, which uses up the already diminished oxygen supply, also encourages growth of obligate anaerobes. Strict anaerobes are present in large numbers in the intestine (95–99% of total bacterial mass), but also in the mouth and genito-urinary tract. The most common infections resulting from abdominal surgery or other gut injury are Enterobacteriaceae and *Bacteroides fragilis.* These are minor components of the gut flora and demonstrate that certain microorganisms more readily produce opportunistic infections than others. Most anaerobes in the normal human flora are non-spore formers and anaerobic infections often occur from this source (Table 4.2). Successful recovery of anaerobic bacteria requires rapid delivery and specimen processing to avoid overgrowth by facultative anaerobes. In addition, if air gets into the sample during transportation to the clinical laboratory the anaerobic organism can lose viability. Special anaerobic containers are used to maintain a moist, anaerobic atmosphere for the specimen during transport. Currently, the most important anaerobic pathogen is *Clostridium difficile,* which is the main cause of antibiotic-associated diarrhoea or even life-threatening pseudomomembranous enterocolitis (see Chapter 15).

Table 4.2. Anaerobic bacteria of clinical importance

Non-spore-formers	Spore-formers
Gram-negative rods Bacteroides (i.e. B. fragilis) Prevotella Porphyromonas Fusobacterium	Clostridium tetani Clostridium perfringens Clostridium difficile
Gram-positive rods Propionibacterium acnes Actinomyces Eubacterium lentum	
Gram-positive cocci Peptostreptococcus Peptococcus	
Gram-negative cocci Veillonella Acidominococcus	

Among Gram-positive aerobic bacteria, *Staphylococcus aureus,* coagulase-negative staphylococci and *Enterococci* are the most prevalent as cause of infections in the ICU. However, other Gram-positive bacteria such as *Corynebacterium* spp. and *Rodococcus equi* can be implicated in opportunistic infections, although a distinction must be carefully made between colonisation and infection. It has been shown that colonisation with either methicillin-susceptible or methicillin-resistant *S. aureus* increases the risk of subsequent infections with the same colonising strains, particularly wound infections and central venous catheter-related bacteraemia [11–13]. *S. aureus* causes several types of infections including pneumonia, bacteraemia and sepsis, and wound infections. Moreover, they continue to be one of the commonest pathogens isolated in ventilator-associated pneumonia and catheter-related bacteraemia (Table 4.1) [14–16]. Among coagulase-negative staphylococci, *S. epidermidis* is the most important species, being a normal commensal at a wide variety of anatomical sites including mucous membranes, the axillae and skin [17]. Coagulase-negative staphylococci cause around 19% of nosocomial ICU infections [18, 19]. They mainly cause neurosurgical shunt and prosthetic joint infections and are, by far, the most common pathogen isolated in catheter-related bacteraemia (Table 4.1). Central venous catheters are indispensable in the treatment of ICU patients, but the use of catheters is associated with a risk of infectious complications. Central venous catheters are the most common source of nosocomial bloodstream infection and it has been estimated that >25,000 episodes occur annually in the United States [20]. In most studies of catheter-acquired infections 30–40% of colonising microorganisms are coagulase-negative staphylococci, with 5%–10% being *S. aureus*, that is microorganisms which are part of the skin flora (Table 4.2) [21, 22]. Nosocomially acquired pathogens are usually less frequently found and include enterococci, *Enterobacter* spp., *P. aeruginosa* and *Candida* spp. at rates of around 5%. For culturing catheters, the most commonly accepted bacteriological technique is the semiquantitative method developed by Maki. Other techniques have been developed, such as shaking a segment of the catheter with a vortex device followed by quantitation of the released bacteria. All staphylococci grow well in blood agar and *S. aureus* is distinguished from coagulase-negative staphylococci by its ability to clot blood plasma.

Finally, *Enterococcus faecalis* and *E. faecium* represent 95% of the infections caused by enterococci. These microorganisms are part of the normal enteric flora of both humans and animals. Enterococci have low pathogenic potential except in patients who are severely ill or immunocompromised; hence reports of enterococcal-caused infections are mainly from ICUs, organ transplant and oncology wards [23, 24]. Enterococci are the second or third most common pathogens causing urinary tract infections, bacteraemia and wound infections.

4.4 Fungal Opportunistic Infections

The habitat of fungi varies depending on the genera and even the species. Among yeasts, *C. albicans*, *C. glabrata* and *C. tropicalis* are part of the commensal flora of the mouth, digestive tract and vagina of humans (*C. albicans* being, by far, the most common). On mucosal surfaces they are kept in low concentrations (usually below 10^4 colony forming units/ml) by the intermicrobial inhibition of commensal bacteria and normally functioning CD4 cells. *C. parapsilosis*, the second most frequent agent of candidaemia in neonates [25] and in adults from Latin America and some other countries such as Spain [26], rarely colonises healthy people, although when it does, the skin seems to be the commonest place.

Most cases of systemic candidiasis are of endogenous origin, with the bulk of evidence pointing to the gut as the most common source, and overgrowth of *Candida* indicated by intense and extensive mucosal colonisation is a necessary prerequisite [27]. This does not impede the possibility of exogenous acquisition from contaminated environmental items, from staff carriers or from other patients through the hands of healthcare workers. Common source outbreaks may also occur [28]. Overgrowth of *Candida* on mucosal surfaces is promoted by very low CD4 cell counts (<200/μl), hyperglycaemia and administration of corticosteroids and antibiotics. In the critical care setting, between one-half and two-thirds of the patients hospitalised for more than a week become colonised by *Candida* and in about 40% multiple non-contiguous sites are affected [29–31].

In contrast to *Candida* spp., neither *C. neoformans* nor moulds are part of the commensal flora of the skin or mucous membranes. They grow as saprobes in decaying organic matter and their spores become easily airborne. *Cryptococcus* is associated with soil rich in bird droppings. Most opportunistic fungi are ubiquitous worldwide and exposure is inevitable unless one is under a protective environment that includes highly efficient air (and possibly water) filtration. At least two-thirds of clinical infections are due to *Aspergillus* spp., particularly *A. fumigatus* and less often *A. flavus*. However, other *Aspergillus* species (*A. terreus*), hyalohyphomycetes [*Fusarium, Pseudallescheria boydii* (*Scedosporium apiospermum*), *Scedosporium prolificans, Paecillomyces, Trichoderma*], *Zygomycetes* (agents of mucormycosis) and several dematiaceous fungi are opportunistic agents of increasing relevance.

Aspergillus spp. and less frequently other moulds can colonise the tracheobronchial tree of patients with chronic obstructive pulmonary disease. Some studies have revealed that *Aspergillus* can be cultured from the sputum of about 2–7% of patients with asthma, chronic bronchitis or bronchiectasis and up to 60% of patients with cystic fibrosis, without evidence of invasive infection [32–36]. In the critical care setting, mould colonisation, almost always of the respiratory tract and due to *Aspergillus*, can be demonstrated in up to 4% of patients. Detection usually occurs after prolonged ICU stay (>2 weeks), and again, chronic obstructive pulmonary disease and prior corticosteroid therapy are the most important risk factors in colonised or infected patients [37]. Outbreaks of infection can occur, usually associated with hospital construction or renovation works, contamination of air-handling systems, or other environmental reservoirs [38].

The reservoir and mode of transmission of *Pneumocystis jirovecii* have not been fully established. However, evidence provided by the use of sensitive PCR techniques has strongly suggested that *P. jirovecii* is carried in the upper and lower respiratory tract by 20–30% of healthy people and 10–40% of patients with different chronic lung disorders [39, 40]. There is also increasing evidence that this fungus can be transmitted, probably by the airborne route, from infected patients to immunosuppressed or immunocompetent hosts [41, 42]. The latter could be the natural reservoir of the organism.

With the exception of the geographically restricted dimorphic fungi that require rich media supplemented with blood and prolonged incubation periods, most fungi are not fastidious and can be isolated from primary mycological (and even bacteriological) cultures in less than 5 days. A few organisms, such as *P. jirovecii*, cannot be cultured at all. The demonstration of fungal elements in clinical specimens requires specific stains. Gram staining is inappropriate for most fungi, except *Candida* spp., which appear as Gram-positive. Specific stains include periodic acid-Schiff, Gomori metenamine-silver and calcofluor white, the last two being able to reveal the wall of all fungi, including *P. jirovecii*. The capsule of *C. neoformans* can be viewed by India ink examination of CSF in ≥50% of patients with meningitis. Isolation of *Candida* and *C. neoformans* from blood can be accomplished by using routine continuously monitored blood culture systems with regular 5-day incubation protocols, although a sensitivity no higher than 50% is to be expected in systemic infection. However, a positive blood culture should always be interpreted as indicative of true fungaemia. Several serological tests for the diagnoses of invasive fungal infection are available. In patients with cryptococcal meningitis, detection of the capsular antigen in CSF is an extremely sensitive and specific test. Serial twice weekly surveillance of galactomannan antigen in blood has proved to be a very sensitive and specific approach for the diagnoses of aspergillosis in neutropenic haematological patients, but sensitivity is greatly diminished in non-neutropenic individuals. Specificity is reduced in neonates, and false-positive results may be due to the administration of piperacillin-tazobactam or amoxicillin-clavulanate. Detection in blood of (1,3)-β-D-glucan may serve as a panfungal test because it may become positive in many fungal infections except those due to *Zygomycetes* and *C. neoformans*. When used serially in high-risk haematological patients it seems to be very specific with a moderate to high sensitivity (55–87%) [43–45]. However, there are serious doubts about the specificity of this test in critically ill patients [46]. Detection in blood of antigens and/or antibodies against *Candida* continues to be plagued with questions concerning performance [47]. The most reliable tests seem to be those based on the finding of mannan/anti-mannan antibodies [48] or antibodies to *C. albicans* germ tubes [49], although further prospective evaluation is required. PCR techniques seem to have a good sensitivity and specificity, particularly for *Aspergillus*, but they are still in-house non-standardised procedures.

4.5 Viral Opportunistic Infections

Viruses are not a common cause of ICU-acquired infection, except for RSV virus in neonatal units, where up to 70% of cases may be hospital-acquired [50]. The risk of nosocomial outbreaks of respiratory virus, particularly influenza or RSV, is always a threat when there is increased circulation of these agents in the community (usually during the winter or spring) [51]. Some Hesperviridae (CMV, herpes simplex 1, and human herpesvirus 6) can reactivate in non-severely immunosuppressed critically ill patients, although a possible link with clinical disease has only been suggested for CMV. HHV-6 has been detected by PCR in the serum of 54% of critically ill patients with multiple organ failure [52], and HSV-1 can be found in the throat or lower respiratory secretions of about 20% of patients intubated for more than a week [53]. Similarly, CMV can be detected in blood or respiratory secretions in up to 35% of patients staying in the unit 10 days or more, particularly in those with sepsis. In this context, CMV has been associated with increased morbidity and mortality, and even with clinical disease, usually pneumonia, although the real frequency of organ damage has not been accurately established [54–56].

The diagnosis of viruses can be achieved by culture or rapid antigen detection and gene amplification techniques. Serology is usually not helpful to provide a timely diagnosis. For respiratory viruses, nasal swab or lavage specimens, sputum, tracheal aspirates and bronchoalveolar lavage fluid may be appropriate samples.

References

1. Haddadin AS, Fappiano SA, Lipsett PA (2002) Methicillin resistant *Staphylococcus aureus* (MRSA) in the intensive care units. Postgrad Med J 78:385–92
2. Reuter S, Sigge A, Wiedeck H, et al. (2002) Analysis of transmission pathways of *Pseudomonas aeruginosa* between patients and tap water outlets. Crit Care Med 30:2222–8
3. Pittet D, Dharan S, Touveneau S, et al.(1999) Bacterial contamination of the hands of hospital staff during routine patient care. Arch Inter Med 159:821–6
4. Richards MJ, Edwards JR, Culver DH, et al. (2000) Nosocomial infections in combined medical-surgical intensive care units in the United States. Infect Control Hosp Epidemiol 21:510–15
5. Richards MJ, Edwards JR, Culver DH, et al. (1999) Nosocomial infections in medical intensive care units in the United States. National Nosocomial Infections Surveillance System. Crit Care Med 27:887–92
6. Sanders WE Jr, Sanders CC (1997) *Enterobacter* spp.: pathogens poised to flourish at the turn of the century. Clin Microbiol Rev 10:220–41
7. Trouillet JL, Chastre J, Vuagnat A, et al. (1998) Ventilator-associated pneumonia caused by potentially drug-resistant bacteria. Am J Respir Crit Care Med 157:531–9
8. Babini GS, Livermore DM (2000) Antimicrobial resistance among *Klebsiella* spp. collected from intensive care units in Southern and Western Europe in 1997–1998. J Antimicrob Chemother 45:183–9
9. Vila J (1998) Mechanisms of antimicrobial resistance in *Acinetobacter baumannii*. Rev Med Microbiol 9:87–97
10. Rello J, Sa-Borges M, Correa H, et al. (1999) Variations in etiology of ventilator-associated pneumonia around four treatment sites: Implications for antimicrobial prescribing practices. Am J Resp Crit Care Med 160:608–13
11. Perl TM, Cullen JJ, Wenzel RP, et al. (2002) Intranasal mupirocin to prevent postoperative *Staphylococcus aureus* infections. N Engl J Med 346:1871–7
12. Kluytmans J, van Belkum A, Verbrugh H (1997) Nasal carriage of *Staphylococcus aureus:* epidemiology, underlying mechanisms, and associated risks. Clin Microbiol Rev 10:505–20
13. Pujol M, Pena C, Pallares R, et al. (1996) Nosocomial *Staphylococcus aureus* bacteremia among nasal carriers of methicillin-resistant and methicillin-susceptible strains. Am J Med 100:509–16
14. Chastre J, Fagon JY (2002) Ventilator-associated pneumonia. Am J Resp Crit Care Med 165:867–903
15. Edmond MB, Wallace SE, McClish DK, et al. (1999) Nosocomial bloodstream infections in United States hospitals: a three-year analysis. Clin Infect Dis 29:239–44
16. Lowy FD (1998) *Staphylococcus aureus* infections. N Engl J Med 339:520–32
17. von Eiff C, Peters G, Heilmann C (2002) Pathogenesis of infections due to coagulase-negative staphylococci. Lancet Infect Dis 2:675–85
18. Vincent JL, Bihari DJ, Suter PM, et al. (1995) The prevalence of nosocomial infection in intensive care units in Europe. Results of the European Prevalence of Infection in Intensive Care (EPIC) Study. EPIC International Advisory Committee. JAMA 274:639–44
19. Spencer RC (1996) Predominant pathogens found in the European Prevalence of Infection in Intensive Care Study. Eur J Clin Microbiol Infect Dis 15:281–5
20. Raad I (1998) Intravascular-catheter-related infections. Lancet 351:893–8
21. Renaud B, Brun-Bruissson C (2001) Outcomes of primary and catheter-related bacteremia: a cohort and case-control study in critically ill patients. Am J Resp Crit Care Med 163:1584–90
22. Lorente L, Villegas J, Martín MM, et al. (2004) Catheter-related infection in critically ill patients. Intensive Care Med 30:1681–4
23. Bonten MJ, Willems R, Weinstein RA (2001) Vancomycin-resistant enterococci: why are they here, and where do they come from? Lancet Infect Dis 1:314–25
24. Hayden MK (2000) Insights into the epidemiology and control of infection with vancomycin-resistant enterococci. Clin Infect Dis 31:1085–65
25. Roilides E, Farmaki E, Evdoridou J, et al. (2004) Neonatal candidiasis: analysis of epidemiology, drug susceptibility, and molecular typing of causative isolates. Eur J Clin Microbiol Infect Dis 23:745–750
26. Pemán J, Cantón E, Gobernado M and the Spanish ECMM Working Group on Candidaemia (2005) Eur J Clin Microbiol Infect Dis 24:23–30
27. Nucci M, Anaissie E (2001) Revisiting the source of candidemia: skin or gut? Clin Infect Dis 33:1959–1967
28. Pfaller MA (1996) Nosocomial candidiasis: emerging species, reservoirs, and modes of transmission. Clin Infect Dis 22(Suppl 2):89–94
29. Petri MG, König J, Moeck HP, et al. (1997) Epidemiology of invasive mycosis in ICU patients: a prospective multicenter study in 435 non-neutropenic patients. Intensive Care Med 23:317–325
30. Olaechea PM, Palomar M, León-Gil C, et al. and the EPCAN Study Group (2004) Economic impact of Candida colonization and Candida infection in the critically ill patient. Eur J Clin Microbiol Infect Dis 23:323–330
31. Charles PE, Dalle F, Aube H, et al. (2004) Candida spp. colonization in critically ill medical patients: a prospective study. Intensive Care Med 31:393–400
32. Kahanpää A (1972) Bronchopulmonary occurrence of fungi in adults. Acta Pathol Microbiol Scand Sect B (Suppl 227):21–147
33. Yu VL, Muder RR, Poorsattar A (1986) Significance of isolation of Aspergillus from the respiratory tract in diagnosis of invasive pulmonary aspergillosis. Am J Med 81:249–254
34. Bakare N, Rickerts V, Bargon J, et al.(2003) Prevalence of

Aspergillus fumigatus and other fungal species in the sputum of adult patients with cystic fibrosis. Mycoses 46:19–23
35. Uffredi ML, Mangiapan G, Cadranel J, et al. (2003) Significance of *Aspergillus fumigatus* isolation from respiratory specimens of nongranulocytopenic patients. Eur J Clin Microbiol Infect Dis 22:457–462
36. Soubani AO, Khanchandani G, Ahmend HP (2004) Clinical significance of lower respiratory tract Aspergillus culture in elderly hospitalized patients. Eur J Clin Microbiol Infect Dis 23:491–494
37. Garnacho-Montero J, Amaya-Villar R, Ortiz-Leyba C, et al. (2005) Isolation of *Aspergillus* spp. from the respiratory tract in critically ill patients: risk factors, clinical presentation and outcome. Crit Care 9:191–199
38. Lutz BD, Jin J, Rinaldi MG, Wickes BL, et al. (2003) Outbreak of invasive Aspergillus infection in surgical patients, associated with a contaminated air-handling system. Clin Infect Dis 37:786–793
39. Sing A, Roggenkamp A, Autenrieth IB, Heesemann J (1999) *Pneumocystis carinii* carriage in immunocompetent patients with primary pulmonary disorders as detected by single or nested PCR. J Clin Microbiol 37:3409–3410
40. Medrano FA, Montes-Cano M, Conde M, et al. (2005) *Pneumocystis jirovecii* in general population. Emerg Infect Dis 11:245–249
41. Miller RF, Ambrose HE, Wakefield AE (2001) *Pneumocystis carinii* f. sp. *hominis* DNA in immunocompetent health care workers in contact with patients with *P. carinii* pneumonia. J Clin Microbiol 39:3877–3882
42. Rabodonirina M, Vanhems P, Couray-Targe S, et al. (2004) Molecular evidence of interhuman transmission of *Pneumocystis pneumonia* among renal transplant recipients hospitalized with HIV-infected patients. Emerg Infect Dis 10:1766–1773
43. Odabasi Z, Mattiuzzi G, Estey E, et al. (2004) β-D-glucan as a diagnostic adjunct for invasive fungal infection: validation, cutoff development, and performance in patients with myelogenous leukemia and myelodysplastic syndrome. Clin Infect Dis 39:199–205
44. Kawazu M, Kanda Y, Nannya Y, et al. (2004) Prospective comparison of the diagnostic potential of real-time PCR, double-sandwich enzyme-linked immunosorbent assay for galactomannan, and a (1→3)-β-D-glucan test in weekly screening for invasive aspergillosis in patients with hematological disorders. J Clin Microbiol 42:2733–2744
45. Pazos C, Pontón J, del Palacio A (2005) Contribution of (1→3)-β-D-glucan chromogenic assay to diagnosis and therapeutic monitoring of invasive aspergillosis in neutropenic adult patients: a comparison with serial screening for circulating galactomannan. J Clin Microbiol 43:299–305
46. Digby J, Kalbfleisch J, Glenn A, et al. (2003) Serum glucan levels are not specific for presence of fungal infections in intensive care unit patients. Clin Diagn Lab Immunol 10:882–885
47. Stevens DA (2002) Diagnosis of fungal infections: current status. J Antimicrob Chemother 49 (Suppl S1):11–19
48. Sendid B, Poirot JL, Tabouret M, et al. (2002) Combined detection of mannanaemia and antimannan antibodies as a strategy for the diagnosis of systemic infection caused by pathogenic Candida species. J Med Microbiol 51:433–442
49. Moragues MD, Ortiz N, Iruretagoyena JR, et al. (2004) Evaluation of a new commercial test (*Candida albicans* IFA IgG) for the serodiagnosis of invasive candidiasis. Enferm Infecc Microbiol Clin 22:83–88
50. Thorburn K, Kerr S, Taylor N, et al. (2004) RSV outbreak in a pediatric intensive care unit. J Hosp Infect 57:194–201
51. Oliveira EC, Lee B, Colice GL (2003) Influenza in the intensive care unit. J Intens Care Med 80–91
52. Desachy A, Ranger-Rogez S, François B, et al. (2001) Reactivation of human herpesvirus type 6 in multiple organ failure syndrome. Clin Infect Dis 32:197–203
53. Bruynseels P, Jorens PG, Demey HE, et al. (2003) Herpes simplex virus in the respiratory tract of critical care patients: a prospective study. Lancet 362:1536–1541
54. Papazian L, Fraise A, Garbe L, et al. (1996) Cytomegalovirus: an unexpected cause of ventilator-associated pneumonia. Anesthesiology 84:280–287
55. Heininger A, Jahn G, Engel C, et al. (2001) Cytomegalovirus infections in nonimmnosuppressed critically ill patients. Crit Care Med 29:541–547
56. Jaber S, Chanques G, Borry J, et al. (2005) Cytomegalovirus infection in critically ill patients: associated factors and consequences. Chest 127:233–241

Chapter 5

Infections in Critically Ill Solid Organ Transplant Recipients

5

O. Len, J. Gavaldà, A. Pahissa

5.1 Introduction

In recent years, advances in surgical techniques, immunosuppressant drugs, diagnostic tests and preventive strategies against a large number of pathogens have achieved considerably lower infection rates among recipients of a solid organ transplant. Certain opportunistic infections such as cytomegalovirus (CMV) and *Pneumocystis jiroveci* have undergone an important reversal in the past decade. Nevertheless, the appearance of new pathogens and the escalation of antibiotic resistance have altered the spectrum of the microorganisms involved and, consequently, infection management in the transplant patient. Nosocomial infection, in particular hospital-acquired bacterial infection, is presently the main source of infection following transplantation. Up to 53% of infections in a group of heart transplant recipients were considered to be hospital-acquired and 63% of them were bacterial [1]. In liver transplant recipients, 82% of all febrile episodes in a 2-year period were described as nosocomial in origin, with 62% of bacterial etiology [2].

Intensive care units are an integral part of the management of patients receiving a solid organ transplant. Nevertheless, they represent the most common source of nosocomial infection, with an incidence several times higher than that of other hospitalization areas. The vulnerability of transplant recipients to opportunistic infections enhanced by the risk of nosocomial infection in ICUs makes these patients a diagnostic and therapeutic challenge.

5.2 Risk Factors

Classically, the risk of infection is considered to be highest in the first 6 months after solid organ transplantation. It is logical that new prophylactic and immunosuppressive practices may delay this critical period and modify the risk factors for infection. Although the overall incidence of infection and CMV disease are approximately 10 times more frequent in the early period (first 6 months after transplantation), the incidence of other opportunistic infections is nearly as frequent in the late period as in the early period. These data suggest that the critical risk period for opportunistic infections must be redefined and extended, particularly in certain high-risk patients: those suffering from acute rejection, those with relapsing CMV disease or previous fungal and/or bacterial infection, liver recipients with a choledochal jejunostomy, and lung transplant recipients [3].

5.2.1 Pretransplant Period

5.2.1.1 Use of Antibiotics

Because of the underlying diseases leading to transplantation, transplant recipients are immunodepressed hosts who have received antibiotics frequently, sometimes for long periods of time. This antibiotic exposure can lead to the onset of infections caused by resistant bacteria. Quinolone prophylaxis for spontaneous bacterial peritonitis in cirrhotic patients has been associated with a higher risk of infection caused by quinolone-resistant Gram-positive cocci and enterobacteria.

Another relevant factor is the production of extended-spectrum beta-lactamases (ESBL) by Gram-negative bacilli. Most ESBLs are mutants of TEM or SHV-1 that lead to hydrolysis of penicillins and other beta-lactams. In addition, 30% of these bacteria also express quinolone resistance. These enzymes have been found most often in *Klebsiella pneumoniae*, although they are also seen in other Gram-negative bacilli.

Another example illustrating the development of resistance due to antibiotic administration is the emergence of vancomycin-resistant enterococci. Once colonization has occurred, they are difficult to eradicate. The use of vancomycin, as well as third-generation cephalosporins and metronidazole, has been associated with the acquisition of this type of bacteria. The number and duration of the antibiotics administered during the pretransplant period in liver recipients correlate significantly with the risk of posterior infection by a vancomycin-resistant enterococcus [4].

Previous colonization of the lungs by *Pseudomonas aeruginosa* or *Burkholderia cepacia* species with multiple antibiotic resistance is associated with high morbidity and mortality in the immediate post-transplantation period. A 1-year survival rate of 34% has been reported among these patients, and this has meant that some hospitals refuse to consider them eligible for transplantation [5].

5.2.1.2
Duration of Hospitalization

A lengthy hospital stay is not only an indirect indicator of poor post-transplantation clinical progress, but also involves an increased risk of colonization by a resistant nosocomial microorganism. In liver transplant recipients, it was found that nasal carrier status for *Staphylococcus aureus* is a predictor of invasive infection by this microorganism [6]. We should mention that 46% of these patients were already carriers before transplantation and prolonged hospitalization was related with acquisition of methicillin resistance [7]. This also occurs with the appearance of ESBL-producing *Klebsiella pneumoniae* strains and vancomycin-resistant enterococci [4].

5.2.1.3
Immunosuppression

Liver transplantation is considered as first-line treatment for fulminant liver failure. Multiorgan failure together with the administration of immunosuppressive medication puts these patients at risk for opportunistic infections, such as invasive aspergillosis, in the immediate post-transplantation period [8]. The use of azathioprine and corticosteroids to treat idiopathic pulmonary fibrosis in lung transplantation has been correlated to a higher incidence of CMV disease [9].

5.2.1.4
Renal Failure

Uremia causes several defects in the host defense mechanisms, such as chemotaxis, complement activation, opsonization, and cellular immunity, which can increase susceptibility to infection, not only among renal transplantation patients. Renal failure, particularly the need for replacement therapy prior to transplantation, identifies patients at risk of invasive aspergillosis [10] and other types of infections, which can increase mortality [11].

5.2.2
Surgical Factors and Type of Transplantation

It is evident that the site, severity, and type of bacterial and fungal infection during the post-transplant period will be influenced by the anatomic barriers affected and the specific surgical complications in each type of transplantation.

Liver transplantation involves complications related to the biliary tree and vascular anastomoses. Thrombosis of the hepatic artery will lead to hepatic infarction and formation of a biloma, which can be infected or not. Although the clinical presentation is usually acute or fulminant, it can also be occult, manifesting as an unexplained fever or recurrent bacteremia. Bile composition is altered after liver transplantation due to cholesterol supersaturation and the formation of biliary sludge, which can predispose the patient to develop cholangitis. Another factor that favors this process is placement of a Kher tube to protect the biliary suture, predisposing the patient to microbial colonization. Furthermore, liver transplant recipients are exposed to invasive candidiasis [12] originating from an endogenous source and facilitated by deficiencies in reticuloendothelial function and translocation of the microorganism through the intestine.

Urinary tract and surgical wound infections are the most common nosocomial infections in renal transplant recipients. They occur in more than 50% of patients during the first 3 months and often lead to bacteremia. Contributing factors are diabetes mellitus, renal failure, malnutrition, and prolonged urinary catheter use.

Lung transplant recipients are especially susceptible to nosocomial bacterial lung infection, particularly during the first month. Loss of mucociliary clearance and the cough reflex, postoperative pain, and donor tracheal colonization are factors that contribute to the high risk of postoperative pneumonia in lung transplant recipients.

In an epidemiological study done as part of RESITRA (Transplant Infection Study Network), 291 heart transplant recipients were followed-up for 2 years and 49% of these patients developed 1 to 10 episodes of infection. The predominant etiology was bacterial (53%), followed by viral (41%), fungal (4%), and other (2%) causes. Lower respiratory tract infection was the most frequent (23.4%), followed by bacteremia (9.6%), and surgical wound infection (5.5%). Nevertheless, the pathogen identified most often was CMV (23%) [13].

The characteristics that predispose to infection among patients who receive a small intestine transplant include the inherent lack of sterility of this kind of surgery and the more intense immunosuppression required to prevent rejection. Virtually all these patients experience at least one infection episode, and those who receive a multiorgan transplant or colon segment are the ones most highly exposed to infection [14]. Bacterial translocation predisposes a patient to peritonitis or intra-abdominal abscesses. Hence, selective intestinal decontamination can be highly beneficial.

5.2.3 Post-transplant Period

5.2.3.1 Immunosuppression

Defense mechanisms altered by immunosuppressive medication can influence a patient's susceptibility to a specific kind of opportunistic pathogen. Corticoids mainly affect T-lymphocyte activation by inhibiting the release of IL-2 and other related cytokines. Indiscriminate use of these drugs in early transplantation programs was related to an increase in fungal infection. In addition, corticoids have nonspecific anti-inflammatory activity and inhibit leukocyte migration. This leads to accelerated replication of hepatitis B virus (HBV) and human herpesvirus 8 (HHV-8) [15].

The therapeutic effect of cyclosporine and tacrolimus is exerted by inhibition of T-lymphocyte activation after blocking transcription of IL-2, IL-3 and interferon gamma [16]. Cyclosporine use has been associated with a higher incidence of Kaposi's sarcoma. Tacrolimus is 30–100 times more potent than cyclosporine and is significantly associated with a lower incidence of episodes of acute rejection and steroid-resistant rejection. Interestingly, one study reported fewer episodes of CMV infection associated with this drug [17]. This fact can be explained by the reduced need for corticoids, due to the lower rejection rate. When mycophenolate mofetil, an ester of mycophenolic acid derived from the *Penicillium brevicompactum* fungus, is associated with tacrolimus therapy, the tacrolimus dose can be reduced, resulting in a lower incidence of nephrotoxicity and neurotoxicity. Mycophenolic acid blocks the production of guanosine nucleotides, leading to selective inhibition of B- and T-lymphocyte proliferation. Its use has been associated with a higher incidence of CMV infection and a lower incidence of *Pneumocystis jiroveci* pneumonia [18]. Treatment with anti-T-lymphocyte monoclonal antibodies and antithymocytic globulin has been linked to a higher incidence and severity of post-transplantation CMV disease. Likewise, the use of OKT3, more common in the past, increased the frequency of infections caused by herpes simplex virus, *Aspergillus* spp., *Pneumocystis jiroveci*, and *Mycobacterium tuberculosis* as well as post-transplantation lymphoproliferative disease [19].

5.2.3.2 Immunomodulating Viruses

Herpesvirus. Herpesviruses exhibit a wide variety of immunosuppressive and immunomodulating characteristics that facilitate superinfections by other opportunistic pathogens and promote oncogenesis and rejection. Cytomegalovirus induces the production of immunosuppressive cytokines that alter lymphocyte and macrophage function. Moreover, these alterations persist once the acute infection has resolved, even up to 60 months later [20]. In addition, CMV is related to rejection, since it modifies the expression of Class I and II major histocompatibility antigens [21, 22]. CMV infection or disease has been associated with increased fibrosis or chronic severe hepatitis due to hepatitis C virus (HCV) and subsequent graft failure in HCV-infected liver transplant recipients [23]. To date, it is unknown whether CMV mediates these events by inducing increased immunosuppression or directly enhancing HCV replication. CMV infection, therefore, has a potential impact on both patient and graft outcome [24].

Human herpesvirus 6 is recognized as an important pathogen in solid organ transplantation. It mainly infects CD4+ T lymphocytes by inhibiting their proliferative capacity, and induces the production of immunomodulatory cytokines such as IL-1 [25]. The presence of HHV-6 is considered an independent predictive factor of invasive fungal infection and mortality in solid organ transplants [26] and an activating factor for the replication of other viruses such as CMV [27]. CMV, furthermore, favors infection by other opportunistic pathogens, such as *Pneumocystis jiroveci* and fungi, and Gram-negative bacteria in lung transplant patients [10].

Gamma herpesviruses, such as Epstein-Barr (EB) and HHV-8, are not directly immunosuppressants, but they are potentially oncogenic [28]. In cases of failure of the specific cytotoxic T-cell response against EB, uncontrolled replication of infected B-lymphocytes occurs, which can lead to a spectrum of entities from polyclonal hyperplasia to B-cell lymphoma. HHV-8 is the cause of Kaposi's sarcoma in solid organ recipients [29]. This virus codes for specific genes in the genome of the host's cells, and thereby promotes angiogenesis, inhibits apoptosis, and counteracts the host's defense mechanisms [30].

Hepatotropic Viruses. In HBsAg-positive recipients, the main cause of death during the early post-transplant period is sepsis. In a series of 23 liver recipients transplanted for cirrhosis secondary to HBV infection, 11 died due to sepsis, 90% of them in the first 3 months [31]. Recurrent HCV infection in the post-transplant period increases the incidence of infections, particularly those dependent on cellular immunity [10, 32].

5.3 Infectious Complications in Critically Ill Transplant Recipients

5.3.1 Bacteremia

The overall incidence of bacteremia in solid organ transplant recipients is around 16%, with some differences according to the type of transplantation: 8% in kidneys, 9% in heart, 10.5% in lung, 11% in liver, and 23% in pancreas [33, 34]. The crude mortality is nearly 10% and is associated with isolation of Gram-negative bacilli and a pulmonary source [33]. In addition, bacteremia is more severe in heart and liver transplant recipients than in kidney recipients [34]. The sources of bacteremia also differ according to the type of transplantation: pneumonia in heart and lung transplantation, urinary tract in kidney transplantation, biliary tree and intra-abdominal in liver transplantation, and surgical wound and urinary tract in pancreas transplantation. In any case, the most frequent overall source of bacteremia is intravascular catheter-related infection, occurring in 39% of cases. The vast majority of these episodes are hospital-acquired.

In kidney transplantation, bacteremia in the post-transplant period is usually caused by Gram-negative aerobic bacilli such as *Escherichia coli.* It has recently been estimated that 7% of bacteremia in kidney transplantation is related to the presence of diabetes mellitus and acute rejection episodes [35]. More than 50% of all cases of bacteremia in this type of transplantation can occur 1 year after transplantation. This appears to be closely related to the return to hemodialysis. *Staphylococcus aureus* is the pathogen mostly often implicated.

In liver transplantation, bacteremia follows the surgical procedure, with an incidence of 11.5% [36]. In about half the cases, the abdomen is the main portal of entry and up to 75% occur in the first 2 months. Reports in the late 1980s indicated that 50% of bacteremia cases were due to Gram-negative bacilli [37]. However, with the current advances in surgical techniques, the main source of bacteremia is now intravascular stents. In a study in which bacteremia was responsible for 45% of febrile episodes in liver transplant recipients admitted to the ICU, the origin was an intravascular catheter in 29% of the episodes, followed by pneumonia (18%) and a biliary origin (18%) [38]. The risk factors associated with bacteremia in this population are mycophenolate mofetil use and the existence of acute rejection [36].

Pneumonia due to Gram-negative bacilli is the main cause of bacteremia in heart transplantation [33]. Other causes of bacteremia identified in these patients include pseudoaneurysms, mediastinitis, and infections due to mechanical assistance devices, in which infection by Gram-positive cocci, particularly *S. aureus,* predominates.

In a study performed among small intestine transplant recipients, 72% of the patients developed at least one episode of bacteremia. Vascular accesses were responsible for infection in 43% of the episodes and 62% of the cases were caused by Gram-positive cocci [14].

Lastly, bacteremia in the donor does not appear to involve any risk for the development of bacteremia in the recipient or for survival when appropriate prophylaxis targeting the specific microorganism is performed. In a study carried out within RESITRA, 15.2% (32/211) of donors with infection at the time of transplantation had positive blood cultures; pneumonia due to *Pseudomonas aeruginosa* developed in only one recipient of a liver graft at 2 days following the procedure [39].

5.3.2 Central Nervous System Infections

Up to 8% of transplant patients may present important neurological sequelae or central nervous system lesions. Infection is the etiology in up to 22% of cases [40]. The incidence of cerebral abscesses in this population has been estimated at 1% for liver transplantation, 0.36% for renal transplantation, and 1% for heart and heart-lung transplantation. Most cases have a fungal etiology, with invasive aspergillosis being the causative pathogen in 90% [41]. The risk factors for the development of this severe complication include those indicating a poor clinical progress after transplantation, such as the presence of bacterial infections, renal failure with or without replacement therapy, and CMV disease [10]. Other pathogens may be implicated, including *Cryptococcus neoformans,* mucoral fungi (e.g., *Rhizopus* spp.), and dematiaceous fungi (e.g., *Alternaria* spp.). Mucoral fungi generally appear in the first 30 days post-transplantation, whereas dematiaceous fungi and *C. neoformans* appear at a median of 21 months [40]. It has been well established that the bimodal presentation of *Aspergillus* spp. is related to various risk factors [10]. This microorganism rarely affects the brain alone; generally there is concomitant lung involvement. Thus, biopsy of cerebral lesions would only be indicated in the absence of lung involvement. *Nocardia* spp. and *T. gondii* are also implicated in cerebral abscess. These infections are usually diagnosed in a stable post-transplantation phase and appear to be more frequent in heart transplantation [41]. Pyogenic abscesses, such as mycotic aneurysms, particularly those due to *S. aureus,* are uncommon and occur primarily in patients with endocarditis.

Meningitis and bacteremia are often caused by *Listeria monocytogenes*, which usually presents at a late stage during the post-transplant period, since cotrimoxazole prophylaxis administered in the early post-transplantation phase prevents this complication. Despite the frequency of CMV disease in patients receiving a solid organ transplant, it is rarely a primary pathogen in CNS infection. Similarly, the incidence of encephalitis due to herpes simplex virus does not appear to be higher than among the general population [42]. Among the components of the family of herpesviruses, HHV-6 has the highest affinity for the central nervous system. In transplant patients, HHV-6 encephalitis manifests as alterations of consciousness ranging from confusion to coma, seizures, and headache rather than as focal alterations. The diagnosis is made by PCR analysis of the virus in cerebrospinal fluid [43]. On many occasions, altered mental status in the early post-transplantation period is attributed to immunosuppressant medication. Nevertheless, it is well demonstrated that lowering the dose of immunosuppressant medication can suffice to reverse the manifestations of HHV-6 infection, which could mean that the alteration may be due to the virus and not to the medication in some cases [44].

5.3.3 Pneumonia

The risk of pneumonia in lung transplantation is up to four times higher than in patients with other transplanted organs, with an incidence of nearly 40%. In RESITRA, it was observed that 40% of pneumonia cases in these patients were recorded during the first month and 31% were related to mechanical ventilation. A bacterial etiology was responsible for 78% of the episodes in which the etiology could be established, with *P. aeruginosa* (48%) and *S. aureus* (16%) being the most frequent microorganisms [45]. The differential diagnosis of pneumonia during the first 15 days after the lung implantation is mainly with preservation lesions or acute rejection. When antifungal prophylaxis is not given, the incidence of invasive pulmonary aspergillosis may be high; in this population it is related to colonization before [10] or after [46] transplantation. Nevertheless, initiation of preventive measures such as nebulized deoxycholate [47] or liposomal [48] amphotericin B is effective for controlling the problem.

In liver transplantation, the origin of pulmonary infiltrates is associated with the diagnosis of pneumonia in 38% of cases [49]. Another study conducted as part of RESITRA showed a 12.7% incidence of pneumonia, with 67% of episodes reported in the first month and 29% related to mechanical ventilation. Gram-negative bacilli (*Acinetobacter baumannii, Pseudomonas aeruginosa* and *Escherichia coli*) were the main cause of pneumonia (82%) [50].

The incidence of pneumonia in heart transplant recipients is 15% [51], with mortality as high as 30% [52]. In this population, 64% of the episodes occur in the first month after transplantation and 43% are associated with mechanical ventilation. According to the latest data reported by the RESITRA investigators, the etiology in these episodes was predominantly bacterial (88%), with *P. aeruginosa, A. baumannii* and *S. aureus* being the main agents. Only 1 of the 44 episodes reported in 292 transplants was due to CMV [51].

With regard to renal transplantation, the incidence of pneumonia reported in the latest studies is 4.6% [53]. Unlike the other types of solid organ transplantation, only 34% occur in the first month after the procedure.

Diagnosis. In solid organ transplant recipients in critical condition, the etiology of pulmonary infiltrates must be diagnosed as soon as possible. In some cases, the radiological findings can assist the diagnosis, with the presence of nodules suggesting fungal or *M. tuberculosis* infection [54]. It should be kept in mind that because of the therapeutic implications of lung transplantation, acute rejection can also have a nodular appearance. Nevertheless cavitation of the nodules is a typical sign of fungal infection. Bacterial pneumonia presents as alveolar infiltrates, whereas *P. jiroveci*, CMV and other herpesviruses present as interstitial or reticulonodular infiltrates. Isolation of *P. jiroveci*, *Legionella* spp., *Nocardia* spp., *M. tuberculosis* or *Cryptococcus* spp. provides the diagnosis of lung infection. However, culture of sputum and respiratory secretions is diagnostic in 20–35% of cases and blood culture in only 6–10% [45, 50, 51, 53]. In one reported series of liver transplant recipients with pneumonia admitted to the ICU, blood cultures were positive in 40% [55]. When the diagnosis is not achieved with noninvasive tests, fibrobronchoscopy with bronchoalveolar lavage (BAL) must be done, preferably in patients with diffuse pulmonary infiltrates. If the patient has nodular involvement, fine-needle aspiration biopsy (FNAB) is superior to BAL [56]. Transbronchial biopsy has additional value for the diagnosis of rejection in lung transplant recipients. Open biopsy should be reserved for patients with progressive involvement refractory to antibiotic therapy, in whom BAL and FNAB have not been diagnostic.

5.3.4 Surgical Wound Infections

Hospital-acquired infection of the surgical wound in solid organ recipients is associated with increased morbidity, including longer hospital stay and graft loss in patients with kidney or pancreas transplants. Surgical wound infection in kidney transplant recipients is usually caused by staphylococci or Gram-negative bacilli. Staphylococcal infections are associated with superficial and early involvement, whereas those caused by Gram-negative bacilli appear later and cause deep infection that can lead to bacteremia, graft loss or even the death of the patient. Prolonged urinary catheterization, wall hematoma formation following surgery, and repeat surgery are risk factors for this condition in renal transplantation [57]. However, improvements in the surgical technique and adequate antibiotic prophylaxis have decreased this problem [35].

Sternotomy infection occurs in 2–20% of heart and lung transplant recipients. The microorganisms involved are Gram-positive cocci, enterobacteria and *P. aeruginosa*. These infections can extend toward the mediastinum and cause mediastinitis in 2–9% of patients receiving these organs. In patients colonized by antibiotic-resistant *P. aeruginosa* receiving a lung transplant for cystic fibrosis, the problem can become extremely serious. Even when the infected lung is removed during the procedure, residual colonization of the oropharynx and paranasal sinuses may be the source of future infections. Aerosolized colistin sodium may be useful to promote the emergence of sensitive microbes in cystic fibrosis candidates with pan-resistant isolates of *Pseudomonas* spp. before transplantation [5].

Surgical wound infection is particularly important in pancreas transplantation, with a reported incidence of 30% [58]. Deep infection of the surgical bed can lead to pancreatic graft loss, with a 1-year survival of 16–20% [58]. Infection is favored by the predisposition to ischemia inherent to the low vascularization of the pancreas and the release of gastric juices in the surgical bed. The predominant microorganisms in this condition are *S. epidermidis* and *C. albicans*. Infection due to the latter is favored by high urinary colonization in diabetic patients, advanced age, retroperitoneal position of the pancreas, and a lack of catheterized drainage. This type of infection is mainly observed in the first month post-transplantation.

A recent study conducted within RESITRA reported that the incidence of surgical wound infection in liver transplantation is around 4.7% of patients, with an associated mortality of 4.2%. In most cases, the etiology is polymicrobial with a predominance of Gram-positive cocci. Analysis of the risk factors associated with this entity found that surgical prophylaxis with first- and second-generation cephalosporins is associated with 6.5-fold greater risk of surgical bed infection. In patients with biliary-enteric bypasses the risk is 2.9-fold higher [59].

5.4 Important Microorganisms in Transplantation Infection in a Critical Recipient

5.4.1 Fungal Infections

The latest data indicate that the incidence of invasive fungal disease in critically ill transplant patients in our setting is about 2.2% [60]. The most common invasive fungal infections in this population are aspergillosis and candidiasis, whereas cryptococcosis, zygomycosis, dematiaceous fungi, and *P. jiroveci* are less frequent. The incidence of aspergillosis and invasive candidiasis according to the type of transplantation is shown in Table 5.1 [60].

Table 5.1. Incidence of invasive aspergillosis and candidiasis by type of transplantation

%	Heart	Liver	Pancreas	Lung	Kidney
Aspergillosis	0.4	0.8	0.7	3.9	0.2
Candidiasis	1.2	1.7	13.6	1.9	0.8

5.4.1.1 *Aspergillosis*

Invasive aspergillosis remains an important cause of morbidity and mortality in solid organ transplantation. This infection shows some common characteristics and risk factors, and others that differ according to the type of transplantation. Although the incidence has gradually decreased over time, mortality continues to be high: about 76% overall and 95% in cases affecting the central nervous system [10].

Epidemiology. The presentation of invasive aspergillosis follows a bimodal pattern with some characteristic risk factors in each case [10]. In 57% of the episodes, the disease manifests during the first 3 months after transplantation and is associated with the variables that define a more seriously ill patient in the postoperative period, such as the need for vasoactive drugs for more than 24 h after surgery, the development of renal failure with or without the need for replacement therapy, more than two episodes of bacterial infection, and CMV disease [10]. Lung transplantation has the highest incidence of invasive aspergillosis among solid organ recipients [10, 60]. In this population, colonization in the 6 months before transplantation has been identified as an independent risk factor for the development of this disease [10]. Colonization is frequent in patients with cystic fibrosis and the characteristic presentation of the disease in these patients is ulcerative tracheobronchitis. Local inflammation of the bronchial suture may act as a trigger for the development of *Aspergillus* infection that can lead to suture dehiscence or fistula formation. In liver transplantation, HCV infection is independently associated with the development of aspergillosis after the 3rd month post-transplantation [10]. Some studies have shown that the evolution of the graft is slightly poorer in these patients with respect to non-hepatitis C virus transplants, partially due to the high recurrence rate of hepatitis C virus in the graft [61]. Regarding the immunomodulator role of HCV, a documented clinical experience has shown a higher number of infectious complications in transplanted patients with HCV infection [62]. Again, immunologic studies in these patients showed a significant decrease in circulating CD4 populations and a lower response to mitogenic stimulation [63]. In all cases, the lung is the portal of entry; hence *Aspergillus* infection occurs very rarely in an intra-abdominal location or in the surgical wound.

Diagnosis. Early diagnosis of invasive aspergillosis is essential to lower the associated mortality. Culture of sputum or BAL specimens detects the fungus in approximately 50% of cases; hence, culturing may follow vascular invasion. High-resolution CT may be suggestive of the disease as soon as the symptoms develop and before cultures are positive [64]. The images known as the halo sign (area of low attenuation around a nodular lesion due to edema or bleeding around an ischemic area) and crescent sign (air around a lung nodule due to contraction of infarcted tissue, a marker of good evolution), although more frequent in neutropenic patients, are highly suggestive of this entity [65]. Serological tests such as galactomannan antigen determined by ELISA have shown high sensitivity and specificity in the diagnosis of invasive aspergillosis among high-risk oncohematologic patients with neutropenia. However, the usefulness of this strategy in solid organ transplant patients has not been determined and should not be relied upon [66]. Depending on the type of lesion, its location, and the level of acquired experience, CT-guided puncture should be considered, with analysis of the specimens obtained by staining, culture and cytology techniques [67].

Prophylaxis. The use of amphotericin B deoxycholate at a low dose of 6 mg in nebulized form, supported by pharmacokinetic studies showing that high, steady levels are achieved for at least 24 h in lung transplant recipients without chronic rejection (Fig. 5.1) [68], is associated with a lower incidence of fungal infection due to *Aspergillus* spp. [47] in lung transplant patients. The role of the azole antifungals has not been proven and they may reduce the incidence of aspergillosis while increasing the incidence of emerging fungi [69]. Recently, it has been shown that oral itraconazole may be useful as prophylaxis in a subset of heart transplant recipients at a high risk of invasive aspergillosis [70]. In a further step ahead, nebulized liposomal amphotericin B administered three times per week during the first 3 months, once per week up to the 6th month and every 15 days thereafter, also supported by pharmacokinetic and clinical studies done by our group in Hospital Vall d'Hebron, has demonstrated excellent efficacy and safety [48]. This approach is currently being extrapolated to high-risk oncohematologic patients with similar efficacy and safety [71].

Treatment. Although it is not always possible, an attempt should be made to reduce immunosuppression first. With regard to antifungal options, a review of the literature shows that liposomal amphotericin B has lower associated toxicity (particularly renal toxicity with concomitant tacrolimus administration), a higher

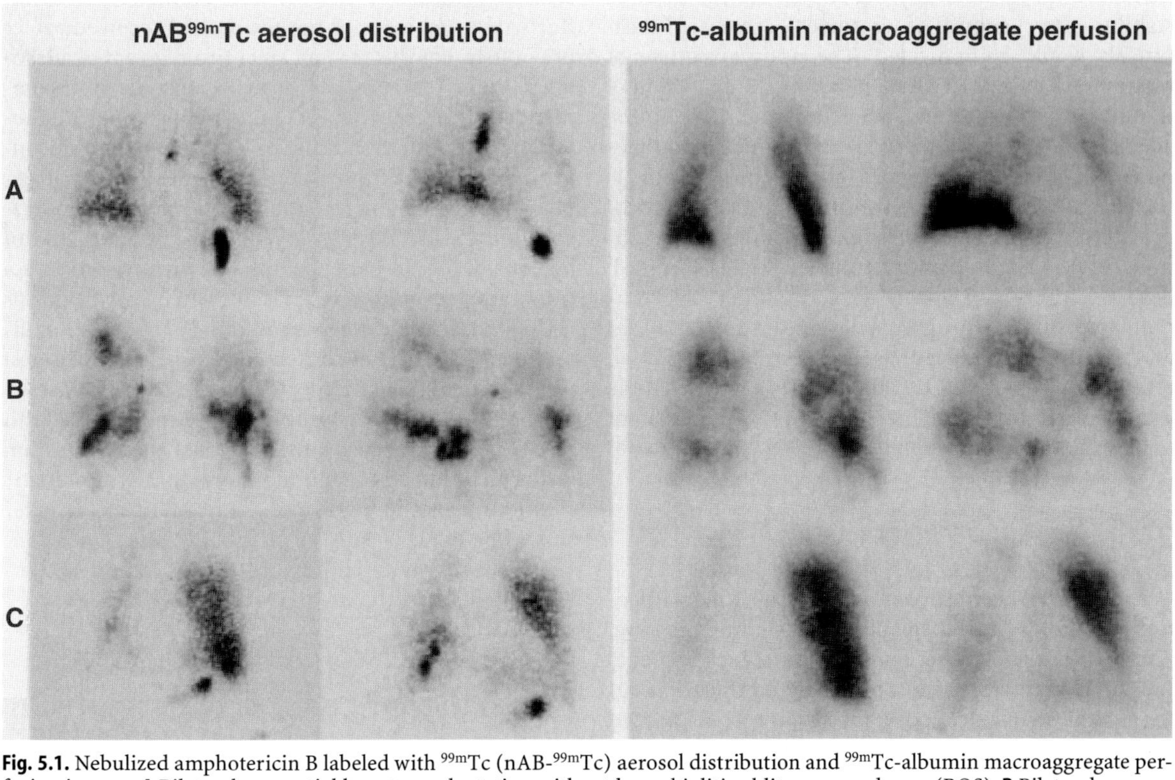

Fig. 5.1. Nebulized amphotericin B labeled with ^{99m}Tc (nAB-^{99m}Tc) aerosol distribution and ^{99m}Tc-albumin macroaggregate perfusion images. **A** Bilateral sequential lung transplantation without bronchiolitis obliterans syndrome (BOS). **B** Bilateral sequential lung transplantation with BOS. **C** Single left-lung transplant

success rate and a lower mortality risk as compared to deoxycholate amphotericin B [72]. Voriconazole also presents better response, higher survival and fewer adverse effects than deoxycholate amphotericin B [73, 74]. The role of intravenous itraconazole must still be elucidated with regard to efficacy and the high number of pharmacological interactions with immunosuppressant drugs. Nevertheless, the oral formulation of itraconazole could be useful in long-term therapy. Caspofungin is approved for use as rescue therapy in patients with a lack of response or intolerance to the first-line treatment. The poor results of existing treatments has encouraged the practice of combining drugs to seek synergistic effects: azoles plus echinocandins or polyenes plus echinocandins, although there is no definitive data about the efficacy and safety of this approach [75, 76].

Surgery should be indicated in patients with massive hemoptysis or hemoptysis secondary to a lesion near large vessels, in paranasal sinus disease, when a single cavitated lung lesion progresses despite appropriate antifungal treatment, and in patients with infiltration of the pericardium, large vessels, bone, or subcutaneous thoracic tissue while under treatment. In our opinion, the treatment of choice is liposomal amphotericin at doses of 5 mg/kg/day or higher. In a recent study, the Cochrane group questioned the role of voriconazole in this setting [77]. In cases of therapeutic failure (progression by the end of the 1st week or stability after 1 month of treatment), associated antifungals would be indicated. The optimal course of treatment is unknown and depends on the extension of the disease, the response, and the patient's immune status. A logical sequence would be to initiate intravenous treatment at least until disease progression is halted and, subsequently, continue with a period of oral formulation to treat possible microfoci for a maximum of 6–12 months after complete remission [66]. Several authors have shown that early surgery substantially improves the prognosis of these patients [78]. In an experimental model of aspergillosis, Gavaldà et al. recently demonstrated that the efficacy of intravenous amphotericin treatment increases with the addition of nebulized liposomal amphotericin [79].

5.4.1.2 Candidiasis

Candidiasis is the most common invasive fungal infection in solid organ transplantation excluding the lung. The highest incidence is found in pancreas recipients [60]. In general, it is a hospital-acquired infection, although the source depends on the type of transplanted organ. Whereas in liver transplant recipients the source is endogenous (usually the intestine), in patients receiving a heart or lung transplant, it may be exogenous (from the donor) [80]. Intra-abdominal infection is most commonly observed in patients undergoing organ transplantation in this cavity. The risk factors include excessively long surgery, retransplantation, considerable transfusion support requirements, renal failure, and CMV infection [12]. However, the incidence of invasive disease caused by *Candida* spp. has declined with the advances in surgical technique and immunosuppressant drugs. In pancreas transplantation, *Candida* infection manifests predominantly as surgical wound infection or candidemia. In lung transplantation, the bronchial suture can be affected, resulting in wound dehiscence and mediastinitis. The anastomosis is particularly vulnerable because of the decreased blood supply and presence of foreign material. The population to be targeted for prophylaxis, the best drug for this purpose, and the course of treatment are still uncertain. In many hospitals, fluconazole is used as prophylaxis for liver and pancreas recipients. Nevertheless, universal prophylaxis should be considered with caution based on the potential appearance of azole-resistant *Candida* spp. [81] and selection of intrinsically resistant fungi such as *Aspergillus* spp. Hence, the use of prophylaxis mainly in high-risk patients may be the most advisable strategy.

With regard to the treatment, we assume that *C. krusei* is intrinsically resistant to fluconazole and that *C. glabrata* develops secondary resistance. However, resistance rates may differ between countries and be influenced by whether or not the patient received azoles previously. For this reason, an antifungigram of all isolated fungi that produce invasive disease is recommended. At present, we recommend liposomal amphotericin B at a dose of 3 mg/kg/day rather than fluconazole because of its broader spectrum and its lower pharmacological interactions with immunosuppressors. If the risk of toxicity is very high, caspofungin can be considered. In patients with catheter-related infection, catheter removal is advisable when *C. parapsilosis* is isolated, an infective focus is found at the catheter insertion point, there are criteria of sepsis, and in cases of persistent candidemia or lack of clinical response by 72 h after initiating appropriate treatment [82]. With respect to candiduria, most are cases of colonization rather than infection, and therefore only symptomatic candiduria should be treated. Removal of the catheter should be done as early as possible. Washes with conventional amphotericin B are not currently recommended [83].

5.4.1.3 Pneumocystis jiroveci

Most *P. jiroveci* infections are considered reactivations of an endogenous infection acquired in childhood. However, it has been shown to be present in more than

50% of the air samples collected from hospital rooms where patients with *P. jiroveci* infection are staying [84]. In the absence of prophylaxis, lung transplant recipients are at greater risk for developing disease due to this microorganism. The infection usually presents between the 3rd and 6th month after transplantation. Later cases occur in patients who receive more intense immunosuppression due to rejection [85].

Coexistence of this infection with CMV or bacterial infection is not rare, particularly in lung transplant patients. However, prophylaxis with co-trimoxazole is very effective and therefore recommended in all solid organ transplants. The duration of prophylaxis is usually the first 6 months in heart, kidney and liver transplantation. A minimum of 12 months would be recommended in lung transplantation. These limits have been established on the basis of the decreased risk of the disease after the first 6 months post-transplantation. However, patients who receive greater immunosuppression because of late rejection should continue or reinitiate co-trimoxazole prophylaxis [86]. Prophylaxis with this drug is also effective against *Nocardia* spp., *Listeria* spp., *Toxoplasma gondii* and *Legionella* spp. In addition, the adverse effects are minimal: skin rash in 1% and leukopenia in 3%. In patients with sulfamide allergy, nebulized pentamidine every month is an alternative approach.

5.4.1.4 Cryptococcosis

An average of 2.8% and up to 5% of organ transplant patients develop *Cryptococcus neoformans* infection. In a study performed in Spain from September 2003 to February 2005, there were no cases of cryptococcosis during a follow-up of 2,615 solid organ recipients [60]. However, there are important geographical variations. Cryptococcosis is a significant opportunistic infection in the USA, with some centers reporting a rate of up to 5% in transplant recipients. Most cases occur 6 months after transplantation. Overall mortality in transplant recipients with cryptococcosis ranges from 20% to 42% and the rate approaches 50% in patients with central nervous system infection [87].

Combination therapy with amphotericin B and flucytosine has been shown to render CSF cultures negative within 2 weeks in 55–85% of patients with cryptococcal meningitis. These data, however, are derived primarily from hosts other than organ transplant recipients. The response of the infection to antifungal therapy in organ transplantation has not been well characterized. Approaches to the management of *C. neoformans* infection in transplant patients have mainly been extrapolated from studies in HIV patients. Treatment practices vary widely, particularly with regard to the duration of antifungal maintenance therapy for cryptococcosis after organ transplantation. Generally, life-long suppressive therapy is not used; however, the optimal duration of therapy and the risk of relapse upon discontinuation of antifungal agents is still uncertain [88]. Prophylaxis with fluconazole is not indicated, due to the low incidence of the disease and its unpredictable appearance throughout the post-transplant period.

5.4.1.5 Zygomycosis

Infections caused by Zygomycetes are very rare: 0.3% in liver transplantation, 0.4% in kidney and 0.8% in lung. The incidence has increased in recent years because of the use of voriconazole antifungal prophylaxis in some populations [68]. Lung involvement is evident in only 25% of reported cases. Other infection sites are the paranasal sinuses, brain, skin, and gastrointestinal tract [89]. Up to 72% of cases are due to *Rhizopus* spp. Other species include *Cunninghamella* spp., *Mucor* spp., and *Absidia corymbifera*. This infection occurs in the first 6 months after transplantation, usually coinciding with an increase in immunosuppression to treat rejection. It is also observed more often among patients with diabetes mellitus. Lung presentation occurs in the form of nodules or a cavitation without a fluid/air level. In these cases, the treatment should consist of decreased immunosuppression, surgical resection and administration of liposomal amphotericin B at a dose of 10 mg/kg/day or, recently, posaconazole, with the peculiarity of its exclusively oral administration route [90].

5.4.1.6 Dematiaceous Fungi

Pigmented fungi are being increasingly recognized as pathogens in patients receiving a solid organ transplant [91]. This is because of improvements in microbiological diagnostic techniques and a growing immunodepressed population at risk of acquiring an opportunistic infection. Most of these infections occur in the late post-transplantation period. Nevertheless, up to 21% present within the first 3 months with disseminated disease (predominantly cerebral abscesses). Cutaneous involvement is frequent, with treatment consisting of surgical resection and itraconazole at 400 mg/day for no less than 6 months. The mortality is higher than 80% in cases of pulmonary or disseminated disease, partly because of a high resistance to amphotericin B and azoles [92].

5.4.2 Bacterial Infections

5.4.2.1 *Staphylococcus aureus*

Methicillin-resistant *S. aureus* (MRSA) has become one of the main bacterial etiologies in solid organ transplant infections. Catheter infection is the main source and up to 42% of bacteremia cases are due to this microorganism, but it can also cause surgical wound infections, nosocomial pneumonia, intra-abdominal abscesses, and endocarditis. These infections occur in the early post-transplantation period, 53% within the first 30 days [93]. More than half the cases occur in the ICU. The mortality of bacteremia due to MRSA depends on the origin of the infection. It can be as high as 86% in the case of pneumonia versus only 6% in catheter infection, regardless of the APACHE II score [93]. These data underscore the pathogenicity and virulence of MRSA in solid organ transplant patients. This infection significantly correlates to prior colonization [6]. Nevertheless, attempts to eradicate carrier status have not been shown to be effective in decreasing the incidence of the disease. Glycopeptides have been the treatment of choice, but the development of linezolid has provided a useful alternative [94].

5.4.2.2 *Extended-Spectrum Beta-Lactamase-Producing Enterobacteria*

In general, enterobacteria produce intra-abdominal infection, respiratory infection and bacteriemia in the transplant population. Specifically, *Klebsiella* spp. is the fourth cause of hospital-acquired pneumonia, mainly in relation with mechanical ventilation [95]. Antibiotic resistance mediated by beta-lactamase production continues to increase [96]. In fact, an outbreak of ESBL-producing *E. coli* in a transplant unit has been reported [97]. The production of these enzymes confers resistance to the cephalosporins and beta-lactamase inhibitors and, additionally, through other mechanisms, to quinolones and aminoglycosides. Some authors have suggested restricting the use of third-generation cephalosporins in these patients to prevent the development of resistance [98]. Isolation of these cases reduces the possibility of transmission between patients. Carbapenems are the treatment of choice for these infections [96].

5.4.2.3 *Enterococci*

Vancomycin-resistant *E. faecium* in solid organ transplantation seems to be an isolated problem in some centers in the USA where an incidence of 10–16% has been documented in liver transplant patients. The infection is commonly intra-abdominal and occurs within the first month after transplantation [99]. The risk factors for the development of this infection in liver transplant patients include carrier status, previous treatment with vancomycin, biliary complications, prolonged ICU hospitalization, repeat surgery, and primary graft dysfunction [100]. Mortality can be as high as 50%. Antibiotic therapy should be based on the use of quinupristin-dalfopristin or linezolid [101].

5.4.2.4 *Legionellosis*

The incidence of legionellosis in solid organ transplantation is 2–9% [102], with the main source being deposits of contaminated water from cooling systems. Outbreaks originating in humidifiers or ice-making machines have also been described in this population [103]. Pneumonia is the main clinical manifestation of infection, although cases of pericarditis, cellulitis, and peritonitis have been reported. *Legionella* is difficult to culture; hence, the diagnosis currently relies on determination of the urinary antigen. In order to avoid the interactions of macrolides with tacrolimus or cyclosporine, the treatment of choice in solid organ recipients is levofloxacin.

5.4.3 Viral Infections

5.4.3.1 *Cytomegalovirus*

Cytomegalovirus infection occurs in the majority of solid-organ transplant recipients, primarily in the first 3 months post-transplantation, when immunosuppression is most intense. CMV can be transmitted to transplant recipients via infected donor organs or cellular blood products, the former being the primary source of CMV infection after solid-organ transplantation, then denominated primary infection. Secondary infection or reactivation infection develops when endogenous latent virus is reactivated in a CMV-seropositive individual following transplantation. Superinfection or reinfection occurs when a seropositive recipient receives latent, infected cells from a seropositive donor. In the immunosuppressed solid-organ transplant recipient, CMV has three major effects: (1) it causes infectious diseases syndromes (see below); (2) it has been implicated in causing increased immunosuppression, which may explain the frequent association of CMV with other opportunistic infections, such as fungal and *Pneumocystis* infections; and (3) it has been associated with acute or chronic allograft rejection. However, the variables that hasten the progression of allograft injury have not been fully defined. CMV infection, therefore, has a potential impact on both patient and graft outcome [104].

Nonetheless, recent advances have led to decreases in the associated morbidity and mortality of this complication. CMV infection, defined as isolation of the virus or detection of CMV viral proteins or DNA/messenger RNA in any body fluid or tissue, can progress to CMV disease, either as a viral syndrome or organ disease (pneumonia, digestive disease, hepatitis, encephalitis, retinitis, nephritis, cystitis, myocarditis, or pancreatitis) [105]. Interestingly, CMV shows a predilection for transplanted organs in the case of focal disease. The diagnosis of focal disease requires CMV detection in the affected tissue with histopathologic methods and/or culture, rather than by PCR, given the low positive predictive value of the latter [105].

The strategies to fight this infection are based on prophylaxis and preemptive treatment, and, lastly, treatment of the disease itself. Thus, transplant patients should be monitored to detect CMV infection, either through antigenemia assay or real-time PCR, depending on the criteria of the microbiology laboratory of each center [106]. Monitoring is done in blood, although there is no universally accepted threshold value at which treatment is indicated. This will depend on the patient's risk status and the experience of each hospital. Real time PCR has an advantage over antigenemia assay in patients with leukopenia of less than 1,000 elements/μl, in whom antigenemia may not be evaluable; nevertheless, this situation is uncommon in solid organ recipients. Monitoring should be done weekly while the patient is hospitalized and adjusted to the follow-up visits thereafter. Once treatment is started, weekly monitoring is advisable. Increases in CMV in the course of treatment may indicate resistance, but underdosing of ganciclovir should be excluded. Persistent CMV replication may also indicate resistance depending on the viral load, which should be repeated within a minimum of 10 – 15 days.

CMV infection develops in 30 – 80 % of patients who undergo a solid organ transplantation. The incidence and presence of CMV disease varies according to the type of transplantation, the associated risk factors, and the preventive strategies used [107]. A recent study in renal transplantation has shown changes in the risk factors associated with CMV infection as a result of continuing progress in the transplantation field. Thus, in addition to the known risk factors (donor/recipient CMV serological mismatch, presence of rejection episodes and use of antilymphocytic drugs) there are others, such as simultaneous pancreas transplantation, use of cyclosporine but not tacrolimus, donor age greater than 60, and the development of viral diseases other than CMV; in contrast, rapamycin use has a protective effect [108]. Disease development is more frequent, and usually more severe, in intestine, pancreas, and lung transplantation than in liver, heart and kidney. Intestinal transplants are most highly affected, since they contain considerable lymphoid tissue.

The highest risk is between the 1st and 6th month, with a maximum incidence between the 2nd and 3rd month. In primary infection, the recipient's lack of specific immunity allows considerable CMV replication that is usually associated with symptomatic infection, sometimes extremely severe, with an early onset and greater tendency to recur, whereas in reactivation the recipient's humoral and cellular immunity decrease the incidence and severity of the disease [109]. Transplantation of a seropositive organ to a seronegative recipient is the main risk factor for CMV disease and has been observed in all types of transplantation. Administration of antilymphocytic or antithymocytic globulins or OKT3 monoclonal antibodies leads to the production and secretion of cytokines that trigger the inflammatory cascade and strongly stimulate CMV replication. Other risk factors include high corticoid dose, high CMV viral load, coinfection with other herpesviruses (particularly HHV-6), and the use of mycophenolate mofetil at doses of 3 g or more for immunosuppressive therapy. Nonetheless, it is difficult to identify the adverse gastrointestinal effects of this drug at this dose [110].

CMV serological status should be determined in all solid organ donors and recipients (latent infection) prior to transplantation. In seronegative recipients of an organ from a seronegative or unknown donor it is advisable, but can be difficult, to assure that transfusion support is CMV-seronegative or filtered to prevent transmission. All seronegative recipients from a seropositive donor should receive prophylaxis followed by monitoring with antigenemia or real-time PCR and preemptive ganciclovir therapy if necessary. In this population, our group applies prophylaxis with intravenous ganciclovir at a dose of 5 mg/kg/12 h while patients are hospitalized, and valganciclovir 900 mg every 24 h at discharge and up to day 100 post-transplantation. After this period the patient is monitored by antigenemia or real-time PCR at each medical visit up to the 6th month. If necessary, valganciclovir at 900 mg/12 h is given until antigenemia tests are negative. Preemptive therapy with intravenous ganciclovir or valganciclovir, depending on whether or not the patients is hospitalized, is also recommended when antilymphocytic antibodies are used for treating corticoid-resistant rejection or as induction immunosuppression [111].

In patients with a risk of primary infection undergoing lung, pancreas, or intestine transplants, the risk of CMV disease is extremely high; hence universal prophylaxis followed by monitoring and preemptive therapy is the best strategy regardless of the recipient/donor CMV serological status. Our group prolongs ganciclovir or valganciclovir exposure up to 100 days post-transplantation, since the first manifestation of infection in these patients can be severe (pneumonitis, enteritis), without prior warning by increased viral load. We believe it is important to assure that the patient has passed the immediate postoperative period before having to confront possible CMV disease. Monitoring should also be performed weekly, but in this case up to the 6th month and every 2 weeks thereafter up to 1 year after transplantation or until the risk of graft dysfunction, which would imply intense immunosuppression, has passed. In the remaining seropositive patients, prevention is based on anticipated treatment guided by antigenemia or PCR testing. Recommended prophylaxis is oral valganciclovir at 900 mg/24 h [112] or intravenous ganciclovir at 6 mg/kg/day if the patient does not tolerate oral intake, up to a maximum of 3 months and always adjusted according to kidney function. The use of anti-CMV hyperimmune gamma globulin as prophylaxis is highly controversial [113]. It has been widely applied by different groups, although there are no definitive studies demonstrating its efficacy. The treatment of choice for CMV disease is ganciclovir at a dose of 5 mg/kg/12 h. In the event of severe ganciclovir resistance or leukopenia, the option would be foscarnet at 60 mg/kg/8 h [111]. Valganciclovir may be useful in mild disease [114]. The duration of treatment is not well established; hence the risk of recurrence.

5.4.3.2 Herpes Simplex Virus

Most solid organ recipients present early mucositis as a consequence of reactivation of latent herpes simplex. Visceral or disseminated infection is rare, but can have a fulminant course without adequate antiviral treatment. Onset occurs in the first month after transplantation. Mortality due to this complication can be higher than 70%, depending on the series [115]. In lung transplantation the presence of herpes simplex in the respiratory tract can be associated with pneumonitis [116]. Doses similar to those applied in cases of encephalitis should be used to treat the visceral infection.

5.4.3.3 Varicella-zoster Virus

Depending on the series, the geographical area, and whether the infection occurs in adults or children, seronegativity to varicella-zoster virus varies from 5% to 70% [117]. These patients are susceptible to developing primary infection by donor transmission. Visceral dissemination can be a cause of death when it leads to hepatitis, pneumonitis, pancreatitis, gastroenteritis or meningoencephalitis. On occasions, pain precedes the onset of the cutaneous lesions, and this can delay the diagnosis and worsen the prognosis.

5.4.3.4 Human Herpesvirus 6 and 7

A growing body of evidence suggests that the most important effects of HHV-6 and HHV-7 reactivation on the outcome of liver transplantation may be mediated indirectly by their interactions with CMV. Documented coinfection among these three herpesviruses in clinical syndromes that were classically ascribed to be solely caused by CMV has raised substantial interest in the potential role of HHV-6 and HHV-7 as copathogens in the direct and indirect illnesses caused by CMV [118].

Most infections by HHV-6 are reactivations of latent virus; however, there are proven cases of donor transmission. Onset occurs between the 2nd and 3rd month after transplantation. Clinical symptoms vary from myelosuppression to interstitial pneumonia or fever of unknown origin. HHV-6 is a highly neurotropic virus; hence the patient can present with encephalitis or simply with behavioral changes. Due to the prevalence of this virus in the general population, PCR determination for the diagnosis of active infection is not fully established. HHV-6 is sensitive to ganciclovir and foscarnet and resistant to acyclovir.

5.4.3.5 Human Herpesvirus 8

Kaposi's sarcoma is a tumor of multicentric origin, composed of endothelium-lined vascular spaces and spindle-shaped cells. The incidence of Kaposi's sarcoma in transplant recipients is 400–500 times greater than that in the general population, and is rising within the transplant population, currently comprising more than 5% of all de novo neoplasms in this group. The exact pathogenesis is still unknown, but DNA sequences from human herpesvirus 8 (HHV-8) are present in the different clinical variants of Kaposi's sarcoma. Risk factors associated with the development of these tumors post-transplantation include the geographical origin of the patient, HSV-8 infection before and after transplantation, and the immunosuppressive regimen used, but the importance of each factor remains to be determined [119].

5.4.3.6 Epstein-Barr Virus

Epstein-Barr virus infection in transplantation recipients may cause mild symptoms such as malaise, fever, headache, and sore throat but may also be associated with post-transplantation lymphoproliferative disease (PTLD), which is a significant cause of morbidity and mortality in transplant recipients [120]. The term PTLD acknowledges the fact that these lesions are heterogeneous and may not meet the diagnostic criteria for lymphoma. In contrast with CMV, optimal preventive and treatment strategies for EB virus-related PTLD remain elusive and are not definitive. Recent experimental and clinical data, however, demonstrate a promising role for immunotherapy in preventing and treating PTLD [121]. Moreover, it seems that ganciclovir may have a role as preventive agent for the lymphoproliferative disease.

References

1. Waser M, Maggiorini M, Luthy A, Laske A, vor Sequesser L, Mohassi P, et al. (1994) Infectious complications in 100 consecutive heart transplant recipients. Eur J Clin Microbiol Infect Dis 13:12–18
2. Chang FY, Singh N, Gayowski T, Wagener MM, Marino IR (1998) Fever in liver transplant recipients: changing spectrum of etiologic agents. Clin Infect Dis 26:59–65
3. Carrido RS, Aquado JM, Diaz-Pedrache C, Len O, Montejo M, Moreno A, et al. (2006) A review of critical periods for opportunistic infection in the new transplantation era. Transplantation 82:1457–1462
4. Linden PK, Miller CB (1999) Vancomycin-resistant enterococci: the clinical effect of a common nosocomial pathogen. Diagn Microbiol Infect Dis 33:113–120
5. Bauldoff GS, Nunley DR, Manzetti JD, Dauber JH, Keenan RJ (1997) Use of aerosolized colistin sodium in cystic fibrosis patients awaiting lung transplantation. Transplantation 64:748–753
6. Chang FY, Singh N, Gayowski T, Drenning SD, Wagener MM, Marino IR (1998) *Staphylococcus aureus* nasal colonization and association with infections in liver transplant recipients. Transplantation 65:1169–1172
7. Chang FY, Singh N, Gayowski T, Wagener M, Marino IR (1998) *Staphylococcus aureus* nasal colonization in patients with cirrhosis: prospective assessment of association with infections. Infect Control Hosp Epidemiol 19:328–332
8. Grems JJ, Hiatt JR, Klein AS, Hart J, El-Khoury G, Winston D, et al. (1998) Disseminated aspergillosis complicating orthotopic liver transplantation for fulminant hepatic failure refractory to corticosteroid therapy. Transplantation 46:479–481
9. Milstone AP, Brumble LM, Loyd JE, Ely EW, Roberts JR, Pierson RN 3rd, et al. (2000) Active CMV infection before lung transplantation: risk factors and clinical implications. J Heart Lung Transplant 19:744–750
10. Gavalda J, Len O, San Juan R, Aguado JM, Fortun J, Lumbreras C, et al. (2005) Risk factors for invasive aspergillosis in solid-organ transplant recipients: a case-control study. Clin Infect Dis 41:52–59
11. Gayowsksi T, Marino IR, Singh N, Doyle H, Wagener MM, Fung JJ, et al. (1998) Orthotopic liver transplantation in high-risk patients: risk factors associated with mortality and infectious morbidity. Transplantation 65:499–504
12. Singh N (2003) Fungal infections in the recipients of solid organ transplantation. Infect Dis Clin North Am 17:113–134
13. Muñoz P, Muñoz V, Fogueda M, Blanes M, Cuervas-Mons V, Moreno A, et al. (2005) Infectious complications after heart transplantation. Results of a prospective national network in Spain (RESITRA). 45th Interscience Conference on Antimicrobial Agents and Chemotherapy, Washington, December 2005; Abstract K-1567, p 357
14. Kusne S, Furukawa H, Abu-Elmagd W, Irish W, Rakela J, Fung J et al. (1996) Infectious complications after small bowel transplantation in adults: an update. Transplant Proc 28:2761–2762
15. Hudnall SD, Rady PL, Tyring SK, Fish JC (1999) Hydrocortisone activation of human herpesvirus 8 viral DNA replication and gene expression in vitro. Transplantation 67:648–652
16. Ochiai TA, Nakajima K, Nagata M, Suzuki T, Asano T, Uematsu T, et al. (1987) Effect of a new immunosuppressive agent, FK506 on heterotopic cardiac allotransplantation in the rat. Transplant Proc 19:1284–1286
17. The U.S. Multicenter FK506 Liver Study Group (1994) A comparison of tacrolimus (FK506) and cyclosporine for immunosuppression in liver transplantation. N Engl J Med 331:1110–1115
18. Paterson DL, Singh N, Panebianco A, Wannstedt CF, Wagener MM, Gayowski T, et al. (1998) Infectious complications occurring in liver transplant recipients receiving mycophenolate mofetil. Transplantation 66:593–598
19. Singh N (1997) Infections in solid organ transplant recipients. In: Wenzel RP (ed) Prevention and control of nosocomial infections. Williams and Wilkins, Baltimore, MD, p 1100
20. Roenhorst HW, Beelen JM, Middeldorp JM, Schirm J, Teggess AM, The TH (1985) Maintenance of cytomegalovirus (CMV) latency and host immune responses of long term renal allograft survivors. II. Secondary CMV infections associated with impaired in vitro proliferative responses to mitogens, allogeneic lymphocytes and CMV infected cells. Clin Exp Immunol 61:72–79
21. Grattan MT, Moreno-Cabral CE, Starnes VA, Oyer PE, Stinson EB, Shumway NE (1989) Cytomegalovirus infection is associated with cardiac allograft rejection and atherosclerosis. JAMA 261:3561–3566
22. Reinke P, Fietze E, Ode-Hakim S, Prosch S, Lippert J, Ewert R, et al. (1994) Late acute renal allograft rejection and symptomless cytomegalovirus infection. Lancet 344:1737–1738
23. Razonable RR, Burak KW, van Cruijsen H, Brown RA, Charlton MR, Smith TF, et al. (2002) The pathogenesis of hepatitis C virus is influenced by cytomegalovirus. Clin Infect Dis 35:974–981
24. de Otero J, Gavalda J, Murio E, Vargas V, Calico I, Llopart L, et al. (1998) Cytomegalovirus disease as a risk factor for graft loss and death after orthotopic liver transplantation. Clin Infect Dis 26:865–870
25. Singh N, Carrigan DR (1996) Human herpesvirus-6 in transplantation: an emerging pathogen. Ann Intern Med 124:1065–1071
26. Dockrell DH, Mendez JC, Jones M, Harmsen WS, Ilstrup DM, Smith TF, et al. (1999) Human herpesvirus 6 seronegativity before transplantation predicts the occurrence of fungal infection in liver transplant recipients. Transplantation 67:399–403
27. Dockrell DH, Prada J, Jones MF, Patel R, Badley AD, Harmsen WS, et al. (1997) Seroconversion to human herpesvirus 6 following liver transplantation is a marker of cytomegalovirus disease. J Infect Dis 176:1135–1140
28. Lee H, Locker J, Nalesnik M, Reyes J, Jaffe R, Alashari M, et al. (1995) The association of Epstein-Barr virus with smooth muscle tumors occurring after organ transplantation. N Engl J Med 332:19–25
29. Alkan S, Karcher DS, Ortiz A, Khalil S, Akhtar M, Ali MA (1997) Human herpesvirus-8 Kaposi's sarcoma-associated herpesvirus in organ transplant patients with immunosuppression. Br J Haematol 96:412–414
30. Boshoff C, Weiss RA (1998) Kaposi's sarcoma-associated herpesvirus. Adv Cancer Res 75:57–86
31. Eason JD, Freeman RB, Rohrer RJ, Lewis WD, Jenkins R,

Dienstag J, et al. (1994) Should liver transplantation be performed for patients with hepatitis B? Transplantation 57:1588–1593
32. Singh N, Gayowski T, Wagener MM, Marino IR (1996) Increased infections in liver transplant recipients with recurrent hepatitis C virus hepatitis. Transplantation 61:402–406
33. Moreno A, Cervera C, Rovira M, Uriburu C, Almela M, De la Camara R, et al. (2005) Bloodstream infection in transplant patients in Spain. 45th Interscience Conference on Antimicrobial Agents and Chemotherapy, Washington, December 2005; Abstract K-1563, p 356
34. Wagener MM, Yu VL (1992) Bacteremia in transplant recipients: a prospective study of demographics, etiologic agents, risk factors, and outcomes. Am J Infect Control 20:239–247
35. Moreno A, Cervera C, Cofán F, Marco F, Linares L, Alorda C, et al. (2005) Risk factors for the development of bacteremia in renal transplant recipients. 45th Interscience Conference on Antimicrobial Agents and Chemotherapy, Washington, December 2005; Abstract K-1564, p 356
36. Cervera C, Moreno A, Puig de la Bellacasa J, Cisteró P, Navasa M, Lumbreras C, et al. (2005) Risk factors for the development of bacteremia in liver transplant recipients. 45th Interscience Conference on Antimicrobial Agents and Chemotherapy, Washington, December 2005; Abstract K-1565, p 356
37. George DL, Arnow PM, Fox AS, Baker AL, Thistlethwaite JR, Emond JC, et al. (1991) Bacterial infection as a complication of liver transplantation: epidemiology and risk factors. Rev Infect Dis 13:387–396
38. Singh N, Chang FY, Gayowski T, Wagener M, Marino IR (1999) Fever in liver transplant recipients in the intensive care unit. Clin Transplant 13:504–511
39. Len O, Gavaldà J, Puigfel Y, Alvarez M, Alvarez M, Gentil M, et al. (2005) Donor infection and transmission to the recipient of a solid allograft. A prospective study from RESITRA. 45th Interscience Conference on Antimicrobial Agents and Chemotherapy, Washington, December 2005; Abstract K-1805, p 359
40. Bonham CA, Dominguez EA, Fukui MB, Paterson DL, Pankey GA, Wagener MM, et al. (1998) Central nervous system lesions in liver transplant recipients: prospective assessment of indications for biopsy and implications for management. Transplantation 66:1596–1604
41. Selby R, Ramirez CB, Singh R, Kleopoulos I, Kusne S, Starzl TE, et al. (1997) Brain abscess in solid organ transplant recipients receiving cyclosporine-based immunosuppression. Arch Surg 132:304–310
42. Singh N, Yu VL, Gayowski T (1994) Central nervous system lesions in adult liver transplant recipients: clinical review with implications for management. Medicine 73:110–118
43. Wang FZ, Linde A, Hagglund H, Testa M, Locasciulli A, Ljungman P (1999) Human herpesvirus 6 DNA in cerebrospinal fluid specimens from allogeneic bone marrow transplant patients: does it have clinical significance? Clin Infect Dis 28:562–568
44. Singh N, Paterson DL (2000) Encephalitis caused by human herpesvirus-6 in transplant recipients: relevance of a novel neurotropic virus. Transplantation 69:2474–2479
45. Gavalda J, Lama R, Varela A, Vicente JL, Peña F, Gaudo J, et al. (2005) Pneumonia after lung transplantation in the XXI century: a multicenter prospective study. 45th Interscience Conference on Antimicrobial Agents and Chemotherapy, Washington, December 2005; Abstract K-1558, p 354
46. Cahill BC, Hibbs JR, Savik K, Juni BA, Dosland BM, Edin-Stibbe C, et al. (1997) Aspergillus airway colonization and invasive disease after lung transplantation. Chest 112:1160–1164
47. Monforte V, Roman A, Gavalda J, Bravo C, Tenorio L, Ferrer A, et al. (2001) Nebulized amphotericin B prophylaxis for Aspergillus infection in lung transplantation: study of risk factors. J Heart Lung Transplant 20:1274–1281
48. Monforte V, Gavalda J, Roman A, Lopez R, Bravo C, Pou L, et al. (2004) Pharmacokinetics and efficacy of nebulized ambisome in lung transplantation. 44th Interscience Conference on Antimicrobial Agents and Chemotherapy, Washington, November 2004; Abstract M-1042, p 419
49. Singh N, Falestiny M, Rogers P, Reed MJ, Pularski J, Norris R, et al. (1998) Pulmonary infiltrates in the intensive care unit: predictors and outcome. Chest 114:1129–1136
50. Valera B, Bernardos A, Porras F, Fortun J, Lumbreras C, Len O, et al. (2005) Pneumonia after liver transplantation in the XXI century: a multicenter prospective study. 45th Interscience Conference on Antimicrobial Agents and Chemotherapy, Washington, December 2005; Abstract K-1560, p 355
51. Jimenez-Jambrina M, Hernandez A, Cordero E, Gurgui M, Alonso L, Blanes M, et al. (2005) Pneumonia after heart transplantation in the XXI century: a multicenter prospective study. 45th Interscience Conference on Antimicrobial Agents and Chemotherapy, Washington, December 2005; Abstract K-1561, p 355
52. Cisneros JM, Muñoz P, Torres-Cisneros J, Gurgui M, Rodriguez-Hernandez MJ, Aguado JM, et al. (1998) Pneumonia after heart transplantation: a multiinstitutional study. Clin Infect Dis 27:324–331
53. Valera B, Gentil MA, San-Juan R, Aznar J, Beneyto MI, Marcos MA, et al. (2005) Pneumonia after kidney transplantation in the XXI century: a multicenter prospective study. 45th Interscience Conference on Antimicrobial Agents and Chemotherapy, Washington, December 2005; Abstract k-1559, p 355
54. Paterson DL, Singh N, Gayowski T, Marino IR (1998) Pulmonary nodules in liver transplant recipients. Medicine 77:50–58
55. Singh N, Gayowski T, Wagener MM, Marino IR (1999) Pulmonary infiltrates in liver transplant recipients in the intensive care unit. Transplantation 67:1138–1144
56. Clark BD, Vezza PR, Copeland C, Wilder AM, Abati A (2002) Diagnostic sensitivity of bronchoalveolar lavage versus lung fine needle aspirate. Mod Pathol 15:1259–1265
57. Lapchik MS, Castelo Filho A, Pestana JO, Silva Filho AP, Wey SB (1992) Risk factors for nosocomial urinary tract and postoperative wound infections in renal transplant patients: a matched pair case control study. J Urology 147:994–998
58. Everett JE, Wahoff DC, Statz C, Gillingham KJ, Gruessner A, Gruessner RW, et al. (1994) Characterization and impact of wound infection after pancreas transplantation. Arch Surg 129:1310–1316
59. Asensio A, Ramos A, García-Navarro M, Gavalda J, Quijano Y, Lopez-Medrano F (2005) Effect of antibiotic prophylaxis on the risk of surgical site infection in orthotopic liver transplant. 45th Interscience Conference on Antimicrobial Agents and Chemotherapy, Washington, December 2005; Abstract K-1812, p 360
60. Gavaldà J, Len O, Rovira M, Borrell N, Cámara R, Cisneros J, et al. (2005) Epidemiology of invasive fungal infections in solid organ and hematopoietic stem cell transplant recipients: a prospective study from RESITRA. 45th Interscience Conference on Antimicrobial Agents and Chemotherapy, Washington, December 2005; Abstract M-990, p 428
61. Loinaz C, Lumbreras C, Moreno E, Colina F, Fuertes A, Go-

mez R, et al. (2001) Liver transplantation and hepatitis C virus. Results in a Spanish center since 1989. Hepatogastroenterology 48:1435–1442

62. Singh N, Gayowski T, Wagener MM, Marino IR (1996) Increased infections in liver transplant recipients with recurrent hepatitis C virus hepatitis. Transplantation 61:402–406
63. Corell A, Morales JM, Mandrono A, Munoz MA, Andres A, Fuertes A, et al. (1995) Immunosuppression induced by hepatitis C virus infection reduces acute renal transplant rejection. Lancet 346:1497–1498
64. Stevens DA (2002) Diagnosis of fungal infections: current status. J Antimicrob Chemother 49 Suppl 1:11–19
65. Heussel CP, Kauczor HU, Heussel G, Fischer B, Mildenberger P, Thelen M (1997) Early detection of pneumonia in febrile neutropenic patients: use of thin-section CT. AJR Am J Roentgenol 169:1347–1353
66. Gavalda J, Ruiz I; Grupo de Estudio de Micologia Medica (MICOMED); Grupo de Estudio de Infeccion en el Transplante (GESITRA); Sociedad Española de Enfermedades Infecciosas y Microbiologia Clinica (SEIMC) (2003) Guidelines for the treatment of infection due to *Aspergillus* spp. Enferm Infecc Microbiol Clin 21:571–578
67. Nosari A, Anghilieri M, Carrafiello G, Guffanti C, Marbello L, Montillo M, et al. (2003) Utility of percutaneous lung biopsy for diagnosing filamentous fungal infections in hematologic malignancies. Haematologica 88:1405–1409
68. Monforte V, Roman A, Gavalda J, López R, Pou L, Simo M, et al. (2003) Nebulized amphotericin B concentration and distribution in the respiratory tract of lung-transplanted patients. Transplantation 75:1571–1574
69. Chamilos G, Marom EM, Lewis RE, Lionakis MS, Kontoyiannis DP (2005) Predictors of pulmonary zygomycosis versus invasive pulmonary aspergillosis in patients with cancer. Clin Infect Dis 41:60–66
70. Munoz P, Rodriguez C, Bouza E, Palomo J, Yanez JF, Dominguez MJ, et al. (2004) Risk factors of invasive aspergillosis after heart transplantation: protective role of oral itraconazole prophylaxis. Am J Transplant 4:636–643
71. Ruiz I, Molina I, Gavalda J, Bueno J, Barrenetxea C, Zuazu J, et al. (2005) Safety and tolerability of nebulized liposomal amphotericin B in hematologic patients. 45th Interscience Conference on Antimicrobial Agents and Chemotherapy, Washington, December 2005; Abstract M-977, p 425
72. Bowden R, Chandrasekar P, White MH, Li X, Pietrelli L, Gurwith M, et al. (2002) A double-blind, randomized, controlled trial of amphotericin B colloidal dispersion versus amphotericin B for the treatment of invasive aspergillosis in immunocompromised patients. Clin Infect Dis 35: 359–366
73. Herbrecht R, Denning DW, Patterson TF, Bennett JE, Greene RE, Oestmann JW, et al. (2002) Voriconazole versus amphotericin B for primary therapy of invasive aspergillosis. N Engl J Med 347:408–415
74. Denning DW, Ribaud P, Milpied N, Caillot D, Herbrecht R, Thiel E, et al. (2002) Efficacy and safety of voriconazole in the treatment of acute invasive aspergillosis. Clin Infect Dis 34:563–571
75. Perea S, González G, Fothergill AW, Kirkpatrick WR, Rinaldi MG, Patterson TF (2002) In vitro interaction of caspofungin acetate with voriconazole against clinical isolates of *Aspergillus* spp. Antimicrob Agents Chemother 46:3039–3041
76. Arikan S, Lozano-Chiu M, Paetznick V, Rex J (2002) In vitro synergy of caspofungin and amphotericin B against *Aspergillus* and *Fusarium* spp. Antimicrob Agents Chemother 46:245–247
77. Jorgensen KJ, Johansen HK, Gotzsche PC (2006) Flaws in design, analysis and interpretation of Pfizer's antifungal trials of voriconazole and uncritical subsequent quotations. Trials 7:3
78. Caillot D, Mannone L, Cuisenier B, Couaillier JF (2001) Role of early diagnosis and aggressive surgery in the management of invasive pulmonary aspergillosis in neutropenic patients. Clin Microbiol Infect 7 (Suppl 2):54–61
79. Gavalda J, Martin MT, Lopez P, Gomis X, Ramirez JL, Rodriguez D, et al. (2005) Efficacy of nebulized liposomal amphotericin B in treatment of experimental pulmonary aspergillosis. Antimicrob Agents Chemother 49:3028–3030
80. Kanj SS, Welty-Wolf K, Madden J, Tapson V, Baz MA, Davis RD, et al. (1996) Fungal infections in lung and heart-lung transplant recipients, report of 9 cases and review of the literature. Medicine 75:142–156
81. Fortun J, Lopez-San Roman A, Velasco JJ, Sanchez-Sousa A, de Vicente E, Nuno J, et al. (1997) Susceptibility of *Candida glabrata* strains with reduced susceptibility of azoles in four liver transplant patients with invasive candidiasis. Eur J Clin Microbiol Infect Dis 16:314–318
82. Gavalda J, Ruiz I (2003) Guidelines for the treatment of invasive fungal infection. Invasive fungal infection by *Candida* spp. Invasive Fungal Infection Study Group (MICOMED) and Infection in Transplantation Study Group (GESITRA) of the Spanish Society for Infectious Diseases and Clinical Microbiology (SEIMC). Enferm Infecc Microbiol Clin 21:498–508
83. Pappas PG, Rex JH, Sobel JD, Filler SG, Dismukes WE, Walsh TJ, et al. Infectious Diseases Society of America (2004) Guidelines for treatment of candidiasis. Clin Infect Dis 38:161–189
84. Olsson M, Sukura A, Lindberg L, Linder E (1996) Detection of *Pneumocystis carinii* DNA by filtration of air. Scand J Infect Dis 28:279–282
85. Arend SM, Westendorp RG, Kroon FP, van't Wout JW, Vandenbroucke JP, van Es LA, et al. (1996) Rejection treatment and cytomegalovirus infection as risk factors for *Pneumocystis carinii* pneumonia in renal transplant recipients. Clin Infect Dis 22:920–925
86. Gordon SM, LaRosa SP, Kalmadi S, Arroliga AC, Avery RK, Truesdell-LaRosa L, et al. (1999) Should prophylaxis for *Pneumocystis carinii* pneumonia in solid organ transplant recipients ever be discontinued? Clin Infect Dis 28:240–246
87. Vilchez RA, Fung J, Kusne S (2002) Cryptococcosis in organ transplant recipients: an overview. Am J Transplant 2:575–580
88. Singh N, Lortholary O, Alexander BD, Gupta KL, John GT, Pursell KJ, et al. (2005) Antifungal management practices and evolution of infection in organ transplant recipients with *Cryptococcus neoformans* infection. Transplantation 80:1033–1039
89. Singh N, Gayowski T, Singh J, Yu VL (1995) Invasive gastrointestinal zygomycosis in a liver transplant recipient: case report and review of zygomycosis in solid-organ transplant recipients. Clin Infect Dis 20:617–620
90. van Burik JA, Hare RS, Solomon HF, Corrado ML, Kontoyiannis DP (2006) Posaconazole is effective as salvage therapy in zygomycosis: a retrospective summary of 91 cases. Clin Infect Dis 42:e61–65
91. Singh N, Chang FY, Gayowski T, Marino IR (1997) Infections due to dematiaceous fungi in organ transplant recipients: case report and review. Clin Infect Dis 24:369–374
92. Husain S, Alexander BD, Munoz P, Avery RK, Houston S, Pruett T, et al. (2003) Opportunistic mycelial fungal infections in organ transplant recipients: emerging importance of non-Aspergillus mycelial fungi. Clin Infect Dis 37:221–229

93. Singh N, Paterson DL, Chang FY, Gayowski T, Squier C, Wagener MM, et al. (2000) Methicillin-resistant *Staphylococcus aureus:* the other emerging resistant gram-positive coccus among liver transplant recipients. Clin Infect Dis 30:322–327
94. Shorr AF, Kunkel MJ, Kollef M (2005) Linezolid versus vancomycin for *Staphylococcus aureus* bacteraemia: pooled analysis of randomized studies. J Antimicrob Chemother 56:923–929
95. Bouza E, Cercenado E (2002) *Klebsiella* and *Enterobacter:* antibiotic resistance and treatment implications. Semin Respir Infect 17:215–230
96. Paterson DL (2002) Serious infections caused by enteric gram-negative bacilli: mechanisms of antibiotic resistance and implications for therapy of gram-negative sepsis in the transplanted patient. Semin Respir Infect 17:260–264
97. Paterson DL, Singh N, Rihs JD, Squier C, Rihs BL, Muder RR (2001) Control of an outbreak of infection due to extended-spectrum beta-lactamase-producing *Escherichia coli* in a liver transplantation unit. Clin Infect Dis 33:126–128
98. Rahal JJ, Urban C, Horn D, et al. (1998) Class restriction of cephalosporin use to control total cephalosporin resistance in nosocomial Klebsiella. JAMA 280:1233–1237
99. Newell KA, Millis JM, Arnow PM, Bruce DS, Woodle ES, Cronin DC, et al. (1998) Incidence and outcome of infection by vancomycin-resistant *Enterococcus* following orthototic liver transplantation. Transplantation 65:439–442
100. Papanicolaou GA, Myers BR, Meyers J, Mendelson MH, Lou W, Emre S, et al. (1996) Nosocomial infections with vancomycin-resistant *Enterococcus faecium* in liver transplant recipients: risk factors for acquisition and mortality. Clin Infect Dis 23:760–766
101. Lundstrom TS, Sobel JD (2004) Antibiotics for gram-positive bacterial infections: vancomycin, quinupristin-dalfopristin, linezolid, and daptomycin. Infect Dis Clin North Am 18:651–668
102. Chow JW, Yu VL (1998) Legionella: a major opportunistic pathogen in transplant recipients. Semin Respir Infect 13:132–139
103. Bangsborg JM, Uldum S, Jensen JS, Bruun BG (1995) Nosocomial legionellosis in three heart-lung transplant patients: case reports and environmental observations. Eur J Clin Microbiol Infect Dis 14:99–104
104. Patel R, Paya C (1997) Infections in solid-organ recipients. Clin Microbiol Rev 10:86–124
105. Ljungman P, Griffiths P, Paya C (2002) Definitions of cytomegalovirus infection and disease in transplant recipients. Clin Infect Dis 34:1094–1097
106. Razonable RR, Paya CV, Smith TF (2002) Role of the laboratory in diagnosis and management of cytomegalovirus infection in hematopoietic item cell and solid organ transplant recipients. J Clin Microbiol 40:746–752
107. Paya C, Razonable RR (2003) Cytomegalovirus infection after solid transplantation. In: Bowden RA, Ljungman P, Paya CV (eds) Transplant infections, 2nd edn. Lippincott Williams and Wilkins, Philadelphia, p 298
108. San Juan R, Lumbreras C, Aguado JM, Montejo M, Pumarola T, Rufi G, et al. (2005) Impact of new transplantation practices in the development of *cytomegalovirus* disease after renal transplantation: a prospective study of the Spanish Network of Infection in Transplantation (RESITRA). 45th Interscience Conference on Antimicrobial Agents and Chemotherapy, Washington, December 2005; Abstract V-1395, p 487
109. Emery VC, Hassan-Walker AF, Burroughs AK, Griffiths PD (2002) Cytomegalovirus replication dynamics in CMV-naïve and experienced immunocompromised hosts. J Infect Dis 185:1723–1728
110. Hambach L, Stadler M, Dammann E, Ganser A, Hertenstein B (2002) Increased risk of complicated CMV infection with the use of mycophenolate mofetil in allogeneic stem cell transplantation. Bone Marrow Transplant 29:903–906
111. Torre-Cisneros J, Fortun J, Aguado JM, de la Camara R, Cisneros JM, Gavalda J, et al. (2005) Consensus document from GESITRA-SEIMC on the prevention and treatment of cytomegalovirus infection in transplanted patients. Enferm Infecc Microbiol Clin 23:424–437
112. Paya C, Humar A, Domínguez E, Washburn K, Blumberg E, Alexander B, et al. (2004) Efficacy and safety of valganciclovir vs oral ganciclovir for prevention of cytomegalovirus disease in solid organ transplant recipients. Am J Transplant 4:611–620
113. Vrtovec B, Thomas CD, Radovancevic R, Frazier OH, Radovancevic B (2004) Comparison of intravenous ganciclovir and cytomegalovirus hyperimmune globulin preemptive treatment in cytomegalovirus-positive heart transplant recipients. J Heart Lung Transplant 23:461–465
114. Len O, Gavaldà J, Ruiz I, Aguado JM, Borrell N, Cervera C, et al. (2005) Efficacy of valganciclovir in the treatment of cytomegalovirus disease in solid organ transplantation. A prospective study from RESITRA. 45th Interscience Conference on Antimicrobial Agents and Chemotherapy, Washington, December 2005; Abstract V-600, p 473
115. Kusne S, Schwartz M, Breinig MK, Dummer JS, Lee RE, Selby R, et al. (1991) Herpes simplex virus hepatitis after solid organ transplantation in adults. J Infect Dis 163:1001–1007
116. Holt ND, Gould FK, Taylor CE, Harwood JF, Freeman R, Healy MD, et al. (1997) Incidence and significance of noncytomegalovirus viral respiratory infection after adult lung transplantation. J Heart Lung Transplant 16:416–419
117. Kusne S, Pappo O, Manez R, Pazin G, Carpenter B, Fung JJ, et al. (1995) Varicella zoster virus hepatitis and a suggested management plan for prevention of VZV infection in adult transplant recipients. Transplantation 60:619–621
118. Razonable RR, Brown RA, Humar A, Covington E, Alecock E, Paya CV; PV16000 Study Group (2005) Herpesvirus infections in solid organ transplant patients at high risk of primary cytomegalovirus disease. J Infect Dis 192:1331–1339
119. Munoz P, Alvarez P, de Ory F, Pozo F, Rivera M, Bouza E (2002) Incidence and clinical characteristics of Kaposi sarcoma after solid organ transplantation in Spain: importance of seroconversion against HHV-8. Medicine (Baltimore) 81:293–304
120. Preiksaitis JK (2004) New developments in the diagnosis and management of posttransplantation lymphoproliferative disorders in solid organ transplant recipients. Clin Infect Dis 39:1016–1023
121. Oertel SH, Verschuuren E, Reinke P, Zeidler K, Papp-Vary M, Babel N, et al. (2005) Effect of anti-CD 20 antibody rituximab in patients with post-transplant lymphoproliferative disorder (PTLD). Am J Transplant 5:2901–2906

Chapter 6

HIV in the Intensive Care Unit

P. Castro, J.M. Nicolás, J.M. Gatell

6.1 Introduction

Human immunodeficiency virus (HIV) infection (types 1 and 2) is an increasing problem worldwide. The latest data, estimated by the Joint United Nations Program on HIV/AIDS and the World Health Organization, have shown a rise in the number of cases, reaching the highest level ever not only in developing countries but also in the industrialized world. In 2005 the total number of adults living with HIV, newly infected and who died due to acquired immunodeficiency syndrome (AIDS) was 38.0 million (1.9 million, 4.2 million and 2.6 million in North America, western and central Europe, respectively) [1]. At some point in their lives, some of these people will need critical care. Before the use of highly active antiretroviral therapy (HAART) regimens, most intensive care unit (ICU) admissions were due to AIDS-related illnesses. However, changes in epidemiology have increased AIDS-unrelated diagnoses in the ICU, which is why the title of the chapter in the first edition of this book ("AIDS in the Intensive Care Unit") has been changed to "HIV in the Intensive Care Unit." In order to provide optimal care, it is essential that intensivists be familiar with the different problems that may appear in an HIV patient requiring ICU admission and they must know about the potential use of antiretroviral therapy, its secondary effects, and potential drug-drug interactions.

6.2 Epidemiology of HIV-Infected Patients in the ICU

6.2.1 Historical Evolution

Since the diagnosis of the first cases of HIV infection in 1981, there have been great changes in the epidemiology of these patients in the ICU. Changes in admission and mortality rates, as well as in the diagnoses and the characteristics of the patients, have been reported in different studies, particularly after the introduction of HAART [2].

At the beginning of the epidemic the highest rates of mortality [up to 69 %, mainly due to *Pneumocystis jiroveci* pneumonia (PCP)] and shorter long-term survival (7 months) were observed [3]. Consequently ICU care was often considered futile in AIDS patients and their admission to the ICU decreased. With the appearance of advances in HIV care such as the use of corticosteroids in PCP, and the decrease in mortality rates, the rates of ICU

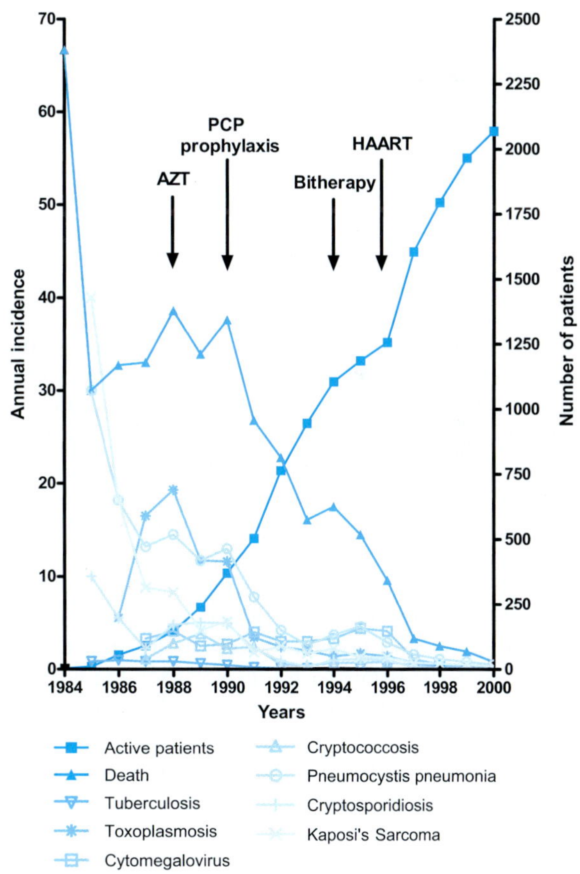

Fig. 6.1. Evolution of number of active patients (*right axis*), and annual incidence of death and opportunistic infections in the Hospital Clinic of Barcelona from 1984 to 2000 (*left axis*). Note the progressive increase in the number of active patients and the decrease in the annual incidences of death and opportunistic infections with the introduction of the different advances in HIV infection management

admission increased, together with a proportional rise in mortality [4, 5].

The main causes of ICU admission were, at that time, opportunistic infections (OI) in very immunocompromised patients. Respiratory failure (in up to 90% of the patients) typically because of PCP [6] was the most frequent complication with slight increases in the rate of non-pulmonary diagnoses in the mid-1990s such as sepsis, toxoplasma encephalitis, cardiomyopathy and acute renal failure [7–12].

The use of HAART (defined in general as the use of at least three antiretroviral drugs of at least two classes) since 1996 has led to a decline in the morbidity and mortality associated with HIV infection and a decrease in the incidence of OI, independently of the use of antimicrobial prophylaxis (Fig. 6.1) [13–16]. Accordingly, the percentage of AIDS-related admissions to hospital has decreased [16] and these changes have also influenced the trends of ICU admission.

6.2.2 Admission Rates

In the HAART era the rate of hospitalized HIV-infected patients admitted to the ICU varies from 4% to 12% [16–19], with controversial data regarding the variations in this rate. While some series have found a decrease [20], others have described an increase [16, 19, 21]. This increase may have different explanations. Firstly, a rise in the total number of HIV admissions to hospital due to the increase in the number of HIV cases has been reported (Fig. 6.1) [21]. Secondly, there is an increasing proportion of late diagnoses of HIV infection which often present as an AIDS-related life-threatening event [22]. There has also been an increase in AIDS-unrelated causes of admission among patients on HAART, due to the treatment itself or to the improvement in life expectancy of these patients. Moreover, treating physicians have greater confidence in the outcome of HIV-infected patients due to better therapeutic options [21]. Finally HAART "availability" neither means the "universality" nor precludes the "efficacy" of HAART. There are people who do not have access to treatment, and people under treatment who do not have the correct control of their infection. In some studies during the HAART era, 60% of admitted patients without HAART fulfilled criteria for receiving this treatment [21]. Variations in patient populations, differing ICU admission standards and variable clinical practices limit the conclusions of comparing results across different studies.

6.2.3 Characteristics of Patients

The epidemic characteristics of HIV-infected patients admitted to the ICU have also changed. Different studies have reported differences in the ethnic and risk factors of these patients after the introduction of HAART. In American ICUs there has been an increase in the number of intravenous drug users and African Americans infected by HIV [20, 21], while in European ICUs there has been an increase in foreigners from areas of higher rates of HIV infection [19]. These increases, however, reflect the changes in the epidemic in the community, since these populations show greater increases in new cases of HIV infection with a lower probability of receiving HAART [1, 17, 23]. Patients are also significantly more likely to be admitted from the emergency (45%) than from the hospitalization ward [19].

Finally, there is an increase in the proportion of "late testers," that is, patients newly diagnosed with HIV infection in the ICU, often in the context of an AIDS-related event [19, 22].

6.2.4 Diagnoses

The spectrum of reasons why an HIV-infected patient can be admitted to an ICU has widened since the introduction of HAART and the lengthening in survival and life expectancy. Diagnoses on admission nowadays may or may not be related to very different aspects of HIV infection (Table 6.1).

Table 6.1. Causes of ICU admission in HIV-infected patients

Related to HIV infection
Related to immunosuppression (AIDS related): opportunistic infections (PCP, tuberculosis, etc.), malignancies (Kaposi's sarcoma, non-Hodgkin lymphoma, etc.) (see Table 6.4)
Unknown HIV infection
Related to HIV treatment
Direct adverse events: lactic acidosis, hypersensitivity reactions, toxic hepatitis
Long-term effects (due to increase in cardiovascular risk factors): ischemic cardiopathy, stroke
Immune reconstitution inflammatory syndromes: tuberculosis, PCP, *Cryptosporidium* and *Microsporidium*, multifocal leukoencephalopathy
Drug-drug interactions
Related to HIV risk factors
Related to HBV and/or HCV liver disease: gastrointestinal bleeding, hepatic encephalopathy
Related to illicit drug abuse: intoxication, endocarditis, soft tissue infections
Unrelated to HIV infection
Traumatism, post-transplantation[a]

ICU intensive care unit, *HIV* human immunodeficiency virus, *AIDS* acquired immunodeficiency syndrome, *PCP Pneumocystis jiroveci* pneumonia, *HBV* hepatitis B virus, *HCV* hepatitis C virus

[a] HIV patients are now included in transplantation lists due to the improvement in their life prognosis

Respiratory failure is still the most important cause of ICU admission, although the percentage of pulmonary diagnoses has declined to 30–40%, particularly due to a decrease in the incidence of PCP down to 3–20%, depending on the series [17–21, 24] (Table 6.2). As this is an important cause of mortality even today (mortality rates of 55% of PCP in the ICU have been reported in recent studies [25]), its decrease is thought to be one of the most notable causes of mortality decline.

On the other hand, severe bacterial infections leading to sepsis are increasing in frequency [11, 16, 24, 26], being the most common site of infection in the lungs [18, 24].

The biggest differences are found in the significant increase of AIDS-unrelated events due to the introduction of HAART [2, 21, 24], although some studies disagree with this observation [19]. It is now common to diagnose acute severe secondary effects of HAART such as lactic acidosis or hypersensitivity reactions; long-term adverse events that have also been related to HAART such as acute myocardial infarction or stroke; comorbidities related to HIV risk-factors such as cirrhosis complications (hepatic encephalopathy, gastrointestinal bleeding), and overdoses in drug addicts, among others.

Finally, with the improvement in their prognosis, we also see HIV-infected patients being admitted because of HIV-unrelated pathologies, similar to HIV-uninfected patients, with traumatisms, community-acquired infections, and complications during the postoperative and even post-transplantation courses [27].

Table 6.2 shows the causes of admission referred to in articles in which they have been analyzed after the introduction of HAART.

6.2.5 Mortality Rates

Evidence of improved ICU survival of HIV patients in the HAART era has been reported, with the published rates of mortality ranging between 20% and 40%. The

Table 6.2. Reasons for ICU admission of HIV-infected patients in the HAART era

	Study [reference]					
	Khouli [17]	Casalino [24]	Narasmihan [21]	Vincent [19]	Afessa [18]	Morris [20]
Interval	1997–1999	1996–1999	2001	1998–2000	1995–1999	1996–1999
Number of patients	242	230	63	236	169	354
Use of HAART (%)	45	28	52	50.4	ne	25.1
CD4 count (median cells/mm³)	85	150.6[a]	–	–	45	64
<200 cells/mm³ (%)			56	70.7		
Mortality (%)						
In-ICU	30	20		25		
In-hospital	39		29		29.6	29
Diagnosis category (%)						
AIDS-related	60	37	33	49.5		37.7
Respiratory failure	30	31.7	22		38.5	40.7
PCP	14	10	3	19	14	10.7
Bacterial pneumonia				20		8.7
Asthma			3		4	
Sepsis	13	22.6	16		15	11.9
Neurologic disease	18	23.9	10		16.6	12.4
Toxoplasma encephalitis		11		14		
Hematologic	4					
AIDS-related tumors				9.7		
Kaposi's sarcoma			2			
AIDS-unrelated						
GI/liver/pancreas disease	14		11		8.9	7.3
Cardiovascular disease	11	2.6	3		8.1	9.9
Drug overdose	5		11		6.5	1.1
Renal disease	5		13		3.5	
Metabolic disease			5		1.7	1.7
Diabetes mellitus				0.8		
ARV side effects				3		
Lactic acidosis				0.8		
Cytopenia				0.4		
Renal failure				1.2		
Toxicodermia				0.4		
Postoperation					1.7	4.2
Trauma					1.1	3.7

ICU intensive care unit, *HIV* human immunodeficiency virus, *HAART* highly active antiretroviral therapy, *AIDS* acquired immunodeficiency syndrome, *PCP Pneumocystis jiroveci* pneumonia, *GI* gastrointestinal, *ARV* antiretroviral

[a]Should be mean instead of median

most important reason for a general decrease in mortality with respect to the pre-HAART era compared to historical series seems to be an increase in non-AIDS-related diagnoses, which are associated with a better survival. However, some recent studies did not find any differences between mortality rates in the era just prior to and after HAART. The differences may be attributable to variations in ICU utilization for HIV-infected patients, hospital characteristics, geographic location and data interpretation.

6.2.6 Prognostic Factors

Different studies have identified several factors associated with poor outcome in HIV-infected patients in the ICU. These factors do not seem to have changed over the years and are the same as those in the pre-HAART era, probably due to the fact that AIDS-related admissions use to have worse prognosis and imply a real or virtual absence of HAART.

Although numerous factors have been related to higher mortality rates (age, prehospitalization functional status, number of previous OI, HIV disease stage, time since AIDS diagnosis, weight loss, etc.), the most consistent mortality predictors on multivariate analysis in recent studies have been the need for mechanical ventilation [17, 20, 24], PCP, especially if requiring mechanical ventilation and, above all, if complicated with pneumothorax (mortality near 100%) [20], low serum albumin [7, 10, 17, 18, 26, 28, 29], HIV-related illness [17, 20], APACHE II score > 17 [26], and a high SAPS II score [19, 24]. Other factors such as a poor preadmission functional status are more debatable [30]. Although it has been found that a higher CD4 cell count could be associated with a better prognosis in some studies [19], others have not demonstrated this relationship or have only found a shorter long-term survival when this count is low [10, 18, 20, 21].

The use of HAART as a prognostic factor is also controversial. Some studies have found survival to be significantly improved in HAART patients but the association is lost on multivariate analysis. One possible explanation is that HAART may act by influencing other variables that have a strong relationship have survival in the model (for example HAART patients have a significantly higher serum albumin level and CD4 cell count) [20]. However, it is of note that one study found that the mortality on admission with PCP under HAART was lower than without HAART (25 vs. 63%), independently of its effect on CD4 cell count, HIV RNA level, overall health status, and PCP disease severity [25]. In this case, explanations for a possible survival benefit with HAART may include decreased HIV viral fitness, an attenuated rise in viral titers during PCP, anti-*Pneumocystis* properties of protease inhibitors (PIs), or that patients on HAART differed from those without HAART. In the latter case, people not receiving HAART reportedly do not usually have prophylaxis for OI [17].

However, several recent studies did not find HAART influenced mortality (either in-ICU or in-hospital), the need for mechanical ventilation or the length of stay [17, 21]. Different study designs (retrospective and prospective, comparison of historical cohorts, etc.) may explain, in part, this controversy but the main reason seems to be the type of patient included. On one hand, the proportion of patients under HAART in each study is low and variable, always under the proportion in the general infected population (25–50%) [17–21, 24]. On the other hand, the retrospective nature of most of the studies makes it impossible to determine whether HAART was effective in a specific patient or if HAART was really being performed before admission. In fact, when viral load or CD4 cell count are analyzed in these studies, no significant differences are found between patients with or without HAART [17, 24]. One study showed that of admitted patients under HAART, 35% had failed to respond [19]. As suggested by Masur, "correct" comparisons should be made between patients who had achieved a sustained response to HAART and those who had not [31]. Usually, when an AIDS-related event is the cause of ICU admission, the patient probably is not receiving HAART (due to unknown HIV-infection, lack of access to health care or voluntarily) or does not respond to the regimen (due to resistance, lack of compliance or intolerance). In the latter case, the evolution of the patient can be expected to be similar to that of a subject without HAART.

In any case, the availability of HAART has been clearly associated with an improvement in long-term survival after ICU discharge. Three-month survival has improved up to 94% from 85% among ICU survivors [19, 20, 24]. This is probably because all survivors, up to 95% in some series, begin or restart HAART rapidly during the first weeks following ICU discharge [19, 24]. Other factors associated with long-term survival are AIDS at ICU admission [24].

Therefore, the short-term survival of HIV-infected patients admitted to the ICU is primarily dependent on acute illness severity, independently of previous use of HAART if AIDS-related, while long-term survival is closely dependent on HIV disease-related variables, including the availability of HAART.

6.3 HIV-Related Causes of ICU Admission

6.3.1 Admission Related to HIV Immunosuppression

Known as AIDS-related admissions (Tables 6.1, 6.3, 6.4) [32], they were the most important cause of admission to the ICU of HIV-infected patients until the HAART era. Moreover, although they have decreased as a cause of ICU admission, they continue to be present: among others new diagnoses, lack of access to health care, and treatment failures due to drug-resistant virus are all causes of acquisition of OI in the HAART era. The acute therapy recommended is shown in Table 6.5 [33].

Special attention should be given to the possibility of OI developing resistance to current therapies, such as sulphonamide-resistant PCP [34, 35] or ganciclovir-resistant cytomegalovirus [36].

6.3.2 Unknown HIV Infection

A particular situation is when an HIV-infected patient who does not know that he or she is infected is admitted to the ICU. Since HIV infection is asymptomatic early in its course when there is relatively normal immune function, patients with unsuspected HIV infection may develop both HIV-unrelated illness which may require ICU admission and, later, events related to HIV infection. The ICU clinician should suspect an unknown underlying HIV infection when an OI appears in a patient with no apparent cause of immunosuppression, although risk factors for HIV may not be evident. In fact, it has been described that in the HAART era there is a growing proportion of patients diagnosed on the appearance of an AIDS-related event [22].

A more uncommon, although possible, situation is an acute HIV infection as a cause of ICU admission. An estimated 40–90% of patients with acute HIV infection experience symptoms of acute retroviral syndrome [37]. Some of these, if severe, may need ICU care: meningoencephalitis, Guillain-Barré syndrome, etc. [38]. Clinicians should consider the etiologic diagnosis of patients who experience a compatible clinical syndrome and who report recent high risk behavior.

Table 6.3. Classification system for HIV-infected adolescents (≥13 years) and adults

CD4+ T-lymphocyte categories		Clinical categories A	B	C (AIDS)
1	≥500/mm³ (≥29%)	A1	B1	C1
2	200–499/mm³ (14–28%)	A2	B2	C2
3	<199/mm³ (<14%) (AIDS)	A3	B3	C3

HIV human immunodeficiency virus, *AIDS* acquired immunodeficiency syndrome

Table 6.4. Clinical categories of HIV infection in adolescents and adults

Category A: one or more of the conditions listed below:
- Asymptomatic HIV infection
- Persistent generalized lymphadenopathy
- Acute (primary) HIV infection with accompanying illness or history of acute HIV infection

Category B: one or more of the conditions listed below:
- Bacillary angiomatosis
- Oropharyngeal candidiasis (thrush)
- Vulvovaginal candidiasis when it is persistent, frequent or poorly responsive to therapy
- Cervical dysplasia (moderate or severe)/cervical carcinoma in situ
- Constitutional symptoms, such as fever (38.5 °C) or diarrhea lasting longer than 1 month
- Oral hairy leukoplakia
- Herpes zoster (shingles), involving at least two distinct episodes or more than one dermatome
- Idiopathic thrombocytopenic purpura
- Listeriosis
- Pelvic inflammatory disease, particularly if complicated by tubo-ovarian abscess
- Peripheral neuropathy
- Other symptomatic conditions attributed to HIV infection or indicative of a defect in cell-mediated immunity that are not included in clinical category C

Category C: one or more of the conditions listed below:
- Candidiasis of bronchi, trachea, or lungs
- Candidiasis, esophageal
- Cervical cancer, invasive
- Coccidioidomycosis, disseminated or extrapulmonary
- Cryptococcosis, extrapulmonary
- Cryptosporidiosis, chronic intestinal (longer than 1 month's duration)
- Cytomegalovirus disease (other than liver, spleen, or nodes)
- Cytomegalovirus retinitis (with loss of vision)
- Encephalopathy, HIV-related
- Herpes simplex: chronic ulcer(s) (greater than 1 months' duration); or bronchitis, pneumonitis, or esophagitis
- Histoplasmosis, disseminated or extrapulmonary
- Isosporiasis, chronic intestinal (greater than 1 month's duration)
- Kaposi's sarcoma
- Lymphoma, Burkitt's (or equivalent term)
- Lymphoma, immunoblastic (or equivalent term)
- Lymphoma, primary, of brain
- *Mycobacterium avium* complex or *M. kansasii*, disseminated or extrapulmonary
- *Mycobacterium* tuberculosis, any site (pulmonary or extrapulmonary)
- *Mycobacterium*, other species or unidentified species, disseminated or extrapulmonary
- *Pneumocystis jiroveci* pneumonia
- Pneumonia, recurrent
- Progressive multifocal leukoencephalopathy
- Salmonella septicemia, recurrent
- Toxoplasmosis of brain
- Wasting syndrome due to HIV

HIV human immunodeficiency virus

Table 6.5. Acute therapy of severe AIDS-related opportunistic infections that may need ICU admission[a,b]

Infection	Treatment of choice	Alternative therapy[c]	Notes
Pneumocystis jiroveci pneumonia	Trimethoprim-sulfamethoxazole (TMP/SMX): 15–20 mg/kg/day TMP and 75–100 mg/kg/day SMX i.v. q6 h or q8 h for 3 weeks	Pentamidine 3–4 mg/kg i.v. qd for 3 weeks	If $PaO_2 < 70$ mmHg at room air, addition of corticosteroids (prednisolone 40 mg/12 h, e.g., 5 days, 40 mg/24 h days 6–10 and 20 mg/24 h days 11–21) is recommended
Toxoplasma gondii encephalitis	Pyrimethamine 200 mg po ×1, then 50 mg (<60 kg) to 75 mg (≥60 kg) po qd and sulfadiazine 1,000 mg (<60 kg) to 1,500 mg (≥60 kg) po q6 h for at least 6 weeks	Pyrimethamine 200 mg po ×1, then 50 mg (<60 kg) to 75 mg (≥60 kg) po qd and clindamycin 600 mg i.v. or po q6 h for at least 6 weeks	Folinic acid should be used with pyrimethamine to minimize hematologic toxicity (10–20 mg po qd)
Cryptosporidiosis	HAART		
Microsporidiosis	HAART *Enterocytozoon bieneusi*: fumagillin 60 mg po qd Others: albendazole 400 mg po bid	Itraconazole 400 mg po qd (for *Trachipleistophora* or *Brachiola*)	
Mycobacterium tuberculosis	Isoniazid (INH) 5 mg/kg (max: 300 mg) po qd and rifampin 10 mg/kg (max: 600 mg) po qd or rifabutin 300 mg po qd and pyrazinamide (PZA) 30 mg/kg po qd and ethambutol (EMB) 15–25 mg/kg po qd for 8 weeks		When liver disease is present, if moderate avoid PZA, if severe avoid INH and PZA Evaluate presence of drug-resistant agents
Mycobacterium avium complex	Clarithromycin 500 mg po bid and ethambutol 15 mg/kg po qd and rifabutin 200 mg po qd	Azithromycin 600 mg po qd and ethambutol 15 mg/kg po qd and rifabutin 200 mg po qd	
Bacterial pneumonia[d]	Extended-spectrum cephalosporin and a macrolide or quinolone		Adjustment by antibiogram should be done
Salmonellosis	Ciprofloxacin 400 mg i.v. bid at least 4–6 weeks[e]	Third generation cephalosporin (ceftriaxone or cefotaxime) i.v.	
Campylobacter jejuni	Ciprofloxacin 400 mg i.v. bid at least 2 weeks	Azithromycin 500 mg po qd at least 2 weeks	Consider addition of an aminoglycoside in bacteremic patients
Shigellosis	Fluoroquinolone i.v. or po for 2 weeks	Azithromycin 500 mg po on day 1, then 250 mg po qd for 2 weeks	TMP-SMX is an alternative in the United States
Bartonella (*henselae* and *quintana*)	CNS infections: doxycycline 100 mg i.v. or po q12 h Non-CNS infections: erythromycin 500 mg i.v. or po qd or doxycycline 100 mg i.v. or po q12 h	Azithromycin 600 mg po qd or Clarithromycin 500 mg po bid	
Candidiasis (mucosal)			
Oropharyngeal	Fluconazole 100 mg po qd or itraconazole oral solution 200 mg po qd for 1–2 weeks	Clotrimazole 10 mg po 5 times/day or nystatin suspension 4–6 ml qid or 1–2 flavored tablets 4–5 times daily for 1–2 weeks	When fluconazole refractory, amphotericin B may be used
Esophageal	Fluconazole 100 mg (up to 400 mg) po or i.v. qd or itraconazole oral solution 200 mg po qd for 2–3 weeks	Voriconazole 200 mg po or i.v. bid for 2–3 weeks	When fluconazole refractory, amphotericin B or caspofungin may be used
Cryptococcus neoformans	Amphotericin B (deoxycholate 0.7 mg/kg or liposomal 4 mg/kg) i.v. qd and/or flucytosine 25 mg/kg po qd for 2 weeks	Fluconazole 400–800 mg/day (po or i.v.) and flucytosine 25 mg/kg po qd for 4–6 weeks	Consolidation therapy is necessary with fluconazole 400 mg po qd for 8 weeks or until CSF cultures are sterile Repeated lumbar puncture may be indicated as adjunctive therapy when intracranial pressure is > 20 cmH_2O

Table 6.5. (*Cont.*)

Infection	Treatment of choice	Alternative therapy[c]	Notes
Histoplasma capsulatum	Amphotericin B (deoxycholate 0.7 mg/kg or liposomal 4 mg/kg) i.v. qd for 3–10 days or until clinically improved in disseminated forms and for 12–16 weeks in meningitis	Itraconazole 400 mg i.v. qd for disseminated forms	Chronic maintenance therapy with itraconazole 200 mg po qd is necessary
Coccidiodomycosis			
Meningeal	Fluconazole 400–800 mg i.v. or po qd	Intrathecal amphotericin B	
Non-meningeal	Amphotericin B deoxycholate 0.5–1 mg/kg i.v. qd until clinical improvement ± fluconazole 400–800 mg i.v.		A total dose of 500–1,000 mg is usually necessary
Invasive aspergillosis	Voriconazole 400 mg i.v. or po q12 h for 2 days, then 200 mg q12 h	Amphotericin B (deoxycholate 1 mg/kg/day or lipid formulation 5 mg/kg/day) i.v.	Duration of treatment based on clinical response
Cytomegalovirus (esophagitis, colitis, pneumonitis or neurological disease)	Ganciclovir i.v. or foscarnet i.v. for 3–4 weeks or until signs and symptoms have resolved	Valganciclovir po may be used when there is good oral absorption in esophagitis or colitis	Preemptive treatment of patients with cytomegalovirus viremia without evidence of organ involvement is not recommended
Herpes simplex			
Severe mucocutaneous infection	Acyclovir 5 mg/kg i.v. q8 h. After lesions began to regress, change to po treatment with famciclovir, valacyclovir or acyclovir	Foscarnet 120–200 mg/kg i.v. in 2–3 divided doses until clinical response	
Encephalitis	Acyclovir 10 mg/kg i.v. q8 h for 2–3 weeks		
Varicella zoster virus			
Primary infection (chickenpox)	Acyclovir 10 mg/kg i.v. q8 h for 7–10 days. After lesions begin to regress, change to treatment po with famciclovir, valacyclovir or acyclovir		
Extensive cutaneous lesion or visceral involvement	Acyclovir 10 mg/kg i.v. q8 h until cutaneous and visceral disease is clearly resolved		
Penicilliosis	Amphotericin B 0.6 mg/kg i.v. for 2 weeks followed by itraconazole po 400 mg/day for 10 weeks		
Leishmaniasis	Pentavalent antimony 20 mg/kg i.v. or i.m. qd for 3–4 weeks	Amphotericin B (deoxycholate 0.5–1.0 mg/kg i.v. qd for total dose of 1.5–2 g or lipid formulation 2–5 mg/kg i.v. qd for 10 days)	Severely neutropenic patients may need granulocyte macrophage colony stimulating factor
Paracoccidioidomycosis	Amphotericin B	Itraconazole 100–200 mg po qd	
Isospora belli	TMP/SMX (160/800) po or i.v. qd for 10 days	Pyrimethamine 50–75 mg po qd	Folinic acid should be used with pyrimethamine to minimize hematologic toxicity (10–20 mg po qd)

AIDS acquired immunodeficiency syndrome, *ICU* intensive care unit, *i.v.* intravenous, *q "n" h* every "*n*" hour, *qd* daily, *po* oral, *HAART* highly active antiretroviral therapy, *bid* twice a day, *CNS* central nervous system, *CSF* cerebrospinal fluid, *i.m.* intramuscular

[a] Only opportunistic infections that are usually the cause of ICU admission and their severe forms are shown. Treatment of mild-to-moderate cases is not discussed here

[b] Some opportunistic infections require chronic maintenance therapy or secondary prophylaxis after the acute phase until immunosuppression is resolved

[c] The second option of treatment is depicted. More alternatives may be possible

[d] Empiric therapy

[e] If CD4 T cell count $<200/mm^3$ and/or bacteremia

6.3.3 Admissions Related to HIV Treatment

6.3.3.1 Direct Adverse Events

HIV-infected patients sometimes receive a large amount of medicines, many associated with substantial adverse effects. In addition to the classical syndromes such as the Steven-Johnsons syndrome associated with sulphonamides, the increased use of antiretroviral agents has introduced new risks and potential critical illness, some of which may be relevant to the ICU clinician. Table 6.6 depicts some of the most common serious and potentially life-threatening adverse events related to the different antiretroviral therapy.

Although the clinical spectrum is wide, adverse events usually present with cutaneous and systemic symptoms and biochemical abnormalities such as an elevation in transaminases and, in some cases, they may be confused with other clinical problems that should be ruled out. Adverse events are usually associated with some risk factors and management usually includes support therapy and discontinuation of

Table 6.6. Potentially life-threatening events related to antiretroviral therapy that may require ICU admission

Adverse Event	Related drug	Symptoms	Frequency	Risk Factors	Management	Notes
Acute toxic hepatitis	NVP	Abrupt onset of flu-like symptoms (nausea, vomiting, myalgia, fatigue), abdominal pain, jaundice, fever Skin rash (50%) May progress to fulminant hepatic failure	1–5%	Higher CD4 T cell count at initiation. Female gender Elevated ALT or AST at baseline Previous liver disease (HBV, HCV, alcoholic). HIV negative (postexposure prophylaxis)	Support therapy Discontinue ART Discontinue all other hepatotoxic agents	Greatest risk within first weeks of therapy (since 18 weeks) Other causes of hepatitis should be ruled out Hepatic injury may progress despite treatment discontinuation Do not rechallenge patient with offending agent
Lactic acidosis	NRTIs (d4T, ddI, ZDV)	Insidious onset months after treatment with non-specific gastrointestinal prodrome (nausea, anorexia, abdominal pain), weight loss and fatigue. Multiorgan failure (respiratory, hepatic, ...) progressively appears Increased lactate (>5 mmol), metabolic acidosis with increased anion gap, elevated serum transaminases	1–25 cases/ 1000 patients/year Mortality up to 50–70%, especially if serum lactate >10 mmol	Combination of ddI + d4T, HU or ribavirin. Long duration of NRTI use Female gender Obesity Pregnancy Impaired creatinine clearance Nadir CD4 cell count < 250 cells/mm^3	Support therapy Fluid hydration Discontinue ART Thiamine, riboflavin and l-carnitine have been assayed	It may be accompanied by hepatic steatosis, pancreatitis or myopathy (mitochondrial toxicities) Asymptomatic hyperlactatemia Technique for obtaining lactate must be correct Do not rechallenge patient with offending agent
Pancreatitis	ddI (± d4T, HU, RBV or TDF)	Weeks to months after initiating treatment, post-prandial abdominal pain, nausea, vomiting and increased serum amylase and lipase	ddI 1–7% ddI+HU, RBV, d4T or TDF increase frequency	History of pancreatitis Alcoholism Hypertriglyceridemia Concomitant use of ddI with d4T, HU, RBV or TDF	Support therapy Discontinue ART	May appear in the context of lactic acidosis
Acute neuropathy	d4T	Rapidly progressive ascending demyelinating polyneuropathy (Guillain-Barré like) with motor weakness months after initiation of ART Respiratory paralysis may develop Creatine phosphokinase can be markedly increased	Rare	Prolonged d4T use Pregnancy?	Support therapy Discontinue ART Plasmapheresis, corticosteroid, immunoglobulin, carnitine, acetycarnitine have been assayed	May appear in the context of lactic acidosis Recovery can take months and some symptoms may be irreversible Do not rechallenge patient with offending agent

Table 6.6. *(Cont.)*

Adverse Event	Related drug	Symptoms	Frequency	Risk Factors	Management	Notes
Stevens-Johnson Syndrome	NNRTI. Also APV, f-APV, ABC, ZDV, ddI, IDV, LPV/r, ATV	First few days to weeks after initiation of therapy skin eruption appears also involving the mucosa, which may evolve to blisters and necrosis Usually presents with fever, tachycardia, malaise, myalgia and arthralgia	NVP: 0.3–1%. EFV and DLV: 0.1%. Excepcional for other drugs	NVP Female gender Ethnical predisposition (Black, Asian, Hispanic) Use of corticosteroids	Support therapy Discontinue ART Discontinue other possible agents Local wound care Empiric broad-spectrum antimicrobial therapy if superinfection is suspected Corticosteroid and intravenous immunoglobulin have been assayed	Do not rechallenge patient with offending agent
Hypersensitivity reaction	ABC	Acute onset of high fever, diffuse skin rash, malaise, nausea, headache, myalgia, chills, diarrhea, vomiting, abdominal pain, dyspnea, arthralgia and respiratory symptoms If continues hypotension, respiratory distress due to acute interstitial pneumonitis and vascular collapse may appear Rechallenge reactions are generally worse and mimic anaphylaxis	2–9%	HLA-B*5701 HLA-DR7 HLA-DQ3 Being naïve	Support therapy Discontinue ART	First reaction usually initiates by 10th day of treatment (90% within 6 weeks) Rechallenge reactions begin within hours Other causes must be ruled out (viral infections...) Usually resolves in 48 hours. Do not rechallenge patient with offending agent

ART antiretroviral therapy, *ICU* intensive care unit, *NVP* nevirapine, *ALT* alanine transferase, *AST* aspartate transferase, *HBV* hepatitis B virus, *HCV* hepatitis C virus, *NRTI* nucleoside/nucleotide reverse transcriptase inhibitors, *NNRTI* non-nucleoside reverse transcriptase inhibitor, *PI* protease inhibitor, *APV* amprenavir, *f-APV* fosamprenavir, *ABC* abacavir, *ZDV* zidovudine, *ddI* didanosine, *IDV* indinavir, *LPV/r* lopinavir/ritonavir, *ATV* atazanavir, *3TC* lamivudine, *FCT* emtricitabine, *d4T* stavudine, *TDF* tenofovir, *HU* hydroxyurea, *RBV* ribavirin

HAART. Afterwards, it is recommended not to rechallenge the patient with the offending agent [39–48].

Table 6.7 presents other adverse events associated with HAART that, although not so severe, intensivists should be aware of.

6.3.3.2 Long-Term Effects

Patients receiving HAART, especially PIs, are subject to metabolic complications, including lipid abnormalities (hypertriglyceridemia, hypercholesterolemia) and glucose abnormalities (glucose intolerance, insulin resistance and type 2 diabetes mellitus). The combination of increasing age, due to a decrease in mortality, the cardiovascular risk apparently associated with HIV infection itself and these metabolic disturbances may influence the development of atherosclerosis syndromes such as coronary and cerebrovascular disease, some of which may require ICU admission [49–54]. Nonetheless, HAART was introduced for HIV-infected patients a relatively short time ago and the results of studies still remain controversial.

6.3.3.3 Immune Reconstitution Inflammatory Syndrome

In a small proportion of HIV-infected patients a paradoxical clinical deterioration may develop shortly after the initiation of HAART, usually associated with fever, due to restoration of the capacity to raise an inflammatory immune response against both infectious and non-infectious antigens. This phenomenon is known as the immune reconstitution inflammatory syndrome (IRIS). Four criteria have been postulated to establish the diagnosis: (1) diagnosis of AIDS; (2) treatment with HAART leads to an increase in CD4 T count and a decrease in HIV-1 viral load (although sometimes IRIS appears before the changes can be demonstrated); (3) appearance of symptoms consistent with an infectious/inflammatory condition while on HAART; and (4) the symptoms cannot be explained by a newly acquired infection, by the expected clinical course of previously recognized infectious agents or by therapeutic side effects. IRIS has been described for a wide variety of pathogens and situations: *Mycobacterium avium complex*, *M. tuberculosis*, *Bartonella henselae*, *Cryptococcus neoformans* (meningitis and lymphadenitis), *Pneumo-*

Table 6.7. Adverse events of antiretroviral drugs and need for dose adjustment in case of renal or hepatic insufficiency

Class/agent	Toxicity	Adjustment in RI	Adjustment in HI
NRTI	Lactic acidosis with hepatic steatosis		
Abacavir (ABC)	Hypersensitivity reaction	No	No
Didanosine (ddI)	Pancreatitis, peripheral neuropathy, nausea, diarrhea	Yes	No
Emtricitabine (FTC)	Minimal toxicity	Yes	No
Lamivudine (3TC)	Minimal toxicity	Yes	No
Stavudine (d4T)	Peripheral neuropathy, lipodystrophy, rapidly progressive ascending neuromuscular weakness, pancreatitis, hyperlipidemia	Yes	No
Tenofovir (TDF)	Asthenia, headache, diarrhea, nausea, vomiting, flatulence, renal insufficiency and acute tubular necrosis	Yes	No
Zalcitabine (ddC)	Peripheral neuropathy, stomatitis, pancreatitis	Yes	No
Zidovudine (AZT)	Myelosuppression (macrocytic anemia or neutropenia), GI intolerance, headache, insomnia, asthenia	Yes	No
Trizivir (AZT+3TC+ABC)	Same as its components separately	Yes	No
Truvada (TDF+FTC)	Same as its components separately	Yes	No
NNRTI	Rash, increased transaminase levels		
Delavirdine (DLV)	Headache	No	Use with caution
Efavirenz (EFV)	Central nervous system symptoms (dizziness, somnolence, insomnia, abnormal dreams, hallucinations, amnesia, agitation, confusion)	No	Use with caution
Nevirapine (NVP)	Stevens-Johnson syndrome, acute toxic hepatitis	No	Avoid use if severe HI
PI	Hyperlipidemia, hyperglycemia, fat maldistribution and possible increased bleeding episodes in patients with hemophilia		
Amprenavir (APV)	GI intolerance, rash, transaminase elevation, oral paresthesias	No	Yes
Atazanavir (ATV)	Indirect hyperbilirubinemia, prolonged PR interval	No	Yes
Fosamprenavir (f-APV)	Skin rash, GI intolerance, headache, transaminase elevation	No	Yes
Indinavir	Nephrolithiasis, GI intolerance, indirect hyperbilirubinemia, dizziness, rash, thrombocytopenia, hemolytic anemia	No	Yes
Lopinavir+ritonavir (LPV/r)	GI intolerance, asthenia, elevated serum transaminases	No	Use with caution
Nelfinavir (NFV)	GI intolerance (diarrhea), elevated serum transaminases	No	Use with caution
Ritonavir (RTV)	GI intolerance, paresthesias (circumoral and extremities), elevated serum transaminases	No	Use with caution
Saquinavir (SQV)	GI intolerance, headache, elevated serum transaminases	No	Use with caution
Tipranavir (TPV)	Hepatotoxicity, rash	No	Use with caution
Fusion inhibitors			
Enfuvirtide (T20)	Local injection site reactions (injectable), hypersensitivity reaction	No	No

RI renal insufficiency, *HI* hepatic impairment, *NRTI* nucleoside reverse transcriptase inhibitors, *NNRTI* non-nucleoside reverse transcriptase inhibitors, *PI* protease inhibitors, *GI* gastrointestinal

cystis jirovecii, toxoplasmosis, cytomegalovirus, herpesvirus, varicella-zoster virus, hepatitis C and B virus, progressive multifocal leukoencephalopathy (JC virus), and Kaposi sarcoma, among others. Most of these agents have been proven to be present before starting HAART, but in some cases IRIS appears against microbes that have not been previously clinically recognized. This syndrome usually appears from 10 to 180 days after the initiation of HAART, but some cases have been reported to occur several months later [55, 56].

IRIS is important in the ICU for two reasons: in some cases the inflammatory response is so high as to be life-threatening and requires ICU admission. This is the case, especially, of respiratory failure related to paradoxical worsening of PCP, or intracranial hypertension after *C. neoformans* meningitis [57]. On the other hand, distinguishing IRIS from OI treatment failure, a superimposed infection or drug toxicity is challenging to the intensivist.

Anti-inflammatory agents, usually corticosteroids or non-steroidal drugs in the case of a mild reaction, have been the suggested treatment for IRIS [55]. However, the most important thing is the recognition of this syndrome, allowing continuation of HAART and treatment of OI, thereby avoiding unnecessary changes or addition of treatments if superinfections or therapeutic failure have been ruled out.

Table 6.8. Common interactions between antiretroviral drugs and intensive care unit medications

Agent	Antiretroviral[a]	Interaction
Antiarrhythmics		
Amiodarone	IDV, RTV, TPV	Increased cardiac effects
Flecainide, propafenone, quinidine	LPV/r, RTV, TPV	Increased cardiac effects
Diltiazem	ATV, f-APV	Increased cardiac effects
Anticonvulsants: carbamazepine, phenobarbital, phenytoin	PIs, NNRTI	Potential increase in anticonvulsant effect, potential decrease in ARV effect
Antifungal: voriconazole, ketoconazole	NNRTI, PIs	Potential increase in ARV effect, potential decrease in antifungal effect
Anti-mycobacterial		
Rifampin	PIs, NNRTI	Decreased ARV levels
Clarithromycin	NNRTI, PIs	Increased clarithromycin levels
Ergotamine	PIs	Increased ergotamine effect
Gastrointestinal drugs		
Cisapride	PIs, EFV, DLV	Increased cisapride levels
Proton pump inhibitors	ATV, DLV	Decreased ARV levels
H_2-receptor antagonists	ATV, f-APV	Decreased ARV levels
Methadone	NNRTI, APV, f-APV, RTV, LPV/r, NFV, SQV, ddI	Opiate withdrawal
Metronidazole	APV, LPV/r, RTV	Disulfiram-like reaction
Psychotropic: midazolam/triazolam	PIs, DLV, EFV	Increased sedative effects
Sildenafil	PIs, DLV	Increased sildenafil effect
Warfarin	DLV, EFV	Increased anticoagulant effect

PIs protease inhibitors, *NNRTI* non-nucleoside reverse transcriptase inhibitors, *IDV* indinavir, *RTV* ritonavir, *TPV* tipranavir, *LPV/r* lopinavir/ritonavir, *ATV* atazanavir, *f-APV* fosamprenavir, *EFV* efavirenz, *DLV* delavirdine, *NFV* nelfinavir, *SQV* saquinavir, *ddI* didanosine

[a] These are the most common antiretrovirals that interact with each drug. However, other antiretrovirals and other drugs present multiple interactions. Information about drug-drug interactions is available on the following websites, among others: www.hiv-druginteractions.org, *www.depts.washington.edu/hivaids/drug*, *www.actis.org*, www.medscape.com/druginfo/druginterchecker/, www.interaccioneshiv.com (website in Spanish)

6.3.3.4 Interactions

Any patient receiving HAART may develop drug interactions (Table 6.8). Although it is unusual for one of these to lead a patient to ICU admission, these interactions should be taken into account to avoid iatrogenic damage [2, 58–60].

6.4 HIV-Unrelated Causes of ICU Admission

With life expectancy increasing among HIV-infected individuals, other usual pathologies requiring ICU support may lead to hospitalization. Causes of ICU admission unrelated to HIV infection are similar to those among non-HIV-infected individuals of similar age and demographics, and their management, response to treatment and prognosis are similar to those in individuals without HIV infection who have the same illness.

6.5 HAART in the ICU

Since the introduction of HAART has demonstrated such benefits, the question has now been raised as to what role antiretroviral therapy should have in the ICU. Intensivists may find three possible scenarios: patients without HAART presenting an OI and, therefore, criteria to initiate this therapy; patients on HAART who must discontinue this therapy; and finally patients on HAART who may continue treatment. Nowadays much of what is done is based on physicians' experience rather than data from controlled studies [61]. Consultation with a specialist in the management of HIV patients and a pharmacist is of great help.

6.5.1 Initiating HAART in the ICU

When a naïve HIV patient (a patient who has never received antiretroviral therapy) presents an OI, etiologic treatment should be started (Table 6.5). Some authors also advise the initiation of HAART at this time since the improvement in immune function would potentially contribute to a faster resolution of OI and thus reduce the risk for a second OI. This benefit has been best demonstrated in OI for which limited or no effective therapies are available: cryptosporidiosis, microsporidiosis, progressive multifocal leukoencephalopathy and Kaposi sarcoma. In these cases, the early benefits of potent HAART outweigh the risks, and should therefore be started as soon as possible [33, 62–64].

However, initiation of HAART concurrent with the diagnosis of an OI has some potential problems, which may be magnified in the ICU setting. Firstly, the number of antiretrovirals available in an intravenous or liquid presentation is limited, restricting potential receivers. Moreover, experience with administration by nasogastric tube or in patients with erratic gastrointestinal absorption is scarce, and patients may be exposed to subtherapeutic drug levels, leading to potential selection of resistance mutations. Using more drugs may add potential toxicity (Table 6.7), make it difficult to distinguish the etiology of an adverse event when it appears, and expose the patient to a large number of drug interactions between OI therapies and antiretroviral therapy (Table 6.8). Furthermore, in the acute situation it may be difficult to predict patient compliance thereafter. Finally, there is the risk of the appearance of IRIS.

In any case, no randomized controlled trials have demonstrated that initiating HAART will improve the outcome of patients treated with specific therapy for acute OI, and whether initiating HAART in critically ill patients with HIV infection improves mortality. Nonetheless, neither has it been demonstrated that the initiation of antiretroviral therapy in the setting of an acute OI worsens the prognosis or treatment of that OI. Therefore, the question about whether to initiate HAART in the ICU remains unanswered.

6.5.2 Discontinuing HAART in the ICU

When a patient on HAART is admitted to the ICU, interruption of treatment may become necessary when the situation precludes oral therapy or when the cause of admission is related to HIV therapy. Changing HAART for alternative regimes is more difficult than initiating HAART in a naïve patient, because of overlapping toxicities, previous drug resistance, or difficulty in administering the most suitable drug [61]. When HAART is discontinued, all components should be discontinued simultaneously, since mono- or bitherapy may favor the development of resistance. If possible, exceptions should be made with some antiretrovirals. On one hand, non-nucleoside reverse transcriptase inhibitors (NNRTI) (efavirenz or nevirapine) have a long half-life with detectable plasma levels up to 21 days or more after discontinuation. If they are discontinued simultaneously with the other drugs of a regimen, "functional monotherapy" is performed thereby, increasing the risk of selection of resistance mutations [65]. That is why some experts recommend stopping the NNRTI first before the other antiretroviral drugs, although the optimal interval is not known [39]. On the other hand, patients with hepatitis B coinfection who are receiving emtricitabine, lamivudine or tenofovir, which have antihepatitis B activity, may develop an exacerbation of hepatitis when these drugs are stopped [66].

6.5.3 Maintaining HAART in the ICU

Sometimes an HIV patient under HAART can be admitted to the ICU for a reason that permits treatment continuation. In that case, maintaining treatment may have some problems: difficulty in administering the drug, poor drug absorption leading to development of resistance, and, especially, multiple drug interactions between antiretroviral drugs and other normally used drugs in the ICU (Table 6.8). Moreover, treatment will have to be adjusted to renal and hepatic function if necessary when they are altered, especially NRTI in renal impairment (Table 6.7). However, there are also benefits: the risk of mutations is reduced when treatment is incorrectly discontinued and a decrease in the CD4 T cell count is avoided with a rise in viral load, which could be deleterious and induce even an acute retroviral syndrome [67, 68]. Thus, in practical terms, HAART should be continued whenever possible [61].

6.6 Conclusion

HAART has led to a substantial reduction in the mortality and morbidity due to HIV infection. The main consequence of this change is a wider variety of reasons leading to ICU admission, with an increase of AIDS-unrelated admissions. However, intensivists will need to continue treating AIDS-related events in patients "without" HAART (never initiated or with therapeutic failure) but must also be familiar with the influence of HAART in HIV management, being able to recognize side effects, potential drug-drug interactions and how to start or to stop this therapy if necessary. Therefore HIV-infected patients will be an even greater challenge to clinicians in the ICU.

References

1. UNAIDS/WHO (2005) AIDS epidemic update: December 2005. http://www.unaids.org
2. Morris A, Masur H, Huang L (2006) Current issues in critical care of the human immunodeficiency virus-infected patient. Crit Care Med 34:42–49
3. Wachter RM, Luce JM, Turner J, et al. (1986) Intensive care of patients with the acquired immunodeficiency syndrome.

Outcome and changing patterns of utilization. Am Rev Respir Dis 134:891–896

4. Wachter RM, Luce JM, Safrin S, et al. (1995) Cost and outcome of intensive care for patients with AIDS, *Pneumocystis carinii* pneumonia, and severe respiratory failure. JAMA 273:230–235
5. Gallant JE, Chaisson RE, Moore RD (1998) The effect of adjunctive corticosteroids for the treatment of *Pneumocystis carinii* pneumonia on mortality and subsequent complications. Chest 114:1258–1263
6. Rogers PL, Lane HC, Henderson DK, et al. (1989) Admission of AIDS patients to a medical intensive care unit: causes and outcome. Crit Care Med 17:113–117
7. De Palo VA, Millstein BH, Mayo PH, et al. (1995) Outcome of intensive care in patients with HIV infection. Chest 107: 506–510
8. Lazard T, Retel O, Guidet B, et al. (1996) AIDS in a medical intensive care unit: immediate prognosis and long-term survival. JAMA 276:1240–1245
9. Rosen MJ, Clayton K, Schneider RF, et al. (1997) Intensive care of patients with HIV infection: utilization, critical illnesses, and outcomes. Pulmonary Complications of HIV Infection Study Group. Am J Respir Crit Care Med 155: 67–71
10. Nickas G, Wachter RM (2000) Outcomes of intensive care for patients with human immunodeficiency virus infection. Arch Intern Med 160:541–547
11. Rosenberg AL, Seneff MG, Atiyeh L, et al. (2001) The importance of bacterial sepsis in intensive care unit patients with acquired immunodeficiency syndrome: implications for future care in the age of increasing antiretroviral resistance. Crit Care Med 29:548–556
12. Leifeld L, Rockstroh J, Skaide S, et al. (2000) Indication, outcome and follow up of intensive care in patients with HIV-infection. Eur J Med Res 5:199–202
13. Paul S, Gilbert HM, Ziecheck W, et al. (1999) The impact of potent antiretroviral therapy on the characteristics of hospitalized patients with HIV infection. AIDS 13:415–418
14. Palella FJ, Jr, Delaney KM, Moorman AC, et al. (1998) Declining morbidity and mortality among patients with advanced human immunodeficiency virus infection. HIV Outpatient Study Investigators. N Engl J Med 338:853–860
15. Kaplan JE, Hanson D, Dworkin MS, et al. (2000) Epidemiology of human immunodeficiency virus-associated opportunistic infections in the United States in the era of highly active antiretroviral therapy. Clin Infect Dis 30 Suppl 1:S5–14
16. Nuesch R, Geigy N, Schaedler E, Battegay M (2002) Effect of highly active antiretroviral therapy on hospitalization characteristics of HIV-infected patients. Eur J Clin Microbiol Infect Dis 21:684–687
17. Khouli H, Afrasiabi A, Shibli M, et al. (2005) Outcome of critically ill human immunodeficiency virus-infected patients in the era of highly active antiretroviral therapy. J Intensive Care Med 20:279–285
18. Afessa B, Green B (2000) Clinical course, prognostic factors, and outcome prediction for HIV patients in the ICU. The PIP (pulmonary complications, ICU support, and prognostic factors in hospitalized patients with HIV) study. Chest 118:138–145
19. Vincent B, Timsit JF, Auburtin M, et al. (2004) Characteristics and outcomes of HIV-infected patients in the ICU: impact of the highly active antiretroviral treatment era. Intensive Care Med 30:859–866
20. Morris A, Creasman J, Turner J, et al. (2002) Intensive care of human immunodeficiency virus-infected patients during the era of highly active antiretroviral therapy. Am J Respir Crit Care Med 166:262–267
21. Narasimhan M, Posner AJ, DePalo VA, et al. (2004) Intensive care in patients with HIV infection in the era of highly active antiretroviral therapy. Chest 125:1800–1804
22. Castilla J, Sobrino P, De La FL, et al. (2002) Late diagnosis of HIV infection in the era of highly active antiretroviral therapy: consequences for AIDS incidence. AIDS 16:1945–1951
23. Hamers FF, Downs AM (2004) The changing face of the HIV epidemic in western Europe: what are the implications for public health policies? Lancet 364:83–94
24. Casalino E, Wolff M, Ravaud P, et al. (2004) Impact of HAART advent on admission patterns and survival in HIV-infected patients admitted to an intensive care unit. AIDS 18:1429–1433
25. Morris A, Wachter RM, Luce J, et al. (2003) Improved survival with highly active antiretroviral therapy in HIV-infected patients with severe *Pneumocystis carinii* pneumonia. AIDS 17:73–80
26. Alves C, Nicolas JM, Miro JM, et al. (2001) Reappraisal of the aetiology and prognostic factors of severe acute respiratory failure in HIV patients. Eur Respir J 17:87–93
27. Miro JM, Laguno M, Moreno A, et al. The Hospital Clinic OLT in HIV Working Group (2006) Management of end stage liver disease (ESLD): What is the current role of orthotopic liver transplantation (OLT)? J Hepatol 44 Suppl 1:S140–S145
28. Wachter RM, Russi MB, Bloch DA, et al. (1991) *Pneumocystis carinii* pneumonia and respiratory failure in AIDS. Improved outcomes and increased use of intensive care units. Am Rev Respir Dis 143:251–256
29. Bedos JP, Dumoulin JL, Gachot B, et al. (1999) *Pneumocystis carinii* pneumonia requiring intensive care management: survival and prognostic study in 110 patients with human immunodeficiency virus. Crit Care Med 27:1109–1115
30. Casalino E, Mendoza-Sassi G, Wolff M, et al. (1998) Predictors of short- and long-term survival in HIV-infected patients admitted to the ICU. Chest 113:421–429
31. Masur H (2002) Acquired immunodeficiency syndrome in the intensive care unit: will human immunodeficiency virus-related admissions continue to decline? Am J Respir Crit Care Med 166:258–259
32. Anonymous (1992) 1993 revised classification system for HIV infection and expanded surveillance case definition for AIDS among adolescents and adults. MMWR Recomm Rep 41:1–19
33. Benson CA, Kaplan JE, Masur H, et al. (2004) Treating opportunistic infections among HIV-exposed and infected children: recommendations from CDC, the National Institutes of Health, and the Infectious Diseases Society of America. MMWR Recomm Rep 53:1–112
34. Helweg-Larsen J, Benfield TL, Eugen-Olsen J, et al. (1999) Effects of mutations in *Pneumocystis carinii* dihydropteroate synthase gene on outcome of AIDS-associated *P. carinii* pneumonia. Lancet 354:1347–1351
35. Kovacs JA, Gill VJ, Meshnick S, et al. (2001) New insights into transmission, diagnosis, and drug treatment of *Pneumocystis carinii* pneumonia. JAMA 286:2450–2460
36. Baldanti F, Paolucci S, Parisi A, et al. (2002) Emergence of multiple drug-resistant human cytomegalovirus variants in 2 patients with human immunodeficiency virus infection unresponsive to highly active antiretroviral therapy. Clin Infect Dis 34:1146–1149
37. Kinloch-de Loes S, de Saussure P, Saurat JH, et al. (1993) Symptomatic primary infection due to human immunodeficiency virus type 1: review of 31 cases. Clin Infect Dis 17:59–65
38. Huang ST, Lee HC, Liu KH, et al. (2005) Acute human im-

munodeficiency virus infection. J Microbiol Immunol Infect 38:65 – 68
39. Bartlett JG, Lane HC, Panel on Clinical Practices for Treatment of HIV Infection convened by the DHHS (2005) Guidelines for the use of antiretroviral agents in HIV-1-infected adults and adolescents. http://AIDSinfo.nih.gov
40. Falco V, Rodriguez D, Ribera E, et al. (2002) Severe nucleoside-associated lactic acidosis in human immunodeficiency virus-infected patients: report of 12 cases and review of the literature. Clin Infect Dis 34:838 – 846
41. Martinez E, Blanco JL, Arnaiz JA, et al. (2001) Hepatotoxicity in HIV-1-infected patients receiving nevirapine-containing antiretroviral therapy. AIDS 15:1261 – 1268
42. Lonergan JT, Behling C, Pfander H, et al. (2000) Hyperlactatemia and hepatic abnormalities in 10 human immunodeficiency virus-infected patients receiving nucleoside analogue combination regimens. Clin Infect Dis 31:162 – 166
43. Miller KD, Cameron M, Wood LV, et al. (2000) Lactic acidosis and hepatic steatosis associated with use of stavudine: report of four cases. Ann Intern Med 133:192 – 196
44. Hewitt RG (2002) Abacavir hypersensitivity reaction. Clin Infect Dis 34:1137 – 1142
45. Fagot JP, Mockenhaupt M, Bouwes-Bavinck JN, et al. (2001) Nevirapine and the risk of Stevens-Johnson syndrome or toxic epidermal necrolysis. AIDS 15:1843 – 1848
46. Carr A, Cooper DA (2000) Adverse effects of antiretroviral therapy. Lancet 356:1423 – 1430
47. Bonnet F, Bonarek M, Morlat P, et al. (2003) Risk factors for lactic acidosis in HIV-infected patients treated with nucleoside reverse-transcriptase inhibitors: a case-control study. Clin Infect Dis 36:1324 – 1328
48. Claessens YE, Chiche JD, Mira JP, et al. (2003) Bench-to-bedside review: severe lactic acidosis in HIV patients treated with nucleoside analogue reverse transcriptase inhibitors. Crit Care 7:226 – 232
49. Bozzette SA, Ake CF, Tam HK, et al. (2003) Cardiovascular and cerebrovascular events in patients treated for human immunodeficiency virus infection. N Engl J Med 348: 702 – 710
50. Friis-Moller N, Sabin CA, Weber R, et al. (2003) Combination antiretroviral therapy and the risk of myocardial infarction. N Engl J Med 349:1993 – 2003
51. Holmberg SD, Moorman AC, Williamson JM, et al. (2002) Protease inhibitors and cardiovascular outcomes in patients with HIV-1. Lancet 360:1747 – 1748
52. Martinez E, Domingo P, Galindo MJ, et al. (2004) Risk of metabolic abnormalities in patients infected with HIV receiving antiretroviral therapy that contains lopinavir-ritonavir. Clin Infect Dis 38:1017 – 1023
53. Martinez E, Casamitjana R, Conget I, et al. (1998) Protease inhibitor-associated hyperinsulinaemia. AIDS 12:2077 – 2079
54. Martinez E, Gatell J (1998) Metabolic abnormalities and use of HIV-1 protease inhibitors. Lancet 352:821 – 822
55. Shelburne SA, III, Hamill RJ, Rodriguez-Barradas MC, et al. (2002) Immune reconstitution inflammatory syndrome: emergence of a unique syndrome during highly active antiretroviral therapy. Medicine (Baltimore) 81:213 – 227
56. Cheng VC, Yuen KY, Chan WM, et al. (2000) Immunorestitution disease involving the innate and adaptive response. Clin Infect Dis 30:882 – 892
57. Wislez M, Bergot E, Antoine M, et al. (2001) Acute respiratory failure following HAART introduction in patients treated for *Pneumocystis carinii* pneumonia. Am J Respir Crit Care Med 164:847 – 851
58. Piscitelli SC, Gallicano KD (2001) Interactions among drugs for HIV and opportunistic infections. N Engl J Med 344:984 – 996
59. Kotb R, Vincent I, Dulioust A, et al. (2006) Life-threatening interaction between antiretroviral therapy and vinblastine in HIV-associated multicentric Castleman's disease. Eur J Haematol
60. Fantoni M, Autore C, Del Borgo C (2001) Drugs and cardiotoxicity in HIV and AIDS. Ann N Y Acad Sci 946:179 – 199
61. Soni N, Pozniak A (2001) Continuing HIV therapy in the ICU. Crit Care 5:247 – 248
62. Foudraine NA, Weverling GJ, van Gool T, et al. (1998) Improvement of chronic diarrhoea in patients with advanced HIV-1 infection during potent antiretroviral therapy. AIDS 12:35 – 41
63. Murdaca G, Campelli A, Setti M, et al. (2002) Complete remission of AIDS/Kaposi's sarcoma after treatment with a combination of two nucleoside reverse transcriptase inhibitors and one non-nucleoside reverse transcriptase inhibitor. AIDS 16:304 – 305
64. Tantisiriwat W, Tebas P, Clifford DB, et al. (1999) Progressive multifocal leukoencephalopathy in patients with AIDS receiving highly active antiretroviral therapy. Clin Infect Dis 28:1152 – 1154
65. Mackie NE, Fidler S, Tamm N, et al. (2004) Clinical implications of stopping nevirapine-based antiretroviral therapy: relative pharmacokinetics and avoidance of drug resistance. HIV Med 5:180 – 184
66. Sellier P, Clevenbergh P, Mazeron MC, et al. (2004) Fatal interruption of a 3TC-containing regimen in a HIV-infected patient due to re-activation of chronic hepatitis B virus infection. Scand J Infect Dis 36:533 – 535
67. Kilby JM, Goepfert PA, Miller AP, et al. (2000) Recurrence of the acute HIV syndrome after interruption of antiretroviral therapy in a patient with chronic HIV infection: A case report. Ann Intern Med 133:435 – 438
68. Zavascki AP (2005) Severe acute hepatitis due to retroviral rebound syndrome after discontinuation of highly active antiretroviral therapy. J Infect (in press)

Chapter 7

Fungal Infections

7

R.A. Barnes, J. Sinha

7.1 Introduction

Fungal infections are a significant problem and represent a major cause of morbidity and mortality in a variety of patients. Improvements in supportive care and widespread use of antimicrobial agents have resulted in an expanding population of at-risk patients. This trend not only concerns severely compromised hosts such as transplant recipients, neutropenic and HIV-positive patients, but also non-compromised patients on surgical and medical intensive care units, burns and neonatal units with specific risk factors for infection.

Many studies have identified an increase in the incidence of fungal infection over the last decade with a major impact on outcomes in critically ill patients. The National Nosocomial Infections Surveillance (NNIS) programme has provided nationwide information from the USA for the past two decades [1]. Data from 1980–1990 show that nosocomial infections increased from 2.0 to 3.8 infections per 1,000 patients discharged during that period and that critical care patients were at highest risk. The studies also demonstrate differences between community-acquired endemic fungi such as *Histoplasma capsulatum* and *Blastomyces dermatidis* which are restricted to specific geographical locations and nosocomial infections with *Candida* and *Aspergillus* spp. that prevail in large health-care facilities and largely account for the increasing problem [2]. Population-based surveillance has identified a cumulative incidence of invasive mycotic infection of 178.3 per million per year, with *Candida* accounting for 72.8 per million per year of this [3]. Whilst human immunodeficiency virus infection was an important contributing factor in this population (being an underlying factor in 47%) other studies have confirmed the extent of the problem [4].

Surveillance of fungal infection in Europe is less comprehensive but nosocomial infection in the ICU appears similar to NNIS data [5, 6]. The EPIC study comprised a single day point prevalence study of over 1,400 intensive care units (ICUs) in western Europe. Fungal isolates were reported from 17% of patients of whom half were receiving antifungal treatment [7]. Yeasts were reported as the major causative organism [8]. Many of these may have represented colonisation rather than infection, highlighting problems in diagnosis, but there is no doubt that fungi have emerged as significant nosocomial pathogens in critically ill patients. Population-based surveillance reported substantial increases in invasive candidosis over this period, from 6.8 to 13.7 per million population in England and Wales [9].

7.2 *Candida* Infections

Yeasts account for 11% of all bloodstream infections in the ICU [1] and 8–15% of nosocomial septicaemias in the USA [10]. Rates from Europe suggest that candidaemia rose from 4.7 cases per 1,000 patient days to 7.4 cases between 1987 and 1990 [11]. An incidence of 1 candidaemia per 500 admissions has been documented in medical and surgical ICUs [12] and *Candida* accounted for 8% of blood culture isolates from a tertiary neonatal ICU [13]. Intensive care treatment is an independent risk factor for fungaemia even when other risk factors are taken into account. Candidaemia has a substantial impact on mortality and although some improvements in survival have been achieved attributable mortality remains high [5, 14]. This is higher than other nosocomial bloodstream infections. In one large study, candidaemia was the only bloodstream pathogen that independently influenced outcome of nosocomial infection in ICU patients [15].

Much has been made of the marked "pathogen shift" with a significant decrease in the proportion of *C. albicans* infections (falling from around 90% to 30–50% of all yeast blood culture isolates) over the last 5–10 years coinciding with the emergence of non-*albicans* species such as *C. tropicalis, C. parapsilosis, C. glabrata* and *C. krusei* [16]. The widespread use of azoles has been implicated [17–19]. Interestingly, this pathogen shift has not been noted within ICUs [5] and appears to be confined to haematology and transplant patients in whom azole prophylaxis use is high. Ongoing surveillance is required to monitor trends. There is a generally accepted hierarchy of pathogenicity of *Candida* species with *C. albicans* at the top of the league and *C. glabrata* bringing up the rear. Nonetheless, even less virulent forms of candidosis can have significant implications for morbidity in critically ill patients and may be more refractory to treatment.

7.2.1 Risk Factors for Candidosis

Candida are ubiquitous yeasts that colonise our skin and mucosal surfaces. *C. albicans* is part of the endogenous flora of the oropharynx and gastrointestinal tract of normal healthy individuals and may colonise skin surfaces in small numbers. Other *Candida* spp. may colonise hospitalised patients and the hands of healthcare workers allowing horizontal spread and the potential for hospital-acquired infection.

Many studies have identified risk factors for invasive disease but since these factors are common to most critical care patients they lack discrimination and are of limited usefulness in identifying high-risk patients. Use of central venous catheters, colonisation, broad-spectrum antibiotics and haemodialysis are independent risk factors for disseminated infection [20] but are common to many hospitalised patients. Better understanding of risk factors for individual groups and knowledge of which risk factors are predictors of mortality [21] will enable more rational use of preventative measures. Obviously degree and duration of neutropenia is a significant factor in classically immunocompromised patients [22] whilst operative time, retransplantation, reoperation and cytomegalovirus infection are relevant to liver and solid organ transplant recipients [23]. In neonates, low birth weight is the major factor whilst on medical and surgical ICUs length of stay, severity of illness, peritonitis and pancreatitis [24, 25] may be more useful predictors of invasive *Candida* infection than other commonly cited risk factors.

In all risk groups, *Candida* colonisation is an independent risk factor for infection and precedes invasive disease in most cases. However, more than 50% of ICU patients will become colonised during hospitalisation and distinguishing infection from colonisation may be difficult. Risk of infection increases with the number of sites colonised and is dependent on the colonising species. One study demonstrated that 15% of patients colonised with *C. albicans* at one site developed fungaemia rising to 17% when two or more sites were colonised, and patients colonised with *C. tropicalis* at one site had a 58% risk of subsequent fungaemia rising to 100% when two or more sites were colonised with this species [26]. Further studies in surgical ICU patients have confirmed this trend [27] and advocate the use of a candidal colonisation index to assess the degree of colonisation. A ratio of ≥ 0.5 (representing the number of distinct sites colonised with the same strain over the number of sites tested) has been shown to have a positive predictive value of 66% for determining infection, and sensitivity can be further increased if quantitative culture is applied [28].

Many risk factors involve altered host defences that allow fungal overgrowth, whilst others provide a portal of entry through translocation across mucosal surfaces or direct invasion via intravenous lines or wounds.

Raised gastric pH due to sedation, antacids, H_2 antagonists and exocrine abnormalities may lead to *Candida* overgrowth in the bowel. Widespread use of broad-spectrum antibiotic agents compounds this. Severity of illness, splanchnic ischaemia, impaired gut mobility or ileus will contribute to translocation of yeasts through the bowel mucosa. Total parenteral nutrition is a risk factor over and above the presence of the central line and intravenous lipids promote fungal growth.

7.2.2 Immune Response to *Candida*

Candida contain immunodominant mannoproteins on their cell walls capable of binding to CD14 and stimulating a proinflammatory T-helper (Th1) cytokine response such that acute fungaemia may present as profound sepsis. Conversely, exposure to fungal mannoproteins may result in a downregulatory response associated with anti-inflammatory (Th2) cytokines and persistent fungal infection. This chronic form is more likely to be associated with other causes of monocyte deactivation following immunosuppression, trauma/surgery, immaturity, head-injury or sepsis ("second-hit phenomena"). The application of this Th1/Th2 paradigm to human infection is far from clear [29, 30] but patterns of T cell cytokine production may predict which patients are at risk of infection following immunocompromise or trauma. Critically ill patients frequently display signs of immuneparesis [31]. Mechanisms of this are poorly understood but probably involve dysregulated monocyte function and a switch from Th1 proinflammatory pathways to the Th2 anti-inflammatory pathways that may facilitate fungal infection and persistence in these patient groups. The theory that virulent fungi may modulate and thereby evade host immunity through the inability of the host to mount a proinflammatory T cell cytokine response is substantiated by animal models [32, 33] and anecdotal evidence in humans [34]. Lymphocytes from neonates show a marked reduction in their capacity to inhibit growth of *C. albicans* [35].

Humoral responses are important in determining recovery from fungal infection and a variety of antibodies to *Candida* have been identified [36, 37] but appear to be of little value in identifying at-risk patients in the ICU. Antibody responses to immunodominant highly conserved heat-shock proteins [38] or cell wall protein determinants [39] may be more relevant in protecting the host from infection.

7.2.3 Clinical Presentation

Candidal infection in critically ill patients presents non-specifically. Fever, moderate leucocytosis and fever that fail to respond to broad spectrum antimicrobial agents may be the only clinical signs and some of these may be absent in immunocompromised individuals or those undergoing haemfiltration. Fever is present in up to 80% of individuals and leucocytosis occurs in only 50% [40]. Acute phase proteins responses are elevated. A rising C-reactive protein (CRP) level in the absence of any other identified cause should alert the clinician to the possibility of yeast infection [41, 42].

Candidaemia is defined as the isolation of any *Candida* species from at least one blood culture specimen [20] and is commonly line-associated. The concept of benign candidaemia (i.e. fungaemia that requires line-removal only and forgoes the need for systemic antifungal treatment) is flawed [43]. It is well recognised that even transient candidaemia requires both line removal and a course of antifungal treatment if metastatic complications and excessive mortality are to be avoided. This applies regardless of the species involved as "non-pathogenic" species of *Candida* cannot be identified accurately in critically ill hosts.

Acute dissemination can occur to multiple organs with the formation of microabscesses. Skin and muscle may be involved with the development of a characteristic erythematous papular rash [44]. Dissemination to other non-contiguous organs may be more difficult to identify [45]. Retinal lesions and ophthalmitis are relatively rare occurring in only 9–15% of ICU patients [46, 47], and routine examination for ophthalmitis has little clinical benefit [48]. Skin lesions and septic arthritis are similarly infrequently reported. The reticuloendothelial system is the commonest site for dissemination but microabscesses within the liver and spleen are often only be detected at autopsy. Intra-abdominal candidosis occurs following leakage of commensal gut yeasts into the peritoneal cavity following gastrointestinal perforation or abdominal surgery. Frequently this is a transient phenomenon that is rapidly cleared provided effective surgical repair is achieved. A continued abdominal focus due to recurrent perforation or anastomotic breakdown may lead to invasive disease and disseminate into the bloodstream [49].

Renal candidosis may be difficult to distinguish from colonisation of the urinary tract in catheterised patients. Candiduria is a frequent finding in catheterised patients and is consistent with colonisation. Funguria in patients with urological pathology or which persists despite changes of urinary catheters is strongly predictive of infection [50, 51]. Similarly funguria in neonates requires further investigation and should prompt suprapubic urine aspiration and surveillance cultures for other sites of colonisation. Persistent isolation requires investigation by renal ultrasound for detection of echogenic renal fungal balls or abscesses [52].

Other organ involvement is also difficult to identify clinically. Candidal pneumonia is a rare condition associated with a high mortality rate. The condition may arise following haematogenous dissemination and presents as miliary lesions throughout the lung fields, or may occur as a primary condition following aspiration of oropharyngeal contents, presenting as a patchy, haemorrhagic bronchopneumonia [53]. Isolation from bronchoscopic specimens has poor predictive value due to the high rates of colonisation in mechanically ventilated patients and should not be used as the sole criterion to initiate treatment [54]. Diagnosis depends on histological demonstration of fungus within the tissues [55].

7.2.4 Diagnosis

The non-specific clinical features of invasive candidal infections mean that demonstration of fungi in clinical specimens must be combined with good clinical acumen. Serology has a relatively small role to play but molecular techniques are under increasing scrutiny.

Historically, blood cultures are insensitive markers of candidaemia [56] but recent changes in automated culture systems utilising large volume, lytic methods have greatly improved detection rates and largely obviated the need for specialised systems such as semi-quantitative lysis centrifugation cultures [57].

A wide variety of antigens are known to circulate in candidosis but most attention has focused on the detection of circulating cell wall mannan [58], although evaluation in critically ill patients is limited. Beta-(1,3)-D-glucan, a characteristic fungal cell wall constituent, can be rapidly detected in invasive fungal infection using a modification of the chromogenic limulus lysate test [59, 60]. False positive and negative results occur for all these immunoassays such that a single result cannot be interpreted in isolation. Careful evaluation of all these tests is required in parallel to assess the diagnostic clinical utility in different patient groups [61].

Molecular techniques have opened the way for rapid and sensitive diagnosis of a variety of opportunist pathogens but progress with the detection of fungal DNA by the polymerase chain reaction (PCR) has been hampered by problems with extracting fungal DNA from human samples and with contamination of specimens [62]. A variety of *Candida* genes have been identified as targets for amplification [63–65] and a "universal" fungal primer to amplify highly conserved multicopy ribosomal DNA can be used to detect a wide range of fungal pathogens [66]. Studies related to ICU patients are limited but do suggest potential for rapid diagnosis of yeast infection and identification to species level [67, 68]. Larger studies to compare various methods and confirm the usefulness of this approach in the rapid diagnosis of infection in critically ill patients are needed [69].

7.2.5 Treatment

Several phases of treatment have been proposed [70] representing a continuum of therapy of increasing intensity. Prophylaxis is reserved for severely immunocompromised patients such as liver transplant patients and those with prolonged neutropenia. Randomised studies have suggested that azoles are superior to topical agents in the prevention of superficial and systemic infections and fluconazole is most frequently used in this situation. Several studies have shown a decrease in superficial and systemic candidosis with the use of fluconazole prophylaxis patients with haematological malignancy [71] and high-risk liver transplant patients [72]. Whilst systematic review may seem to suggest that all ICU patients benefit from antifungal prophylaxis [73] most studies concentrate on selected subgroups of critically ill patients with multiple risk factors for infection [74]. Concerns that overuse of azole agents will contribute to the pathogen shift and emergence of resistance should be balanced against evidence of benefit in selected groups. Critically ill patients may have several risk factors for *Candida* infection but the incidence of infection remains low and widespread chemoprophylaxis is not justified [75], although high risk patient groups can be identified who may benefit from prophylaxis or pre-emptive therapy [76]. Currently, fluconazole prophylaxis should be considered for ICU patients who have necrotizing pancreatitis [77–83], recurrent abdominal perforation/anastomotic breakdown [84, 85], or oesophageal rupture [86].

Pre-emptive therapy represents the most logical approach to treatment of fungal infection in the ICU. It involves identifying patients likely to have fungal infection through evaluation of risk factors and surveillance of colonising flora. Typical patients for consideration of pre-emptive therapy are as follows:

- Criteria for pre-emptive therapy:
  - Persistent pyrexia and leucocytosis and grossly elevated CRP
  - Persistent funguria or repeated isolation from abdominal drain specimens
  - Patients colonised with *C. tropicalis*
  - Patients colonised with other yeast species at two or more non-contiguous sites

Empirical therapy is associated with the management of neutropenic fever but may occasionally be used in other ICU patients considered to be at extreme risk but in whom there is no direct evidence of fungal infection.

Definitive therapy is reserved for patients with conclusive evidence of invasive disease in the form of fungaemia, histological evidence of invasion or isolation from another sterile site. All patients with candidaemia and evidence of deep fungal infection should be treated with a systemic antifungal agent at an appropriate dose [87].

Traditionally the treatment options for invasive candidal infections were limited to fluconazole or amphotericin B deoxycholate. Recently, newer delivery methods for polyenes, new triazole derivatives and new classes of drugs such as the echinocandins have broadened the choices.

Amphotericin deoxycholate has excellent fungicidal activity but use is limited by toxicity, which is frequently severe, and results in increased mortality [88]. Newer formulations such as lipid-associated and liposomal polyenes can reduce adverse events but not eliminate them completely. Even liposomal amphotericin, which has the best side-effect profile of all available polyenes, is associated with some nephrotoxicity which can translate into greater length of hospitalisation [89]. Other strategies such as continuous infusions [90] or heat treated amphotericin may abrogate side effects but clinical data are limited [91].

A large number of new antifungal agents some utilising novel targets or new preparations of existing drugs have appeared in recent years. The practical choice of which antifugal agent to use in adult critical care patients lies between lipid amphotericin B preparations, fluconazole, voriconazole or caspofungin [92].

The triazoles block ergosterol synthesis by inhibiting cytochrome P450 enzymes. Itraconazole and voriconazole have a broader spectrum of activity and are active against *Candida* and *Aspergillus* spp. and other filamentous and dimorphic fungi. Until recently the lack of an intravenous preparation limited the usefulness of itraconazole in critically ill patients. Experience of use in the ICU setting remains limited. Fluconazole has been widely used and randomised controlled trials support its use in the treatment of yeast infections in ICU patients showing equivalent efficacy and a superior safety profile compared to amphotericin B [47, 93, 94]. It can be used safely in neonates [95] where the pharmacokinetics after oral administration parallel those after intravenous dosing [96]. The spectrum of activity of fluconazole is more limited and whilst active against most *C. albicans* strains, some non-albicans species (*C. krusei*) are intrinsically resistant and some (*C. glabrata*) rapidly acquire resistance. Yet other species such as *C. tropicalis* show variable dose-dependent susceptibility patterns. Resistance may develop due to a number of mechanisms, notably mutations in the cytochrome P450 enzymes (which confer cross-resistance to other azole drugs) or the presence of an efflux pump mechanism (which may be selective for fluconazole or cause loss of susceptibility to other azoles). Resistant *C. albicans* strains are reported only after prolonged courses of treatment and are rare in non-HIV infected patients. Resistance in non-*albicans* strains is rarely seen in azole naïve populations and fluconazole remains a very useful drug for the treatment of candidal infection in critically ill patients who have not received prophylaxis with azoles [5]. Failure of fluconazole therapy is usually due to inadequate dosage or duration of therapy [97]. Dosages of 400 mg/day (6 mg/kg/day in neonates) are recommended in the UK but higher dosages may be needed in hypercatabolic patients particularly those receiving continuous renal replacement therapy which will remove the drug effectively [98, 99]. Dosages of 800 mg/day can be used safely [92, 100] and haemofiltration [98] or continuous peritoneal dialysis [101] are not necessarily an indication for dose reduction. Nevertheless, debate continues on whether fluconazole should be used as a first-line agent in empirical treatment of documented yeast infections before speciation and susceptibility is available [42]. Voriconazole and posaconazole are the two latest triazole compounds in clinical use. Voriconazole has a broad spectrum of activity against both moulds and yeasts including fluconazole resistant *C .krusei*. However, for most other candidal infections, susceptibility mirrors fluconazole [102] and there is little real advantage in ICU patients in whom azole resistance is known to be low. It is available in both intravenous and orl forms, has excellent bioavailability and a relatively low incidence of side effects although drug interactions may limit use in the ICU. It is licensed for primary treatment for invasive aspergillosis where improved survival and tolerability have been demonstrated when compared to conventional amphotericin B. Posaconazole has a similar spectrum of activity but is available in an oral formulation only and shows promise for both prophylaxis and treatment. The role of these new triazoles in the ICU is unclear [103]. Voriconazole has been compared to conventional amphotericin B [104] and shown to be less toxic but offers little advantage over fluconazole at the present time. Even in the event of a massive increase in non-*albicans* infections and the emergence of resistant strains in the ICU setting, it is unlikely that another triazole would be chosen unless the mechanisms of resistance had been determined.

Echinocandins represent a new class of antifungal drug, which block fungal cell wall synthesis by non-competitive inhibition of the enzyme beta-(1,3)-D-glucan synthase, a target unique to the fungal cell. They have good activity against *Candida* and *Aspergillus* spp., but *Cryptococcus neoformans* are resistant. Activity against the 'cyst' but not 'trophozoite' form of *Pneumocystis jiroveci* has also been reported but clinical activity is doubtful. Caspofungin is a semisynthetic lipopeptide that has been licensed for the treatment of invasive *Candida* infections and is preferable to conventional amphotericin B in the treatment of candidaemia [105]. Activity against candidal biofilms [106] has been demonstrated. It is also an alternative to amphotericin as an empirical antifungal choice [107]. Caspofungin can also be used against invasive aspergillosis in patients refractory or intolerant to other therapies. It is not extensively metabolised within the body and is excreted by hydrolysis and chemical degradation. The drug is rapidly active, has a good safety profile and the prospect of interaction with other drugs and emerging resistance is low. It is only available in intravenous form and given 50 mg once daily, after an initial dose of 70 mg. Dose reduction is not necessary in elderly patients or in cases of moderate renal impairment or patients receiving renal support but caution is advised in patients with severe hepatic dysfunction. Anidulafungin and micafungin are also echinocandins with a similar spectrum of activity to caspofungin [108].

Amphotericin B has fungicidal activity against most moulds and yeasts and resistance is rare. Increased morbidity and mortality associated with amphotericin B toxicity means that conventional amphotericin B is rarely indicated in critically ill patients now that viable alternatives are available [109].

Up to 90 % of patients experience immediate infusion-related adverse events, which include headache, fever, chills, muscle and joint pains, gastrointestinal symptoms and hypotension. More serious side effects are related to nephrotoxicity, with reported rates ranging from 15 % to 90 %. Nephrotoxicity is manifested by a reduction in glomerular filtration rate, increasing creatinine levels and renal tubular acidosis resulting in severe electrolyte loss and a rising creatinine. Dosages of 1 mg/kg/day are generally used for empirical treatment but 0.7 mg/kg/day is usually adequate for most yeast infections (although *C. lusitaniae* may acquire resistance). The entrapment of amphotericin B within a lipid carrier formulation has been shown to reduce early reactions and nephrotoxicity. A variety of liposomes and lipid complexes have been developed to carry the insoluble amphotericin B within a biodegradable vesicle or lipid bilayer. Liposomes are vesicles consisting of an aqueous environment surrounded by a sphere of phospholipid bilayers. Changing characteristics such as size, electrical charge, permeability and lipid composition can alter the biological and pharmacological properties of the liposomes. Three commercial preparations are available: amphotericin B lipid complex (Abelcet), or ABLC, consists of amphotericin complexed with lipid bilayers in a 'ribbon-like' structure. Amphotericin colloidal dispersion (Amphocil), or ABCD, consists of a lipid complex in a disc-like structure. Finally, liposomal amphotericin (AmBisome), or L-AmB, is the only formulation that contains true liposomal structures [110]. The pharmacokinetics of the different licensed preparations depend on the size, charge, stability and clearance lipid complex/liposome. The increased selectivity of the lipid preparations for fungal ergosterol is thought to account for the decreased toxicity associated with these products but efficacy is not necessarily increased. The improved therapeutic index that has been reported comes from the ability to administer much higher dosages of the drug and through uptake by macrophages and concentration at sites of infection [111]. Following intravenous administration, uptake of the lipid-complexed formulations of amphotericin B appears to be primarily by the reticuloendothelial system, although plasma lipoproteins may also have a role to play. Hence, lipid formulations achieve higher tissue concentrations in the spleen, liver and lungs and relatively lower levels in the kidney, heart and brain. The three lipid formulations appear to have different incidences of side effects. L-AmB appears to have the lowest incidence of early reactions (reported at c. 5–20%), despite having the fastest infusion rate of all three preparations. ABLC and ABCD appear to have a roughly equivalent incidence of early reactions as conventional amphotericin B. All three lipid formulations have a lower rate of nephrotoxicity [89], although all products may be associated with a risk of anaphylaxis. Allergic reactions may be more common with L-AmB infusions (reported rate c. 2%), including rash, flushing, bronchospasm, rigors and back pain. Dose-to-dose equivalence has not been demonstrated and dosage recommendations should be followed for each type of preparation.

Other antifungal drugs may have a role in infections in critical care patients: The pyrimidine analogue flucytosine has a limited spectrum of activity confined mainly to yeast species and resistance can develop rapidly. The drug is myelosuppressive but may be useful in combination with other antifungal agents in the treatment of cryptococcal meningitis, candidal peritonitis and endocarditis [112].

Terbinafine is an allylamine compound widely used for the treatment of superficial dermatophyte infections. However, in vitro susceptibility data suggests it may have a broader spectrum of activity and could be of use in the treatment of candidosis and other systemic mycoses. Synergy with azole and amphotericin has been demonstrated but clinical benefit is anecdotal [113, 114].

Chemotherapy alone is likely to be unsuccessful if other measures to control a focus of infection are not taken. Removal of potentially infected intravascular catheters should be advised [5, 87] and surgical procedures such as repair of abdominal leakage may be necessary. Other adjunctive therapies have advocated the use of biological response modifiers such as cytokines, antibodies and growth factors to modulate the immune system in cases of fungal infection [115, 116]. The importance of a proinflammatory response in the elimination of opportunist fungal infection has already been discussed. Targeting essential heat-shock proteins in fungal cells and walls is a recent approach [117]. Clinical data are limited but it is likely these modalities and antifungal agents may act synergically [118–120]. Increasing understanding of innate immune recognition of fungal pathogens may lead to new methods of modifying host responses to improve outcome [121].

With the recent increase of available antifungal therapeutic agents, rational protocols for antifungal usage on ICUs need to be developed and implemented [76] (Fig. 7.1).

7.2.6 Prevention

Preventative strategies should target both exogenous and endogenous sources of infection.

It is recognised that horizontal transmission of yeasts can occur from patient to patient and via the hands of health care workers representing a potent source of infection. Up to 75% of nursing staff carry *Candida* on their hands with *C. parapsilosis* the most frequent species isolated [122]. This species has been implicated in outbreaks particularly on neonatal units. Hand hygiene and attention to aseptic technique can reduce transmission of yeasts [123].

Genomic analysis of strains shows that patients may become colonised with multiple strains simultaneously and several different modes of transmission may be involved. DNA typing methods comparing patient strains generally reveal patient-unique strains although instances of cross-infection may be demonstrated occasionally [124]. Reduction of endogenous fungal carriage may also reduce the colonisation load and prevent infection via the skin, gut and mucous membranes. Selective decontamination of the digestive tract including non-absorbable antifungal agents such as nystatin and amphotericin has been suggested [125] and is advocated in many liver transplant [126] and neonatal units [127].

Attention to infection control combined with rational use of antibacterial agents should be central to any preventative strategy. Intravenous longlines provide an important portal of entry for exogenous infection and often serve as a focus of infection through seeding of the line and biofilm formation. Adherence to aseptic techniques and protocols for line insertion and mainte-

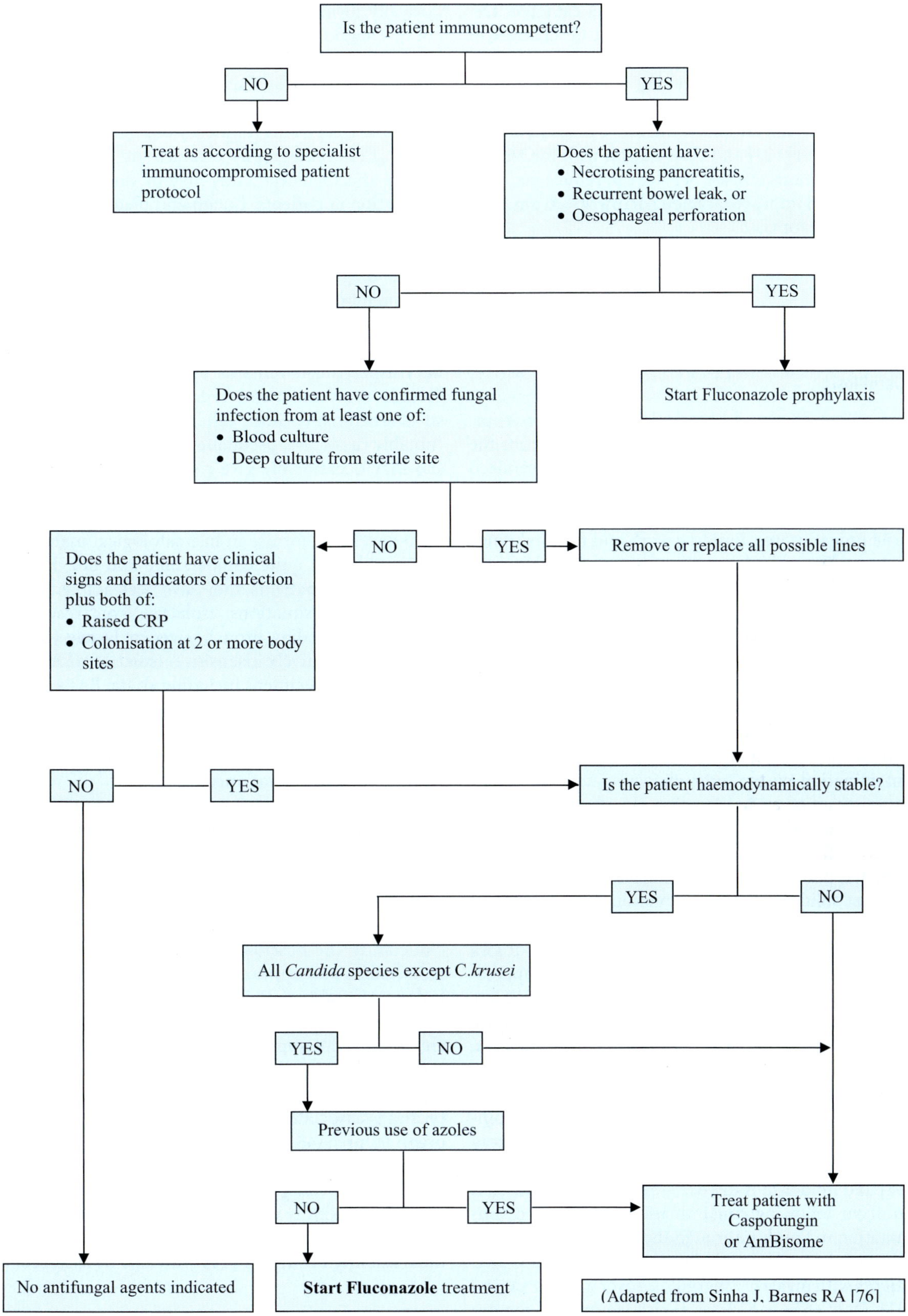

Fig. 7.1. Protocol for rational use of antifungal agents in the ICU

nance are important. Similarly, urinary catheters frequently become colonized and should be changed if yeasts are present in the urine. Persistent funguria requires investigation and screening of the renal tract to detect fungal balls.

Broad spectrum antibiotic therapy will result in fungal overgrowth [128] and close liaison with the Microbiology/Infectious Disease Service can reduce inappropriate use and improve targeted narrow spectrum therapy when appropriate.

7.3 Other Fungal Infections

7.3.1 Aspergillosis

Aspergillosis in non-neutropenic ICU patients is uncommon; a rate of 1.3% has been reported from the NNIS study and this includes immunocompromised patients [1]. *Aspergillus* species are ubiquitous environmental fungi and disease follows exposure to airborne fungal spores. Building work and hospital renovation can generate large quantities of dust that contaminate patient care areas and this has been associated with outbreaks of invasive disease [129]. Air sampling is an insensitive way of detecting this: it is often carried out only after clusters of cases appear; this is generally many weeks after the contamination has occurred and a source is rarely documented. Awareness of the problem is crucial and high-risk patients should be nursed away from areas where the potential for dust contamination exists. Outbreaks associated with building construction and renovation can affect ICUs [130], and contamination of air filters [132] and false ceiling spaces [132] have given rise to clusters of cases amongst ventilated patients and liver transplant patients [133]. Amongst solid organ transplantation, liver transplant patients represent a high risk group for invasive aspergillosis [134]. Whilst neutropenia remains a major risk factor, changing epidemiology and immunosuppressive regimens has resulted in many cases occurring late in the transplant period after neutropenia has resolved, often in association with graft-versus-host disease, newer immunomodulating agents and corticosteroid usage [135].

Aspergillosis can occur in apparently immunocompetent hosts [136] and has been associated with steroid inhalers [137], topical application of corticosteroids [138] and influenza A disease [139]. Cutaneous disease can occur following contamination of wounds or implantation in the skin through the use of contaminated splints or dressings [140]. One study identified 37 ICU patients with invasive aspergillosis over a 2-year period [141]. Only 46% had classical risk factors and the authors conclude that immunoparesis associated with the critically ill may be a significant predisposing factor [142]. Diagnosis of invasive aspergillosis is difficult; many cases remain undiagnosed during life and are only revealed at autopsy. Clinical signs and symptoms are non-specific and refractory fever may be the only manifestation. Despite the frequency of pulmonary involvement, chest radiography changes are frequently unhelpful and the chest X-ray may be normal in a large proportion of patients. Cough and pleuritic chest pain are common symptoms in non-ventilated patients. CT and MRI scanning of the chest has greatly improved the clinical diagnosis, and the presence of single or multiple enhancing nodules with cavitation, air crescent formation or the early CT-halo sign are strongly suggestive of filamentous fungal infection of which pulmonary aspergillosis remains by far the most common. Pleural involvement and wedge-shaped infarcts are also characteristic. Since other opportunist infections (notably fusariosis, pseudallerischiosis, and nocardiosis) may occasionally give rise to similar CT appearances, diagnostic bronchoalveolar lavage and antigen testing are useful. Consensus diagnostic criteria have been developed for use in haematological malignancy [143]. Although quite cumbersome and not designed for critically ill patients, they have been applied usefully within ICU situations. Isolation from respiratory specimens including bronchoalveolar lavage (BAL) is specific but relatively insensitive. Isolation of *Aspergillus* spp. from specimens including sputa, BALs and endotracheal aspirates has a positive predictive value of 82% in BMT patients [144]. This is less sensitive in other patient groups (e.g. ICU patients where colonisation without invasion is not uncommon).

Dissemination to any organ can occur but the brain, liver and skin are common sites. In the brain, disseminated lesions may present as areas of infarction. Embolic cerebrovascular accidents are rare in thrombocytopenic patients following transplantation, and CNS infarction, particularly multiple lesions, should alert the clinician to the possibility of invasive fungal disease. Skin lesions may appear as ecthyma gangrenosum-like lesions. Mortality remains high although there is some evidence that early initiation of high-dose amphotericin (before the appearance of pulmonary infiltrates) improves outcome. Nonetheless, invasive aspergillosis in ICU patients is an independent predictor of mortality, and is associated with a longer ICU stay and multiorgan failure [143].

High-resolution CT scans of the chest are now considered the investigation of choice in the diagnosis of IPA. The proximity of lesions to major structures such as the pulmonary artery, the risk of haemorrhage and the feasibility of surgery [145] can also be assessed.

7.3.2 Cryptococcal Infection

Cryptococcal infections are generally restricted to patients with profound cellular immunodeficiency such as HIV disease but a proportion occurs in apparently normal hosts. Systemic spread from a primary focus usually involves the central nervous system. Meningitis or meningoencephalitis is the typical presentation but primary pulmonary, cutaneous [146] or prostatic [147] disease can occur. Raised intracranial pressure is associated with a poor response to treatment and increased morbidity and mortality [148]. The disease may follow a chronic relapsing course [149] but care should be taken to distinguish disease progression from immune reconstitution inflammatory syndrome in HIV positive patients who have recently commenced highly active retroviral treatment [150]. Diagnosis is made by detection of the cryptococcal antigen in blood and cerebrospinal fluid, and treatment with amphotericin B plus flucytosine is usually effective [87]. Patients with continued immunosuppression require long-term secondary prophylaxis with triazoles to prevent relapse.

7.3.3 *Pneumocystis jiroveci (carinii)*

Pneumocystis jiroveci (previously *carinii*) pneumonia is associated with HIV disease [151], post-transplant immunosuppression and other cellular immunodeficiencies. Patients on high dose corticosteroids and those with low CD4 counts due to vasculitic disease such as Wegener's granulomatosis are also at risk [152]. Highly active retroviral treatment has reduced opportunistic infection in HIV but the impact on ICU admissions from pneumocystic infection has been less noticeable [153]. Infection usually presents as an interstitial pneumonitis but features can vary considerably. Progressive dyspnoea and a dry cough are the commonest presenting symptoms but *Pneumocystis carinii* pneumonia (PCP) can also present as a fulminant infection mimicking bacterial sepsis. Fever is usually, but not invariably, present. Chest radiographs show interstitial or acinar infiltrates but may be normal in the early stages [154]. Hypoxia is a feature in more than 90% of patients at presentation and may worsen rapidly on exercise and as the patient progresses to respiratory failure. Extrapulmonary pneumocystosis has occasionally been reported.

Induced sputum examination has proved useful in the HIV-positive setting but the differential diagnosis tends to be wider in transplant patients and the fungal load is less such that bronchoalveolar lavage is the preferred diagnostic procedure in this group. Diagnosis depends on demonstration of the organism in the BAL fluid using a variety of staining and immunofluorescence techniques. Molecular diagnosis by PCR is highly sensitive and specific but the test is not rapidly available at every centre and so has a limited role in clinical management.

Trimethoprim-sulphamethoxazole (TMP-SMZ, 20 mg/kg trimethoprim) remains the treatment of choice for PCP. It may take several days for a response to become apparent. Patients can be switched to oral therapy after 7–10 days if responding. Pentamidine, clindamycin-primaquine and atovaquone are all suitable agents for patients unable to tolerate TMP-SMZ. The addition of corticosteroids is beneficial in the treatment of severe PCP in AIDS but efficacy has not been evaluated fully outside of this risk group.

7.3.4 Emerging Fungal Infections

A variety of emerging pathogens have been reported as causes of infections in critical care patients, and may cause life-threatening disseminated systemic infections in immunocompromised patients. Non-*Candida* yeasts including *Rhodotorula rubra, Malassezia furfur, Trichosporon beigelii* and *Pichia anomala* are rare causes of line-associated infection [155]. *Malassezia furfur* is a lipophilic yeast whose presence may go undetected unless culture medium is overlaid with olive oil to permit growth from clinical specimens. It is a recognised pathogen in neonatal units and is associated with central venous lines and lipid infusions [156]. Recently it was implicated in an outbreak of folliculitis in an adult intensive care unit [157]. Moulds such as *Fusarium* spp. and the mucorales can cause syndromes similar to aspergillosis and *Scedosporium apiospermum* (*Pseudallescheria boydii*) infection may follow near-drowning incidents [158, 159]. Voriconazole may be indicated in these emerging mould infections [160].

7.4 Conclusion

Fungi are supreme opportunist pathogens, capable of adapting to change and taking advantage of compromised patients. Their ability to colonise, infect and immunomodulate make them significant pathogens within the ICU.

Regular surveillance is essential to monitor epidemiological trends and pathogen shifts. Evidence-based effective preventative measures and prompt diagnosis and rational treatment of these infections will improve outcomes in critically ill patients.

References

1. Beck-Sague CM, Jarvis WR, and the National Nosocomial Infections Surveillance System (1993) Secular trends in the epidemiology of nosocomial fungal infections in the United States, 1980–1990. J Infect Dis 167:1247–1251
2. Jarvis WR (1995) Epidemiology of nosocomial fungal infections with emphasis on Candida species. Clin Infect Dis 20:1526–1530
3. Rees JR, Pinner RW, Hajjeh RA, Brandt ME, Reingold AL (1998) The epidemiological features of invasive mycotic infections in the San Franscisco Bay area 1992–1993: Results of a population-based laboratory active surveillance. Clin Infect Dis 27:1138–1147
4. Nicolle LE, Rotstein C, Bourgault AM, et al. (1998) Invasive fungal infections in Canada from 1992 to 1994. Can J Infect Dis 9:347–352
5. Kibbler CC, Seaton S, Barnes RA, Gransden WR, Holliman RE, Johnson EM, Perry JD, Sullivan DJ, Wilson JA (2003) Management and outcome of blood stream infections due to Candida species in England and Wales. J Hosp Infect 54:18–24
6. Tortorano AM, Biraghi E, Astolfi A, et al. and the FIMUA Candidaemia Study Group (2002) European Confederation of Medical Mycology (ECMM) prospective survey of candidaemia: report from one Italian region. J Hosp Infect 51:297–304
7. Vincent J-L, Bihari DJ, Suter PM, et al. (1995) The prevalence of nosocomial infection in intensive care units in Europe: Results of the European Prevalence of Infection in Intensive Care (EPIC) study. J Am Med Assoc 274:639–644
8. Spencer RC (1996) Predominant pathogens found in the European prevalence of infection in intensive care study. Eur J Clin Microbiol Infect Dis 15:281–285
9. Lamagni TL, Evans BG, Shigematsu M, Johnson EM (2001) Emerging trends in the epidemiology of invasive mycoses in England and Wales (1990–9). Epidemiol Infect 126: 397–414
10. Pfaller M, Wenzel R (1992) Impact of the changing epidemiology of fungal infections in the 1990's. Eur J Clin Microbiol Infect Dis 11:287–291
11. Voss A, Le Noble JLML, Lunel FMV, Foudraine NA, Meis JFGM (1997) Candidemia in intensive care unit patients: Risk factors for mortality. Infection 25:8–11
12. Nolla-Salas J, Sitges-Serra A, Leon-Gil C, et al. (1997) Candidemia in non-neutropenic critically ill patients: Analysis of prognostic factors and assessment of systemic antifungal therapy. Intensive Care Med 23:23–30
13. Ronnestad A, Abrahamsen TG, Gaustad P, Finne PH (1998) Blood culture isolates during 6 years in a tertiary neonatal intensive care unit. Scand J Infect Dis 30:245–251
14. Wey SB, Mori M, Pfaller MA, Woolson RF, Wenzel RP (1989) Risk factors for hospital acquired candidemia. A matched case-control study. Archiv Int Med 149:2349–53
15. Pittet D, Li N, Woolson RF, Wenzel RP (1997) Microbiological factors influencing the outcome of nosocomial bloodstream infections. A six year, validated, population based model. Clin Infect Dis 24:1068–78
16. Price MF, LaRocca MT, Gentry LO (1994) Fluconazole susceptibilities of Candida species and distribution of species recovered from blood cultures over a 5-year period. Antimicrob Agents Chemother 38:1422–1424
17. Wingard JR, Merz WG, Rinaldi MG (1991) Increase in *Candida krusei* infection among patients with bone marrow transplantation and neutropenia treated prophylactically with fluconazole. N Engl J Med 325:1274–1277
18. Wingard JR, Merz WG, Rinaldi MG, et al. (1993) Association of *Torulopsis glabrata* infections with fluconazole prophylaxis in neutropenic bone marrow transplant patients. Antimicrob Agents Chemother 37:1847–1849
19. Odds FC (1996) Epidemiological shifts in opportunistic and nosocomial Candida infections: Mycological aspects. Int J Antimicrob Agents 6:141–144
20. Vincent J-L, Anaissie E, Bruining H, et al. (1998) Epidemiology, diagnosis and treatment of systemic Candida infection in surgical patients under intensive care. Intensive Care Med 24:206–216
21. Fraser VJ, Jones M, Dunkel J, et al. (1992) Candidemia in a tertiary care hospital: Epidemiology, risk factors, and predictors of mortality. Clin Infect Dis 15:414–421
22. Jantunen E, Ruutu P, Niskanen L, et al. (1997) Incidence and risk factors for invasive fungal infections in allogeneic BMT recipients. Bone Marrow Transplant 19:801–808
23. Collins LA, Samore MH, Roberts MS, et al. (1994) Risk factors for invasive fungal infections complicating othotopic liver transplantation. J Infect Dis 170:644–52
24. Petri MG, Konig J, Moecke HP, et al. (1997) Epidemiology of invasive mycosis in ICU patients: A prospective multicenter study in 435 non-neutropenic patients. Intensive Care Med 23:317–325
25. Calandra T, Bille J, Schneider R, Mossiman F, Francoli P (1989) Clinical significance of Candida isolated from the peritoneum in surgical patients. Lancet ii:1437–1440
26. Voss A, Hollis RJ, Pfaller MA, Wenzel RP, Doebbeling BN (1994) Investigation of the sequence of colonization and candidemia in nonneutropenic patients. J Clin Microbiol 32:975–980
27. Garbino J, Pittet D (1997) Candida infections in the ICU. Clin Intensive Care 8:187–200
28. Pittet D, Monod M, Suter PM, Frenk E, Auckenthaler R (1994) Candida colonization and subsequent infections in critically ill surgical patients. Ann Surg 220:751–758
29. Romagnani S (1997) The Th1/Th2 paradigm. Immunol Today 18:263–266
30. Allen JE, Maizels RM (1997) Th1-Th2: Reliable paradigm or dangerous dogma? Immunol Today 18:387–392
31. Kox WJ, Volk T, Kox SN, Volk H-D (2000) Immunomodulatory therapy in sepsis. Intensive Care Med 26:S124–128
32. Cenci E, Mencacci A, Spaccapelo R, et al. (1995) T helper type 1 (TH1) and TH2-like responses are present in mice with gastric candidiasis and protective immunity is associated with TH1 development. J Infect Dis 171:1279–1288
33. Romani L, Cenci E, Mencacci A, et al. (1993) Gamma-interferon modifies CD4+ subset expression in murine candidiasis. Infect Immun 60:4950–4952
34. Poynton CH, Barnes RA, Rees J (1998) Interferon gamma in the treatment of deep-seated fungal infection in acute leukemia. Clin Infect Dis 26:239–240
35. Shareef MJ, Myers TF, Mathews HL, Witek-Janusek L (1999) Reduced capacity of neonatal lymphocytes to inhibit the growth of *Candida albicans*. Biol Neonate 75: 31–39
36. Freidank H, Thiel L, Henninger S (1994) Comparison of immunodiffusion and counterimmunoelectrophoresis in demonstrating precipitating antibodies against *Candida* and *Aspergillus* antigens. Mycoses 37(Suppl 1):79–83
37. Weis C, Kappe R, Sonntag H-G (1997) Western blot analysis of the immune response to *Candida albicans* antigens in 391 long-term intensive care patients. Mycoses 40:153–157
38. Matthews RC, Maresca B, Burnie JP, et al. (1998) Stress proteins in fungal diseases. Med Mycol 36(Suppl):45–51
39. Martinez JP, Gil ML, Lopez-Ribot JL, LaJean Chaffin W (1998) Serologic response to cell wall mannoproteins and proteins of *Candida albicans*. Clin Microbiol Rev 11:121–141

40. Pittet D, Garbino J (1995) Fungal infections in the critically ill. Curr Opin Crit Care 1:369–380
41. Flanagan PG, Barnes RA (1998) Fungal infections in the intensive care unit. J Hosp Infect 38:163–177
42. Ronnestad A, Abrahamsen TG, Gaustad P, Finne PH (1999) C-reactive protein (CRP) response patterns in neonatal septicaemia. APMIS 107:593–600
43. Henderson VJ (1996) Emerging and reemerging microbial threats. Nosocomial fungal infections. Archiv Surg 131: 330–337
44. Walsh TJ, Chanock SJ (1997) Laboratory diagnosis of invasive candidiasis: a rationale for complementary use of culture- and non-culture based detection systems. Int J Infect Dis 1(Suppl 1):S11–S19
45. Dean DA, Burchard KW (1996) Fungal infections in surgical patients. Am J Surg 171:374–382
46. Donahue SP, Greven CM, Zuravleff JJ, et al. (1994) Intraocular candidiasis in patients with candidemia: clinical implications derived from a prospective, multicenter study. Ophthamology 101:1302–1309
47. Rex JH, Bennett JE, Sugar AM, Pappas PG, et al. (1994) A randomized trial comparing fluconazole with amphotericin B for the treatment of candidemia in patients without neutropenia. N Engl J Med 331:1325–1330
48. Rodriguez-Adrian LJ, King RT, Tamayo-Derat LG, et al. (2003) Retinal lesions as clues to disseminated bacterial and candidal infections – Frequency, natural history, and etiology. Medicine 82:187–202
49. Calandra T (1997) Candida infection in the intensive care unit. Curr Opin Crit Care 3:335–41
50. Nassoura Z, Ivatury RR, Simon RJ, Jabbour N, Stahl WM (1993) Candiduria as an early marker of disseminated infection in critically ill surgical patients: the role of fluconazole therapy. J Trauma 35:290–294
51. Ng BB, Telenti A, King B, Steckelberg JM, Wilson WR (1993) Candidemia from a urinary tract source: microbiological aspects and clinical significance. Clin Infect Dis 17:662–666
52. Bryant K, Maxfield C, Rabalais G (1999) Renal candidiasis in neonates with candiduria. Paediatr Infect Dis J 18: 959–963
53. Haron E, Vartivarian S, Anaissie E, Dekmezian R, Bodey GP (1993) Primary Candida pneumonia: Experience at a large cancer center and review of the literature. Medicine 72:137–142
54. Rello J, Esandi M-E, Diaz E, et al. (1998) The role of Candida sp isolated from bronchoscopic samples in nonneutropenic patients. Chest 114:146–149
55. Bauer TT, Torres A (1999) Candida pneumonia. Clin Intensive Care 10:33–39
56. Geha DJ, Roberts DT (1994) Laboratory detection of fungaemia. Clin Lab Med 14:83–97
57. Wilson ML, Davis TE, Mirrett S, et al. (1993) Controlled comparison of the BACTEC high-blood-volume fungal medium, BACTEC Plus 26 aerobic blood culture bottle, and 10 milliliter isolator blood culture system for detection of fungemia and bacteremia. J Clin Microbiol 31:865–871
58. Sendid B, Tabouret M, Poirot JL, et al. (1999) New enzyme immunoassays for sensitive detection of circulating *Candida albicans* mannan and antimannan antibodies: Useful combined test for diagnosis of systemic candidiasis. J Clin Microbiol 37:1510–1517
59. Odabasi Z, Mattiuzzi G, Estey E, et al. (2004) Beta-D-glucan as a diagnostic adjunct for invasive fungal infections: Validation, cutoff development, and performance in patients with acute myelogenous leukemia and myelodysplastic syndrome. Clin Infect Dis 39:199–205
60. Pickering JW, Sant HW, Bowles CAP, Roberts WL, Woods GL (2005) Evaluation of a (1→3)-beta-D-glucan assay for diagnosis of invasive fungal infections. J Clin Microbiol 43:5957–5962
61. Mitsutake K, Miyazaki T, Tashiro T, et al. (1996) Enolase antigen, mannan antigen, Cand-Tec antigen, and beta-glucan in patients with candidemia. J Clin Microbiol 34: 1918–1921
62. Loeffler J, Hebart H, Bialek R, et al. (1999) Contaminations occurring in fungal PCR assays. J Clin Microbiol 37: 1200–1202
63. Crampin AC, Matthews RC (1993) Application of the polymerase chain reaction to the diagnosis of candidosis by amplification of a HSP 90 gene fragment. J Med Microbiol 39:233–238
64. Kan VL (1993) Polymerase chain reaction for the diagnosis of candidemia. J Infect Dis 168:779–783
65. Burgener-Kairuz P, Zuber J-P, Jaunin P, et al. (1994) Rapid detection and identification of *Candida albicans* and *Torulopsis* (*Candida*) *glabrata* in clinical specimens by species-specific nested PCR-amplification of a cytochrome P-450 lanosterol-alpha-demethylase (L1A1) gene fragment. J Clin Microbiol 32:1902–1907
66. Einsele H, Hebart H, Roller G, et al. (1997) Detection and identification of fungal pathogens in using molecular probes. J Clin Microbiol 35:1353–1360
67. White PL, Barnes RA, Shetty A (2003) Detection and identification of Candida species using nested PCR and the Light Cycler™ system. J Med Microbiol 52:229–238
68. White PL, Archer AE, Barnes RA (2005) A comparison of non-culture based methods for the diagnosis of systemic fungal infections with an emphasis on invasive Candida infections. J Clin Microbiol 43:2181–2187
69. Chryssanthou E, Klingspor L, Tollemar J, et al. (1999) PCR and other non-culture methods for diagnosis of invasive Candida infections in allogeneic bone marrow and solid organ transplant recipients. Mycoses 42:239–247
70. British Society for Antimicrobial Chemotherapy Working Party (1994) Management of deep Candida infection in surgical and intensive care unit patients. Intensive Care Med 20:522–528
71. Uzun O, Anaissie EJ (1995) Antifungal prophylaxis in patients with haematological malignancies: a reappraisal. Blood 86:2063–2072
72. Tollemar J (1999) Prophylaxis against fungal infections in transplant recipients: Possible approaches. Biodrugs 11: 309–318
73. Playford EG, Webster AC, Sorrell TC, Craig JC (2006) Antifungal agents for preventing fungal infections in non-neutropenic critically ill patients. The Cochrane Database of Systematic Reviews Issue 1, art. no.: CD004920.pub2. DOI: 10.1002/14651858.CD004920.pub2
74. Pelz RK, Hendrix CW, Swoboda SM, et al. (2001) Double-blind placebo-controlled trial of fluconazole to prevent candidal infections in critically ill surgical patients. Ann Surg 233:542–548
75. Rex JH, Sobel JD (2001) Prophylactic antifungal therapy in the intensive care unit. Clin Infect Dis 32:1191–1200
76. Sinha J, Barnes RA (2003) Fungal infections in critical care: the appropriate use of antifungal agents. Br J Intensive Care Med 13:89–98
77. Gotzinger P, Sautner T, Spittler A (2000) Severe acute pancreatitis causes alterations in HLA-DR and CD14 expression on peripheral blood monocytes independently of surgical treatment. Eur J Surg 166:628–632
78. Beger HG, Bittner R, Block S, Buchler M (1986) Bacterial contamination of pancreatic necrosis – a prospective clinical study. Gastroenterology 91:433–438
79. Grewe M, Tsiotos GG, de-Leon EL, Sarr MG (1999) Fungal infection in acute necrotizing pancreatitis. J Am Coll Surg 188:408–414

80. Gotzinger P, Wamser P, Barlan M, et al. (2000) Candida infection of local necrosis in severe acute pancreatitis is associated with increased mortality. Shock 14:320–323
81. Hoerauf A, Hammer S, Muller-Myhsok B, Rupprecht H (1998) Intra-abdominal Candida infection during acute necrotizing pancreatitis has a high prevalence and is associated with increased mortality. Crit Care Med 26:2010–2015
82. Butturini G, Salvia R, Bettini R, et al. (2001) Infection prophylaxis in necrotising pancreatitis: an old challenge with new perspectives. J Hosp Infect 49:4–8
83. Shrikhande S, Friess H, Issenegger C, et al. (2000) Fluconazole penetration into the pancreas. Antimicrob Agents Chemother 44:2569–2571
84. Calandra T, Schneider R, Bille J, Mosimann F, Francioli P (1989) Clinical significance of Candida isolated from peritoneum in surgical patients. Lancet 2:1437–1440
85. Eggimann P, Francioli P, Bille J, et al. (1999) Fluconazole prophylaxis prevents intra-abdominal candidiasis in high-risk surgical patients. Crit Care Med 27:1066–1072
86. Bauer TM, Dupont V, Zimmerli W (1996) Invasive candidiasis complicating spontaneous esophageal perforation (Boerhaave syndrome). Am J Gastroenterol 91:1248–1250
87. Denning DW, Kibbler CC, Barnes RA (2003) British Society for Medical Mycology proposed standards of care for patients with invasive fungal infections. Lancet Infect Dis 3:230–240
88. Harbarth S, Burke JP, Lloyd JF, et al. (2002) Clinical and economic outcomes of conventional amphotericin B-associated nephrotoxicity. Clin Infect Dis 35:e120–7
89. Ullman AJ, Sanz MA, Tramarin A, et al. (2006) Prospective study of amphotericin B formulations in immunocompromised patients in four European countries. Clin Infect Dis 43:e279–283
90. Imhof A, Walter RB, Schaffner A (2003) Continuous infusion of escalated doses of amphotericin B deoxycholate: An open-label observational study. Clin Infect Dis 36:943–951
91. Lewis RE, Wiederhold NP, Prince RA, Kontoyiannis DP (2006) In vitro pharmacodynamics of rapid versus continuous infusion of amphotericin B deoxycholate against Candida species in the presence of human serum albumin. J Antimicrob Chemother 57:288–293
92. Edwards JE Jr, Bodey GP, Bowden RA, et al. (1997) International conference for the development of a consensus on the management and prevention of severe candidal infections. Clin Infect Dis 25:43–62
93. Rex JH, Pappas PG, Karchmer AW, et al. (2003) A randomized and blinded multicenter trial of high-dose fluconazole plus placebo versus fluconazole plus amphotericin B as therapy for candidemia and its consequences in nonneutropenic subjects. Clin Infect Dis 36:1221–8
94. Pappas PG, Rex JH, Sobel JD, et al. (2004) Guidelines for treatment of candidiasis. Clin Infect Dis 38:161–89
95. Huttova M, Hartmanova I, Kralinsky K, et al. (1998) Candida fungemia in neonates treated with fluconazole: Report of forty cases. Pediatr Infect Dis J 17:1012–1015
96. Nahata MC, Tallian KB, Force RW (1999) Pharmacokinetics of fluconazole in young infants. Eur J Drug Metabol Pharmacokinet 24:155–157
97. Flanagan PG, Barnes RA (1997) Hazards of inadequate fluconazole dosage to treat deep-seated or systemic *Candida albicans* infection. J Infect 35:295–297
98. Pittrow L, Penk A (1999) Dosage adjustment of fluconazole during continuous renal replacement therapy (CAVH, CVVH, CAVHD, CVVHD). Mycoses 42:17–19
99. Muhl E, Martens T, Iven H, Rob P, Bruch HP (2000) Influence of continuous veno-venous haemodiafiltration and continuous veno-venous haemofiltration on the pharmacokinetics of fluconazole. Eur J Clin Pharmacol 56:671–678
100. Martins M, Rex JH (1996) Resistance to antifungal agents in the critical care setting: problems and perspectives. New Horizons 4:338–344
101. Wong S-F, Leung MP, Chan M-Y (1997) Pharmacokinetics of fluconazole in children requiring peritoneal dialysis. Clin Therapeutics 19:1039–1047
102. Pfaller M, Diekema DJ, Rinaldi M, et al. (2005) Results from the ARTEMIS DISK Global Antifungal Surveillance Study: A 6.5-year analysis of the worldwide susceptibility of yeasts to fluconazole and voriconazole using standardized disk diffusion testing. J Clin Microbiol 43:5848–5859
103. Graybill JR (2005) Voriconazole for candidosis: an important addition? Lancet 366:1413–4
104. Kullberg BJ, Sobel JD, Ruhnke M, et al. (2005) Voriconazole versus a regimen of amphotericin B followed by fluconazole for candidaemia in non-neutropenic patients: a randomised non-inferiority trial. Lancet 366 (9495): 1435–1442
105. Duarte JM, Betts R, Rotstein C, et al. (2002) Comparison of caspofungin and amphotericin B for invasive candidiasis. N Engl J Med 347:2020–2029
106. Bachmann SP, VandeWalle K, Ramage G, et al. (2002) In vitro activity of caspofungin against *Candida albicans* biofilms. Antimicrob Agents Chemother 46(11):3591–6
107. Walsh TJ, Teppler H, Donowitz GR, et al. (2004) Caspofungin versus liposomal amphotericin B for empirical antifungal therapy in patients with persistent fever and neutropenia. N Engl J Med 351:1391–1402
108. Ostrosky-Zeichner L, Kontoyiannis D, Raffalli J, et al. (2005) International, open-label, noncomparative, clinical trial of micafungin alone and in combination for treatment of newly diagnosed and refractory candidemia. Eur J Clin Microbiol Infect Dis 24:654–61
109. Harbarth S, Burke JP, Lloyd JF, et al. (2002) Clinical and economic outcomes of conventional amphotericin B-associated nephrotoxicity. Clin Infect Dis 35:e120–e127
110. Wong-Beringer A, Jacobs RA, Guglielmo BJ (1998) Lipid formulations of amphotericin B: Clinical efficacy and toxicity (review). Clin Infect Dis 27:603–618
111. Adler-Moore JP, Proffitt RT (1993) Development, characterization, efficacy and mode of action of AmBisome, a unilamellar liposomal formulation of amphotericin B. J Liposome Res 3:429–450
112. Pappas G, Rex JH, Sobel JD, et al. (2004) Guidelines for treatment of candidiasis. Clin Infect Dis 38:161–168
113. Ghannoum MA, Elewski B (1999) Successful treatment of fluconazole-resistant oropharyngeal candidiasis by a combination of fluconazole and terbinafine. Clin Diagn Lab Immunol 6:921–923
114. Howden BP, Slavin MA, Schwarer AP, Mijch AM (2003) Successful control of disseminated *Scedosporium prolificans* infection with a combination of voriconazole and terbinafine. Eur J Clin Microbiol 22:111–113
115. Stevens DA, Walsh TJ, Bistoni F, et al. (1998) Cytokines and mycoses. Med Mycol 36(Suppl 1):174–172
116. Stevens DA, Kullberg BJ, Brummer E, et al. (2000) Combined treatment: antifungal drugs with antibodies, cytokines or drugs. Med Mycol 38:305–315 Suppl
117. Matthews RC, Rigg G, Hodgetts S, et al. (2003) Preclinical assessment of the efficacy of Mycograb, a human recombinant antibody against fungal HSP90. Antimicrob Agents Chemother 47:2208–16
118. Mencaci A, Cenci E, Bacci A, Bistoni F, Romani L (2000) Host immune reactivity determines the efficacy of combination immunotherapy and antifungal chemotherapy in candidiasis. J Infect Dis 181:686–694
119. Romani L (2001) Host immune reactivity and antifungal chemotherapy: The power of being together. J Chemother 13:347–353

120. Matthews RC, Burnie JP (2005) Human recombinant antibody to HSP90: A natural partner in combination therapy. Curr Mol Med 5:403 - 411
121. Netea MG, Van der Meer JWM, Sutmuller RP, Adema GJ, Kullberg BJ (2005) From the Th1/Th2 paradigm towards a toll-like receptor/T-helper bias. Antimicrob Agents Chemother 49:3991 - 3996
122. Strasbaugh LJ, Sewell DL, Ward TT, et al. (1994) High frequency of yeast carriage on the hands of hospital personnel. J Clin Microbiol 32:2299 - 2300
123. Pfaller MA (1994) Epidemiology and control of fungal infection. Clin Infect Dis 19 Suppl 1:S1–S6
124. Pfaller MA, Messer SA, Houston A, et al. (1998) National epidemiological of mycoses survey: A multicentre study of strain variation and antifungal susceptibility among isolates of Candida species. Diagn Microbiol Infect Dis 31:289 - 296
125. Lingnau W, Berger J, Javorsky F, et al. (1998) Changing bacterial ecology during a five year period of selective intestinal decontamination. J Hosp Infect 39:195 - 206
126. Arnow PM, Carandang GC, Zabner R, Irwin ME (1996) Randomized controlled trial of selective bowel decontamination for prevention of infections following liver transplantation. Clin Infect Dis 22:997 - 1003
127. Damjanovic V, Connolly CM, van Saene HKF, et al. (1993) Selective decontamination with nystatin for control of a Candida outbreak in a neonatal intensive care unit. J Hosp Infect 24:245 - 259
128. Van Saene R, Fairclough S, Petros A (1998) Broad- and narrow-spectrum antibiotics: A different approach. Clin Microbiol Infect 4:56 - 57
129. Manuel RJ, Kibbler CC (1998) The epidemiology and prevention of invasive aspergillosis. J Hosp Infect 39:95 - 10
130. Harvey IM, Leadbeatter S, Peters TJ, et al. (1988) An outbreak of disseminated aspergillosis associated with an intensive care unit. Commun Med 10:306 - 313
131. Pittet D, Huguenin T, Dharan S, et al. (1996) Unusual cause of lethal pulmonary aspergillosis in patients with chronic obstructive pulmonary disease. Am J Respir Crit Care Med 154:541 - 544
132. Humphreys H, Johnson EM, Warnock DW, et al. (1991) An outbreak of aspergillosis in a general ICU. J Hosp Infect 18:167 - 177
133. Fitzpatrick F, Prout S, Gilleece A, Fenelon LE, Murphy OM (1999) Nosocomial aspergillosis during building work – A multidisciplinary approach. J Hosp Infect 42: 170 - 171
134. Singh N, Paterson DL (2005) Aspergillus infections in transplant recipients. Clin Microbiol Rev 18:44
135. Singh N (2003) Impact of current transplantation practices on the changing epidemiology of infections in transplant recipients. Lancet Infect Dis 3:156 - 161
136. Hovenden JL, Nicklason F, Barnes RA (1991) Invasive aspergillosis in non-immunocompromised patients. Br Med J 302:583 - 584
137. Fairfax AJ, David V, Douce G (1999) Laryngeal aspergillosis following high dose inhaled fluticasone therapy for asthma. Thorax 54:860 - 861
138. Lewis MB, Henderson B (1999) Invasive intracranial aspergillosis secondary to intranasal corticosteroids. J Neurol Neurosurg Psychiatry 67:416 - 417
139. Funabiki Y, Ishii K, Kusaka S, et al. (1999) Aspergillosis following influenza a infection. Jpn J Geriatr 36:274 - 278
140. Munn S, Keane F, Child F, Philpott-Howard J, Du Vivier A (1999) Primary cutaneous aspergillosis. Br J Dermatol 141:378 - 380
141. Vandewoude KH, Blot SI, Benoit D, Colardyn F, Vogelaers D, (2004) Invasive aspergillosis in critically ill patients: attributable mortality and excesses in length of ICU stay and ventilator dependence. J Hosp Infect 56:269 - 276
142. Kox WJ, Volk T, Kox SN, Volk H-D (2000) Immunomodulatory therapy in sepsis. Intensive Care Med 26:S124 - 128
143. Ascioglu S, Rex JH, Pauw B, et al. (2002) Defining opportunistic invasive fungal infections in immunocompromised patients with cancer and hematopoietic stem cell transplants: an international consensus. Clin Infect Dis 34:7 - 14
144. McWhinney PHM, Kibbler CC, Hamon MD, et al. (1993) Progress in the diagnosis and management of aspergillosis in bone marrow transplantation: 13 years experience. Clin Infect Dis 17:397 - 404
145. Yeghen T, Kibbler CC, Prentice HG, et al. (2000) Management of invasive pulmonary aspergillosis in hematology patients: A review of 87 consecutive cases at a single institution. Clin Infect Dis 31:859 - 868
146. Bellosta M, Gaviglio MR, Mosconi M, et al. (1999) Primary cutaneous cryptococcosis in an HIV-negative patient. Eur J Dermatol 9:224 - 226
147. Caballes RL, Caballes RA (1999) Primary cryptococcal prostatitis in an apparently uncompromised host. Prostate 39:119 - 122
148. Park MK, Hospenthal DR, Bennett JE (1999) Treatment of hydrocephalus secondary to cryptococcal meningitis by use of shunting. Clin Infect Dis 28:629 - 633
149. Yip SKH, Cheng C, Wong MYC, et al. (1998) Cryptococcal prostatic abscess in an immunocompromised patient: A case report and review of the literature. Ann Acad Med Singapore 27:873 - 876
150. Lortholary O, Fontanet A, Memain N, et al. (2006) Incidence and risk factors of immune reconstitution inflammatory syndrome complicating HIV-associated cryptococcosis in France. AIDS 19:1043 - 1049
151. Miguez-Burbano MJ, Flores M, Ashkin D, et al. (2006) Non-tuberculous mycobacteria disease as a cause of hospitalization in HIV-infected subjects. Int J Infect Dis 10:47 - 55
152. Sneller MC (1995) Wegener's granulomatosis. J Am Med Assoc 273:1288 - 1291
153. Palacios R, Hidalgo A, Reina C, et al. (2006) Effect of antiretroviral therapy on admissions of HIV-infected patients to an intensive care unit. HIV Med 7:193 - 196
154. Opravil M, Marincek B, Fuchs WA, et al. (1994) Shortcomings of chest radiography in detecting *Pneumocystis carinii* pneumonia. J Acquir Immun Defic Syndr 7:39 - 45
155. Klein NC, Gill MV, Cunha BA (1996) Unusual organisms causing intravenous line infections in compromised hosts: II. Fungal infections. Infect Dis Clin Pract 5:303 - 310
156. Gueho E, Boekhout T, Ashbee HR, et al. (1998) The role of *Malassezia* species in the ecology of human skin and as pathogens. Med Mycol Suppl 36:220 - 229
157. Archer-Dubon C, Icaza-Chivez ME, Orozco-Topete R, et al. (1999) An epidemic outbreak of *Malassezia* folliculitis in three adult patients in an intensive care unit: A previously unrecognized nosocomial infection. Int J Dermatol 38:453 - 456
158. Wilichowski E, Christen H-J, Schiffmann H, et al. (1996) Fatal *Pseudallescheria boydii* panencephalitis in a child after near-drowning. Pediatr Infect Dis J 15:365 - 370
159. Kowacs PA, Silvado CES, de Almeida SM, et al. (2004) Infection of the CNS by *Scedosporium apiospermum* after near drowning. Report of a fatal case and analysis of its confounding factors. J Clin Pathol 57:205 - 207
160. Chakraborty A, Workman MR, Bullock PR (2005) *Scedosporium apiospermum* brain abscess treated with surgery and voriconazole – Case report. J Neurosurg 103:83 - 87

8 Using Protocols To Improve the Outcomes of Critically Ill Patients with Infection: Focus on Ventilator-Associated Pneumonia and Severe Sepsis

S.T. Micek, M.H. Kollef

Translating the results of research into clinical practice in critically ill patients is a challenging endeavor and often a slow, complex process. The literature is replete with evidence-based guidelines for the prevention and treatment of infections in critically ill patients aimed to standardize care, reduce costs, and improve patient outcomes [1–4]. Despite the widespread publicity of such documents, non-adherence to guidelines is readily apparent and directly impacts patient morbidity and mortality [5–7]. Explanations for the lack of guideline adherence include disagreement with interpretation of clinical trials, limited evidence in support of specific pharmacologic or non-pharmacologic treatment strategies, and simply the hesitancy to change practices at the beside.

One method that has proven to be successful in the transfer of research advancements to clinical practice within individual medical centers is recognition of the need for quality improvement, involvement of esteemed multidisciplinary staff to champion an intervention, followed by mass education, assessment of the intervention's impact on patient and hospital endpoints, and finally feeding back findings related to the process. Examples of successful quality improvement initiatives focused on development and implementation of treatment pathways or protocols in critically ill patients include weaning from mechanical ventilation [8–10], ICU sedation [11, 12], and intensive insulin therapy [13]. This chapter describes the impact of protocols for the management of patients with ventilator-associated pneumonia (VAP) and severe sepsis.

8.1 Ventilator-Associated Pneumonia (VAP)

The antimicrobial management of VAP is a balancing act of providing appropriate initial treatment in a timely manner with broad-spectrum therapy based on the knowledge of the local pathogens and susceptibility rates, avoiding unnecessary antimicrobials through the use of protocols to change from broad- to narrow-spectrum therapy of anti-infective treatment after 48–72 h of therapy based on culture results and susceptibilities, and using a short course of treatment. This "de-escalation" strategy attempts to unify these principles into a single approach that will optimize patient outcomes while minimizing the emergence of antibiotic resistant pathogens.

Failure to provide treatment with an appropriate initial antimicrobial regimen for VAP has resulted in significantly higher rates of septic shock and hospital mortality [14–16]. Additionally, treatment delays of greater than 24 h after meeting diagnostic criteria for VAP have been associated with statistically higher rates of bacteremia and in-hospital mortality [17]. Importantly, adjusting an initial inappropriate VAP treatment regimen according to culture and sensitivity does not result in outcomes equal to patients treated with antimicrobial therapy that is active from the outset of therapy [14, 15]. In an effort to optimize the likelihood of prescribing an initial appropriate regimen for clinically suspected VAP, the ATS/IDSA evidence-based guideline recommends a combination of antimicrobials targeting the most common bacterial pathogens associated with early- and late-onset infection [2]. It is important to recognize that the predominant pathogens associated with hospital-acquired infections, including VAP, may vary between hospitals as well as among specialized units within individual hospitals [18, 19]. Therefore, clinicians should be aware of the prevailing bacterial pathogens in their hospitals and their associated antimicrobial susceptibilities when prescribing a combination therapy regimen as endorsed by the ATS/IDSA guidelines.

The benefits of a guideline for VAP management was tested in a clinical setting by Ibrahim et al., who conducted a before-and-after study evaluating the impact of a VAP treatment guideline on initial administration of appropriate antimicrobial therapy [20]. In the particular medical ICU where the protocol was implemented, *Pseudomonas aeruginosa* and methicillin-resistant *Staphylococcus aureus* (MRSA) were the most common causes of VAP based on historical data. Consequently, the protocol dictated the combination of imipenem-cilastatin, ciprofloxacin, and vancomycin be prescribed initially as this regimen provided in vitro coverage for >90% of *P. aeruginosa* and 100% of MRSA isolates. In cases that had a bacterial pathogen identified, patients managed via the protocol were statistically more likely to receive initial appropriate treatment compared to those treated prior to implementation (94.2% vs. 48%; $p<0.001$). Similarly, Wood and colleagues found a high percentage (76%) of trauma ICU patients with VAP were prescribed appropriate initial coverage after altering their clinical pathway based on historical pathogen incidence [21]. Patients received ampicillin/sulbactam if they were diagnosed with early VAP (through day 7 of hospitalization) and cefepime plus vancomycin for late VAP (after day 7). This was chosen due to the low incidence of *P. aeruginosa, Acinetobacter baumannii*, and MRSA as a cause of early VAP.

Modification of an initial, appropriate broad spectrum antibiotic regimen using a de-escalation strategy should occur based on the results of the patient's clinical response and microbiologic testing. This includes decreasing the number and spectrum of antibiotics and shortening the duration of therapy administered if there are signs of clinical improvement or a causative organism has been identified. Rello and colleagues examined the impact of a VAP treatment protocol incorporating de-escalation principles in 115 patients [22]. Per treatment protocol, patients demonstrating clinical improvement 48 h after initiation of broad-spectrum antimicrobials were subject to streamlining therapy. The approach included narrowing to a single agent if *P. aeruginosa* was not identified; focusing the antimicrobial spectrum of activity based on susceptibility data, i.e., changing from combination therapy to monotherapy for *P. aeruginosa;* and limiting the course of therapy to 5 days in patients remaining afebrile for 48 h. Under this protocol, de-escalation occurred in 31.4% of the patients. The de-escalation practice pattern that evolved under the auspices of the protocol was predominantly in patients with early VAP vs. late VAP (40.7% vs. 12.5%; odds ratio 4.81; 95% confidence interval 1.7–13.6) and in patients with multi-susceptible pathogen isolation compared to multi-resistant organisms (49.3% vs. 2.7%; $p<0.05$).

The implementation of formal clinical monitoring [i.e., clinical pulmonary infection score (CPIS)] into clinical pathways recommending de-escalation therapy for VAP has been evaluated by several investigators. Singh and colleagues attempted to reduce the emergence of resistance by limiting the number of antibiotics and duration of antibiotic therapy in patients having a low likelihood of VAP as indicated by a CPIS ≤ 6 [23]. Patients with the clinical diagnosis of VAP (not uniformly diagnosed via quantitative cultures of BAL) but with CPIS 6 were randomized to conventional therapy determined by the treating physician or to ciprofloxacin monotherapy. Per study protocol, patients in the ciprofloxacin monotherapy group had treatment discontinued on day 3 if the CPIS remained 6, whereas therapy was permitted to continue in the conventional therapy group. Patients in the ciprofloxacin monotherapy group had significantly shorter courses of antibiotic therapy (3 days vs. 10 days; $p=0.0001$), significantly less development of antimicrobial resistance or subsequent superinfection (15% vs. 35%; $p=0.017$), and shorter ICU lengths of stay (median 4 days vs. 9 days; $p=0.04$) with no observed difference in 30-day all cause mortality (13% vs. 31%; $p=0.06$).

Or do we want to say a slight trend to improvement in 30-day all cause mortality?

Ibrahim et al. conducted a pre-/post-protocol study that evaluated a clinical guideline for clinically diagnosed VAP employing the goals of de-escalation therapy and promoted a 7-day course of antimicrobial therapy in responding patients with uncomplicated VAP (i.e., absence of empyema or secondary bacteremia) [20]. The guideline incorporated in this trial dictated that antibiotic treatment had to be de-escalated via two modalities: (1) narrowing of therapy 24–48 h into treatment based on the availability of culture results and the patient's clinical course and (2) subsequent recommendation of a 7-day course of therapy. Use of antibiotic treatment beyond 7 days was only encouraged for patients with clinical parameters that remained abnormal or consistent with persistent infection. Upon implementation of the clinical guideline, 98% of patients had one or two antibiotics discontinued by 48 h of treatment. The duration of treatment was significantly shorter during the post-protocol period compared with the pre-protocol period (8.6 ± 5.1 days vs. 14.8 ± 8.1 days, $p<0.001$). Additionally, there were fewer secondary infections due to antibiotic resistant organisms during the clinical guideline phase. No differences in clinical outcome measures including in-hospital mortality or ICU and hospital lengths of stay were observed.

In a study by Micek and colleagues, patients with clinically diagnosed VAP were randomly assigned to have the duration of antibiotic therapy determined by the clinical judgment of the treating physician (standard therapy) or by a formalized discontinuation policy [24]. Patients assigned to the discontinuation group were monitored during the weekday by a clinical pharmacist who made recommendations to stop one or more antibiotics if a non-infectious etiology for pulmonary infiltrates was identified or if all of the following criteria were met: (1) temperature $<38.3\,^{\circ}C$, (2) white blood cell count $<10\times10^3$ or decreased 25% from peak value, (3) improvement or lack of progression on chest X-ray, (4) absence of purulent sputum, and (5) $PaO_2 : FiO_2$ ratio >250. Eighty-nine percent of patients in the discontinuation group had at least one antibiotic discontinued within 48 h of recommendation. The overall duration of treatment was significantly shorter in the discontinuation group compared to standard therapy

(6.0 ± 4.9 days vs. 8.0 ± 5.6 days, $p = 0.001$). No differences were observed with respect to in-hospital mortality, ICU and hospital length of stay, the duration of mechanical ventilation, or the acquisition of a second episode of VAP.

The implementation of VAP treatment protocols incorporating the administration of broad-spectrum empiric antimicrobial therapy based on patient risk factors, serial assessment of clinical markers used to monitor response to empiric therapy, institution of locally developed and clinician accepted guidelines designed to minimize the number and duration of antibiotics in the face of positive cultures and/or clinical improvement optimizes patient outcomes while preventing the emergence of antibiotic resistance.

8.2 Severe Sepsis

The unscrambling of the complex pathophysiology associated with severe sepsis has made much progress and current understanding of this process is no longer rudimentary [25, 26]. Novel drug entities and new therapeutic strategies targeting these pathways have demonstrated efficacy in reducing patient mortality [27–29]. The challenge for clinicians is the integration of these pharmacotherapies to confer the recognized survival benefit into critical care practice. The Surviving Sepsis Campaign has teamed with the Institute for Healthcare Improvement to create the Severe Sepsis Bundles, which are designed in an effort to optimize the timing, sequence, and goals of the individual elements of care as delineated in the Surviving Sepsis Guidelines [1]. The creation of comprehensive treatment protocols integrating goal-directed hemodynamic stabilization, early, appropriate antimicrobial therapy, and associated adjunctive severe sepsis therapies initiated in the emergency department and continued in the intensive care unit has been reported in several retrospective and prospective, observational trials.

The significance of early, aggressive volume resuscitation and hemodynamic stabilization was demonstrated in a randomized, controlled, single-center trial in patients that presented to the emergency department with signs of the systemic inflammatory response syndrome (SIRS) and hypotension as published by Rivers et al. [27]. Administration of crystalloids, red blood cell transfusions, vasopressors and inotropes based on aggressive monitoring of intravascular volume and a tissue oxygen marker within 6 h of presentation to the emergency department resulted in a 16% decrease in absolute 28-day mortality. The major differences in treatment between the intervention and control groups were in the volume of intravenous fluids received, the number of patients transfused packed red blood, the use of dobutamine, and the presence of a dedicated study team for the first 6 h of care. Equally important as rapid hemodynamic stabilization is the administration of appropriate initial antimicrobial treatment of patients with severe sepsis. Several investigations have found appropriate therapy to be an important determinant of patient outcome [30–32], with early administration possibly playing a pivotal role [33].

The implementation of treatment pathways mimicking the interventions of the well-scripted, carefully performed procedures employed by Rivers et al. has been put into practice in the clinical setting. Trzeciak et al. described the results of incorporating clinical research into a real-life setting whereby the emergency department and ICUs at an academic medical center collaborated in a therapeutic quality initiative focused on implementing early goal-directed therapy (EGDT) [34]. Upon institution of a hospital-specific, EGDT protocol, 91% of patients managed met central venous pressure (CVP), mean arterial pressure (MAP), and central venous oxygen saturation goal ($SCVO_2$) endpoints within a median of 6 h of presentation. Similarly, Shapiro et al. have described the creation of the Multiple Urgent Sepsis Therapies (MUST) protocol, a multidisciplinary collaborative that combines all sepsis bundle elements, including EGDT and early, appropriate antimicrobial therapy [35]. Key to the successful implementation of a complex process of care such as the MUST protocol is the massive education initiative associated with each endeavor. Such labors include training classes for emergency department and intensive care unit physicians and nurses, bedside reference guides, educational websites, protocol summary posters, and ultimately a sepsis order set specific to individual hospital capabilities, such as computerized physician order entry systems.

Several studies have detailed the impact of adopting severe sepsis protocols on treatment processes and patient outcomes. Micek and colleagues compared 60 patients presenting to the emergency department who were managed prior to the implementation of the standardized order set (before-group) that focused on intravenous fluid administration and the appropriateness of initial antimicrobial therapy and 60 patients treated after the roll out of the protocol (after-group) (Figs. 8.1, 8.2) [36]. Patients in the after-group received statistically more intravenous fluids while in the emergency department (3,789 ± 1,730 ml vs. 2,825 ± 1,624 ml; $p = 0.002$), they were more likely to receive intravenous fluids greater than 20 ml/kg of body weight prior to vasopressor administration (88.3% vs. 58.3%; $p < 0.001$), and consequently were less likely to require vasopressor administration at the time of transfer to the intensive care unit (71.7% vs. 100%; $p < 0.001$). Additionally, a statistically greater number of patients in the after-group were more likely to receive a blood transfusion

UNLESS THE WORD SPECIFIC IS WRITTEN AFTER A DRUG ORDER BY TRADE NAME, A GENERIC EQUIVALENT DRUG APPROVED BY THE PHARMACY AND THERAPEUTICS COMMITTEE MAY BE DISPENSED IN ACCORDANCE WITH THE MEDICAL STAFF BYLAWS.

PLEASE CHECK (✔) THE APPROPRIATE BOX □ AND FILL IN THE BLANK(S) AS NEEDED. IF YOU DO NOT NEED AN ORDER, DRAW A LINE THROUGH IT AND INITIAL.

DATE	TIME	Microbiologic Diagnosis
		Obtain the following cultures: □ Blood (peripheral) x 2 sets □Urine □ Respiratory Secretions □ Stool C. difficile toxin □ Other ______
		Antimicrobial Therapy (To be initiated within 3 hours of presentation)
		Medications: for probable type of Infection **Patient's weight (kg):______ Patient's height:______** **Community Acquired Pneumonia (CAP)** Choose one: □ Ceftriaxone 1 gram IVPB NOW and Q24 hours plus Azithromycin 500 mg IVPB NOW and Q24 hours PCN/Cephalosporin Allergy □ Moxifloxacin 400 mg IVPB NOW and Q24 hours **Healthcare Associated Pneumonia (HCAP)** Choose one: □ Cefepime 1 gram IVPB NOW and Q8 hours plus Gentamicin 5 mg/kg IVPB NOW and Q24 hours □ Piperacillin/Tazobactam 4.5 grams IVPB NOW and Q6 hours plus Gentamicin 5 mg/kg IVPB NOW and Q24 hours □ Cefepime 1 gram IVPB NOW and Q8 hours plus Ciprofloxacin 400mg IVPB NOW and Q8 hours □ Piperacillin/Tazobactam 4.5 grams IVPB NOW and Q6 hours plus Ciprofloxacin 400mg IVPB NOW and Q8 hours PCN/Cephalosporin Allergy □ Aztreonam 2 grams IVPB NOW and Q8 hours plus Gentamicin 5 mg/kg IVPB NOW and Q24 hours And: □ Vancomycin 20mg/kg=______mg IVPB NOW and Q12 hours (rounded to nearest 250mg; max single dose = 2 gm) **Intra-abdominal Infection** Choose one: □ Cefepime 1 gram IVPB NOW and Q8 hours plus Metronidazole 500mg IVPB NOW and Q8 hours □ Ciprofloxacin 400mg IVPB NOW and Q8 hours plus Metronidazole 500mg IVPB NOW and Q8 hours □ Piperacillin/Tazobactam 4.5 grams IVPB NOW and Q6 hours **Urinary Tract Infection** Choose one: □ Ceftriaxone 1 gram IVPB NOW and Q24 hours (community-acquired) □ Cefepime 1 gram IVPB NOW and Q8 hours (healthcare-acquired) PCN/Cephalosporin Allergy □ Ciprofloxacin 400 mg IVPB NOW and Q12 hours Other: ______ *** All doses are based on CrCl > 75 ml/min, dose adjustments may be needed after 24 hours**
		MD:______ Telephone #/Pager # ______

Fig. 8.1. Protocol

(20 % vs. 6.7 %; $p=0.032$) as a result of a significantly increased $SCVO_2$ monitoring (48.3 % vs. 1.7 %; $p<0.001$). Patients in the after-group were also more likely to be treated with an appropriate initial antimicrobial regimen (86.7 %% vs. 71.7 %; $p=0.043$) compared to patients in the before-group. As a result of the aggressive management initiated in the emergency department and continued in the intensive care unit, patients managed via the severe sepsis order sets had a shorter hospital length of stay (12.1±9.2 days vs. 8.9±7.2 days; $p=0.038$), and a lower risk for 28-day mortality (48.3 % vs. 30.0 %; $p=0.040$).

Shapiro et al. evaluated the implementation and outcomes of the Multiple Urgent Sepsis Therapies (MUST) protocol compared to historical controls in an academic medical center [37]. During the first 6 h (resuscitation phase) of therapy, patients managed via the protocol group received significantly more intravenous fluids (4,107±2,590 ml vs. 2,871±1,773 ml; $p=0.001$), were more likely to receive vasopressors (80 % vs. 45 %; $p=0.001$) and had a significant improvement in appropriate antibiotic coverage compared to historical controls (97 % vs. 88 %; $p=0.05$). Additionally, non-statistically significant increases in red blood cell transfusion

UNLESS THE WORD SPECIFIC IS WRITTEN AFTER A DRUG ORDER BY TRADE NAME, A GENERIC EQUIVALENT DRUG APPROVED BY THE PHARMACY AND THERAPEUTICS COMMITTEE MAY BE DISPENSED IN ACCORDANCE WITH THE MEDICAL STAFF BYLAWS.

PLEASE CHECK (✔) **THE APPROPRIATE BOX □ AND FILL IN THE BLANK(S) AS NEEDED. IF YOU DO NOT NEED AN ORDER, DRAW A LINE THROUGH IT AND INITIAL.**

INITIATE THE FOLLOWING STANDARDIZED ORDERS FOR ALL PATIENTS IN SEVERE SEPSIS OR SEPSIS-INDUCED HYPOPERFUSION (SYSTOLIC BLOOD PRESSURE < 90 MMHG [AFTER A CRYSTALLOID FLUID CHALLENGE OF 20-30 ML/KG OVER 30 MINUTES] OR A BLOOD LACTATE CONCENTRATION OF ≥ 4 MMOL/L)

DATE	TIME	ORDERS
		Admission Status: □ **Inpatient** **Recommended Admit Location: 83ICU or 89ICU or 84ICU if surgical patient**
		Diagnosis: **1.)** __________ **2.)** __________ **3.)** __________
		Early Goal-Directed Therapy (To be initiated within 6 hours of presentation)
		Procedures: 1.) Arterial Catheterization 2.) Central Venous Catheterization (subclavian or internal jugular) 3.) Central Venous Pressure Transducer Set-up
		IV Fluids Choose One: □ 0.9 NS 500 ml IV over 30 minutes, repeat until central venous pressure (CVP) 8-12 mmHg or 12-15 in mechanically ventilated patients □ Other
		Vasopressors: If the mean arterial pressure remains < 65 mmHg despite achieving a CVP of 8-15 mmHg, initiate vasopressor therapy. It may be necessary to employ vasopressors early as an emergency measure in patients with septic shock □ Dopamine 10 mcg/kg/min, titrate to a mean arterial pressure (MAP) of 65-90 mmHg □ Norepinephrine 5 mcg/min, titrate to a mean arterial pressure (MAP) of 65-90 mmHg
		Tissue Perfusion Assessment □ Obtain central venous oxygen saturation ($S_{CV}O_2$) q 30 minutes until ≥ 70% □ Continuous central venous oxygen saturation ($S_{CV}O_2$) monitoring until ≥ 70%
		Transfusion Therapy: If central venous oxygen saturation is < 70% despite a CVP of 8-15 mmHg and the addition of vasopressors, the patient should be transfused with packed red blood cells to achieve a hematocrit ≥ 30%. Separate order should be written.
		Inotropic Therapy: If central venous pressure, mean arterial pressure and hematocrit have been optimized, and the central venous oxygen saturation remains < 70%, consider inotropic therapy. □ Dobutamine 2.5 mcg/kg/min, titrate by 2.5 mcg/kg/min to a central venous oxygen saturation ($S_{CV}O_2$) q 30 minutes until ≥ 70% (max dose 20 mcg/kg/min)
		MD:__________ **Telephone #/Pager #** __________

Fig. 8.2. Protocol

(30% vs. 18%; $p=0.7$) and dobutamine administration (14% vs. 4%; $p=0.06$) were observed in patients treated via the protocol. The intensified approach to early resuscitation dictated by the protocol in combination with other therapies resulted in a 9.1% absolute risk reduction in 28-day mortality (20.3% vs. 29.4%; $p=0.3$).

In a study by Kortgen and colleagues, the effects of standard operating procedure (SOP) for treatment of severe sepsis and septic shock were compared to those in control patients managed prior to the introduction of the pathway [38]. Cohorts of 30 patients each were compared. Patients receiving therapy under the auspices of the SOP were statistically more likely (all p values <0.05) to be treated with dobutamine (40% vs. 6.7%), hydrocortisone (100% vs. 43.3%), drotrecogin alfa (activated) (23.3% vs. 0%), and insulin infusions (100% vs. 60%) within 24 h of initial organ failure. These differences, in combination with other fundamental therapies including goal-directed volume resuscitation and lung-protective ventilation strategies, and antimicrobial therapy resulted in a statistically lower 28-day mortality rate amongst patients managed with the SOP (27% vs. 53%, $p<0.05$), with a relative risk reduction of 50% (95% CI 1.2%–74.7%).

Gao et al. evaluated the outcomes of patients who manifested a severe sepsis syndrome after hospital admission in terms of whether compliance with sepsis care bundles occurred during their management [39]. The sepsis care bundles provided recommendations for the management of intravenous fluids, blood transfusions, antibiotics, and vasopressors. There was an overall compliance of 52% with the sepsis bundles for this population. Despite being comparable in terms of baseline demographics and severity of illness, the compliant patients had a statistically lower risk of hospital mortality compared to the non-compliant patients (29% vs. 55%; $p=0.045$).

In summary, the initial management of patients with septic shock and VAP appears to be critical in terms of determining outcome. Institution of standardized physician order sets, or some other systematic approach, for the management of patients with severe infections appears to consistently improve the delivery of recommended therapies and as a result may improve patient outcomes. Given that physician order sets expose patients to no additional risks, and are associated with little to no acquisition costs, their implementation should become the standard of care for the management of septic shock and VAP.

References

1. Dellinger RP, Carlet JM, Masur H, et al. (2004) Surviving sepsis campaign guidelines for management of severe sepsis and septic shock. Crit Care Med 32(3):858–73
2. Guidelines for the management of adults with hospital-acquired, ventilator-associated, and healthcare-associated pneumonia. Am J Respir Crit Care Med 171(4):388–416
3. Mandell LA, Bartlett JG, Dowell SF, File TM, Jr, Musher DM, Whitney C (2003) Update of practice guidelines for the management of community-acquired pneumonia in immunocompetent adults. Clin Infect Dis 37(11):1405–33
4. Kollef MH (1999) The prevention of ventilator-associated pneumonia. N Engl J Med 340(8):627–34
5. Bodi M, Rodriguez A, Sole-Violan J, et al. (2005) Antibiotic prescription for community-acquired pneumonia in the intensive care unit: impact of adherence to Infectious Diseases Society of America guidelines on survival. Clin Infect Dis 41(12):1709–16
6. Menendez R, Torres A, Zalacain R, et al. (2005) Guidelines for the treatment of community-acquired pneumonia: predictors of adherence and outcome. Am J Respir Crit Care Med 172(6):757–62
7. Rello J, Lorente C, Bodi M, Diaz E, Ricart M, Kollef MH (2002) Why do physicians not follow evidence-based guidelines for preventing ventilator-associated pneumonia? A survey based on the opinions of an international panel of intensivists. Chest 122(2):656–61
8. Ely EW, Baker AM, Dunagan DP, et al. (1996) Effect on the duration of mechanical ventilation of identifying patients capable of breathing spontaneously. N Engl J Med 335(25): 1864–9
9. Kollef MH, Shapiro SD, Silver P, et al. (1997) A randomized, controlled trial of protocol-directed versus physician-directed weaning from mechanical ventilation. Crit Care Med 25(4):567–74
10. Horst HM, Mouro D, Hall-Jenssens RA, Pamukov N (1998) Decrease in ventilation time with a standardized weaning process. Arch Surg 133(5):483–8; discussion 8–9
11. Brook AD, Ahrens TS, Schaiff R, et al. (1999) Effect of a nursing-implemented sedation protocol on the duration of mechanical ventilation. Crit Care Med 27(12):2609–15
12. Kress JP, Pohlman AS, O'Connor MF, Hall JB (2000) Daily interruption of sedative infusions in critically ill patients undergoing mechanical ventilation. N Engl J Med 342(20): 1471–7
13. Van den Berghe G, Wouters P, Weekers F, et al. (2001) Intensive insulin therapy in critically ill patients. N Engl J Med 345(19):1359–67
14. Kollef MH, Ward S (1998) The influence of mini-BAL cultures on patient outcomes: implications for the antibiotic management of ventilator-associated pneumonia. Chest 113(2):412–20
15. Luna CM, Vujacich P, Niederman MS, et al. (1997) Impact of BAL data on the therapy and outcome of ventilator-associated pneumonia. Chest 111(3):676–85
16. Alvarez-Lerma F (1996) Modification of empiric antibiotic treatment in patients with pneumonia acquired in the intensive care unit. ICU-Acquired Pneumonia Study Group. Intensive Care Med 22(5):387–94
17. Iregui M, Ward S, Sherman G, Fraser VJ, Kollef MH (2002) Clinical importance of delays in the initiation of appropriate antibiotic treatment for ventilator-associated pneumonia. Chest 122(1):262–8
18. Babcock HM, Zack JE, Garrison T, Trovillion E, Kollef MH, Fraser VJ (2003) Ventilator-associated pneumonia in a multi-hospital system: differences in microbiology by location. Infect Control Hosp Epidemiol 24(11):853–8
19. Namias N, Samiian L, Nino D, et al. (2000) Incidence and susceptibility of pathogenic bacteria vary between intensive care units within a single hospital: implications for empiric antibiotic strategies. J Trauma 49(4):638–45; discussion 45–6
20. Ibrahim EH, Ward S, Sherman G, Schaiff R, Fraser VJ, Kollef MH (2001) Experience with a clinical guideline for the treatment of ventilator-associated pneumonia. Crit Care Med 29(6):1109–15
21. Wood GC, Mueller EW, Croce MA, Boucher BA, Hanes SD, Fabian TC (2005) Evaluation of a clinical pathway for ventilator-associated pneumonia: changes in bacterial flora and the adequacy of empiric antibiotics over a three-year period. Surg Infect 6(2):203–13
22. Rello J, Vidaur L, Sandiumenge A, et al. (2004) De-escalation therapy in ventilator-associated pneumonia. Crit Care Med 32(11):2183–90
23. Singh N, Rogers P, Atwood CW, Wagener MM, Yu VL (2000) Short-course empiric antibiotic therapy for patients with pulmonary infiltrates in the intensive care unit. A proposed solution for indiscriminate antibiotic prescription. Am J Respir Crit Care Med 162(2):505–11
24. Micek ST, Ward S, Fraser VJ, Kollef MH (2004) A randomized controlled trial of an antibiotic discontinuation policy for clinically suspected ventilator-associated pneumonia. Chest 125(5):1791–9
25. Hotchkiss RS, Karl IE (2003) The pathophysiology and treatment of sepsis. N Engl J Med 348(2):138–50
26. Annane D, Bellissant E, Cavaillon JM (2005) Septic shock. Lancet 365(9453):63–78
27. Rivers E, Nguyen B, Havstad S, et al. (2001) Early goal-directed therapy in the treatment of severe sepsis and septic shock. N Engl J Med 345(19):1368–77
28. Annane D, Sebille V, Charpentier C, et al. (2002) Effect of treatment with low doses of hydrocortisone and fludrocortisone on mortality in patients with septic shock. JAMA 288(7):862–71
29. Bernard GR, Vincent J-L, Laterre P-F, et al. (2001) Efficacy and safety of recombinant human activated protein C for severe sepsis. N Engl J Med 344(10):699–709
30. Harbarth S, Garbino J, Pugin J, Romand JA, Lew D, Pittet D (2003) Inappropriate initial antimicrobial therapy and its

effect on survival in a clinical trial of immunomodulating therapy for severe sepsis. Am J Med 115(7):529–35

31. Garnacho-Montero J, Garcia-Garmendia JL, Barrero-Almodovar A, Jimenez-Jimenez FJ, Perez-Paredes C, Ortiz-Leyba C (2003) Impact of adequate empirical antibiotic therapy on the outcome of patients admitted to the intensive care unit with sepsis. Crit Care Med 31(12):2742–51
32. Micek ST, Isakow W, Shannon W, Kollef MH (2005) Predictors of hospital mortality for patients with severe sepsis treated with Drotrecogin alfa (activated). Pharmacotherapy 25(1):26–34
33. Vyas D, Javadi P, DiPasco PJ, Buchman TG, Hotchkiss RS, Coopersmith CM (2005) Early antibiotic administration but not antibody therapy directed against IL-6 improves survival in septic mice predicted to die on basis of high IL-6 levels. Am J Physiol Regul Integr Comp Physiol 289(4): R1048–53
34. Trzeciak S, Dellinger RP, Abate NL, et al. (2006) Translating research to clinical practice: a 1-year experience with implementing early goal-directed therapy for septic shock in the emergency department. Chest 129(2):225–32
35. Shapiro NI, Howell M, Talmor D (2005) A blueprint for a sepsis protocol. Acad Emerg Med 12(4):352–9
36. Micek ST, Roubinian N, Heuring T, et al. (2006) A before-after study of a standardized hospital order set for the management of septic shock. Crit Care Med (in press)
37. Shapiro NI, Howell MD, Talmor D, et al. (2006) Implementation and outcomes of the Multiple Urgent Sepsis Therapies (MUST) protocol. Crit Care Med 34(4):1025–32
38. Kortgen A, Niederprum P, Bauer M (2006) Implementation of an evidence-based "standard operating procedure" and outcome in septic shock. Crit Care Med 34(4):943–9
39. Gao F, Melody T, Daniels DF, Giles S, Fox S (2005) The impact of compliance with 6-hour and 24-hour sepsis bundles on hospital mortality in patients with severe sepsis: a prospective observational study. Crit Care 9(6):R764–70

Chapter 9

Microbial Surveillance in the Intensive Care Unit 9

S. Blot, P. Depuydt, K. Vandewoude

9.1 Introduction

Nosocomial infections occur approximately three to six times more frequently in patients admitted to ICUs than in patients residing in general wards [1]. The prevalence of nosocomial infection in critically ill patients is about 20%, depending on the type of admission diagnosis and underlying conditions predisposing to microbial colonization and infection [2]. Despite all the efforts taken in infection control, the incidence of nosocomial infection in ICUs has increased over the past 3 decades. There are several reasons for this trend. Together with the widespread use of invasive techniques disrupting the host's anatomical barriers, more patients are receiving immunosuppressive therapy, decreasing humoral and cellular defense against microorganisms. And, thirdly, improved emergency and supportive care has resulted in better acute phase survival, but simultaneously has led to a growing number of long-term ICU residents. All these factors result in a pool of patients extremely vulnerable to nosocomial infection, grouped in units with a high workload and a degree of urgency which results in a suboptimal compliance with standard infection control measures.

Along with the threat of nosocomial infection goes the emergence of antimicrobial resistance [3]. Over time, for most bacterial species, sensitive strains have been replaced by resistant ones, and the patterns of resistance have increased in complexity, often with geographic variability [4]. The onward march of antimicrobial resistance is a major challenge to the adequate treatment of infections in the ICU. Both infections and antimicrobial resistance negatively impact outcome through increased morbidity and mortality. The higher mortality in antimicrobial-resistant infection appears to be mainly due to an increased risk of inappropriate initial antimicrobial therapy, which has been identified as an important predictor for an unfavorable outcome in numerous recent studies [5–7]. Apart from this human cost, resistance imposes an increased health-economic burden due to the additional hospital stay and the higher cost of broad-spectrum antibiotics [8–11].

Several mechanisms are involved in the appearance and spread of multi-drug-resistant (MDR) organisms in the hospital and community. These include: (1) acquisition of resistance by a sensitive strain due to de novo mutation, genetic transfer or overt expression of resistance already present in the population; (2) differential selection of a resistant subpopulation; (3) introduction of a resistant organism in a previously sensitive population; and (4) horizontal transmission of an MDR strain in the hospital. Whereas the first and second mechanisms essentially are driven by selection pressure due to antibiotic use, the last two phenomena can be contained by imposing barrier precautions or the identification of a possible point source of contamination. Timely control of an endemic spread of MDR strains requires early detection by an efficacious microbial surveillance program [12]. As such, microbial ecology data both on a health care facility level (hospital or ICU) and on a larger (community) scale by microbial surveillance have gained importance both for effective treatment of infection and to avoid the advance of antimicrobial resistance.

9.2 Type and Aim of Surveillance Systems

Microbial surveillance in the ICU can be defined as the continual, systematic collection, analysis, and interpretation of microbiological data essential for the planning, implementation, and evaluation of infection control practice either on an individual or a unit level. Site-specific infection density rates can be calculated by using the number of patients at risk, total patient days, days of indwelling urinary catheterization, central venous catheter days, or days on mechanical ventilation. Trends in infection rates are important indicators of quality control and are often used for benchmarking. Microbial surveillance, however, has a larger scope than the – often post hoc – registration of infection rates. While the diagnosis of infection is based on microbiological sampling of clinically relevant sites (e.g., sputum, urine, wounds), examination of the colonization status should take into account nose, mouth and perineum as reservoirs of potentially MDR bacteria. For example, sampling of nose and perineum is rarely significant for diagnosis of infection, but may be of particular value to detect epidemiologically important microorganisms such as, respectively, methicillin-resistant *Staphylococcus aureus* (MRSA), vancomycin-resistant enterococci (VRE) or multiresistant gram-negative strains. A surveillance system that takes into consideration colonization as well as clinically indicated culture samples is a much more powerful tool for infection management and control. In addition to retrospective quality control, routine surveillance allows early detection of outbreaks with epidemiologically important microorganisms and provides data for the appropriate empirical antimicrobial therapy. Conceptually, this should contribute to better individual patient outcomes, as well as to a reduction in antimicrobial selection pressure by selection of agents with a judiciously targeted spectrum of activity. In this chapter the focus is on microbial surveillance and how it can benefit clinical practice, on top of the mere registration of infections.

Three major purposes can be recognized for microbial surveillance in the ICU. Firstly, surveillance is a cornerstone in infection control. Secondly, it can be used to control antimicrobial prescription patterns and therefore as a tool to limit the emergence of resistance. Finally, surveillance cultures can be used to guide empirical antimicrobial therapy. An up-to-date knowledge of locally prevailing antimicrobial drug resistance is an essential prerequisite for an appropriate initial antibiotic selection. Whether surveillance aiming at the colonization status of the individual patient can be used for the individual tailoring of the empirical therapy remains controversial. As the first two objectives are generally accepted and implemented, these are briefly discussed, while more attention is given to the value of surveillance cultures in optimizing empirical therapy.

9.2.1
Active Surveillance To Steer Infection Control

In the hospital, microbial surveillance is a potentially useful tool in tackling the problem of infection caused by MDR bacteria at different levels.

Firstly, microbial surveillance programs to detect contamination of hospital equipment, such as the presence of *Pseudomonas* or *Legionella* species in an aqueous environment (ventilator circuits, tap water, aerosols), should allow early control of this iatrogenic source of infection.

Secondly, microbial surveillance is helpful in the early detection of outbreaks of infection caused by MDR bacteria, after which barrier precautions can be rapidly implemented to limit further spread. The success of this strategy depends both on the quality of the surveillance (i.e., number and sensitivity of surveillance cultures) and on the mechanisms of dispersal of resistance. Thus, MDR pathogens, for which horizontal transmission is the main contributing factor of dissemination, are most likely to be controlled by this strategy. Examples of these are MRSA, *Candida* species and VRE. In contrast, multi-drug resistance acquired by expression of drug resistance coding genes widely dispersed within a microbial species is more likely to be contained by measures aimed to reduce selection pressure by antibiotic restriction. An example is carbapenem resistance in *Acinetobacter* species through expression of carbapenemases [13]. Control of MRSA serves as the best known example of the application of microbial surveillance guiding barrier precautions to dam dispersal [14–17]. It should be noted, however, that several authors reported failure of this strategy to control nosocomial spread of MRSA [18, 19], while others reported relapsing rates of spread after cessation of intensive surveillance [20], and only limited data exist on long-term control in endemic settings. A "search and destroy" strategy, consisting of searches for MRSA carriers coupled with attempts at decolonization, e.g., by applying nasal mupirocin, is the subject of ongoing controversy [21].

It has become apparent that endemicity for MDR strains such as MRSA in the hospital environment is maintained to a certain extent by a steady influx of colonized patients (the infection often previously acquired in health care related settings). In such endemic settings, screening at admission should be considered in patients referred from other hospitals or long-term care facilities, or after previous exposure to antibiotics such as fluoroquinolones, which are known risk factors for harbouring MDR strains [22]. Early identification of colonization by MRSA could allow prevention of spread in the hospital by strict barrier precautions. On a larger scale, countries with a very low to sporadic prevalence of MRSA, such as the Netherlands and Denmark, so far seem to have effectively used screening of patients referred from abroad as a barrier to keep the MRSA problem outside their hospitals.

Similarly and more recently, VRE infection control has received considerable attention, with several studies highlighting the potential as well as the limitations of microbial surveillance guided barrier precautions in containing VRE dissemination. For example, a new occurrence of VRE in an Italian ICU invoked an active surveillance program directing the intensification of infection control measures with successful control of further dispersal [23]. Even when endemicity has been established, an active surveillance program combined with contact precautions has been shown to effectively limit spread of VRE [24]. It should be noticed that the great majority of patients colonized with VRE are detected by surveillance cultures and go undetected by routine clinical cultures [24, 25], although even an active surveillance program may still miss a significant number of cases [26]. Otherwise, surveillance and barrier precautions can be impracticable in regions of high prevalence of asymptomatic VRE carriers (such as many parts of Europe); an alternative approach is to target barrier precautions on epidemic strains of VRE identified by molecular typing [27].

Finally, microbial surveillance appears to be a useful monitoring tool to assess the impact of educational infection control programs implemented in order to prevent the spread of resistance or particular types of nosocomial infection such as catheter-related bacteremia or ventilator-associated pneumonia [28–30].

9.2.2 Controlling the Advance of Resistance

As excessive antibiotic use is a major culprit for the ever increasing emergence of antibiotic resistance, microbial surveillance should not be limited to the microbial flora but should also focus on antimicrobial prescription, enabling detection of trends in antibiotic prescription. Simultaneous monitoring of both local microbial ecology and antimicrobial use may provide insights into the ever changing dynamics of resistance. In this way the impact of antimicrobial policies such as selective digestive decontamination, antibiotic cycling, formulary-based restrictions and de-escalation strategies can be prospectively evaluated [31–33]. An example of this is provided by a recent study in which restriction of fluoroquinolone use in one of four teaching hospitals resulted in a 20% reduction of MRSA isolation in routine clinical samples, as compared to the three hospitals that served as a control; however, due to increased use of cephalosporins, an increased number of infections with extended-beta lactamase producing Enterobacteriaceae was noticed [34]. Retrospectively, pattern recognition in epidemiology of resistance could allow the linking of trends to changing practice in antimicrobial prescription. While these surveillance systems provide valuable information for evaluating and guiding antibiotic policies, real time monitoring antibiotic prescription on the scale of the individual ICU may directly impact clinical practice. Thus, surveillance of antibiotic treatment by an infectious diseases consultant or a clinical pharmacist could avoid or limit inappropriate or inadvertent prolonged use of broad spectrum antimicrobials [35]. Furthermore, a policy of antibiotic restriction limits the emergence of fungal overgrowth, resulting in unnecessary prescription of antifungals [36].

9.2.3 Surveillance Cultures as a Guide for Empirical Antimicrobial Therapy

At the community level, microbial surveillance, through the collection of data from several ICUs over a geographic region, is important for charting and monitoring the dispersal of newly emerging MDR strains (such as VRE, penicillin-resistant *Streptococcus pneumoniae* and *Staphylococcus aureus* with intermediate vancomycin susceptibility). This surveillance provides vital information on which to base treatment policies, and by which to assess their effectiveness. Information obtained from surveillance should be used to regularly update local guidelines for empirical antibiotic therapy in community-acquired as well as nosocomial infection.

In severe infection such as nosocomial pneumonia and bloodstream infection, the odds on a favorable outcome by antimicrobial therapy are largest during the first hours or days of the clinical syndrome, and rapidly decline thereafter; therefore initial therapy must be chosen on an empirical basis, since the microbiological results of diagnostic cultures become available not until after 24–48 h [5–7].

Increasing antimicrobial resistance has driven the development of new strategies to maximize the likelihood of appropriate initial antimicrobial therapy without falling into an indistinct and undue use of broad spectrum drugs. In the example of ventilator-associated pneumonia, it has been acknowledged since the landmark paper of Trouillet et al. that clinical risk factors, such as a prolonged intubation of >1 week and prior antibiotic exposure, increase the risk of infection caused by MDR microorganisms and subsequently should trigger the institution of a larger spectrum antibiotic [37]. However, it has since been observed that the locally prevailing microbial ecology is to a large extent indicative for the etiology in ventilator-associated pneumonia (VAP), with 'overruling' of the clinical risk profile in local circumstances of high MDR endemicity [38]. As a consequence, general literature based guidelines about empirical therapy in severe infection such as hospital-acquired pneumonia should be translated into local surveillance based guidelines.

To take this concept one step further, an intriguing strategy is to target empirical antibiotic therapy according to colonization status of the individual patient. Knowledge of colonization or previous infection with an MDR strain should be taken into account in empirical antibiotic choice, but otherwise the issue is whether a systematic screening of ICU patients for MDR colonization could be predictive for the microbial etiology of the infectious episode. Two earlier studies failed to identify a significant predictive value of colonization status for the etiology of subsequent infection, in casu

VAP. In the pioneering study of Hayon et al., colonization cultures predicted VAP etiology in only one-third to two-thirds of the cases and the subsequent study of Bouza et al. in cardiosurgical patients found only one episode of pneumonia caused by a prior identified pathogen [39, 40]. Both studies, however, had a low sampling frequency, and part of the poor prediction may be due to the lengthy intervals between surveillance cultures and subsequent infection, precluding the detection of relevant changes in microbial colonization. Interestingly, three recent publications have boosted interest in individual patient surveillance. Firstly, Blot et al. found in a retrospective study of bacteremia caused by MDR gram-negative bacilli that prediction of the bacteremic pathogen in surveillance cultures (of any site) was associated with significantly more appropriate antibiotic therapy within the first 24 h as well as 48 h following bacteremia [41]. In a subsequent study, the authors observed a significant contribution of surveillance cultures to an adequate early antibiotic therapy in a subgroup of patients at risk for VAP caused by MDR bacteria [42]. Secondly, a remarkably high predictive value of tracheal surveillance cultures on the etiology of subsequent, microbiologically proven, VAP was observed in a French study [43]. Finally, surface cultures predicted catheter colonization and infection with an accuracy of 71% and 66% respectively in a recent study by Bouza et al. [44].

The major limitation of a surveillance strategy to anticipate individual infectious etiology is the cost and workload imposed, since frequent sampling is mandatory. In the study of Bouza for example, 3,712 surface cultures were necessary to anticipate 15 catheter infections in 130 patients. The cost-effectiveness of such a policy should be addressed in a randomized controlled trial. In a multicenter approach, such a design would be hampered by the variability of ecology and resistance patterns between participating centers, whereas in a single center setting, it may be ethically unacceptable to blind the treating physician in the control, 'non-surveillance' arm for the results of surveillance cultures in the active, 'surveillance' arm. As surveillance is primarily detected at early identification of MDR colonization, one can expect that the cost-benefit ratio can be most relevant in health care settings with a high risk of the acquisition of an MDR ecology, i.e., tertiary ICUs with high endemicity of such strains, or alternatively within subsets of patients at the highest risk for infection caused by MDR bacteria.

9.3 Conclusion

Microbial surveillance contributes to control of the spread of nosocomial infections and MDR microorganisms in particular. Routine surveillance allows early detection of MDR outbreaks. It also permits the evaluation of the impact of antibiotic strategies or infection control measures on local endemicity of MDR problem pathogens or on more subtle trends in microbial ecology. Microbial surveillance can also be mentioned as a promising tool to guide empirical antimicrobial therapy, based upon up-to-date information on both local ecology and individual colonization status. The value of routine surveillance strongly depends on the sampling frequency of cultures. However, the cost-benefit ratio of frequent sampling is questionable, even in high risk patient populations such as the critically ill. Therefore, the potential benefit of a surveillance strategy can be commensurate with the incidence of the more difficult-to-treat MDR infections.

References

1. Daschner F (1985) Nosocomial infections in intensive care units. Intensive Care Med 11:284–287
2. Vincent JL, Bihari DJ, Suter PM, et al. (1995) The prevalence of nosocomial infection in intensive care units in Europe. Results of the European Prevalence of Infection in Intensive Care (EPIC) Study. EPIC International Advisory Committee. JAMA 274:639–644
3. Schaberg DR, Culver DH, Gaynes RP (1991) Major trends in the microbial etiology of nosocomial infection. Am J Med 91:72S–75S
4. Hanberger H, Diekema D, Fluit A, et al. (2001) Surveillance of antibiotic resistance in European ICUs. J Hosp Infect 48:161–176
5. Kollef M (2003) Appropriate empirical antibacterial therapy for nosocomial infections: getting it right the first time. Drugs 63:2157–2168
6. Blot SI, Vandewoude KH, Hoste EA, Colardyn FA (2002) Effects of nosocomial candidemia on outcomes of critically ill patients. Am J Med 113:480–485
7. Harbarth S, Garbino J, Pugin J, Romand JA, Lew D, Pittet D (2003) Inappropriate initial antimicrobial therapy and its effect on survival in a clinical trial of immunomodulating therapy for severe sepsis. Am J Med 115:529–535
8. Blot SI, Depuydt P, Annemans L, et al. (2005) Clinical and economic outcomes in critically ill patients with nosocomial catheter-related bloodstream infections. Clin Infect Dis 41:1591–1598
9. Carmeli Y, Eliopoulos G, Mozaffari E, Samore M (2002) Health and economic outcomes of vancomycin-resistant enterococci. Arch Intern Med 162:2223–2228
10. Carmeli Y, Troillet N, Karchmer AW, Samore MH (1999) Health and economic outcomes of antibiotic resistance in *Pseudomonas aeruginosa*. Arch Intern Med 159:1127–1132
11. Niederman MS (2001) Impact of antibiotic resistance on clinical outcomes and the cost of care. Crit Care Med 29:N114–120
12. Bonten MJ, Mascini EM (2003) The hidden faces of the epidemiology of antibiotic resistance. Intensive Care Med 29:1–2
13. Pournaras S, Markogiannakis A, Ikonomidis A, et al. (2006) Outbreak of multiple clones of imipenem-resistant *Acinetobacter baumannii* isolates expressing OXA-58 carbapenemase in an intensive care unit. J Antimicrob Chemother 57:557–561

14. Jernigan JA, Clemence MA, Stott GA, et al. (1995) Control of methicillin-resistant *Staphylococcus aureus* at a university hospital: one decade later. Infect Control Hosp Epidemiol 16:686–696
15. Boyce JM (1995) Strategies for controlling methicillin-resistant *Staphylococcus aureus* in hospitals. J Chemother 7 Suppl 3:81–85
16. Garner JS (1996) Guideline for isolation precautions in hospitals. The Hospital Infection Control Practices Advisory Committee. Infect Control Hosp Epidemiol 17:53–80
17. Hartstein AI, Denny MA, Morthland VH, LeMonte AM, Pfaller MA (1995) Control of methicillin-resistant *Staphylococcus aureus* in a hospital and an intensive care unit. Infect Control Hosp Epidemiol 16:405–411
18. Zafar AB, Butler RC, Reese DJ, Gaydos LA, Mennonna PA (1995) Use of 0.3% triclosan (Bacti-Stat) to eradicate an outbreak of methicillin-resistant *Staphylococcus aureus* in a neonatal nursery. Am J Infect Control 23:200–208
19. Rao N, Jacobs S, Joyce L (1988) Cost-effective eradication of an outbreak of methicillin-resistant *Staphylococcus aureus* in a community teaching hospital. Infect Control Hosp Epidemiol 9:255–260
20. Back NA, Linnemann CC, Jr, Staneck JL, Kotagal UR (1996) Control of methicillin-resistant *Staphylococcus aureus* in a neonatal intensive-care unit: use of intensive microbiologic surveillance and mupirocin. Infect Control Hosp Epidemiol 17:227–231
21. Herwaldt LA (1999) Control of methicillin-resistant *Staphylococcus aureus* in the hospital setting. Am J Med 106:11S-18S; discussion 48S–52S
22. Garau J, Xercavins M, Rodriguez-Carballeira M, et al. (1999) Emergence and dissemination of quinolone-resistant *Escherichia coli* in the community. Antimicrob Agents Chemother 43:2736–2741
23. Peta M, Carretto E, Barbarini D, et al. (2006) Outbreak of vancomycin-resistant *Enterococcus* spp. in an Italian general intensive care unit. Clin Microbiol Infect 12:163–169
24. Calfee DP, Giannetta ET, Durbin LJ, Germanson TP, Farr BM (2003) Control of endemic vancomycin-resistant Enterococcus among inpatients at a university hospital. Clin Infect Dis 37:326–332
25. Ostrowsky BE, Venkataraman L, D'Agata EM, Gold HS, DeGirolami PC, Samore MH (1999) Vancomycin-resistant enterococci in intensive care units: high frequency of stool carriage during a non-outbreak period. Arch Intern Med 159:1467–1472
26. D'Agata EM, Gautam S, Green WK, Tang YW (2002) High rate of false-negative results of the rectal swab culture method in detection of gastrointestinal colonization with vancomycin-resistant enterococci. Clin Infect Dis 34:167–172
27. Mascini EM, Troelstra A, Beitsma M, et al. (2006) Genotyping and preemptive isolation to control an outbreak of vancomycin-resistant *Enterococcus faecium*. Clin Infect Dis 42:739–746
28. Walder B, Pittet D, Tramer MR (2002) Prevention of bloodstream infections with central venous catheters treated with anti-infective agents depends on catheter type and insertion time: evidence from a meta-analysis. Infect Control Hosp Epidemiol 23:748–756
29. Eggimann P, Pittet D (2002) Overview of catheter-related infections with special emphasis on prevention based on educational programs. Clin Microbiol Infect 8:295–309
30. Safdar N, Crnich CJ, Maki DG (2005) The pathogenesis of ventilator-associated pneumonia: its relevance to developing effective strategies for prevention. Respir Care 50:725–739; discussion 739–741
31. Colardyn F (2005) Appropriate and timely empirical antimicrobial treatment of ICU infections – a role for carbapenems. Acta Clin Belg 60:51–62
32. Rello J, Vidaur L, Sandiumenge A, et al. (2004) De-escalation therapy in ventilator-associated pneumonia. Crit Care Med 32:2183–2190
33. Merz LR, Warren DK, Kollef MH, Fraser VJ (2004) Effects of an antibiotic cycling program on antibiotic prescribing practices in an intensive care unit. Antimicrob Agents Chemother 48:2861–2865
34. Charbonneau P, Parienti JJ, Thibon P, et al. (2006) Fluoroquinolone use and methicillin-resistant *Staphylococcus aureus* isolation rates in hospitalized patients: a quasi experimental study. Clin Infect Dis 42:778–784
35. Lemmen SW, Becker G, Frank U, Daschner FD (2001) Influence of an infectious disease consulting service on quality and costs of antibiotic prescriptions in a university hospital. Scand J Infect Dis 33:219–221
36. Blot S, Vandewoude K (2004) Management of invasive candidiasis in critically ill patients. Drugs 64:2159–2175
37. Trouillet JL, Chastre J, Vuagnat A, et al. (1998) Ventilator-associated pneumonia caused by potentially drug-resistant bacteria. Am J Respir Crit Care Med 157:531–539
38. Rello J, Sa-Borges M, Correa H, Leal SR, Baraibar J (1999) Variations in etiology of ventilator-associated pneumonia across four treatment sites: implications for antimicrobial prescribing practices. Am J Respir Crit Care Med 160:608–613
39. Bouza E, Perez A, Munoz P, et al. (2003) Ventilator-associated pneumonia after heart surgery: a prospective analysis and the value of surveillance. Crit Care Med 31:1964–1970
40. Hayon J, Figliolini C, Combes A, et al. (2002) Role of serial routine microbiologic culture results in the initial management of ventilator-associated pneumonia. Am J Respir Crit Care Med 165:41–46
41. Blot S, Depuydt P, Vogelaers D, et al. (2005) Colonization status and appropriate antibiotic therapy for nosocomial bacteremia caused by antibiotic-resistant gram-negative bacteria in an intensive care unit. Infect Control Hosp Epidemiol 26:575–579
42. Depuydt PO, Blot SI, Benoit DD, et al. (2006) Antimicrobial resistance in nosocomial bloodstream infection associated with pneumonia and the value of systematic surveillance cultures in an adult intensive care unit. Crit Care Med 34:653–659
43. Michel F, Franceschini B, Berger P, et al. (2005) Early antibiotic treatment for BAL-confirmed ventilator-associated pneumonia: a role for routine endotracheal aspirate cultures. Chest 127:589–597
44. Bouza E, Munoz P, Burillo A, et al. (2005) The challenge of anticipating catheter tip colonization in major heart surgery patients in the intensive care unit: are surface cultures useful? Crit Care Med 33:1953–1960

Use of Anti-infective Therapy in Critically Ill Patients

II

Chapter 10

Antimicrobial Prophylaxis in the Intensive Care Unit

10

A.M. Bal, I.M. Gould

Patients in intensive care units (ICUs) are at high risk of developing nosocomial infections. These include nosocomial respiratory infections that are usually ventilator acquired, urinary tract infections secondary to catheterization and bloodstream infections secondary to line colonization. Infections in intensive care lead to significant morbidity and mortality. As most of these infections, particularly if acquired after more than 48 h stay in the hospital, are caused by hospital acquired organisms resistant to commonly used antibiotics, their treatment is expensive, prolonged and carries the risk of adverse effects. Hence, prevention of hospital-acquired infections in intensive care settings is extremely important. If effective, such measures have the potential to prevent mortality and morbidity, prevent the spread of infections from one patient to another, decrease the risk of emergence of drug resistant organisms by limiting the use of antibiotics for therapeutic purposes, lead to fewer days of stay in the intensive care and decrease cost. This review summarizes antibiotic and antifungal prophylaxis in intensive care settings.

In general, although antibiotic prophylaxis is always tempting, there are very few well-established indications for it outwith the perioperative situation. In particular, the use of any regimen that adds to the already established burden of intensive therapeutic use has to be viewed with extreme caution. In this context it may well be useful to differentiate short-term use for cessation of outbreaks [such as methicillin-resistant *Staphylococcus aureus* (MRSA) or extended spectrum β lactamase (ESBL) producing gram negative bacilli] from prevention of the inevitable sporadic infection that occurs in all ICUs. The former is outwith the scope of this chapter.

10.1 Ventilator-Associated Pneumonia

Nosocomial pneumonia accounts for the vast majority of deaths due to nosocomial infections. Mortality rates are particularly high for ventilator-associated pneumonia (VAP). By definition, nosocomial pneumonias are caused by organisms not present or not incubating at the time of hospital admission. Pneumonia usually develops more than 48–72 h after hospital admission. The etiology of VAP depends upon the type of disease: mild, moderate, or severe, presence or absence of risk factors and the time of onset of pneumonia. Box 10.1 lists the common causative organisms of VAP.

Guidelines for empirical antibiotic therapy have been formulated keeping in mind the target organisms mentioned in the table and their predicted antibiotic susceptibility patterns. Prophylactic regimes for pneumonia have also used antibiotics that are broadly active against this group of microorganisms especially those that are associated with pneumonia early in the intensive care stay. The value of antibiotic regimens for prevention of pneumonia has however been debated. Prophylactic strategies take into account the pathogenesis of VAP.

Nosocomial pneumonias most commonly develop as a result of microaspiration of oropharyngeal secretions. In patients who are intubated, secretions pool around the cuff of the endotracheal tube. These secretions make their way to the lower respiratory tract as a result of alterations in the diameter of the airway lumen. Consequently, most prophylactic regimes have targeted decolonization of the upper airway with the use of topical antibiotics. These have included oral paste, oral suspensions and, sometimes, nebulized antibiotics.

In some patients, aspiration of gastric secretions may lead to aspiration pneumonia. Organisms that col-

Box 10.1. Causative organisms of hospital acquired pneumonia.

Causative organisms
S. aureus
MRSA
Streptococcus pneumoniae
Hemophilus influenzae
Klebsiella pneumoniae
Klebsiella spp.
Enterobacter cloacae
Enterobacter spp.
Pseudomonas aeruginosa
Acinetobacter
Stenotrophomonas maltophilia
Burkholderia cepacia

onize the stomach can potentially lead to pneumonia if they find their way into the alveoli as a result of aspiration. However, the gastric reservoir hypothesis has not been universally accepted. Isolates from gastric secretion have rarely been found to cause pneumonia. Nevertheless, selective digestive decontamination (SDD) of the upper gastrointestinal tract has been used to eradicate microorganisms in the stomach.

A third route of infection in the lungs is haematogenous dissemination from distant sources of infection such as the urinary tract. Prophylaxis for infections acquired through this route target the initial focus of infection.

The Centers for Disease Control and Prevention and Healthcare Infection Control Practices Advisory Committee recommends several measures for prevention of health care associated pneumonia [1]. The broad categories include staff education, microbiological surveillance, prevention of transmission of organisms and modifying the risk factors associated with infections. Unfortunately, no definitive recommendations could be made about systemic antimicrobial prophylaxis as the issue remains unresolved. The two main routes for antibiotic intervention are parenteral and topical. The latter is aimed at decontaminating the digestive tract that is thought to be the source of most infections.

Sirvent and colleagues [2] carried out a randomized controlled clinical trial to study the efficacy of antimicrobial prophylaxis for the prevention of VAP in patients with head injury requiring more than 72 h of ventilation. Fifty patients in the study group received two 1.5-g doses of intravenous cefuroxime 12 h apart while 50 patients in the control group did not receive cefuroxime. Twelve patients in the study group and 25 patients in the control group developed pneumonia and the difference was statistically significant. However, there was no overall difference in mortality between the two groups. In another prospective trial, Krueger and colleagues [3] studied the usefulness of antibiotic prophylaxis with intravenous ciprofloxacin and topical gentamicin and polymyxin applied to the nostrils, mouth and stomach in intensive care patients. Patients were randomized to receive either the antibiotics or placebo. The incidence of pneumonia was significantly lower in the antibiotic group as compared to the placebo group. Although the overall mortality in the two groups was not different, significantly fewer patients with the acute physiology and chronic health evaluation (APACHE) score between 20 and 29 in the antibiotic group died. However, the patients with these mid-range APACHE scores were not randomized at study entry and hence the study was not specifically designed to test the role of antibiotic intervention in this subset. In contrast to the two reports, de La Cal et al. [4] reported a significant reduction not only in the incidence of pneumonia but also in mortality rates (9.4% in patients receiving SDD compared to 27.8% in those receiving placebo) in critically ill burn patients who were treated for SDD. The predominant finding of this study was a reduction in the incidence of primary endogenous pneumonia. The median time of onset of primary endogenous pneumonia was 3 days and it appeared to coincide with the sharp fall in survival rates for patients on placebo. However, the use of broad-spectrum antibiotics for reasons other than treating pneumonia could have affected the outcome of this study.

Several reports showing a favourable trend in reducing the rates of infection associated with the use of topical antibiotics have been published. Silvestri et al. [5] studied the usefulness of oral vancomycin gel for the prevention of MRSA pneumonia. Patients who received oral vancomycin had a reduced incidence of secondary lower respiratory tract infection with MRSA. However, the number of patients in this study was relatively small, 42 in each group. Pugin and colleagues [6] reported a beneficial effect of oropharyngeal decontamination with topical polymyxin, neomycin and vancomycin as compared to placebo in decreasing the incidence of VAP by a factor of 5 without an effect on overall mortality. Similar observations were made by Bergmans and colleagues [7]. Using topical gentamicin, colistin and vancomycin for oropharyngeal decolonization, they found a beneficial effect in eradicating colonization of the oropharynx in the antibiotic group as compared to the placebo group and a second control group that did not receive any topical medication or placebo. However, mortality was not affected.

Liberati et al. [8] did a meta-analysis on the efficacy of topical antibiotics and efficacy of a combination of topical and systemic antibiotics. Seventeen trials were included in each of the two groups. The authors concluded that a combination of topical and systemic antibiotics led to a reduction in the incidence of pneumonia and a significant decrease in mortality rates attributable to pneumonia while the use of topical antibiotics reduced the incidence of pneumonia but did not affect mortality. Safdar and colleagues [9] did a meta-analysis to ascertain the use of SDD in liver transplant patients and found that although the incidence of gram negative infections was reduced, there was little change in the overall incidence of infection and no reduction in mortality. In another recently published review [10], it was suggested that SDD lowers mortality in settings where MRSA and VRE are not endemic but should be considered experimental in areas where these infections are prevalent.

Another method of antibiotic delivery is administration of the drug via a nebulizer with the aim of preventing biofilm formation in the lumen of the endotracheal tube. Adair et al. [11] compared nebulized gentamicin with parenteral cefotaxime or cefuroxime for prevention of biofilm formation. Each of the three groups comprised 12 patients. Microbial biofilms of common pathogens including *Staphylococcus aureus*, enterococci, Enterobacteriaceae and *Pseudomonas* species and related organisms were found on seven endotracheal tubes in the cefotaxime group and eight in the cefuroxime group. None of the biofilms in the gentamicin group contained these organisms. The authors suggested that by preventing the formation of biofilms, nebulized gentamicin might be beneficial in prevention of nosocomial pneumonia. However, there was no direct evidence to establish any clinically significant association between decreased incidence of pneumonia and the use of nebulized gentamicin. The numbers compared also appear to be small.

Prophylactic use of antibiotics for a prolonged period could however be harmful. In a retrospective study carried out by Hoth and colleagues [12], use of prophylactic antibiotics for more than 48 h was associated with later diagnosis of the first episode of pneumonia, a higher incidence of infection with resistant gram-negative organisms and a higher likelihood of antibiotic related complications.

General recommendations for antibiotic prophylaxis have therefore been difficult. Reports have often been contradictory and this could be due to differences in clinical settings, local differences in organisms and their susceptibility profiles, and the nature of the study designs. At the same time, one should acknowledge the difficulty in designing such studies involving patients who are critically ill and have a variety of illnesses ranging in severity. Many such patients may need antibiotic intervention for reasons other than prophylaxis and this could have an effect on the outcome. Moreover, there is a possibility of a reporting bias wherein only those studies that show a beneficial trend get reported. Notably, benefits in prevention of pneumonia did not translate into benefits in terms of overall survival in most reports in the literature. However, prophylaxis could be beneficial in a small subgroup of patients as suggested in Krueger's report [3] and more studies are needed to identify such groups. In absence of reports showing clear benefits, it is difficult to formulate guidelines as regards prophylactic strategies for the prevention of pneumonia. These drawbacks cited above were acknowledged in the guidelines on the management of hospital-acquired pneumonia formulated by the joint committee of the American Thoracic Society and Infectious Diseases Society of America [13]. These guidelines do not recommend the routine use of systemic antibiotics for the purpose of prophylaxis until more data become available. Routine use of oral antibiotics for SDD was also discouraged particularly in settings with a high incidence of multidrug resistant pathogens. Others [14] have criticized this latter verdict quoting reports from various ICUs including those where the use of SDD helped eradicate ESBL producing strains of *Klebsiella pneumoniae* [15, 16].

Amidst the controversies, it is well known that ICUs are genesis units for new antimicrobial resistant pathogens with implications for the whole hospital. The initial selection of multiresistant strain is due to the intense high antibiotic use seen in most intensive units. In this context a word of caution; the European strategy for antibiotic prophylaxis survey of antibiotic use in European ICUs showed that those units with the highest antibiotic use were those that routinely used SDD (D. Monnet, personal communication). We therefore feel that routine use of SDD should be avoided until more robust evidence based data are available.

10.2 Catheter Related Urinary Tract Infections

Urinary tract infections secondary to catheter placements are the commonest nosocomial infections encountered. Such infections can lead to bacteraemia that can then seed other organ systems. The two main objectives of prophylactic strategies to prevent catheter associated urinary tract infections are:

1. Prevention of bacteriuria
2. Prevention of complications of bacteriuria

Antimicrobial prophylaxis involves:

1. Use of catheters impregnated with antimicrobial agents
2. Use of topical antimicrobial agents in the urinary tract
3. Use of parenteral antibiotics

The use of silver impregnated catheters has been a matter of debate. While some studies have shown favourable trends in the incidence of urinary tract infections, others have failed to show a beneficial effect. Bologna et al. [17] reported no significant difference between standard latex catheters and those impregnated with silver agents. In the study reported by Riley and colleagues [18], the rate of bacteriuria was 11.4% in the study group compared with 12.9% in the control group. Staphylococcal infections were higher in patients who had a silver impregnated catheter in place. Other studies have reported significantly lower rates of infections with the use of silver catheters but this has not been a consistent finding in intensive care patients. Hence, use of such catheters is not routinely recommended. Catheters impregnated with rifampicin and minocycline have also been used to prevent the occurrence of urinary tract infection. Darouiche and colleagues [19] conducted a trial on patients undergoing radical prostatectomy. Patients were randomized to receive a silicone catheter (control group) or a silicone catheter impregnated with rifampicin and minocycline. At day 7 and day 14, patients in the study group had a significantly lower incidence of bacteriuria than those in the control group. Johnson, Kuskowski and Wilt [20] recently published the results of their systematic review on the use of bladder catheters impregnated with antimicrobials and concluded that such catheters can prevent bacteriuria for a short duration. A comparison between the individual trials found large variability in the magnitude of beneficial outcome.

The commonest route of entry of organisms in the catheterized urinary tract is the space between the urethral mucosa and the catheter. Use of topical agents should theoretically decrease the risk of acquiring infections through this route. In practice, however, this effect has not been demonstrated and, in fact, has been associated with an increased risk of infection. In a randomized trial, Huth and colleagues [21] demonstrated that application of silver sulfadiazine to the urethral meatus had no significant effect on the rate of bacteriuria.

Patients often receive antibiotics for various other reasons and this fact can diminish the chances of urinary tract infection at least in the first few days of catheterization. In general, use of any antimicrobial agent solely for the purpose of preventing bacteriuria should be discouraged as it is of unproven benefit and will inevitably lead to the emergence of resistant organisms.

10.3 Bloodstream Infections

Bacteraemia in patients in intensive care is usually secondary to a primary source of infection, most frequently, intravascular catheters. Catheter related bacteraemia has mortality in the range of 12–25% for each episode [22]. Various prophylactic strategies have been used to decrease the incidence of catheter-associated bacteraemia. The three widely used strategies include:

1. Use of antiseptic dressings applied on the catheter insertion site designed to prevent the colonization of the catheter by the organisms colonizing the skin at the insertion site
2. Use of prophylactic antibiotic into the lumen of the catheter as line locks
3. Use of intravascular catheters impregnated with antiseptic or antibiotics

Antiseptic impregnated dressings have been used to prevent colonization of the catheters but conflicting reports exist as regards their efficacy. In a paediatric cardiac intensive care setting, patients were randomized to receive a transparent polyurethane insertion site dressing (control group, $N=71$) or a chlorhexidine gluconate-impregnated sponge dressing covered by transparent polyurethane dressing (study group, $N=74$). While the rate of catheter colonization was decreased in the study group, the rate of bloodstream infection was not different between the two groups [23]. An important variable that could affect the outcome is the site of catheter placement. Mimoz and colleagues [24] evaluated the efficacy of chlorhexidine gluconate-benzalkonium chloride-benzyl alcohol solution (CBBS) with a 10% solution of povidone-iodine. The CBBS was more effective than povidone-iodine in reducing the incidence of central venous catheter induced sepsis but there was no difference in the incidence of sepsis due to arterial catheters.

A number of studies have assessed the use of antiseptic or antibiotic impregnated catheters in decreasing the incidence of bacteraemia. Osma and colleagues [25] recently reported the data on use of impregnated catheters in critically ill patients. One hundred and thirty-three patients were randomly chosen to receive a standard triple lumen catheter ($N=69$) or a catheter impregnated with chlorhexidine and silver sulfadiazine ($N=64$). The mean duration of catheter insertion was 8.9 and 11.7 days respectively. At the time of removal, 14 catheters in each group were found to be colonized. Four cases of bloodstream infection were detected in the antiseptic impregnated catheter group and one case in standard catheter group. No evidence of benefit was thus detected in this study. Others have shown a beneficial effect of chlorhexidine and silver sulfadiazine-impregnated catheters. Maki et al. [26] showed that these catheters were less likely to be colonized and 5 times less likely to give rise to bloodstream infections. The differences in observations could be due to the length of time for which the catheters were placed in situ. While the median duration of catheter placement was more than 7 days in the study carried out by Osma et al., the average duration of catheterization was only 6 days in Maki's study. A meta-analysis has shown that the decrease in the risk of bloodstream infection secondary to the use of catheters impregnated with antimicrobial agents is only seen for the first week after catheter placement. If used for longer duration, there is no data to suggest any benefit [27].

In patients who need long term vascular access, tunnelling of catheters has been a standard practice to reduce the rate of catheter sepsis. Darouiche and colleagues [28] compared the strategy of catheter tunnelling with the use of antibiotic-impregnated vascular device in patients requiring long-term access. The likelihood of colonization was the same in the two groups of patients and bloodstream infection was less likely in the antibiotic-impregnated catheter group. However, because the antibiotic-impregnated catheters were in place for a shorter length of time than the tunnelled catheters (mean duration 30.2 vs. 43.8 days), a direct evaluation of the long-term efficacy of impregnated catheters in decreasing the risk of colonization or infection was not possible.

In another study done in Spain, 228 patients were randomized to receive rifampicin and minocycline impregnated catheters and 237 patients received non-impregnated catheters. Cultures were taken from skin at the site of catheter insertion, catheter tip, subcutaneous segment, catheter hub, peripheral blood and infusate. The outcome measures included catheter related bloodstream infection (CRBSI) and infection related complications such as pus at the site of insertion. The infection related complications decreased from 8.6 to 5.7 per 1,000 catheter days while CRBSI rate decreased from 5.9 to 3.1, thus showing a favourable trend with the use of impregnated catheters. The rate of catheter tip colonization was 24 in the control group and 10.4 in the antibiotic impregnated group. However, an increase in colonization with *Candida* species was observed in the latter group. The 30-day mortality was not found to be different [29].

In a study that compared the use of chlorhexidine and silver sulfadiazine impregnated catheters with rifampicin and minocycline impregnated catheters, catheter colonization was three times less likely and CRBSIs were 12 times less likely in the latter group [30]. The use of rifampicin and minocycline impregnated catheters has also been found to be cost effective [31]. The decrease in cost has been calculated to be equal to $196 per chlorhexidine catheter used [32].

Garland et al. [33] conducted a prospective, double-blind randomized trial to assess the benefits of using vancomycin line locks in critically ill neonates with newly placed central lines. The infants were randomized to receive either vancomycin line locks or saline locks 2–3 times daily. Two out of 42 patients in the vancomycin group and 13 out of 43 in the control group developed CRBSI. The difference was significant and no cases of vancomycin resistant staphylococci or enterococci were recorded. The use of vancomycin-ciprofloxacin-heparin and vancomycin-heparin line locks was compared to heparin line locks alone in a group of immunocompromised children [34]. The use of antibiotic containing solutions significantly reduced the complications associated with tunnelled lines.

However, there are a number of problems associated with inferring data from these studies and making recommendations. McConnell and colleagues [35] did a systematic analysis of the reports suggesting reduced risk of infection associated with the use of antibiotic impregnated catheters. The authors found several flaws relating to study design. These included inconsistent definitions, confounding factors (such as allowance for exchange of catheters over a guide wire or use of therapeutic antibiotics through the catheters), inadequate statistical methods and lack of clinically relevant endpoints such as overall mortality. Other drawbacks of impregnated catheters are the risk of adverse effect due to the antimicrobial agents. Lupus like syndrome has been reported due to the use of minocycline [36]. A case of anaphylactic shock has also been reported following the use of such catheters [37]. Emergence of resistance to rifampicin and minocycline secondary to their use in catheters has also been a matter of concern [35] though direct evidence to this effect is lacking. The strategy of using antibiotic line locks is usually discouraged because of the risk of acquiring resistant organisms. Line locks can be used with some justification in special situations such as in patients who experience frequent episodes of catheter related bloodstream infections and must have the line in place.

At present, there is not enough evidence to support routine use of impregnated catheters or line locks for prevention of CRBSIs. Although in theory the principle is attractive, its use has not been convincingly demonstrated. Until supported by unequivocal evidence, we feel it is premature to use such catheters routinely given the fact that there is a definite chance of emergence of drug resistant organisms and selection of organisms that are less susceptible to the agents used for impregnating the catheters. They definitely should not be used where the catheter is expected to be in place for less than one week.

10.4 Antifungal Prophylaxis

Invasive fungal infections are a significant cause of morbidity and mortality in patients in ICUs. Because of high mortality, fewer therapeutic options and lack of adequate data showing benefits of treatment, prevention of fungal infections should be considered important. The usual source of fungal bloodstream infections is colonization of central venous catheters with yeasts, and in many cases removal of the lines following colonization would prevent subsequent infection. Host associated risk factors for invasive fungal infections include diabetes mellitus, use of total parenteral nutrition, haemodialysis, prior use of broad-spectrum antibiotics [38], recurrent gastrointestinal tract perforations and acute pancreatitis [39]. The azole group of antifungal agents are commonly used for prophylaxis in critically ill patients. Both fluconazole and itraconazole have been reported to decrease the incidence of fungal colonization and infection and decrease the mortality attributed to fungal infection. However, effects on the overall mortality are questionable [40]. The newer antifungal agents including the newer azoles and echinocandins may prove to be useful in the future [41]. In a meta-analysis of trials reported by Cruciani et al. [42], prophylaxis with ketoconazole or fluconazole was associated with reduced incidence of candidaemia, reduced attributable mortality due to fungal infections and also reduced overall mortality. However, it is often difficult to distinguish fungal colonization from fungal infection and, as a result, the outcome could not be ascertained with certainty.

Petri and colleagues [43] reported a prospective epidemiological study of invasive fungal infections in patients in ICU and found that while colonization was common (64%) invasive infection is extremely rare. Indeed, not even a single case of *Candida* pneumonia was found in 435 patients included in their report. In the absence of any clear benefit, it should be remembered that antifungal prophylaxis is associated with significant cost, adverse effects, drug interactions, likelihood of generating resistance, and a shift to fungal species such as *Candida glabrata* and *C. krusei* that are often resistant to commonly used azoles. Importantly, therapeutic options for resistant fungal species are limited.

Antifungal prophylaxis may be of benefit to only a select group of patients and such groups should be clearly identified before instituting prophylaxis. These may include critically ill patients with the aforementioned risk factors. Paphitou et al. [38] found that patients with risk factors had a higher rate of invasive candidiasis than those without (16.6% vs. 5.1%). At present, it is not recommended for general use in intensive care patients. However, there is a need to differentiate the use of antifungal agents for prophylaxis versus their use as pre-emptive agents in febrile neutropenic patients not responding to antibiotics. In such situations, pre-emptive use of fluconazole or amphotericin in neutropenic patients may be of benefit in decreasing mortality rates in patients with haematology malignancies.

References

1. Tablan OC, Anderson LJ, Besser R, Bridges C, Hajjeh R, CDC, et al. (2004) Guidelines for preventing health-care-associated pneumonia, 2003: recommendations of CDC and the Healthcare Infection Control Practices Advisory Committee. MMWR Recomm Rep 53:1–36
2. Sirvent JM, Torres A, El-Ebiary M, Castro P, de Batlle J, Bonet A (1997) Protective effect of intravenously administered cefuroxime against nosocomial pneumonia in patients with structural coma. Am J Respir Crit Care Med 155:1729–1734
3. Krueger WA, Lenhart FP, Neeser G, Ruckdeschel G, Schreckhase H, Eissner HJ, et al. (2002) Influence of combined intravenous and topical antibiotic prophylaxis on the incidence of infections, organ dysfunctions, and mortality in critically ill surgical patients: a prospective, stratified, randomized, double-blind, placebo-controlled clinical trial. Am J Respir Crit Care Med 166:1029–1037
4. de La Cal MA, Cerda E, Garcia-Hierro P, van Saene HK, Gomez-Santos D, Negro E, et al. (2005) Survival benefit in critically ill burned patients receiving selective decontamination of the digestive tract: a randomized, placebo-controlled, double-blind trial. Ann Surg 241:424–430
5. Silvestri L, van Saene HK, Milanese M, Fontana F, Gregori D, Oblach L, et al. (2004) Prevention of MRSA pneumonia by oral vancomycin decontamination: a randomised trial. Eur Respir J 23:921–926
6. Pugin J, Auckenthaler R, Lew DP, Suter PM (1991) Oropharyngeal decontamination decreases incidence of ventilator-associated pneumonia. A randomized, placebo-controlled, double-blind clinical trial. JAMA 265:2704–2710
7. Bergmans DC, Bonten MJ, Gaillard CA, Paling JC, van der Geest S, van Tiel FH, et al. (2001) Prevention of ventilator-associated pneumonia by oral decontamination: a prospective, randomized, double-blind, placebo-controlled study. Am J Respir Crit Care Med 164:382–388
8. Liberati A, D'Amico R, Pifferi S, Torri V, Brazzi L (2004) Antibiotic prophylaxis to reduce respiratory tract infections and mortality in adults receiving intensive care. Cochrane Database Syst Rev (1):CD000022
9. Safdar N, Said A, Lucey MR (2004) The role of selective digestive decontamination for reducing infection in patients undergoing liver transplantation: a systematic review and meta-analysis. Liver Transpl 10:817–827
10. de Jonge E (2005) Effects of selective decontamination of digestive tract on mortality and antibiotic resistance in the intensive-care unit. Curr Opin Crit Care 11:144–149
11. Adair CG, Gorman SP, Byers LM, Jones DS, Feron B, Crowe M, et al. (2002) Eradication of endotracheal tube biofilm by nebulised gentamicin. Intensive Care Med 28:426–431
12. Hoth JJ, Franklin GA, Stassen NA, Girard SM, Rodriguez RJ, Rodriguez JL (2003) Prophylactic antibiotics adversely affect nosocomial pneumonia in trauma patients. J Trauma 55:249–254
13. American Thoracic Society, Infectious Diseases Society of America (2005) Guidelines for the management of adults with hospital-acquired, ventilator-associated, and healthcare-associated pneumonia. Am J Respir Crit Care Med 171:388–416
14. Silvestri L, van Saene HK, de la Cal MA, Gullo A (2006) Adult hospital and ventilator-associated pneumonia guidelines: eminence- rather than evidence-based. Am J Respir Crit Care Med 173:131–133
15. Brun-Buisson C, Legrand P, Rauss A, Richard C, Montravers F, Besbes M, et al. (1989) Intestinal decontamination for control of nosocomial multiresistant gram-negative bacilli. Study of an outbreak in an intensive care unit. Ann Intern Med 110:873–881
16. Taylor ME, Oppenheim BA (1991) Selective decontamination of the gastrointestinal tract as an infection control measure. J Hosp Infect 17:271–278
17. Bologna RA, Tu LM, Polansky M, Fraimow HD, Gordon DA, Whitmore KE (1999) Hydrogel/silver ion-coated urinary catheter reduces nosocomial urinary tract infection rates in intensive care unit patients: a multicenter study. Urology 54:982–987
18. Riley DK, Classen DC, Stevens LE, Burke JP (1995) A large randomized clinical trial of a silver-impregnated urinary catheter: lack of efficacy and staphylococcal superinfection. Am J Med 98:349–356
19. Darouiche RO, Smith JA Jr, Hanna H, Dhabuwala CB, Steiner MS, Babaian RJ, et al. (1999) Efficacy of antimicrobial-impregnated bladder catheters in reducing catheter-associated bacteriuria: a prospective, randomized, multicenter clinical trial. Urology 54:976–981
20. Johnson JR, Kuskowski MA, Wilt TJ (2006) Systematic review: antimicrobial urinary catheters to prevent catheter-associated urinary tract infection in hospitalized patients. Ann Intern Med 144:116–126
21. Huth TS, Burke JP, Larsen RA, Classen DC, Stevens LE (1992) Randomized trial of meatal care with silver sulfadiazine cream for the prevention of catheter-associated bacteriuria. J Infect Dis 165:14–18
22. Centers for Disease Control and Prevention (CDC) (2005)

Reduction in central line-associated bloodstream infections among patients in intensive care units – Pennsylvania, April 2001–March 2005. MMWR Morb Mortal Wkly Rep 54:1013–1016

23. Levy I, Katz J, Solter E, Samra Z, Vidne B, Birk E, et al. (2005) Chlorhexidine-impregnated dressing for prevention of colonization of central venous catheters in infants and children: a randomized controlled study. Pediatr Infect Dis J 24:676–679
24. Mimoz O, Pieroni L, Lawrence C, Edouard A, Costa Y, Samii K, et al. (1996) Prospective, randomized trial of two antiseptic solutions for prevention of central venous or arterial catheter colonization and infection in intensive care unit patients. Crit Care Med 24:1818–1823
25. Osma S, Kahveci SF, Kaya FN, Akalin H, Ozakin C, Yilmaz E, et al. (2006) Efficacy of antiseptic-impregnated catheters on catheter colonization and catheter-related bloodstream infections in patients in an intensive care unit. J Hosp Infect 62:156–162
26. Maki DG, Stolz SM, Wheeler S, Mermel LA (1997) Prevention of central venous catheter-related bloodstream infection by use of an antiseptic-impregnated catheter. A randomized, controlled trial. Ann Intern Med 127:257–266
27. Walder B, Pittet D, Tramer MR (2002) Prevention of bloodstream infections with central venous catheters treated with anti-infective agents depends on catheter type and insertion time: evidence from a meta-analysis. Infect Control Hosp Epidemiol 23:748–756
28. Darouiche RO, Berger DH, Khardori N, Robertson CS, Wall MJ Jr, Metzler MH, et al. (2005) Comparison of antimicrobial impregnation with tunneling of long-term central venous catheters: a randomized controlled trial. Ann Surg 242:193–200
29. Leon C, Ruiz-Santana S, Rello J, de la Torre MV, Valles J, Alvarez-Lerma F, et al. (2004) Benefits of minocycline and rifampin-impregnated central venous catheters. A prospective, randomized, double-blind, controlled, multicenter trial. Intensive Care Med 30:1891–1899
30. Darouiche RO, Raad II, Heard SO, Thornby JI, Wenker OC, Gabrielli A, et al. (1999) A comparison of two antimicrobial-impregnated central venous catheters. Catheter Study Group. N Engl J Med 340:1–8
31. Marciante KD, Veenstra DL, Lipsky BA, Saint S (2003) Which antimicrobial impregnated central venous catheter should we use? Modeling the costs and outcomes of antimicrobial catheter use. Am J Infect Control 31:1–8
32. Veenstra DL, Saint S, Sullivan SD (1999) Cost-effectiveness of antiseptic-impregnated central venous catheters for the prevention of catheter-related bloodstream infection. JAMA 282:554–560
33. Garland JS, Alex CP, Henrickson KJ, McAuliffe TL, Maki DG (2005) A vancomycin-heparin lock solution for prevention of nosocomial bloodstream infection in critically ill neonates with peripherally inserted central venous catheters: a prospective, randomized trial. Pediatrics 116: e198–205
34. Henrickson KJ, Axtell RA, Hoover SM, Kuhn SM, Pritchett J, Kehl SC, et al. (2000) Prevention of central venous catheter-related infections and thrombotic events in immunocompromised children by the use of vancomycin/ciprofloxacin/heparin flush solution: A randomized, multicenter, double-blind trial. J Clin Oncol 18:1269–1278
35. McConnell SA, Gubbins PO, Anaissie EJ (2003) Do antimicrobial-impregnated central venous catheters prevent catheter-related bloodstream infection? Clin Infect Dis 37:65–72
36. Masson C, Chevailler A, Pascaretti C, Legrand E, Bregeon C, Audran M (1996) Minocycline related lupus. J Rheumatol 23:2160–2161
37. Oda T, Hamasaki J, Kanda N, Mikami K (1997) Anaphylactic shock induced by an antiseptic-coated central venous (correction of nervous) catheter. Anesthesiology 87:1242–1244
38. Paphitou NI, Ostrosky-Zeichner L, Rex JH (2005) Rules for identifying patients at increased risk for candidal infections in the surgical intensive care unit: approach to developing practical criteria for systematic use in antifungal prophylaxis trials. Med Mycol 43:235–243
39. Calandra T, Marchetti O (2004) Clinical trials of antifungal prophylaxis among patients undergoing surgery. Clin Infect Dis 39 Suppl 4:S185--192
40. Castagnola E, Machetti M, Bucci B, Viscoli C (2004) Antifungal prophylaxis with azole derivatives. Clin Microbiol Infect 10 Suppl 1:86–95
41. Ostrosky-Zeichner L (2004) Novel approaches to antifungal prophylaxis. Expert Opin Investig Drugs 13:665–672
42. Cruciani M, de Lalla F, Mengoli C (2005) Prophylaxis of Candida infections in adult trauma and surgical intensive care patients: a systematic review and meta-analysis. Intensive Care Med 31:1479–1487
43. Petri MG, Konig J, Moecke HP, Gramm HJ, Barkow H, Kujath P, et al. (1997) Epidemiology of invasive mycosis in ICU patients: a prospective multicenter study in 435 non-neutropenic patients. Paul-Ehrlich Society for Chemotherapy, Divisions of Mycology and Pneumonia Research. Intensive Care Med 23:317–325

11 Antifungal Therapy in the Intensive Care Unit

J.A. Paiva, J.M. Pereira

11.1 Introduction

Candidemia and systemic candidiasis were considered rare diseases until the 1950s, and by 1964 only 48 cases of disseminated candidiasis had been described. Endemic mycoses such as coccidiomycosis, blastomycosis and histoplasmosis, described in the early twentieth century, remained a medical curiosity for a long time.

Fungal diseases have become clinically important in the last 3 decades and *Candida* has emerged as one of the most important pathogens. In the 1970s, the incidence of disseminated candidiasis was two cases per 1,000 hospital discharges. The NNIS study (USA) demonstrated that the nosocomial fungal infection rate doubled from 2.0 to 3.8 infections per 1,000 hospital discharges from 1980 to 1990 [1]. The proportion of nosocomial fungal infections rose from 6.4% to 10.4% over the same period and the highest rates were found in intensive care units (ICUs), and oncological, cardiac surgery and especially burns wards [2]. The EPIC study [3] showed that fungi were the fifth most frequent pathogen after Enterobacteriaceae, *Staphylococcus aureus*, *Pseudomonas aeruginosa* and coagulase negative *Staphylococcus* and that 17% of all ICU patients had deep fungal infections. Although the number may be overestimated, 50% of patients in whom fungi were isolated were receiving antifungals, showing that the isolation was diagnosed as being clinically significant. Recently, Martin et al. [4] reported an increase of 207% in the number of cases of sepsis caused by fungal organisms, from 5,231 cases in 1979 to 16,042 cases in 2000.

Candida spp. are the predominant cause of fungal infection in critically ill patients, accounting for 85.6% of fungal isolates in the NNIS survey and for 78% of all fungal infections in 1990 in the USA. However, the incidence of aspergillosis has also increased in the last 20 years and other fungi like *Fusarium*, *Mucor*, *Trichosporum* and *Cryptococcus* are emerging as a significant problem.

Not only is the incidence increasing but also the attributable mortality of these infections is also marked, varying in different studies from 25% to 60% [5, 6]. An elegant study in a teaching hospital showed that the attributable mortality from nosocomial candidemia was 38% [7]. Morbidity is also marked, with a median length of stay longer than compared controls.

11.2 The Antifungal Armamentarium

There are mainly five classes of antifungal agents: allylamines, flucytosine, azoles, polyene antibiotics and echinocandins. The allylamines such as terbinafine and griseofulvin are primarily effective against dermatophyte infections, so they will not be dealt with in this chapter. The antifungal effects of azoles, allylamines and polyene antibiotics are directed primarily against ergosterol and its synthesis [8], as ergosterol is the main sterol of the fungal cell membrane and has a fundamental function in cell proliferation. Echinocandins, a new class of antifungals, act by inhibition of cell wall glucan synthesis (Fig. 11.1).

Flucytosine or 5-fluorocytosine is a synthetic fluorinated pyrimidine which inhibits fungal DNA and RNA protein synthesis. The enzyme cytosine permease transports it into a susceptible cell and the enzyme cytosine deaminase transforms it to either 5-fluorouracil, which inhibits DNA synthesis, or floxuridine, which inhibits thymidylate synthetase. Cytosine deaminase is present in fungal cells but not in human cells, although the intestinal flora can convert the parent compound into 5-fluoruracil [9–11]. Flucytosine is a fungistatic

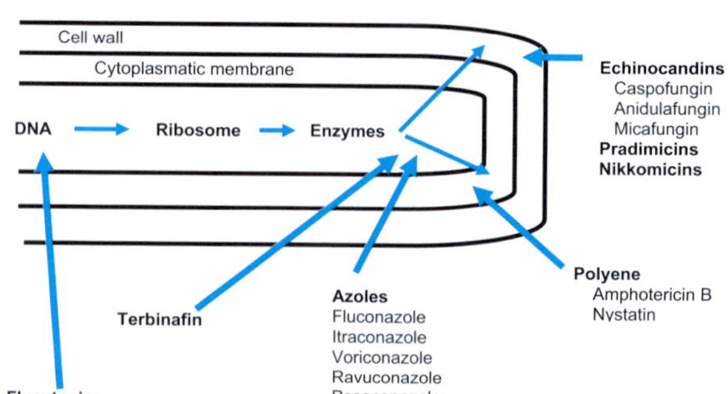

Fig. 11.1. Action of the antifungal agents

agent with a narrow spectrum of activity – most *Candida* spp., *Cryptococcus neoformans* and some molds. Many fungi demonstrate primary or acquired resistance. Approximately 10% of *Candida albicans*, 20% of *Candida tropicalis* and 2% of *Cryptococcus neoformans* are resistant to flucytosine from the onset of treatment with MIC above 16 mg/l [12] and the development of resistance during treatment is common [13]. Therefore, it should not be used as monotherapy in *Candida* spp. infections. *Coccidioides immitis*, *Blastomyces dermatitidis* and *Pseudallescheria boydii* are resistant to flucytosine and *Aspergillus* spp. show variable susceptibility [14]; acquired resistance during treatment is frequent. Flucytosine may be used in combination with amphotericin B for systemic candidiasis and cryptococcosis, as synergism has been described between these two drugs [15–17], and this therapeutic combination is often well tolerated [18]. Nevertheless, there is no conclusive proof of the benefit of this association. Indications for its use might be: (a) in neonates, because of the 45% incidence of meningitis; (b) in endophthalmitis, endocarditis, suppurative thrombophlebitis or meningitis; (c) in *Candida lusitaniae* and *Candida glabrata* infections; and (d) if the patient is critically ill and deteriorating. There were also reports of successful treatment of candidiasis and cryptococcosis with flucytosine in combination with fluconazole or itraconazole, but further comparative trials are required before these combinations can be advocated [12, 19].

Flucytosine is well absorbed after oral administrations and similar serum concentrations are obtained following oral and parenteral administration. Its half-life is 3–6 h in patients with normal renal function and, as its protein binding is only 12%, it has a high penetration into organs, body fluids and cerebrospinal fluid [14], with tissue concentrations usually exceeding 50% of simultaneous blood concentrations [20]. In adults with normal renal function, an oral dose of 25 mg/kg administered 6-hourly results in peak serum levels of 30–80 mg/l at 1–2 h [20, 21]. There is a slight accumulation of the drug during the first 4 days of treatment and then peak concentrations remain constant. Most textbooks state that if renal function is normal, the initial dose should be 50–150 mg/kg given in four divided doses at 6-h intervals. If there is renal dysfunction, the initial dose should be reduced to 25 mg/kg and subsequent doses and intervals adjusted to achieve peak serum concentrations of 70–80 mg/l and a trough of 30–40 mg/l (Table 11.1). However, these proposed doses are based on those needed to achieve penetration into the cerebrospinal fluid, and flucytosine at 25 mg/kg/day at 12-h intervals should be adequate to maintain serum levels above MIC for most susceptible *Candida* [19, 22]. In small infants, as half-life is prolonged, intervals should be increased to 24 h [21].

Table 11.1. Doses and dose intervals of flucytosine according to renal function

Creatinine clearance (ml/min)	Individual dose (mg/kg)	Dose interval (h)
>40	25.0–37.5	6
20–40	25.0–37.5	12
10–20	25.0–37.5	>24

The main adverse effects consist of granulocytopenia and thrombocytopenia, rashes and gastrointestinal toxicity, namely nausea, vomiting and diarrhea; mild changes in liver function occur in around 10% of patients [20]. Bone marrow suppression occurs frequently in patients with AIDS and its use should be avoided in these patients. Myelotoxicity appears to be concentration dependent, although this adverse reaction may be due to the production of fluorouracil from enterobacillary flucytosine metabolism in the gut, rather than to parent compound [23]. The hematological and hepatic abnormalities usually resolve if treatment is discontinued; however, liver necrosis has been rarely reported in patients receiving flucytosine as contributing directly to death. Due to its potentially teratogenic effects, it is contraindicated during pregnancy [11]. Serum creatinine must be monitored at least twice weekly and dosages appropriately adjusted. Blood counts and liver function tests must be performed regularly. Special caution must be taken when flucytosine is used with other nephrotoxic or myelosuppressive drugs. The use of this drug requires facilities for monitoring serum concentration [24], especially when used in association with amphotericin B or in patients with renal failure [21, 25]. Optimal and minimum serum concentrations for efficacy are not known, but toxicity occurs when blood levels exceed 100 mg/l for 2 or more weeks [11] or when it is used in combination with amphotericin B [11, 14, 26–28].

The azoles are classified as imidazoles (miconazole and ketoconazole) and triazoles. These can be divided into first generation (fluconazole and itraconazole) and second generation (voriconazole, posaconazole, ravuconazole).

The antifungal azoles target ergosterol biosynthesis by inhibiting the fungal cytochrome P450-dependent enzyme, lanosterol 14-α-demethylase. This demethylation step is dependent on the activation of cytochrome P450, a heme protein containing one molecule of protoporphyrin IX, which is the terminal oxidase of the hepatic microsomial oxidase system and has an important role in the synthesis and degradation of many substances. The interaction of azoles with heme iron of the cytochrome P450 inhibits the cytochrome activation and the enzyme function with a consequent depletion of ergosterol, the principal sterol in the fungal cell membrane [8, 29]; this depletion results in a breakdown of normal cellular function, increases cell membrane permeability and inhibits cell replication [30–34]. The triazoles have a greater affinity for fungal P450-dependent enzymes than the imidazoles and thus exhibit greater antifungal activity and a lower toxicity profile.

The oral absorption of fluconazole is good, even almost complete, and, unlike itraconazole, it is not altered by the presence of food or gastric acidity. Therefore, identical serum concentrations are attained after both oral and parenteral administration [35]. Peak plasma concentration is related to the dose, with a linear relationship [36], and occurs within 2–4 h after oral administration [29]. After repeated dosing, serum levels increase and a steady state is reached after about 14 days. Its protein binding is weak (about 12% of the drug), 80% is excreted by the kidney in unchanged active form and it has a prolonged half-life (20–30 h) that allows once daily dosing [37–39]. Therefore, dosages must be adjusted in renal failure and monitoring of serum levels is recommended, trying to maintain them at 6–20 μg/ml [40]. The normal recommended dose should be given on day one, followed by a daily dose that should be reduced by 50% if the creatinine clearance is between 11 and 50 ml/min. Dialysis removes 50% of the drug and a dose must be administered after each dialysis [41]. Empirical fluconazole should be administered at a daily dose of 800 mg for critically ill patients receiving continuous venovenous hemodialysis (CVVHD) or continuous venovenous hemodiafiltration (CVVHDF) with a combined ultrafiltration and dialysate flow rate of 2 l/h and at a daily dose of 400 mg for patients receiving continuous venovenous hemofiltration (CVVHF). The dose may be decreased to 400 mg/day (CVVHD or CVVHDF) or to 200 mg/day (CVVHF) if the species is not *Candida glabrata* and the fluconazole MIC is ≤8 mg/l [42]. Fluconazole is widely and evenly distributed throughout the body [19] with constant levels achieved within 1 h [43]. It penetrates well into cerebrospinal fluid, where drug concentration may reach 60–80% of the serum level [44, 45]. Bone is the place where concentrations are lowest and therefore higher doses should be used to treat bone fungal infections and also to treat muscle and central nervous system infections by *Cryptococcus neoformans*, *Coccidioides immitis* and *Histoplasma capsulatum* [38, 46]. The dosage of fluconazole is, nevertheless, still a matter of debate: while the most widely used is 5 mg/kg/day, some centers prefer the use of a higher dose in the critically ill patient, namely 10 mg/kg/day. This question will be dealt with later in this chapter.

Fluconazole is a fungistatic agent active against most *Candida* species, *Cryptococcus neoformans*, *Coccidioides immitis*, *Histoplasma capsulatum*, *Paracoccidioides brasiliensis*, *Sporothrix shenckii* and *Blastomyces dermatiditis* [29, 37]. It is ineffective against *Aspergillus* and *Mucor* species. *Candida glabrata* is frequently resistant to fluconazole and it has virtually no activity against *Candida krusei*, which has intrinsic resistance to the drug [47–49]. The widespread use of fluconazole in repeated low-dose courses, as prophylaxis or therapy, has resulted in acquired fungal resistance. Fluconazole-resistant strains of *Candida albicans* have become more and more common among patients with AIDS [50, 51] and more recently in non-HIV patients [52–54]. The SCOPE program showed that the level of resistance of *Candida albicans* to fluconazole was 9.6%, varying between 2.9% and 15.5% with geographical location [48].

Fluconazole is generally well tolerated. Nausea and vomiting are the most common side effects, but they seldom cause discontinuation of treatment [11, 37]. Elevation of hepatic enzymes occurs in a small percentage of individuals, but treatment should only be discontinued if there is symptomatic hepatitis or laboratory signs of persistent hepatic dysfunction, which are rare [11, 29, 55–57]. Stevens-Johnson syndrome has been described in AIDS and cancer patients, although a causal relationship has not been clearly established. The drug should be discontinued if bullous lesions or erythema multiform develop [21, 43]. Azoles interfere with the elimination of drugs metabolized by the hepatic cytochrome P450. The sedative effect of midazolam, the anticoagulant effect of warfarin, the hypoglycemic effect of sulfonylureas, the anticonvulsant effect of phenytoin and carbamazepine and the effects of theophylline, cisapride and cyclosporine may be increased by the azoles; on the other hand rifampicin accelerates clearance of fluconazole (Table 11.2) [21, 43, 58, 59].

Itraconazole is a weak base and requires an acid environment for absorption. Absorption after oral administration is variable and incomplete and its hepatic excretion is complex, particularly in the critically ill patient [60]. Serum concentrations are markedly lower when gastric acid is reduced and capsules are used. Absorption is enhanced if we use liquid formulation or if we use an acid agent such as a cola beverage with the capsules [21]. Unfortunately, it has only recently been approved for parenteral use. Doses used range from 200 mg to 400 mg/day. Peak plasma concentration after a 200-mg dose averages 0.3 μg/ml and it is three to five times higher after 7–10 days of treatment. In other words, serum levels may take up to 1 week to reach therapeutic levels and that is why a load dose should be used and serum levels should be monitored, knowing that good levels are above 2 μg/ml and ideal levels above 8 μg/ml [61]. The half-life is dependent on the dose and duration of administration and varies from 15 to 42 h [62]. Ninety-nine percent of the drug binds to proteins [37] and, unlike fluconazole, it penetrates very poorly into cerebrospinal fluid [63], although tissue concentrations in the brain, kidney, liver, lung and skin

Table 11.2. Drug interactions of antifungal agents

Antifungal	Drugs	Effect
Amphotericin B	Aminoglycosides	Nephrotoxicity
	Cyclosporin	Nephrotoxicity
	Corticosteroids	Hypokalemia/long QT
	Astemizole	Hypokalemia/long QT
	Terfenadine	Hypokalemia/long QT
	Digoxin	Hypokalemia/long QT
Fluconazole and itraconazole	Cisapride	Arrhythmia
	H_1 receptor antagonism	Arrhythmia
	Aminophiline	Arrhythmia
	Cyclosporin	Nephrotoxicity
	Lovastatin	Rhabdomyolysis
	Astemizole	Drug increased levels
	Carbamazepine	Drug increased levels
	Tacrolimus	Drug increased levels
	Triazolam	Drug increased levels
	Warfarin	Drug increased levels
Fluconazole	Sulfonylureas	Drug increased levels
	Phenytoin	Drug increased levels
	Rifampicin	Drug increased levels
	Rifabutin	Drug increased levels
	Midazolam	Drug increased levels
	Tacrolimus	Drug increased levels
	Saquinavir	Drug increased levels
Itraconazole (Itra)	Busulfan	Drug increased levels
	Calcium channel blockers	Drug increased levels
	Digoxin	Drug increased levels
	Midazolam	Drug increased levels
	Rifampicin	Drug increased levels
	Vincristine	Drug increased levels
	H_2-receptor antagonism	Itra diminished absorption
	Proton pump inhibitors	Itra diminished absorption
	Sucralfate	Itra diminished absorption
	Rifampicin	Itra diminished levels
	Phenobarbitone	Itra diminished levels
	Phenytoin	Itra diminished levels
Voriconazole	Cyclosporin	Drug increased levels
	Tacrolimus	Drug increased levels
	Warfarin	Drug increased levels
	Statins	Drug increased levels
	Benzodiazepines	Drug increased levels
	Calcium channel blockers	Drug increased levels
	Sulfonylureas	Drug increased levels
	Protease inhibitors	Drug increased levels
	Rifampin	Voriconazole diminished levels
	Carbamazepine	Voriconazole diminished levels
	Long-acting barbiturates	Voriconazole diminished levels
	Terfenadine	Voriconazole diminished levels
	Cisapride	Voriconazole diminished levels
	Phenytoin	Voriconazole diminished levels
	Omeprazole	Voriconazole increased levels
	Non-nucleotide RTI	Voriconazole increased levels

are two to five times greater than in plasma [64]. It has the ability to reach high intracellular concentrations, particularly in the immune cells, namely the alveolar macrophages [65]. It is metabolized by the liver and excreted in the feces; therefore no drug adjustments are necessary in renal failure and dialysis does not remove the drug [11, 66]. Severe infections should be treated with a loading dose of 300 mg twice daily for 3–4 days, followed by 200–400 mg/day. Its use in critically ill patients is, however, hampered by the absence, until very recently, of a parenteral formulation [67].

Itraconazole is a fungistatic agent active against *Aspergillus* species [68]; European studies report response rates of 63–70% for aspergillosis and the response is better in pulmonary than in disseminated aspergillosis. It is also active against many *Candida* species, and isolates that are resistant to fluconazole are not necessarily cross-resistant to itraconazole [69], such as is the case with some *Candida krusei* and *Candida glabrata* [47]. However, strains of *Candida* spp. which are highly resistant to fluconazole often have reduced susceptibility to itraconazole and even the newer azoles, as the SCOPE program has shown [48, 70, 71].

Itraconazole is also well tolerated, but can cause nausea, vomiting, abdominal discomfort and epigastric pain, constipation, dizziness, pruritus and allergic rashes. These effects are usually self-limited [21, 43]. Hypokalemia may occur after prolonged therapy and hepatic function should be monitored as plasma transaminase elevation may occur. At high doses, hypertension has been described. It is contraindicated in patients with known hypersensitivity to azole derivatives or with severe hepatic impairment and in pregnancy [21]. Drug interactions are similar to those described for fluconazole and are summarized in Table 11.2.

Recently, a second generation of azoles was introduced into clinical practice. Voriconazole, posaconazole and ravuconazole are the three main new triazole drugs to be introduced in this family of antifungals.

Voriconazole has demonstrated a broad-spectrum in vitro activity against numerous isolates of *Candida* spp., *Cryptococcus neoformans*, *Scedosporium* spp., *Trichosporon* spp., *Aspergillus* spp. including amphotericin B resistant clinical isolates, *Blastomyces dermatitidis*, some *Fusarium* isolates, *Coccidioides immitis* and *Histoplasma capsulatum*. It was also found to have good in vitro activity against dermatophytes. It is inactive against *Mucor* and *Rhizopus*.

The recommended IV dose is 6 mg/kg every 12 h for two doses, then 4 mg/kg every 12 h. Once oral medication can be tolerated by the patient, the oral formulation should be administered (200 mg every 12 h for patients weighing over 40 kg and 100 mg every 12 h for patients weighing less). Voriconazole may be administered orally or as an intravenous infusion over 1–2 h [72]. The oral bioavailability is approximately 96%.

Following oral administration, peak plasma levels are reached in 1–2 h. Peak concentrations and area under the curve are reduced by 34% and 24%, respectively, when the drug is administered with high-fat meals. The absorption of oral voriconazole is not dependent upon gastric pH. It is metabolized by the cytochrome P450 system and the majority of the metabolized drug is excreted in the urine. Voriconazole exhibits moderate binding to plasma proteins, estimated as 58% [73]. Tissue and CSF levels exceed those of trough plasma levels severalfold [72].

In patients with mild to moderate hepatic insufficiency, a single oral dose of voriconazole resulted in increases in AUC approximately 3.2 times higher than in normal subjects; therefore, after the standard loading dose, only half of the recommended maintenance dose should be used in these patients. There are no data available in patients with severe hepatic impairment [73]. No dose adjustment is necessary for oral administration of voriconazole in patients with renal dysfunction. However, cyclodextrin, the vehicle of the intravenous formulation, will accumulate in patients with moderate renal insufficiency. Therefore, the intravenous formulation should not be used in patients with a creatinine clearance rate <50 ml/min [73] or for patients receiving any form of renal replacement therapy [42]. Although oral formulations are not contraindicated, there are few data about dosing for patients receiving continuous renal replacement therapy [74] and, on the basis of pharmacokinetics data, no dose reduction is recommended in these patients [42].

As a cytochrome P450 inhibitor, voriconazole is subject to many drug interactions. Concomitant use of drugs such as rifampin, carbamazepine, long-acting barbiturates, cisapride, rifabutin, terfenadine and astemizole is contraindicated [72]. Voriconazole increases plasma concentrations of cyclosporin, tacrolimus warfarin, statins, benzodiazepines, calcium channel blockers, and sulfonylureas. Omeprazole and non-nucleotide reverse transcriptase inhibitors may inhibit voriconazole metabolism and consequently increase serum levels (Table 11.2).

Visual disturbances, including blurring and photophobia, occurred in at least 20% of subjects in clinical studies of voriconazole. These reactions were transient and typically resolved in spite of continued voriconazole. Patients should be cautioned to avoid driving at night while taking voriconazole and, as photosensitivity has occurred with voriconazole, patients should be advised to stay out of strong, direct sunlight while on voriconazole. The other most common adverse events in clinical trials were fever, nausea, vomiting, chills and abnormal liver function tests. Adverse reactions occurring rarely during the infusion of voriconazole included flushing, fever, diaphoresis, tachycardia, dyspnea, dizziness, nausea, pruritus and rash [73]. Serum levels should be below 6 μg/ml at day 3 to avoid serious side effects.

Ravuconazole is structurally similar to fluconazole and is only available in an oral formulation. It has a long terminal half-life of approximately 100 h [75–77] and has been well tolerated in single doses of 800 mg/day and 400 mg/day for up to 14 days, with headache being the most reported adverse event [76]. Ravuconazole has a broad spectrum of activity against pathogenic fungi including *Aspergillus* spp., *Candida* spp., *Cryptococcus neoformans* and *Trichosporon* spp. [77–82]. The activity of ravuconazole against *Candida* spp. was comparable to that of voriconazole, with the exception of *Candida glabrata* where ravuconazole is less active [82].

Posaconazole, an analogue of itraconazole, has a good oral bioavailability and an estimated half-life of 22 h [83]. In vitro studies demonstrate that posaconazole has a broad spectrum activity against *Aspergillus* spp., *Candida* spp., including strains resistant to fluconazole, *Cryptococcus neoformans*, *Trichosporon* spp., *Zygomycetes* and dermatophytes [82, 84–86]. It seems to be ten times more potent than itraconazole against *Aspergillus* spp.

Amphotericin B is a polyene naturally recovered from *Streptomyces nodosus* in 1953 and commercially available since 1956. It binds to ergosterol, the principal sterol in the membrane of susceptible fungal cells, causing impairment of membrane barrier function, loss of cell constituents, metabolic disruption and cell death. In addition to its membrane permeabilizing effects, the drug can cause oxidative damage to fungal cells [12, 87]. It has minimal cutaneous or mucosal absorption, namely minimal absorption from the gastrointestinal tract. After intravenous administration, levels are proportional to the dose and rate of infusion. Peak serum concentrations are 1.2 and 2.4 mg/ml after intravenous administration of 0.5 and 1 mg/kg, respectively, and the peak mean serum concentrations increase when the infusion rate is increased [88, 89]. Its metabolism is complex. Plasma initial half-life is 24 h but elimination half-life reaches 15 days. After 12 h, less than 10% remains in the blood; it is widely distributed in tissues, mainly to the liver (24–41%), lungs (2–6%), kidney (0.6–2%) and spleen (0.7–1.6%) and much less to adipose tissue or muscle. It is slowly degraded and plasma levels remain detectable 7–8 weeks after treatment is stopped and the drug has been detected for longer than 1 year in liver, kidney and spleen. Serum concentrations do not reflect tissue concentrations and serum and tissue concentrations have an unclear relationship to either toxicity or efficacy – therefore measuring drug levels is rarely of clinical value [90]. Protein binding is high (90–95%), it enters serous cavities, but penetration into cerebrospinal fluid is poor [43]. Only a small part of the compound is eliminated through the kidneys and biliary tract; therefore renal or hepatic impairment has little effect on serum drug levels and dialysis does not modify blood levels [11]. As it is not a water-soluble compound, a carrier must be used for clinical use. In its conventional form, deoxycholate and a buffer are added to amphotericin B, producing a colloidal suspension dispersion suitable for intravenous administration when suspended in a 5% glucose solution [91].

Amphotericin B may be fungistatic or fungicidal, depending on the concentration obtained and the susceptibility of the fungus, but it has the widest spectrum of activity amongst all the antifungals, with a fungicidal effect against *Candida* species, *Aspergillus* species, *Blastomyces dermatidis*, *Coccidioides immitis*, *Cryptococcus neoformans*, *Histoplasma capsulatum*, *Paracoccidioides brasiliensis* and *Sporothrix schenckii*. It is effective in certain forms of mucormycosis, hyalophomycosis and phaeohyphomycosis, but often ineffective in pseudallescheriasis and trichosporonosis and some fusariosis. Treatment failure attributable to the development of amphotericin resistance is rare. *Candida lusitaniae* is resistant to amphotericin B [92] and resistant strains of *Candida guillermondii*, *Candida tropicalis* and *Candida krusei*, with alterations in the cell membrane, including reduced amounts of ergosterol, have been isolated during treatment. Susceptibility to amphotericin B varies among *Aspergillus* species, being less in *Aspergillus terreus* [93]. However, overall emergence of resistance during treatment is rare [12, 13]. It has been the drug of choice for severe invasive fungal infections in the last 30 years due to its very broad fungicidal activity against *Candida* spp. and *Aspergillus* spp. [22, 94]. In clinical studies, response rates were 55% for *Aspergillus* spp., 55–65% for *Candida* spp. and 75% for *Cryptococcus neoformans* [7, 95]. *Candida* with higher MIC to amphotericin B are difficult to treat and one should aim for serum levels of 1–2.5 μg/ml [13].

Adverse effects of amphotericin B deoxycholate may be divided into infusion-related or acute and dose-related or late (Table 11.3). The peak frequency of fever, rigors and other infusion-related reactions, caused by production of TNF and PgE by macrophages [96], occurs on the 1st to 3rd day of therapy and subsequently declines, generally subsiding after 1 week of therapy even without treatment [97, 98]. Longer infusion times are associated with a reduction in the incidence of infusion-related toxicities. Normochromic, normocytic anemia accompanies most 2–3 week courses of amphotericin B, with a decrease in hematocrit by as much as 35%, occurring secondary to decreased production of erythropoietin rather than to diminished bone marrow production; this effect is reversible when the drug is discontinued [99]. Nephrotoxicity is the most significant toxic effect of amphotericin B administration; and about 80% of the patients receiving the drug show some degree of renal impairment, although it is generally reversible, especially in those submitted to a cumulative dose higher than 0.5–1 g, with sodium depletion, older than 30 years old, with abnormal baseline renal function and under other nephrotoxic drugs [100]. It manifests as azotemia, decreased urinary concentration ability, renal tubular acidosis, symptomatic hypokalemia or renal magnesium wasting [101]. Signs of nephrotoxicity usually occur within the first 4 days of starting a course of treatment. An adequate assessment of patients before, during and after therapy may help reduce this toxicity [102]. Preventive measures consist of: avoiding salt depletion, use of concomitant antibiotics with sodium salts, loading with 0.9% saline prior to infusion of amphotericin B [101] and use of pentoxifylline [103]. Monitoring for increased serum creatinine, hypokalemia and hypomagnesemia should occur daily during the first weeks of therapy. Nephrotoxicity is usually reversible by increasing sodium loading, reducing dose, increasing dosing interval with total dose reduction or temporarily suspending the treatment when serum creatinine reaches approximately 3 mg/dl. Recommendations for the prevention and management of nephrotoxicity are summarized in Table 11.4. Interactions of the drug are shown in Table 11.2.

Due to these adverse effects, the maximal tolerable dose of amphotericin B deoxycholate is usually 0.6–1.0 mg/kg/day. Although recent work suggests the efficacy of lower dose regimens of 0.3–0.7 mg/kg/day [104, 105], there is also the knowledge that the maximal tolerable doses may sometimes be suboptimal for clinical success. Pharmacy has tried to resolve this problem by combining amphotericin in lipid-based formulations to reduce the toxicity of the conventional com-

Table 11.3. Adverse effects of amphotericin B

Frequency	Dose-related	Infusion-related
Common	Renal failure (30%) Kaliuria Magnesuria Anemia	Fever (30–90%) Rigors (30–75%) Nausea (4–60%) Vomiting Diarrhea
Uncommon	Bronchospasm Hypotension	Headache Thrombophlebitis Myalgia Arthralgia
Rare	Asystole Bradycardia Thrombocytopenia Neutropenia Malignant hyperthermia Ventricular fibrillation Acute liver failure Seizures Flushing/rash Hearing loss	

Table 11.4. Recommendations for the prevention and management of amphotericin B nephrotoxicity

Dose test	1 mg amphotericin B Infuse test dose over 10 – 30 min without premedication
Maintenance dose	250 – 1,000 ml normal saline prior to infusion Infusion 0.5 – 1.0 mg/kg in 0.1 mg/ml D5 %W Do not use solutions containing electrolytes Administer entire desired maintenance dose on first day Circumstances for gradual dose escalation: Test dose reaction History of prior amphotericin intolerance Suboptimal cardiopulmonary function Renal impairment Indolent fungal disease Options if creatinine increases: Increase sodium loading Increase dosing interval with total dose reduction Temporary suppression of treatment (if serum creatinine ≥ 30 mg/l)
Duration	Infuse daily dose over 1 h if < 0.9 mg/kg and Cr Cl < 25 mg/min Infuse daily dose over 2 h if ≥ 1 mg/kg Infuse daily dose over 4 – 6 h if Cr Cl > 25 mg/min or hyperkalemia
Medications	Premedicate for first three doses or 1 week; if no reactions omit – Fever: hydrocortisone 25 – 50 mg IV/infusate or acetaminophen, paracetamol or ibuprofen – Nausea: diphenydramine 25 – 50 mg PO or IV Add 1,000 U heparin for infusion through peripheral line Meperidine 25 – 50 mg IV every 15 min × 3, as needed for rigors If rigors are predictable, add meperidine 20 – 30 min before infusion

pound, especially nephrotoxicity, as they do not contain deoxycholate, which is responsible for direct tubular toxicity [106 – 110]. Three formulations have been developed that differ in the way amphotericin B interacts with the lipid and therefore have different properties, but all can be given at doses significantly higher than amphotericin deoxycholate with fewer side effects [111, 112]. The lipid compounds are less toxic, equally less nephrotoxic and with maximum tolerated doses higher than that of amphotericin B deoxycholate [25]. Moreover, nephrotoxicity is less common with the lipid compounds as renal function may be improved or stabilized when they are substituted [25, 113]. This is particularly important in critically ill patients who are susceptible to many other causes of renal failure, like trauma, sepsis, drugs, etc. Nevertheless, the doses recommended for the three formulations are: amphotericin B lipid complex (5 mg/kg/day), amphotericin B colloidal dispersion (4 mg/kg/day) and liposomal amphotericin B (1 – 3 mg/kg/day). Remember that when equivalent doses are compared with conventional amphotericin B, concentrations in serum lipid formulations are lower, probably because of accumulation in the liver and in the spleen [114]. In spite of the lack of a properly controlled trial comparing these formulations with the parent compound, preclinical and clinical studies suggest that lipid-based formulations are likely to be as effective as conventional amphotericin B [25] and their adverse events are the same but significantly rarer, especially nephrotoxicity. In addition, 40 – 60 % of the patients in which fungal infection was refractory to amphotericin B deoxycholate may respond to lipid-based formulations.

The pharmacokinetics of the lipid-based amphotericin B formulations are related to its molecular structures. Amphotericin B lipid-complex is rapidly and significantly taken up by the reticuloendothelial system, resulting in lower plasma levels and higher tissue penetration, namely in the lungs, liver and spleen, than conventional amphotericin B; in other words it has a lower area under the curve and higher volume of distribution [108, 110, 115, 116]. The lower plasma levels partially justify the lower incidence of nephrotoxicity of this compound [109]. It is well tolerated and infusion-related side effects, such as chills, fever, nausea and tremor, are the most frequent adverse events [113, 117].

Plasma levels of amphotericin B colloidal dispersions are also lower than those of deoxycholate, but a fair proportion are rapidly taken up by phagocytosis by the liver, which acts as a reservoir that slowly releases the drug [118]. Lung tissue concentrations are lower than those of amphotericin B lipid complex [119]. The incidence of nephrotoxicity is also lower than for deoxycholate amphotericin B [120] and the incidence of hepatotoxicity is also low [121]. The most frequent adverse events are infusion-related, namely fever and chills, with a frequency that justifies pre-medication [122 – 124].

The small size of liposomal amphotericin B molecule leads to a low reticuloendothelial uptake, low distribution into tissues and therefore higher plasma and area under the curve levels [107]. It is well tolerated, with a low nephrotoxicity and a very low incidence of infusion-related side effects. The most frequent adverse events are hypokalemia and increase in liver enzymes [125]. A recent randomized, double-blind, multicenter trial showed that liposomal amphotericin B is as effective as deoxycholate amphotericin B for empirical antifungal therapy in patients with fever and neutropenia and it is associated with fewer breakthrough fungal infections, less infusion-related toxicity and less nephrotoxicity [126]. A study by Walsh et al. showed that doses of 7.5 – 15 mg/kg/day of liposomal amphotericin B were safe and well tolerated.

The three lipid formulations have a reduced propensity for causing toxicity but, considering positive but limited efficacy data and cost, should be reserved for special situations that are discussed below or for second line therapy [127]. They were shown to be as effective as the conventional compound, but there are no controlled, randomized studies available comparing the three preparations [116, 128] and the articles published addressing this issue reached no conclusion and lack consistency [129].

The new antifungal echinocandins (caspofungin, micafungin, anidulafungin) are inhibitors of the fungal cell wall β-(1,3)-D-glucan synthetase enzyme complex. They have a large molecular weight and this presumably explains their poor oral absorption; therefore they should only be used intravenously. As they have a half-life of 10 – 18h h, once a day usage is appropriate. The precise degradation pathways are not fully understood, but almost all drug is degraded by non-oxidative pathways in the liver, and the metabolites, which have no antifungal activity, are excreted in the bile and feces. Therefore there is no need to adjust the dose in patients with renal impairment. On the other hand, a reduced dose should probably be given to patients with significant hepatic dysfunction (50% daily dose after a standard loading dose) [130]. None of the compounds can be dialysed, and so no adjustment is necessary for patients who need renal replacement treatment [131]. They are concentrated in the liver, spleen and gut, are present in equal concentrations in plasma and lung and in lower concentrations in other tissues, such as urine, cerebrospinal fluid and vitreous.

The echinocandin antifungal spectrum is restricted to *Candida* spp. and *Aspergillus* spp. with few exceptions. They are not active at clinically relevant concentrations against *Zygomycetes*, *Cryptococcus neoformans*, *Fusarium* spp. and *Trichosporon* spp. [131]. All three compounds are fungicidal in vitro and in vivo against most isolates of *Candida* spp. and fungistatic against *Aspergillus* spp. [131]. Minimum inhibitory concentrations of all three are much lower than for amphotericin B and fluconazole against all common *Candida* spp. except *Candida parapsilosis* and *Candida guillermondii*, for which they are similar. Interestingly, echinocandins have a postantifungal effect [131].

They are highly active against *Pneumocystis carinii* but have only modest activity against *Coccidioides immitis*, *Blastomyces dermatididis*, *Scedosporium spp.*, *Paecilomyces variotii* and *Histoplasma capsulatum*.

The adverse events and toxic effects of the echinocandins are few. The most frequent adverse effects are: headache (3% with micafungin and about 15% with caspofungin), fever (arises in about 35% of the patients treated with caspofungin [132 – 134]), hepatotoxicity, phlebitis, histamine release and hemolysis (clinically significant hemolytic anemia seems to be rare in clinical studies).

Since echinocandins are poor substrates for the cytochrome P450 enzymes and are not substrates for intestinal or tissue P-glycoprotein, fewer drug interactions are described. Slight increases in caspofungin clearance have been seen with powerful inducers of inhibitors of hepatic metabolism, such as efavirenz, phenytoin, nevirapine, nelfinavir, carbamazepine and dexamethasone, so a slight increase in daily dose of caspofungin (70 mg/day) is appropriate [131]. A slightly reduced exposure to tacrolimus (20%) was seen with coadministration of caspofungin, and monitoring of tacrolimus concentrations is recommended [135]. Cyclosporin and caspofungin seem to interact, resulting in raised caspofungin concentrations but no change in cyclosporin serum levels [131]. No interactions were noted with other antifungals such as itraconazole and amphotericin B [136].

No drug interactions have been described with micafungin and other highly protein-bound compounds including warfarin, diazepam, salicylic acid and methotrexate. Results of a combination study of anidulafungin and cyclosporin in healthy volunteers showed a slight increase in exposure to anidulafungin [131].

Other antifungal strategies may also be useful. Immunomodulators may be important adjuncts for the therapy of invasive mycosis. This is not a surprise, as it is well known that both adequate number and function of granulocytes and intact cell-mediated immunity are essential to a good outcome. In the prophylactic setting, the American Society of Clinical Oncology recommended that G-CSF and GM-CSF should be used in patients with more than a 40% chance of acquiring a fungal infection [137]. Another study showed that in non-neutropenic patients with acute traumatic brain injury and cerebral hemorrhage the prophylactic administration of G-CSF was associated with decreased risk of bacteremia, but did not alter the incidence of other nosocomial infections, length of stay or mortality in this patient group [138]. In the therapeutic setting, some in vitro studies have proven that G-CSF, GM-CSF and interferon gamma may be better than the first two recombinant cytokines in their ability to improve immune function against fungi [139]. These agents may therefore be used in persistently neutropenic patients with proven severe fungal infection [140].

11.3 Therapy of Fungal Infections

Candida spp. cause the huge majority of fungal infections, approximately 85%. Other fungi, namely *Aspergillus*, *Mucor*, *Fusarium*, *Trichosporum* and *Cryptococcus* are also a cause of infection in the ICU, but usually in the immunocompromised patient [95].

The gold standard of diagnosis for *Candida* spp. infection is the presence of positive blood cultures and histological evidence from culture of tissue sample obtained from at least one internal organ, but most diagnoses are based on presumptive criteria and clinical suspicion is undoubtedly the key to diagnosis and to an adequate therapeutic decision. The *Candida* genus includes more than 150 species and 11 of them have already been isolated in the human. Although *Candida albicans* remains the most prevalent species, there has been a clear shift towards non-*albicans* species [48, 71, 141], namely *Candida tropicalis*, *Candida parapsilosis*, *Candida krusei* (particularly in neutropenic patients) and *Candida glabrata* (especially in patients with solid tumors). Six multicenter surveys showed that 42–50% of systemic fungal infections were caused by non-*albicans* species [71, 142–146]. The SENTRY, epidemiology and fungal susceptibility programs performed in the USA, Canada and South America demonstrated that 47% of the candidemias were caused by non-*albicans* species and that *Candida parapsilosis*, *Candida glabrata* and *Candida tropicalis* caused almost 40% [70]. A species very similar to *albicans* has also been described, first in oropharyngitis in HIV patients and more recently in HIV negative patients: *Candida dubliniensis* [147]. This increase in the incidence of non-*albicans Candida* species in the ICU is in part due to the pressure caused by the frequent use of fluconazole [148–155]. This shift has enormous clinical and therapeutic relevance as some species show some particularities. For instance, *Candida tropicalis* shows a higher invasive capacity as 50–60% of the colonized patients develop disseminated candidiasis; *Candida parapsilosis* is associated with total parenteral nutrition and with central venous catheter infection by this species is often not preceded by colonization and it may be less susceptible to killing by amphotericin B; *Candida lusitaniae* [156] may be resistant *ab initio* or easily develops resistance to amphotericin B and, less often, to fluconazole; *Candida glabrata* is commonly resistant to fluconazole or resistance may emerge; *Candida krusei* is virtually always intrinsically resistant to this drug and *Candida dubliniensis* is sometimes resistant to fluconazole but susceptible to other azoles.

Aspergillus is an important pathogen in the neutropenic patient and in all those receiving immunosuppressive treatment for cancer or transplantation. It may also cause disease in HIV-infected patients and in patients with chronic obstructive pulmonary disease, bronchiectasis, lung carcinoma, sarcoidosis or tuberculosis or in patients who were submitted to long-term corticotherapy [20, 157–160].

Mucormycosis (zygomycosis) is seldom seen in normal patients, as the major risk factors are uncontrolled diabetes mellitus, other forms of metabolic acidosis, burns and malignant hematological disorders [12, 20]. *Fusarium* spp. are increasingly recognized as a cause of infection in neutropenic cancer patients and burns and trauma patients [20]. Disseminated trichosporonosis was reported in bone marrow and solid organ transplants, in neutropenic hematological oncological patients after chemotherapy and in AIDS patients; localized deep infections may occur in immunocompetent patients as a complication of cataract extraction, insertion of prosthetic heart valves, intravenous drug abuse, peritoneal dialysis and topical steroid treatment [20, 161]. *Pseudallescheria* infection may occur in patients with structural lung disease, immunosuppression and following trauma [20, 162]. *Cryptococcus neoformans* can cause disease in normal individuals, but a high proportion of human infections occur in immunocompromised patients, especially in persons with impairment of T-cell mediated immunological function, such as the HIV patient [12, 20].

11.4 When To Start Antifungal Therapy

As the diagnosis is difficult and usually presumptive, deciding when to start antifungal therapy is problematic and, given the high morbidity and mortality associated with fungal infections, the British Society of Antimicrobial Chemotherapy Working Party analyzed the four broad approaches to the use of antimicrobial therapy: prophylaxis, pre-emptive therapy, empirical therapy and definitive therapy [49].

Prophylaxis is not indicated in the ICU or in the surgical setting and concerns about the selection of less susceptible *Candida* spp. have limited this approach [22, 49]. Safran [156] showed that 22% of the patients in a surgical ICU treated with fluconazole had secondary fungal infections frequently resistant to fluconazole and this finding was associated with high mortality (44% vs. 9%). Even the use of antifungal agents, together with antibacterial agents, as oral nonabsorbable antimicrobials to decontaminate the gastrointestinal tract did not prove to result in any difference in survival in trauma patients and patients under prolonged mechanical ventilation [163, 164]. Nevertheless, although not recommended in the ICU setting, prophylaxis may be beneficial in a subgroup of patients at high risk of infection [165], such as the neutropenic, the bone marrow transplant, the lung transplant with history of fungal infection and the fulminant liver failure or liver transplant recipient patient [94, 165]. For all these cases, fluconazole is the drug of choice and it should be used for the least time to prevent the selection of azole-resistant organisms.

Pre-emptive therapy is the treatment of individual patients thought to be at high risk of developing deep candidiasis, identified by clinical or laboratory markers to prevent the disease. The British Working Party does not recommend this approach as there is no proof of its value [22, 49, 94], but they consider that patients at particular high-risk might be considered for this kind of therapy [49]. Some studies showed that subsets of critically ill patients in which the incidence of fungal infections is particularly high might benefit from the use of pre-emptive therapy. Such is the case for patients with extensive burns [166], patients on extracorporeal membrane oxygenation systems or on left ventricular assist devices [167, 168], patients with pancreatitis or those submitted to gastrointestinal surgery [164]. Eggimman et al. showed in a randomized, prospective, double-blind, placebo-controlled study that fluconazole may prevent colonization and invasive intra-abdominal *Candida* infections in high-risk surgical patients [169].

Empirical therapy is the treatment of patients thought to have established deep candidiasis without microbiological, histological or serological confirmation. As fungal diagnosis is difficult, empirical therapy is and will continue to be necessary on some occasions. The Working Party proposed the following indications for empirical therapy: (a) clinically unstable or deteriorating premature neonate with skin breaks from which *Candida* has been grown or positive urine microscopy or culture for yeast was found; (b) candiduria in high-risk patients with deteriorating clinical status; and (c) patients with prosthetic valve endocarditis likely to be due to *Candida* even with negative blood cultures [49]. Some authors suggest that anti-*Candida* therapy should also be started in patients with peritonitis caused by intestinal perforation below the duodenum, especially in cancer patients, immunosuppressed patients, when the perforation was not diagnosed for more than 24 h, was hospital-acquired or occurred in patients with unstable conditions, hepatic cirrhosis or pancreatitis or required a second unplanned abdominal surgery [165]. Antifungal therapy is also frequently started empirically in burnt patients with skin invasion, candiduria in certain clinical settings (Table 11.5), two or more sites colonized by *Candida* in a high-risk patient and persistent fever unresponsive to broad-spectrum antibiotics in a high-risk patient.

The neutropenic patient is an example of these high-risk patients. Amphotericin B deoxycholate is the standard agent in refractory neutropenic fever. The use of liposomal amphotericin B and itraconazole in this setting were also approved by the FDA. Recently, Walsh et al. [170] showed in a large, prospective, randomized, multicenter, open-label study that voriconazole did not fulfil the protocol-defined criteria for noninferiority to liposomal amphotericin B for empirical antifungal therapy in patients with neutropenia and persistent fever (26% vs. 30.6%). Indeed, in high risk patients, voriconazole was similar to liposomal amphotericin B. This second generation azole was superior in reducing breakthrough fungal infections (1.9% vs. 5%), infusion related toxicity and nephrotoxicity. Hepatotoxicity was similar in both groups. Voriconazole use was also associated with a reduction in mean duration of hospitalization by 1 day in all patients and by 2 days in high risk patients and this difference was statistically significant. Voriconazole, according to this data, seems to be a suitable alternative to amphotericin B for empirical antifungal therapy in refractory neutropenic fever.

Table 11.5. Candiduria plus any of these conditions should be considered high probability of invasive candidiasis and therefore a reason for antifungal therapy

Candiduria plus:	Piuria
	Pseudo-hyphae in urine
	Fever and signs of pyelonephritis
	Tubular casts with *Candida*
	Persistent candiduria even after changing urinary catheter
	Candida tropicalis
	Candida in other sites
	Abdominal and urological surgery or procedure
	Liver or renal transplant
	Diabetes mellitus

Caspofungin was compared to liposomal amphotericin B in this setting in a large, prospective, randomized, multicenter, double-blind study published by Walsh et al. [171] 2 years ago. Caspofungin was as effective as amphotericin B concerning the overall favorable response (33.9% vs. 33.7%), but in a high risk population caspofungin did better than amphotericin B although the difference was not statistically significant (43.2 vs. 37.7%). The authors observed a significantly higher rate of successful treatment of baseline fungal infections with the use of caspofungin. No difference was found concerning breakthrough fungal infection and resolution of fever in the setting of neutropenia. Caspofungin seems to be an effective alternative to the standard treatment and generally better tolerated, but at a much higher cost when compared to amphotericin B deoxycholate.

Definitive therapy is the treatment of established deep candidiasis, which requires microbiological or histological evidence of fungal infection. The diagnosis of deep candidiasis is established by any of these: (a) at least one positive blood culture in an at risk patient or with acute clinical signs and symptoms compatible with the infection; (b) *Candida* isolated from any sterile site except urine; (c) positive yeast microscopy from a sterile specimen; and (d) histological evidence of yeast or mycelial forms in tissue from at risk patients [49].

There are few cases in which antifungal therapy is started as definitive therapy. What usually happens in the intensive care setting is that you have to identify the patients at risk of developing fungal infection. The conditions associated with an increased risk [2, 172–174] are stated in Table 11.6. *Candida* colonization typically precedes infection with genotypically, identical *Candida* strains. Thus the *Candida* reservoir is clearly endogenous and colonization is an independent risk factor and also a prerequisite for *Candida* infection [175, 176]. Pittet et al. proposed the "*Candida* colonization index" to identify patients who should be put under early antifungal therapy [175]. The index is the ratio of the number of non-blood distinct sites colonized by *Candida* spp. to the total number of sites cultured and it was shown to predict the development of candidemia. A threshold ≥0.5 accurately identified the infected patients. One must therefore maintain a high level of clinical suspicion for all these at risk patients in order to identify patients at an early stage with suspected fungal infection. In the face of clinical suspicion the following steps must be taken: (a) reassess risk factors for *Candida* infection; (b) assess the intensity of *Candida* colonization; (c) perform two sets of blood cultures per day on two consecutive days; (d) obtain cultures of all relevant specimens, according to the clinical scenario, namely respiratory specimens, urine, cerebrospinal fluid, wound, etc.; (e) exclude other possible causes of fever: (f) perform chest teleradiography or chest CT scan if there is suspicion of fungal pneumonia; and (g) assess sites of hematogenous dissemination: endophthalmitis (optic fundus examination) and septic thrombophlebitis.

Table 11.6. Conditions associated with an increased risk of *Candida* infection

Conditions
Immunosuppressive therapy
HIV infection
Malignancy
Major surgery, especially abdominal
Trauma
Burns
Malnutrition
Solid or bone marrow transplant
Neutropenia
High severity score
Hepatic dysfunction
Peritonitis
Acute pancreatitis
Advanced age
Broad spectrum antibiotics (number and duration)
Total parenteral nutrition
Mechanical ventilation
Hemodialysis
Invasive procedures
Long stay in the ICU

11.5 Which Antifungal Agent?

The choice of the antifungal for empirical therapy of candidiasis is based on the condition of the patient, namely immune status and hemodynamic condition, and the species of *Candida* that is colonizing that specific patient or is more prevalent in that particular unit.

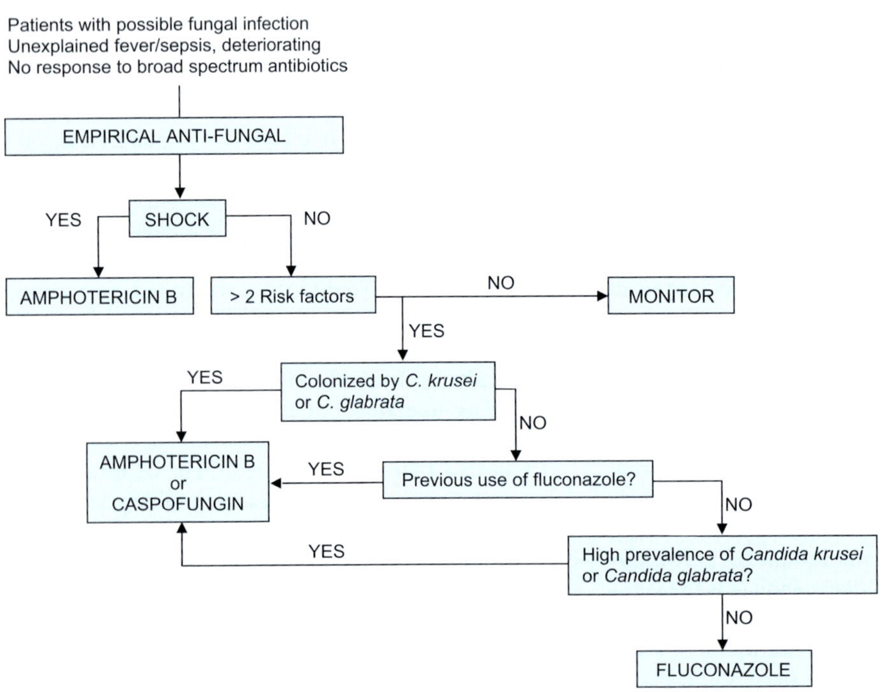

Fig. 11.2. Algorithm for empirical antifungal therapy

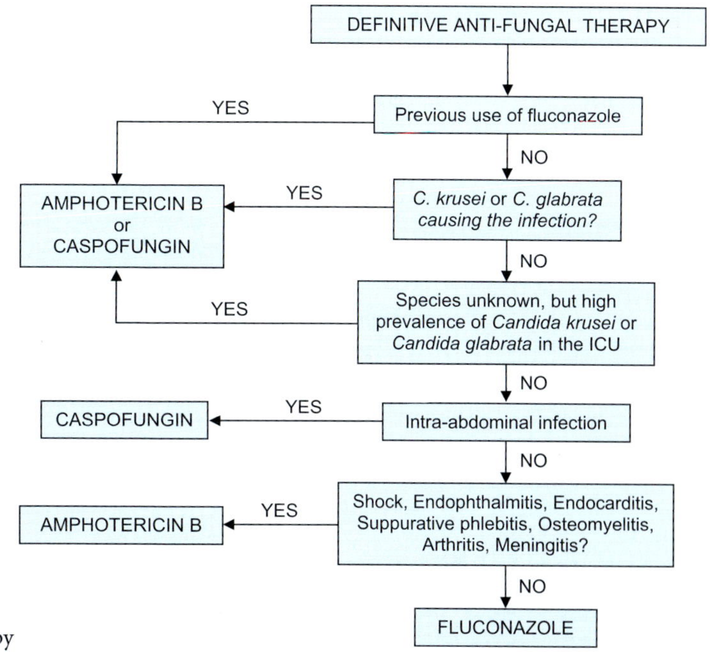

Fig. 11.3. Algorithm for definitive antifungal therapy

In hemodynamically stable patients, not colonized by *Candida glabrata* or *Candida krusei* and who were not previously treated with azoles and in units where these species are not prevalent, fluconazole may be used. If one of these conditions is not satisfied, amphotericin B or caspofungin should be preferred (Fig. 11.2).

The choice of the antifungal agent for definitive therapy is based on the identity of the fungus and the condition of the patient (Fig. 11.3). The currently available systemic antifungal agents useful in the intensive care setting are amphotericin B (deoxycholate and lipid formulations), fluconazole, caspofungin and voriconazole, while itraconazole and flucytosine are less often useful and used.

In the past, patients with candidemia thought to have a low risk of developing a disseminated candidiasis were left untreated. This was based on the belief that *Candida* was a "benign pathogen" and that candidemia was often transient, beliefs that were defended in the late 1960s [177, 178]. Clinical practice proved this strategy to be wrong and *Candida* spp. to be a serious pathogen with high morbidity and mortality. Our capacity to determine prognostic signs or to predict patients with candidemia that would progress to disseminated candidiasis is poor; in fact, retrospective studies have shown an error rate of around 30% in defining a population of candidemic patients who do not require treatment [179]. Besides, less toxic antifungals and ways of decreasing the toxicity of amphotericin B were developed. All this generated the clear consensus that all candidemia should and must be treated [180]. Table 11.7 summarizes the therapeutic strategies for *Candida* fungal infections.

At least four studies [181–184] showed that, in stable non-neutropenic patients, fluconazole may be considered as an alternative to amphotericin B for first-line therapy of candidemia [165], unless it is caused by fluconazole-resistant yeasts like *Candida krusei* or *Candida glabrata* or if the patient had previously been or is at the moment under fluconazole or any other azole therapy. Fluconazole showed the same efficacy but was significantly better tolerated and produced a lower incidence of nephrotoxicity, namely in the Rex et al. study [184], the largest study of candidemia in non-neutropenic patients that compared fluconazole 400 mg/day with amphotericin B 0.6 mg/kg/day. Similar results were found in the neutropenic cancer patient [181]; side effects occurred in 5–12% for fluconazole and in 35–44% for amphotericin B. According to these results, fluconazole could be considered as the drug of choice for *Candida* infection, but this conclusion must be treated with caution as the number of non-*albicans* species, namely those intrinsically resistant and those with acquired resistance to fluconazole, are increasing [94, 144]. Fluconazole is clearly the best agent in two specific situations: infections caused by *Candida lusitaniae* [185] and urinary tract candidiasis, due to its high urinary concentrations [49], while penetration of amphotericin B into the urine is poor. Candiduria is a frequent problem in the ICU, but the majority of cases do not require any treatment apart from catheter and other urinary tract prosthetic materials change or removal [186, 187]; this measure is highly successful, 87–93% at 8 weeks, in clearing funguria [188]. Nevertheless, funguria may also be an early marker of disseminated infection in the critically ill patient [189]. Table 11.5

Table 11.7. Therapeutic strategies for *Candida* infection in the ICU

Infection	Agent of choice	Alternative
Candidemia	Fluconazole 400–800 mg/day or amphotericin B 0.5–1.0 mg/kg/day	Caspofungin
Candidemia in neutropenic patient	Amphotericin B 0.7–1.0 mg/kg/day or Liposomal amphotericin B 3–6 mg/kg/day or caspofungin	Fluconazole 6–12 mg/kg/day
Endophthalmitis	Amphotericin B 1.0 mg/kg/day ± flucytosine	Fluconazole 400–800 mg/day
Endocarditis	Amphotericin B 1.0 mg/kg/day ± flucytosine	Fluconazole 6–12 mg/kg/day or Liposomal amphotericin B 3 mg/kg/day or caspofungin
Meningitis	Amphotericin B 1.0 mg/kg/day ± flucytosine	Fluconazole 400–800 mg/day
Suppurative phlebitis	Amphotericin B 0.5–1.0 mg/kg/day ± flucytosine	Fluconazole 400–800 mg/day
Osteomyelitis/arthritis	Amphotericin B 0.5–1.0 mg/kg/day	Fluconazole 6 mg/kg/day
Pericarditis	Amphotericin B 0.5–0.7 mg/kg/day	Fluconazole 400 mg/day
Peritonitis and intra-abdominal infection	Fluconazole 200–400 mg/day or Caspofungin	Amphotericin B 0.5–1.0 mg/kg/day
Esophagitis	Fluconazole 200 mg/day on 1st day → 100 mg/day	Itraconazole 200 mg/day or Voriconazole 4 mg/kg/day or caspofungin or amphotericin B 0.3–0.7 mg/kg/day
Wound infection	Fluconazole 400 mg/day	Amphotericin B 0.5–0.7 mg/kg/day
Cystitis	Fluconazole 200 mg/day	
Pyelonephritis	Fluconazole 200–400 mg/day	Amphotericin B 0.3–0.7 mg/kg/day
Oropharyngeal	Fluconazole 100–200 mg/day	Itraconazole 200 mg/day

summarizes the conditions and situations in which we treat candiduria [190, 191], using catheter change and fluconazole 200–400 mg/day. If candiduria is persistent after this, we use irrigation with 5–10 mg of amphotericin B with an intravesical dwell time of 2 hours, once or twice daily for 2 days. Bladder irrigation is more effective when the drug concentration is 50 mg/l rather than 10 mg/l [192].

The use of caspofungin for invasive candidiasis was compared with amphotericin B by Mora-Duarte et al. [139]. In this study, caspofungin showed a significantly higher response rate than amphotericin B (80% vs. 65%), particularly if the patient had intra-abdominal abscesses (75 vs. 33%). Caspofungin performed better than amphotericin B in non-*albicans Candida* infections and the authors registered a similar rate of relapse 6–8 weeks after treatment. Fewer side effects were observed with the use of caspofungin (2.8 vs. 16.5%), including nephrotoxicity and hypokalemia. According to these results, caspofungin seems to be a good alternative to amphotericin B for invasive candidiasis, with fewer side effects but more costly.

In non-*albicans Candida* infections, a recent study [140] showed a better, although not statistically significant, response with caspofungin than amphotericin B. These results, in addition to those from the Mora-Duarte et al. [139] study, raise the possibility that caspofungin can be considered the first choice for non-*albicans Candida* infections.

There is limited experience with voriconazole for invasive candidiasis. In a comparative, randomized, multicenter study published by Kullberg et al. [137], voriconazole was shown to be non-inferior to a regimen of amphotericin B followed by fluconazole in the treatment of candidemia in non-neutropenic patients, with successful outcome in 41% of patients in both groups. Additionally, clearance of *Candida* from the bloodstream with voriconazole was as rapid as with amphotericin B. More patients on voriconazole failed treatment before the end due to adverse events, especially those that were not drug-related, but there were significantly fewer serious adverse events and cases of renal toxicity in the voriconazole group than in the amphotericin B/fluconazole group. For *Candida albicans*, *Candida parapsilosis* and *Candida glabrata*, successful response rates were similar between both groups, but for *Candida tropicalis* (32% vs. 6%) and for *Candida krusei* (25% vs. 0%), the proportion of patients responding to voriconazole was substantially higher. Voriconazole was also tested in a small group of patients ($n=52$) with invasive candidiasis refractory or intolerant to other antifungals [193]. In this study, voriconazole showed an overall response rate of 56% and the response rates by species were generally similar among the different *Candida* spp., notably in patients infected with *Candida krusei* (70%). There were no differences in response related to previous azole exposure, and toxicity associated with voriconazole use was similar to other studies. Although there is limited data, voriconazole provides an important new treatment option for candidemia.

In esophagitis, peritonitis, wound infection and pyelonephritis by *Candida*, fluconazole may be the preferred drug. There are, however, some doubts about the optimal dose of fluconazole, namely 5 mg/kg/day or 10 mg/kg/day. A study by Graninger et al. [194] showed higher cure rates when the higher dose was used: 83% vs. 60%. Some authors recommend that treatment should be started with a higher dose, for instance 600–800 mg/day IV, for 3 days and then followed by 400 mg/day IV or orally [22]. Although 5 mg/kg/day is the usual dose, at least patients on hemodiafiltration and catabolic patients should receive a higher dose [194–196]. A higher dose should also be used for catabolic patients. It is worth mentioning the fact that fluconazole has also been shown to be effective in the treatment of chronic disseminated candidiasis, even after prior amphotericin B therapy and that it can be useful for maintenance therapy after response to amphotericin B therapy [197, 198]. In the liver transplant setting, as the azoles, through their effect on hepatic microsomial function, inhibit the metabolism of cyclosporine and tacrolimus, doses of fluconazole should be limited to 200–400 mg/day and safety and efficacy of these doses in this setting have been demonstrated, including in patients with severe allograft dysfunction [199, 200].

Amphotericin B should be preferred in any clinically unstable, deteriorating patient, in patients with high-grade candidemia or in patients with hematogenous deep-organ infections, like severe endophthalmitis, suppurative phlebitis, endocarditis, pericarditis, osteomyelitis and meningitis. It may be used alone or in association with flucytosine [19, 49, 94, 165, 201], but the use of this agent requires facilities for monitoring serum concentrations and seems to be only justified in patients with high-grade persistent fungemia or perhaps with infection in sites where penetration of amphotericin B is far from ideal such as vegetations, meninges and vitreous. In the case of endophthalmitis, amphotericin B IV is usually enough, but if lesions are expansive or close to the macula, flucytosine should be added; consultation with an ophthalmologist is mandatory in all cases and in large, progressive or symptomatic lesions the use of 5 mg amphotericin B intravitreal and partial vitrectomy may be needed and may even be sight-saving procedures. There are very few data on the efficacy of azole treatment for hematogenous candidal endophthalmitis, although its use is documented in 96 patients and 108 eyes with a response rate of about 90%, with 200–400 mg/day of fluconazole for 6–8 weeks [202], and some series also suggest its efficacy [203, 204]. However, two animal studies [205, 206] and one clinical study [207] have shown less satisfactory results.

During the past 2 decades, invasive aspergillosis has emerged worldwide as an important cause of nosocomial and community-acquired infection among a wide spectrum of immunocompromised patients, including patients undergoing cancer chemotherapy, hematopoietic stem-cell transplantation (HSCT), or solid-organ transplantation and patients with advanced HIV infection. The overall mortality rate for invasive aspergillosis remains dramatically high, approaching 90% in populations of profoundly immunocompromised patients.

The therapeutic options available to treat invasive aspergillosis are limited to a small arsenal of antifungal compounds. For the past 4 decades, deoxycholate amphotericin B has been considered to be the standard antifungal agent for treatment of invasive aspergillosis in severely immunocompromised patients. Several recent studies have indicated that the overall response rate to treatment is less than 40% and may be as low as 10–15% among patients undergoing allogenic HSCT. However, the usefulness of deoxycholate amphotericin B is hampered by dose-limiting nephrotoxicity and acute infusion-related toxicity.

The lipid formulations of amphotericin B are associated with less toxicity at higher dosages; however, their overall efficacy at current therapeutic dosages may be similar to that of deoxycholate amphotericin B in the primary treatment of invasive aspergillosis. They should, however, be used in patients infected by fungi with high MICs to amphotericin B, such as *Mucorales*, *Fusarium* and most *Aspergillus*. These forms have, as we have stated before, a higher therapeutic index, owing to reduced toxicity and to organ distribution, resulting in targeting the drug to the reticular endothelial system and sites of inflammation, such as liver, spleen and lung [208]. Although the clinical significance of the difference in the tissue distribution of several compounds is not totally known, it seems to be an important treatment outcome. For instance, using lipid complex amphotericin B obtains the highest concentration in the lung [209]. Recently a large study showed that patients with life-threatening mycosis were successfully treated with lipid complex amphotericin B (5 mg/kg/day) after failure of or intolerance to the conventional formulation [113]. In a randomized, multicenter study in neutropenic patients with documented or suspected fungal infections, liposomal amphotericin B (5 mg/kg/day) was superior to amphotericin B (1 mg/kg/day) in terms of efficacy and safety [128].

Voriconazole is another option in the treatment of invasive aspergillosis. Herbrecht et al. [210] demonstrated in a large, randomized, unblinded, multicenter study comparing voriconazole and deoxycholate amphotericin B, that initial treatment with voriconazole led to better responses (52.8% vs. 31.6%) and improved survival (70.8% vs. 57.9%). Voriconazole-treated patients had significantly fewer severe drug-related adverse events. Four more studies showed that voriconazole was associated with a significant percentage of success (45–58%) as salvage or primary therapy for invasive aspergillosis.

The role of caspofungin in the treatment of invasive aspergillosis was assessed by Kartsonis et al. [211] in a

Table 11.8. Therapeutic strategies for non-*Candida* fungal infections in the ICU

Infection	Agent of choice	Alternative
Invasive acute aspergillosis	Voriconazole or Liposomal amphotericin B 5 mg/kg/day	Voriconazole + caspofungin Amphotericin B + caspofungin
Cerebral aspergillosis	Voriconazole	Liposomal amphotericin B 5 mg/kg/day
Aspergillus invasive sinusitis	Liposomal amphotericin B 3–5 mg/kg/day	Voriconazole
Cryptococcus meningitis	Amphotericin B 0.7 mg/kg/day ± flucytosine	Fluconazole 400–800 mg/day
Cryptococcus meningitis in AIDS	Amphotericin B 0.7 mg/kg/day + flucytosine 100–150 mg/kg/day or liposomal amphotericin B 5 mg/kg/day (6 weeks)	Amphotericin B 0.7 mg/kg/day (2 weeks) → fluconazole 400 mg/day (8 weeks) then 200 mg/day or fluconazole 800 mg/day
Pulmonary cryptococcosis	Amphotericin B 0.5–0.7 mg/kg/day	Fluconazole 400 mg/day (4–6 weeks)
Mucormycosis	Complex lipid or liposomal amphotericin B ≥5 mg/kg/day (8 weeks) + reversion predisposing conditions + aggressive surgery	
Fusarium	Complex lipid or liposomal amphotericin B 5 mg/kg/day	Voriconazole
Trichosporonosis	Fluconazole 800–1,200 mg/day	Complex lipid or liposomal amphotericin or voriconazole
Pseudallescheria infection	Voriconazole	Fluconazole 800–1200 mg/day or itraconazole
Scedosporium infection	Voriconazole	

non-comparative, small, open label, multicenter study with 48 patients with invasive *Aspergillus* spp. infection refractory or intolerant to deoxycholate amphotericin B or a lipid formulation. Forty percent of the patients refractory to at least one antifungal agent and 27% of the patients refractory to multiple antifungal agents responded favorably. Most of the patients (80%) intolerant to a polyene exhibited a favorable response. Some case reports confirmed that caspofungin seems to be an effective and well tolerated alternative for the salvage treatment of invasive aspergillosis [212, 213].

Table 11.8 describes the therapeutic strategies for non-*Candida* fungal infections. Amphotericin B is the drug of choice for almost all these infections except pseudallescheriosis and perhaps trichosporonosis. In fact, amphotericin B resistant *Trichosporon beigelii* has been described and *Pseudallescheria boydii* is often resistant to that drug. However, the lipid formulations result in better tissue distribution in liver, spleen and lungs than deoxycholate and therefore may be active against infections where effective concentrations of amphotericin B are not readily achievable, such as those caused by *Aspergillus* spp., *Fusarium* spp. and *Mucorales*.

Although in vitro studies indicated some antagonism between fluconazole and amphotericin B [214], this effect may not be relevant in vivo [215] and, although there are no definitive data to support combination therapy, it has been used by some in severely acutely ill patients with systemic mycosis and septic shock or even in transplant patients [20, 215].

The results of in vitro studies and animal models suggest that combination therapy with azoles and echinocandins may have additive activity against *Aspergillus* species. For instance, in an experimental invasive pulmonary aspergillosis model, the association of ravuconazole with micafungin was studied by Petraitis et al. [216]. This combination led to a significant reduction in mortality, residual fungal burden and serum galactomannan antigenemia. Interestingly, no toxicity was observed with the echinocandin-triazole combination.

Marr et al. [217] evaluated the outcome of patients with aspergillosis who experienced failure of initial therapy with amphotericin B formulations and received a combination of voriconazole and caspofungin ($n=16$ patients) for salvage therapy which was associated with an improved 3-month survival rate. According to these results, the authors claimed that randomized trials are warranted to validate this association as primary treatment of invasive aspergillosis.

11.6 When To Stop Antifungal Therapy?

The duration of therapy is also a matter of debate. For the most severe invasive mycosis it should be at least 4 weeks [49]. In severe forms, in very critically ill patients it should be even longer, around 8 weeks, although the intensity of dosing can often be decreased after the first 2 weeks of therapy [49]. For hematogenous candidiasis, immunosuppressed patients should be treated for at least 10–14 days and immunocompetent patients for at least 5 days after the disappearance of all symptoms and signs of infection [20]. In the neutropenic, it must be continued throughout the duration of neutropenia. In the case of endophthalmitis, therapy must be continued until at least 10 days after the ocular lesion has resolved [19]. The rate of visceral seeding following candidemia in solid organ transplant recipients is significantly higher than that for the general population, exceeding 50% at some centers, and therefore therapy must be continued for at least 2 weeks after the last positive blood culture and clinical response has occurred [165].

Maintenance of therapy is only indicated in patients with persistent presence of foreign material infected with *Candida* which cannot be removed, such as vascular grafts, artificial joints or ventriculoperitoneal shunts. In the case of impossibility of removal, lifelong therapy with antifungal agents should be performed, usually with fluconazole 100–200 mg/day. If the agent is resistant to fluconazole, intermittent amphotericin B or itraconazole should be used, depending on susceptibility tests. However, patients with candidemia should be followed for at least 3 months after the initial episode, as most late complications occur during this period [218, 219].

11.7 Conclusions

The antifungal armamentarium has recently been enlarged by a new triazole and a new class of drugs – the echinocandins. Two new triazoles and two new echinocandins will soon be entering the clinical arena.

We now have drugs that act on several sites of fungal structure and metabolism: (1) inhibition of nucleic acid synthesis, (2) the cytoplasmic membrane, and (3) the fungal cell wall.

This variety of antifungal drugs allows us to individualize the choice of therapy for invasive fungal infections, based on: (1) the infecting pathogens; (2) host factors, such as organ dysfunction and immune status; (3) toxicity profile of the drug; and (4) concurrent drugs.

Figure 11.4 summarizes an algorithm of selection of the antifungal drug.

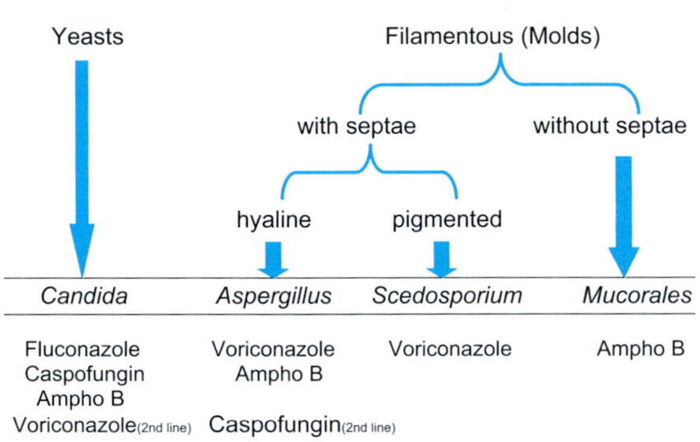

Fig. 11.4. Algorithm of selection of the antifungal drug

References

1. Beck-Sague C, Jarvis WR (1993) Secular trends in the epidemiology of nosocomial fungal infections in the United States, 1980–1990. J Infect Dis 167:1247
2. Fridkin SK, Jarvis WR (1996) Epidemiology of nosocomial fungal infections. Clin Microbiol Rev 9:499
3. Vincent JL, Bihari DJ, Suter PM, et al. (1995) The prevalence of nosocomial infection in intensive care units in Europe (EPIC). JAMA 274:639
4. Martin GS, Mannino MS, Eaton S, et al. (2003) The epidemiology of sepsis in the United States from 1979 through 2000. N Engl J Med 308:1546
5. Jarvis WR (1995) Epidemiology of nosocomial fungal infections, with emphasis on *Candida* species. Clin Infect Dis 20:1526
6. Pittet (1993) Nosocomial blood stream infections. In: Wenzel (RP) Prevention and control of nosocomial infections, 2nd edn. Williams and Wilkins, Baltimore, p 512
7. Wey SB, Motomi M, Pfaller MA, et al. (1988) Hospital acquired candidemia: the attributable mortality and excess length of stay. Arch Intern Med 148:2642
8. Elewski BE (1993) Mechanisms of action of systemic antifungal agents. J Am Acad Dermatol 28:S28
9. Johnson E (1999) Mycological activity of antifungal agents. In: Vincent JL (ed) The management of fungal in the ICU. The Liposome Company, London, p 43
10. Hoeprich PD (1989) Chemotherapy for systemic mycosis. Prog Drug Res 33:317
11. Terrell CL, Hughes CE (1992) Antifungal agents used for deep-seated mycotic infections. Mayo Clin Proc 67:69
12. Richardson MD, Warnock DW (1997) Antifungal drugs. In: Fungal infections – diagnosis and management, 2nd edn. Blackwell Science, Oxford, p 21
13. Iwata K (1992) Drug resistance in human pathogenic fungi. Eur J Epidemiol 8:407
14. Bennett JE (1977) Flucytosine. Ann Intern Med 86:319
15. Benson JM, Nahata MC (1988) Clinical use of systemic antifungal agents. Clin Pharm 7:424
16. Medoff G, Comfort M, Kobayashi GS (1971) Synergistic action of amphotericin B and 5-flucytosine against yeast-like organisms. Proc Soc Exp Biol Med 138:571
17. Beggs WH, Andrews FA, Sarosi GA (1981) Combined action of amphotericin B and 5-flucytosine on pathogenic yeasts susceptible to either drug alone. Chemotherapy 27:247
18. Francis P, Walsh TJ (1992) Evolving role of flucytosine in immunocompromised patients: new insights into safety, pharmacokinetic and antifungal therapy. Clin Infect Dis 15:1003
19. Anaissie E, Solomkin JS (1994) Fungal infection. In: Willmore DW, Cheung LY, Harken AH (eds) Care of the surgical patient. New York Scientific American Medical 1. American College of Surgeons, New York
20. Hastings M, Wolff M (1999) Current treatment of fungal infections in the ICU. In: Vincent JL (ed) The management of fungal in the ICU. The Liposome Company, London, p 55

21. Richardson MD, Kokki M (1998) Therapeutic guidelines in systemic fungal infections. Current Medical Literature, London
22. Vincent JL, Anaissie E, Bruining H, et al. (1998) Epidemiology, diagnosis and treatment of systemic *Candida* infection in surgical patients under intensive care. Int Care Med 24:206
23. Schafer-Korting M (1993) Pharmacokinetic optimization of oral antifungal therapy. Clin Pharmacokinet 25:329
24. British Society for Antimicrobial Chemotherapy Working Party on Fungal Infections (1991) Laboratory monitoring of antifungal chemotherapy. Lancet 35:1577
25. Viscoli C, Castagnola E (1999) Advantages and disadvantages of current therapy. In: Vincent JL (ed) The management of fungal in the ICU. The Liposome Company, London, p 71
26. Stamm AM, Diasio RB, Dismukes WE, et al. (1987) Toxicity of amphotericin B plus flucytosine in 194 patients with cryptococcal meningitis. Am J Med 83:236
27. Dellamonica P, Fournier JP, Garraffo R, et al. (1985) Contribution à la surveillance des traitments comportant de la 5-flucytosine. Pathol Biol 33:642
28. Bennett JE, Dismukes WE, Duma RJ, et al. (1979) A comparison of amphotericin B alone and combined with flucytosine in the treatment of cryptococcal meningitis. N Engl J Med 201:126
29. Como JA, Dismukes WE (1994) Oral azoles as systemic antifungal therapy. N Engl J Med 330:263
30. Lavrijsen KLM, van Hout JMG, van Dick DMJ, et al. (1990) Induction potential of fluconazole toward drug-metabolizing enzymes in rat. Antimicrob Agents Chemother 36:1799
31. Joly V, Bolard J, Yeni P (1992) *In vitro* models for studying toxicity of antifungal agents. Antimicrob Agents Chemother 36:1799
32. van den Bossche H, Marichal P, Le Jeune L, et al. (1993) Effects of itraconazole on cytochrome P450-dependent sterol 14-alpha-demethylation and reduction of 3-ketosteroids in *Cryptococcus neoformans*. Antimicrob Agents Chemother 37:2101
33. Kramer KM, Tesquet D, Johnson AL, Johnston LH (1998) Budding yeast RSI1/APC2, a novel gene necessary for initiation of anaphase, encodes an APC subunit. EMBO J 17:498
34. Goa KL, Barradell LB (1995) Fluconazole – an update of its pharmacodynamic, pharmacokinetic properties and therapeutic use in major superficial and systemic mycosis in immunocompromised patients. Drugs 50:658
35. Blum RA, D'Andrea DT, Fiorentino BM, et al. (1991) Increased gastric pH and the bioavailability of fluconazole and ketoconazole. Ann Intern Med 114:755
36. Anaissie EJ, Kontoyiannis DP, Huls C, et al. (1995) Safety, plasma concentrations and efficacy of high-dose fluconazole in invasive mould infections. J Infect Dis 172:599
37. Saag MS, Dismukes WE (1988) Azole anti-fungal agents: emphasis on new triazoles. Antimicrob Agents Chemother 32:1
38. Fischman AJ, Alpert NM, Livni E, et al. (1993) Pharmacokinetics of 18 F-labeled fluconazole in healthy human subjects by positron emission tomography. Antimicrob Agents Chemother 37:1270
39. Humphrey MJ, Jevons S, Tarbit MH (1985) Pharmacokinetic evaluation of UK-49858, a metabolically stable triazole antifungal drug, in animals and humans. Antimicrob Agents Chemother 28:648
40. Graybill JR (1989) New antifungal agents. Eur J Clin Microbiol Infect Dis 8:402
41. Toon S, Ross CE, Gokal R, Rowland M (1990) An assessment of the effects of impaired renal function and hemodialysis on the pharmacokinetics of fluconazole. Br J Clin Pharmacol 29:221
42. Trotman RL, Williamson JC, Shoemaker DM, et al. (2005) Antibiotic dosing in critically ill adult patients receiving continuous renal replacement therapy. Clin Infect Dis 41:1159
43. Silvestri L, Mur Laffon D, Gullo A (1998) Antifungal agents. In: van Saene HKF, Silvestri L, de la Cal MA (eds) Infection control in the intensive care unit. Springer, Milan, p 50
44. Tucker RM, William PL, Arathon EG, et al. (1988) Pharmacokinetics of fluconazole in cerebrospinal fluid and serum in human coccidioidal meningitis. Antimicrob Agents Chemother 32:369
45. Arndt CAS, Walsh TJ, McCully CL, et al. (1988) Fluconazole penetration into cerebrospinal fluid: implications for treating fungal infections of the central nervous system. J Infect Dis 157:178
46. Berry AJ, Rinaldi MJ, Graybill JR (1992) Use of high-dose fluconazole as salvage therapy for cryptococcal meningitis in patients with AIDS. Antimicrob Agents Chemother 36:690
47. Nguyen MH, Yu CY (1998) Voriconazole against fluconazole-susceptible and resistant *Candida* isolates: *in vitro* efficacy compared with that of itraconazole and ketoconazole. J Antimicrob Chemother 42:253
48. Pfaller MA, Jones RN, Messer SAA, et al. (1998) National surveillance of nosocomial bloodstream infections due to *Candida albicans*: frequency of occurrence and antifungal susceptibility in the SCOPE Program. Diagn Microbiol Infect Dis 31:327
49. British Society for Antimicrobial Chemotherapy Working Party on Fungal Infections (1994) Management of deep *Candida* infection in surgical and intensive care units. Intensive Care Med 20:522
50. Sanglard D, Ischer F, Monod M, et al. (1996) Susceptibilities of *Candida albicans* multidrug transporter mutants to various antifungal agents and other metabolic inhibitors. Antimicrob Agents Chemother 40:2300
51. Hernaez ML, Gil C, Pla J, et al. (1998) Induced expression of the *Candida albicans* multidrug resistance gene CDR1 in response to fluconazole and other antifungals. Yeasts 14:517
52. White MH, Bowden RA, Sandler ES, et al. (1998) Randomized, double-blind clinical trial of amphotericin B colloidal dispersion versus amphotericin B in the empirical treatment of fever and neutropenia. Clin Infect Dis 271:296
53. Marr KA, Lyons CN, Rustad T, et al. (1998) Rapid, transient fluconazole resistance in *Candida albicans* is associated with increased mRNA levels of CDR. Antimicrob Agents Chemother 42:2584
54. Moran GP, Sanglard D, Donnelly SM, et al. (1998) Identification and expression of multidrug transporters responsible for fluconazole resistance in *Candida dubliniensis*. Antimicrob Agents Chemother 42:1819
55. Bronstein JA, Gros P, Hernandez E, et al. (1997) Fatal acute hepatitis necrosis due to dose-dependent fluconazole hepatotoxicity. Clin Infect Dis 25:1266
56. Muñoz P, Moreno S, Berenguer J, et al. (1991) Fluconazole related hepatotoxicity in patients with acquired immunodeficiency syndrome. Arch Intern Med 151:1020
57. Hay RJ (1993) Risk/benefit of modern antifungal therapy: focus on hepatic reactions. J Am Acad Dermatol 29:S50
58. Albengres E, Le Fouet H, Tillement JP (1998) Systemic antifungal agents. Drug Saf 18:83
59. Michalets EL (1998) Update: clinically significant cytochrome P450 drug interactions. Pharmacotherapy 18:84

60. Barone JA, Koh JA, Bierman RH, et al. (1993) Food interaction and steady-state pharmacokinetics of itraconazole in healthy male volunteers. Antimicrob Agents Chemother 37:778
61. Daneshmend TK, Warnock DW (1983) Clinical pharmacokinetics of systemic antifungal drug. Pharmacokinet 8:17
62. Hardin TC, Graybill JR, Fetchick R, et al. (1998) Pharmacokinetics of itraconazole following oral administration to normal volunteers. Antimicrob Agents Chemother 32: 1310
63. Perfect JR, Savani DV, Durack DT (1985) Penetration of imidazoles and triazoles into cerebrospinal fluid of rabbits. J Antimicrob Chemother 16:81
64. van Cutsem J, van Gerven F, Janssen PA (1987) Activity of orally, topically and parenterally administered itraconazole in the treatment of superficial and deep mycosis: animal models. Rev Infect DIs 9:S15
65. Perfect JR, Savani DV, Durack DT (1993) Uptake of itraconazole by alveolar macrophages. Antimicrob Agents Chemother 37:903
66. Walsh TJ, Pizzo A (1988) Treatment of systemic fungal infections: recent progress and current problems. Eur J Clin Microbiol Infect Dis 7:460
67. Denning DW, Lee JY, Hosteler JS, et al. (1994) NIAID Mycosis Study Group: Multicenter trial of oral itraconazole therapy for invasive aspergillosis. Am J Med 7:460
68. De Pauw BE, Meis JF (1998) Progress in fighting systemic fungal infection in hematological neoplasia. Support Cancer Center 6:31
69. Johnson EM, Davey KG, Szekely A, et al. (1995) Itraconazole susceptibilities of fluconazole susceptible and resistant isolates of five *Candida* species. J Antimicrob Chemother 36:787
70. Pfaller MA, Jones RN, Doern GV, et al. (1998) International surveillance of bloodstream infections due to *Candida* species: frequency of occurrence and antifungal susceptibilities of isolates collected in 1997 in the United States, Canada and South America for the SENTRY Program. J Clin Microbiol 36:1886
71. Pfaller MA, Jones RN, Messer SA, Edmond MB, et al. (1998) National surveillance of nosocomial bloodstream infections due to species of *Candida* other than *Candida albicans*: frequency of occurrence and antifungal susceptibility in the SCOPE program. Diagn Microbiol Infect Dis 30:121
72. Groll AH, Gea-Banacloche JC, Glasmacher A, et al. (2003) Clinical pharmacology of antifungal compounds. Infect Dis Clin North Am 17:159
73. Bland SE (2002) Voriconazole. Pharmacotherapy Perspectives Nov/Dec:32
74. Robatel C, Rusca M, Padoin C, et al. (2004) Disposition of voriconazole during continuous veno-venous hemodiafiltration in a single patient. J Antimicrob Chemother 54:269
75. Neely MN, Ghannoum MA (2000) The exciting future of antifungal therapy. Eur J Clin Microbiol Infect Dis 19:897
76. Ernst EJ (2001) Investigational antifungal agents. Pharmacotherapy 21:65S
77. Moore CB, Walls CM, Denning DW (2000) In vitro activity of the new triazole BMS-207147 against *Aspergillus* species in comparison with itraconazole and amphotericin B. Antimicrob Agents Chemother 44:441
78. Diekema DJ, Pfaller MA, Messer SA, et al. (1999) In vitro activities of BMS-207147 against over 600 contemporary clinical bloodstream isolates of *Candida* species from the SENTRY antimicrobial surveillance programme in North America and Latin America. Antimicrob Agents Chemother 43:2236
79. Fung-Tome JC, Huczko E, Minassian B, et al. (1998) In vitro activity of a new oral triazole: BMS-207147. Antimicrob Agents Chemother 42:313
80. Hata K, Kimura J, Miki H, et al. (1996) In vitro and in vivo antifungal activities of ER-30346, a novel oral triazole with a broad antifungal spectrum. Antimicrob Agents Chemother 40:2237
81. Yamazumi T, Pfaller MA, Messer SA, et al. (2000) In vitro activities of ravuconazole against 541 clinical isolates of *Cryptococcus neoformans*. Antimicrob Agents Chemother 44:2883
82. Pfaller MA, Messer SA, Hollis RJ, et al. (1998) In vitro susceptibilities of *Candida* bloodstream isolates to the new triazole antifungal agents BMS-207147, Sch 56592 and voriconazole. Antimicrob Agents Chemother 42:3242
83. Ezzet F, Wexler D, Courtney R, et al. (2001) The pharmacokinetics of posaconazole in neutropenic oncology patients (Abstract A 26). In: Abstracts of 41st Interscience Conference on Antimicrobial Agents and Chemotherapy. Edited by American Society for Microbiology, Chicago, p 4
84. Sheehan DJ, Hitchcock CA, Sibley CM (1999) Current and emerging azole antifungal agents. Clin Microbiol Rev 12:40
85. Law D, Moore CB, Denning DW (1997) Activity of SCH 56592 compared with those of fluconazole and itraconazole against *Candida* spp. Antimicrob Agents Chemother 41:2310
86. Pfaller MA, Messer SA, Jones RN (1997) Activity of a new triazole, Sch 56592, compared with those of four other antifungal agents tested against clinical isolates of *Candida* spp. and *Saccharomyces cerevisiae*. Antimicrob Agents Chemother 41:233
87. Kerridge D (1998) Polyene macrolides antibiotics. In: van den Bossche H, Mackenzie DWR, Cauwenbergh G (eds) *Aspergillus* and aspergillosis. Plenum Press, New York, p 147
88. Fields BT Jr, Bates JH, Abernathy RS (1970) Amphotericin B serum concentrations during therapy. Appl Microbiol 19:955
89. Atkinson AJ Jr, Bennett JE (1978) Amphotericin B pharmacokinetics. Antimicrob Agents Chemother 13:271
90. van Burik JA, Bowden RA (1995) Standard antifungal treatment, including role of alternative modalities to administer amphotericin B. In: Meunier F (ed) Invasive fungal infections in cancer patients. Bailliere Tindall, London, p 89
91. Brajtburg J, Powderly WG, Kobayashi GS, et al. (1990) Amphotericin B delivery systems. Antimicrob Agents Chemother 34:381
92. Bodey GP (1991) Antifungal agents. In: Bodey GP (ed) Candidiasis: pathogenesis, diagnosis and treatment. Raven Press, New York, p 371
93. Pfaller MA, Messer SA, Hollis RJ, et al. (2002) Antifungal activities of posaconazole, ravuconazole and voriconazole compared to those of itraconazole and amphotericin B against 239 clinical isolates of *Aspergillus* spp. and other filamentous fungi: report from SENTRY antimicrobial surveillance program, 2000. Antimicrob Agents Chemother 46:1032
94. Flanagan PG, Barnes RA (1998) Fungal infections in the intensive care unit. J Hosp Infect 38:163
95. Warnock DW (1995) Fungal complications of transplantations: diagnosis, treatment and prevention. J Antimicrob Chemother 36:73
96. Chia JKS, McManus EJ (1990) *In vitro* tumor necrosis factor induction assay for analysis of febrile toxicity associated with amphotericin B preparations. Antimicrob Agents Chemother 34:906
97. Grasela TH, Goodwin SD, Walawandu MK, et al. (1990)

Prospective surveillance of intravenous amphotericin B use patterns. Pharmacotherapy 10:341

98. Gelfand JA, Kimball K, Burke JF, et al. (1988) Amphotericin B treatment of human mononuclear cells *in vitro* results in secretion of tumour necrosis factor and interleukin-1. Clin Res 36:456A
99. Lin AC, Goldwasser E, Bernard EM, et al. (1990) Amphotericin B blunts erythropoietin response to anemia. J Infect Dis 161:348
100. Gallis HA, Drew RH, Pickard WW (1990) Amphotericin B: 30 years of clinical experience. Rev Infect DIs 12:308
101. Branch RA (1988) Prevention of amphotericin B induced renal impairment: a review on the use of sodium supplementation. Arch Intern Med 148:2389
102. Miano-Mason TM (1997) Mechanisms and management of amphotericin B-induced nephrotoxicity. Cancer Pract 5:176
103. Khoo SH, Bond J, Denning DW (1994) Administering amphotericin B: a practical approach. J Antimicrob Chemother 33:203
104. Solomkin JS, Flohr A, Simmons RL (1982) *Candida* infections in surgical patients: dose requirements and toxicity of amphotericin B. Ann Surg 195:177
105. Medoff G (1987) Controversial areas of antifungal chemotherapy: short-course and combination therapy with amphotericin B. Rev Infect DIs 9:403
106. Laenders AC, de Marie S (1996) The use of lipid formulations of amphotericin B for systemic fungal infections. Leukemia 10:1570
107. Mehta J (1997) Do variations in molecular structure affect the clinical efficacy and safety of lipid-based amphotericin B preparations? Leuk Res 21:183
108. Wingard JR (1997) Efficacy of amphotericin B lipid complex injection (ABLC) in bone marrow transplant recipients with life threatening systemic mycosis. BMT 19:343
109. Luke RG, Boyle JA (1998) Renal effects of amphotericin B lipid complex. Am J Kidney Dis 31:780
110. Rap R, Gubbins PO (1998) Amphotericin B lipid complex. Ann Pharmacother 31:1174
111. Tang CM, Bowler ICJW (1997) Do the new lipid formulations of amphotericin B really work? Clin Micro Infect 16:98
112. White MN, Bowden RA, Sandler ES, et al. (1998) Randomized, double-blind clinical trial of amphotericin B colloidal dispersion versus amphotericin B in the empirical treatment of fever and neutropenia. Clin Infect Dis 27:296
113. Walsh TJ, Hiemenz JW, Seibel NL, et al. (1998) Amphotericin B lipid complex for invasive fungal infections: analysis of safety and efficacy in 556 cases. Clin Infect Dis 26:1383
114. Garbino J, Pittet D (1997) *Candida* infections in the intensive care unit. Clin Intensive Care 8:187
115. Adedoyin A, Bernard JF, Swenson CE, et al. (1997) Pharmacokinetic profile of Abelcet (amphotericin B lipid complex injection): combined experience from phase I and phase II studies. Antimicrob Agents Chemother 41: 2201
116. Anaissie E, White M, Uzon O, et al. (1995) Amphotericin B lipid complex versus amphotericin B for the treatment of invasive candidiasis: a prospective randomized, multicenter trial. Programs and abstracts of the 35th Interscience Conference on Antimicrobials Agents and Chemotherapy 30: Abst LM21
117. Goff DA, Sierawski SJ (1998) A clinical and economic analysis of amphotericin B lipid complex (ABLC; Abelcet) vs. amphotericin B. Programs and abstracts of the 38th Interscience Conference on Antimicrobials Agents and Chemotherapy
118. Fielding RM, Smith PC, Wang LH, et al. (1991) Comparative pharmacokinetics of amphotericin B after administration of a novel colloidal delivery system, ABCD, and a conventional formulation to rats. Antimicrob Agents Chemother 35:1208
119. Taylor RL, Williams DM, Craven PC, et al. (1982) Amphotericin B in liposomes: a novel therapy for histoplasmosis. Am Rev Respir Dis 125:610
120. Oppenheim BA, Herbrecht R, Kusne S (1995) The safety and efficacy of amphotericin B colloidal dispersion in the treatment of invasive mycosis. Clin Infect Dis 21:1145
121. Dupont B (1999) Clinical efficacy of amphotericin B colloidal dispersion against infections caused by *Candida* spp. Chemotherapy 45 (Suppl 1):27
122. Anaissie EJ, Mattiuzzi GN, Miller CB, et al. (1998) Treatment of invasive fungal infections in renally impaired patients with amphotericin B colloidal dispersion. Antimicrob Agents Chemother 42:606
123. Herbrecht R (1997) Safety of amphotericin B colloidal dispersion. Eur J Clin Microbiol Infect Dis 16:74
124. Gurwith M, Mamelok R, Pietrelli L, et al. (1999) Renal sparing by amphotericin B colloidal dispersion: clinical experience in 572 patients. Chemotherapy 45 (Suppl 1):39
125. Meunier F, Prentice HG, Ringden O (1991) Liposomal amphotericin B (Ambisome): safety data from a phase II/III clinical trial. J Antimicrob Chemother 28:83
126. Walsh TJ, Fingers RW, Arndt CAS, et al. (1999) Liposomal amphotericin B for empirical therapy in patients with persistent fever and neutropenia. N Eng J Med 340:764
127. Slain D (1999) Lipid-based amphotericin B for the treatment of fungal infections. Pharmacotherapy 19:306
128. Laenders AC, Daenen S, Jansen RLH, et al. (1998) Liposomal amphotericin B in the treatment of documented and suspected neutropenia-associated invasive fungal infections. Br J Haematol 103:20
129. Clarck AD, Mackenreich S, Tansey PJ, et al. (1998) A comparative analysis of lipid-complexed and liposomal amphotericin B preparations in haematological oncology. Br J Haematol 103:198
130. Holland S, Stone J, Li S, et al. (2001) Effect of hepatic insufficiency on the pharmacokinetics of caspofungin. In: Program and Abstracts of the 41st Interscience Conference on Antimicrobial Agents and Chemotherapy 2001. Edited by American Society for Microbiology, Chicago: Abst A-14
131. Denning DW (2003) Echinocandin antifungal drugs. Lancet 362:1142
132. Villanueva A, Arathoon EG, Noriega LM, et al. (2001) A randomized double-blind study of caspofungin versus amphotericin for the treatment of candidal esophagitis. Clin Infect Dis 33:1529
133. Arathon EG, Gotuzzo E, Noriega LM, et al. (2002) Randomized, double-blind, multicenter study of caspofungin versus amphotericin B for treatment of oropharyngeal and esophageal candidiasis. Antimicrob Agents Chemother 46:451
134. Villanueva A, Gotuzzo E, Arathon EG, et al. (2002) A randomized double-blind study of caspofungin versus fluconazole for the treatment of esophageal candidiasis. Am J Med 113:294
135. Holland S, Stone J, Li S, et al. (2001) Drug interactions between caspofungin and tacrolimus. In: Program and Abstracts of the 41st Interscience Conference on Antimicrobial Agents and Chemotherapy. Edited by American Society for Microbiology, Chicago
136. Del Poeta M, Cruz MC, Cardenas ME, et al. (2000) Synergistic antifungal activities of bafilomycin A(1), fluconazole and the pneumocandin MK-0991/caspofungin ace-

tate with calcineurin inhibitors FK506 and L-685,818 against *Cryptococcus neoformans*. Antimicrob Agents Chemother 44:739

137. Kullberg BJ, Sobel JD, Ruhnke M, et al. (2005) Voriconazole versus a regimen of amphotericin B followed by fluconazole for candidemia in non-neutropenic patients: a randomized non-inferiority trial. The Lancet 366:1435
138. Heard SO, Fink MP, Gamelli RL, et al. (1998) Effect of prophylactic administration of recombinant human granulocyte colony stimulating factor (filgrastim) on the frequency of nosocomial infections in patients with acute brain injury or cerebral hemorrhage. Crit Care Med 26:748
139. Mora-Duarte J, Betts R, Rotstein C, et al. (2002) Comparison of caspofungin and amphotericin B for invasive candidiasis. N Engl J Med 347:2020
140. Colombo AL, Perfect JR, DiNubile M, et al. (2003) Global distribution and outcomes for *Candida* species causing invasive candidiasis: results from an international randomized double-blind study of caspofungin versus amphotericin B for the treatment of invasive candidiasis. Eur J Clin Microbiol Infect Dis 22:470
141. Voss A, le Noble JL, Verduyn Lunel FM, et al. (1996) Candidemia in intensive care units: risk factors for mortality. Infection 25:130
142. Diaz E, et al. (1998) Nosocomial candidemia risk factors. Intensive Care Med 24 (Suppl 1):S143
143. Nguyen MH, Peacock JE Jr, Morris AJ, et al. (1996) The changing face of candidemia: emergence of non-*Candida albicans* species and antifungal resistance. Am J Med 100:617
144. Rex JH, Bennett JE, Sugar AM, et al. (1995) Intravascular catheter exchange and duration of candidemia. Clin Infect Dis 21:994
145. Wingard JR (1995) Importance of *Candida* species other than *Candida albicans* as pathogens in oncology patients. Clin Infect Dis 20:115
146. Meunier F, Aoun M, Bitar N (1992) Candidemia in immunocompromised patients. Clin Infect Dis 14:S120
147. Kirkpatrick WR, Revankar SG, McAtee RK, et al. (1998) Detection of *Candida dubliniensis* in oropharyngeal samples from human immunodeficiency virus-infected patients in North America by Primary CHROMagar *Candida* screening and susceptibility testing of isolates. J Clin Microbiol 300:7
148. Safran DB, Dawson E (1997) The effect of empiric and prophylactic treatment with fluconazole on yeast isolates in a surgical trauma intensive care unit. Arch Surg 132:1184
149. Blinkhorn RJ, Adelstein D, Spagnuolo PJ (1989) Emergence of a new opportunistic pathogen, *Candida lusitaniae*. J Clin Microbiol 27:236
150. Warnock DW, Burke JF, Cope NJ, et al. (1988) Fluconazole resistance in *Candida glabrata*. Lancet 1310
151. Gleason TG, May AK, Caparelli D, et al. (1997) Emerging evidence of selection of fluconazole-tolerant fungi in surgical intensive care units. Arch Surg 132:1197
152. van den Bossche H, Marichal P, Odds FC, et al. (1992) Characterization of an azole-resistant *Candida glabrata* isolate. Antimicrob Agents Chemother 36:2602
153. Viscoli C, Girmenia C, Marinus A, et al. (1999) Candidemia in cancer patients: a prospective, multicenter surveillance study by the invasive fungal infection group of the EORTC. Clin Infect Dis 28:1071
154. Wingard JR, Merz WG, Rinaldi MG, et al. (1991) Increase in *Candida krusei* infection among patients with BMT and neutropenia treated prophylactically with fluconazole. N Engl J Med 325:1274
155. Seidenfeld SM, Cooper BH, Smith JW, et al. (1983) Amphotericin B tolerance: a characteristic of *Candida parapsilosis* not shared by other *Candida* species. J Infect Dis 147:116
156. Merz WG (1984) *Candida lusitaniae*: frequency of recovery, colonization, infection and amphotericin B resistance. J Clin Microbiol 20:1194
157. Fisher BD, Dixon DM (1999) Invasive aspergillosis: progress in early diagnosis and treatment. Am J Med 5:131
158. Walsh TJ, Dixon DM (1989) Nosocomial aspergillosis: environmental microbiology, hospital epidemiology, diagnosis and treatment. Eur J Epidemiol 1989:131
159. Wald A, Leisenring W, van Burik JA, et al. (1997) Epidemiology of *Aspergillus* infections in a large cohort of patients undergoing bone marrow transplantation. J Infect Dis 175:1459
160. Rello J, Esandi ME, Mariscal D, et al. (1998) Invasive pulmonary aspergillosis in patients with chronic obstructive pulmonary disease: report of eight cases and review. Clin Infect Dis 26:1473
161. Walsh TJ, Melcher GP, Rinaldi MG, et al. (1990) *Trichosporum beigelii*, an emerging pathogen resistant to amphotericin B. B J Clin Microbiol 28:1616
162. Lutwick LI, Galgiani JN, Johnson RH, et al. (1976) Visceral fungal infections due to *Pseudallescheria boydii. In vitro* drug sensitivity studies. Am J Med 61:632
163. Gastinne H, Wolff M, Delatour F, Faurisson F, et al. (1992) A controlled trial in intensive care units of selective decontamination of the digestive tract with nonabsorbable antibiotics. The French Group on selective decontamination of the digestive tract. N Engl J Med 326:594
164. Quinio B, Albanese J, Bues-Charbit M, et al. (1996) Selective decontamination of the digestive tract in multiple trauma patients. A prospective, double-blind, randomized, placebo-controlled study. Chest 109:762
165. Edwards JE Jr, Bodey GP, Bowden RA, et al. (1997) International conference for the development of a consensus on the management and prevention of severe *Candida* infections. Clin Infect Dis 25:43
166. Dubé MP, Heseltine PNR, Rinaldi MG, et al. (1994) Fungemia and colonization with nystatin resistant *Candida rugosa* in a burn unit. Clin Infect Dis 18:77
167. Burket JS, Bartlett RH, Hyde KV, et al. (1999) Nosocomial infections in adult patients undergoing extracorporeal membrane oxygenation. Clin Infect Dis 28:828
168. Goldstein DJ, El-Amir NG, Ashton RCJ, et al. (1995) Fungal infections in left ventricular assist device recipients. ASAID J 41:873
169. Eggimann P, Francioli P, Bille J, et al. (1999) Fluconazole prophylaxis prevents intra-abdominal candidiasis in high-risk surgical patients. Crit Care Med 27:1066
170. Walsh TJ, Pappas P, Winston DJ, et al. (2002) Voriconazole compared with liposomal amphotericin B for empirical antifungal therapy in patients with neutropenia and persistent fever. N Engl J Med 346:225
171. Walsh TJ, Teppler H, Donowitz GR, et al. (2004) Caspofungin versus liposomal amphotericin B for empirical antifungal therapy in patients with persistent fever and neutropenia. N Engl J Med 351:1391
172. Wenzel RP (1995) Nosocomial candidemia: risk factors and attributable mortality. Clin Infect Dis 20:1531
173. Wright WL, Wenzel RP (1997) Nosocomial candida: Epidemiology, transmission and prevention. Infect Dis Clin North Am 11:411
174. Rello J, Diaz E (1999) Epidemiology and aetiology of fungal infections in the ICU. In: Vincent JL (ed) Management of fungal in the ICU. The Liposome Company, London, p 11

175. Pittet D, Monod M, Suter PM, et al. (1994) *Candida* colonization and subsequent infections in critically ill surgical patients. Ann Surg 230:751
176. Petri MG, Konig J, Moecke HP, et al. (1997) Epidemiology of invasive mycosis in ICU patients: a prospective multicenter study in 435 non-neutropenic patients. Intensive Care Med 23:317
177. Ellis CA, Spivack ML (1967) The significance of candidemia. Ann Intern Med 67:511
178. Toala P, Schroeder SA, Daly AK, et al. (1970) *Candida* at Boston City Hospital. Clinical and epidemiological characteristics and susceptibility to eighth antimicrobial agents. Arch Intern Med 126:983
179. Fraser VJ, Jones M, Dunkel J, et al. (1992) Candidemia in a tertiary care hospital: epidemiology, risk factors and predictors of mortality. Clin Infect Dis 15:414
180. Edwards JE Jr (1991) Invasive *Candida* infections – evolution of a fungal pathogen. N Engl J Med 324:1060
181. Anaissie E, Darouiche RO, Abi-Said D, et al. (1996) Management of invasive *Candida* infections: results of a prospective randomized, multicenter study of fluconazole versus amphotericin B and review of the literature. Clin Infect Dis 23:964
182. Anaissie EJ, Vartivarian SE, Abi-Said D, et al. (1996) Fluconazole versus amphotericin B in the treatment of hematogenous candidiasis: a matched cohort study. Clin Infect Dis 101:170
183. Nguyen MH, Peacock JE Jr, Tanner DC, et al. (1995) Therapeutic approaches in patients with candidemia. Evaluation in a multicenter prospective observational study. Arch Intern Med 155:2429
184. Rex JH, Bennett JE, Sugar AM, et al. (1994) A randomized trial comparing fluconazole and amphotericin B for the treatment of candidemia in patients with neutropenia. N Engl J Med 331:1325
185. van't Wout JW (1996) Fluconazole treatment of candidal infections caused by non-albicans *Candida* species. Eur J Clin Microbiol Infect Dis 15:238
186. Ang BSP, Telenti A, King B, et al. (1993) Candidemia from a urinary tract source: microbiological aspects and clinical significance. Clin Infect Dis 17:662
187. Sobel JD (1999) Management of asymptomatic candiduria. Int J Antimicrob Agents 11:285
188. Potasman I, Castin A, Moskovitz B, et al. (1997) Oral fluconazole for *Candida* urinary tract infection. Urol Int 59:252
189. Nassoura Z, Ivatury RR, Simon RJ, et al. (1993) Candidemia as an early marker of disseminated infection in the critically surgical patient: the role of fluconazole therapy. Trauma 35:290
190. Fisher JF, Newman CL, Sobel JD (1995) Yeasts in the urine: solution for a budding problem. Clin Infect Dis 20:183
191. Leu HS, Huang CT (1995) Clearance of funguria with short-course anti-fungal regimens: prospective, randomized, controlled study. Clin Infect Dis 20:1152
192. Nerbit SA, Katz LE, McClain BW, et al. (1999) Comparison of two concentrations of amphotericin B bladder irrigation in the treatment of funguria in patients with indwelling urinary catheters. Am J Health Syst Pharm 56:872
193. Ostrosky-Zeichner L, Oude Lashof AML, Kullberg BJ, et al. (2003) Voriconazole salvage treatment of invasive candididasis. Eur J Clin Microbiol Infect Dis 22:651
194. Graninger W, Presterie E, Schneeweiss B, et al. (1992) Treatment of *Candida albicans* fungemia with fluconazole. J Infect 26:133
195. Pittrow L, Penk A (1999) Dosage adjustments of fluconazole during continuous renal replacement therapy (CAVH, CVVH, CAVHD, CVVHD). Mycosis 42:17
196. Moody SB, Sveska KJ (1993) Fluconazole dosing in renal impairment: a drug usage evaluation. Hosp Formul 28: 499
197. Kaufman CA, Bradley SE, Ross SC, et al. (1991) Hepatosplenic candidiasis. Successful treatment with fluconazole. Am J Med 91:137
198. Anaissie EJ, Bodey GP, Kantarjian H, et al. (1991) Fluconazole therapy for chronic disseminated candidiasis in patients with leukemia and prior amphotericin B therapy. Am J Med 91:142
199. Hadley S, Karchmer AW (1995) Fungal infections in solid organ transplant recipients. Infect Dis Clin North Am 9:1045
200. Hibberd PL, Rubin RH (1994) Clinical aspects of fungal infection in organ transplant recipients. Clin Infect Dis 19 (Suppl 1):S33
201. Pittet D, Anaissie E, Solomkin JS (1996) When to start antifungal therapy in the non-neutropenic critically ill patient. In: Vincent JL (ed) Yearbook of intensive care and emergency medicine. Springer-Verlag, Berlin, p 964
202. Penk A, Pittrow L (1998) Status of fluconazole in the therapy of endogenous *Candida* endophthalmitis. Mycosis 41 (Suppl 2):41
203. del Palacio A, Cuetara MS, Ferro M, et al. (1993) Fluconazole in the management of endophthalmitis in disseminated candidiasis of heroin addicts. Mycosis 36:193
204. Akler ME, Velland M, McNealy DM, et al. (1995) Use of fluconazole in the treatment of *Candida* endophthalmitis. Clin Infect Dis 20:657
205. Filler SG, Cusllip MA, Mayer CL, et al. (1991) Comparison of fluconazole and amphotericin B for the treatment of disseminated candididasis and endophthalmitis in rabbits. Antimicrob Agents Chemother 35:288
206. Savani DV, Perfect JR, Cobo LM, et al. (1987) Penetration of new azole compounds into the eye and efficacy in experimental *Candida* endophthalmitis. Antimicrob Agents Chemother 31:6
207. Nomura J, Ruskin J (1993) Failure of therapy with fluconazole for *Candida* endophthalmitis. Clin Infect Dis 17:888
208. Adler-Moore JP, Profitt RT (1993) Development, characterization, efficacy and modes of action of (Ambisome) a unicellular liposomal formulation of amphotericin B. J Liposomal Res 3:429
209. Wong-Beringer A, Jacobs RA, Guglielmo BJ (1998) Lipid formulation of amphotericin B: clinical efficacy and toxicities. Clin Infect Dis 27:603
210. Herbrecht R, Denning DW, Patterson TF, et al. (2002) Voriconazole versus amphotericin B for primary therapy of invasive aspergillosis. N Engl J Med 347:408
211. Kartsonis NA, Saah AJ, Lipka CJ, et al. (2005) Salvage therapy with caspofungin for invasive aspergillosis: results from the caspofungin compassionate use study. J Infect 50:196–205
212. Taccone FS, Marechal L, Meuleman N, et al. (2003) Caspofungin salvage therapy in a neutropenic patient with probable invasive aspergillosis: a case report. Support Cancer Center 11:742
213. Maertens JA, et al. (2002) Caspofungin for aspergillosis (intolerant or refractory). In: Abstracts of the 42nd Interscience Conference on Antimicrobial Agents and Chemotherapy. Edited by American Society for Microbiology, Chicago
214. Scheven M, Senf L (1994) Quantitative determination of fluconazole-amphotericin B antagonism for *Candida albicans* by agar-diffusion. Mycosis 37:205
215. Sugar AM, Hitchcock CA, Troke PF, Picard M (1995)

Combination therapy of murine invasive candidiasis with fluconazole and amphotericin B. Antimicrob Agents Chemother 19:598

216. Petraitis V, Petraitiene R, Sarafandi AA, et al. (2003) Combination therapy in treatment of experimental pulmonary aspergillosis: synergistic interaction between an antifungal triazole and an echinocandin. Clin Infect Dis 187:1834
217. Marr KA, Boeckh M, Carter RA, et al. (2004) Combination antifungal therapy for invasive aspergillosis. Clin Infect Dis 39:797
218. Donahue SP, Greven CM, Zuravleff JJ, et al. (1994) Intraocular candidiasis in patients with candidemia: clinical implications derived from a prospective multicenter study. Ophthalmology 101:1302
219. von Eiff M, Fahrenkamp A, Roos N, Fegeler W, van de Loo J (1990) Hepatosplenic candidiasis – a late manifestation of *Candida* septicemia. Mycosis 33:283

12 Dose Adjustment and Pharmacokinetics of Antibiotics in Severe Sepsis and Septic Shock

J.A. Roberts, J. Lipman

12.1 General

Prescription of antibiotics in critically ill patients is a complex process that requires ongoing patient health evaluation to account for the dynamic sepsis disease process. Pathophysiological changes such as organ dysfunction, fluid shifts and altered immune status are common, and are able to reduce the efficacy of anti-infective treatments. Throughout this chapter, dosing of antibiotics that are commonly used in critically patients with sepsis or septic shock will be discussed. The importance of knowledge of the pharmacokinetic and pharmacodynamic principles of each class will be discussed, and how to optimise these parameters and therefore augment patient responses.

12.1.1 Sepsis

The older definitions of sepsis [1] (a systemic inflammatory response syndrome (SIRS) triggered by an overwhelming infection) have recently been refined [1, 2]. Severe sepsis occurs upon failure or dysfunction of at least one organ. Septic shock is defined by hypotension in the setting of severe sepsis which is unresponsive to fluid resuscitation. While much research has been directed at cellular targets to limit the associated inflammatory and coagulation cascades including interleukins, cytokines and tumour necrosis factor-alpha (TNF-α) [3], none of these interventions have been found to be as important or effective as optimal antibiotic therapy [3–8]. However, the appropriate prescription of antibiotics requires a detailed knowledge of the pathophysiological and subsequent pharmacokinetic changes that occur throughout the course of sepsis [9, 10].

12.1.1.1 Pathophysiological Changes in Sepsis That Can Affect Drug Distribution

Brief Pathophysiology of Sepsis Without Organ Dysfunction

The pathogenesis of sepsis appears highly complex [2, 3, 11, 12]. Endotoxins from bacteria or fungi stimulate the production of various endogenous mediators [13]. These mediators may affect the vascular endothelium directly or indirectly, resulting in either vasoconstriction or vasodilatation with maldistribution of blood flow, endothelial damage and increased capillary permeability. This capillary leak syndrome results in fluid shifts from the intravascular compartment to the interstitial space [14, 15] which is known as ‘third spacing’. This would increase the volume of distribution (Vd) of water-soluble drugs which decreases their serum drug concentration.

Increased Creatinine Clearance in Critically Ill Patients Without Renal Dysfunction

Patients often present with hypotension from the inflammatory response associated with sepsis. Standard initial management involves administration of intravenous fluids to elevate blood pressure. If hypotension persists, inotropic agents (some of which may be “inoconstrictors”) are prescribed. It is therefore not surprising that patients with sepsis often have higher than normal cardiac indices [11, 16, 17]. In the absence of significant organ dysfunction, often there is an increased renal preload and consequently increased creatinine and drug clearance [18–20].

Previous studies have reported that critically ill patients with normal serum creatinine levels may have high creatinine clearance [21, 22]. This phenomenon is most likely to result from the clinical interventions used to reverse hypotension as described above. The implications of the high creatinine clearance, which is probably related to high renal (and hepatic) blood flow, will result in supranormal clearance of renally cleared drugs. This increase in clearance is the major reason for the different dosing requirements between ICU and

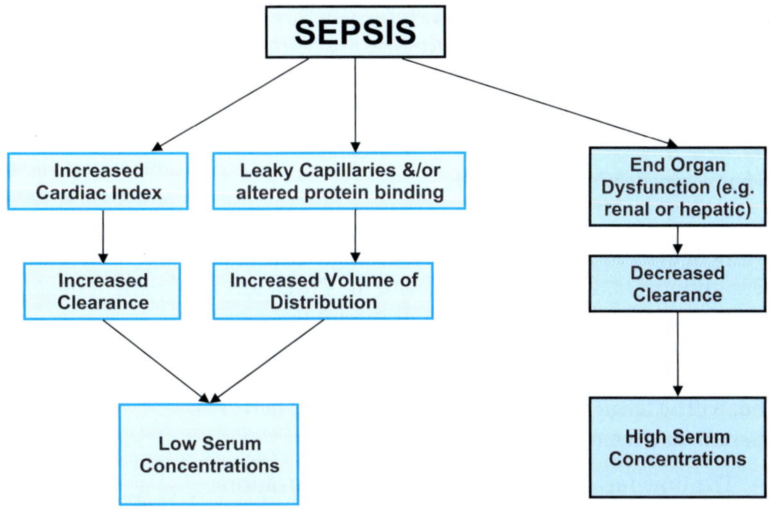

Fig. 12.1. Schematic representation of the basic pathophysiological changes that can occur during sepsis and their subsequent pharmacokinetic effects

non-ICU patients [23, 24]. A similar scenario probably occurs for hepatically cleared antibiotics.

Pathophysiology of Sepsis Causing Organ Dysfunction

As sepsis progresses, significant myocardial depression can occur which leads to a decrease in organ perfusion [16]. Myocardial insufficiency and abnormalities of the macrovascular circulation are compounded by failure of the microcirculation. This induces end-organ microvascular alterations which may progress to multiple organ dysfunction syndrome (MODS) [25]. This often includes renal and/or hepatic dysfunction. There is a consequent decrease in antibiotic clearance, which prolongs elimination half-life and may increase antibiotic concentrations and/or lead to the accumulation of metabolites [26].

Figure 12.1 schematically identifies the pharmacokinetic changes that can occur due to the altered pathophysiology during sepsis.

Determining Renal Function in Critically Ill Patients with Sepsis

Accurate knowledge of renal function is a critical factor in drug and antibiotic dosing as most antibiotics are primarily eliminated by this means. If renal dysfunction occurs in a critically ill patient with sepsis, calculation of the efficiency of the kidney can be problematic. Accepted norms for calculating creatinine clearance (as a marker of renal function) in 'normal' ward patients such as the Cockroft-Gault method [27] and the Modified Diet in Renal Disease (MDRD) study [28] have been reported to lose their accuracy in critically ill patients [29]. As such, the most effective way to calculate renal function remains using either an 8-, 12- or 24-h creatinine clearance collection [30–32]. If acute renal failure occurs such that the patient needs intermittent haemodialysis or continuous renal replacement therapy (CRRT), a new variable is introduced. Chapter 13 discusses the altered dosing of antibiotics that is necessary in these patients.

12.1.2 Applied Clinical Pharmacology

To achieve 'ideal' treatment of an infection, it is necessary to optimise the possible interactions between the host, the pathogen, and the antibiotic [33]. This task becomes more difficult in critically ill patients, where recommended antibiotic regimens have been derived from volunteer studies or other patient groups who were not critically ill. Therefore, consideration of the effect of the pathophysiological changes, caused by sepsis, on the pharmacokinetic and pharmacodynamic parameters of the antibiotic is necessary. Further, since the physiology of these patients may change over a relatively short period of time, ongoing evaluations of sickness severity are indicated to allow timely adjustment of antibiotic dosing.

12.1.2.1 Pharmacokinetic Considerations

Pharmacokinetics (PK) refers to the study of concentration changes of a drug over a given time period. The primary PK parameters of importance to antibiotics include:

- Volume of distribution (Vd)
- Clearance (CL)
- Half-life ($T_{1/2}$)
- The peak serum concentration achieved by a single dose (C_{max})
- The lowest concentration during a dosing period (C_{min})
- The area under the serum concentration time curve (AUC).

These factors can be used to determine whether appropriate concentrations of the antibiotic are being delivered to the target area [34].

12.1.2.2
Pharmacodynamic Considerations

Pharmacodynamics (PD) relate PK parameters (measures of drug exposure) and pharmacologic effect [35]. For antibiotics, PD parameters relate the PK factors to the ability of the antibiotic to kill or inhibit the growth of the infective organism. This interaction can be referred to as "pharmacokinetics-pharmacodynamics" but will be termed "pharmacodynamics" (PD) here. PD parameters include:

- The time for which a drug's serum concentration remains above the minimum inhibitory concentration (MIC) for a dosing period (T>MIC)
- The ratio of the maximum serum antibiotic concentration (C_{max}) to MIC (C_{max}/MIC)
- The ratio of the area under the concentration time curve during a 24-h time period (AUC_{0-24}) to MIC (AUC_{0-24}/MIC) (see Fig. 12.2).

Pharmacodynamically, the rate and extent of an antibiotic's bactericidal activity is dependent on the interaction between drug concentrations at the site of infection, bacterial load, phase of bacterial growth and the MIC of the pathogen [34]. It follows that a change in any of these factors will affect the PD profile of the antibiotic against a particular pathogen and may affect the outcome of therapy. Developing dosing regimens that maximise the rate of response in patients with sepsis is important for accelerating patient recovery and minimising the development of antibiotic resistance [34, 36]. Effective antibiotic therapy is essential to optimise patient outcomes [5–8, 37].

12.1.3
Kill Characteristics of Different Antibiotic Classes

Pharmacodynamically, different antibiotic classes appear to have different types of kill characteristics on bacteria (Fig. 12.2, Table 12.1). An understanding of these pharmacodynamic properties is important as it enables appropriate dose adjustment for unique patient cases.

These kill characteristics have been determined from in vitro studies and describe the PK measurements that represent optimal bactericidal activity [34]. The β-lactam group of antibiotics have a time-dependent (or concentration-independent) kill characteristic with T>MIC the best predictor of efficacy [38]. As such, maintaining the concentration of these antibiot-

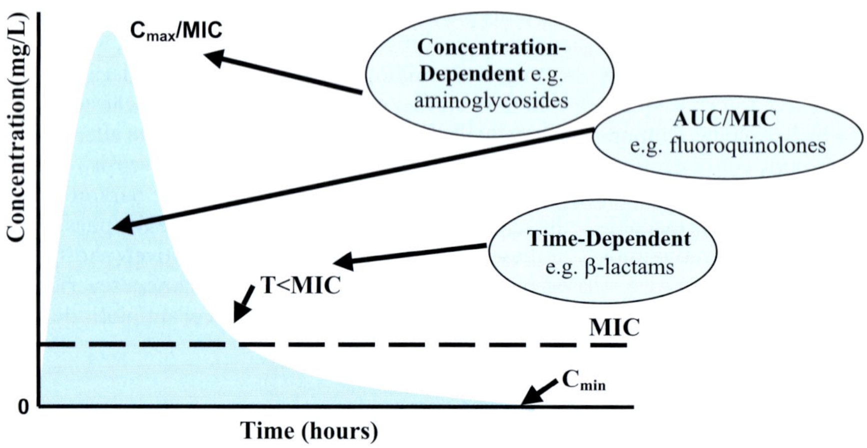

Fig. 12.2. Pharmacokinetic and pharmacodynamic parameters of antibiotics on a concentration vs. time curve

Table 12.1. Pharmacodynamic properties that correlate with efficacy of selected antibiotics

Antibiotics	Aminoglycosides Metronidazole Fluoroquinolones Telithromycin Daptomycin Quinupristin/dalfopristin	Fluoroquinolones Aminoglycosides Azithromycin Tetracyclines Glycopeptides Tigecycline Quinupristin/dalfopristin Linezolid	β-Lactams Carbapenems Linezolid Erythromycin Clarithromycin Lincosamides
PD kill characteristics	Concentration-dependent	Concentration-dependent with time dependence	Time-dependent
Optimal PD parameter	C_{max}: MIC	AUC_{0-24}: MIC	T>MIC

ics above the MIC of the infective pathogen will ensure optimal efficacy. In contrast, aminoglycosides have a concentration-dependent (or time-independent) kill characteristic where effect is determined by C_{max}/MIC [39]. Fluoroquinolones are more complex, and were initially reported to be C_{max}/MIC dependent, although subsequent studies have also found that AUC_{0-24}/MIC is important [40, 41] (Table 12.2). The pharmacodynamic parameters associated with efficacy for other antibiotics are described in Table 12.1.

12.1.3.1 Post-Antibiotic Effect

Most antibiotics demonstrate a post-antibiotic effect (PAE). PAE refers to the continued suppression of bacterial growth for prolonged periods when drug concentrations fall below the MIC of the bacteria [42]. β-Lactams demonstrate a modest PAE against Gram positive organisms but no PAE (except carbapenems) against Gram negative organisms [42, 43]. Aminoglycosides demonstrate a significant PAE (>3 h) the duration of which is concentration-dependent [39, 44–50]. Fluoro-

Table 12.2. General PK characteristics of various antibiotics and possible changes that can occur during fluid shifts in critically ill patients

Antibiotic class	Vd (l/kg)	Increased Vd with fluid shifts?	Decreased C_{max} with fluid shifts?	Serum $T_{1/2}$ (h)	Protein binding	Altered CL in sepsis?	TDM required?
Aminoglycosides [69, 249, 250]	0.2–0.3 (consistent with extracellular water)	Yes	Yes	2–3	Low	Varies proportionately with renal function	Yes – to ensure high C_{max} and adequate CL [78, 98, 99] [96, 97, 100]
β-Lactams [22, 23, 104, 105, 251, 252]	Variable but consistent with extracellular water	Yes	Yes	0.5–2 (except ceftriaxone [102])	Low (except ceftriaxone and oxacillin)	Varies proportionately with renal function (some exceptions)	No
Carbapenems [140]	Variable but consistent with extracellular water	Yes	Yes	1 (except ertapenem 4 h)	Low (except ertapenem)	Varies proportionately with renal function	No
Vancomycin [163]	0.2–1.25 (consistent with extracellular water)	Yes	Yes	4–6	30–55%	Varies proportionately with renal function	Yes – to ensure serum trough concentrations >15 mg/L [164]
Teicoplanin [165–167]	0.9–1.6	Yes	Yes	80–160	90%	Varies proportionately with renal function	Yes – to ensure therapeutic concentrations reached
Tigecycline [206, 207, 253]	7–10	Unlikely	Unlikely	37–66	73–79%	May decrease with cholestasis	No
Quinupristin/dalfopristin [224, 254, 255]	quinupristin = 0.45 dalfopristin = 0.24	Yes	Yes	1.3–1.5	quinupristin (23–32%) dalfopristin (50–56%)	Varies proportionately with renal function	No
Daptomycin [256–258]	0.09 (consistent with extracellular water)	Yes	Yes	5.8–11.6	92%	Varies proportionately with renal function	No
Telithromycin [212–214, 259]	2.7–2.9	Unknown	?No	10–13	60–70%	Varies proportionately with renal function	No
Clindamycin [228–230, 260–263]	0.6–1.2	No	Yes	1.5–5	65–90%	Decreased hepatic clearance	No
Linezolid [234–236]	0.5–0.6	Yes	Yes	3.5–7	31%	Slightly decreased clearance	No

quinolones also possess a prolonged PAE [51, 52]. Interestingly, the PAE of an antibiotic can change in states of altered immune function, such as neutropenia [53–55] or in critically ill patients with sepsis although this has not been widely characterised for all antibiotics. A reduction in leukocyte count has been shown to reduce the efficacy of aminoglycosides (see Sect. 2.1.3.2).

12.1.3.2
Post-β-Lactamase Inhibitor Effect

Post-β-lactamase inhibitor effect (PLIE) refers to a period of continued suppression of bacterial growth after removal of a β-lactamase inhibitor (also known as suicide inhibitor) [56]. It has been shown to occur in vitro for amoxicillin plus clavulanate [56] and more recently ceftazidime plus sulbactam [57]. It is thought that a β-lactam and suicide inhibitor (e.g. clavulanate or sulbactam) may be combined to utilise this PLIE in extended-spectrum β-lactamases (ESBLs), to enable reduced β-lactam doses [56]. However, to date there is scarce evidence of the clinical effects of PLIE itself.

12.1.3.3
Inoculum Effect

The inoculum effect refers to the presence of high initial concentrations of bacteria (initially seen with *E. coli*). These elevated concentrations confer higher MICs and reduced bactericidal activity of third generation beta-lactams [58]. This is thought to be due to a production of beta-lactamases [59] for which other broad spectrum β-lactams, including fourth generation cephalosporins, may have added efficacy [60–62]. This is largely an academic observation though, because in clinical practice, the identification of bacterial load may be difficult and thus dose changes are not indicated at this time. However, the importance of effective broad spectrum antibiotic therapy is given credence.

12.2
Antibiotic Classes

Below, aminoglycosides, β-lactams, glycopeptides, fluoroquinolones and other various antibiotics used in critically ill patients with sepsis and septic shock will be considered. General PK and PD characteristics will be considered for each of these classes. The clinical application and dosing implications of these properties for critically ill patients will also be addressed.

12.2.1
Aminoglycosides

Aminoglycosides are an older class of antibiotics that include gentamicin, tobramycin and amikacin.

12.2.1.1
Pharmacokinetics

- General (see Table 12.2)

The debate of aminoglycoside dosing continues because of the narrow therapeutic index of these drugs. There is accumulating evidence to show that administering aminoglycosides as a once daily dose is associated with less nephro- and ototoxicity than the same total dose administered in small, multiple doses [63–68]. It is therefore considered that the troughs – or more specifically the area under the concentration-time curve – are more closely correlated with the well-documented adverse renal and ototoxic effects of these drugs [63–68]. Monitoring of serum aminoglycoside concentrations is essential for minimising these adverse effects. The serum half life ($T_{1/2}$) of aminoglycosides will increase in renal impairment as they are excreted unchanged almost entirely by glomerular filtration [69].

12.2.1.2
Pharmacodynamic Principles of Aminoglycosides

The kill characteristic of the aminoglycosides is concentration dependent [44–50, 70–72]. Experimentally, a high peak concentration of an aminoglycoside antibiotic provides a better, faster killing effect on standard bacterial inocula. In a retrospective study, Moore et al. [39] demonstrated quite unequivocally that a high peak concentration of aminoglycoside relative to the MIC for the infecting organism was a major determinant of the clinical response. Aminoglycosides also exhibit a significant PAE which can prevent bacterial regrowth for prolonged periods should drug concentrations fall below the MIC [39, 42, 44–50, 68].

Clarification of these properties of aminoglycosides: (1) high widely spaced doses causing less toxicity than smaller more frequent doses; (2) high doses producing better kill curves; and (3) the post-antibiotic effect, led to the development of single daily dosing for aminoglycoside antibiotics [73, 74]. It has now been shown in prospective human clinical trials [68, 75–78] and numerous meta-analyses [64–67] that this recommendation is valid, i.e. large, single, daily doses (or more correctly, extended interval dosing – EIAD) aminoglycosides produce less toxicity and comparable if not superior clinical outcomes.

12.2.1.3
Aminoglycoside Dosing in Critically Ill Patient with Sepsis

Effect of 'Third-Spacing'

The problem of patient variability in peak aminoglycoside serum concentrations has been observed in critically ill patients [69, 79–89]. In sepsis without organ dysfunction there is typically increased aminoglycoside clearance [48, 86, 87, 89]. An increase in aminoglycoside Vd has been noted in patients with sepsis, due to the processes described above [14, 15, 90], and with patient sickness severity, measured by APACHE II score [91]. Importantly, the critically ill patient with a high APACHE II score and normal renal function will not only have lower trough concentrations, but also lower peak concentrations compared with a patient who has a lower APACHE II score. The effect of sickness severity on aminoglycoside concentrations, resulting in a change in Vd in an individual patient during the course of therapy, may explain, at least in part, the wide variability of dosages needed to achieve therapeutic concentrations as reported in published studies [79–89].

Effect of Organ Dysfunction

The value of once-daily dosing in this population has been studied [53] and randomised trials comparing once-daily and multiple-daily dosing of aminoglycoside have been performed with co-administration of a β-lactam antibiotic. These studies were subjected to a meta-analysis which found no significant differences in efficacy between once-daily and multiple-daily dosing [92], although reduced toxicity from once-daily dosing has been shown [93]. Until there are further studies suggesting otherwise the evidence supports the administration of high dose (7 mg/kg if normal renal function; amikacin requires 28 mg/kg) once-daily aminoglycosides be administered.

In our experience, if the patient has supranormal renal function and is eliminating the drug rapidly such that nomogram or trough-level monitoring suggests doses higher than 7 mg/kg are required, increasing the frequency rather than the dose should be considered. The C_{max}:MIC ratio conferred by 7 mg/kg is often ~10 and maximises bacterial killing. Higher doses are thought to have no additional effect. It is possible that administration at 18-hourly intervals may be appropriate while supranormal renal function is present. If the patient has renal impairment, doses of 3–5 mg/kg 24-hourly may be required. Should therapeutic drug monitoring determine that the patient is not excreting this low-dose aminoglycoside, then the dose should be maintained and a longer interval between dosing be selected (36- or 48-hourly dosing). Monitoring by trough levels should occur in this situation, although alternate therapeutic agents should be considered.

Effect of Neutropenia

The aminoglycoside PAE has been demonstrated in Gram positive and negative organisms [54, 94]. In vitro studies have shown enhanced bacterial phagocytosis by leukocytes after exposure to aminoglycosides which has been termed the post-antibiotic leukocyte enhancement (PALE) [95]. It follows that in a critically ill patient with neutropenia or a low leukocyte count (as shown in animal models [54]), that aminoglycosides may have decreased efficacy. This has been supported by data that shows that as the absolute neutrophil count decreases, higher bactericidal activity is required [55] and this may be obtained by increasing the aminoglycoside dose (C_{max}) although more research into this area is required. The value of once-daily dosing in this population has been studied [53] and randomised trials comparing once-daily and multiple-daily dosing of aminoglycoside have been performed with co-administration of a β-lactam antibiotic. These studies were subjected to a meta-analysis which found no significant differences in efficacy between once-daily and multiple-daily dosing [92], although there is reduced toxicity from once-daily dosing [93]. Until there are further studies suggesting otherwise the evidence supports the administration of high dose (7 mg/kg if normal renal function) once-daily aminoglycosides be given with a broad spectrum β-lactam antibiotic to critically ill patients with sepsis that have a low leukocyte count.

12.2.1.4
Monitoring of Aminoglycosides in Critically Ill Patients with Sepsis

In 'normal' ward patients there are various methods for monitoring aminoglycoside dosing. Due to the prevalent adverse effects of nephrotoxicity and ototoxicity numerous methods of aminoglycoside monitoring exist:

1. Trough levels
2. Published nomograms
3. Bayesian computer software

In patients with renal function within the reference range, 24-h dosing using published nomograms could be used [96, 97]. Alternate methods of monitoring aminoglycosides after once-daily dosing have also been successfully suggested [78, 98, 99] including using Bayesian methods which have shown reduced toxicity profiles [96, 97, 100]. If altered Vd is suspected, or dosing is used that does not follow convention, then ensuring trough levels are < 0.5 mg/l prior to subsequent dosing is recommended to ensure that the patient is eliminating the aminoglycoside appropriately.

12.2.1.5
Summary of Aminoglycoside Dosing in Critically Ill Patients with Sepsis

Aminoglycosides should be initially dosed at 7 mg/kg (amikacin – 28 mg/kg) to enable a high C_{max}:MIC ratio with drug clearance monitored by using either published nomograms [90] or trough serum concentrations if renal dysfunction is suspected. Such dosing should enable a C_{max}:MIC >10 which maximises the PAE and bacterial killing [42, 90, 101]. Subsequent doses should be individualised [90]. If drug or creatinine clearance is reduced, then maintenance of doses to maximise the C_{max}:MIC ratio at extended intervals is recommended, even if that requires 36- or 48-hourly dosing. Careful monitoring of therapy is recommended to reduce the incidence of nephrotoxicity and/or ototoxicity.

12.2.2
β-Lactam Antibiotics

The β-lactam group of antibiotics consists of penicillins, cephalosporins, carbapenems and monobactams. Carbapenems will be considered separately because of different pharmacodynamic properties.

12.2.2.1
Pharmacokinetics

- General (see Table 12.2)

β-Lactam antibiotics include many compounds and variability certainly exists (e.g. ceftriaxone has a longer $t_{1/2}$ – 5.8–8.7 h in adults – and high protein binding – >80% [102]). In conventional bolus dosing regimes, serum concentrations of these antibiotics fall to low levels between doses [22, 103, 104]. Renal elimination of these drugs is often linearly related to creatinine clearance, so serum concentrations will increase in the presence of renal dysfunction [105–107] except for those β-lactams that have significant biliary clearance (e.g. ceftriaxone and oxacillin). In contrast, low serum concentrations of these antibiotics can occur in the acute phase of sepsis due to enhanced cardiac and renal (and possibly hepatic) function resulting in high drug clearance [22, 104].

12.2.2.2
Pharmacodynamic Principles of β-Lactam Antibiotics

Kill characteristics of β-lactam antibiotics differ significantly from those of aminoglycosides. In-vivo animal experiments have demonstrated that β-lactams have a slow continuous kill characteristic that is almost entirely related to the time for which concentrations in tissue and serum exceed a certain threshold (generally the MIC) of the infecting organism (T>MIC) [14]. Once the concentration of the antibiotic falls below this threshold, any remaining bacteria multiply almost immediately [44–49, 70, 71, 108]. This may also facilitate the development of antibiotic resistance, particularly if the serum concentrations fall below the threshold for more than half the dosing interval [109]. It has been proposed that, in the absence of any PAE, the serum concentration of a β-lactam antibiotic should exceed the MIC for the respective organism for 90–100% of the dosing interval [110]. Animal and in vitro studies show that β-lactams do confer a PAE on Gram positive staphylococci, streptococci and enterococci while only carbapenems have demonstrated a PAE against Gram negative organisms [36, 38, 43, 94, 111–115]. Other studies have demonstrated maximum killing of bacteria at 4–5 times MIC, with still higher concentrations providing no added efficacy [116, 117]. As such, it has been proposed that concentrations of β-lactam antibiotics should be maintained at 4–5 times the MIC for extended periods during each dosing period [45–47]. It is noteworthy that bolus dosing (for example, of cephalosporins) produces unnecessary peak and low trough concentrations below MIC for much of the dosing interval [22, 104, 118, 119]. It follows that an improved PD profile is obtained with either more frequent dosing [104, 110] or continuous infusions [104, 108, 110, 111, 116, 118–125].

12.2.2.3
β-Lactam Dosing in Critically Ill Patients with Sepsis

Effect of 'Third-Spacing' on β-Lactam Dosing

It is increasingly apparent that the PK of the β-lactam antibiotics in the critically ill patient with sepsis is different from those in other patients [126, 127]. Some studies have shown an increased Vd [9, 22, 128], which may cause β-lactam concentrations to be lower than expected. Joukhadar et al. [10] showed that an increased Vd in patients with septic shock results in unbound piperacillin concentrations that can be 5–10 times lower in the extracellular fluid of subcutaneous tissue compared with serum levels after a piperacillin bolus dose. The effect of more frequent dosing or continuous infusion is unclear and as such dose adjustment from increased Vd is not routinely performed.

Effect of Organ Dysfunction on β-Lactam Dosing

Sepsis without organ dysfunction can lead to increased β-lactam clearance and result in lower serum concentrations than expected [22, 48, 86, 87, 89, 104, 116, 118–120, 126, 127]. High β-lactam clearance has been demonstrated in several other studies [22, 104, 116, 118–120]. One inclusion criterion common to many of these studies was normal serum creatinine. In two of these studies it was shown that the clearance of cefepime and, more recently, cefpirome is linearly related to creatinine clearance [22, 104]. As such, creatinine clearance was reported to be an independent predictor of antibiotic clearance. PK-PD modelling found that the $T>$MIC could be predicted by creatinine clearance, and that serum concentrations of these antibiotics were low when using a standard dosing regimen [22, 104]. As a result, dosing adjustment according to increased renal function is an important PK consideration to ensure optimal therapy that complies with β-lactam PD properties. This may require increased dosing, or preferably increased frequency of dosing, to ensure $T>$MIC is maximised. Preliminary data suggests clinical and bacteriologic superiority when administering ceftriaxone by continuous infusion compared with bolus dosing of ceftriaxone in patients with sepsis [129].

In severe sepsis with renal and/or hepatic dysfunction, reduced β-lactam clearance can occur. Consequently, serum drug concentrations may be elevated to higher than expected concentrations. Dependent on the infective organism and toxicity profile of the β-lactam, dose reduction, in line with product information, may be indicated.

Administration of β-Lactams by Continuous Infusion

Administration by continuous infusion optimises the PD profile of β-lactams [103, 108, 110, 117, 130]. Numerous studies have compared administration of β-lactams by continuous infusion with bolus dosing [108, 116, 131–133]. The results have largely shown comparable therapeutic efficacy with other literature purporting improved patient survival, decreased length of stay in ICU and decreased resources expended on patient therapy when continuous infusion is used [7, 134]. Four previous studies have compared the clinical outcome of continuous infusion and intermittent bolus dosing of a β-lactam antibiotic [126, 129, 132, 135]. Of these studies, only Roberts et al. [129] found a clinical difference which suggested clinical and bacteriologic superiority of administering ceftriaxone 2-g as a continuous intravenous infusion compared to a once-daily bolus dose. Further research is required to quantify the clinical utility of administering β-lactams as a continuous infusion. Continuous infusion has also shown a reduction in the total daily dose of drug required, shorter duration of treatment [120] and decreased nursing time for antibiotic administration, and a possible reduction in the formation of resistant bacteria [118, 136]. These have also been validated in cost-analyses. Disadvantages of continuous infusion have also been documented and include drug stability for 24-h infusions (e.g. meropenem may only be stable for a maximum 8 h requiring a new infusion to be made when a bolus would normally be administered [137, 138]), and the requirement for an intravenous line to be permanently designated for the continuous infusion because of possible drug-drug intravenous compatibility issues.

Effect of Neutropenia on β-Lactam Dosing

Severe sepsis may also lead to an immune system dysfunction evident by the presence of neutropenia. Previous studies with *K. pneumoniae* have suggested that neutropenia may not reduce the antibacterial effect of β-lactams significantly, but may enable a relapse of infection when antibiotic therapy is ceased [35, 139]. It follows that critically ill patients may require β-lactam therapy until the patient's white cell count normalises.

12.2.2.4 *Summary of β-Lactam Dosing in Critically Ill Patients with Sepsis*

β-Lactam antibiotics will often require dosing different to that suggested by studies in healthy volunteers. More frequent dosing or continuous infusion of the antibiotic is suggested if there is organ dysfunction and/or 'third spacing'. The required dose for continuous infusion is generally less than that required for the intermittent bolus dose.

12.2.3 Carbapenems

Carbapenem antibiotics include meropenem, imipenem and panipenem.

12.2.3.1 *Pharmacokinetics*

- General (see Table 12.2)

Carbapenems are a separate class of β-lactam antibiotics that possess good Gram negative and Gram positive activity. Like other β-lactams, these antibiotics typically have a minimal side effect profile [140]. Increased seizure activity has been noted with imipenem and as a result it has been recorded as a potential adverse event for all carbapenems, particularly in infants, elderly patients and those with renal dysfunction [141–144]. Due to instability, imipenem is typically combined with cilastatin and betamipron is combined with panipenem as a renal protectant [145]. These adjuncts have higher protein binding and may accumulate in patients with renal failure, the significance of which is unknown [140]. In conventional bolus dosing regimens, serum concentrations of carbapenems fall to low concentrations between doses. Renal elimination of these drugs is directly related to creatinine clearance, so serum concentrations will accumulate with renal dysfunction if dosing adjustments are not made [140, 146–148].

12.2.3.2 *Pharmacodynamic Principles of Carbapenems*

Kill characteristics of carbapenems are similar to other β-lactam antibiotics and show time-dependent killing [110]. However, in vitro models have shown that carbapenems require a reduced percentage of T>MIC for bacteriostatic activity (20%) and bactericidal activity (40%) [149] which may relate to the carbapenem PAE [113].

12.2.3.3 *Carbapenem Dosing in Critically Ill Patients with Sepsis*

Effect of 'Third-Spacing' on Carbapenem Dosing

As with other β-lactam antibiotics, the PK of the carbapenems changes in the critically ill patient with sepsis. Specifically, carbapenems demonstrate decreased $T_{1/2}$ and increased Vd, and CL [140, 150, 151], which will result in reduced C_{max} and T>MIC. The clinical effect of more frequent dosing or continuous infusion is unclear and as such dose adjustment from increased Vd is not presently indicated.

Effect of Organ Dysfunction on Carbapenem Dosing

As with aminoglycosides and other β-lactams, in sepsis without organ dysfunction, increased clearance can occur resulting in lower serum concentrations of carbapenems. Higher dosing or more frequent dosing may thus be indicated for critically ill patients with sepsis without organ dysfunction.

Administration of Carbapenems by Continuous Infusion

Administration by continuous infusion to maximise T>MIC remains a topical issue for carbapenems. Some research has shown meropenem to be unsuitable for 8-h infusions in a tropical country, where room temperature is 32–37°C [152], and that it spontaneously degrades in saline solutions after less than 6 h at normal room temperature(25°C) [153]. Other research has shown adequate stability for 8-h infusions to be administered [137, 138] and up to 12 h in a cold pouch [154]. Intermittent 3-h infusions have also been utilised in previous studies [155]. Some preliminary data suggests clinical superiority of administration by continuous infusion in critically ill patients [156]; however, further studies are needed. Thus, while the apparent need for more frequent dosing or administration by continuous infusion is reduced from this in vitro data, concentration-related toxicity can be avoided [38, 149] and pharmacoeconomic advantages from reduced total daily dose may still be conferred [157]. Optimisation of the PD profile of carbapenems has been shown previously by the use of extended infusions [138, 158, 159] although to date only improved in vitro efficacy has been reported [138, 160]. Further research to determine the clinical efficacy of administering carbapenems as a continuous infusion is required.

Effect of Neutropenia on Carbapenem Dosing

As with other β-lactams, the impaired immune function of the critically ill patient will most likely have little effect in changing the MIC breakpoints and no dose adjustment is indicated at this time, although it would be prudent to at least continue therapy until the neutropenia has normalised.

12.2.3.4 *Summary of Carbapenem Dosing in Critically Ill Patients with Sepsis*

Carbapenems have pharmacodynamic properties different to other β-lactam antibiotics because of the decreased T>MIC required for activity. Thus, while more frequent dosing or continuous infusion of the antibiotic will optimise the pharmacodynamic profile, it is recommended only when there is organ dysfunction and/or significant 'third spacing'.

12.2.4 Glycopeptides

Glycopeptide antibiotics include vancomycin and teicoplanin.

12.2.4.1 *Pharmacokinetics*

- General (see Table 12.2)

Vancomycin is predominantly renally eliminated and while it has been associated with self-limiting nephrotoxicity, particularly during co-administration of other nephrotoxins [161, 162], its potential to cause nephrotoxicity has been debated [163]. However, Fernandez de Gatta et al. [164] found a relationship between vancomycin exposure and nephrotoxicity and provided evidence that therapeutic drug monitoring (TDM) of vancomycin led to a reduced incidence of nephrotoxicity [164].

Teicoplanin has a similar Vd to vancomycin but a much longer $T_{1/2}$ in patients with normal renal function [165–167]. It is highly protein bound and predominantly renally eliminated. A decrease in albumin level or binding has been found to increase the Vd and apparent clearance of teicoplanin [166]. TDM of teicoplanin is not necessary to avoid toxicity, but can be helpful in certain patient groups to ensure therapeutic concentrations are present [167].

12.2.4.2
Pharmacodynamic Principles of Glycopeptides

The specific interpretation of the PD properties of glycopeptides are not fully understood. Vancomycin will be preferentially discussed as representative of the glycopeptides due to its prevalent usage. Vancomycin is well known to induce PAE and has PD properties in common with both aminoglycosides and β-lactams. Some data suggests that the bactericidal activity of vancomycin is time-dependent [168–170]. Similar results have been obtained for teicoplanin in a rabbit endocarditis model [171]. Interestingly, an in vitro study [172] found no difference in rates of killing of S. *aureus* by vancomycin when given as various forms of continuous infusion and bolus dosing suggesting that $T>$MIC is not the categorical PD factor. C_{max}:MIC was found to be the PD factor correlated with efficacy in a non-neutropenic mouse peritonitis model for *S. pneumoniae* and *S. aureus,* suggesting that glycopeptides might show concentration-dependent killing against some organisms [173]. Whether this PD effect is primarily due to the presence of neutrophils in this model is unknown.

Other studies have proposed that AUC_{0-24}:MIC is the most important PK-PD parameter correlating with efficacy [35, 174]. As such, the optimal dosing regimen for administration of vancomycin remains unknown: continuous infusion or bolus dosing. Wysocki et al. [175] specifically compared continuous infusion and intermittent dosing of vancomycin in 160 patients, and found no significant difference in clinical efficacy. However, recently Rello et al. [176] described a suggestion of clinical superiority of continuous infusion of vancomycin in a subset of patients treated for ventilator-associated pneumonia caused by methicillin-resistant *Staphylococcus aureus.* Thus, while the economic advantages of reduced dosage of vancomycin by continuous infusion have been described [175], the clinical relevance of this remains unclear.

12.2.4.3
Glycopeptide Dosing in Critically Ill Patients with Sepsis

Effect of 'Third-Spacing' on Glycopeptide Dosing

Sepsis without organ dysfunction will cause an increased Vd and an increased rate of renal excretion of vancomycin. As a consequence, in our experience we have found that higher doses than those conventionally recommended (similar to paediatric doses of 40 mg/kg/day [177]) may be needed to optimise serum concentrations.

Effect of Organ Dysfunction on Glycopeptide Dosing

Glycopeptide clearance varies proportionately with creatinine clearance [174]. Thus higher doses are required if there is supranormal renal function. However, with renal dysfunction there will be reduced CL and drug accumulation [161, 162, 178]. As a result, diligent monitoring of trough vancomycin serum concentrations (recommended concentration 15–20 mg/l) is currently recommended to ensure efficacy of dose by following the $T>$MIC PD property [179]. For teicoplanin, when there is no renal impairment dosing at 6 mg/kg 12-hourly for three doses, followed by 6 mg/kg 24-hourly thereafter, is recommended. Serum concentration monitoring is indicated only when high doses (12 mg/kg/day) are used or to avoid toxicity. Current practice suggests that teicoplanin concentrations be maintained above 10 mg/l (15–20 mg/l for endocarditis) [174].

Administration of Glycopeptides By More Frequent Dosing or Continuous Infusion

Adequate vancomycin trough concentrations can be maintained by dosing 6-, 8- or 12-hourly or by continuous infusion although the optimal dosing regimen for vancomycin remains unresolved because of the lack of definitive evidence of PD efficacy and evidence linking concentrations to either outcome or toxicity [169, 179]. The ongoing debate on the optimal administration of vancomycin [169, 172, 175, 176, 180] demonstrates the need for further research in this area.

Effect of Neutropenia on Glycopeptide Dosing

Improved outcomes from dosing glycopeptides by continuous infusion may particularly be found in critically ill patients with neutropenia. Some research has shown that AUC_{0-24}/MIC is the most important PD parameter in animal neutropenic models [174], while C_{max}:MIC has been shown in non-neutropenic models [173]. Thus, more frequent dosing or continuous infusion may have advantages in neutropenic patients although more research in this area is required.

Penetration of Glycopeptides into Solid Organs

Vancomycin poorly penetrates into solid organs, particularly the lung [181, 182]. Thus, if the sepsis is thought to emerge from a lung focus, the co-prescription of rifampicin as dual therapy has been suggested [181]. Therapy with rifampicin as a single agent is not recommended due to its propensity to cause bacterial resistance [183], and the potential for drug interactions from CYP3A4 induction must always be considered. Alternatively, high dose vancomycin (aiming for trough concentrations ≥20 mg/l) has been advocated [183] for sepsis originating in solid organs. Of course, other antibacterial agents do provide better penetration of the epithelial lining fluid of the lung and thus therapy with either fusidic acid [184], linezolid [185], tigecycline [186] or televancin [187] may be preferred.

We believe that teicoplanin does not add many clinical advantages and that newer drugs in production will take its place as vancomycin substitutes.

12.2.4.4
Summary of Glycopeptide Dosing in Critically Ill Patients with Sepsis

The pharmacodynamic properties of vancomycin are not fully understood at this time. To optimise dosing of vancomycin in critically ill patients with sepsis, maintenance of trough levels of at least 15–20 mg/l are required. Teicoplanin must have loading doses to ensure therapeutic concentrations are rapidly obtained (6–10 mg/kg doses 12-hourly for three doses followed by 6 mg/kg 24-hourly thereafter). Dose adjustments for variations in renal function may also be required.

12.2.5
Fluoroquinolones

Fluoroquinolone antibiotics include ciprofloxacin, moxifloxacin, levofloxacin and gatifloxacin. These are a relatively new class of antibiotics and, to date, less research has been committed to moxifloxacin, levofloxacin and gatifloxacin. As such where information is not available on these antibiotics, information known of ciprofloxacin will be used.

12.2.5.1
Pharmacokinetics

- General (see Table 12.3)

All fluoroquinolones have extensive distribution characteristics and achieve good extracellular and intracellular concentrations with excellent penetration of neutrophils and lymphocytes [188].

12.2.5.2
Pharmacodynamic Principles of Fluoroquinolones

Fluoroquinolones display largely concentration-dependent kill characteristics but also some time-dependent effects. Previous research has suggested that achieving a C_{max}:MIC ratio of 10 for ciprofloxacin is the critical variable in predicting bacterial eradication [189]. Forrest et al. [40] studied ciprofloxacin in critically ill patients and concluded that achieving an AUC_{0-24h}:MIC greater than 125 is associated with a successful clinical outcome. This result is necessary for Gram negative organisms with Gram positive organisms requiring an AUC_{0-24hr}:MIC of 30 [40, 190–192], although fluoroquinolones should not be used as single agent treatment of Gram positive infections. Inappropriate low dosing of ciprofloxacin has also been associated with the emergence of resistant bacterial strains (particularly enterococci, *Pseudomonas* and MRSA) [193–195]. For Gram negative bacteria, this may occur when AUC_{0-24h}: MIC < 100 [196, 197]. Therefore, AUC_{0-24h}: MIC and C_{max}: MIC are PD variables that require close attention for optimal fluoroquinolone usage. The dose recommended to achieve these pharmacodynamics for ciprofloxacin is 400 mg IV 8-hourly in adults and this need not be changed during sepsis unless renal dysfunction occurs [198, 199]. Pharmacodynamic analysis has shown that this maximum dose has a 55% probability of achieving the AUC target of 125 [200] and as such larger doses or different dosing regimens may be used in the future. There is growing evidence for increased dosing of levofloxacin in critically

Table 12.3. General PK characteristics of fluoroquinolone antibiotics and possible changes that can occur during fluid shifts in critically ill patients

Fluoroquinolone	Vd (l/kg)	Increased Vd with fluid shifts?	Decreased C_{max} with fluid shifts?	Serum $T_{1/2}$ (h)	Protein binding	Altered CL in sepsis with renal dysfunction?	Normal dose	Dose adjustment in renal dysfunction?
Ciprofloxacin [264–266]	1.2–2.7	No	Yes	3 (4–5 h in the elderly)	20–40%	No	IV 400 mg 8-hourly	Dose reduction in severe renal dysfunction
Levofloxacin [267, 268]	0.92–1.36	?No	Yes	6–8.9	24–38%	Yes	500–750 mg daily	(a) CrCL = 20–49 ml/min → 250–500 mg daily; (b) CrCL is 10–19 ml/min → 250–500 mg 48-hourly
Moxifloxacin [268–270]	2.45–3.55	No	Yes	9.3–15.6	39–52%	No	400 mg daily	No
Gatifloxacin [264, 271]	1.98–2.31	No	Yes	6.5–9.6	20%	Yes	400 mg daily	CrCL ≤ 40 ml/min → 400 mg initial dose followed by 200 mg 24-hourly

ill patients with sepsis (1,000 mg daily) [201, 202], and with more safety and efficacy data, further increases in recommended doses may occur for other fluoroquinolone antibiotics as well.

12.2.5.3
Fluoroquinolone Dosing in Critically Ill Patients with Sepsis

Effect of 'Third-Spacing' on Fluoroquinolone Dosing

All fluoroquinolone antibiotics demonstrate good tissue penetration [199]. PK studies with ciprofloxacin in adult patients with severe sepsis and intra-abdominal sepsis [199] have shown that the Vd of ciprofloxacin is not altered with fluid shifts, or over time, since it distributes intracellularly and binds to structures therein. This characteristic is also maintained for the infant less than 12 months old [21], where body water content is greater than in older children and adults. Thus, while dose adjustments for altered Vd are not required in critically ill patients, dose adjustments may be necessary in enhanced or reduced renal function.

Effect of Organ Dysfunction on Fluoroquinolone Dosing

Ciprofloxacin is metabolised in liver to multiple metabolites although dose adjustment and dose adjustment is recommended by the product information [203] with renal dysfunction to prevent accumulation of drug and metabolites [204]. Other research by Jones et al. [205] has shown impaired ciprofloxacin clearance in renal impairment only when the patient had concomitant bowel or liver pathology suggesting that accumulation will only occur when at least two elimination pathways are compromised. The authors recommended that in critically ill patients with sepsis and acute renal impairment, dose adjustment is only necessary if the patient also has intra-abdominal disease.

Levofloxacin and gatifloxacin are only moderately lipophilic and are predominantly renally cleared. Dosage reductions for renal impairment can be made as described in Table 12.3. However, at this time there is no recommendation for higher dosing should the patient develop supranormal renal function.

Moxifloxacin requires no dose reduction in renal impairment or mild hepatic impairment. Dosing in severe hepatic impairment has not been investigated at this time.

12.2.5.4
Summary of Fluoroquinolone Dosing in Critically Ill Patients with Sepsis

Bolus dosing optimises the pharmacodynamic properties of fluoroquinolones enabling a C_{max}:MIC ratio of 10 to be achieved. Administration of adequate doses is essential to prevent development of resistant organisms. Dose adjustment in critically ill patients with sepsis is only required in renal impairment for levofloxacin, gatifloxacin and ciprofloxacin.

12.2.6
Tigecycline

Tigecycline is a member of the glycylcyclines, which are novel tetracyclines with Gram positive and gram negative activity.

12.2.6.1
Pharmacokinetics

- General (see Table 12.2)

Tigecycline has shown rapid and extensive penetration into body tissues that is reflected by its large Vd (7–10 l/kg). It was shown to have 74% penetration into inflammatory fluid in an inflammatory blister fluid model [206]. It is primarily eliminated by biliary excretion with only 15% of the dose eliminated unchanged in urine [207].

12.2.6.2
Pharmacodynamic Principles of Tigecycline

Tigecycline displays time-dependent killing against *Strepotoccus pneumoniae*, *Haemophilus influenzae* and *Neisseria gonorrhea* [208] but AUC_{0-24}/MIC is more likely to be correlated with efficacy [206, 209]. This is because of its long half-life and prolonged PAE. However, more research into the pharmacodynamic principles of tigecycline is suggested to clarify this.

12.2.6.3
Tigecycline Dosing in Critically Ill Patients with Sepsis

Effect of 'Third-Spacing' on Tigecycline Dosing

No evidence exists to support altered dosing in patients with 'third spacing'. However, there is little experience with tigecycline in critically ill patients with sepsis and more information may later emerge regarding this issue.

Effect of Organ Dysfunction on Tigecycline Dosing

Dose adjustment in renal failure is not required with tigecycline. However, as most of the dose (59%) is eliminated in faeces, careful consideration of dose reduction may be necessary if the patient develops severe renal impairment or significant cholestasis.

12.2.6.4
Summary of Tigecycline Dosing in Critically Ill Patients with Sepsis

Tigecycline should be reserved for infections caused by multi-resistant organisms. While a higher (100 mg loading dose then 50 mg 12-hourly) and lower dosing regimen (50 mg loading dose then 25 mg 12-hourly) has been previously trialled [210], the superior clinical and bacteriologic success of the higher dosing regimen suggests that it may be more suitable for critically ill patients with sepsis. Again, however, as this is a new antibiotic, subsequent study may result in changes to recommended dosing.

12.2.7
Telithromycin

Telithromycin is the first ketolide marketed and has properties very similar to macrolide antibiotics.

12.2.7.1
Pharmacokinetics

- General (see Table 12.2)

Telithromycin has been shown to have good extracellular penetration with good levels in respiratory tissues [211], sites of inflammation (blister fluids 38% above plasma [212]) and in neutrophils [213]. However, poor penetration in muscle and adipose [214] has been shown.

12.2.7.2
Pharmacodynamic Principles of Telithromycin

Telithromycin displays concentration-dependent killing [215, 216] with C_{max}:MIC ratio the parameter most predictive of a successful outcome. Telithromycin also exhibits long postantibiotic effects and postantibiotic sub-MIC effects enabling once-daily dosing [215, 216].

12.2.7.3
Telithromycin Dosing in Critically Ill Patients with Sepsis

Effect of 'Third-Spacing' on Telithromycin Dosing

No evidence exists to support altered dosing in patients with 'third spacing', and current evidence suggests no dose adjustments are required in patients based on weight [217]. However, this is a new drug and information may later emerge regarding this issue.

Effect of Organ Dysfunction on Telithromycin Dosing

If a patient develops renal impairment, dose adjustment may be required. In moderate to severe renal impairment (CrCL 30 ml/min), doses should be halved (800 mg 24-hourly reduced to 400 mg 24-hourly) [217]. No dose adjustment is required in hepatic disease [213].

Drug Interactions of Telithromycin

Telithromycin is a strong inhibitor of the metabolic enzyme CYP3A4 and should be used with caution with midazolam and triazolam (potential to prolong Q-Tc), HMG-CoA reductase inhibitors or 'statins' (risk of myopathy), digoxin, metoprolol and theophylline (elevated drug levels). Phenytoin and other enzyme inducers may reduce telithromycin levels. Telithromycin is only available in oral dosage form and is recommended at 800 mg daily for 7–10 days for community acquired pneumonia.

12.2.7.4
Summary of Telithromycin Dosing in Critically Ill Patients with Sepsis

Telithromycin should be predominantly used for multi-resistant organisms. Its utility in sepsis may be reduced at this time because it is only available in an oral dosage form.

12.2.8
Daptomycin

Daptomycin is a novel lipopolypetide antimicrobial agent with good activity against most Gram positive pathogens. While it was discovered 20 years ago, it has been marketed only recently and only few clinical studies have been performed which provide data on toxicity.

12.2.8.1
Pharmacokinetics

- General (see Table 12.2)

In healthy patients, daptomycin demonstrates linear pharmacokinetic properties and is primarily renally eliminated. No studies have been done in patients under 18 years at this time. Cl is highly correlated with creatinine clearance (CrCL) and dosing should be adjusted in line with this. Early trials correlated muscle weakness, myalgia and marked increases in creatinine phosphokinase (CPK) with 12-hourly dosing [218], and it is thus now recommended for 24-hourly dosing. Dosing is recommended at 4 mg/kg/24 h by intravenous administration.

12.2.8.2 Pharmacodynamic Principles of Daptomycin

C_{max}:MIC is the PD parameter associated with clinical efficacy [219]. Daptomycin has a prolonged PAE of 2–6 h in MSSA and MRSA [220] and 1–2.5 h in *S. pneumoniae* [219]. However, in a murine neutropenic thigh-infection model this increased to 8.8–10.8 h from 4.8–5.5 h respectively [219].

12.2.8.3 Daptomycin Dosing in Critically Ill Patients with Sepsis

Effect of 'Third-Spacing' on Daptomycin Dosing

Distribution is likely to be limited to the extracellular fluid spaces, so third spacing will result in reduced C_{max}. It distributes rapidly into inflammatory fluid (blister study in volunteers) but does not reach the plasma concentrations, probably due to differences in the protein content of this fluid [221].

Effect of Organ Dysfunction on Daptomycin Dosing

If a patient develops moderate to severe renal impairment (CrCl < 30 ml/min), then the frequency should be extended to 48 hourly dosing [222]. The effect of reduced serum albumin levels in hepatic impairment, on unbound daptomycin concentration, remains unknown but patients should be monitored for changes in CPK if this occurs.

Effect of Low Serum Calcium on Daptomycin

It has been suggested that daptomycin requires the presence of free calcium ions in a growth medium to demonstrate its activity against Gram positive organisms [223], and the effect this may have in humans with low serum calcium is unknown. If the patient with sepsis presents with low serum calcium levels, this should be corrected and the patient's clinical response to daptomycin should be carefully monitored.

12.2.8.4 Summary of Daptomycin Dosing in Critically Ill Patients with Sepsis

Information about the optimal dosing and possible toxicities of daptomycin is still accumulating. In critically ill patients, even less is known and careful monitoring of the patient is necessary should daptomycin be prescribed. Initial administration at 4 mg/kg as a single 24-hourly dose is recommended with extended frequency of dosing indicated for renal impairment. Special considerations for use include altered serum calcium or albumin. Daptomycin should be reserved for serious infections caused by MRSA, VRE and MRSE that do not respond to vancomycin.

12.2.9 Quinupristin/Dalfopristin

Quinupristin/dalfopristin (Q/D) is a combination of two injectable streptogramins with demonstrated efficacy against multi-resistant Gram positive organisms.

12.2.9.1 Pharmacokinetics

- General (see Table 12.2)

In vitro studies have shown significant CYP3A4 inhibition by Q/D, and care should be exercised when administering other drugs that are also inhibitors or substrates for, or inducers of, this enzyme system [224]. Q/D has shown a significant PAE against *Enterococcus faecium* (0.2–3.2 h) [225].

12.2.9.2 Pharmacodynamic Principles of Quinupristin/Dalfopristin

Q/D is thought to have concentration-dependent efficacy. Aeschlimann and Ryback [225] demonstrated this in vitro by showing that 99.9 % killing of isolates of vancomycin-resistant *Enterococcus faecium* (VREF) was best correlated with a high ratio of Q/D concentration to minimum bactericidal concentration (MBC). Some authors have suggested that AUC_{0-24}/MIC is the primary parameter correlated with efficacy [226].

12.2.9.3 Quinupristin/Dalfopristin Dosing in Critically Ill Patients with Sepsis

Effect of Organ Dysfunction on Quinupristin/ Dalfopristin Dosing

Hepatic dysfunction may result in altered metabolism of Q/D or may cause unpredictable effects to other CYP3A4 metabolised drugs from unknown inhibition.

12.2.9.4 Summary of Quinupristin/Dalfopristin in Critically Ill Patients with Sepsis

Little information exists aiding dosing of quinupristin/dalfopristin in critically ill patients with sepsis. If it is believed that penetration to the infection site may be impaired, then co-administration with another antibiotic (e.g. linezolid or a glycopeptide) is recommended [227]. Q/D is recommended to be dosed at 7.5 mg/kg intravenous administration 8-hourly for VREF and 7.5 mg/kg intravenous administration 12-hourly for complicated skin and skin structure infections with *Staphylococcus aureus* (methicillin-susceptible) [224].

12.2.10 Clindamycin (as a Representative of the Lincosamides)

The lincosamide antibiotics include clindamycin and lincomycin.

12.2.10.1 *Pharmacokinetics*

- General (see Table 12.2)

Clindamycin is widely distributed throughout the body and achieves therapeutic concentrations in most body compartments [228–230]. It is extensively hepatically metabolised and renally cleared [228] with a $T_{1/2}$ that may increase in hepatic dysfunction [231].

Lincomycin has similar properties to clindamycin although distribution into tissues may not be as wide as clindamycin [232]. While lincomycin is also extensively hepatically metabolised [233], its $T_{1/2}$ is prolonged in both severe renal and hepatic impairment [233].

12.2.10.2 *Pharmacodynamic Principles of Lincosamides*

T>MIC has been determined to be the pharmacodynamic factor correlated with efficacy. Free drug levels of lincosamides should exceed the MIC of the infective pathogen for at least 40–50% of the dosing interval [226].

12.2.10.3 *Lincosamide Dosing in Critically Ill Patients with Sepsis*

Effect of 'Third-Spacing' on Lincosamide Dosing

Third spacing is unlikely to have a major clinical effect on lincosamide pharmacokinetics. While this may result in a reduced C_{max}, the effect on T>MIC should be limited as lincosamides already have extensive distribution throughout the body.

12.2.10.4 *Effect of Organ Dysfunction on Lincosamide Dosing*

Alterations in renal function are unlikely to affect clindamycin pharmacokinetics. However, lincomycin clearance may be affected, as previously shown in severe renal impairment [233]. Hepatic dysfunction is likely to affect the clearance of both clindamycin and lincomycin [231, 233] and dose reductions should be considered in severe renal impairment.

12.2.10.5 *Summary of Lincosamides in Critically Ill Patients with Sepsis*

Lincosamides represent an excellent therapeutic choice for suspected/confirmed anaerobic infections in critically ill patients with sepsis due to their extensive distribution characteristics. Standard doses should be used for clindamycin (1,200–2,700 mg in three- or four-divided doses) unless significant hepatic impairment is present. Lincomycin dosing (600 mg to 2.4 g 8-hourly dependent on severity of infection) should be reduced in the presence of either significant renal or hepatic impairment.

12.2.11 Linezolid

Linezolid is the first of a new class of antimicrobials called the oxazolinediones.

12.2.11.1 *Pharmacokinetics*

- General (see Table 12.2)

Linezolid has a Vd consistent with total body water and a $T_{1/2}$ of 3.5–6.0 h [234]. It widely distributes into tissues including inflammatory fluids, extracellular lining fluid and CSF [235, 236]. Linezolid is mostly metabolised and then renally cleared although no dose adjustment is recommended in renal dysfunction [237] or hepatic dysfunction [235].

12.2.11.2 *Pharmacodynamic Principles of Linezolid*

In animal models, T>MIC was the major predictor of efficacy with *S. pneumoniae* in a murine thigh infection model [238] and a rat pneumonia model [239]. In both models T>MIC of 40–45% was the best predictor of outcome. Subsequent animal models using *S. pneumoniae*, *S. aureus* and pneumococci have predicted that an AUC_{0-24}/MIC ratio of 50–80 correlates well with efficacy [240]. A 600-mg 12-hourly dose should achieve this ratio in humans against susceptible organisms with MICs up to 2–4 mg/l. There is some information to suggest that maximal *S. aureus* killing may occur when T>MIC for 100% of the dosing interval [35].

12.2.11.3 *Linezolid Dosing in Critically Ill Patients with Sepsis*

Effect of 'Third-Spacing' on Linezolid Dosing

Third spacing is likely to result in increased Vd and a decreased C_{max} but this should not be clinically significant.

Effect of Organ Dysfunction on Linezolid Dosing

Hepatic dysfunction is not likely to alter the dosing schedule for linezolid, as metabolism occurs non-enzymatically [235]. No data in severe hepatic dysfunction is currently available. Dose adjustment in renal failure is also not recommended at this time, even though accumulation of metabolites has been shown [235, 237].

Potential Drug Interactions Associated with Linezolid

Although linezolid undergoes non-enzymatic metabolism, it has been shown to affect warfarin activity by decreasing the mean international normalised ratio (INR) by 10% in healthy volunteers [241]. Warfarin should be carefully dosed in such patients.

Linezolid is a reversible non-selective inhibitor of monoamine oxidase (MAO) [235]. As such it may have potential drug interactions with drugs that inhibit MAO resulting in an increased vasopressor response. In critical care units, ongoing blood pressure monitoring reduces the significance of this interaction. Linezolid may also contribute to serotonin syndrome if co-administered with sympathomimetic amines (e.g. pseudoephedrine) or tyramine (as found in mature cheese, soya beans and yeast extracts). This interaction may be more problematic in critical care units as a ventilated patient with concurrent prescription of muscle relaxants may not display the classical symptoms of serotonin syndrome such as confusion, delirium, restlessness and tremor.

Myelosuppression and Linezolid

In the majority of patients, linezolid is safe and well tolerated for up to 28 days at 600 mg twice daily [242]. Evidence exists that therapy longer than 14 days can rarely cause reversible myelosuppression [243], although a causal relationship has not been established. As such patients prescribed linezolid should have complete blood counts ordered weekly if 2 or more weeks treatment is indicated [242].

12.2.11.4 Summary of Linezolid in Critically Ill Patients with Sepsis

Linezolid is the first oxazolidinone released and is suitable for the treatment of Gram positive infections. No evidence exists for dosing other than 600 mg 12-hourly exists in critically ill patients at this time, even those with third-spacing or renal and/or hepatic dysfunction.

12.3 Duration of Antibiotic Therapy for Critically Ill Patients with Sepsis

Little data exists to rationally guide duration of antibiotic treatment in critically ill patients. However, increasing awareness of the risks of prolonged courses of broad spectrum agents has led internationally to a trend towards shortening the length of treatment. Most courses of antibiotics in ICU are given for an empirical duration based upon site of infection and pathogen. Some data exist to modify durations based upon clinical response.

The Infectious Disease Society of America (IDSA) guidelines on management of Community Acquired Pneumonia (CAP) in adults [244] suggests that length of treatment should be guided by clinical factors, such as response, severity, and co-morbidities. Specifically, they note that pneumonia caused by *Streptococcus pneumoniae* should be treated until the patient has been afebrile for at least 72 h. Similar recommendations are made for management of neutropenic patients with cancer [244], based upon duration of fever and neutrophil count.

Evidence based data to guide duration of treatment are sparse. Singh et al. [245] examined the effect of a 3-day course of ciprofloxacin as compared to standard antibiotic treatment for 10–21 days for ICU patients with pulmonary infiltrates, but thought to have a low risk of pneumonia. They documented no difference in mortality and a lower length of stay in the short duration group. Antimicrobial resistance and superinfection rates were higher in the group receiving standard treatment. A French study examined the effects of an 8-day antibiotic course compared with 15 days in the management of ventilator associated pneumonia [246]. A total of 401 patients were enrolled, and no difference in mortality, duration of mechanical ventilation, or length of stay was noted. The authors did comment on a higher recurrence rate of pulmonary infections in patients with *P. aeruginosa* managed with the shorter course; this was not associated with unfavourable outcomes. Denneson et al. examined the resolution of infectious parameters in 27 patients with diagnosed VAP [247]. They determined that maximum resolution occurs in the first 6 days of treatment, whilst acquired colonisation with resistant pathogens appears primarily in the second week. Based on this data the authors hypothesised that a 1-week course of antibiotics may be sufficient to treat VAP whilst decreasing the rate of emergence of resistant bacteria.

The Surviving Sepsis Campaign [248] published antibiotic treatment guidelines in 2004. These guidelines recommend a typical 7- to 10-day course of antibiotic therapy that should be guided by microbiological results and clinical response.

In summary, whilst there is little evidence to guide the clinician in deciding the optimal duration of treatment of infections in the critically ill, there is a move to decrease the duration of antibiotic therapy. Increasing awareness of the emergence of multi-resistant pathogens is leading to reluctance to engage in protracted courses of broad spectrum antibiotics, and whilst this appears to be supported by the data, larger clinical trials are urgently required.

12.4 Conclusion

Current antibiotic regimens have mostly been derived from trials with patients who are not critically ill with conditions such as sepsis. In order to optimise antibiotic regimens in patients with sepsis, the pathophysiological effects of SIRS need consideration, in conjunction with knowledge of the different kill characteristics of the various antibiotic classes. The end result will be doses and regimens that are more appropriate for use in critically ill with sepsis that may differ from more common antibiotic prescribing practices.

Certain antibiotics can have a high Vd, hence leading to low C_{max} during sepsis. It follows then that underdosing may occur if a high peak is needed (e.g. aminoglycosides).

The Vd of antibiotics that distribute primarily into extravascular water, namely aminoglycosides, vancomycin and, to a lesser extent, β-lactams, changes with clinical severity, so dosing may need to be altered during the course of illness, something not described for non-critically ill patients.

Some patients with serum creatinine within the normal range can have higher than normal drug clearances, thereby producing low serum concentrations. If a drug needs to have a minimum serum concentration maintained (e.g. β-lactams), a high drug clearance will lead to underdosing for renally excreted drugs. In other words when creatinine clearance is high, the renal clearance of these drugs will be high. In relation to the aminoglycosides this means that not only are large doses required to be administered, but because of high creatinine clearances these antibiotics may also need dosing even more frequently than every 24 h. As discussed above, all β-lactams should, in such patients, be dosed more frequently than suggested in non-sepsis patients. In view of renal clearance of the fluoroquinolones, in the presence of high creatinine clearances we can assume fluoroquinolone clearance is also high. If this were to be true these antibiotics would also need to have higher daily doses than proposed in the standard literature.

Treatment of sepsis remains a significant challenge given persisting high mortality and morbidity rates. Data suggests that effective antibiotic therapy remains the most important intervention available to the clinician. In treating sepsis, a clinician must be aware of the impact of the various pathophysiological and subsequent pharmacokinetic changes that can occur during sepsis. In this article we have described the common antibiotic classes and the PD features that must be recognised to optimise clinical efficacy. Facilitation of these PD parameters will optimize antibiotic therapy in septic patients, and augment therapeutic outcomes.

References

1. Bone RC, Balk RA, Cerra FB, Dellinger RP, Fein AM, Knaus WA, Schein RM, Sibbald WJ (1992) Definitions for sepsis and organ failure and guidelines for the use of innovative therapies in sepsis. The ACCP/SCCM Consensus Conference Committee. American College of Chest Physicians/ Society of Critical Care Medicine. Chest 101:1644–1655
2. Calandra T, Cohen J (2005) The international sepsis forum consensus conference on definitions of infection in the intensive care unit. Crit Care Med 33:1538–1548
3. Rice TW, Bernard GR (2005) Therapeutic intervention and targets for sepsis. Annu Rev Med 56:225–248
4. Hugonnet S, Harbarth S, Ferriere K, Ricou B, Suter P, Pittet D (2003) Bacteremic sepsis in intensive care: temporal trends in incidence, organ dysfunction, and prognosis. Crit Care Med 31:390–394
5. Garnacho-Montero J, Garcia-Garmendia JL, Barrero-Almodovar A, Jimenez-Jimenez FJ, Perez-Paredes C, Ortiz-Leyba C (2003) Impact of adequate empirical antibiotic therapy on the outcome of patients admitted to the intensive care unit with sepsis. Crit Care Med 31:2742–2751
6. Harbarth S, Garbino J, Pugin J, Romand JA, Lew D, Pittet D (2003) Inappropriate initial antimicrobial therapy and its effect on survival in a clinical trial of immunomodulating therapy for severe sepsis. Am J Med 115:529–535
7. Kollef MH, Sherman G, Ward S, Fraser VJ (1999) Inadequate antimicrobial treatment of infections: a risk factor for hospital mortality among critically ill patients. Chest 115:462–474
8. MacArthur RD, Miller M, Albertson T, Panacek E, Johnson D, Teoh L, Barchuk W (2004) Adequacy of early empiric antibiotic treatment and survival in severe sepsis: experience from the MONARCS trial. Clin Infect Dis 38:284–288
9. Kieft H, Hoepelman AI, Knupp CA, van Dijk A, Branger JM, Struyvenberg A, Verhoef J (1993) Pharmacokinetics of cefepime in patients with the sepsis syndrome. J Antimicrob Chemother 32 Suppl B:117–122
10. Joukhadar C, Frossard M, Mayer BX, Brunner M, Klein N, Siostrzonek P, Eichler HG, Muller M (2001) Impaired target site penetration of beta-lactams may account for therapeutic failure in patients with septic shock. Crit Care Med 29:385–391
11. Parrillo JE (1993) Pathogenetic mechanisms of septic shock. N Engl J Med 328:1471–1477
12. Grocott-Mason RM, Shah AM (1998) Cardiac dysfunction in sepsis: new theories and clinical implications. Intensive Care Med 24:286–295
13. van der Poll T (2001) Immunotherapy of sepsis. Lancet Infect. Dis 1:165–174
14. Nuytinck HK, Offermans XJ, Kubat K, Goris JA (1988) Whole-body inflammation in trauma patients. An autopsy study. Arch Surg 123:1519–1524
15. Gosling P, Sanghera K, Dickson G (1994) Generalized vascular permeability and pulmonary function in patients following serious trauma. J Trauma 36:477–481
16. Parrillo JE, Parker MM, Natanson C, Suffredini AF, Danner RL, Cunnion RE, Ognibene FP (1990) Septic shock in humans. Advances in the understanding of pathogenesis, cardiovascular dysfunction, and therapy. Ann Intern Med 113:227–242
17. Pea F, Porreca L, Baraldo M, Furlanut M (2000) High vancomycin dosage regimens required by intensive care unit patients cotreated with drugs to improve haemodynamics following cardiac surgical procedures. J Antimicrob Chemother 45:329–335
18. Di Giantomasso D, Bellomo R, May CN (2005) The haemodynamic and metabolic effects of epinephrine in experi-

mental hyperdynamic septic shock. Intensive Care Med 31:454–462
19. Di Giantomasso D, May CN, Bellomo R (2002) Norepinephrine and vital organ blood flow. Intensive Care Med 28:1804–1809
20. Di Giantomasso D, May CN, Bellomo R (2003) Norepinephrine and vital organ blood flow during experimental hyperdynamic sepsis. Intensive Care Med 29
21. Lipman J, Gous AG, Mathivha LR, Tshukutsoane S, Scribante J, Hon H, Pinder M, Riera-Fanego JF, Verhoef L, Stass H (2002) Ciprofloxacin pharmacokinetic profiles in paediatric sepsis: how much ciprofloxacin is enough? Intensive Care Med 28:493–500
22. Lipman J, Wallis SC, Rickard CM, Fraenkel D (2001) Low cefpirome levels during twice daily dosing in critically ill septic patients: pharmacokinetic modelling calls for more frequent dosing. Intensive Care Med 27:363–370
23. Lipman J, Wallis SC, Boots RJ (2003) Cefepime versus cefpirome: the importance of creatinine clearance. Anesth Analg 97:1149–1154
24. Pinder M, Bellomo R, Lipman J (2002) Pharmacological principles of antibiotic prescription in the critically ill. Anaesth Intensive Care 30:134–144
25. Marshall JC (2001) Inflammation, coagulopathy, and the pathogenesis of multiple organ dysfunction syndrome. Crit Care Med 29:S99–106
26. Power BM, Forbes AM, van Heerden PV, Ilett KF (1998) Pharmacokinetics of drugs used in critically ill adults. Clin Pharmacokinet 34:25–56
27. Cockroft DW, Gault MH (1976) Prediction of creatinine clearance from serum creatinine. Nephron 16:31–41
28. Levey AS, Bosch JP, Lewis JB, Greene T, Rogers N, Roth D (1999) A more accurate method to estimate glomerular filtration rate from serum creatinine: a new prediction equation. Modification of Diet in Renal Disease Study Group. Ann Intern Med 130:461–470
29. Roberts G, Ibsen P, Teglman C (2005) Renal function in elderly patients grossly overestimated by MDRD approach to renal function estimation. In: Society of Hospital Pharmacists of Australia, 27th Federal Conference. Brisbane, Australia, p 71
30. Pong S, Seto W, Abdolell M, Trope A, Wong K, Herridge J, Harvey E, Kavanagh BP (2005) 12-hour versus 24-hour creatinine clearance in critically ill pediatric patients. Pediatr Res 58:83–88
31. Wells M, Lipman J (1997) Pitfalls in the prediction of renal function in the intensive care unit. A review. S Afr J Surg 35:16–19
32. Wells M, Lipman J (1997) Measurements of glomerular filtration in the intensive care unit are only a rough guide to renal function. S Afr J Surg 35:20–23
33. Nicolau DP (1998) Optimizing antimicrobial therapy and emerging pathogens. Am J Man Care 4:S525–S530
34. Nicolau DP (2003) Optimizing outcomes with antimicrobial therapy through pharmacodynamic profiling. J Infect Chemother 9:292–296
35. Craig WA (2003) Basic pharmacodynamics of antibacterials with clinical applications to the use of b-lactams, glycopeptides, and linezolid. Infect Dis Clin N Am 17:479–501
36. Gudmundsson S, Vogelman B, Craig WA (1986) The in-vivo postantibiotic effect of imipenem and other new antimicrobials. J Antimicrob Chemother 18 Suppl E:67–73
37. Cunha BA (1995) Antibiotic treatment of sepsis. Med Clin North Am 79:551–558
38. Craig WA (1998) Pharmacokinetic/pharmacodynamic parameters: rationale for antibacterial dosing of mice and men. Clin Infect Dis 26:1–10; quiz 11–12
39. Moore RD, Lietman PS, Smith CR (1987) Clinical response to aminoglycoside therapy: importance of the ratio of peak concentration to minimal inhibitory concentration. J Infect Dis 155:93–99
40. Forrest A, Nix DE, Ballow CH, Goss TF, Birmingham MC, Schentag JJ (1993) Pharmacodynamics of intravenous ciprofloxacin in seriously ill patients. Antimicrob Agents Chemother 37:1073–1081
41. Gunderson BW, Ross GH, Ibrahim KH, Rotschafer JC (2001) What do we really know about antibiotic pharmacodynamics. Pharmacotherapy 21:302–318
42. Rodvold KA (2001) Pharmacodynamics of antiinfective therapy: taking what we know to the patient's bedside. Pharmacotherapy 21:319–330
43. Craig WA, Ebert SC (1991) Killing and regrowth of bacteria in vitro: a review. Scand J Infect Dis 74:63–70
44. Vogelman B, Gudmundsson S, Leggett J, Turnidge J, Ebert S, Craig WA (1988) Correlation of antimicrobial pharmacokinetic parameters with therapeutic efficacy in an animal model. J Infect Dis 158:831–847
45. Vogelman B, Craig WA (1986) Kinetics of antimicrobial activity. J Pediatr 108:835–840
46. Vogelman BS, Craig WA (1985) Postantibiotic effects. J Antimicrob Chemother 15 Suppl A:37–46
47. Roosendaal R, Bakker-Woudenberg IA, van den Berghe-van Raffe M, Vink-van den Berg JC, Michel BM (1989) Impact of the dosage schedule on the efficacy of ceftazidime, gentamicin and ciprofloxacin in *Klebsiella pneumoniae* pneumonia and septicemia in leukopenic rats. Eur J Clin Microbiol Infect Dis 8:878–887
48. Bakker-Woudenberg IA, Roosendaal R (1990) Impact of dosage schedule of antibiotics on the treatment of serious infections. Intensive Care Med 16:S229–234
49. Craig W (1984) Pharmacokinetic and experimental data on beta-lactam antibiotics in the treatment of patients. Eur J Clin Microbiol Infect Dis 3:575–578
50. Mouton JW, Vinks AA (2005) Pharmacokinetic/pharmacodynamic modelling of antibacterials in vitro and in vivo using bacterial growth and kill kinetics: the minimum inhibitory concentration versus stationary concentration. Clin Pharmacokinet 44:201–210
51. Turnidge J (1998) Pharmacokinetics and pharmacodynamics of fluoroquinolones. Drugs 58:29–36
52. Lode H, Borner K, Koeppe P (1998) Pharmacodynamics of Fluoroquinolones. Clin Infect Dis 27:33–39
53. Fisman DN, Kaye KM (2000) Once daily dosing of aminoglycoside antibiotics. Infect Dis Clin N Am 14:475–487
54. Kapusnik JE, Hackbarth CJ, Chambers HF, Carpenter T, Sande MA (1988) Single, large, daily dosing versus intermittent dosing of tobramycin fro treating experimental pseudomonas pneumonia. J Infect Dis 158:7–12
55. Klatersky J (1986) Concept of empiric therapy with antibiotic combinations; indications and limits. Am J Med 80:2–12
56. Thorburn CE, Molesworth SJ, Sutherland R, Rittenhouse S (1996) Postantibiotic and post-beta-lactamase inhibitor effects of amoxicillin plus clavulanate. Antimicrob Agents Chemother 40:2796–2801
57. Lavigne JP, Bonnet R, Michaux-Charachon S, Jourdan J, Caillon J, Sotto A (2004) Post-antibiotic and post-beta-lactamase inhibitor effects of ceftazidime plus sulbactam on extended-spectrum beta-lactamase-producing Gram-negative bacteria. J Antimicrob Chemother 53:616–619
58. Kim KS (1985) Efficacy of cefmenoxime in experimental Escherichia coli bacteremia and meningitis. Antimicrob Agents Chemother 28:389–392
59. Levison ME (1995) Pharmacodynamics of antimicrobial agents. Bactericidal and postantibiotic effects. Infect Dis Clin North Am 9:483–495

60. Jauregui L, Matzke D, Scott M, Minns P, Hageage G (1993) Cefepime as treatment for osteomyelitis and other severe bacterial infections. J Antimicrob Chemother 32 Suppl B:141–149
61. Phelps DJ, Carlton DD, Farrell CA, Kessler RE (1986) Affinity of cephalosporins for beta-lactamases as a factor in antibacterial efficacy. Antimicrob Agents Chemother 29: 845–848
62. Hoepelman AI, Kieft H, Aoun M, Kosmidis J, Strand T, Verhoef J, Gillespie SH, Riddell J, Varghese G, Meunier F (1993) International comparative study of cefepime and ceftazidime in the treatment of serious bacterial infections. J Antimicrob Chemother 32 Suppl B:175–186
63. Zhanel GG, Ariano RE (1992) Once daily aminoglycoside dosing: maintained efficacy with reduced nephrotoxicity? Ren Fail 14:1–9
64. Ali MZ, Goetz MB (1997) A meta-analysis of the relative efficacy and toxicity of single daily dosing versus multiple daily dosing of aminoglycosides. Clin Infect Dis 24:796–809
65. Bailey TC, Little JR, Littenberg B, Reichley RM, Dunagan WC (1997) A meta-analysis of extended-interval dosing versus multiple daily dosing of aminoglycosides. Clin Infect Dis 24:786–795
66. Munckhof WJ, Grayson ML, Turnidge JD (1996) A meta-analysis of studies on the safety and efficacy of aminoglycosides given either once daily or as divided doses. J Antimicrob Chemother 37:645–663
67. Barza M, Ioannidis JP, Cappelleri JC, Lau J (1996) Single or multiple daily doses of aminoglycosides: a meta-analysis. BMJ 312:338–345
68. Olsen KM, Rudis MI, Rebuck JA, Hara J, Gelmont D, Mehdian R, Nelson C, Rupp ME (2004) Effect of once-daily dosing vs. multiple daily dosing of tobramycin on enzyme markers of nephrotoxicity. Crit Care Med 32:1678–1682
69. Chambers HE, Sande MA (1996). In: Goodman and Gillman's The pharmacological basis of therapeutics. McGraw Hill, New York, 1103–1121
70. Leggett JE, Fantin B, Ebert S (1989) Comparative antibiotic dose-effect relations at several dosing intervals in murine pneumonitis and thigh-infection models. J Infect Dis 159:281–292
71. Schentag JJ, Smith IL, Swanson DJ, DeAngelis C, Fracasso JE, Vari A, Vance JW (1984) Role for dual individualization with cefmenoxime. Am J Med 77(6A):43–50
72. Bouvier d'Yvoire MJY, Maire PH (1996) Dosage regimens of antibacterials: implications of a pharmacokinetic/pharmacodynamic model. Clin Drug Invest 11:229–239
73. Chan GL (1989) Alternative dosing strategy for aminoglycosides: impact on efficacy, nephrotoxicity, and ototoxicity. DICP 23:788–794
74. Gilbert DN (1991) Once-daily aminoglycoside therapy. Antimicrob Agents Chemother 35:399–405
75. Marik PE, Havlik I, Monteagudo FS, Lipman J (1991) The pharmacokinetic of amikacin in critically ill adult and paediatric patients: comparison of once- versus twice-daily dosing regimens. J Antimicrob Chemother 27 Suppl C:81–89
76. Marik PE, Lipman J, Kobilski S, Scribante J (1991) A prospective randomized study comparing once- versus twice-daily amikacin dosing in critically ill adult and paediatric patients. J Antimicrob Chemother 28:753–764
77. Van der Auwera P, Meunier F, Ibrahim S, Kaufman L, Derde MP, Tulkens PM (1991) Pharmacodynamic parameters and toxicity of netilmicin (6 milligrams/kilogram/day) given once daily or in three divided doses to cancer patients with urinary tract infection. Antimicrob Agents Chemother 35:640–647
78. Prins JM, Buller HR, Kuijper EJ, Tange RA, Speelman P (1993) Once versus thrice daily gentamicin in patients with serious infections. Lancet 341:335–339
79. Mann HJ, Fuhs DW, Awang R, Ndemo FA, Cerra FB (1987) Altered aminoglycoside pharmacokinetics in critically ill patients with sepsis. Clin Pharm 6:148–153
80. Fuhs DW, Mann HJ, Kubajak CA, Cerra FB (1988) Intrapatient variation of aminoglycoside pharmacokinetics in critically ill surgery patients. Clin Pharm 7:207–213
81. Chelluri L, Jastremski MS (1987) Inadequacy of standard aminoglycoside loading doses in acutely ill patients. Crit Care Med 15:1143–1145
82. Chelluri L, Warren J, Jastremski MS (1989) Pharmacokinetics of a 3 mg/kg body weight loading dose of gentamicin or tobramycin in critically ill patients. Chest 95:1295–1297
83. Townsend PL, Fink MP, Stein KL, Murphy SG (1989) Aminoglycoside pharmacokinetics: dosage requirements and nephrotoxicity in trauma patients. Crit Care Med 17:154–157
84. Reed RL, 2nd, Wu AH, Miller-Crotchett P, Crotchett J, Fischer RP (1989) Pharmacokinetic monitoring of nephrotoxic antibiotics in surgical intensive care patients. J Trauma 29:1462–1468; discussion 1468–1470
85. Dasta JF, Armstrong DK (1988) Variability in aminoglycoside pharmacokinetics in critically ill surgical patients. Crit Care Med 16:327–330
86. Dager WE (1994) Aminoglycoside pharmacokinetics: volume of distribution in specific adult patient subgroups. Ann Pharmacother 28:944–951
87. Triginer C, Izquierdo I, Fernandez R, Rello J, Torrent J, Benito S, Net A (1990) Gentamicin volume of distribution in critically ill septic patients. Intensive Care Med 16:303–306
88. Zaske DE, Cipolle RJ, Strate RJ (1980) Gentamicin dosage requirements: wide interpatient variations in 242 surgery patients with normal renal function. Surgery 87:164–169
89. Beckhouse MJ, Whyte IM, Byth PL, Napier JC, Smith AJ (1988) Altered aminoglycoside pharmacokinetics in the critically ill. Anaesth Intensive Care 16:418–422
90. Buijk SE, Mouton JW, Gyssens IC, Verbrugh HA, Bruining HA (2002) Experience with a once-daily dosing program of aminoglycosides in critically ill patients. Intensive Care Med 28:936–942
91. Marik PE (1993) Aminoglycoside volume of distribution and illness severity in critically ill septic patients. Anaesth Intensive Care 21:172–173
92. Hatala R, Dinh TT, Cook DJ (1997) Single daily dosing of aminoglycosides in immunocompromised adults: A systematic review. Clin Infect Dis 24:810–815
93. Barclay ML, Begg EJ, Hickling KG (1994) What is the evidence for once-daily aminoglycoside therapy? Clin Pharmacokinet 27:32–48
94. Craig WA (1993) Post-antibiotic effects in experimental infection models: relationship to in-vitro phenomena and to treatment of infections in man. J Antimicrob Chemother 31 Suppl D:149–158
95. McDonald P, Wetherall B, Pruul H (1981) Postantibiotic leukocyte enhancement: Increased susceptibility of bacteria pretreated with antibiotics to activity of leukocytes. Rev Infect Dis 3:38–44
96. Burton ME, Brater DC, Chen PS, Day RB, Huber PJ, Vasko MR (1985) A Bayesian feedback method of aminoglycoside dosing. Clin Pharmacol Ther 37:349–357
97. Duffull SB, Kirkpatrick CM, Begg EJ (1997) Comparison of two Bayesian approaches to dose-individualization for once-daily aminoglycoside regimens. Br J Clin Pharmacol 43:125–135
98. Begg EJ, Barclay ML, Duffull SB (1995) A suggested ap-

proach to once-daily aminoglycoside dosing. Br J Clin Pharmacol 39:605–609

99. Nicolau DP, Freeman CD, Belliveau PP, Nightingale CH, Ross JW, Quintiliani R (1995) Experience with a once-daily aminoglycoside program administered to 2,184 adult patients. Antimicrob Agents Chemother 39:650–655
100. Kirkpatrick CM, Duffull SB, Begg EJ, Frampton C (2003) The use of a change in gentamicin clearance as an early predictor of gentamicin-induced nephrotoxicity. Ther Drug Monit 25:623–630
101. Kashuba ADM, Nafiziger AN, Drusano GL, Bertino JSJ (1999) Optimizing aminoglycoside therapy for nosocomial pneumonia caused by gram-negative bacteria. Antimicrob Agents Chemother 43:623–629
102. Stoeckel K (1981) Pharmacokinetics of Rocephin, a highly active new cephalosporin with an exceptionally long biological half-life. Chemotherapy 27 Suppl 1:42–46
103. Lipman J, Crewe-Brown HH, Saunders GL, Gous AG (1996) Subtleties of antibiotic dosages–do doses and intervals make a difference in the critically ill? S Afr J Surg 34:160–162
104. Lipman J, Wallis SC, Rickard C (1999) Low plasma cefepime levels in critically ill septic patients: pharmacokinetic modeling indicates improved troughs with revised dosing. Antimicrob Agents Chemother 43:2559–2561
105. Barbhaiya RH, Forgue ST, Gleason CR, Knupp CA, Pittman KA, Weidler DJ, Movahhed H, Tenney J, Martin RR (1992) Pharmacokinetics of cefepime after single and multiple intravenous administrations in healthy subjects. Antimicrob Agents Chemother 36:552–557
106. Lipman J, Wallis S, Boots R (2003) Cefepime versus cefpirome: the importance of creatinine clearance. Anesth Analg 97:1149–1154
107. McKindley DS, Boucher BA, Hess MM, Croce MA, Fabian TC (1996) Pharmacokinetics of aztreonam and imipenem in critically ill patients with pneumonia. Pharmacotherapy 16:924–931
108. Mouton JW, Vinks AA, Punt NC (1997) Pharmacokinetic-pharmacodynamic modeling of activity of ceftazidime during continuous and intermittent infusion. Antimicrob Agents Chemother 41:733–738
109. Fantin B, Farinotti R, Thabaut A, Carbon C (1994) Conditions for the emergence of resistance to cefpirome and ceftazidime in experimental endocarditis due to *Pseudomonas aeruginosa*. J Antimicrob Chemother 33:563–569
110. Turnidge JD (1998) The pharmacodynamics of beta-lactams. Clin Infect Dis 27:10–22
111. Tessier PR, Nicolau DP, Onyeji CO, Nightingale CH (1999) Pharmacodynamics of intermittent- and continuous-infusion cefepime alone and in combination with once-daily tobramycin against *Pseudomonas aeruginosa* in an in vitro infection model. Chemotherapy 45:284–295
112. Drusano GL (2004) Antimicrobial pharmacodynamics: critical interactions of 'bug and drug'. Nat Rev Microbiol 2:289–300
113. Bustamante CI, Drusano GL, Tatem BA, Standiford HC (1984) Postantibiotic effect of imipenem on *Pseudomonas aeruginosa*. Antimicrob Agents Chemother 26:678–682
114. Fantin B, Ebert S, Leggett J, Vogelman B, Craig WA (1991) Factors affecting duration of in-vivo postantibiotic effect for aminoglycosides against gram-negative bacilli. J Antimicrob Chemother 27:829–836
115. Tauber MG, Zak O, Scheld WM, Hengstler B, Sande MA (1984) The postantibiotic effect in the treatment of experimental meningitis caused by Streptococcus pneumoniae in rabbits. J Infect Dis 149:575–583
116. Angus BJ, Smith MD, Suputtamongkol Y, Mattie H, Walsh AL, Wuthiekanun V, Chaowagul W, White NJ (2000) Pharmacokinetic-pharmacodynamic evaluation of ceftazidime continuous infusion vs intermittent bolus injection in septicaemic melioidosis. Br J Clin Pharmacol 50:184–191
117. Mouton JW, den Hollander JG (1994) Killing of Pseudomonas aeruginosa during continuous and intermittent infusion of ceftazidime in an in vitro pharmacokinetic model. Antimicrob Agents Chemother 38:931–936
118. Young RJ, Lipman J, Gin T, Gomersall CD, Joynt GM, Oh TE (1997) Intermittent bolus dosing of ceftazidime in critically ill patients. J Antimicrob Chemother 40:269–273
119. Lipman J, Gomersall CD, Gin T, Joynt GM, Young RJ (1999) Continuous infusion ceftazidime in intensive care: a randomized controlled trial. J Antimicrob Chemother 43:309–311
120. MacGowan AP, Bowker KE (1998) Continuous infusion of beta-lactam antibiotics. Clin Pharmacokinet 35:391–402
121. Burgess DS, Hastings RW, Hardin TC (2000) Pharmacokinetics and pharmacodynamics of cefepime administered by intermittent and continuous infusion. Clin Ther 22:66–75
122. Tam VH, Louie A, Lomaestro BM, Drusano GL (2003) Integration of population pharmacokinetics, a pharmacodynamic target, and microbiologic surveillance data to generate a rational empiric dosing strategy for cefepime against *Pseudomonas aeruginosa*. Pharmacotherapy 23: 291–295
123. Boselli E, Breilh D, Duflo F, Saux MC, Debon R, Chassard D, Allaouchiche B (2003) Steady-state plasma and intrapulmonary concentrations of cefepime administered in continuous infusion in critically ill patients with severe nosocomial pneumonia. Crit Care Med 31:2102–2106
124. Jaruratanasirikul S, Sriwiriyajan S, Ingviya N (2002) Continuous infusion versus intermittent administration of cefepime in patients with Gram-negative bacilli bacteraemia. J Pharm Pharmacol 54:1693–1696
125. Georges B, Archambaud M, Saivin S, Decun JF, Cougot P, Mazerolles M, Andrieu P, Suc C, Houin G, Chabanon G, Virenque C (1999) Continuous versus intermittent cefepime infusion in critical care. [Preliminary results]. Pathol Biol (Paris) 47:483–485
126. Hanes SD, Wood GC, Herring V, Croce MA, Fabian TC, Pritchard E, Boucher BA (2000) Intermittent and continuous ceftazidime infusion for critically ill trauma patients. Am J Surg 179:436–440
127. Gomez CM, Cordingly JJ, Palazzo MG (1999) Altered pharmacokinetics of ceftazidime in critically ill patients. Antimicrob Agents Chemother 43:1798–1802
128. Joynt GM, Lipman J, Gomersall CD, Young RJ, Wong EL, Gin T (2001) The pharmacokinetics of once-daily dosing of ceftriaxone in critically ill patients. J Antimicrob Chemother 47:421–429
129. Roberts J, Boots R, Rickard C, Thomas P, Quinn J, Roberts D, Richards B, Lipman J. (2007) Is continuous infusion of ceftriaxone better than once a day dosing in intensive care? A randomised controlled pilot study. J Antimicrob Chemother (2006 Nov 28; [Epub ahead of print])
130. Fry DE (1996) The importance of antibiotic pharmacokinetics in critical illness. Am J Surg 172:20S-25S
131. Lorente L, Garcia C, Martin M, Mora M (2005) Continuous infusion versus intermitted infusion of ceftazidime for the treatment of pneumonia caused by *Pseudomonas aeruginosa*. In: 25th International Symposium on Intensive Care and Emergency Medicine. Brussels, Belgium: Critical Care, s16
132. Nicolau DP, McNabb J, Lacy MK, Quintiliani R, Nightingale CH (2001) Continuous versus intermittent adminis-

tration of ceftazidime in intensive care unit patients with nosocomial pneumonia. Int J Antimicrob Agents 17: 497–504
133. McNabb JJ, Nightingale CH, Quintiliani R, Nicolau DP (2001) Cost-effectiveness of ceftazidime by continuous infusion versus intermittent infusion for nosocomial pneumonia. Pharmacotherapy 21:549–555
134. Krueger WA, Lenhart FP, Neeser G, Ruckdeschel G, Schreckhase H, Eissner HJ, Forst H, Eckart J, Peter K, Unertl KE (2002) Influence of combined intravenous and topical antibiotic prophylaxis on the incidence of infections, organ dysfunctions, and mortality in critically ill surgical patients: a prospective, stratified, randomized, double-blind, placebo-controlled clinical trial. Am J Respir Crit Care Med 166:1029–1037
135. Georges B, Conil JM, Cougot P, Decun JF, Archambaud M, Seguin T, Chabanon G, Virenque C, Houin G, Saivin S (2005) Cefepime in critically ill patients: continuous infusion vs. an intermittent dosing regimen. Int J Clin Pharmacol Ther 43:360–369
136. Klepser ME, Patel KB, Nicolau DP, Quintiliani R, Nightingale CH (1998) Comparison of bactericidal activities of intermittent and continuous infusion dosing of vancomycin against methicillin-resistant *Staphylococcus aureus* and *Enterococcus faecalis*. Pharmacotherapy 18:1069–1074
137. Krueger WA, Bulitta J, Kinzig-Schippers M, Landersdorfer C, Holzgrabe U, Naber KG, Drusano GL, Sorgel F (2005) Evaluation by Monte Carlo simulation of the pharmacokinetics of two doses of meropenem administered intermittently or as a continuous infusion in healthy volunteers. Antimicrob Agents Chemother 49:1881–1889
138. Thalhammer F, Traunmuller F, El Menyawi I, Frass M, Hollenstein UM, Locker GJ, Stoiser B, Staudinger T, Thalhammer-Scherrer R, Burgmann H (1999) Continuous infusion versus intermittent administration of meropenem in critically ill patients. J Antimicrob Chemother 43:523–527
139. Roosendaal R, Bakker-Woudenberg IA, Van den Berghe JC, van Raafe M, Michel MF (1986) Continuous versus intermittent administration of ceftazidime in experimental *Klebsiella pneumoniae* pneumonia in normal and leukopenic rats. Antimicrob Agents Chemother 30:403–408
140. Mouton JW, Touzw DJ, Horrevorts AM, Vinks AA (2000) Comparative pharmacokinetics of the carbapenems: clinical implications. Clin Pharmacokinet 39:185–201
141. Barrons RW, Murray KM, Richey RM (1992) Populations at risk for penicillin-induced seizures. Ann Pharmacother 26:26–29
142. Day IP, Goudie J, Nishiki K, Williams PD (1995) Correlation between in vitro and in vivo models of proconvulsive activity with the carbapenem antibiotics, biapenem, imipenem/cilastatin and meropenem. Toxicol Lett 76:239–243
143. Laethem T, De Lepeleire I, McCrea J, Zhang J, Majumdar A, Musson D, Rogers D, Li S, Guillaume M, Parneix-Spake A, Deutsch P (2003) Tissue penetration by ertapenem, a parenteral carbapenem administered once daily, in suction-induced skin blister fluid in healthy young volunteers. Antimicrob Agents Chemother 47:1439–1442
144. Norrby SR, Newell PA, Faulkner KL, Lesky W (1995) Safety profile of meropenem: international clinical experience based on the first 3125 patients treated with meropenem. J Antimicrob Chemother 36 Suppl A:207–223
145. Naganuma H, Tokiwa H, Hirouch Y (1991) Nephroprotective effect and its mechanism of betamipron: I. Relationships of renal transport. Chemotherapy (Jpn) 39:166–177
146. Gibson TP, Demetriades JL, Bland JA (1985) Imipenem/cilastatin: pharmacokinetic profile in renal insufficiency. Am J Med 78:54–61
147. Leroy A, Fillastre JP, Etienne I, Borsa-Lebas F, Humbert G (1992) Pharmacokinetics of meropenem in subjects with renal insufficiency. Eur J Clin Pharmacol 42:535–538
148. Konishi K, Suzuki H, Saruta T, Hayashi M, Deguchi N, Tazaki H, Hisaka A (1991) Removal of imipenem and cilastatin by hemodialysis in patients with end-stage renal failure. Antimicrob Agents Chemother 35:1616–1620
149. Drusano GL (2003) Prevention of resistance: a goal for dose selection for antimicrobial agents. Clin Infect Dis 36:S42–50
150. Novelli A, Adembri C, Livi P, Fallani S, Mazzei T, De Gaudio AR (2005) Pharmacokinetic evaluation of meropenem and imipenem in critically ill patients with sepsis. Clin Pharmacokinet 44:539–549
151. Kitzes-Cohen R, Farin D, Piva G, De Myttenaere-Bursztein SA (2002) Pharmacokinetics and pharmacodynamics of meropenem in critically ill patients. Int J Antimicrob Agents 19:105–110
152. Jaruratanasirikul S, Sriwiriyajan S (2003) Stability of meropenem in normal saline solution after storage at room temperature. Southeast Asian J Trop Med Public Health 34:627–629
153. Viaene E, Chanteux H, Servais H, Mingeot-Leclercq MP, Tulkens PM (2002) Comparative stability studies of antipseudomonal beta-lactams for potential administration through portable elastomeric pumps (home therapy for cystic fibrosis patients) and motor-operated syringes (intensive care units). Antimicrob Agents Chemother 46: 2327–2332
154. Kuti JL, Nightingale CH, Knauft RF, Nicolau DP (2004) Pharmacokinetic Properties and Stability of continuous-Infusion Meropenem in Adults with Cystic Fibrosis. Current Therapeutics 26:493–501
155. Jaruratanasirikul S, Sriwiriyajan S, Punyo J (2005) Comparison of the pharmacodynamics of meropenem in patients with ventilator-associated pneumonia following administration by 3-hour infusion or bolus injection. Antimicrob Agents Chemother 49:1337–1339
156. Lorente L, Huidobro S, Martín M, Mora M (2005) Meropenem administration by intermittent infusion versus continuous infusion for the treatment of nosocomial pneumonia. Crit Care 9:P38
157. Kotapati S, Nicolau DP, Nightingale CH, Kuti JL (2004) Clinical and economic benefits of a meropenem dosage strategy based on pharmacodynamic concepts. Am J Health Syst Pharm 61:1264–1270
158. Craig WA, Ebert SC (1992) Continuous infusion of beta-lactam antibiotics. Antimicrob Agents Chemother 36: 2577–2583
159. Kuti JL, Capitano B, Nicolau DP (2002) Cost-effective approaches to the treatment of community-acquired pneumonia in the era of resistance. Pharmacoeconomics 20: 513–528
160. Keil S, Wiedemann B (1997) Antimicrobial effects of continuous versus intermittent administration of carbapenem antibiotics in an in vitro dynamic model. Antimicrob Agents Chemother 41:1215–1219
161. Elting LS, Rubenstein EB, Kurtin D, Rolston KV, Fangtang J, Martin CG, Raad, II, Whimbey EE, Manzullo E, Bodey GP (1998) Mississippi mud in the 1990 s: risks and outcomes of vancomycin-associated toxicity in general oncology practice. Cancer 83:2597–2607
162. Riley HD, Jr. (1970) Vancomycin and novobiocin. Med Clin North Am 54:1277–1289
163. Cunha BA (1995) Vancomycin. Med Clin North Am 79:817–831

164. Fernandez de Gatta MD, Calvo MV, Hernandez JM, Caballero D, San Miguel JF, Dominguez-Gil A (1996) Cost-effectiveness analysis of serum vancomycin concentration monitoring in patients with hematologic malignancies. Clin Pharmacol Ther 60:332–340
165. Brogden RN, Peters DH (1994) Teicoplanin. A reappraisal of its antimicrobial activity, pharmacokinetic properties and therapeutic efficacy. Drugs 47:823–854
166. Barbot A, Venisse N, Rayeh F, Bouquet S, Debaene B, Mimoz O (2003) Pharmacokinetics and pharmacodynamics of sequential intravenous and subcutaneous teicoplanin in critically ill patients without vasopressors. Intensive Care Med 29:1528–1534
167. Wilson AP (2000) Clinical pharmacokinetics of teicoplanin. Clin Pharmacokinet 39:167–183
168. Larsson AJ, Walker KJ, Raddatz JK, Rotschafer JC (1996) The concentration-independent effect of monoexponential and biexponential decay in vancomycin concentrations on the killing of *Staphylococcus aureus* under aerobic and anaerobic conditions. J Antimicrob Chemother 38:589–597
169. Saunders NJ (1994) Why monitor peak vancomycin concentrations? Lancet 344:1748–1750
170. Lowdin E, Odenholt I, Cars O (1998) In vitro studies of pharmacodynamic properties of vancomycin against *Staphylococcus aureus* and *Staphylococcus epidermidis*. Antimicrob Agents Chemother 42:2739–2744
171. Chambers HF, Kennedy S (1990) Effects of dosage, peak and trough concentrations in serum, protein binding, and bacterial rate on efficacy of teicoplanin in a rabbit model of endocarditis. Antimicrob Agents Chemother 47:2018–2021
172. Duffull SB, Begg EJ, Chambers ST, Barclay ML (1994) Efficacies of different vancomycin dosing regimens against *Staphylococcus aureus* determined with a dynamic in vitro model. Antimicrob Agents Chemother 38:2480–2482.
173. Knudsen JD, Fuursted K, Raber S, Espersen F, Frimodt-Moller N (2000) Pharmacodynamics of glycopeptides in the mouse peritonitis model of *Streptococcus pneumoniae* or *Staphylococcus aureus* infection. Antimicrob Agents Chemother 44:1247–1254
174. Rybak MJ (2006) The pharmacokinetic and pharmacodynamic properties of vancomycin. Clin Infect Dis 42 Suppl 1:S35–39
175. Wysocki M, Delatour F, Faurisson F, Rauss A, Pean Y, Misset B, Thomas F, Timsit JF, Similowski T, Mentec H, Mier L, Dreyfuss D (2001) Continuous versus intermittent infusion of vancomycin in severe Staphylococcal infections: prospective multicenter randomized study. Antimicrob Agents Chemother 45:2460–2467
176. Rello J, Sole-Violan J, Sa-Borges M, Garnacho-Montero J, Munoz E, Sirgo G, Olona M, Diaz E (2005) Pneumonia caused by oxacillin-resistant *Staphylococcus aureus* treated with glycopeptides. Crit Care Med 33:1983–1987
177. Gous AG, Dance MD, Lipman J, Luyt DK, Mathivha R, Scribante J (1995) Changes in vancomycin pharmacokinetics in critically ill infants. Anaesth Intensive Care 23:678–682
178. Matzke GR, McGory RW, Halstenson CE, Keane WF (1984) Pharmacokinetics of vancomycin in patients with various degrees of renal function. Antimicrob Agents Chemother 25:433–437
179. MacGowan AP (1998) Pharmacodynamics, pharmacokinetics, and therapeutic drug monitoring of glycopeptides. Ther Drug Monit 20:473–477
180. James JK, Palmer SM, Levine DP, Rybak MJ (1996) Comparison of conventional dosing versus continuous-infusion vancomycin therapy for patients with suspected or documented gram-positive infections. Antimicrob Agents Chemother 40:696–700
181. Bodi M, Ardanuy C, Olona M, Castander D, Diaz E, Rello J (2001) Therapy of ventilator-associated pneumonia: the Tarragona strategy. Clin Microbiol Infect 7:32–33
182. Cruciani M, Gatti G, Lazzarini L, Furlan G, Broccali G, Malena M, Franchini C, Concia E (1996) Penetration of vancomycin into human lung tissue. J Antimicrob Chemother 38:865–869
183. Lipman J (2005) Is the end-game penetration (of the airway)? Crit Care Med 33:1654–1655
184. Turnidge J (1999) Fusidic acid pharmacology, pharmacokinetics and pharmacodynamics. Int J Antimicrob Agents 12 Suppl 2:S23–34
185. Conte JE, Golden JA, Kipps J, Zurlinden E (2002) Intrapulmonary pharmacokinetics of linezolid. Antimicrob Agents Chemother 26:1475–1480
186. Peterson LR (2005) Antimicrobial activity and pharmacokinetics/pharmacodynamics of the novel glycylcycline, tigecycline. Diagn Microbiol Infect Dis 52:163–164
187. Reyes N, Skinner R, Kaniga K, Krause KM, Shelton J, Obedencio GP, Gough A, Conner M, Hegde SS (2005) Efficacy of telavancin (TD-6424), a rapidly bactericidal lipoglycopeptide with multiple mechanisms of action, in a murine model of pneumonia induced by methicillin-resistant *Staphylococcus aureus*. Antimicrob Agents Chemother 49:4344–4346
188. Smith RP, Baltch AL, Franke MA, Michelsen PB, Bopp LH (2000) Levofloxacin penetrates human monocytes and enhances intracellular killing of *Staphylococcus aureus* and *Pseudomonas aeruginosa*. J Antimicrob Chemother 45:483–488
189. Preston SL, Drusano GL, Berman AL (1998) Pharmacodynamics of levofloxacin: a new paradigm for early clinical trials. JAMA 279:125–129
190. Piddock LJ, Dalhoff A (1993) Should quinolones be used in the treatment of bacterial infections in neutropenic patients? J Antimicrob Chemother 32:771–774
191. Nix DE, Spivey JM, Norman A, Schentag JJ (1992) Dose-ranging pharmacokinetic study of ciprofloxacin after 200-, 300-, and 400-mg intravenous doses. Ann Pharmacother 26:8–10
192. Goss TF, Forrest A, Nix DE, Ballow CH, Birmingham MC, Cumbo TJ, Schentag JJ (1994) Mathematical examination of dual individualization principles (II): The rate of bacterial eradication at the same area under the inhibitory curve is more rapid for ciprofloxacin than for cefmenoxime. Ann Pharmacother 28:863–868
193. Zhou J, Dong Y, Zhao X, Lee S, Amin A, Ramaswamy S, Domagala J, Musser JM, Drlica K (2000) Selection of antibiotic-resistant bacterial mutants: allelic diversity among fluoroquinolone-resistant mutations. J Infect Dis 182:517–525
194. MacGowan A, Rogers C, Bowker K (2000) The use of in vitro pharmacodynamic models of infection to optimize fluoroquinolone dosing regimens. J Antimicrob Chemother 46:163–170
195. Hyatt JM, Schentag JJ (2000) Pharmacodynamic modeling of risk factors for ciprofloxacin resistance in *Pseudomonas aeruginosa*. Infect Control Hosp Epidemiol 21: S9–11
196. Thomas JK, Forrest A, Bhavnani SM, Hyatt JM, Cheng A, Ballow CH, Schentag JJ (1998) Pharmaco-dynamic evaluation of factors associated with the development of bacterial resistance in acutely ill patients during therapy. Antimicrob Agents Chemother 42:521–527
197. Schentag JJ (1999) Antimicrobial action and pharmacokinetics/pharmacodynamics: the use of AUIC to improve efficacy and avoid resistance. J Chemother 11:426–439

198. Lipman J, Scribante J, Gous AG, Hon H, Tshukutsoane S (1998) Pharmacokinetic profiles of high-dose intravenous ciprofloxacin in severe sepsis. The Baragwanath Ciprofloxacin Study Group. Antimicrob Agents Chemother 42:2235–2239
199. Gous A, Lipman J, Scribante J, Tshukutsoane S, Hon H, Pinder M, Mathivha R, Verhoef L, Stass H (2005) Fluid shifts have no influence on ciprofloxacin pharmacokinetics in intensive care patients with intra-abdominal sepsis. Int J Antimicrob Agents 26:50–55
200. Sun HK, Kuti JL, Nicolau DP (2005) Pharmacodynamics of antimicrobials for the empirical treatment of nosocomial pneumonia: a report from the OPTAMA Program. Crit Care Med 33:2222–2227
201. Graninger W, Zeitlinger M (2004) Clinical applications of levofloxacin for severe infections. Chemotherapy 50 Suppl 1:16–21
202. Viale P, Pea F (2003) What is the role of fluoroquinolones in intensive care? J Chemother 15 Suppl 3:5–10
203. MIMS Australia (2005) Ciproxin(R) Product Information. In: E Donohoo (ed) MIMS Online. CMP Medica Australia Pty Ltd, St Leonards, NSW
204. Hoffken G, Lode H, Prinzing C, Borner K, Koeppe P (1985) Pharmacokinetics of ciprofloxacin after oral and parenteral administration. Antimicrob Agents Chemother 27:375–379
205. Jones EM (1997) The pharmacokinetics of intravenous ciprofloxacin 400 mg 12 hourly in patients with severe sepsis: the effect of renal function and intra-abdominal disease. J Antimicrob Chemother 40:121–124
206. Meagher AK, Ambrose PG, Grasela TH, Ellis-Grosse EJ (2005) Pharmacokinetic/pharmacodynamic profile for tigecycline-a new glycylcycline antimicrobial agent. Diagn Microbiol Infect Dis 52:165–171
207. Muralidharan G, Micalizzi M, Speth J, Raible D, Troy S (2005) Pharmacokinetics of tigecycline after single and multiple doses in healthy subjects. Antimicrob Agents Chemother 49:220–229
208. Petersen PJ, Jacobus NV, Weiss WJ, Sum PE, Testa RT (1999) In vitro and in vivo antibacterial activities of a novel glycylcycline, the 9-t-butylglycylamido derivative of minocycline (GAR-936). Antimicrob Agents Chemother 43:738–744
209. Meagher AK, Ambrose PG, Grasela TH, Ellis-Grosse EJ (2005) The pharmacokinetic and pharmacodynamic profile of tigecycline. Clin Infect Dis 41 Suppl 5:S333–340
210. Postier RG, Green SL, Klein SR, Ellis-Grosse EJ, Loh E (2004) Results of a multicenter, randomized, open-label efficacy and safety study of two doses of tigecycline for complicated skin and skin-structure infections in hospitalized patients. Clin Ther 26:704–714
211. Muller-Serieys C, Andrews J, Vacheron F, Cantalloube C (2004) Tissue kinetics of telithromycin, the first ketolide antibacterial. J Antimicrob Chemother 53:149–157
212. Namour F, Sultan E, Pascual MH, Lenfant B (2002) Penetration of telithromycin (HMR 3647), a new ketolide antimicrobial, into inflammatory blister fluid following oral administration. J Antimicrob Chemother 49:1035–1038
213. Kasbekar N, Acharya PS (2005) Telithromycin: the first ketolide for the treatment of respiratory infections. Am J Health Syst Pharm 62:905–916
214. Gattringer R, Urbauer E, Traunmuller F, Zeitlinger M, Dehghanyar P, Zeleny P, Graninger W, Muller M, Joukhadar C (2004) Pharmacokinetics of telithromycin in plasma and soft tissues after single-dose administration to healthy volunteers. Antimicrob Agents Chemother 48: 4650–4653
215. Odenholt I, Lowdin E, Cars O (2001) Pharmacodynamics of telithromycin In vitro against respiratory tract pathogens. Antimicrob Agents Chemother 45:23–29
216. Jacobs MR, Bajaksouzian S, Appelbaum PC (2003) Telithromycin post-antibiotic and post-antibiotic sub-MIC effects for 10 Gram-positive cocci. J Antimicrob Chemother 52:809–812
217. Shi J, Montay G, Chapel S, Hardy P, Barrett JS, Sack M, Marbury T, Swan SK, Vargas R, Leclerc V, Leroy B, Bhargava VO (2004) Pharmacokinetics and safety of the ketolide telithromycin in patients with renal impairment. J Clin Pharmacol 44:234–244
218. Tally FP, Zeckel M, Wasilewski MM, Carini C, Berman CL, Drusano GL, Oleson FB, Jr. (1999) Daptomycin: a novel agent for Gram-positive infections. Expert Opin Investig Drugs 8:1223–1238
219. Safdar N, Andes D, Craig WA (2004) In vivo pharmacodynamic activity of daptomycin. Antimicrob Agents Chemother 48:63–68
220. Pankuch GA, Jacobs MR, Appelbaum PC (2003) Postantibiotic effects of daptomycin against 14 staphylococcal and pneumococcal clinical isolates. Antimicrob Agents Chemother 47:3012–3014
221. Wise R, Gee T, Andrews JM, Dvorchik B, Marshall G (2002) Pharmacokinetics and inflammatory fluid penetration of intravenous daptomycin in volunteers. Antimicrob Agents Chemother 46:31–33
222. Schriever CA, Fernandez C, Rodvold KA, Danziger LH (2005) Daptomycin: a novel cyclic lipopeptide antimicrobial. Am J Health Syst Pharm 62:1145–1158
223. Andrew JH, Wale MC, Wale LJ, Greenwood D (1987) The effect of cultural conditions on the activity of LY146032 against staphylococci and streptococci. J Antimicrob Chemother 20:213–221
224. MIMS Australia (2005) Synercid IV (R), Product Information. In: E Donohoo (ed) MIMS Online. CMP Medica Australia Pty Ltd, St Leonards, NSW
225. Aeschlimann JR, Rybak MJ (1998) Pharmacodynamic analysis of the activity of quinupristin-dalfopristin against vancomycin-resistant *Enterococcus faecium* with differing MBCs via time-kill-curve and postantibiotic effect methods. Antimicrob Agents Chemother 42:2188–2192
226. Craig WA (2001) Does the dose matter? Clin Infect Dis 33 Suppl 3:S233–237
227. De Gaudio AR, Di Filippo A (2003) What is the role of streptogramins in intensive care? J Chemother 15 Suppl 3:17–21
228. Fass RJ, Saslaw S (1972) Clindamycin: clinical and laboratory evaluation of parenteral therapy. Am J Med Sci 263:368–382
229. Nagar H, Berger SA, Hammar B, Gorea A (1989) Penetration of clindamycin and metronidazole into the appendix and peritoneal fluid in children. Eur J Clin Pharmacol 37:209–210
230. Mueller SC, Henkel KO, Neumann J, Hehl EM, Gundlach KK, Drewelow B (1999) Perioperative antibiotic prophylaxis in maxillofacial surgery: penetration of clindamycin into various tissues. J Craniomaxillofac Surg 27:172–176
231. Avant GR, Schenker S, Alford RH (1975) The effect of cirrhosis on the disposition and elimination of clindamycin. Am J Dig Dis 20:223–230
232. Gwilt PR, Smith RB (1986) Protein binding and pharmacokinetics of lincomycin following intravenous administration of high doses. J Clin Pharmacol 26:87–90
233. Bellamy HM Jr, Bates BB, Reinarz JA (1967) Lincomycin metabolism in patients with hepatic insufficiency: effect of liver disease on lincomycin serum concentrations. Antimicrob Agents Chemother 7:36–41

234. Stalker DJ, Jungbluth GL, Hopkins NK, Batts DH (2003) Pharmacokinetics and tolerance of single- and multiple-dose oral or intravenous linezolid, an oxazolidinone antibiotic, in healthy volunteers. J Antimicrob Chemother 51:1239–1246
235. MacGowan AP (2003) Pharmacokinetic and pharmacodynamic profile of linezolid in healthy volunteers and patients with Gram-positive infections. J Antimicrob Chemother 51 Suppl 2:ii17–25
236. Boselli E, Breilh D, Rimmele T, Djabarouti S, Toutain J, Chassard D, Saux MC, Allaouchiche B (2005) Pharmacokinetics and intrapulmonary concentrations of linezolid administered to critically ill patients with ventilator-associated pneumonia. Crit Care Med 33:1529–1533
237. Brier ME, Stalker DJ, Aronoff GR, Batts DH, Ryan KK, O'Grady M, Hopkins NK, Jungbluth GL (2003) Pharmacokinetics of linezolid in subjects with renal dysfunction. Antimicrob Agents Chemother 47:2775–2780
238. Andes D, van Ogtrop ML, Craig W (1998) Pharmacodynamic activity of a new oxazolidinone linezolid in an animal infection model. In: 38th Interscience Conference on Antimicrobial Agents and Chemotherapy. San Diego, CA: American Society for Microbiology, 3
239. Gentry-Nielsen MJ, Olsen KM, Preheim LC (2002) Pharmacodynamic activity and efficacy of linezolid in a rat model of pneumococcal pneumonia. Antimicrob Agents Chemother 46:1345–1351
240. Andes D, van Ogtrop ML, Peng J, Craig WA (2002) In vivo pharmacodynamics of a new oxazolidinone (linezolid). Antimicrob Agents Chemother 46:3484–3489
241. Azie NE, Stalker DJ, Jungbluth GL, Sisson T, Adams G (2000) Effect of linezolid on CYP2C9 using racemic warfarin as a probe. Abstract PI-81. Clinical Pharmacology and Therapeutics 69:P21
242. French G (2003) Safety and tolerability of linezolid. J Antimicrob Chemother 51 Suppl 2:ii45–53
243. Gerson SL, Kaplan SL, Bruss JB, Le V, Arellano FM, Hafkin B, Kuter DJ (2002) Hematologic effects of linezolid: summary of clinical experience. Antimicrob Agents Chemother 46:2723–2726
244. Bartlett JG, Dowell SF, Mandell LA, File Jr TM, Musher DM, Fine MJ (2000) Practice guidelines for the management of community-acquired pneumonia in adults. Infectious Diseases Society of America. Clin Infect Dis 31:347–382
245. Singh N, Rogers P, Atwood CW, Wagener MM, Yu VL (2000) Short-course empiric antibiotic therapy for patients with pulmonary infiltrates in the intensive care unit. A proposed solution for indiscriminate antibiotic prescription. Am J Respir Crit Care Med 162:505–511
246. Chastre J, Wolff M, Fagon JY, Chevret S, Thomas F, Wermert D, Clementi E, Gonzalez J, Jusserand D, Asfar P, Perrin D, Fieux F, Aubas S (2003) Comparison of 8 vs 15 days of antibiotic therapy for ventilator-associated pneumonia in adults: a randomized trial. JAMA 290:2588–2598
247. Dennesen PJ, van der Ven AJ, Kessels AG, Ramsay G, Bonten MJ (2001) Resolution of infectious parameters after antimicrobial therapy in patients with ventilator-associated pneumonia. Am J Respir Crit Care Med 163:1371–1375
248. Dellinger RP, Carlet JM, Masur H, Gerlach H, Calandra T, Cohen J, Gea-Banacloche J, Keh D, Marshall JC, Parker MM, Ramsay G, Zimmerman JL, Vincent JL, Levy MM (2004) Surviving Sepsis Campaign guidelines for management of severe sepsis and septic shock. Crit Care Med 32:858–873
249. Pharmacia Australia (2005) Product Information: Gentamicin Injection BP (R), gentamicin sulphate. In. Rydalmere NSW,
250. Mangione A, Schentag JJ (1980) Therapeutic monitoring of aminoglycoside antibiotics: an approach. Ther Drug Monit 2:159–167
251. Levitt DG (2003) The pharmacokinetics of the interstitial space in humans. BMC Clinical Pharmacology 3:3–32
252. Swabb EA, Singhvi SM, Leitz MA, Frantz M, Sugerman A (1983) Metabolism and pharmacokinetics of aztreonam in healthy subjects. Antimicrob Agents Chemother 24: 394–400
253. Rubinstein E, Vaughan D (2005) Tigecycline: a novel glycylcycline. Drugs 65:1317–1336
254. Bernard E, Bensoussan M, Bensoussan F, Etienne S, Cazenave I, Carsenti-Etesse E, Le Roux Y, Montay G, Dellamonica P (1994) Pharmacokinetics and suction blister fluid penetration of a semisynthetic injectable streptogramin. Eur J Clin Microbiol Infect Dis 13:768–771
255. Chant C, Rybak MJ (1995) Quinupristin/dalfopristin (RP 59500): a new streptogramin antibiotic. Ann Pharmacother 29:1022–1027
256. Dvorchik B, Sica D, Gehr T (2002) Pharmacokinetics and safety of single-dose daptomycin in subjects with graded renal insufficiency and end-stage renal disease. In: Interscience Conference on Antimicrobial Agents and Chemotherapy. San Diego
257. Dvorchik BH, Brazier D, DeBruin MF, Arbeit RD (2003) Daptomycin pharmacokinetics and safety following administration of escalating doses once daily to healthy subjects. Antimicrob Agents Chemother 47:1318–1323
258. Woodworth JR, Nyhart EH, Jr., Brier GL, Wolny JD, Black HR (1992) Single-dose pharmacokinetics and antibacterial activity of daptomycin, a new lipopeptide antibiotic, in healthy volunteers. Antimicrob Agents Chemother 36:318–325
259. Nguyen M, Chung EP (2005) Telithromycin: The first ketolide antimicrobial. Clin Ther 27:1144–1163
260. DeHaan RM, Metzler CM, Schellenberg D, Vandenbosch WD (1973) Pharmacokinetic studies of clindamycin phosphate. J Clin Pharmacol 13:190–209
261. Gordon RC, Regamey C, Kirby WM (1973) Serum protein binding of erythromycin, lincomycin, and clindamycin. J Pharm Sci 62:1074–1077
262. Mann HJ, Townsend RJ, Fuhs DW, Cerra FB (1987) Decreased hepatic clearance of clindamycin in critically ill patients with sepsis. Clin Pharm 6:154–159
263. Rovers JP, Ilersich AL, Einarson TR (1995) Meta-analysis of parenteral clindamycin dosing regimens. Ann Pharmacother 29:852–858
264. MICROMEDEX T (1974–2005) Micromedex Healthcare Series. In: DRUGDEX Evaluations. Thomson Micromedex, Greenwood Village, Colorado
265. Bennett WM, Aronoff GR, Golper TA, et al. (1994) Drug prescribing in renal failure. American College of Physicians, Philadelphia
266. Brittain DC, Scully BE, McElrath MJ, Steinman R, Labthavikul P, Neu HC (1985) The pharmacology of orally administered ciprofloxacin. Drugs Exp Clin Res 11:339–341
267. Chien SC, Wong FA, Fowler CL, Callery-D'Amico SV, Williams RR, Nayak R, Chow AT (1998) Double-blind evaluation of the safety and pharmacokinetics of multiple oral once-daily 750-milligram and 1-gram doses of levofloxacin in healthy volunteers. Antimicrob Agents Chemother 42:885–888
268. Chien SC, Chow AT, Natarajan J, Williams RR, Wong FA, Rogge MC, Nayak RK (1997) Absence of age and gender effects on the pharmacokinetics of a single 500-milligram oral dose of levofloxacin in healthy subjects. Antimicrob Agents Chemother 41:1562–1565

269. Stass H (1999) Distribution and Tissue Penetration of Moxifloxacin. Drugs 58:229–230
270. Stass H, Dalhoff A, Kubitza D, Schuhly U (1998) Pharmacokinetics, safety, and tolerability of ascending single doses of moxifloxacin, a new 8-methoxy quinolone, administered to healthy subjects. Antimicrob Agents Chemother 42:2060–2065
271. Nakashima M, Uematsu T, Kosuge K, Kusajima H, Ooie T, Masuda Y, Ishida R, Uchida H (1995) Single- and multiple-dose pharmacokinetics of AM-1155, a new 6-fluoro-8-methoxy quinolone, in humans. Antimicrob Agents Chemother 39:2635–2640

Prescription of Antimicrobial Agents in Patients Undergoing Continuous Renal Replacement Therapy

R. Freebairn, J. Cohen, J. Lipman

13.1 Introduction

The prescription of antibiotics to critically ill patients is an extremely common intervention. Early and appropriate antimicrobial administration has been repeatedly shown to improve mortality in septic patients [1–7]. However, whilst the choice of drug class will normally be influenced by numerous factors such as the likely organism, the current unit flora, and the patient's co-morbidities, the dose prescribed will usually be a standard one, perhaps modified by an estimated glomerular filtration rate (GFR) or a suggested "dialysis dose". Yet, in the critically ill, a host of factors may influence the therapeutic level of prescribed antibiotics. These include increased volumes of distribution, changes in protein binding and increased extrarenal and renal losses all of which may contribute to lower than predicted drug levels when the usual patient dosage regimens are used [8]. The problem becomes more complex when renal failure supervenes. The addition of renal replacement therapy, restoration of renal function during recovery and alterations in volume of distribution may all lead to lowered tissue levels of antibiotics, with the potential to increase morbidity and mortality through inadequate antibiotic activity [9, 10]. Whilst pharmacokinetic and pharmacodynamic principles of antibiotic dosing are receiving increased interest [11], the recent widespread uptake of renal replacement therapies in the ICU has exposed a hole in our knowledge of the correct dosage adjustments to make when employing such strategies.

Altered dosing regimes are necessary when patients with renal failure require antibiotic therapy. There is a plethora of guidelines describing dosage adjustment in the presence of chronic renal impairment including whilst on dialysis. However, most of these refer to intermittent or peritoneal dialysis. While these serve as immediately accessible guides, the application of these to the critically ill with acute renal failure undergoing continuous or frequent intermittent renal replacement techniques may be hazardous.

There are a multiplicity of renal replacement techniques and daily dialysis "doses" with little consensus on appropriate dose, optimal techniques or even definitions [12, 13]. ICU patients need distinct and data-based dosages taking into account specific co-morbidities and current treatment regimens [14]. Dosages based on cookbook formulae for "dialysis" are often "a pure gamble" [15].

Whenever practicable, antibiotic dosing regimens should be monitored by analysis of serum drug levels. This is particularly relevant in renal failure and in the critically ill, where elevated levels may precipitate worsening renal clearance, further increasing the antibiotics toxicity. Underdosage may result in resistance developing [16]. Knowledge of serum antibiotic levels provides evidence that therapeutically useful levels are attained and that the safety profile of the drug is maintained. These parameters differ between different antibiotic classes. Unfortunately, apart from a very few antibiotics with a toxic profile, antibiotic assays are not routinely available outside of research facilities.

Whereas aminoglycoside and glycopeptide dosage intervals are greatly simplified by routine monitoring of concentrations, other antibiotics are not measured, and toxic levels may only be apparent with the onset of a complication such as seizures. Guidance to doses and dosing intervals is well established in chronic renal failure; however, occasionally with very severe infections, such as endocarditis and meningococcal septicaemia treated with penicillin, the narrow line between ensuring effectiveness and toxicity is best managed by introducing synergy with a second antibiotic.

13.1.1 Indications for Renal Replacement Therapy

Discussion of the indications for renal replacement therapy (RRT) and continuous RRT (CRRT) are beyond the scope of this chapter. While current recommendations include fluid overload, hyperkalaemia, severe acidosis, and uraemic pericardial effusions in the presence of acute renal failure, irrespective of indication, optimal timing of initiation of CRRT remains controversial [17, 18].

13.2 Definitions

13.2.1 Acute Renal Failure

There are multiple definitions and limited consensus on the nomenclature of acute renal failure [13]. A pragmatic approach provided by Bellomo et al. utilises a classification scheme based upon GFR and urine output [13]. Antibiotic dosage requirements fall if renal clearance declines. The addition of CRRT has a variable influence on clearance, which is dependent upon the antibiotic type, patient comorbidity, and the actual technique used.

13.2.2 Renal Replacement Therapy

The ambiguity surrounding the type and style of RRT in part arises from evolution of techniques. It is only recently that the dedicated propriety CRRT machines have become commonplace in intensive care units. Prior to this many hybrid techniques had been devised, adopted either during transition from arteriovenous systems, the modification of intermittent dialysis techniques, or the fusion of both [12, 17, 19, 20]. The multiple systems deliver different doses of dialysis and filtration through a variety of filter membranes [21]. The applicability of pharmacokinetic data collected using one system to another was unknown, and marked differences in clearances have occurred when CRRT parameters have been altered [20]. The uniformity of propriety machines and filters has reduced the chaos, but the additional hybrid techniques such as slow low-efficiency daily dialysis (SLEDD) introduces yet another set of variables [20, 22]. Standardized nomenclature using total daily dialysis dose and total daily filtration dose may reduce ambiguity [13, 23, 24]. To be useful in guiding antibiotic prescribing, descriptions in the presence of RRT need to include details of all these variables.

13.3 Fundamental Antibiotic Pharmacokinetics

13.3.1 Volume of Distribution

The volume of distribution (Vd) is the apparent volume into which a drug distributes. Volume of distribution does not relate to an anatomical volume, as is demonstrated by metronidazole and ciprofloxacin having volumes of distribution of greater than 1 litre per kilogram of body weight. This means these drugs distribute much more widely than plasma volume.

Drugs with a high volume of distribution require less frequent dosing, even in the presence of a high clearance. With high clearances, although the drug is completely cleared from that volume of plasma, a large volume of distribution means that the subsequent fall in concentration is small. Therefore the dose of drug required to replace the cleared antibiotic is small and replacement doses need not be as given frequently. Renal replacement therapy has a less marked effect upon kinetics in this class of drug.

Volumes of distributions in critically ill patients vary from those of healthy volunteers [25, 26]. These changes are unpredictable, and alter over time in relation to deteriorations and improvements in patients' condition and in response to other medications being administered [25, 27–29]. In sepsis, and burns, for example, Vd is usually increased, which has implications for antimicrobial dosing regimes [26, 30]. Normal loading antibiotic doses may require augmentation, while in renal failure subsequent doses are given less frequently. An increased Vd due to critical illness and fluid overload at the onset of oliguria, however, would dictate that the normal loading antibiotic doses should at least remain unchanged if not increased, while subsequent doses are given less frequently.

13.3.2 Half-life

Half-life ($t_{1/2}$) is the time required to change the amount of drug in the blood by one-half during its (the drugs') elimination. Recommendations on suitable antibiotic dosage intervals during RRT or acute renal failure are based on estimations of the half-life ($t_{1/2}$). Half-life, clearance and volume of distribution are mathematically coupled, such that increases in the volume of distribution with a constant clearance will result in a longer half-life of the antibiotic. Changes during acute and recovery phases of illness alter antibiotic volume of distribution [10]. In addition to interpatient variability, titration of other treatments over time, such as weaning haemodynamic support, may influence antibiotic pharmacokinetics [31, 32].

13.3.3 Clearance

Total clearance while receiving RRT is the sum of clearance by RRT system, residual renal clearances and nonrenal clearance (such as metabolism by liver or loss through biliary excretion). Clearance in renal failure even whilst on RRT is likely to be less than normal healthy kidneys and thus $t_{1/2}$ will be prolonged. Therefore dosage intervals more often need to be increased in patients who are RRT dependent. However, implementation of RRT for indications other than oliguric renal failure may result in higher than expected clearances. Drugs that are rapidly cleared by CRRT may need to be increased [8].

Typically levofloxacin, aminoglycosides, glycopeptides, most of the beta-lactams and fluconazole have prolonged $t_{1/2}$ on RRT and need prolonged dosage intervals, whereas ceftriaxone, clindamycin, macrolides, metronidazole, itraconazole, amphotericin B, acyclovir, rifampicin and ciprofloxacin have substantial non-renal clearances and $t_{1/2}$ during RRT is only marginally increased. As previously mentioned the proportion of non-renal clearances may increase in the presence of renal failure.

The volume of blood/serum/ plasma cleared by the renal replacement per hour is the sum of the product of the filtration rate and the sieving coefficient, and the product of the dialysis rate and the saturation coefficient. An additional amount may be also be cleared by absorption on to the membrane.

Total body clearance per day is the sum of the clearance by continuous RRT filtration, absorption and dialysis clearance per day and the total daily renal and non-renal clearance of the drug. Time off dialysis will obviously decrease daily clearances.

13.3.4 The Sieving Coefficient

The sieving coefficient describes the fraction of drug eliminated from the plasma into the filtrate. The calculation of sieving coefficient is made by dividing the filtration drug concentration by the plasma concentration using samples taken simultaneously during elimination phase. A sieving coefficient of 1 represents unfettered passage of drug from the blood to the filtrate, with no retention by the filtering process.

The degree of protein binding inversely affects the sieving coefficient. Some antibiotics are highly protein bound and hence have a very low sieving coefficient.

For many antibacterials this reduction is not a significant issue, but some, such as ceftriaxone and dicloxacillin, are highly bound to albumin, while others are highly bound to other proteins, such as clindamycin to alpha-1-acid glycoprotein. Not only are free concentrations diminished but also such drugs are retained by the protein and thus not easily eliminated by renal replacement techniques. With these antibiotics the recommended regimes for use in anuric patients may be appropriate, with no adjustment in dose or frequency required if extracorporal renal replacement therapy is introduced.

Complicating this issue, particularly in the critically ill, is that of changes in protein binding. This may be due to displacement by other medications, hyperbilirubinaemia, acidosis or reductions in circulating plasma protein levels. Drugs with a high sieving coefficient may have their clearances increased as a result of this phenomenon [33, 34].

Sieving coefficients may also be altered when predilution and postdilution ratios are varied [35, 36]. In a study comparing different pre-dilution to post-dilution ratios the sieving coefficient for vancomycin decreased with decreasing pre-dilution while its clearance increased.

Higher sieving coefficients greater than one are only possible in some circumstances and represent an active process. Such occurrences reflect either protein clearance, precipitation, or filter electrostatic interactions.

While the sieving coefficient is specific to the drug and membrane, clearances achieved by extracorporal systems are dependent on system design and flow rates through the system. The clearance in theory can be calculated from the filtration rate multiplied by the sieving coefficient. When dialysis is incorporated the saturation coefficient can be calculated from the dialysate concentration divided by the blood concentration. However, the saturation coefficient is dependent upon the filter size and flow rates. At high flow rates with small filter sizes contact time may be inadequate to achieve equilibrium, with a resultant drop in the saturation coefficient. Saturation coefficients are therefore expressed within certain flow and filter size parameters. Reducing blood flow rates encourages more complete equilibration of dialysate with blood and thus improves the saturation coefficient. It does not necessarily improve clearance.

13.4 Determinants of Antibiotic Clearance in CRRT

13.4.1 Patient Specific Factors

Critical illness, multi-organ dysfunction and, in particular, renal failure induce numerous physiological changes that can impact upon antibiotic levels. Alterations in total body water, volume of distribution, plasma protein levels, acid-base status, and vital organ function will all impact upon antibiotic pharmacokinetics. Thus several factors need to be taken into account when prescribing in this patient group.

13.4.1.1 Residual Renal Function

Most antibiotics are cleared from the blood stream by the kidneys and excreted largely unchanged in urine. Thus oliguria induces accumulation. While oliguria is common, many patients have some degree of residual renal function. This residual renal function may be insufficient to maintain physiologic homeostasis, but the presence or absence of such function may have a large effect on the clearance of antibiotic and other medications. A standard CRRT using 2,000 ml/h of combined filtration and dialysis produces a maximum 33 ml/min clearance. An additional glomerular filtration of

10–15 ml/min, while small in itself, represents a 30% increase in total clearance. If antibiotic levels are to be aimed towards a therapeutic target, fluctuations of this magnitude make acquiring the target from fixed RRT formulae extremely rare.

Patients receiving RRT for indications other than oliguric acute renal failure, such as blood purification strategies in sepsis, or early in renal failure in an attempt to preserve renal function, present a complex conundrum. Significant intrinsic renal function may be preserved, and the addition of filtration or dialysis to patients with preserved renal function may require increased dosing of antibiotic [37, 38]. The evidence does not support this indication for CRRT and appropriate antibiotic dose regimes with this indication are unknown.

Unfortunately estimation of residual renal function is often impracticable to measure. Unstable creatinine kinetics from variable urine output and creatinine production in critically ill patients make accurate estimation of glomerular filtration rate (GFR) unreliable. Plasma creatinine may be influenced by factors such as drugs and feeding, masking changes in renal function, and prediction equations are inaccurate in unstable ICU patients [39].

13.4.1.2 *Non-Renal Clearance*

In the presence of renal failure non-renal mechanisms of drug elimination may increase. Increased proportions of clearance of a number of antibiotics due to non-renal mechanisms have been previously reported in anuric patients and patients receiving CRRT [40–43]. Non-renal clearance and tissue distribution may not be constant during acute renal failure [44]. For example, although renal clearance of imipenem falls, non-renal clearance may provide 90 ml/min in acute renal failure, while non-renal clearance is only 50 ml/min as end stage renal failure develops [45]. Similarly at the onset of acute renal failure normal non-renal clearance of vancomycin is preserved [46]. However with time, non-renal clearance decreases, eventually approaching the clearance observed in patients with chronic failure. In some circumstances, such as high fluid losses in burns or the use of vasoactive substances to augment cardiac output, clearances may be increased above that expected from renal function [47]. Thus timing, other organ dysfunction and co-morbidity may all influence the degree of non-renal clearance.

13.4.1.3 *Extrinsic Losses*

In addition to the normal mechanisms of drug clearance (largely hepatic), patients with critical illness may have high insensible or wound losses that may clear significant volume of antibiotic. Debridement or ongoing fluid losses into dressings or drains may increase significantly "clearances" of antibiotics. Fluctuations in losses over time may alter antibiotic tissue levels. The fluid losses, with progressive renal dysfunction, followed by the addition of CRRT may result in widely inconsistent and unpredictable levels of antibiotics.

13.4.1.4 *Plasma Protein Level*

While the use of albumin as a resuscitation fluid does not improve outcome, the addition of plasma protein may alter the characteristics of antibiotic clearances. Sieving coefficients are altered by the plasma protein level [34]. The toxicity of amikacin is related to the circulating albumin level [48]. If plasma protein levels are not accounted for, both clearance and plasma levels may be altered.

13.4.2 Renal Replacement Technique Specific

13.4.2.1 *General Comments*

The pharmacokinetics of drugs in critically ill patients on CRRT depends on many factors. There is a complex interaction between the patient, the drug and the type of renal replacement therapy. The drug factors include molecular size, protein binding, charge and volume of distribution. Concomitant medications may alter binding and volume of distribution and thus clearance.

The factors relevant in the renal replacement therapy include the type and size of filter used, adsorption of drug onto the filter, the blood flow rate, the ultrafiltration rate, the rate of predilution, and the rate of countercurrent dialysis, as well as the total duration of therapy.

The procedure chosen varies with the patients' needs and local policy, resources and experience. However, subtle changes in technique may profoundly alter clearance and thus antibiotic dosage requirement.

13.4.2.2 *Filtration Vs. Dialysis*

Continuous veno-venous haemofiltration (CVVHF) antibiotic clearance is by convection. The sieving coefficient and ultrafiltration rate are considerably more significant than molecular size. Conversely, removal by continuous haemodialysis (CVVHD) is a diffusive process that is molecular weight sensitive and thus better suited to removal of molecules below 500 Da. Consequently clearance of antibiotics with larger molecular weights such as glycopeptides (>1,100 Da) may be more efficient with CVVHF than CVVHD.

At any filtration rate, clearance is most efficient for antibiotics with the highest sieving coefficients. These include aminoglycosides, carbapenems, metronidazole and vancomycin, all have sieving coefficients between 0.9 and 1. Cefuroxime, cefotaxime, and ceftazidime also have moderately high sieving coefficients, 0.9, 0.62, and 0.86, respectively, and are efficiently cleared by haemofiltration. Antibiotics with the highest sieving coefficients are also most influenced by changes in the filtration rate.

Most antibiotics other than vancomycin and teicoplanin are of low molecular weight and are also easily removed by diffusion during CVVHD. Consequently most antibiotics are readily cleared by CVVHDF, and once creatinine clearances approach 35 ml/min, there may be little need to extend dosage intervals for standard doses for fear of toxicity. Antibiotics such as glycopeptides and aminoglycosides can, and should, be monitored with titration of dosage regimes accordingly.

13.4.2.3 Exchange Rates

Many regimes utilise a 33-ml/min exchange rate, but this may vary. Addition of dialysis to CVVHDF is often accompanied by a reduction in filtration rates to keep the total exchange at 33 ml/min. High volumes of exchange such as with high volume filtration may significantly increase antibiotic clearance [35]. However, clearances may also alter with the mode of RRT. Vancomycin has increased clearance with filtration compared to dialysis [49]. Thus exchanging a 33 ml/min filtration rate for a 16.5 ml/min filtration and16.5 ml/min dialysis rate may not produce identical clearances. Predilution volumes also alter filtration clearances with maximal vancomycin clearance achieved when one-third of replacement fluid was given pre-filter [35]. Optimal clearances seem to be achieved with one-third of replacement fluid given pre-filter. Thus acute renal failure patients treated with CRRT should receive a vancomycin starting dose similar to that of patients with normal renal function and then levels monitored.

As a general rule severely infected patients with poor renal function or who are dependent on renal replacement should receive normal antibiotic doses given less frequently. Whenever possible these patients' antibiotic levels should be monitored by troughs and post-administration peaks to avoid toxicity. While ideally, this should be all antibiotics, in reality commercial assays are only available for aminoglycosides and glycopeptides.

13.4.2.4 Membrane

Membrane properties vary between manufacturers, with a wide variety of polymers, pore width, and membrane structures available as a commercial filter. Many antibiotics appear to be unaffected by the type of membrane [36, 50, 51]. However, the clearance of other antibiotics appears membrane dependent, with AN69 membranes achieving lower clearances of ceftriaxone and ceftazidine [52, 53]. In some circumstances clearance is membrane dependent only [54]. Cefpirome clearance appears filtration and membrane independent during filtration. However, cefpirome clearance was improved with increasing dialysis rates across polyacrylnitrile membranes (while unaffected if a polyamide filter was used [54]).

13.4.2.5 Duration of Therapy

Continuous methods may simply deliver the dose of dialysis over the entire day, while alternative methods (SLEDD, daily IHD) deliver equivalent doses over a shorter period. Dosing regimes for IHD and CRRT cannot necessarily be extrapolated for critically ill patients treated with renal replacement hybrids such as slow low-efficiency dialysis (SLED), sustained low-efficiency daily dialysis (SLEDD), and extended daily dialysis (EDD) [20, 22, 55].

Dosing data in the newer forms of haemodialysis are even more limited than other forms of RRT. The extent of drug removal can vary immensely between each dialysis approach and unique characteristics concerning each patient's ability to store and remove it [22]. Repeated frequent intermittent haemodialysis or filtration may alter intrinsic clearance and sieving or saturation coefficients thus changing antibiotic dosing needs.

In clinical practice, circuit failures such as clotted filters require replacement, and both diagnostic and therapeutic procedures (e.g. CT scan, tracheostomy) interrupt "continuous" RRT. The accumulated intervals produce fluctuating daily doses of CRRT, impacting upon antibiotic clearance, and confounding time based antibiotic dosing schedules. Thus time off dialysis complicates antibiotic clearances and hence dosing even further.

13.4.2.6 Absorption to Membranes

While filtered and dialysed clearance can be accounted for by measurement of losses in the filtrated and dialysed volume produced, losses due to absorption on the membrane are more difficult to establish [36]. However, in some circumstances, particularly if filters are changed frequently, drug may be absorbed to the membrane filter. The clinical relevance of this currently unclear.

13.4.3 Antibiotic Specifics

The goal of drug administration is to achieve adequate effects with minimal or no adverse effects. It would be ideal to be able to measure infection-site antibiotic concentrations (e.g. for lung infections pulmonary parenchymal levels, for soft tissue infections interstitial levels, etc.) and correlate these to clinical outcome. Whilst this has recently become a possibility in isolated research units, clinical utility is still unidentified. Therefore more surrogate endpoints of antibiotic dosing have to be utilised clinically until this tool becomes more routine. Understanding of, and thereby utilising, the relationship between the pharmacodynamic and pharmacokinetic properties of the various classes of antibiotics helps to determine the optimal dosage regimen and predicting which pharmacokinetic parameter should correlate best with clinical efficacy [56]. Parameters to consider include: peak drug concentration, time above the minimum inhibitory concentration (MIC), the area under the serum concentration time curve and the area under the inhibitory curve (AUC/MIC or AUIC) [56]. The pharmacodynamics of antibiotics relate to the time course of drug activity and the mode of action on bacteria ('kill characteristics') [56]. This includes the post-antibiotic effect (PAE) and other persisting drug effects.

β-Lactams have a characteristic slow continuous (time-dependent) kill characteristic. The cephalosporin and penicillins are dependent on levels being maintained above MIC (sometimes 5×MIC) [56]. This contrasts with the kill characteristic of aminoglycosides, which is concentration dependent. A high peak concentration of an aminoglycoside provides a better, faster killing effect on standard bacterial inocula. All aminoglycosides exhibit a significant post-antibiotic effect (PAE) – the continued suppression of bacterial growth despite zero serum concentration of antibiotic. The duration of this effect is variable and dependent on several factors, the most important of which is the preceding peak, i.e. is concentration dependent. PAE is much more pronounced in aminoglycosides than other antibiotics, and more pronounced with Gram-negative bacilli than with other bacteria.

The efficacy of aminoglycosides (such as gentamicin) is dependent upon peak concentrations. Increases in volumes of distribution (from volume overload and leaking capillaries), changes in protein binding and protein concentrations may all lower the peak level seen in the critically ill patient with acute failure. There is a natural tendency to lower the doses of renally toxic antibiotics in the presence of acute renal failure. However, sometimes standard doses of antibiotics should be administered, accounting for the increased volume of distribution. The presence of acute renal failure for the aminoglycosides and the glycopeptides should mandate the measurement of levels at frequent intervals. Repeated doses should not be given until the level falls below the recommended trough for these antibiotics.

13.5 Specific Issues with Antibiotic Dosing During CRRT

13.5.1 Aminoglycosides

Aminoglycosides have a narrow therapeutic window and unpredictable pharmacokinetics in the critically ill. Renal hypoperfusion from any cause, and sepsis, even without overt shock, increases the risk of aminoglycoside renal toxicity. For patients undergoing CRRT individualised dosing regimes guided by repeated serum aminoglycoside measurements are appropriate [57, 58]. Increased toxicity of prolonged elevated levels of aminoglycosides in patients with renal failure receiving large once daily doses may be reduce aminoglycoside value [59]. Aminoglycoside-related hearing loss is multifactorial, is worsened by renal failure, and may progress despite discontinuing the antibiotic [60, 61].

13.5.2 Glycopeptides

As glycopeptides have proportionally high renal clearances, acute renal failure dramatically extends $t_{1/2}$. While membranes previously used for IHD did not remove vancomycin, the high flux membranes employed for CRRT effectively clear much of the vancomycin. Serum levels should guide dosing [35].

13.5.3 Beta-Lactam Antibiotics

In-vivo animal experiments have demonstrated that the kill characteristics of β-lactam antibiotics differ significantly from those of aminoglycosides. β-Lactams have a slow continuous kill characteristic. Bacterial killing, therefore, is almost entirely related to the time for which levels in tissue and plasma exceed a certain threshold. As these antibiotics have a large therapeutic ratio due to their low toxicity rate even at high doses, it has been suggested that levels should be kept sometimes up to five times the MIC [56].

β-Lactam antibiotics are widely used in the critically ill. However, adverse central nervous system effects including confusion, psychosis, myoclonus and seizures have not infrequently been implicated with antibiotics usage in renal failure [61–64]. β-Lactam antibiotics induce convulsions by interfering with gamma-aminobutyric acid (GABA) pathways. Brain antibiotic levels are increased by uraemia, further increasing the risk of toxicity [61].

13.6 Special Considerations

13.6.1 Antibiotic Combinations

For a variety of reasons antibiotics are combined with other substances to enhance efficacy. Such examples are cotrimoxazole, where two antibacterial agents combined cause two breaks in a vital microbial pathway, imipenem, where cilastatin reduces the toxicity produced by the renal metabolism of imipenem, and clavulanic acid or sulbactam, where the additive reduces the β-lactamase activity, and thus broadens the spectrum of the antibacterial agent used.

13.6.1.1 Imipenem

Imipenem, a broad spectrum carbapenem antibiotic, is presented in fixed combination with cilastatin [65]. Imipenem can be metabolized by dipeptidase, dehydropeptidase I, located at the lumenal surface of the renal proximal tubular cells. Cilastatin inhibits the metabolism of imipenem, therefore lowering the dosage requirement, thus reducing tubular toxicity. Renal clearance is by glomerular filtration and active tubular secretion for both imipenem and cilastatin [66]. With increasing renal dysfunction, the half-life of imipenem is controlled by a metabolic clearance pathway which is unaffected by cilastatin [66], imipenem metabolites as well as imipenem. While imipenem is effectively cleared, cilastatin is not easily removed by intermittent haemodialysis or CRRT. The doses of imipenem recommended for patients with end stage renal failure, however, will lead to underdosing and inadequate antibiotic therapy during RRT [45]. High imipenem doses inevitably result in a marked accumulation of cilastatin. However, high doses of the carbapenem may be required during continuous RRT [67–69]. As the pharmacokinetic properties of the co-drugs differ, care must be taken with imipenem/cilastatin (and panipenem/betamipron) to prevent accumulation [70]. Other carbapenems which do not require co-drugs, such as meropenem, may be preferred and have less risk of neurotoxicity at high doses [71].

13.6.1.2 Beta-Lactamase Inhibitors

Beta-Lactamase inhibitors have similar complexities. Renal clearance, volume of distribution and protein binding differ between the three commonly used beta-lactamase inhibitors. When choosing combinations of beta-lactam antibiotic and beta-lactamase inhibitor, it is important to ensure that not only are the pharmacokinetic properties of drug and inhibitor similar, but that they remain similar under changing pathophysiological conditions, including clearance by extracorporeal techniques [72]. Kinetics of piperacillin, in combination with the beta-lactamase inhibitor tazobactam, have been studied in volunteers and patients in relatively stable conditions. The piperacillin-tazobactam combination at a ratio of 8:1 has ideal pharmacokinetic properties in normal or slightly impaired renal function. However, in RRT dependent patients, while the fixed drug preparations can be used initially the piperacillin dosage needs to be increased relative to that of tazobactam to prevent accumulation of tazobactam [73]. Use of supplemental doses of piperacillin alone should be considered.

13.6.2 Metabolites

While many of the antibiotics accumulate in the presence of renal dysfunction, accumulation may lead to increased clearance by metabolism or by other pathways. For example, the 15% of metabolised ciprofloxacin will increase metabolites themselves which may accumulate and reach levels that have either therapeutic or adverse effects. These metabolites have varied clearances by filtration. Addition of continuous RRT following accumulation of a drug does not guarantee that the adverse effect of the drug will be removed.

13.7 Final Comments

Inadequate or inappropriate antibiotics increase morbidity and mortality in the critically ill [2, 16, 56, 74]. The optimal pharmacokinetic profile to achieve adequate antimicrobial activity varies with antibiotic type, the minimum inhibitory concentration of the antibiotic, the specific strain of microbe, and the site of infection [75]. While accumulation often occurs in acute renal failure, increased volumes of distribution, non-renal clearance and the addition of RRT may contribute to produce sub-therapeutic antibiotic levels. Guidelines for antibiotic dosing in critically ill patients are included in Table 13.1. Consideration must be given to the technique used, which may vary between different studies.

Table 13.1. Recommended doses for "standard" RRT regimes (usually 33 ml/min exchange rates)

	CVVHD Dose	Interval	Notes	CVVH Dose	Interval	Notes	SLEDD Dose	Interval	Notes
Benzylpenicillin									
Ampicillin									
Flucloxacillin	4 g	8 h	[76]	4 g	8 h	[76]			
Cephazolin	2 g	12 h		2 g	12 h		15–20 mg/kg	Each dialysis	[77]
Cefuroxime	750 mg	12 hrly	[78]	750 mg	12 hrly	[78]			
Ceftriaxone	2 g	12 h	[10, 79]	2 g	12 h	[10, 79]			
Ceftazidime	2 g	8 g		2 g	8 h	[80]			
Cefpirome				1 g	12 h	[81]			
Cefipime	1 g	12 g	[82]	1 g	12 h	[82]			MI [51]
Imipenem/cilastatin	1 g	24 hrly	[68]	1 g	24 h	[68]			
Meropenem	1 g	8 hrly	[69]	1 g	8 hrly	[69]			
Piperacillin/tazobactam	4.5 g	8 hrly	D [73, 83]	4.5 g	8 hrly	D [73, 83]			
Gentamicin	7 mg/kg	SAM	[84–86]	7 mg/kg	SAM	[84–86]	7 mg/kg	SAM	[85, 86]
Tobramycin		SAM			SAM			SAM	
Amikacin		SAM			SAM			SAM	
Ciprofloxacin	400–600 mg	24 h	[41, 87]	600–800 mg	24 h	[41, 88]			
Moxifloxacin	400 mg	24 h	[89]						
Clindamycin	600–900 mg	8 h		600–900 mg	8 h				
Levofloxacin	250–400 mg	24 h	MB-PS [41, 88]	250–400 mg	24 h	MB-PS [41, 88]			
Linezolid	600 mg	12 h	[42]	600 mg	12 h	[90]			
Vancomycin	450 mg	12 h SAM	[91] SAM	25	SAM	X	25 mg/kg	SAM	[22]
Teicoplanin	800 mg	SAM	[92]	800 mg	SAM	[92]	800 mg	SAM	[92]
Amphotericin									
Lipid complex									
Liposomal	0.4 mg/kg	24 h		0.4 mg/kg	Daily				
Doxycholate									
Metronidazole	500 mg	8 hrly	[93]	500 mg	8 hrly	[93]	500 mg	8 hrly	[93]
Acyclovir	5–7.5 mg/kg	24 h	[94]	5–7.5 mg/kg	24 h	[94]			
Fluconazole	800 mg	24 h	[95]	500–800 mg	24 h	[95] F10			
Fluconazole	500–600 mg	12 hrly	[8]	500–600 mg	12 hrly	[8]			

MB there may be significant binding of drug to membrane, *MI* membrane independent, no difference between PS and AN69 membranes, *DD* dual drug therapy accumulation of one of the components may be a problem (tazobactam, cilastatin), *F1* lower clearances at filtration of 1,000 ml/h, *SAM* serum antibiotic level monitoring recommended

Concerns of toxicity may influence clinicians to restrict doses or antibiotic combinations, which may result in non-optimal antibiotic use. Equally problematic is that the complexity of managing the critically ill may hide significant unrecognized adverse effects. For example, it is possible that the diagnosis of a metronidazole induced peripheral nerve toxicity in critically ill patients with renal failure would be obscured by the presence of uraemia and non-specific critical illness polyneuropathy [61]. Other accumulation effects such as neurological toxicity from cephalosporin may go unrecognisable in the sedated patient, and may be of little or no clinical consequence. Accumulation of antibiotics may affect the central or peripheral nervous system, including the auditory system, and the kidneys. These are outlined in Table 13.2.

Table 13.2. Potential adverse effects of accumulation of antibiotics in the critically ill

Adverse effect on:	Antibiotic group
Central nervous system	Beta-lactams [61, 63]
	Including carbapenems [71]
	Quinolones [96]
	Aminoglycosides
	Antivirals [97]
Ototoxicity	Cephalosporins [98]
	Aminoglycosides [99, 100]
	Macrolides [100, 101]
	Glycopeptides [60]
Peripheral nervous system	Penicillins [100]
	Aminoglycosides [99]
	Metronidazole [100]
	Cindamycin [100]
	Glycopeptides [60, 102]
Renal (tubular or interstitial nephritis)	Penicillin [103, 104]
	Cephalosporin [105, 106]
	Aminoglycosides [99]
	Glycopeptides [60]
Other	Quinolones (tendons) [107]

13.8 Summary and Conclusions

The clinician confronted with a patient on RRT requiring antibiotic therapy must consider the effect of patient, machine, and drug variables.

The important patient variables include volume of distribution, changes in plasma protein levels, and the effects of residual renal function. Volumes of distribution are often increased in the critically ill, especially in sepsis and burns. A patient with a high Vd at the onset of oliguria may require an increased loading dose, and a reduction in dose frequency.

Low plasma protein levels will be relevant when considering drugs that are normally highly protein bound, such as ceftriaxone and dicloxacillin. An increase in free drug concentration caused by hypoalbuminaemia will lead to an increased clearance on RRT. Similarly, drug toxicity may increase.

The effect of residual renal function must also be considered. In the ICU setting RRT may be employed without oliguria and in patients with a significant remaining intrinsic function. Dosage adjustments in this group are difficult to estimate.

Machine variables relate to the type and duration of therapy. With convection based techniques clearance will be dependent primarily upon ultrafiltration rate and sieving coefficient. Conversely, with a diffusive process, molecular weight becomes a more important factor. With either process, the clinician should attempt to take into account the effect of unplanned treatment interruptions - for surgery, or diagnostic procedures for example.

With regard to drug characteristics, the pharmacodynamics and kill characteristics of the antibiotic being used must be considered. Aminoglycosides, for example, that rely on upon peak concentrations to achieve bacterial killing, will have a different dose adjustment to β-lactams that have time dependent kill characteristics.

It is apparent that renal failure and the use of RRT in the critically ill patient add a significant degree of complexity to the prescription of antibiotics.

As the use of RRT increases throughout intensive care there is as yet little good data to guide the clinician in making the necessary dose adjustments to antibiotic regimes. Currently available guidelines are often based upon non-critically ill patients in chronic dialysis programs and their relevance to the ICU setting is questionable. Monitoring of antibiotic levels gives the most useful clinical information at present, but its availability is limited to only a few compounds.

The need for good quality data to guide clinicians in this field is urgent. At present the best advice appears to be to measure antibiotic levels where possible, and in the case of published dialysis dose adjustments to remember that "one size does not fit all".

References

1. Kollef MH, Sherman G, Ward S, Fraser VJ (1999) Inadequate antimicrobial treatment of infections: a risk factor for hospital mortality among critically ill patients. Chest 115:462–474
2. Garnacho-Montero J, Garcia-Garmendia JL, Barrero-Almodovar A, Jimenez-Jimenez FJ, Perez-Paredes C, Ortiz-Leyba C (2003) Impact of adequate empirical antibiotic therapy on the outcome of patients admitted to the intensive care unit with sepsis. Crit Care Med 31:2742–2751
3. MacArthur RD, Miller M, Albertson T, Panacek E, Johnson D, Teoh L, Barchuk W (2004) Adequacy of early empiric antibiotic treatment and survival in severe sepsis: experience from the MONARCS trial. Clin Infect Dis 38:284–288
4. Ibrahim EH, Sherman G, Ward S, Fraser VJ, Kollef MH (2000) The influence of inadequate antimicrobial treatment of bloodstream infections on patient outcomes in the ICU setting. Chest 118:146–155
5. Valles J, Rello J, Ochagavia A, Garnacho J, Alcala MA (2003) Community-acquired bloodstream infection in critically ill adult patients: impact of shock and inappropriate antibiotic therapy on survival. Chest 123:1615–1624
6. Harbarth S, Garbino J, Pugin J, Romand JA, Lew D, Pittet D (2003) Inappropriate initial antimicrobial therapy and its effect on survival in a clinical trial of immunomodulating therapy for severe sepsis. Am J Med 115:529–535
7. Micek ST, Isakow W, Shannon W, Kollef MH (2005) Predictors of hospital mortality for patients with severe sepsis treated with Drotrecogin alfa (activated). Pharmacotherapy 25:26–34
8. Yagasaki K, Gando S, Matsuda N, Kameue T, Ishitani T, Hirano T, Iseki K (2003) Pharmacokinetics and the most suitable dosing regimen of fluconazole in critically ill patients receiving continuous hemodiafiltration. Intensive Care Med 29:1844–1848
9. Eckhardt A, Borner K, Keller F, Zellner D (1997) Dosage adjustment of antiinfective therapy in patients with renal impairment. Int J Clin Pharmacol Ther 35:99–102
10. Joynt GM, Lipman J, Gomersall CD, Young RJ, Wong EL, Gin T (2001) The pharmacokinetics of once-daily dosing of ceftriaxone in critically ill patients. J Antimicrob Chemother 47:421–429
11. Roberts J, Lipman J (2006) Antibacterial dosing in Intensive Care: Pharmacokinetics, degree of disease and pharmacodynamics of sepsis. Clin Pharmacokinet 45:755–773
12. Freebairn RC, Lipman J (1993) Renal replacement therapy for the critically ill – precarious progress. Part I. Definitions and physiological aspects. S Afr J Surg 31:114–120
13. Bellomo R, Ronco C, Kellum JA, Mehta RL, Palevsky P (2004) Acute renal failure – definition, outcome measures, animal models, fluid therapy and information technology needs: the Second International Consensus Conference of the Acute Dialysis Quality Initiative (ADQI) Group. Crit Care 8:R204–212
14. Dager WE (2006) Filtering out important considerations for developing drug-dosing regimens in extended daily dialysis. Crit Care Med 34:240–241
15. Kroh UF (2001) Pharmacokinetic studies in patients on continuous renal replacement therapies. Intensive Care Med 27:629–630
16. Zhou J, Dong Y, Zhao X, Lee S, Amin A, Ramaswamy S, Domagala J, Musser JM, Drlica K (2000) Selection of antibiotic-resistant bacterial mutants: allelic diversity among fluoroquinolone-resistant mutations. J Infect Dis 182: 517–525
17. Bellomo R, Ronco C (1998) Indications and criteria for ini-

tiating renal replacement therapy in the intensive care unit. Kidney Int Suppl 66:S106–109
18. Palevsky PM (2005) Renal replacement therapy I: indications and timing. Crit Care Clin 21:347–356
19. Waldrop J, Ciraulo DL, Milner TP, Gregori D, Kendrick AS, Richart CM, Maxwell RA, Barker DE (2005) A comparison of continuous renal replacement therapy to intermittent dialysis in the management of renal insufficiency in the acutely III surgical patient. Am Surg 71:36–39
20. Marshall MR, Ma T, Galler D, Rankin AP, Williams AB (2004) Sustained low-efficiency daily diafiltration (SLEDD-f) for critically ill patients requiring renal replacement therapy: towards an adequate therapy. Nephrol Dial Transplant 19:877–884
21. Freebairn RC, Lipman J (1993) Renal replacement therapy for the critically ill-precarious progress. Part II. Technical aspects and clinical application. S Afr J Surg 31:147–151
22. Kielstein JT, Czock D, Schopke T, Hafer C, Bode-Boger SM, Kuse E, Keller F, Fliser D (2006) Pharmacokinetics and total elimination of meropenem and vancomycin in intensive care unit patients undergoing extended daily dialysis. Crit Care Med 34:51–56
23. Schiffl H, Lang SM, Fischer R (2002) Daily hemodialysis and the outcome of acute renal failure. N Engl J Med 346:305–310
24. Kopple JD, Jones MR, Keshaviah PR, Bergstrom J, Lindsay RM, Moran J, Nolph KD, Teehan BP (1995) A proposed glossary for dialysis kinetics. Am J Kidney Dis 26:963–981
25. Dorman T, Swoboda S, Zarfeshenfard F, Trentler B, Lipsett PA (1998) Impact of altered aminoglycoside volume of distribution on the adequacy of a three milligram per kilogram loading dose. Critical Care Research Group. Surgery 124:73–78
26. Beckhouse MJ, Whyte IM, Byth PL, Napier JC, Smith AJ (1988) Altered aminoglycoside pharmacokinetics in the critically ill. Anaesth Intensive Care 16:418–422
27. Belzberg H, Zhu J, Cornwell EE, 3rd, Murray JA, Sava J, Salim A, Velmahos GC, Gill MA (2004) Imipenem levels are not predictable in the critically ill patient. J Trauma 56:111–117
28. Wong PY, Zhu M, Li RC (2000) Pharmacokinetic and pharmacodynamic interactions between intravenous ciprofloxacin and oral ferrous sulfate. J Chemother 12:286–293
29. Ronchera-Oms CL, Tormo C, Ordovas JP, Abad J, Jimenez NV (1995) Expanded gentamicin volume of distribution in critically ill adult patients receiving total parenteral nutrition. J Clin Pharm Ther 20:253–258
30. Pittrow L, Penk A (1999) Special pharmacokinetics of fluconazole in septic, obese and burn patients. Mycoses 42 Suppl 2:87–90
31. Zaske DE, Strate RG, Kohls PR (1991) Amikacin pharmacokinetics: wide interpatient variation in 98 patients. J Clin Pharmacol 31:158–163
32. Lugo G, Castaneda-Hernandez G (1997) Relationship between hemodynamic and vital support measures and pharmacokinetic variability of amikacin in critically ill patients with sepsis. Crit Care Med 25:806–811
33. Hansen E, Bucher M, Jakob W, Lemberger P, Kees F (2001) Pharmacokinetics of levofloxacin during continuous veno-venous hemofiltration. Intensive Care Med 27:371–375
34. Ittner KP, Roth G, Gruber M, Pawlik M, Taeger K (2005) Clearance of moxifloxacin during continuous haemofiltration (CVVHF) in vitro. J Antimicrob Chemother 56:360–364
35. Uchino S, Cole L, Morimatsu H, Goldsmith D, Bellomo R (2002) Clearance of vancomycin during high-volume haemofiltration: impact of pre-dilution. Intensive Care Med 28:1664–1667
36. Choi G, Gomersall CD, Lipman J, Wong A, Joynt GM, Leung P, Ramsay SJ, Ho OM (2004) The effect of adsorption, filter material and point of dilution on antibiotic elimination by haemofiltration an in vitro study of levofloxacin. Int J Antimicrob Agents 24:468–472
37. Dailly E, Kergueris MF, Pannier M, Jolliet P, Bourin M (2003) Population pharmacokinetics of imipenem in burn patients. Fundam Clin Pharmacol 17:645–650
38. Lipman J, Wallis SC, Boots RJ (2003) Cefepime versus cefpirome: the importance of creatinine clearance. Anesth Analg 97:1149–1154, table of contents
39. Wells M, Lipman J (1997) Measurements of glomerular filtration in the intensive care unit are only a rough guide to renal function. S Afr J Surg 35:20–23
40. Jones EM, McMullin CM, Hedges AJ, Lovering AM, White LO, Reeves DS, MacGowan AP (1997) The pharmacokinetics of intravenous ciprofloxacin 400 mg 12 hourly in patients with severe sepsis: the effect of renal function and intra-abdominal disease. J Antimicrob Chemother 40:121–124
41. Malone RS, Fish DN, Abraham E, Teitelbaum I (2001) Pharmacokinetics of levofloxacin and ciprofloxacin during continuous renal replacement therapy in critically ill patients. Antimicrob Agents Chemother 45:2949–2954
42. Brier ME, Stalker DJ, Aronoff GR, Batts DH, Ryan KK, O'Grady M, Hopkins NK, Jungbluth GL (2003) Pharmacokinetics of linezolid in subjects with renal dysfunction. Antimicrob Agents Chemother 47:2775–2780
43. Vos MC, Vincent HH, Yzerman EP (1992) Clearance of imipenem/cilastatin in acute renal failure patients treated by continuous hemodiafiltration (CAVHD). Intensive Care Med 18:282–285
44. Tegeder I, Schmidtko A, Brautigam L, Kirschbaum A, Geisslinger G, Lotsch J (2002) Tissue distribution of imipenem in critically ill patients. Clin Pharmacol Ther 71:325–333
45. Tegeder I, Bremer F, Oelkers R, Schobel H, Schuttler J, Brune K, Geisslinger G (1997) Pharmacokinetics of imipenem-cilastatin in critically ill patients undergoing continuous venovenous hemofiltration. Antimicrob Agents Chemother 41:2640–2645
46. Macias WL, Mueller BA, Scarim SK (1991) Vancomycin pharmacokinetics in acute renal failure: preservation of nonrenal clearance. Clin Pharmacol Ther 50:688–694
47. Walstad RA, Aanderud L, Thurmann-Nielsen E (1988) Pharmacokinetics and tissue concentrations of ceftazidime in burn patients. Eur J Clin Pharmacol 35:543–549
48. Contreras AM, Ramirez M, Cueva L, Alvarez S, de Loza R, Gamba G (1994) Low serum albumin and the increased risk of amikacin nephrotoxicity. Rev Invest Clin 46:37–43
49. Jeffrey RF, Khan AA, Prabhu P, Todd N, Goutcher E, Will EJ, Davison AM (1994) A comparison of molecular clearance rates during continuous hemofiltration and hemodialysis with a novel volumetric continuous renal replacement system. Artif Organs 18:425–428
50. Joy MS, Matzke GR, Frye RF, Palevsky PM (1998) Determinants of vancomycin clearance by continuous venovenous hemofiltration and continuous venovenous hemodialysis. Am J Kidney Dis 31:1019–1027
51. Isla A, Gascon AR, Maynar J, Arzuaga A, Toral D, Pedraz JL (2005) Cefepime and continuous renal replacement therapy (CRRT): in vitro permeability of two CRRT membranes and pharmacokinetics in four critically ill patients. Clin Ther 27:599–608
52. Matzke GR, Frye RF, Joy MS, Palevsky PM (2000) Determinants of ceftriaxone clearance by continuous venovenous hemofiltration and hemodialysis. Pharmacotherapy 20: 635–643
53. Matzke GR, Frye RF, Joy MS, Palevsky PM (2000) Determi-

nants of ceftazidime clearance by continuous venovenous hemofiltration and continuous venovenous hemodialysis. Antimicrob Agents Chemother 44:1639–1644
54. Phillips GJ, Davies JG, Olliff CJ, Kingswood C, Street M (1998) Use of in vitro models of haemofiltration and haemodiafiltration to estimate dosage regimens for critically ill patients prescribed cefpirome. J Clin Pharm Ther 23:353–359
55. Kumar D, Arora A, Singh NP, Kohli R, Kar P, Das BC (2005) Hepatitis G virus infection in hemodialysis patients from urban Delhi. Ren Fail 27:87–93
56. Pinder M, Bellomo R, Lipman J (2002) Pharmacological principles of antibiotic prescription in the critically ill. Anaesth Intensive Care 30:134–144
57. Buijk SE, Mouton JW, Gyssens IC, Verbrugh HA, Bruining HA (2002) Experience with a once-daily dosing program of aminoglycosides in critically ill patients. Intensive Care Med 28:936–942
58. Denaro CP, Ravenscroft PJ (1987) Usefulness of estimating individual pharmacokinetic data for aminoglycoside therapy in seriously ill patients. Aust N Z J Med 17:526–532
59. Hatala R, Dinh T, Cook DJ (1996) Once-daily aminoglycoside dosing in immunocompetent adults: a meta-analysis. Ann Intern Med 124:717–725
60. Chow AW, Azar RM (1994) Glycopeptides and nephrotoxicity. Intensive Care Med 20 Suppl 4:S23–29
61. Chow KM, Szeto CC, Hui AC, Li PK (2004) Mechanisms of antibiotic neurotoxicity in renal failure. Int J Antimicrob Agents 23:213–217
62. Martinez-Rodriguez JE, Barriga FJ, Santamaria J, Iranzo A, Pareja JA, Revilla M, dela Rosa CR (2001) Nonconvulsive status epilepticus associated with cephalosporins in patients with renal failure. Am J Med 111:115–119
63. Herishanu YO, Zlotnik M, Mostoslavsky M, Podgaietski M, Frisher S, Wirguin I (1998) Cefuroxime-induced encephalopathy. Neurology 50:1873–1875
64. Ferrara N, Abete P, Giordano M, Ferrara P, Carnovale V, Leosco D, Beneduce F, Ciarambino T, Varricchio M, Rengo F (2003) Neurotoxicity induced by Cefepime in a very old hemodialysis patient. Clin Nephrol 59:388–390
65. Norrby SR (1985) Imipenem/cilastatin: rationale for a fixed combination. Rev Infect Dis 7 Suppl 3:S447–451
66. Drusano GL (1986) An overview of the pharmacology of imipenem/cilastatin. J Antimicrob Chemother 18 Suppl E:79–92
67. Hashimoto S, Honda M, Yamaguchi M, Sekimoto M, Tanaka Y (1997) Pharmacokinetics of imipenem and cilastatin during continuous venovenous hemodialysis in patients who are critically ill. Asaio J 43:84–88
68. Fish DN, Teitelbaum I, Abraham E (2005) Pharmacokinetics and pharmacodynamics of imipenem during continuous renal replacement therapy in critically ill patients. Antimicrob Agents Chemother 49:2421–2428
69. Kuti JL, Nicolau DP (2005) Derivation of meropenem dosage in patients receiving continuous veno-venous hemofiltration based on pharmacodynamic target attainment. Chemotherapy 51:211–216
70. Mouton JW, Touzw DJ, Horrevorts AM, Vinks AA (2000) Comparative pharmacokinetics of the carbapenems: clinical implications. Clin Pharmacokinet 39:185–201
71. Norrby SR (2000) Neurotoxicity of carbapenem antibiotics: consequences for their use in bacterial meningitis. J Antimicrob Chemother 45:5–7
72. de la Pena A, Derendorf H (1999) Pharmacokinetic properties of beta-lactamase inhibitors. Int J Clin Pharmacol Ther 37:63–75
73. van der Werf TS, Mulder PO, Zijlstra JG, Uges DR, Stegeman CA (1997) Pharmacokinetics of piperacillin and tazobactam in critically ill patients with renal failure, treated with continuous veno-venous hemofiltration (CVVH). Intensive Care Med 23:873–877
74. Lipman J, Wallis SC, Rickard CM, Fraenkel D (2001) Low cefpirome levels during twice daily dosing in critically ill septic patients: pharmacokinetic modelling calls for more frequent dosing. Intensive Care Med 27:363–370
75. Craig WA (2001) Does the dose matter? Clin Infect Dis 33 Suppl 3:S233–237
76. Meyer B, Ahmed el Gendy S, Delle Karth G, Locker GJ, Heinz G, Jaeger W, Thalhammer F (2003) How to calculate clearance of highly protein-bound drugs during continuous venovenous hemofiltration demonstrated with flucloxacillin. Kidney Blood Press Res 26:135–140
77. Sowinski KM, Mueller BA, Grabe DW, Manley HJ, Frye RF, Bailie GR, Marx MA (2001) Cefazolin dialytic clearance by high-efficiency and high-flux hemodialyzers. Am J Kidney Dis 37:766–776
78. Davies SP, Lacey LF, Kox WJ, Brown EA (1991) Pharmacokinetics of cefuroxime and ceftazidime in patients with acute renal failure treated by continuous arteriovenous haemodialysis. Nephrol Dial Transplant 6:971–976
79. Kroh UF, Lennartz H, Edwards DJ, Stoeckel K (1996) Pharmacokinetics of ceftriaxone in patients undergoing continuous veno-venous hemofiltration. J Clin Pharmacol 36:1114–1119
80. Traunmuller F, Schenk P, Mittermeyer C, Thalhammer-Scherrer R, Ratheiser K, Thalhammer F (2002) Clearance of ceftazidime during continuous venovenous haemofiltration in critically ill patients. J Antimicrob Chemother 49:129–134
81. Van der Werf TS, Fijen JW, Van de Merbel NC, Spanjersberg R, Moller AV, Ligtenberg JJ, Tulleken JE, Zijlstra JG, Stegeman CA (1999) Pharmacokinetics of cefpirome in critically ill patients with renal failure treated by continuous veno-venous hemofiltration. Intensive Care Med 25: 1427–1431
82. Malone RS, Fish DN, Abraham E, Teitelbaum I (2001) Pharmacokinetics of cefepime during continuous renal replacement therapy in critically ill patients. Antimicrob Agents Chemother 45:3148–3155
83. Valtonen M, Tiula E, Takkunen O, Backman JT, Neuvonen PJ (2001) Elimination of the piperacillin/tazobactam combination during continuous venovenous haemofiltration and haemodiafiltration in patients with acute renal failure. J Antimicrob Chemother 48:881–885
84. Hickling KG, Begg EJ, Perry RE, Atkinson HC, Sharman JR (1991) Serum aminoglycoside clearance is predicted as poorly by renal aminoglycoside clearance as by creatinine clearance in critically ill patients. Crit Care Med 19:1041–1047
85. Triginer C, Izquierdo I, Fernandez R, Rello J, Torrent J, Benito S, Net A (1990) Gentamicin volume of distribution in critically ill septic patients. Intensive Care Med 16:303–306
86. Hansen M, Christrup LL, Jarlov JO, Kampmann JP, Bonde J (2001) Gentamicin dosing in critically ill patients. Acta Anaesthesiol Scand 45:734–740
87. Wallis SC, Mullany DV, Lipman J, Rickard CM, Daley PJ (2001) Pharmacokinetics of ciprofloxacin in ICU patients on continuous veno-venous haemodiafiltration. Intensive Care Med 27:665–672
88. Bellmann R, Egger P, Gritsch W, Bellmann-Weiler R, Joannidis M, Dunzendorfer S, Wiedermann CJ (2002) Elimination of levofloxacin in critically ill patients with renal failure: influence of continuous veno-venous hemofiltration. Int J Clin Pharmacol Ther 40:142–149
89. Fuhrmann V, Schenk P, Jaeger W, Ahmed S, Thalhammer F (2004) Pharmacokinetics of moxifloxacin in patients un-

dergoing continuous venovenous haemodiafiltration. J Antimicrob Chemother 54:780–784
90. Meyer B, Kornek GV, Nikfardjam M, Karth GD, Heinz G, Locker GJ, Jaeger W, Thalhammer F (2005) Multiple-dose pharmacokinetics of linezolid during continuous venovenous haemofiltration. J Antimicrob Chemother 56:172–179
91. DelDot ME, Lipman J, Tett SE (2004) Vancomycin pharmacokinetics in critically ill patients receiving continuous venovenous haemodiafiltration. Br J Clin Pharmacol 58: 259–268
92. Thalhammer F, Rosenkranz AR, Burgmann H, Graninger W, Hollenstein U, Schenk P, Thalhammer-Scherrer R, Traindl O, Horl WH, Breyer S (1997) Single-dose pharmacokinetics of teicoplanin during hemodialysis therapy using high-flux polysulfone membranes. Wien Klin Wochenschr 109:362–365
93. Lamp KC, Freeman CD, Klutman NE, Lacy MK (1999) Pharmacokinetics and pharmacodynamics of the nitroimidazole antimicrobials. Clin Pharmacokinet 36:353–373
94. Trotman RL, Williamson JC, Shoemaker DM, Salzer WL (2005) Antibiotic dosing in critically ill adult patients receiving continuous renal replacement therapy. Clin Infect Dis 41:1159–1166
95. Muhl E, Martens T, Iven H, Rob P, Bruch HP (2000) Influence of continuous veno-venous haemodiafiltration and continuous veno-venous haemofiltration on the pharmacokinetics of fluconazole. Eur J Clin Pharmacol 56:671–678
96. Bagon JA (1999) Neuropsychiatric complications following quinolone overdose in renal failure. Nephrol Dial Transplant 14:1337
97. Izzedine H, Launay-Vacher V, Deray G (2005) Antiviral drug-induced nephrotoxicity. Am J Kidney Dis 45:804–817
98. Sennesael J, Verbeelen D, Lauwers S (1982) Ototoxicity associated with cephalexin in two patients with renal failure. Lancet 2:1154–1155
99. Duff P (1992) The aminoglycosides. Obstet Gynecol Clin North Am 19:511–517
100. Snavely SR, Hodges GR (1984) The neurotoxicity of antibacterial agents. Ann Intern Med 101:92–104
101. Kroboth PD, McNeil MA, Kreeger A, Dominguez J, Rault R (1983) Hearing loss and erythromycin pharmacokinetics in a patient receiving hemodialysis. Arch Intern Med 143:1263–1265
102. Huang KC, Heise A, Shrader AK, Tsueda K (1990) Vancomycin enhances the neuromuscular blockade of vecuronium. Anesth Analg 71:194–196
103. Schellie SF, Groshong T (1999) Acute interstitial nephritis following amoxicillin overdose. Mo Med 96:209–211
104. Labriola L, Jadoul M, Daudons M, Pirson Y, Lambert M (2003) Massive amoxycillin crystalluria causing anuric acute renal failure. Clin Nephrol 59:455–457
105. Longstreth KL, Robbins SD, Smavatkul C, Doe NS (2004) Cephalexin-induced acute tubular necrosis. Pharmacotherapy 24:808–811
106. Leong CL, Thiruventhiran T (2000) Cefuroxime-induced acute renal failure. Nephron 84:185
107. Khaliq Y, Zhanel GG (2003) Fluoroquinolone-associated tendinopathy: a critical review of the literature. Clin Infect Dis 36:1404–1410

Chapter 14

Methods for Implementing Antibiotic Control in the Intensive Care Unit

A. Sandiumenge

14.1 Introduction

In recent decades, multiresistant pathogens have become established in our institutions, increasing mortality, morbidity, patient length of stay and related economic and social costs [1, 2]. Paradoxically, antibiotics constitute an important part of both the problem and the solution of resistance emergence and development. According to a range of multicenter studies, ICUs are the setting in which antimicrobials are most frequently prescribed. Between 33% and 62.3% of patients admitted to an ICU receive one or more antibiotics [3, 4], and although a causative association is difficult to demonstrate, antimicrobial use is clearly related to the development of antimicrobial resistance [5]. Unfortunately, reducing total antibiotic use in hospitals is difficult to accomplish and is not always efficient [6] in improving antibiotic susceptibilities. In recent years efforts have focused on rationalizing management of the available antimicrobial armory rather than on reducing its total use [7, 8]. Many interventions have been proposed and evaluated to find the best strategy to optimize antibiotic prescription and to reduce resistance rates. In this chapter, we review some of the strategies recommended for antimicrobial control.

14.2 Optimal Use of Antimicrobial Agents

It has been estimated that up to 50% of antibiotic usage in hospital is incorrect for reasons of indication, choice, dosage or duration of therapy. There is evidence that failure to give the appropriate antimicrobial treatment is associated with increases in mortality, length of stay and related costs [9, 10]. Though different, the concepts of adequate (meaning sufficient in terms of dose and frequency of administration) and appropriate antimicrobial therapy (meaning correct in terms of sensitivity in vitro to the targeted organisms) are frequently used interchangeably [11]. However, adequate and appropriate antimicrobial prescription does not always imply optimal therapy. Therapeutic failures have been documented despite adequate and appropriate therapy for severe infections or infections caused by resistant microorganisms in the ICU [12]. Reports on the beneficial effects of combination antibiotic therapy for community-acquired pneumonia (CAP) [13, 14], based on the potential for synergistic bactericidal activity or the immunomodulatory effects of certain agents [15], could extend the definition of optimal therapy beyond the concepts of adequateness and appropriateness of antimicrobial prescription. We could also add that optimal therapy does not necessarily mean effective therapy, because the host defense mechanisms must be "willing and able" to participate in the defense of their own system from the attacking intruder. Experience with immunocompromised patients has demonstrated that optimal antimicrobial therapy does not always guarantee effectiveness.

Clinicians treating critically ill patients should be aware of distinctive pathophysiological characteristics such as variations in extracellular fluid content, mechanical ventilation or in renal or liver function that may influence drug disposition in these sets of patients [16]. As a result, in many cases the peak concentration of the drugs will be lower than the levels expected in non-critically ill patients, and the half life of the administered antibiotic will also be reduced [17–19]. In this setting an increase in the antibiotic dose should be considered in order to achieve the adequate plasma concentration of the antibiotic. The way to optimize delivery of antibiotics depends on the differential pharmacokinetic (relationship between drug concentration and time)/pharmacodynamic (relationship between drug concentration and pharmacologic effect) characteristics of each agent. For concentration-dependent antimicrobials such as fluoroquinolones or aminoglycosides, whose efficacy is mainly related to the C_{max} and AUC/MIC, the least fractioned dosage regimen is preferred, according to toxicity patterns and terminal elimination half life of each antimicrobial [20, 21]. On the other hand, time-dependent antimicrobials such as beta-lactams or vancomycin should reach concentrations above the MIC 40% of the time to achieve optimal bacterial cell killing. To achieve this, it may be necessary to administer the antibiotic as a continuous infusion [22, 23].

Similarly, decreased renal clearance or hepatic failure, other conditions often seen in critically ill patients, may reduce antimicrobial excretion increasing the risk of toxicity. In this setting antimicrobial dosage should be tailored, particularly when renal replacement therapy is required.

Reaching the source of the infection is crucial for adequate antibiotic treatment in critically ill septic patients. Poor penetration of the antibiotic in the infected tissue is associated with decreased treatment effectiveness. Vancomycin's low level of penetration in the lung [24] could explain the poor outcome reported in patients with methicillin resistant *Staphylococcus aureus* (MRSA)-related ventilator-associated pneumonia (VAP) treated with this agent [25]. The timing of initiation and withdrawal of antibiotic therapy may also play an important role in the outcome of critically ill patients with severe infections. A short delay in starting appropriate antibiotic treatment has been associated with a higher mortality rate in hospitalized patients with sepsis [26]. Similarly, shorter antimicrobial treatments have been demonstrated to be as effective as longer ones in the treatment of VAP patients, avoiding the risk of toxicity and the development of resistance [27]. Efforts should be made to administer the adequate antimicrobial therapy at the right time, with the right dose, and for the correct duration, in order to improve patient outcome and to avoid antibiotic-related complications.

14.3 Protocols and Guidelines

Antimicrobial practice guidelines and protocols have emerged as potentially effective strategies for both reducing unnecessary antibiotic administration and optimizing the use of the ones prescribed. The implementation of guidelines or protocols may be confined to an area of the hospital, to a group of practitioners, or to specific clinical conditions. They can be applied to prophylactic, empirical, disease-specific or drug specific use of antimicrobials, and may be implemented in several ways, depending on the particular characteristics of each institution. Computerized antimicrobial guidelines based on patient records are reported to improve antimicrobial-related complications and resistance. Evans et al. [28] reduced antibiotic prescription (67% vs. 73%, $p<0.03$), allergic reactions (6.4% vs. 13%, $p<0.01$), excess drug dosages (16% vs. 36%, $p<0.01$) and antibiotic-susceptibility mismatching (2.2% vs. 18%, $p<0.01$) after implementing a computerized antibiotic guideline for a year. Length of stay in the ICU and hospital and antibiotic costs were also reduced. Non-automated or partially automated systems, usually run by hospital-based quality improvement teams, have demonstrated similar results. Apisarnthanarak et al. [29] reported that the implementation of a less sophisticated multifaceted intervention program of antibiotic control over a 1-year period was highly effective in a 350-bed hospital in a developing country in controlling prescribing practices, antibiotic use rates, bacterial resistance and cost savings. Other initiatives incorporating multidisciplinary teams with pharmacists or infectious disease specialists in the implementation of antibiotic guidelines have also proved their worth in controlling antibiotic use, though they are not always cost-effective [30, 31].

The use of guidelines has become popular worldwide for the treatment of particular clinical conditions such as severe community acquired pneumonia [32] and nosocomial pneumonia [33]. Although a positive impact has been noted on outcome [34], well-controlled studies are still needed to demonstrate a positive impact on antimicrobial usage and resistance in the ICU setting. Despite general acceptance, individual physicians often resist guideline compliance mostly due to a fear of losing clinical autonomy or to the lack of local data on effectiveness [35]. To improve the chances of successful implementation, guidelines should be the result of the combined efforts of physicians, pharmacists, nurses, and other health care practitioners and should be viewed as an adjunct to, rather than a substitute for, a physician's judgment [36], providing an evidence-based approach to practice as well as appropriate feedback and continuous educational programs. Guidelines should not be universal, but should be locally designed, dynamic, institution-specific, multifaceted, and tailored to local susceptibility patterns [37].

14.4 Formulary Restrictions

Restricting the use of certain antimicrobials or antimicrobial classes has been proposed as an effective strategy to control resistance, reduce pharmacy expenses, and avoid adverse drug reactions [38]. Antibiotic restriction programs have been implemented in outbreak situations of microorganisms resistant mostly to broad spectrum agents [6], agents to which resistance has developed rapidly [39, 40], or agents with known toxicity. The implementation of restriction programs varies from institution to institution, but the most frequently used procedure is the requirement of previous authorization by infectious disease specialists [41], which can be obtained through a simple phone call, full written consultation, or more sophisticated automated computer support systems.

However, the implementation of restriction programs in the ICU context has not been uniformly successful. Increases in other non-restricted antimicrobials, ignorance of the complex mechanisms of resistance, or methodological flaws in the implementation of the different restriction policies may explain this failure. Restriction of one antimicrobial can promote a compensatory increase in the use of non-restricted agents, a phenomenon described by Burke as "squeezing the balloon" (constraining one end causes the other end to bulge) [42]. The increase in other non-restricted agents may lead to a rise in total antimicrobial expenditure [43] or promote the development of resistance to the agent used. Rahal et al. [44] reported a 44% decrease in the number of infections caused by cephalosporin-resistant *Klebsiella* after an 80.1% reduction of third-generation cephalosporins in response to an outbreak of this pathogen. However, the same group also reported that the intervention was associated with an unintended 140.6% increase in the use of imipenem and a concomitant 69% increase in infections due to imipenem-resistant *Pseudomonas aeruginosa.*

Few data are currently available on the complexity of factors influencing the development of resistance to an antibiotic or antibiotic class. The theoretical basis for restriction programs is that withholding the use of one antimicrobial would reduce its selective pressure on the exposed microorganisms and curb the development of resistance to the restricted agent. However, it has been recognized that multiresistant organisms can be selected as a result of the use of antimicrobial agents unrelated to the agent of interest. Multiple antimicrobials within the same class or from a different one may be associated with changes in susceptibility to other drugs as a result of genetic linkage of resistance determinants that encode resistance to multiple classes of antibiotics. Several examples have been described in the literature, demonstrating the complexity of the interactions between antimicrobial agents and resistant organisms. It has been reported the association between cephalosporins or agents with potent activity against anaerobic bacteria with colonization by vancomycin-resistant *Enterococcus* [45, 46]. Similarly reports on how decreased resistance of Enterobacteriaceae and *P. aeruginosa* to aminoglycosides has been associated with decreases in cephalosporin use are also available in the literature [47]. Therefore, before implementing a restriction program, the use of multiple agents, similar and dissimilar, should be considered in evaluations of susceptibility trends.

Restriction policies have been increasingly implemented, but always as a response to outbreaks of multiresistant pathogens, along with other infection control measures. Their impact in non-outbreak situations has not yet been comprehensively studied.

14.5 Cycling and Mixing

Antibiotic cycling or rotation involves the scheduled substitution of a single antimicrobial or a class of antimicrobials with another agent or class that exhibits a comparable spectrum of activity. The principle underpinning this strategy is that withdrawal of a class of antibiotics for a pre-determined period will limit the selective pressure exerted by those agents, curbing resistance rates to the drug withdrawn; so when it is reintroduced at a later date, its efficacy will remain intact.

During the last 2 decades, several studies of antimicrobial rotation have been performed. The results are controversial, in terms of microbiological susceptibility [48–55], antimicrobial prescribing practices [56, 57], and clinical outcomes [49, 54, 56, 58] (Table 14.1). However, the evaluation of this strategy is hampered by ambiguities in the definition of the notion of cycling. Cycling/rotation of antibiotics means that the antimicrobial restricted in one cycle should be reintroduced at a later time. This should not be confused with scheduled changes of antibiotics without repeating the process [59–61]. Similarly, other important methodological issues are not clearly defined, meaning that it is difficult to extrapolate the results of cycling trials to other settings. Most cycling trials published to date are implemented as a reactive measure to an outbreak of resistant pathogens (mostly Gram-negative microorganisms), in small, homogeneous sets of patients confined in closed units (mostly ICUs) where pathogens are exposed to heavy antimicrobial pressure. Whether cycling may be effective in preventing the emergence of antimicrobial resistance in a different setting where resistance rates are low and stable has yet to be proved. Similarly, the data available on cycling have not been able to provide answers to practical questions such as what antimicrobials should be cycled, in what order, and for how long. Although some authors have limited the definition of cycling to alternating agents of different classes [64], early studies on antimicrobial cycling have shown that resistance to a particular agent can be controlled by alternating agents of similar class. There is no consensus on the optimal duration of antimicrobial cycling; in the existing literature antimicrobial cycle duration ranges from 1 to 51 months and may be determined on the bases of the local microbiological flora or a preset time period. According to mathematical modeling [62, 63], the dynamics of resistance are driven by the replacement of resistant strains by new admissions. For this reason (mean ICU stay is between 1 and 2 weeks), successful interventions in ICUs should show measurable results within a few weeks or months.

Table 14.1. Summary of antimicrobial cycling studies

Reference	Primary objective	Site	Baseline period/ control group	Cycled agent (time) Cycle order (roman no.)	Clinical outcome	Microbiological outcome	Concomitant intervention/outcomes
Gerding et al. 1991 [41]	Impact of cycling on bacterial susceptibility to GEN	Institution-wide	GEN (3m) I	AMK (26m) II GEN (12m) III AMK (27m) IV GEN (51m) V	NR	↓ GEN R during AMK period and again during GEN periods	Moving to another hospital
Kollef et al. 2000 [49]	Impact of cycling on % inadequate antimicrobial treatment	2 ICUs	CAZ (6m) I	CIP (6m) II FEP (5m) III	↓ Mortality in APII> 15		↓ % inadequate treatment for GNB
Grusson et al. 2000 [42][1]	Impact of cycling on: [1]Incidence on VAP due to R GNB	1 ICU	CTX + CIP (24m)	β-Lactam and AG* [1](1m cycles during 24m) [2](same protocol 3 years)	[1]↓VAP < 7 days [2]↓ VAP and VAP < 5 days	[1]↓ incidence MRSA [2]↓ % *Burkholderia cepacia* in VAP	*Restriction CTX and CIP
2005 [51][2]	[2]Long term effect						
Bradley et al. 1999 [43]	Impact of cycling on acquisition of GRE	Hematology Unit	CAZ (4m) I	TZP* (8m) II CAZ* (4m) III		↓% acquisition GRE on TZP period NS GRE on CAZ cycle	*Introduction of infection control measures
Moss et al. 2002 [45]	Impact of cycling on colonization with resistant bacteria	Paediatric ICU	Standard practice (broad spectrum and de-escalation)	IPM (3m) I and IV TZP (3m) II and V CAZ/CLI (3m) III and VI	No change in prevalence BSI	No change in colonization due to R microorganisms	
Tolzis et al. (2002) [46]	Impact of cycling on colonization by GNB	2 Neonatal ICU	Unrestricted antibiotic use in side-by-side unit	GEN TZP CAZ (1m cycles during 24m)	–	No effect in decreasing the reservoir of R GNB	
Warren et al. (2004) [47][3] Mertz et al. (2005) [50][4]	Impact of cycling on: [3]Acquisition of enteric colonization/infection with R GNB [4]Antibiotic use patterns	Medical ICU	Baseline observation period (5m)	FEP (4m) I and V FQ (4m) II and VI CBP (4m) III and VII TZP (4m) VIII	[3]↑Intensive Care Unit LOS during cycling No significant changes in VAP, BSI or mortality	[3]No changes in acquisition of enteric colonization with R microorganisms	[4]Cycling: ↑ overall antibiotic use. Favors antibiotic heterogeneity
Van Loon et al. (2005) [44]	Impact of cycling on acquisition rate of R GNB to the antibiotic in use	Surgical ICU	NR	FQ (4m) I β-lactams (4 g CFs) (4m) II FQ (4m) III β-Lactam (TZP) (4m) IV	–	↑ Resistant bacteria to the antibiotic in use	Cycling: ↑ overall antibiotic use
Bruno-Murtha et al. (2005) [48]	Feasibility of cycling in community hospital setting	Medical and surgical ward	NR	FQ (3m) I and V BLI (3m) II and VI FQ (3m) III and VII CFs (3m) IV and VIII	No change in nosocomial infections	↓ in the prevalence of GRE and GNB resistant to CAZ	Cycling: ↑ antibiotic use and related cost
Martinez et al. (2006) [69]	Compare cycling vs. mixing of antispseudomonal β-lactams and CIP on acquisition of R GNB	2 Medical ICUs	Medical ICU 1 mixing (4m) ↓ cycling (4m)	Medical ICU 2 cycling (4m) ↓ mixing (4m)	No change in nosocomial infection	↑ acquisition of *Pseudomonas aeruginosa* resistant to selected β-lactams during mixing	

VAP ventilator-associated pneumonia, *R* resistant, *GRE* glycopeptide resistant enterococcus, *GNB* Gram-negative bacteria, *NR* non-reported, *BSI* blood stream infections, *LOS* length of stay, *MRSA* methicillin-resistant *Staphylococcus aureus*, *AMK* amikacin, *CAZ* ceftazidime, *CTX* ceftriaxone, *CIP* ciprofloxacin, *CBP carbapenems*, *QU* quinolones, *CEF* cephalosporins, *VAN* vancomicin, *GEN* gentamicin, *FEP* cefepime, *AG* aminoglycosides, *CL* clindamicin, *TZP* piperacillin/tazobactam, *FQ* fluoroquinolones, *βLI* beta-lactams-beta-lactamase inhibitors, *4gCFs* fourth generation cephalosporins, *IPM* imipenem, *ICU* Intensive Care Unit

Despite many methodological problems, antimicrobial rotation has been proposed as a structured way of introducing antibiotic heterogeneity (that is, the balanced use of the different antimicrobials available) into prescribing practices [57, 64, 65]. Antimicrobial diversity is, according to mathematical models, the most likely way of reducing the selection pressure that leads to antibiotic resistance [66]. However, although global antibiotic use measured at the end of the cycling program may be balanced, the different antimicrobial schedules that compose each cycle can produce substantial disproportions in antibiotic prescription. These periods, of variable duration, in which homogeneous selective antibiotic pressure is imposed, may favor the emergence of resistance. In a 16-month study, van Loon et al. [51] reported that quarterly homogeneous antibiotic exposure alternating quinolones and beta-lactams increased Gram-negative microorganism resistance to the antibiotic in use.

Reports based on mathematical modeling have proposed an alternative antibiotic-use strategy, mixing, in which each patient treated receives one of several antimicrobials used simultaneously, as an effective way to control and prevent resistance [66, 67]. Bergstrom et al. [67] demonstrated that in broad conditions mixing may impose greater heterogeneity than does cycling. This was confirmed in our trial [68], in which implementing a mixing empirical antibiotic therapy for VAP achieved a more heterogeneous antimicrobial pattern than scheduled antibiotic changes in a single ICU. However, clinical trials performed to date have failed to demonstrate the beneficial effects of mixing on resistance that are postulated by theoretical predictions. Martinez et al. [69] reported that a strategy of monthly rotation of anti-*Pseudomona* beta-lactams and ciprofloxacin was more effective than a mixing strategy for controlling the acquisition of *P. aeruginosa* resistant to selected beta-lactams. Our group [68] reported that mixing was inferior to a more individualized approach of antimicrobial therapy based on patient risk factors and previous antibiotic therapy (patient-based period) in controlling potentially resistant Gram-negative microorganisms (Fig. 14.1). An 18% increase in antimicrobial consumption during the mixing period compared with the patient-based period could explain these findings. Several other factors may be responsible for the mismatch between predictions of mathematical models and the clinical practice in cycling and mixing prescription patterns. Different resistant acquisition mechanisms may influence the effect that different antibiotic strategies have on resistant microorganisms [67]. If resistance is acquired by horizontal transfer of genes or accessory elements, the likelihood of hosts acquiring resistance to two antibiotics may be lower with cycling than with mixing. Otherwise, if resistance to two antibiotics is acquired through mutation, cycling would be worse than mixing [70]. On the other hand, low adherence to the antimicrobial prescription patterns reported in some cycling and mixing studies may introduce new variables to the resistance development equations, thus frustrating predictions formulated by mathematical models [51, 68].

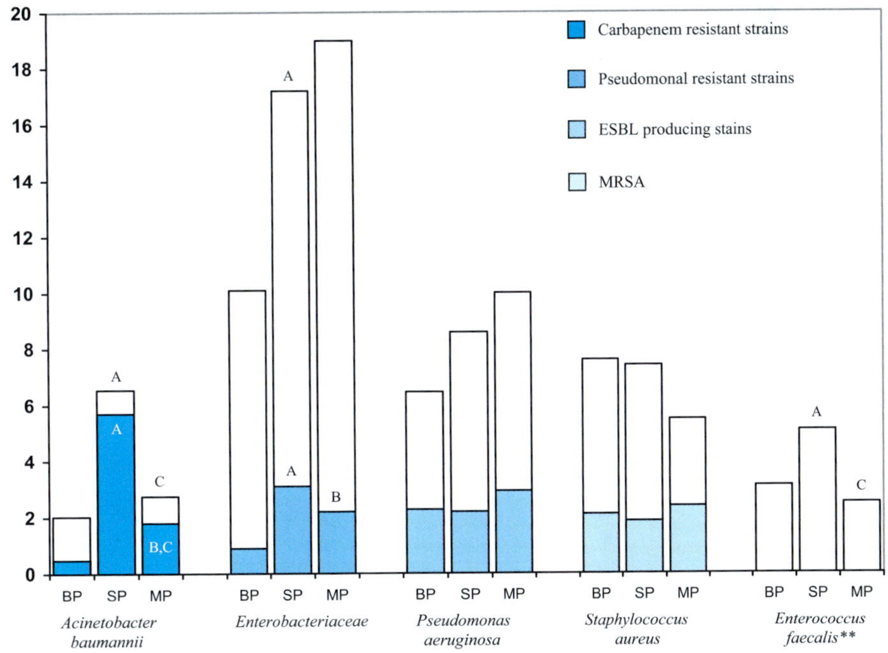

Fig. 14.1. Incidence of patients with clinical isolates of resistant microorganisms. *PB* patient based period, *SP* scheduled changes period, *MP* mixing period. *A* $p < 0.05$ comparing PB with SP; *B* $p < 0.05$ comparing with the PB period with MP; *C* $p < 0.05$ comparing SP with MP. ** <5% of *Enterococcus faecalis* resistant to vancomycin

14.6 De-escalation

De-escalation is a strategy that aims to avoid the overuse of antibiotics while guaranteeing adequate treatment of patients with suspected nosocomial infection. This strategy is a two-step process. The first stage involves the aggressive empirical use of broad-spectrum antimicrobials chosen to cover all likely pathogens. The second stage focuses on simplifying or withdrawing the initial antimicrobial therapy based on microbiological information or on the clinical response observed. (Fig. 14.2)

Failure to administer the correct antimicrobial to a patient with a suspected severe infection has been consistently associated with higher mortality [9, 10]. Initial therapy must be given promptly and should be adequate from the beginning, since modifying an initially inadequate regimen does not improve outcome [9, 71]. In view of the importance of adequate initial antibiotic therapy in critically ill patients with nosocomial infection, de-escalation ensures adequate empirical coverage for all potential pathogens (even those with multidrug resistance) by giving broad-spectrum antimicrobials as first line treatment.

On the other hand, widespread use of broad-spectrum empiric therapy may hasten the emergence of multidrug-resistant pathogens, especially if the pressure exerted by these antimicrobials is prolonged and at suboptimal levels. To minimize the risk of resistance and adverse effects the use of broad-spectrum antimicrobials should be reassessed as soon as microbiological cultures are available or clinical response is evaluated (normally within 48–72 h)

Although no randomized, controlled studies comparing this strategy with other antimicrobial prescription methods have been performed, some authors have evaluated the clinical impact of different de-escalating strategies. Singh et al. [72] used a clinical pulmonary infection scoring system (CPIS) based on clinical, laboratory, microbiological and radiological data in critically ill surgical patients with pulmonary infiltrates to guide the decision process of de-escalating antimicrobial therapy. Although no differences in mortality were reported, reductions in cost, antibiotic usage and antibiotic resistance were observed in the intervention group. Similar findings were reported by Ibrahim et al. [31], who used a clinical guideline consisting of a broad-spectrum antimicrobial empirical therapy for VAP followed by narrowing of antibiotic therapy when a microbiological cause of infection was identified and discontinuation of antibiotic therapy after 7 days if clinical response allowed. Again, no differences in mortality and length of stay were observed, but a higher proportion of patients with adequate therapy and a reduction in the mean duration of therapy was reported.

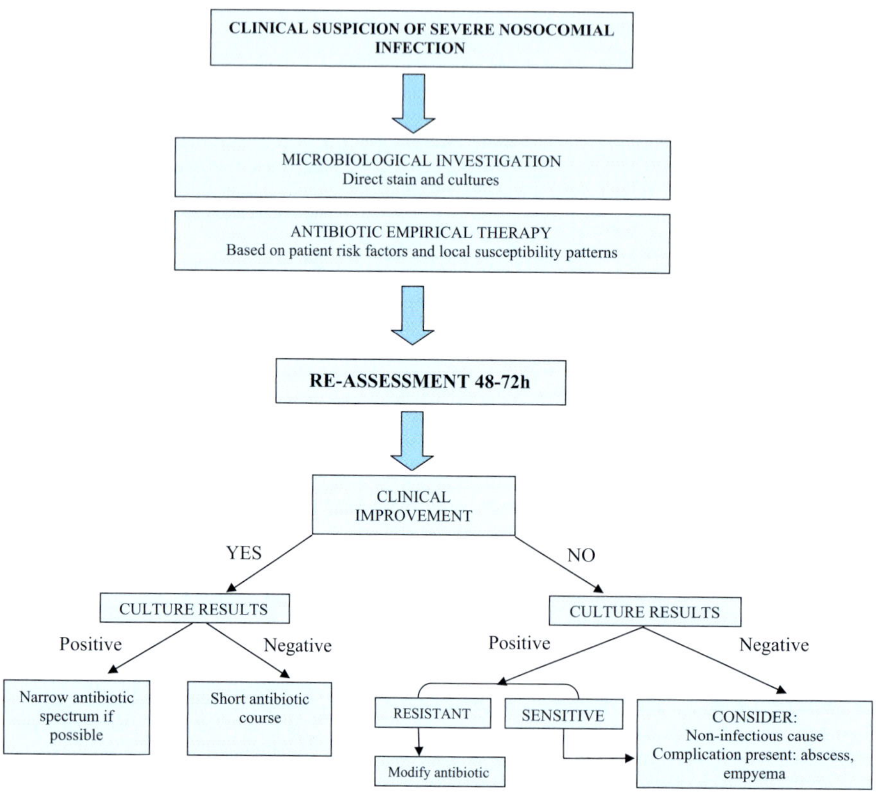

Fig. 14.2. De-escalation scheme

De-escalation was the most important cause of antibiotic modification in our group's experience with 121 VAP episodes [73]. The presence of non-fermenting Gram-negative bacilli and late-onset pneumonia precluded de-escalation in our cohort. The de-escalation rate was not affected by the way in which respiratory samples were taken to guide antibiotic narrowing (i.e., either by quantitative tracheal aspirates or by bronchoscopic techniques).

De-escalation attempts to balance the need for appropriate initial antimicrobial therapy with the need to limit unnecessary antimicrobial exposure. Due to its potential benefits for both the patients and the ICU ecology, this clinical approach has been proposed as a key and responsible strategy for minimizing the development of resistant pathogens and also for containing costs [74].

14.7 Conclusion

Antibiotic use, though important, is only one of the determinants of the complex mechanisms of emergence and development of resistance. Factors related to the patient, the environment and the microorganisms should also be taken into account [75] in our attempts to understand resistance. Controlling all these factors and their complex interactions in the clinical setting is methodologically difficult, a fact that reduces the impact of single interventions on resistance. Predictions formulated by mathematical models able to integrate most of the "known" factors influencing resistance mechanisms have emerged as theoretical solutions to measure different antibiotic/infection control policies. However, these virtual predictions, which hypothesize perfect situations, still have to prove their effectiveness when applied in the imperfect clinical setting. As many authors note, in the clinical setting not even the best planned strategies are always implemented satisfactorily.

Implementation of antimicrobial control studies requires a gigantic effort to control all variables that interfere with the emergence and spread of resistance. Resistant organisms should be characterized phenotypically and genotypically; resistance patterns and their mechanisms should be meticulously identified and monitored; the use of targeted antibiotics should be tightly controlled as well as the implementation of stable infection control methods; and outcome variables should be concisely defined and measured. All this is impossible without the cooperation of a multidisciplinary team and an extensive, continuous education program for all those involved in the management and care of the patient [76].

References

1. Rello J, Rue M, Jubert P, et al. (1997) Survival in patients with nosocomial pneumonia: impact of the severity of illness and the etiologic agent. Crit Care Med 25:1862–1867
2. Carmeli Y, Troillet N, Karchmer AW, et al. (1999) Health and economic outcomes of antibiotic resistance in *Pseudomonas aeruginosa*. Arch Intern Med 159:1127–1132
3. Vincent JL, Bihari DS, Suer PM, et al. (1995) The prevalence of nosocomial infection in intensive care units in Europe. Results of the European prevalence of infection in intensive care (EPIC) study. JAMA 274:639–644
4. Vaque J, Rosello J, Trilla A, et al. (1996) Nosocomial infections in Spain: results of 5 nationwide serial prevalence surveys (EPINE Project, 1990 to 1994). Infect Control Hosp Epidemiol 17:293–297
5. McGowan JE Jr (1987) Is antimicrobial resistance in hospital microorganisms related to antibiotic use? Bull NY Acad Med 63:253–268
6. Cook PP, Catrou PG, Christie JD, et al. (2004) Reduction in broad spectrum antibiotic use is associated with no improvement in hospital antibiogram. J Antimicr Chemother 53:853–859
7. Society for Healthcare Epidemiology of America and Infectious Diseases Society of America Joint Committee on the Prevention of Antimicrobial Resistance (1997) Guidelines for the Prevention of Antimicrobial Resistance in Hospitals. Clin Infect Dis 25: 584–589
8. Goldmann DA, Weinstein R, Wenzel P, et al. (1996) Strategies to prevent and control the emergence and spread of antimicrobial-resistant microorganisms in hospital. A challenge to hospital leadership. JAMA 275:234–240
9. Rello J, Gallego M, Mariscal D, et al. (1997) The value of routine microbiological investigation in ventilator-associated pneumonia. Am J Respir Crit Care Med 156:196–200
10. Rello J, Ollendorf D, Vera-Llonch M, et al. (2002) Epidemiology and outcomes of ventilator-associated pneumonia in a large US database. Chest 122:2115–2121
11. Wunderink R (2004) A long and winding road. Crit Care Med 34:1077–1079
12. Rello J, Jubert J, Valles J (1996) Evaluation of outcome in intubated patients with pneumonia due to *Pseudomonas aeruginosa*. Clin Infect Dis 23:973–978
13. Baddour LM, Yu VL, Lugman KP, et al. (2004) Combination antibiotic therapy lowers mortality among severely ill patients with pneumococcal bacteraemia. Am J Respir Crit Care Med 170:440–444
14. Rello J, Diaz E, Bodi M, et al. (2003) Associations between empirical antimicrobial therapy at the hospital and mortality in patients with severe community-acquired pneumonia. Intensive Care Med 28:1030–1035
15. Pharman MJ (2005) Immunomodulatory effects of antimicrobials in the therapy of respiratory tract infections. Curr Opin Infect Dis 18:125–131
16. Pea F, Pierluigi V, Furlanut M (2005) Antimicrobial therapy in critically ill patients. A review of pathophysiological conditions responsible for altered disposition and pharmacokinetic variability. Clin Pharmacokinet 44:1009–1034
17. Fry DE (1996) The importance of antibiotic pharmacokinetics in critical illness. Am J Surg 172 (Suppl 6A):20S–25S
18. Pinder M, Bellomo R, Lipman J (2002) Pharmacological principles of antibiotic prescription in the critically ill. Anaesth Intensive Care 30:134–144
19. Lugo G, Castañeda-Hernández G (1997) Relationship between hemodynamic and vital support measures and pharmacokinetics variability of amikacin in critically ill patient with sepsis. Crit Care Med 25:806–811

20. Buijk SE, Mouton JW, Gyssens IC, et al. (2002) Experience with a once daily dosing program of aminoglycosides in critically ill patients. Intensive Care Med 28:936–942
21. Olsen KM, Rudis MI, Rebuck JA, et al. (2004) Effect of once-daily dosing vs multiple daily dosing of tobramycin on enzyme markers of nephrotoxicity. Crit Care Med 32:1678–1682
22. Gomez CMH, Cordingly JJ, Palazzo MGA (1999) Altered pharmacokinetics of ceftazidime in critically ill patients. Antimicrog Agents Chemother 43:1798–1802
23. Wysocki M, Thomas F, Wolff MA, et al. (1995) Comparison of continuous with discontinuous intravenous infusion of vancomycin in severe MRSA infection. J Antimicrob Chemother 35:352–354
24. Cruciani M, Gatti G, Lazzarini L et al. (1996) Penetration of vancomycin into human lung tissue. J Antimicrob Chemother 38:865–869
25. Rello J, Torres A, Ricart M, et al. (1994) Ventilator-associated pneumonia by *Staphylococcus aureus*. Comparison of methicillin-resistant and methicillin-sensitive episodes. Am J Respir Crit Care Med 150:1545–1549
26. Meehan TP, Fine MJ, Krumholz HM, et al. (1997) Quality of care, process and outcome in elderly patients with pneumonia. JAMA 278:2080–2084
27. Chastre J, Wolff M, Fagon JY, et al. (2003) Comparison of 8 vs 15 days of antibiotic therapy for ventilator-associated pneumonia in adults. JAMA 290:2588–2598
28. Evans RS, Pestronick SL, Classen DC, et al. (1998) A computer-assisted management program for antibiotics and other antiinfective agents. N Engl J Med 338:232–238
29. Apisarnthanarak A, Danchaivijitr S, Khawacharoenporn T, et al. (2006) Effectiveness of education and an antibiotic-control program in a tertiary care hospital in Thailand. Clin Infect Dis 42:768–775
30. Bailey TC, Ritchie DJ, McMullin ST, et al. (1997) A randomized, prospective evaluation of an interventional program to discontinue intravenous antibiotics at two tertiary care teaching institutions. Pharmacotherapy 17:277–281
31. Ibrahim EH, Ward S, Sherman G, et al. (2001) Experience with a clinical guideline for the treatment of ventilator-associated pneumonia. Crit Care Med 29:1109–1115
32. Niederman MS, Mandel LA, Anzueto A, et al. (2001) Guidelines for the management of adults with community-acquired pneumonia. Diagnosis, assessment of severity, antimicrobial therapy and prevention. Am J Respir Crit Care Med 163:1730–1754
33. Guidelines for the Management of Adults with Hospital-Acquired, Ventilator-Associated and Healthcare-Associated Pneumonia (2005) Am J Respir Crit Care Med 388–416
34. Bodi M, Rodríguez A, Sole-Violan, et al. (2005) Antibiotic prescription for community-acquired pneumonia in the intensive care unit. Impact of adherence to IDSA guidelines on outcome. Clin Infect Dis 41:1709–1716
35. Barclay LP, Hatton RC, Doering PL, et al. (1995) Physicians' perception and knowledge of drug costs: Results of a survey. Formulary 22:231–233
36. Ellrodt AG, Conner L, Riedinger M, et al. (1995) Measuring and improving physician compliance with clinical practice guidelines: A controlled interventional trial. Ann Intern Med 122:277–282
37. Sandiumenge A, Diaz E, Bodi M, et al. (2003) Therapy of ventilator-associated pneumonia. A patient based approach based on the ten rules of "The Tarragona Strategy". Intensive Care Med 29:876–883
38. McGowan JE Jr, Gerdin DN (1996) Does antibiotic restriction prevent resistance? New Horizons 4:370–376
39. Rice LB, Eckstein EC, DeVente J, et al. (1996) Ceftazidime-resistant *Klebsiella pneumoniae* isolates recovered at the Cleveland Department of Veterans Affairs Medical Center. Clin Infect Dis 23:118–124
40. Landman D, Chockalingam M, Quale JM (1999) Reduction in the incidence of methicillin- resistant *Staphylococcus aureus* and ceftazidime-resistant *Klebsiella pneumoniae* following changes in a hospital antibiotic formulary. Clin Infect Dis 28:1062–1066
41. White AC Jr, Atmar RL, Wilson J, et al. (1997) Effects of requiring prior authorization for selected antimicrobials: Expenditures, susceptibilities, and clinical outcomes. Clin Infect Dis 25:230–239
42. Burke JP (1998) Antibiotic resistance-squeezing the Balloon? JAMA 280:1270–1271
43. Rifenburg RP, Paladino JA, Hanson SC, et al. (1996) Benchmark analysis of strategies hospitals use to control antimicrobial expenditures. Am J Health-System Pharmacy 53:2054–2062
44. Rahal JJ, Urban C, Horn D, et al. (1998) Class restriction of cephalosporin use to control total cephalosporin resistance in nosocomial *Klebsiella*. JAMA:1233–1237
45. May AK, Melton SM, McGwin G, et al. (2000) Reduction of vancomycin-resistant enterococcal infections by limitation of broad-spectrum cephalosporin use in trauma and burn intensive care unit. Shock 14:259–264
46. Quale J, Lnadman D, Saurina G, et al. (1996) Manipulation of a hospital antimicrobial formulary to control an outbreak of vancomycin-resistant enterococci. Clin Infect Dis 23:1020–1025
47. Ma MY, Godstein EJ, Friedman MH, et al. (1983) Resistance of gram-negative bacilli as related to hospital use of antimicrobial agents. Antimicrob Agents Chemother 24: 347–352
48. Gerding DN, Larson TA, Hughes RA, et al. (1991) Aminoglycoside resistance and aminoglycoside usage: Ten years of experience in one hospital. Antimicrob Agents Chemother 31:1284–1290
49. Gruson D, Hibert G, Vargas F, et al. (2000) Rotation and restricted use of antibiotics in a medical intensive care unit: Impact on the incidence of ventilator-associated pneumonia caused by antibiotic-resistant Gram negative bacteria. Am J Respir Crit Care Med 162:837–843
50. Bradley SJ, Wilson AL, Allen MC, et al. (1999) The control of hyperendemic glycopeptide-resistant *Enterococcus* spp. on a haematology unit by changing antibiotic usage. J Antimicrob Chemother 43:261–64
51. van Loon H, Vriens M, Fluit A, et al. (2005) Antibiotic rotation and development of Gram-negative antibiotic resistance. Am J Respir Crit Care Med 171:480–487
52. Moss W, Beers C, Johnson E, et al. (2002) Pilot study of antibiotic cycling in a pediatric intensive care unit. Crit Care Med 30:1877–1882
53. Toltzis P, Dul M, Hoyen C, et al. (2002) The effect of antibiotic rotation on colonization with antibiotic-resistant bacilli in a Neonatal Intensive Care Unit. Pediatrics 110:707–711
54. Warren D, Hill G, Merz L, et al. (2004) Cycling empirical antimicrobial agents to prevent emergence of antimicrobial-resistant Gram-negative bacteria among intensive care unit patients. Crit Car Med 32:2450–2456
55. Bruno-Murtha L, Brusch J, Bor D, et al. (2005) A pilot study of antibiotic cycling in the community hospital setting. Infect Control Hospital Epidemiol 26:81–87
56. Kollef MH, Ward S, Sherman G, et al. (2000) Inadequate treatment of nosocomial infections is associated with certain empiric antibiotic choices. Crit Care Med 28:3456–3464
57. Mertz L, Warren D, Kollef M, et al. (2004) Effects on antibiotic cycling program on antibiotic prescribing practices in

an Intensive Care Unit. Antimicrob Agents Chemother 48:2861 - 2865
58. Gruson D, Gilles H, Vargas F, et al. (2003) Strategy of antibiotic rotation: Long-term effect on incidence and susceptibilities of Gram-negative bacilli responsible for ventilator-associated pneumonia. Crit Care Med 31:1908 - 1914
59. Kollef MH, Vlasnik J, Shrpless L, et al. (1997) Scheduled change of antibiotic classes. A strategy to decrease the incidence of ventilator-associated pneumonia. Am J Respir Crit Care Med 156:1040 - 1048
60. Puzniak LA, Mayfield J, Leet T, et al. (2001) Acquisition of vancomycin-resistant enterococci during scheduled antimicrobial rotation in an Intensive Care Unit. Clin Infect Dis 33:151 - 157
61. Raymond DP, Pelletier SJ, Crabtree TD, et al. (2001) Impact of a rotating empiric antibiotic schedule on infectious mortality in an intensive care unit. Crit Care Med 29: 1101 - 1108
62. Lipstich M, Bergstrom C, Levin B (2000) The epidemiology of antibiotic resistance in hospitals: Paradoxes and prescriptions. Proc Natl Acad Sci USA 1938 - 43
63. Bonten M, Austin D, Lipsitch M (2001) Understanding the spread of antibiotic resistant pathogens in hospitals: mathematical models as tools for control. CID 33:1739 - 1746
64. Kollef M (2001) Is there a role for antibiotic cycling in the intensive care unit? Crit Care Med 29:135 - 142
65. Masterson R (2005) Antibiotic cycling: more than it might seem? J Antimicrob Chemother 55:1 - 6
66. Bonhoeffer S, Lipstich M, Levin BR (1997) Evaluating treatment protocols to prevent antibiotic resistance. Proc Natl Acad Sci USA 94:12106 - 12111
67. Bergstrom CT, Lo M, Lipstich C (2004) Ecological theory suggests that antimicrobial cycling will not reduce antimicrobial resistance in hospitals. Proc Natl Acad Sci USA 101:13101 - 13102
68. Sandiumenge A, Diaz E, Rodríguez A, et al. (2006) Impact of diversity of antibiotic use on development of antimicrobial resistance. J Antimicrob Chemother 57:1197
69. Martinez JA, Nicolas JM, Marco F, et al. (2005) Comparison of antimicrobial cycling and mixing in two medical intensive care units. Crit Care Med 34:329 - 335
70. Levin B, Bonten M (2004) Cycling antibiotics may not be good for your health. Proc Natl Acad Sci USA 101: 13101 - 13102
71. Luna CM, Vujacich P, Niderman MS, et al. (1997) Impact of BAL data on the therapy and outcome of ventilator-associated pneumonia. Chest 111:676 - 685
72. Singh N, Rogers P, Atwood CW, et al. (2000) Short course empiric antibiotic therapy for patients with pulmonary infiltrates in the intensive care unit. Am J Respir Crit Care Med 162:505 - 511
73. Rello J, Vidaur L, Sandiumenge A, et al. (2004) De-escalation therapy in ventilator-associated pneumonia. Crit Care Med 32:2183 - 2189
74. Bochud PY, Bonten M, Marchetti O (2004) Antimicrobial therapy for patients with severe sepsis and septic shock: and evidence-based review. Crit Care Med 32:s495 - 512
75. Gould IM (1999) A review of the role of antibiotic policies in the control of antibiotic resistance. J Antimicrob Chemother 43:459 - 465
76. Sandiumenge A, Rello J (2003) Cyclic rotation of antibiotics. Is all that glitters gold? Enferm Infecc Microbiol Clin 21:93 - 100

15 Use of Antibiotics in Pregnant Patients in the Intensive Care Unit

J.-E. Baños, N. Cruz, M. Farré

15.1 Infections and Critical Care in Obstetric Patients

The critically sick pregnant patient is a challenge for the intensive-care physician. Several features, such as physiological changes associated with pregnancy, specific obstetric diseases and the presence of the fetus greatly complicate the assessment and treatment of these patients. The prescription must treat the mother's disease without affecting the fetus [1].

Observational studies have reported that pregnant women take a variety of drugs during pregnancy, including prescription, over-the-counter (OTC) and herbal preparations. Results show that women, in a range of 44 – 96 %, were exposed during pregnancy to at least one drug. An American study, which was carried out between 1996 and 2000 and included 152,531 women, showed that amoxicillin was dispensed to 34,304 women and, in all, more than 90,000 prescriptions were antibiotics [2, 3].

Women can develop an acute illness or pregnancy-induced complications that need intensive drug therapy. Several studies have analyzed obstetric admissions to the ICU [1, 4 – 12]. They conclude that less than 1 % of deliveries are referred to the ICU, mainly for pre-eclampsia, and that maternal mortality may be highly variable, from 0 % in the study of Lapinsky et al. [1] to 20 % in Collop and Sahn's study [8]. Bacterial infections were a significant, although not highly prevalent, cause of admission to the ICU.

Despite infectious diseases not being uncommon during pregnancy and the postpartum period [13, 14], severe infections that need the ICU setting are much less prevalent in this population. Although pneumonia, pyelonephritis and abortion-related infections may be life-threatening, many patients may be treated in regular wards and only severe infections in high-risk patients require critical care. However, it has been shown that infections may account for 24 % of all referral diagnoses [7]. The main causes were sepsis and pneumonia [7, 15, 16].

The characteristics of septic shock in pregnant women have been described in detail by several authors [15 – 17]. The main causes that predispose one to septic shock include pyelonephritis, chorioamnionitis, Stevens-Johnson syndrome, premature rupture of membranes, necrotizing fasciitis, septic abortion and endometritis.

Although the microorganisms that may cause septic shock are mainly Gram-negative bacteria (usually *E. coli*), anaerobes, such as *B. fragilis*, Gram-positive microorganisms, can also be seen [16]. In addition, sexually transmitted infections are particularly relevant for their frequency and significance in pregnancy outcome [18]. Some reviews have examined the relevance of antibiotic treatment to prevent sexually transmitted infections, in order to reduce preterm birth and low birth weight [19]. Both the WHO and CDC have elaborated reference guidelines that recommend drug treatment for sexually transmitted infections in pregnancy [20].

15.2 General Considerations on Antibiotics Use During Pregnancy

Pregnancy always complicates drug treatment. Any drug may be harmful to the mother and also to the fetus so, accordingly, no pharmacological therapy must be initiated unless a clear benefit is expected. Nonetheless, the benefit-risk index recommends active treatment in ICU patients. From the pharmacological point of view, antibiotics are relatively safe drugs when used in pregnant patients with severe infections. Many current antibiotics have been used for at least 30 years and most of them seem to be free of significant teratogenic effects, at least in animals. They are given in short courses, so their adverse effects are rather predictable, but some appreciation of the balance of risks in more serious cases is also needed. However, the understandable reluctance of physicians and pharmaceutical companies to study drugs in pregnant women greatly limits the scientific evidence of the effectiveness and safety of all drugs, including antibiotics, in pregnancy. Three aspects deserve special attention when antibiotic use in pregnant women is considered: the first relates to pharmacokinetic changes induced by pregnancy; the second stresses the potential toxicity to mother and fetus, and the third refers to the effectiveness of antibiotic regimes in obstetric infections.

Pregnancy may change the way in which women handle antimicrobial agents; therefore, some quantitative changes on treatment effects may appear. Most pregnancy-induced effects are of a pharmacokinetic nature. In general, low maternal concentrations have been found after administration of antimicrobials, such as penicillins, cephalosporins, aminoglycosides and erythromycin [21]. The main implications of these findings refer to dosage. For instance, a moderate increase in the dosage of penicillins has been recommended [22, 23]. As a rule, full doses should be used to treat infections in pregnancy and, therefore, treatment regimes should assure that the patient is receiving her right dose. Thus, measurement of blood levels may be needed in some cases when drug pharmacokinetics is influenced by pregnancy. The reason is twofold: first, in order to assure the correct dosage according to the patient and, second, to avoid unnecessary, high blood levels that may be toxic both in the mother and the fetus [13, 24]. Also, the length of treatment should be established by the specific disease and not by the consideration that the patient is pregnant.

In spite of the assertions made in previous paragraphs, a troublesome aspect of antibiotic treatment is its theoretical ability to harm the maternal-fetal unit. Major studies which indicate an association of antibiotic exposure in pregnancy and congenital malformations are lacking [25]. Certain drugs should be avoided, since toxicity may be expected in pregnant women themselves, the fetus, or the neonate. Aminoglycosides, tetracyclines, chloramphenicol and fluoroquinolones must be used with special care in pregnancy [13, 26]. Most authors recognize that tetracyclines and aminoglycosides may have some teratogenic effects [18, 27–29]. Moreover, tetracyclines may have an increased risk of toxicity in the pregnant woman herself [27]. In turn, neonates may be damaged by sulfonamides and chloramphenicol [30]. The withdrawal of these antibiotic drugs is mandatory when the treatment of minor infections by otherwise drug-sensitive bacteria is considered. Nonetheless, these principles may be questioned when severe infection by resistant microorganisms appears.

Obstetric patients admitted to the ICU can be classified into two categories: first, patients with specific obstetric disorders (with approximately 50–80 % of prevalence) and, second, pregnant patients with primarily medical disorders [31]. The most common pregnancy-related infections were chorioamnionitis and puerperal sepsis [32]. The most common unrelated infections, but complicating pregnancy, are respiratory and urinary tract infections [13]. In all, morbidity rates of severe obstetric complications range from 0.8 % to 8.2 %, and mortality rates from 0.02 % to 37 %. The great variability is explained by its different case definition, methodology and especially because of differences in health quality control among countries [33].

Clinical trials showing efficacy of antibiotics in pregnant women are scarce if compared with other areas of drug therapy. This paucity of studies is so important that some textbooks rely on the experience or the personal opinion of the authors [14]. Hence, this chapter will avoid any reference to the specific therapeutics of infections seen in the ICU and will only consider the first two topics described earlier, i.e., the pharmacokinetic changes induced by pregnancy and the safety of antibiotic drugs in the mother and the fetus.

In conclusion, the treatment of maternal infections should follow the general principles of pharmacological therapy in pregnant women. Moreover, drug efficacy ranks first in ICU patients, although the safety of the embryo or fetus should always be considered. Antibiotics must be chosen by susceptibility studies or, more often, by empirical evaluation of the most likely group of microorganisms and their most probable antibiotic susceptibility. Only when this aspect has been considered should embryonic or fetal safety concerns arise [18, 22, 34].

15.3 Pregnancy-Related Pharmacokinetic Changes of Clinical Relevance

Drug pharmacokinetics is mainly affected by pregnancy in two ways. The first concerns the progressive changes in the maternal physiology during pregnancy, which are most evident during the third trimester and the immediate postpartum. These changes affect the absorption, distribution, metabolism and elimination of some drugs. The second way is related to the placental-fetal unit/compartment and modifies the amount of drug crossing the placenta, the fraction metabolized by the placenta and the distribution and elimination of the drug by the fetus [35]. The most relevant changes are observed in drug distribution and in substances predominantly eliminated, unchanged, in urine.

15.3.1 Absorption

Digestive physiology is altered by pregnancy, as shown by a delay in both gastric and intestinal motilities. The increase of plasma progesterone levels during pregnancy accounts for a 30–50 % increase in the gastric and intestinal emptying time. Decreased gastric acid secretion (40 % less than in non-pregnant women) and peptic activity, as well as an increase in mucus secretion, convey an increase in gastric pH. This could influence the ionization of weak acids and bases and may result in unpredictable absorption of orally administered drugs. A recent review examined the differences in oral bioavailability of different drugs, including β-lactamic antimicrobials, between pregnant and non-pregnant women. The results did not show any significant difference in bioavailability during pregnancy [36].

Increased cardiac output during pregnancy increases blood flow to other organs and tissues. Thus, drugs given by the intramuscular route may be more rapidly absorbed. The increase in the pulmonary blood flow could favor alveolar uptake of drugs administered by inhalation [37].

Although the final consequences of these changes are probably of minor importance, the physiological changes that occur in pregnancy theoretically alter drug absorption and should be taken into account [36].

15.3.2 Distribution

The plasma volume expands by approximately 40%, starting around the 6th week of pregnancy, reaching a plateau at 30–34 weeks of gestation. Therefore, the volume of distribution (Vd) of some drugs may be altered [38]. The total mean increase in body water is from 7 to 8.5 l, most of which is extracellular, distributed to the placenta, fetus and amniotic fluid (60%) and maternal tissues (40%). This increase in the apparent Vd can diminish maternal peak serum-drug concentrations (C_{max}) of many drugs. Those drugs that are mainly distributed in water compartments and have a relatively small Vd will show the most important decrease in C_{max}. In consequence, increased drug dosage requirements would be needed to reach similar plasma concentrations [39]. Moreover, the body fat increases by an average of 25% during pregnancy, and, therefore, plasma concentration of drugs which are mainly distributed to fat tissues are decreased [22].

Plasma volume expands faster than albumin production, creating a physiological dilutional hypoalbuminemia, with a decreasing binding capacity. Albumin concentrations decrease during the second trimester and continue to decline throughout pregnancy, reaching concentrations of approximately 70–80% of normal values at the time of delivery [40]. The free fraction of highly protein-bound drugs increases. This increase in free fraction may lead to a decrease in total drug concentrations, because more drug is available to be metabolized by the hepatic enzymes or eliminated from the body. The unbound drug can more easily penetrate tissues and may have a greater effect than expected from total serum levels. The direct determination of free-drug concentrations in critical patients is recommended [22, 35]. These changes can become clinically significant for highly protein-bound drugs with predominant hepatic elimination with a low extraction ratio and/or for those with a narrow therapeutic window [41].

Cardiac output also increases in parallel to plasma volume, with values 30–50% above normal during the third trimester. In addition, pregnancy produces regional blood changes that can affect distribution and elimination. At term, blood flow increases to the uterus and to the kidneys, representing 25% and 20% of cardiac output, respectively.

15.3.3 Hepatic Metabolism

The elevated progesterone and estrogen concentrations observed in pregnancy appear to activate hepatic microsomal enzymes, such as different isoenzymes of cytochrome P450 (CYP) including CYP3A4, CYP 2D6 and CYP 2C9 [36]. This increased hepatic activity can accelerate the biotransformation of the parent drug to active and inactive metabolites. If the drug is being transformed into less active or inactive products, an increased dose of the parent drug or a decreased dosing interval may be necessary. On the other hand, the elimination of other drugs could be reduced by competitive inhibition of microsomal oxidases by progesterone and estradiol. The importance of these changes should be considered for each drug, and no general rule can be applied [22, 35].

15.3.4 Renal Elimination

Renal excretion of drugs is dependent on the glomerular filtration rate, active tubular secretion and/or reabsorption. Renal blood flow and the glomerular filtration rate can increase up to 50% by the 4th month and continue to increase throughout pregnancy when compared with postpartum values [29]. There is limited knowledge on the effect of pregnancy on tubular secretion and/or reabsorption and, therefore, of their relative importance on the renal drug transporters [42].

The consequences of the above-mentioned changes are an important increase in the clearance of substances that are mainly eliminated unchanged in urine. As an example, the clearance of ampicillin doubles during pregnancy, and plasma maximal concentrations are reduced by 60%. An increased dose or a shortened dosing interval may be needed to achieve desired steady-state concentrations [22–35].

15.3.5 Transplacental Passage of Drugs

Many of the pharmacologically active compounds can move bidirectionally across the placenta as a consequence of passive diffusion. Drugs that cross the placenta more easily include small (with low molecular weight), lipophilic, non-ionized molecules and those with a large free fraction or low protein binding. Also, differences in binding capacity between maternal and fetal serum can result in higher fractions of free drug in the fetus (especially if the drug has low protein binding) [23]. Furthermore, some drugs use facilitated diffusion mechanisms, with the assistance of carriers, such as cephalosporins, and would be expected to reach a higher peak of concentration in the fetus than from simple diffusion [43]. The active transport mechanism is too slow and it has received minor attention in scientific reviews.

The placenta increases its surface area and thins as pregnancy advances, these changes being proportional to age and fetal weight. The main effect is an enhancement of transplacental diffusion from the mother to the fetus. The fetal plasma pH is slightly more acidic than the maternal pH, so, therefore, weak bases can be concentrated in the fetus (ion trapping) [35]. An exception are ampicillin and methicillin, strongly acidic antibiotics, which have a complete placental transfer [36]. The equilibrium of maternal-fetal drug concentrations depends on the physicochemical properties of the drug. The time to reach similar maximal concentrations in both sides of the placenta is delayed in the fetus side [35].

The placenta and the fetus are able to metabolize drugs. However, most enzymatic processes are immature in the fetus; thus its contribution to drug elimination is only marginal. Both CYP and uridine diphosphate glucuronosyltransferase isoenzymes (UGT) are present in the fetus, but at very low levels in comparison to the mother. In the fetal liver, CYP 3A7 is the predominant one. The CYP 3A4 levels, the most abundant in adults, are very low in the fetus [44]. The activities of some CYP in the fetus ranged from 1% to 30% of adult values during the pregnant period, and many UGT values ranged from 7.5% to 43% [45].

The overall effect of the above-mentioned pharmacokinetic changes is the decrease by 10–50% of drug concentrations during late pregnancy compared to non-pregnant females. In the early postpartum period, pharmacokinetics remains similar to those seen during the third trimester of pregnancy despite the removal of the placenta and the fetus. The therapeutic implications of these changes should be kept in mind during the postpartum period.

15.4 Antibiotics and Pregnancy

The body of scientific evidence that justifies and guides the rational use of antibiotics in pregnancy is scarce and incomplete due to ethical and legal issues. There are justified reasons for the limited number of clinical studies but, as a consequence, many pharmacological treatments in pregnancy are empirically based and often following clinical and personal experiences as the main criteria to make a choice. Physiological changes during pregnancy could modify pharmacokinetics of the antibiotics, leading to an increase or reduction of plasmatic levels and to toxicity and therapeutic failure, respectively [46].

A brief consideration of some commonly used drugs of each group follows. A detailed review of the general use of antibiotics in pregnancy can be found elsewhere [14, 16, 22, 26, 35, 37, 47, 48]. Table 15.1 shows the United States Food and Drug Administration (FDA) Pharmaceutical Pregnancy Categories.

15.4.1 Penicillins

Penicillins are among the oldest known antibiotics, with approximately 60 years of clinical experience [49]. Penicillins are widely used during all phases of pregnancy, mainly indicated to treat syphilis, pyelonephritis, upper respiratory tract and urinary infections, and for prophylaxis of bacterial endocarditis.

Table 15.1. United States Food and Drug Administration (FDA) Pharmaceutical Pregnancy Categories

Pregnancy Category A	Adequate and well-controlled studies have failed to demonstrate a risk to the fetus in the first trimester of pregnancy (and there is no evidence of risk in later trimesters).
Pregnancy Category B	Animal reproduction studies have failed to demonstrate a risk to the fetus and there are no adequate and well-controlled studies in pregnant women or animal studies have shown an adverse effect, but adequate and well-controlled studies in pregnant women have failed to demonstrate a risk to the fetus in any trimester.
Pregnancy Category C	Animal reproduction studies have shown an adverse effect on the fetus and there are no adequate and well-controlled studies in humans, but potential benefits may warrant use of the drug in pregnant women despite potential risks.
Pregnancy Category D	There is positive evidence of human fetal risk based on adverse reaction data from investigational or marketing experience or studies in humans, but potential benefits may warrant use of the drug in pregnant women despite potential risks.
Pregnancy Category X	Studies in animals or humans have demonstrated fetal abnormalities and/or there is positive evidence of human fetal risk based on adverse reaction data from investigational or marketing experience, and the risks involved in use of the drug in pregnant women clearly outweigh potential benefits.

Several pharmacokinetic studies of penicillins have been performed in pregnant women [47, 50–53]. Most penicillins cross the placenta, but drugs with high protein binding (oxacillin, cloxacillin, dicloxacillin, nafcillin) have a lower ability to cross the placental barrier, resulting in lower fetal tissue and amniotic fluid levels. In contrast, poorly bound penicillins (ampicillin, amoxicillin, methicillin) cross it better and achieve concentrations in the amniotic fluid 0.5–1 times higher than the maternal plasma concentration [35] and can lead to a high concentration in the blood of the newborn [54]. Due to its pharmacokinetic properties (increased blood volume and renal clearance), plasmatic concentration of penicillins can be reduced by up to 50% in pregnant women [23]. Therefore, higher doses could be used to obtain an adequate antibiotic concentration.

In general, β-lactam antibiotics should be considered as probably safe in pregnancy [19]. No adverse effects should be expected in the first trimester. Despite the penicillins' lack of direct toxicity, they are able to cause allergic reactions in the mother and the fetus may be sensitized [13, 54]. The prevalence of allergic reactions is 5–10% in the population [55].

Although little information is available, many clinical studies carried out recently have contributed to additional evidence of penicillin safety and low toxicity. Study reports about phenoxymethylpenicillin, pivampicillin, oxacillin, dicloxacillin, amoxicillin, amoxicillin plus clavulanic acid and ampicillin confirmed the safety of these drugs during pregnancy [49, 56–61]. In fact, there is no evidence of embryotoxic, fetotoxic or teratogenic effects [62]. However, unconditional confidence on new drugs, even if they are from the same β-lactam group, is not recommended and the FDA classifies all penicillins in Category B.

Penicillin G (benzylpenicillin) has been used to treat maternal infections for many years and is the agent of choice for the management of pneumococcal and meningococcal infections. It quickly crosses the placenta and reaches the fetal circulation and the amniotic fluid [63]. At term, maternal serum and amniotic fluid concentrations were equal 60–90 min after i.v. injection and continuous infusions of penicillin G produced similar concentrations in maternal serum, cord serum, and amniotic fluid [64]. Nathan et al. [65] have analyzed the pharmacokinetic properties of benzathine penicillin G (benzathine benzylpenicillin) to treat syphilis in pregnant women in the week prior to delivery. Drug concentrations in maternal and fetal tissues showed a wide variability, so the authors recommended caution when treating pregnant women at this stage due to the risk that altered pharmacokinetics might affect drug efficacy.

Although its early use was associated with an increase in abortion risk, no reports have appeared since 1950 supporting this. There is only one reviewed reference to congenital abnormalities associated with it, but no causal relationship to penicillin G could be shown [50]. In further studies including a large number of pregnant women exposed to penicillin G, no evidence has been found to date suggesting a relationship with major or minor malformations. From these data, it is unlikely that penicillin G should be considered as teratogenic.

Penicillin V (phenoxymethylpenicillin) is used in streptococcal pharyngitis. A study analyzing the pharmacokinetics of penicillin V during the last two trimesters of pregnancy showed faster elimination rates of the drug from the plasma of the pregnant patients compared with non-pregnant women [66]. No evidence was found linking penicillin V and birth defects. Therefore, the probability that penicillin V is teratogenic is very low [47].

Several authors have studied the pharmacokinetic properties of ampicillin in pregnant women [29, 47, 67]. Plasma levels of ampicillin are lower in women during pregnancy than in non-pregnant patients, and this fact is observed throughout the pregnancy [47]. It seems that pregnant women will require higher doses of ampicillin to achieve comparable plasmatic levels [68]. In one study [69], ampicillin pharmacokinetics was compared during and after the pregnancy in the same women. It was shown that pregnancy significantly increased the elimination rate constant, decreased the area under the curve (AUC) by 20% and increased the total body clearance. This antibiotic rapidly crosses the placenta and drug levels, exceeding the minimum inhibitory concentrations (MIC) for most microorganisms, causing intrauterine infections which can be found in fetal blood and amniotic fluid [70]. The drug was given i.v. to women of 15–40 weeks of gestation. When given by infusion to patients at term, the cord to maternal ratios increased over time and approached unity within 2 h. Cord concentrations were higher than 5 mg/l for at least 4 h. Amniotic fluid levels could be detected in 90 min, reaching 20% of peak maternal serum concentrations in 8 h.

Ampicillin has been extensively used in the last half of pregnancy to prevent maternal or fetus infections in at-risk pregnancies like, for instance, premature rupture of membranes [71]. Although it has been linked to congenital heart disease [72], other studies have concluded that it is unlikely that ampicillin is teratogenic [47, 50, 73].

Bacampicillin, a pro-drug of ampicillin, has been poorly studied in pregnant women, but there is no available data linking bacampicillin and birth defects [47].

Amoxicillin is often used to treat bacteriuria in pregnancy [74] and it is also used in the second half of pregnancies in which either the woman or the fetus is at risk for infections because of premature rupture of membranes [75]. Amoxicillin has been administered orally to patients at term [76]. Blood amoxicillin concentrations peaked 4.5 h after administration in both the mother and the fetus, and then rapidly declined. Therefore, it would appear that amoxicillin transfers across the placenta completely.

No birth defect linking amoxicillin has been described [47, 60, 73]; nevertheless, a modification of bowel flora and sensitization could be possible in the neonate. A case report of skin rash has been reported in a neonate after maternal consumption of amoxicillin [60].

Several studies have described the pharmacokinetics of amoxicillin and clavulanic acid for various infections in pregnant women [77, 78]. Both drugs cross the placenta quickly and maternal serum and umbilical cord peak levels occur at 2 h with a fetal:maternal ratio of 0.56. No adverse effects in the fetus or in the newborn linked to the combination have been observed at usual doses (250/500 mg amoxicillin and 125 mg potassium clavulanate t.i.d. for 3–10 days) [47, 61, 79]. Clavulanic acid has no direct toxicity since a study showed no alteration at birth of 556 children exposed to the drug during the first trimester [54], although it has been suggested to avoid its routine use until more evidence is available [13].

The antistaphylococcal penicillins (dicloxacillin, methicillin, oxacillin) cross the placental barrier and reach the fetal circulation and amniotic fluid, but due to their high protein binding (95–97%), the fetal-maternal plasma-concentration ratio is lower compared to other penicillins [80–83]. When methicillin was infused in pregnant women, it reached similar concentrations in the fetal and maternal sera within 30 min, and equilibration occurred within 1 h [84]. No evidence has been found linking congenital defects and dicloxacillin, cloxacillin, methicillin, nafcillin or oxacillin, and these drugs should probably be considered non-teratogenic [47, 73].

The carboxypenicillins (carbenicillin, its derivative carbenicillin indanyl, ticarcillin) are used due to their antipseudomonal activity. Like other penicillins, these drugs are probably safe. There is limited information on the effects of these drugs on pregnancy and therefore they should be reserved to treat severe infections by susceptible bacteria. Carbenicillin crosses the placenta and distributes itself to fetal tissues, but concentrations in amniotic fluid are only a tenth of maternal peak concentrations [84, 85]. Ticarcillin rapidly crosses the placenta and significant drug levels can be found in amniotic fluid and in fetal circulation [86]. No adverse effects on the fetus have been described associated with either carboxypenicillin [47, 73].

The general considerations suggested for carboxypenicillins also apply to ureidopenicillins. Piperacillin, a piperazine derivative of ampicillin, has been used in the last weeks of pregnancy to delay delivery in women with premature rupture of the membranes [87] and for urinary tract infections. When given during pregnancy, piperacillin crosses the placenta rapidly but the fetal:maternal serum level ratio is low [88, 89]. Bourget et al. [90] have studied the pharmacokinetics of the intermittent administration of piperacillin-tazobactam in pregnant women. The kinetic behavior of both drugs was almost identical, with an increase of the Vd and clearance of the combination, probably by a decrease in AUC concentrations. The maternal blood levels were less than the MIC of the target organism at 4 h. Therefore, the authors suggest that continuous infusion is a better option than intermittent administration. Following this assumption, piperacillin-tazobactam should be infused at an hourly rate of 8 mg/min. The transplacental transfer was significant, but not complete, and penetrated the amniotic fluid poorly [91].

The C_{max} after administration of piperacillin was lower in pregnant than in non-pregnant women, whereas the total clearance was faster in the former [89]. Azlocillin has also been studied after i.v. administration in late pregnancy [92]. Concentrations equilibrated between the maternal and fetal compartments 2–3 h after administration. This drug penetrated the amniotic fluid and reached concentrations similar to maternal serum concentrations [35].

No reports linking its use with congenital defects in humans have been described. It was used during 24 and 35 weeks of gestation in women with premature rupture of membranes and no adverse maternal or fetal effects were observed [47, 54].

15.4.2 Cephalosporins

After penicillins, cephalosporins are probably the most prescribed antibiotics during pregnancy. The cephalosporins are largely used in pregnant women, for the prophylaxis of post-cesarean section infections, minor urinary infections, acute pyelonephritis and in cases of bacterial resistance to other antibiotics [93].

This group includes a large number of compounds that may be administered by the oral and/or parenteral route. They are classified in a rather arbitrary way into first, second, third and fourth generation cephalosporins, and this criterion follows the differences in their antibacterial activity.

Cephalosporins may be considered as probably safe, but uncertainty with the newer compounds is a consequence of the scant information available. Some of the injectable cephalosporins are a reasonable choice for treatment of infections in critically ill patients. It has been suggested that some cephalosporins, such as cefamandole, might interfere with vitamin K metabolism and should be avoided [13]. All cephalosporins are classified in Category B by the FDA.

As with penicillins, maternal serum concentrations of cephalosporins are also reduced because of increased renal clearance associated with pregnancy and, therefore, an increase in dosage should be considered [94]. This consideration has special importance when bactericidal concentrations must be attained, as what happens in severe infections. Pharmacokinetic data obtained with cephalosporins showed that maternal serum levels are only a fraction of those obtained in the absence of pregnancy. First-generation cephalosporins do not cross the placenta easily and the fetal serum concentrations rarely exceed 10% of maternal concentrations [95].

The mean serum concentration of cephalexin, cephalotin and cefazolin are all considerably lower in pregnant women when compared with non-pregnant women [37].

Cephalexin is the most widely used cephalosporin during pregnancy and no risk of teratogenicity has been established in women using these antibiotics to date [96]. Cephalotin is a parenteral first-generation cephalosporin widely used during all stages of pregnancy but should be used cautiously in neonatal jaundice because of the risk of kernicterus [62].

Second- and third-generation cephalosporins do a little better at this point, but fetal concentrations are still significantly below maternal levels. An exception to this rule is ceftizoxime [97]. However, transplacental transfer of cephalosporins is also fairly rapid and adequate bactericidal levels are reached in fetal structures [35].

There is no clinical evidence associating the use of cephalosporins during pregnancy and the presence of congenital abnormalities or lethal teratogenic potential [14, 54, 96]. Some animal studies have revealed potential, adverse fetal effects with cephalosporins containing the *N*-methylthiotetrazole side-chain [98]. Some of the second and third cephalosporins have such a side-chain. These reasons have been invoked by some authors to suggest the theoretical advantage of drugs devoid of the *N*-methylthiotetrazole side-chain when indicated during pregnancy [98].

Cefuroxime is a semisynthetic second-generation cephalosporin. It is used by oral and parenteral routes and readily crosses the placenta in late pregnancy. For this reason, it has been used for pyelonephritis. No adverse effects associated with the drug in the newborn have been reported after in utero exposure [54].

Cefepime and ceftriaxone are parenteral cephalosporins of the third generation with high protein-binding and a prolonged half-life. A possible association has been suggested between ceftriaxone (none for cefepime) and cardiovascular defects, but it was not possible to refute other causal concomitant factors such as the mother's disease and concurrently used drugs [54].

Finally, ceftazidime, another parenteral cephalosporin of the third generation, is also considered safe to use during pregnancy [80].

15.4.3 Other β-Lactam Antibiotics

Imipenem, meropenem, ertapenem and aztreonam are other β-lactam antibiotics that may be used in severe infections and could be indicated for use during pregnancy to treat severe pyelonephritis or community-acquired pneumonia, which are not caused by *P. aeruginosa* [99]. Some other β-lactam compounds devoid of antibiotic activity are the β-lactamase inhibitors, such as clavulanic acid (potassium clavulanate), sulbactam and tazobactam. Clavulanic acid and tazobactam have been considered when amoxicillin and piperacillin have been previously reviewed.

Imipenem-cilastatin cross the placenta and their pharmacokinetics during pregnancy has been evaluated [100]. It was shown that after a single dose, plasma concentration in pregnant women was significantly lower than in non-pregnant women, both in early and late pregnancy, and clearance from plasma was faster. Peak amniotic fluid:maternal blood ratios for imipenem-cilastatin were approximately 0.30 and 0.45, respectively [101].

Although no clinical reports describing the use of this antibiotic in the first trimester are available, it seems to be a safe and effective agent during the perinatal period [54]. No reports have been found to describe the use of meropenem in human pregnancy [54]. There is little or no substantiated clinical experience about the use of imipenem in pregnancy and no reports of teratogenicity exist. It is classified in Category C by the FDA [26].

After a single dose of 1 g i.v of aztreonam, detectable concentrations of the antibiotic in fetal serum and amniotic fluid were found. The great majority of studies about the use of aztreonam in pregnant women concluded that the drug is safe [102]. On the other hand, studies performed during the first semester were inconclusive [103]. Therefore, the teratogenic potential of aztreonam has not been well established. It is classified in Category B by the FDA but there is no guarantee that this drug has a safe use, especially in the first 3 months of pregnancy [104].

Ertapenem is a carbapenem agent, introduced in the American market at the end of 2001 and during 2002 in Europe as a parenteral beta-lactam antibiotic. Ertapenem crosses the placental barrier in animal studies without toxicity [105]. No adequate and well-controlled studies in pregnant women were performed, so this drug should be used during pregnancy only if clearly needed. It is also classified in Category B by the FDA.

Meropenem is a broad-spectrum, carbapenem antibiotic, given i.v. There is scarce knowledge about its transplacental transfer and also about its human pregnancy experience. Nevertheless, as a carbapenem-group drug, it is considered safe to be used during the perinatal period (after the 28th week of gestation). The fetal risk before this period is unknown and it is also classified in Category B by the FDA.

15.4.4 Vancomycin

Vancomycin is a useful antibiotic used in pregnancy infections by Gram-positive bacteria when either the organisms are resistant to less toxic anti-infectives (penicillins, cephalosporins) or the patient is allergic to these agents [54]. Vancomycin crosses the placenta and reaches fetal concentrations that are sufficient to treat chorioamnionitis. This antibiotic seems to accumulate in amniotic fluid after repeated administration. The cord concentrations are about 76% of maternal serum levels [106].

Vancomycin administration has been related to the induction of fetal bradycardia. There is one report describing ototoxicity in newborns exposed in utero to the drug. The loss of hearing was recovered after 3–12 months. The renal function of newborns exposed to vancomycin was normal, suggesting the lack of nephrotoxicity [107]. In addition, vancomycin can produce the "red man" syndrome, which is characterized by great histamine liberation after the drug's injection, causing intense uterine contraction; premature labor has been associated with vancomycin use [108]. Therefore, despite the use of vancomycin possibly being useful during the second and third trimesters of pregnancy, there is scarce experience concerning this issue. Moreover, although usual doses of vancomycin do not seem to threaten the fetus, it is classified by the FDA in Category C.

15.4.5 Teicoplanin

Teicoplanin is a glycopeptide antibiotic with a similar molecular structure to that of vancomycin and it is usually indicated for patients who have limited venous access or in whom beta-lactam antibiotics are contraindicated. It is used for the same indications as vancomycin. Despite its long half-life, the incidence of "red man" syndrome is lower than the one described with vancomycin. Until now, there is no safety information regarding the use of teicoplanin during pregnancy and it has still not been approved by the FDA [26].

15.4.6 Fosfomycin

Fosfomycin is indicated against a wide range of common urinary tract pathogens. In pregnant women (28–32 weeks) given a single oral dose of 3 g of fosfomycin, the maximal blood concentrations were lower than those observed in non-pregnant women (20.5 μg/ml at 2 h). Fosfomycin crosses the placenta slowly and reaches concentrations in cord and fetal blood of 50% lower than those in maternal blood. Fosfomycin has been safely used during all trimesters of pregnancy, and no teratogenic effects have been reported [54]. Nevertheless, since adequate and well-controlled studies in humans have not been performed, the FDA classifies it in Category B [109].

15.4.7 Aminoglycosides

In general the aminoglycosides have been used in association with penicillins against *P. aeruginosa* infections during pregnancy. Serum levels of aminoglycosides decreased during pregnancy. The half-life of these drugs is shorter and total body clearance is increased. Aminoglycosides are distributed primarily into extracellular water. Moreover, the increased extracellular fluid during pregnancy increases the Vd and, as a consequence, serum concentrations diminish. Aminoglycosides are also eliminated by the kidney via glomerular filtration, and the increased renal clearance observed in pregnancy contributes to a shorter half-life. Therefore, patients may have increased dosage requirements. Therapeutic drug monitoring, including peak and trough serum concentrations, is needed to ensure adequate dosage [14].

The aminoglycosides cross the placenta and concentrations in fetal plasma are lower than those reached in the mother. The penetration of aminoglycosides in the amniotic fluid is low (30% of maternal serum concentrations), but considerable concentrations of aminoglycosides have been found in fetal renal tissues. The potential ototoxicity is the major concern of its use during pregnancy, which is markedly associated with streptomycin and also with kanamycin [29].

Streptomycin crosses the placenta rapidly and attains concentrations in amniotic fluid and the placenta lower than 50% of those of maternal blood. The use of streptomycin to treat tuberculosis during pregnancy seems safe, but there are a few cases of the eighth cranial-nerve damage in newborns exposed to streptomycin. This ototoxicity included cochlear or vestibular effects [29]. Many reports have associated otoxicity and nephrotoxicity in newborns of mothers exposed to the drug in the first trimester of pregnancy. Although the incidence is probably low, this drug is not recommended in pregnancy [54], so the FDA classifies streptomycin as in Category D.

Gentamicin is the most widely used aminoglycoside, with a preferential use in treating pyelonephritis resistant to beta-lactam agents [93]. During pregnancy, gentamicin plasma concentrations are lower than those in non-pregnant women and could be subtherapeutic in some infections, therefore requiring a dose increase. Gentamicin rapidly crosses the placenta, and maximal cord levels are 34–44% of maternal serum concentrations, peaking 1–2 h after i.m. administration. Amniotic fluid levels are maximal 8 h after treatment. Ototoxicity has not been reported after its use during pregnancy [110, 111], but some studies have shown nephrotoxicity in newborn babies [112]. Gentamicin is classified in Category C by the FDA.

Tobramycin and amikacin cross the placenta and are distributed in most fetal tissues except brain. The highest fetal concentrations are observed in kidney and urine. Cord concentrations at term were 33–50% of maternal serum levels [113]. No reports linking the use of tobramycin or amikacin and congenital defects have been located [23]. As with other aminoglycosides, possible ototoxicity and nephrotoxicity are major concerns when used during pregnancy [13]. It is classified in Category D by the FDA.

The use of any aminoglycoside agent with neuromuscular blockers in myasthenic patients could alter the labor process or even cause respiratory failure. Also, the concomitant use of aminoglycosides and cephalosporins could enhance nephrotoxicity [29]. Therefore, as a general concern, gentamicin should be reserved for restricted indications and administered in the smallest possible dosage during pregnancy [26].

15.4.8 Macrolides

The use of macrolides in pregnant women is limited to treating syphilis and upper-respiratory tract infections in patients with an allergic history to penicillin. Moreover, it has been used to treat toxoplasmosis and urethritis caused by *C. trachomatis* [23].

Erythromycin has been used during pregnancy for the treatment of mycoplasma infections. A randomized, controlled trial in the United States has shown that treatment with erythromycin between 26 and 30 weeks' gestation reduces the incidence of premature rupture of membranes by 10% [19]. Erythromycin concentrations during pregnancy show high variability and it crosses the placenta although the concentrations are very low in fetal plasma (5–19%) [59, 114].

The Collaborative Perinatal Project did not detect any risk of malformation in 230 babies exposed to erythromycin throughout pregnancy [23]. Nevertheless, the Center of Disease Control observed a greater risk of pyloric stenosis in children born from mothers exposed to this drug, while other similar studies showed the opposite [115]. Therefore, until no conclusive results exist, the use of erythromycin in pregnancy should be carefully prescribed and it is classified in Category B by the FDA.

Erythromycin estolate can induce hepatotoxicity in pregnant women. Around 10% of patients treated with this salt during the second trimester of pregnancy have elevated hepatic transaminases. Therefore, erythromycin estolate is contraindicated during pregnancy [116–118].

Spiramycin is used in some countries as the treatment of choice for primary toxoplasmosis in pregnant women. Spiramycin crosses the placenta, and the cord:maternal ratio is approximately 0.5. Moreover, the concentrations in the placenta are 2–4 times higher than those reached in plasma. The drug has not been related to fetal harm or teratogenesis [54, 80].

Clarithromycin is mainly used for the treatment of infections of the upper-respiratory tract, for *H. pylori* eradication and for prophylaxis against *M. avium* in HIV-positive pregnant women. There are some case reports of possible teratogenic effects of clarithromycin. It is associated with spontaneous abortion in humans and, moreover, with cardiovascular abnormalities and palatine cleft in animal studies with rats [26]. Although the evidence is scarce, the drug is not recommended during pregnancy at present [54], and it is classified in Category C by the FDA.

Azithromycin has been used as single-dose therapy for chlamydial infections during pregnancy [14]. The safety of azithromycin during pregnancy has not been fully established, although there are no reports of congenital defects, and it is classified in Category B by the FDA [119].

Roxithromycin (a macrolide derivate from erythromycin) can be used in the treatment of gynecological infections in pregnant women which are caused by chlamydia and *U. urealyticum* [118]. It crosses the placental barrier better than erythromycin and azithromycin. Although no teratogenic effects have been demonstrated, the safety in human beings is not well established yet [26]. It is classified in Category B by the FDA.

Telithromycin is a semisynthetic, erythromycin derivate with enhanced activity against macrolide-resistant streptococci [120]. At present, there are no studies in pregnant women, and teratogenic potential was obtained through animal models. No evidence of teratogenic effects was found and it should be used during pregnancy only if a clear potential benefit could justify its prescription [26]. It is classified in Category C by the FDA.

15.4.9 Nitrofurantoin

Nitrofurantoin crosses the placenta and may induce fetal hemolytic anemia if glucose-6-phosphate dehydrogenase deficiency is present. Its use has not been associated with congenital defects [47, 121]. Nitrofurantoin is classified in Category B by the FDA.

15.4.10 Sulfonamides and Trimethoprim

The main indication to use sulfonamides during pregnancy has been, in recent years, to treat urinary tract infections. These drugs cross the placenta, and fetal concentrations are 70–90% of maternal ones at 2–3 h after administration, and at 2 h equilibrium between maternal and fetal blood is reached [122]. Sulfonamides are teratogenic in some animal species, but most studies have found no association in humans and it is currently believed that they do not seem to have any teratogenic risk [14]. Sulfonamides can displace bilirubin from its albumin-binding sites and, therefore, induce hyperbilirubinemia. This increase could theoretically cause kernicterus in neonates and this risk advises against its use in the third trimester of pregnancy and also in neonates [22, 123]. In addition, sulfonamides could cause hemolytic anemia in newborns deficient in glucose-6-phosphate dehydrogenase [124]. They are classified in Category B by the FDA.

Trimethoprim is mainly used in combination with sulfamethoxazole (cotrimoxazole) to treat urinary infections, and for the prophylaxis of pneumonia caused by *Pneumocystis carinii* in HIV-positive pregnant women. Both substances cross the placenta and reach concentrations in fetal and amniotic fluid similar to those found in maternal plasma. Many studies have shown the ability of this drug to interfere in fetal development, causing palatine cleft, malformation in the urinary tract and in the cardiovascular system [47, 122, 125]. It is classified in Category C by the FDA.

15.4.11 Tetracyclines

Tetracyclines were routinely used for prevention and treatment of obstetric infections until the 1960s, when their overall risks were shown [54]. Tetracyclines cross the placenta, reaching high levels in the fetal blood, despite their poor penetration in amniotic fluid (20% of mother's blood levels). Moreover, concentrations of tetracycline were lower in cord serum in comparison to maternal blood during labor [25].

Tetracyclines can produce adverse effects on fetal teeth and bones, maternal liver toxicity, and congenital defects. Tetracyclines cause yellow discoloration of bone and teeth if administered during the period of development of these tissues. This effect is a consequence of the potent chelating ability of the drug and its deposition in the calcifying bones and teeth as well as the possible destruction of enamel [29].

An association between tetracycline use during pregnancy and liver toxicity has been reported as a rare, but often fatal, event, usually following i.v. dosing of more than 2 g/day and mostly in pregnant women being treated for pyelonephritis [126]. Toxicity and major defects expected by tetracyclines include azotemia, jaundice and acute fatty degeneration in pregnant women. Tetracycline administration has been associated with the appearance of neural-tube defects, palatine cleft, severe congenital cardiovascular abnormalities, hypospadias, inguinal hernia, hypoplasia of limb and clubfoot [28]. Therefore, all tetracyclines are contraindicated during all pregnancy periods [22, 47], especially during the calcification stage of hard tissue; after the 20th week of pregnancy [23]. They are classified in Category D by the FDA.

15.4.12 Lincosamides

Lincosamides have been used as prophylactic therapy prior to cesarean section [54]. Plasma concentrations of clindamycin in pregnancy are similar to those in non-pregnant women. Clindamycin crosses the placenta and reaches cord levels of approximately 50% of that of the maternal blood. The maternal:placenta concentrations ratio is 1 and fetal concentrations are in the therapeutic range [127, 128]. No increased teratogenic risk was observed in 647 babies previously exposed to clindamycin during the first trimester of pregnancy [23].

Lincomycin crosses the placenta, reaching cord levels of about 25% of the maternal serum levels. No effects on the newborn have been observed. The FDA classifies both clindamycin and lincomycin as in Category B agents.

15.4.13 Metronidazole

Metronidazole during pregnancy is restricted to treatment of infections caused by *T. vaginalis* or caused by anaerobic microorganisms [128]. Metronidazole freely crosses the placenta with a cord:maternal plasma ratio of 1 and reaches the fetal blood and amniotic liquid at high concentrations.

The use of metronidazole in pregnancy is controversial. Metronidazole is mutagenic and carcinogenic in bacteria and animals. Several studies have described the safety of metronidazole in pregnancy. In a series of 1,020 women who received metronidazole during the first trimester for treatment of vaginitis, no birth defects attributable to the drug were observed [129]. Similar results have been reported after the analysis of pregnancy outcomes of 1,307 women who received metronidazole between 30 days before and 120 days after the onset of their last normal menstrual period. The use of metronidazole has been associated with a possible teratogenic or cancer-inducing agent in fetuses [29, 130]. Prospective and retrospective studies did not confirm these defects [128, 130]. However, concerns remain and have led to advice against its use in pregnancy.

The manufacturer considers metronidazole to be contraindicated to treat trichomoniasis during the first trimester of pregnancy. It may be used during the second and third trimesters if other alternative therapies have failed [54]. It is classified in Category B by the FDA.

15.4.14 Chloramphenicol

Chloramphenicol freely crosses the placenta, and serum-cord concentrations ranged from 30% to 106% of maternal levels [131]. No reports linking the use of chloramphenicol and congenital defects have been found. Chloramphenicol is metabolized by glucuronoconjugation. In newborns and premature neonates, the immaturity of this metabolic pathway produces high plasma concentrations of the drug that have been associated with the appearance of the "gray baby syndrome" [30]. This syndrome is characterized by cyanosis, paleness, abdominal distension, vomiting and circulatory collapse, resulting in a 50% mortality.

A study based on the Hungarian Case-Control Surveillance of Congenital Abnormalities during a period between 1980 and 1996 did not find any teratogenic risk to fetuses of mothers exposed to this drug during early stages of pregnancy [131]. Nevertheless, the drug should be avoided at term or during the third trimester, but some authors even consider that chloramphenicol is contraindicated during the entire pregnancy [14, 54]. It is classified in Category C by the FDA.

15.4.15 Oxazolidinones

Linezolid is a synthetic, oxazolidinone class, antibacterial agent that is indicated for the treatment of Gram-positive bacteria, including vancomycin-resistant enterococcus in both oral and i.v. formulations. It is mainly used to treat skin and soft tissue infections, pneumonia and bacteriemia [132]. In animal studies, linezolid induced decreased fetal body-weights and reduced ossification of sternebra in rats. There are no adequate and well-controlled studies in pregnant women. Therefore, linezolid should be used during pregnancy only if the potential benefit justifies the potential risk to the fetus [54]. The FDA classifies it as a Category C agent.

15.4.16 Rifampicin

Rifampicin has been used to treat both bacterial infections and tuberculosis. As with other antimycobacterial agents, it crosses the placenta and reaches high levels in fetal plasma. The cord:maternal concentration ratio ranges from 0.12 to 0.33. The risk for fetal malformations is lower than leaving tuberculosis untreated [54]. Like other first-line antituberculosis agents, they are considered by the CDC to be safe for tuberculosis treatment during pregnancy, and no teratogenic effects have been reported with the exception of those related to streptomycin due to an increased risk of ototoxicity in infants [133]. It is classified in Category C by the FDA.

15.4.17 Fluoroquinolones and Quinolones

Fluoroquinolones are widely used to treat ambulatory and severe infections that require hospitalization. These antibiotics are able to cross the placental barrier, but no reports exist about malformations or musculoskeletal anomalies during the first trimester of gestation [29, 134].

Fluoroquinolones have a high affinity for cartilage, and studies in laboratory animals have demonstrated arthropathy of weight-bearing joints after the administration of fluoroquinolones in young animals and during pregnancy [135]. Although there are some cases of arthropathy in children treated with quinolones during pregnancy or childhood, the epidemiological evidence seems to indicate a low risk of congenital malformations. The analysis of human surveys seems to indicate that the frequency of congenital anomalies was not increased during the first-trimester exposure to fluoroquinolones [136]. A recent study following 200 pregnant women exposed to fluoroquinolones (norfloxacin, ciprofloxacin and ofloxacin) has shown a similar rate of major congenital defects to those of the control group (2.2% vs. 2.6%, respectively). There was no clinically significant, musculoskeletal dysfunction in children exposed to fluoroquinolones in the uterus [137]. However, quinolones are contraindicated during pregnancy and until adolescence, the only accepted use being the treatment of lung infections in children with cystic fibrosis.

In pregnant women receiving ciprofloxacin (200 mg i.v. every 12 h), serum concentrations were much lower than those found in non-pregnant patients. This is probably related to an increased renal excretion [138]. Ciprofloxacin crosses the placenta slowly, and its amniotic concentrations are approximately 57% of those obtained in plasma [138].

In the case of pefloxacin, a quinolone mainly eliminated by the hepatic route, the plasma concentrations were similar in pregnant and non-pregnant women. Concentrations of pefloxacin in amniotic fluid were lower than those observed in plasma (70%) [138].

Ofloxacin was administered to 20 pregnant women (19–25 weeks' gestation). Serum and amniotic fluid concentrations were carried out 6 h, 10 h and 24 h after dosing (two 400-mg i.v. doses every 12 h). Maternal blood levels at these times were 0.68, 0.21 and 0.07 μg/ml, whereas amniotic fluid levels were 0.25, 0.15, and 0.13 μg/ml [138].

Levofloxacin is a new, marketed fluoroquinolone. In terms of chemical structure, it is one of the two optical isomers of ofloxacin. Its pharmacokinetic properties should be similar to those of ofloxacin.

Moxifloxacin is an oral synthetic, broad-spectrum, fluoroquinolone anti-infective agent and no reports describing its use during human pregnancy have been located. It is not known if moxifloxacin crosses the human placenta, but its molecular weight is low enough to consider this possibility. In regard to its safety, some reviewers have concluded that, like the other fluoroquinolones, it should be considered contraindicated in pregnancy and, as a rule, safer alternatives are usually available [54]. All of these are classified in Category C by the FDA.

15.4.18 Glycylcyclines

Tigecycline is the first member of a new class of broad-spectrum i.v. antibacterials called glycylcyclines, approved in June 2005 by the FDA, and specifically developed to overcome the two major mechanisms of tetracycline resistance (ribosomal protection and efflux). It is indicated in complicated skin, visceral and severe intra-abdominal infections in adults. It may cause fetal harm when administered to pregnant women. Use of tigecycline during tooth development may cause permanent discoloration of the teeth [139]. Tigecycline is classified in Category D by the FDA.

15.4.19 Polymyxins

Colistin (polymyxin E) is the main representative of the group, with an antimicrobial activity restricted to Gram-negative bacteria. It has been useful during pregnancy only to treat *P. aeruginosa* infections or in the case of cesarean-section prophylaxis, in association with ampicillin. Colistin is classified in Category C by the FDA because of its nephrotoxicity, neurotoxicity, neuromuscular blockade, ataxia, dizziness, convulsions and circumoral paraesthesia. Its use has been superseded by safer antibiotics [140].

References

1. Lapinsky SE, Kruczynski K, Seaward GR, Farine D, Grossman RF (1997) Critical care management of the obstetric patient. Can J Anaesth 44:325–329
2. Glover DD, Amonkar M, Rybeck BF, et al. (2003) Prescription, over-the-counter, and herbal medicine use in a rural, obstetric population. Am J Obstet Gynecol 188:1039–1045
3. Andrade SE, Gurwitz TH, Davis RL, et al. (2004) Prescription drug use in pregnancy. Am J Obstet Gynecol 191:398–407
4. Graham SG, Luxton MC (1989) The requirement for intensive care support for the pregnant population. Anaesthesia 44:581–584
5. Kirshon B, Hinkley CM, Cotton DB, Miller J (1990) Maternal mortality in a maternal-fetal medicine intensive care unit. J Reprod Med 35:25–28
6. Mabie WC, Sibai BM (1990) Treatment in an obstetric intensive care unit. Am J Obstet Gynecol 162:1–4
7. Kilpatrick SJ, Matthay MA (1992) Obstetric patients requiring critical care. A five-year review. Chest 101:1407–1412
8. Collop NA, Sahn SA (1993) Critical illness in pregnancy. An analysis of 20 patients admitted to a medical intensive care unit. Chest 103:1548–1552
9. Monaco TJ Jr, Spielman FJ, Katz VL (1993) Pregnant patients in the intensive care unit: a descriptive analysis. South Med J 86:414–417
10. Lewinsohn G, Herman A, Leonov Y, Klinowski E (1994) Critically ill obstetrical patients: outcome and predictability. Crit Care Med 22:1412–1414
11. Bouvier-Colle MH, Salanave B, Ancel PY, et al. (1996) Obstetric patients treated in intensive care units and maternal mortality. Regional teams for the survey. Eur J Obstet Gynecol Reprod Biol 65:121–125
12. El-Solh AA, Grant BJB (1996) A comparison of severity of illness scoring systems for critically ill obstetrical patients. Am J Resp Crit Care Med 153:A362
13. Wise R (1995) Antibiotics. In: Rubin P (ed) Prescribing in pregnancy, 2nd edn. BMJ Publishing Group, London, pp 29–45
14. Gilstrap LC, Little BB (1999) Antimicrobial agents during pregnancy. In: Gilstrap LC, Little BB (eds) Drugs and pregnancy, 2nd edn. Chapman and Hall, New York, pp 45–75
15. Lee W, Clark SL, Cotton DB, et al. (1988) Septic shock during pregnancy. Am J Obstet Gynecol 159:410–416
16. Gallagher MW, Repke JT, Goldstein PJ (1994) Pharmacologic approach to the critically ill obstetric patient. In: Chernow B (ed) The pharmacologic approach to the critically ill patient. William and Wilkins, Baltimore, pp 847–862
17. Mabie WC, Barton JR, Sibai B (1997) Septic shock in pregnancy. Obstet Gynecol 90:553–561
18. World Heath Organization (2001) Global prevalence and incidence of selected curable sexually transmitted infections: overview and estimates. WHO, Geneva
19. Mullick S, Watson-Jones D, Beksinska M, Mabey D (2005) Sexually transmitted infections in pregnancy: prevalence, impact on pregnancy outcomes, and approach to treatment in developing countries. Sex Trans Infect 81:294–302
20. World Heath Organization (2004) Integrating care for reproductive health, sexually transmitted and other reproductive tract infections; a guide to essential practice. WHO, Geneva
21. Hamod KA, Khouzami VA (1988) Antibiotics in pregnancy. In: Nyebil JR (ed) Drug use in pregnancy, 2nd edn. Lea and Febiger, Philadelphia, pp 29–36
22. Theis JGW, Koren G (1997) Maternal and fetal clinical

pharmacology. In: Speight TM, Holford HG (eds) Avery's drug treatment, 4th edn. Adis, Auckland, pp 75–126
23. Einarson A, Shuhaiber S, Koren G (2001) Effect of antibacterials on the unborn child. Pediatr Drugs 3:803–816
24. Loebstein R, Koren G (2002) Clinical relevance of therapeutic drug monitoring during pregnancy. Ther Drug Monit 24:15–22
25. Folb PI, Dukes MNG (1993) Drug safety in pregnancy. Elsevier, Amsterdam
26. Sá del Fiol F, Gerenutti M, Groppo FC (2005) Antibiotics and pregnancy. Pharmazie 60:483–493
27. Ho JL, Barza M (1985) Chemotherapy of infection. In: Gleicher N (ed) Principles of medical therapy in pregnancy. Plenum Med Book, New York, pp 406–420
28. Czeizel AE, Rockenbauer M (2000) A population-based case-control teratologic study of oral oxytetracycline treatment during pregnancy. Eur J Obstet Gynecol Reprod Biol 88:27–33
29. Niebyl JR (2003) Antibiotics and other anti-infective agents in pregnancy and lactation. Am J Perinatol 20:405–414
30. Johnson TN (2003) The development of drug metabolizing enzymes and their influence on the susceptibility to adverse drug reactions in children. Toxicology 192:37–48
31. Karnard DR, Lapsia V, Krishnan A, et al. (2004) Prognostic factors in obstetric patients admitted to an Indian intensive care unit. Crit Care Med 32:1294–1299
32. Munnur U, Karnard D, Guntupalli KK (2005) Critically ill obstetric patients in an American and Indian public hospital: Comparison of case-mix, organ dysfunction, intensive care requirements, and outcomes. Intensive Care Med 31:1087–1094
33. Minkauskiene M, Nadisauskiene R, Padaiga Z, Makari S (2004) Systematic review on the incidence and prevalence of severe maternal morbidity. Medicina (Kaunas) 40: 299–309
34. Soubra SH, Guntupalli KK (2005) Critical illness in pregnancy: an overview. Crit Care Med 33 (10 Suppl):S248–S255
35. Pacifici GM, Nottoli R (1995) Placental transfer of drugs administered to the mother. Clin Pharmacokinet 28:235–269
36. Anderson GD (2005) Pregnancy-induced changes in pharmacokinetics. A mechanistic-based approach. Clin Pharmacokinet 44:989–1008
37. Loebstein R, Lalkin A, Koren G (1997) Pharmacokinetic changes during pregnancy and their clinical relevance. Clin Pharmacokinet 33:328–343
38. Weller TMA, Rees EN (2000) Antibacterial use in pregnancy. Drug Safety 22:335–338
39. Rubin PC (1986) Prescribing in pregnancy. General principles. BMJ 293:1415–1417
40. Dean M, Stock B, Patterson RJ, et al. (1980) Serum protein binding of drugs during and after pregnancy in humans. Clin Pharmacol Ther 28:253–261
41. Benet LZ, Hoener BA (2002) Changes in plasma protein binding have little clinical relevance. Clin Pharmacol Ther 71:115–121
42. Inui KI, Masuda S, Saito H (2000) Cellular and molecular aspects of drug transport in the kidney. Kidney Int 58:944–958
43. Ostrea EM, Mantaring JB, Silvestre MA (2004) Drugs that affect the fetus and newborn infant via the placenta or breast milk. Pediatr Clin N Am 51:539–579
44. Stevens JC, Hines RN, Gu C, et al. (2003) Developmental expression of the major human hepatic CYP3A enzymes. J Pharmacol Exp Ther 307:573–582
45. Syme MR, Paxton JW, Keelan JA (2004) Drug transfer and metabolism by the human placenta. Clin Pharmacokinetic 43:487–514
46. Preston SL (2004) The importance of appropriate antimicrobial dosing: pharmacokinetic and pharmacodynamic considerations. Ann Pharmacother 38:S14–S18
47. Briggs GG, Freeman RK, Yaffe SJ (1998) Drugs in pregnancy and lactation, 5th edn. William and Wilkins, Baltimore
48. Kullander K, Kallen B (1976) A prospective study of drugs and pregnancy. Acta Obstet Gynecol Scand 55:287–295
49. Czeizel AE, Rockenbauer M, Sorensen HT, Olsen J (2001) A population-based case-control teratologic study of ampicillin treatment during pregnancy. Am J Obstet Gynecol 185:140–147
50. Kunin CM (1966) Clinical pharmacology of the new penicillins. I. The importance of serum protein binding in determining antimicrobial activity and concentration in serum. Clin Pharmacol Ther 7:166–179
51. MacAulay MA, Berg SA, Charles D (1968) Placental transfer of dicloxacillin at term. Am J Obstet Gynecol 102:1162–1168
52. Philipson A (1975) Pharmacokinetics of ampicillins during pregnancy. J Infect Dis 136:370–376
53. Philipson A (1979) Pharmacokinetics of antibiotics in pregnancy and labour. Clin Pharmacokinet 4:297–309
54. Briggs GG, Freeman RK, Jaffe SJ (2005) Drugs in pregnancy and lactation, 7th edn. Williams & Wilkins, Baltimore
55. Shepherd GM (2003) Hypersensitivity reactions to drugs: evaluations and management. Mt Sinai J Med 70:113–125
56. Czeizel AE, Rockenbauer M, Olsen J, Sorensen HT (2000) Oral phenoxymethylpenicillin treatment during pregnancy. Results of a population-based Hungarian case-control study. Arch Gynecol Obstet 263:178–181
57. Dencker BB, Larsen H, Jensen ES, Schonheyder HC, Nielsen GL, Sorensen HT (2002) Birth outcome of 1886 pregnancies after exposure to phenoxymethylpenicillin *in utero*. Clin Microbiol Infect 8:196–201
58. Larsen H, Nielsen GL, Sorensen HT, Moller M, Olsen J, Schonheyder HC (2000) A follow-up study of birth outcome in users of pivampicillin during pregnancy. Acta Obstet Gynecol Scand 79:379–383
59. Czeizel AE, Rockenbauer N, Sorensen HT, Olsen J (1999) A population-based case-control teratologic study of oral erythromycin treatment during pregnancy. Reprod Toxicol 13:531–536
60. Jepsen P, Skriver MV, Floyd A, Lipworth L, Schonheyder HC, Sorensen HT (2003) A population-based study of maternal use of amoxicillin and pregnancy outcome in Denmark. Br J Clin Pharmacol 55:216–221
61. Czeizel AE, Rockenbauer M, Sorensen HT, Olsen J (2001) Augmentin treatment during pregnancy and the prevalence of congenital abnormalities: a population-based case-control teratologic study. Eur J Obstet Gynecol Reprod Biol 97:188–192
62. Pergament E, Schechtman A, Blum K (2004) Antibiotics and pregnancy. Risk newsletter 3:6 1995.www.fetal-exposure.org/ANTIBIOT.html-24/04/2004
63. Wasz-Hockert O, Nummi S, Vuopala S, Jarvinen P (1970) Transplacental passage of azidocillin, ampicillin and penicillin G during early and late pregnancy. Acta Paediatr Scand 206 (Suppl):109–110
64. Woltz J, Zintel H (1945) The transmission of penicillin to amniotic fluid and fetal blood in the human. Am J Obstet Gynecol 49:663–665
65. Nathan L, Bawdon RE, Sidawi JE, Stettler RW, McIntire DM, Wendel GD Jr (1993) Penicillin levels following the administration of benzathine penicillin G in pregnancy. Obstet Gynecol 82:338–342
66. Heikkilä AM, Erkkola RV (1993) The need for adjustment

of dosage regimen of penicillin V during pregnancy. Obstet Gynecol 81:919–921
67. Noschel VH, Peiker G, Schroder S, Meinhold P, Muller B (1982) Untersuchungen zur Pharmakokinetik von Antibiotika und Sulfanilamiden in der Schwangerschaft und unter der Geburt. Zentralbl Gynakol 104:1514–1518
68. Kraybill EN, Chaney NE, McCarthy LR (1980) Transplacental ampicillin: inhibitory concentrations in neonatal serum. Am J Obstet Gynecol 138:793–796
69. Chamberlain A, White S, Bawdon R, Thomas S, Larsen B (1993) Pharmacokinetics of ampicillin and sulbactam in pregnancy. Am J Obstet Gynecol 168:667–673
70. MacAulay MA, Abou-Sabe M, Charles D (1966) Placental transfer of ampicillin. Am J Obstet Gynecol 96:943–950
71. Morales WJ, Angel JL, O'Brien WF, Knuppel RA (1989) Use of ampicillin and corticosteroids in premature rupture of membranes: a randomized study. Obstet Gynecol 173: 721–726
72. Zierler S (1985) Maternal drugs and congenital heart disease. Obstet Gynecol 65:155–165
73. Heinonen OP, Slone D, Shapiro S (1977) Birth defects and drugs in pregnancy. Publishing Sciences Group, Littleton
74. Jakobi P, Neiger R, Merzbach D, Paldi E (1987) Single-dose antimicrobial therapy in the treatment of asymptomatic bacteriuria in pregnancy. Am J Obstet Gynecol 156:1148–1152
75. Mercer BM, Goldenberg RL, Das AF, et al. (2003) What we have learned regarding antibiotic therapy for the reduction of infant morbidity after preterm premature rupture of the membranes. Semin Perinatol 27:217–230
76. Bergogne-Berenzin E, Lambert-Zechovsky N, Rouvillois JL (1979) Etude du passage transplacentaire des beta-lactamines. J Gynecol Obstet Biol Reprod (Paris) 8:359–364
77. Matsuda S (1982) Augmentin treatment in obstetrics and gynaecology. In: Leigh DA, Robinson OPW (eds) Augmentin: Proceedings of an international symposium. Montreux, Switzerland. July 1981. Excerpta Medica 179–191
78. Takase Z, Shirafuji H, Uchida M (1982) Clinical and laboratory studies on BRL25000 (clavulanic acid-amoxicillin) in the field of obstetrics and gynecology. Chemotherapy (Tokyo) 30 (Suppl 2):538–547
79. Pedler SJ, Bint AJ (1985) Comparative study of amoxicillin-clavulanic acid and cephalexin in the treatment of bacteriuria during pregnancy. Antimicrob Agents Chemother 27:508–510
80. Reali A, Ximenes L, Cuzzolin L, Fanos V (2005) Antibiotic therapy in pregnancy and lactation. J Chemother 17:123–130
81. Prigot A, Froix C, Rubin E (1962) Absorption, diffusion, and excretion of new penicillin, oxacillin. Antimicrob Agents Chemother 402–410
82. Depp R, Kind A, Kirby W, Johnson W (1970) Transplacental passage of methicillin and dicloxacillin into the fetus and amniotic fluid. Am J Obstet Gynecol 107:1054–1057
83. MacAulay M, Molloy W, Charles D (1973) Placental transfer of methicillin. Am J Obstet Gynecol 115:58–65
84. Biro L, Ivan E, Elek E, Arr M (1970) Data on the tissue concentration of antibiotics in man. Tissue concentrations of semi-synthetic penicillins in the fetus. Int Z Pharmakol Ther Toxikol 4:321–324
85. Elek E, Ivan E, Arr M (1972) Passage of penicillins from mother to fetus in humans. Int J Clin Pharmacol Ther Toxicol 6:223–228
86. Cho N, Nakayama T, Vehara K, Kunii K (1977) Laboratory and clinical evaluation of ticarcillin in the field of obstetrics and gynecology. Chemotherapy (Tokyo) 25:2911–2923
87. Lockwood CJ, Costigan K, Ghidini A, et al. (1993) Double-blind, placebo-controlled trial of piperacillin prophylaxis in preterm membrane rupture. Am J Obstet Gynecol 169:970–976
88. Brown CEL, Christmas JT, Bawdon RE (1990) Placental transfer of cefazolin and piperacillin in pregnancies remote from term complicated by Rh isoimmunization. Am J Obstet Gynecol 163:938–943
89. Heikkilä A, Erkola R (1991) Pharmacokinetics of piperacillin during pregnancy. J Antimicrob Chemother 28: 419–423
90. Bourget P, Sertin A, Lesne-Hulin A, Fernández H, Ville Y, Van Peborgh P (1998) Influence of pregnancy on the pharmacokinetic behaviour and the transplacental transfer of the piperacillin-tazobactam. Eur J Obstet Gynecol Reprod Biol 76:21–27
91. Brown CEL, Christmas JT, Bawdon RE (1990) Placental transfer of cefazolin and piperacillin in pregnancies remote from term complicated by Rh isoimmunization. Am J Obstet Gynecol 162:549–554
92. Voigt R, Schroder S, Peiker G (1995) Pharmacokinetic studies of azlocillin and piperacillin during late pregnancy. Chemotherapy 31:417–424
93. Christensen B (2000) Which antibiotics are appropriate for treating bacteriuria in pregnancy? J Antimicrob Chemother 46 (Suppl 1):29–34
94. Chow AW, Jewesson PJ (1985) Pharmacokinetics and safety of antimicrobial agents during pregnancy. Rev Infect Dis 7:287–313
95. Graham JE, Oshiro BT, Blanco JD (1992) Limited spectrum (first generation) cephalosporins. Obstet Gynecol Clin North Am 19:449–459
96. Czeizel AE, Rockenbauer M, Sorensen HT, Olsen J (2001) Use of cephalosporins during pregnancy and in the presence of congenital abnormalities: a population-based, case-control study. Am J Obstet Gynecol 184:1289–1296
97. Eriksen NL, Blanco JD (1992) Extended-spectrum (second- and third-generation) cephalosporins. Obstet Gynecol Clin North Am 19:461–474
98. Martens MG (1989) Cephalosporins. Obstet Gynecol Clin North Am 16:291–304
99. Ortiz-Ruiz G, Vetter N, Isaacs R, et al. (2004) Ertapenem versus ceftriaxone for the treatment of the community-acquired pneumonia in adults: combined analysis of two multicentre randomized, double-blind studies. J Antimicrob Chemother 53:59–66
100. Heikkilä A, Renkonen O-V, Erkkola R (1992) Pharmacokinetics and transplacental passage of imipenem during pregnancy. Antimicrob Agents Chemother 36:2652–2655
101. Hirabayashi K, Okada E (1988) Pharmacokinetic and clinical studies of imipenem/cilastatin sodium in the perinatal period. Jpn J Antibiot 11:1797–1804
102. Chimura T, Morisaki N, Funayama T, Matsuo M (1990) Clinical studies on aztreonam in perinatal use. Jpn J Antibiot 43:696–699
103. Bristol-Myers Squibb Company: Azactam: FDA (2004) http://www.fda.gov/cder/foi/label/2002/50580slr033lbl. Pdf searched May 2004.
104. Clark P (1992) Aztreonam. Obstet Gynecol Clin North Am 19:519–528
105. Merck & Co. Inc. (2004) Invanz. FDA www.fda. Gov/medwatch/SAFETY/2004/apr_PI.pdf searched December, 2004
106. Bourget P, Fernandez H, Delouis C, Ribou F (1991) Transplacental passage of vancomycin during the second trimester of pregnancy. Obstet Gynecol 78:908–911
107. Reyes MP, Ostrea EM, Cabinian AE, Schamit C, Rintelmann W (1989) Vancomycin during pregnancy: does it cause hearing loss or nephrotoxicity in the infant? Am J Obstet Gynecol 161:977–981

108. Davey PG, Williams AH (1991) A review of the safety profile of teicoplanin. Antimicrob Chemoter 27:69–73
109. Forrest Pharmaceuticals Monurolβ FDA Label information (2002) http:// www.fda.gov/cder/foi/label/2000/50717SLR004_Monurol_lbl.pdf, searched December 2004
110. Graham JM, Blanco JD, Oshiro BT, Magee KP (1994) Gentamicin levels in pregnant women with pyelonephritis. Am J Perinatol 11:40–41
111. Czeizel AE, Rockenbauer M, Olsen J, Sorensen HT (2000) A teratological study of aminoglycoside antibiotic treatment during pregnancy. Scand J Infect Dis 32:309–313
112. Chang KW, Ng WL (1985) Gentamycin nephropathy in a neonate. Pathology 17:514–515
113. Fernández H, Bourget P, Delouis C (1990) Fetal levels of tobramycin following maternal administration. Obstet Gynecol 76:992–994
114. Philipson A, Sabath LD, Charles D (1976) Erythromycin absorption and elimination in pregnant women. Clin Pharmacol Ther 19:68–77
115. Louik C, Werler MM, Mitchell AA (2002) Erythromycin use during pregnancy in relation to pyloric stenosis. Am J Obstet Gynecol 186:288–290
116. Lewis JH (2000) Drug-induced liver disease. Med Clin North Am 84:1275–1311
117. McCormack WM, George H, Donner A, Kodgis LF, et al. (1977) Hepatotoxicity of erythromycin estolate during pregnancy. Antimicrob Agents Chemother 12:630–635
118. Garland SM, O'Reilly MA (1995) The risks and benefits of antimicrobial therapy in pregnancy. Drug Safety 13:188–205
119. Pfizer Laboratories (2003) Zithromax®. Food and Drug Administration 2003. http://www.fda.gov/cder/foi/label/2004/50670slr021,50693slr008,50730slr011_zithromax_lbl. pdf searched May, 2004
120. Bryskier A (2000) Ketolides-telithromycin, an example of a new class of antibacterial agents. Clin Microbiol Infect 6:661–669
121. Ben David S, Einarson T, Ben David Y, Nulman I, Pastuszak A, Koren G (1995) The safety of nitrofurantoin during the first trimester of pregnancy: meta-analysis. Fund Clin Pharmacol 9:503–507
122. Czeizel AE, Rockenbauer M, Sorensen HT, Olsen J (2001) The teratogenic risk of trimethoprim-sulfonamides: a population-based case-control study. Reprod Toxicol 15: 637–646
123. Ahlfors CE (2000) Unbound bilirubin associated with kernicterus: a historical approach. J Pediatr 137:540–544
124. Perkins RP (1971) Hydrops fetalis and stillbirth in a male glucose-6-phosphate dehydrogenase-deficient fetus possibly due to maternal ingestion of sulfisoxazole: a case report. Am J Obstet Gynecol 111:379–381
125. Hernández-Díaz S, Werler MM, Walker AM, Mitchell AA (2000) Folic acid antagonists during pregnancy and the risk of birth defects. N Engl J Med 30:1608–1614
126. Wenk RE, Gebhart FC, Begahavan BS, Lustgarten JA, McCarthy EF (1981) Tetracycline-associated fatty liver of pregnancy, including possible pregnancy risk after chronic dermatologic use of tetracycline. J Reprod Med 26:135–141
127. Philipson A, Sabath LD, Charles D (1973) Transplacental passage of erythromycin and clindamycin. N Engl J Med 288:1219–1221
128. Sorensen HT, Larsen H, Jensen ES, Thulstrup AM, Schonheyder HC, Nielsen GL, Czeizel A (1999) Safety of metronidazole during pregnancy: a cohort study of risk of congenital abnormalities, preterm delivery and low birth weight in 124 women. J Antimicrob Chemother 44: 854–856
129. Rosa FW, Baum C, Shaw M (1993) Pregnancy outcomes after first trimester vaginitis drug therapy. Obstet Gynecol 82:348–352
130. Piper JM, Mitchelm EF, Ray WA (1993) Prenatal use of metronidazole and birth defects: no association. Obstet Gynecol 82:348–352
131. Czeizel AE, Rockenbauer M (2000) A population-based case-control teratologic study of oral chloramphenicol treatment during pregnancy. Eur J Epidemiol 16:323–327
132. Clemett D, Markham A (2000) Linezolid. Drugs 59:815–827
133. Bothamley G (2001) Drug treatment for tuberculosis during pregnancy: safety considerations. Drug Safety 24: 553–565
134. Chung AM, Reed MD, Blumer JL (2002) Antibiotics and breast feeding: a critical review of the literature. Paediatr Drugs 4:817–837
135. Grady R (2003) Safety profile of quinolone antibiotics in the pediatric population. Pediatr Infect Dis J 22:1128–1132
136. Schaefer C, Amoura-Elefant E, Vial T, et al. (1996) Pregnancy outcome after prenatal quinolone exposure. Evaluation of a case registry of the European Network of Teratology Information Services (ENTIS). Eur J Gynecol Reprod Biol 69:83–89
137. Loebstein R, Addis A, Ho E, et al. (1998) Pregnancy outcome following gestational exposure to fluoroquinolone: a multicenter prospective controlled study. Antimicrob Agents Chemother 42:1336–1339
138. Giamarellou H, Kolohythas E, Petrikkos G, Gazis J, Aravantinos D, Sfikakis P (1989) Pharmacokinetics of three newer quinolones in pregnant and lactating women. Am J Med 87 (Suppl 5A):49S–61S
139. Frampton JE, Curran MP (2005) Tigecycline. Drugs 65: 2623–2635
140. Knothe H, Dette GA (1985) Antibiotics in pregnancy: toxicity and teratogenicity. Infection 13:49–51

Chapter 16

Immunomodulation in Sepsis

G.W. Waterer

16.1 Introduction

Despite all the advances in medical care and technology the mortality rate from severe sepsis has changed little over the past 3 decades [1]. The failure to improve survival from severe sepsis is in part due to the aging population and an increasing number of patients at risk who have substantial comorbidities, including iatrogenic immunosuppression from chemotherapy for malignancy and the variety of immunosuppressive agents now used in a host of chronic autoimmune diseases. However, another substantial contributing factor is that many patients present with, or rapidly develop, sepsis-induced complications for which we have no effective prevention or cure.

In the vast majority of patients with sepsis in whom a pathogen is identified they have usually been treated with appropriate antibiotics. It is therefore extremely unlikely that the mortality rate from sepsis can be improved through the development of newer classes of antibiotics [2]. This is not a new observation; Austrian and Gold reporting in the 1960s that antibiotics had no effect on mortality in the first 48–72 h in patients admitted with bacteremic pneumococcal pneumonia [3].

As antimicrobial approaches seem unlikely to improve the outcome of sepsis, the possibility of modifying the host response has become a major focus of sepsis research. This chapter will focus on previous trials of immunomodulatory agents as well as current agents being trialed and potential agents in the near future.

16.2 The Immune Response in Sepsis

Patients who succumb to sepsis seem to fall into two broad groups. The first group can be loosely categorized as having an excessive immune response to infection, including those who develop septic shock, acute respiratory distress syndrome (ARDS) and multiorgan failure. The second group is patients who can be categorized as having an inadequate host response to infection, including the elderly, alcoholics, diabetics and patients with significant co-morbid illnesses, such as cardiac failure or cirrhosis. In reality these are not two mutually exclusive groups, with substantial overlap existing due to the dynamic changes during the evolution and resolution of sepsis.

The difficulty in balancing the beneficial and the detrimental effects from interfering in the natural history of the immune response to sepsis is a common theme for all immunomodulatory therapy. As shown in Fig. 16.1, the typical response is one of initial exuberant production of proinflammatory cytokines and then a compensatory anti-inflammatory phase (also known as immunoparalysis, endotoxin tolerance or compensatory anti-inflammatory response syndrome). Trying to dampen the proinflammatory phase runs the risk of making the anti-inflammatory phase more extensive, and the duration and severity of immunoparalysis correlates with the risk of death from nosocomial complications [4, 5].

Even when patients are overtly similar, marked variability in the clinical response to the same causative organism is seen. The cause(s) of this significant variability in response to pathogens is multifactorial but clearly has a significant genetic component [6]. Insights into the inheritable risk factors for sepsis are gradually accumulating [7–9] and are a potential hope for the development of interventions in the future.

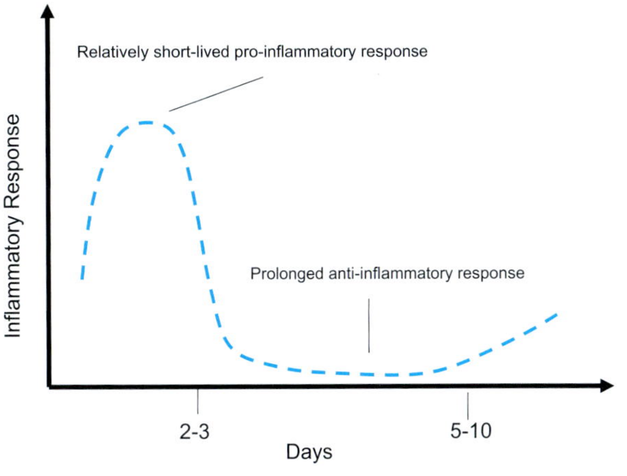

Fig. 16.1. The immune response in sepsis

16.3 Anti-inflammatory Approaches

16.3.1 Anti-TNF Therapies

Tumor necrosis factor (TNF) is a cytokine that for a number of reasons is thought to play a central role in the pathogenesis of sepsis and septic shock. First, TNF concentrations are increased during clinical and experimental sepsis [10–12]; second, increasing concentrations and especially persistence of high concentrations of TNF during sepsis are associated with non-survival [12]; third, endotoxin and bacterial challenge in animals and low-grade endotoxin challenge in humans leads to TNF release [13]; fourth, TNF challenge in animals [14] and humans [15, 16] leads to or simulates sepsis and organ failure; and, fifth, TNF neutralization in experimental sepsis frequently leads to amelioration of sepsis symptoms and increases survival [17–19]. Although these studies clearly underline the pivotal role that TNF plays in the pathogenesis of sepsis, in retrospect it is interesting that there was early data suggesting that in some situations, and particularly in cecal ligation and puncture peritonitis models of sepsis, anti-TNF antibodies actually resulted in increased mortality [20].

Based on the findings of the studies outlined above, drugs against TNF were produced and clinical trials were conducted to test whether inhibiting TNF also improves survival in human sepsis. Early studies of anti-TNF antibodies and TNF-receptor fusion proteins did not lead to the hoped for results in phase III trials [21–26]. However, a meta-analysis of all randomized controlled clinical studies shows that anti-TNF strategies with monoclonal antibodies are effective in increasing survival, with a mean improvement in survival of ~3% [27]. It is striking that most trials show a small, albeit non-significant, increase in survival in patients treated with anti-TNF drugs, suggesting that TNF inhibition has led to beneficial effects in subgroups of patients. The recent positive results with afelimomab targeting patients with sepsis and elevated serum interleukin-6 levels [28] further reinforces the fact that effective reduction in TNF production or effect has therapeutic potential.

A variety of reasons have been suggested for why the effects of these anti-TNF strategies have not produced the dramatic clinical benefit expected from the animal studies. In addition to other reasons, each of these strategies attempted to neutralize already-produced TNF. A more effective strategy may be to suppress or modulate the ongoing production of TNF. In addition, each of these strategies affects the intravascular space predominantly, if not exclusively. Much of the organ dysfunction caused by sepsis may be occurring in spaces without direct intravascular involvement, such as the respiratory epithelium. In addition, the effect of anti-TNF antibodies is only on extracellular or membrane-associated TNF and not intracellular levels.

Two drugs known to reduce TNF production and therefore potential immunomodulatory agents in sepsis are thalidomide and pentoxifylline. Thalidomide shows some promise in an animal *Pseudomonas* sepsis model [29], and can inhibit septic shock in mice [30] and rats [31] injected with endotoxin. LASSBio-468, a thalidomide analogue, also improves survival in mice injected with endotoxin [32].

Pretreatment with pentoxifylline significantly reduces the TNF response to endotoxin in human peripheral blood mononuclear cells and improves survival in endotoxin treated rats [33], but the results when it is given after exposure are unclear. Interestingly pentoxifylline had beneficial effects on coagulation dysfunction after endotoxin injection in rabbits [34], suggesting that it may be able to ameliorate sepsis-induced organ damage. The combination of pentoxifylline and thalidomide has also been shown to reduce mortality from endoxin induced shock in rats [35]. Unlike thalidomide, pentoxifylline has been trialed clinically in neonatal sepsis for nearly a decade, but with inconclusive results largely due to the small number of subjects enrolled and inconsistent methodology amongst the studies [36]. Results have varied from encouragingly positive [37], to a clear trend to worse outcome [38], and much further research is clearly required.

16.3.2 Other Anti-Cytokine Strategies

Given experimental data suggesting IL-1 produces a nearly identical inflammatory response to TNF, this was another logical target for intervention in sepsis. Interleukin-1 receptor antagonist (IL1-RN) is a natural antagonist of IL-1 and showed some promise in animal studies. However, as with anti-TNF trials, the phase III studies of IL1-RN were disappointingly negative [39] after promising early clinical data [40, 41].

Amongst the other failed anti-inflammatory agents trialed to date are prostaglandin antagonists [42, 43], bradykinin antagonists [33] and platelet activating factor antagonists [34, 35]. When taken human clinical trials all have failed to demonstrate any net beneficial effect despite initial promising results in animal studies.

16.3.3 Corticosteroids

With their potent anti-inflammatory action and proven efficacy in a variety of autoimmune diseases, glucocorticoids are an obvious choice of agent to try in patients thought to have an excessive, and deleterious, immune response in sepsis. The use of glucocorticoids in a deliberately immunosuppressive dose in patients with severe sepsis is very different to their increasingly accepted use in lower, physiological replacement doses [44, 45].

The evidence for high dose glucocorticoid therapy in patients with severe sepsis is poor with randomized, controlled trials showing no benefit [46–48]. Pooled analysis of nine randomized, controlled trials showed no beneficial effect of corticosteroids in patients with septic shock [49]. Even more disturbing was a trend to greater mortality in patients receiving corticosteroids, particularly in those who developed secondary infections.

However, recently interest has renewed in their use in the setting of severe community-acquired pneumonia after a small pilot study found a significant survival advantage for patients treated with a continuous hydrocortisone infusion [50]. Although there are problems with this study, notably the absence of any mortality in the treatment group, there is support for high dose glucocorticoids in other respiratory infections such as *Pneumocystis carinii* pneumonia [51, 52] and severe *Varicella* pneumonia [53]. Monton and coworkers [54] also studied the effect of intravenous methylprednisolone on bronchoalveolar lavage fluid (BALF) and serum cytokines in 20 patients with severe nosocomial pneumonia or CAP. The 11 patients who received methylprednisolone had significantly lower serum and BALF cytokine and C-reactive protein levels. There was also a non-significant trend to lower mortality in the steroid treated group (36% vs. 67%).

16.3.4 Macrolide Antibiotics

Although macrolide antibiotics have been used as anti-microbial agents for more than 50 years, recent studies, particularly in pneumonia, have focused attention on their potent immunomodulatory properties. Observational studies by Mufson and Stanek [55], Waterer et al. [56], Martinez et al. [57], Baddour et al. [58] and Weiss et al. [59] have all identified significant mortality reductions in patients with bacteremic pneumococcal pneumonia who received combination antibiotic therapy compared to patients who received monotherapy. Additional observational studies in more general CAP cohorts have also identified outcome benefits of combination therapy over monotherapy [60–63]. While the mechanism is unclear, the most consistent finding is that the key component of combination therapy is the macrolide. This is further supported by a recent study that found that a macrolide was clearly superior to a fluroquinolone as the agent used in combination with a beta-lactam in patients with severe pneumonia [64].

Macrolide antibiotics fairly consistently reduce production of inflammatory cytokines, including TNF, interleukin-1β, interleukin-6, interleukin-8, gamma interferon (IFN-γ) [65], and intercellular adhesion molecule-1 [66, 67]. In both human respiratory epithelial cells [68] and monocytes [69], the reduction in proinflammatory cytokine production is probably via suppression of nuclear factor kappa beta activation. However, given the multitude of effects, macrolides likely act at multiple sites within the inflammatory cascade [70].

Two recent publications have demonstrated a clear survival advantage of clarithromycin therapy in a rabbit-pyelonephritis model of sepsis [71, 72]. Although clarithromycin had no anti-microbial activity against the *Escherichia coli* causing the sepsis, its addition to therapy resulted in a marked increase in survival. The survival benefit was almost equivalent to that of an active bacteriocidal agent (amikacin). Furthermore the increase in survival with administration of clarithromycin was accompanied by a marked decrease in monocyte activation and TNF production compared to control [72]. Earlier work by the same group showed a similar benefit in a rabbit *Pseudomonas*-peritonitis sepsis model [73], demonstrating that the effect was dependent on neither site nor microorganism.

Macrolide antibiotics are now used in a wide range of diseases for their immunomodulatory properties. This list includes diffuse panbronchiolitis, where erythromycin reduces the 5-year mortality rate from 70% to less than 20% [74, 75], cystic fibrosis [76–79], bronchiectasis [80], and obliterative bronchiolitis [77, 81]. With the strength of the clinical data in pneumonia and the supportive animal and basic science data, further studies in patients with severe sepsis are keenly anticipated.

16.3.5 HMG-CoA Reductase Inhibitors

A number of recent retrospective studies have focused attention on the immunomodulatory (as distinct from the cholesterol lowering) properties of HMG-CoA reductase inhibitors (or statins). In patients with bacteremia, use of a statin prior to admission was associated with a substantially lower mortality rate (odds ratio 0.39; CI 95% 0.17, 0.91; $p=0.029$) [82]. Population studies have also suggested a lower risk of severe sepsis in patients taking statins for cardiovascular disease [83, 84]. Statins given after the onset of sepsis also improve survival in mice subjected to cecal ligation and puncture [85].

The exact mechanism by which statins might have beneficial effects in patients is unknown but they clearly can have significant immunological effects [86]. The most likely mechanism is via their ability to prevent NF-kappaB transactivation [87, 88]. Statins also appear to suppress toll-like receptor 2 and 4 expression [89,

90], thereby reducing sensitivity to bacterial antigens, and simvistatin has been shown to modulate chemokine and chemokine receptor expression [91].

There are no current published clinical trials in human subjects, but given the fact that statins are relatively non-toxic, widely available and relatively cheap these are very likely to be conducted over the next few years.

16.4 Immune Stimulation

16.4.1 Granulocyte Colony-Stimulating Factor

The neutrophil, or polymorphonuclear leukocyte (PMN), is a key cell in the host defense against microbial pathogens, particularly against bacteria and fungi. Both alcohol and diabetes, known risk factors for severe sepsis, have been shown to impair PMN function [92, 93]. A logical hypothesis following from this is that improving PMN function may improve the outcome of sepsis.

Granulocyte colony-stimulating factor (G-CSF) is one of a family of glycoproteins that control hematopoiesis [94]. G-CSF has significant effects on PMN function, increasing the response to chemotaxins, enhancing phagocytosis, increasing the respiratory burst, delaying neutrophil apoptosis and increasing bactericidal and fungicidal activity [94, 95]. G-CSF also accelerates the development of PMNs, leading to an increased rate of release from the bone marrow [95]. Due to these properties, G-CSF was an attractive candidate for study in patients with sepsis.

Since PMNs have been implicated in the development of multiorgan dysfunction, including ARDS [96, 97], the potential for harm from G-CSF therapy in some patients also exists. PMNs newly released from the bone marrow appear to preferentially sequester in the lung microvasculature [98], raising further concern about an increased risk of ARDS.

Animal pneumonia models demonstrate both potentials of GCSF treatment. Karzai and colleagues [99] used an endobronchial instillation model to demonstrate that G-CSF had a beneficial effect in *S. aureus* infected rats while *E. coli* infected rats had increased pulmonary injury and mortality with GCSF treatment. A significantly greater drop in peripheral PMN counts in *E. coli* infected rats was consistent with neutrophil mediated lung injury secondary to adherence to endothelium and subsequent degranulation, to which the lung is particularly susceptible [100]. The dose of *E. coli* given was also fivefold greater than the dose of *S. aureus,* raising the possibility that the *E. coli* arm actually produced a model of acute lung injury rather than pneumonia.

The potential pathogen-specific effects of G-CSF are supported by the same research group who confirmed that G-CSF was ineffective in a canine *E. coli* peritoneal sepsis model [101]. However, other researchers have observed G-CSF administration improved survival in animals with Gram negative sepsis [102]. The site of infection may also be important, with suggestions that G-CSF may only be effective for localized extravascular infection where stimulated neutrophils can have a maximum effect [103].

Initial studies of G-CSF in non-neutropenic human patients with pneumonia were encouraging [104]. Nelson et al. [105] conducted a prospective, multicenter, randomized, placebo controlled trial of G-CSF 300 μg/day (for up to 10 days) in 756 patients with community-acquired pneumonia, 380 of whom received active drug. G-CSF appeared to be safe in this population, with even a trend to less ARDS and disseminated intravascular coagulation (DIC), although the numbers of each complication were small. Overall, no significant benefit was demonstrated, and while a trend to better outcome in patients with multilobar pneumonia was found, a subsequent trial looking specifically at multilobar disease did not confirm this benefit [106]. A further follow-up study again in patients with pneumonia and sepsis found no advantage with G-CSF therapy [107], and in a study of non-neutropenic patients with nosocomial pneumonia G-CSF gave no survival advantage [108].

Despite the discouraging results in patients with pneumonia, research has continued trying to define the patient population who will benefit from G-CSF. In rats G-CSF appears to help prevent secondary sepsis after an initial traumatic insult [109]. However, G-CSF appears to increase the likelihood of lung injury in mechanically ventilated rats [110]. Further human studies may well eventuate if a population can be clearly defined in whom G-CSF is likely to beneficial.

16.4.2 Granulocyte-Macrophage Colony-Stimulating Factor

Granulocyte-macrophage colony-stimulating factor (GM-CSF) is another hematopoietic growth factor that has attracted interest as a therapeutic agent in sepsis. Unlike G-CSF, as its name implies GM-CSF has a much greater effect on cells of the monocyte-macrophage lineage [111]. This is particularly pertinent given that monocytes are generally considered to be the primary engine for cytokine production driving the pathogenesis of severe sepsis and septic shock [112–114].

A pilot study of GM-CSF in patients with sepsis-induced respiratory failure found modest improvements in gas exchange and faster ARDS resolution in the treatment group compared to a placebo group [115]. However, Rosenbloom and colleagues [116] conducted a randomized, placebo-controlled, unblinded trial of GM-CSF in 40 non-neutropenic patients with sepsis and found a significantly greater rate of clinical and microbiologic cure or improvement, but no difference in mortality. This was, however, not a typical group of sepsis patients as there was a high percentage (45%) of solid-organ transplant recipients. As these patients are typically still on immunosuppressive therapy, the results are probably not generalizable to 'routine' patients with sepsis. Again further human studies are unlikely to evolve until the patient subgroups most likely to benefit are further defined.

16.5 Conclusion

Despite all the promise the goal of modifying the immune response to improve the outcome of patients with severe sepsis remains elusive. Initial promising animal studies, and phase I and phase II studies have not eventuated into successful phase III trials. Much of the failure may be due to failure to select the right patient group rather than lack of efficacy of the agent. Our current tools for the assessment of immune function in patients with sepsis are crude and until these improve we may not be able to adequately target agents that have the potential to cause harm if used in the wrong situation.

Much of the immediate promise is surprisingly not with expensive, new agents, but with the relatively cheap macrolides and statins. While full clinical trials have not been conducted, the widespread use of these drugs for their traditional indications, their known safety and their low cost make them very appealing agents in sepsis. Only time will tell if they also fail to live up to expectation when assessed rigorously in a proper, randomized, placebo controlled trial. In the meantime research continues to try and define appropriate populations for drugs that have failed the phase III hurdle. As our knowledge of the immunology of sepsis improves and our ability to assess immune individual immune status in a rapid and accurate manner improves drugs such as anti-TNF, antibodies may well see a resurgence of interest and further clinical trials.

References

1. Angus DC, Linde-Zwirble WT, Lidicker J, et al. (2001) Epidemiology of severe sepsis in the United States: analysis of incidence, outcome, and associated costs of care. Crit Care Med 29:1303–1310
2. Simpson JC, Macfarlane JT, Watson J, et al. (2000) A national confidential enquiry into community acquired pneumonia deaths in young adults in England and Wales. British Thoracic Society Research Committee and Public Health Laboratory Service. Thorax 55(12):1040–1045
3. Austrian R, Gold J (1964) Pneumococcal bacteremia with special reference to bacteremic pneumococcal pneumonia. Ann Intern Med 60:759–776
4. Munford RS, Pugin J (2001) Normal responses to injury prevent systemic inflammation and can be immunosuppressive. Am J Respir Crit Care Med 163(2):316–321
5. Muller Kobold AC, Tulleken JE, Zijlstra JG, et al. (2000) Leukocyte activation in sepsis; correlations with disease state and mortality. Intensive Care Med 26(7):883–892
6. Sorensen TI, Nielsen GG, Andersen PK, et al. (1988) Genetic and environmental influences on premature death in adult adoptees. N Engl J Med 318(12):727–732
7. Waterer GW, Wunderink RG (2003) Science review: Genetic variability in the systemic inflammatory response. Crit Care 7(4):308–314
8. Arcaroli J, Fessler MB, Abraham E (2005) Genetic polymorphisms and sepsis. Shock 24(4):300–312
9. Holmes CL, Russell JA, Walley KR (2003) Genetic polymorphisms in sepsis and septic shock: role in prognosis and potential for therapy. Chest 124(3):1103–1115
10. Casey LC, Balk RA, Bone RC (1993) Plasma cytokine and endotoxin levels correlate with survival in patients with the sepsis syndrome. Ann Intern Med 119(8):771–778
11. Debets JM, Kampmeijer R, van der Linden MP, et al. (1989) Plasma tumor necrosis factor and mortality in critically ill septic patients. Crit Care Med 17(6):489–494
12. Dofferhoff AS, Bom VJ, de Vries-Hospers HG, et al. (1992) Patterns of cytokines, plasma endotoxin, plasminogen activator inhibitor, and acute-phase proteins during the treatment of severe sepsis in humans. Crit Care Med 20(2):185–192
13. Michie HR, Manogue KR, Spriggs DR, et al. (1988) Detection of circulating tumor necrosis factor after endotoxin administration. N Engl J Med 318(23):1481–1486
14. Eichenholz PW, Eichacker PQ, Hoffman WD, et al. (1992) Tumor necrosis factor challenges in canines: patterns of cardiovascular dysfunction. Am J Physiol 263(3):H668–675
15. Lenk H, Tanneberger S, Muller U, Ebert J, et al. (1989) Phase II clinical trial of high-dose recombinant human tumor necrosis factor. Cancer Chemother Pharmacol 24(6): 391–392
16. Creaven PJ, Brenner DE, Cowens JW, et al. (1989) A phase I clinical trial of recombinant human tumor necrosis factor given daily for five days. Cancer Chemother Pharmacol 23(3):186–191
17. Beutler B, Milsark IW, Cerami AC (1985) Passive immunization against cachectin/tumor necrosis factor protects mice from lethal effect of endotoxin. Science 229(4716): 869–871
18. Beutler B (1993) Endotoxin, tumor necrosis factor, and related mediators: new approaches to shock. New Horiz 1(1):3–12
19. Tracey KJ, Fong Y, Hesse DG, et al. (1987) Anti-cachectin/TNF monoclonal antibodies prevent septic shock during lethal bacteraemia. Nature 330(6149):662–664
20. Echtenacher B, Falk W, Mannel DN, Krammer PH (1990) Requirement of endogenous tumor necrosis factor/cachectin for recovery from experimental peritonitis. J Immunol 145(11):3762–3766
21. Abraham E, Wunderink R, Silverman H, et al. (1995) Efficacy and safety of monoclonal antibody to human tumor necrosis factor alpha in patients with sepsis syndrome. A randomized, controlled, double-blind, multicenter clinical trial. TNF-alpha MAb Sepsis Study Group. JAMA 273(12): 934–941
22. Cohen J, Carlet J (1996) INTERSEPT: an international, multicenter, placebo-controlled trial of monoclonal antibody to human tumor necrosis factor-alpha in patients with sepsis. International Sepsis Trial Study Group. Crit Care Med 24(9):1431–1440

23. Abraham E, Anzueto A, Gutierrez G, et al. (1998) Double-blind randomised controlled trial of monoclonal antibody to human tumour necrosis factor in treatment of septic shock. NORASEPT II Study Group. Lancet 351(9107): 929–933
24. Fisher CJ Jr, Agosti JM, Opal SM, et al. (1996) Treatment of septic shock with the tumor necrosis factor receptor:Fc fusion protein. The Soluble TNF Receptor Sepsis Study Group. N Engl J Med 334(26):1697–1702
25. Reinhart K, Wiegand-Lohnert C, Grimminger F, et al. (1996) Assessment of the safety and efficacy of the monoclonal anti-tumor necrosis factor antibody-fragment, MAK 195F, in patients with sepsis and septic shock: a multicenter, randomized, placebo-controlled, dose-ranging study. Crit Care Med 24(5):733–742
26. Abraham E, Glauser MP, Butler T, et al. (1997) p55 Tumor necrosis factor receptor fusion protein in the treatment of patients with severe sepsis and septic shock. A randomized controlled multicenter trial. Ro 45-2081 Study Group. JAMA 277(19):1531–1538
27. Reinhart K, Karzai W (2001) Anti-tumor necrosis factor therapy in sepsis: update on clinical trials and lessons learned. Crit Care Med 29(7 Suppl):S121–125
28. Panacek EA, Marshall JC, Albertson TE, et al. (2004) Efficacy and safety of the monoclonal anti-tumor necrosis factor antibody F(ab')2 fragment afelimomab in patients with severe sepsis and elevated interleukin-6 levels. Crit Care Med 32(11):2173–2182
29. Giamarellos-Bourboulis EJ, Bolanos N, Laoutaris G, et al. (2005) Immunomodulatory intervention in sepsis by multidrug-resistant *Pseudomonas aeruginosa* with thalidomide: an experimental study. BMC Infect Dis 5:51
30. Moreira AL, Wang J, Sarno EN, et al. (1997) Thalidomide protects mice against LPS-induced shock. Braz J Med Biol Res 30(10):1199–1207
31. Schmidt H, Rush B, Simonian G, et al. (1996) Thalidomide inhibits TNF response and increases survival following endotoxin injection in rats. J Surg Res 63(1):143–146
32. Alexandre-Moreira MS, Takiya CM, de Arruda LB, et al. (2005) LASSBio-468: a new achiral thalidomide analogue which modulates TNF-alpha and NO production and inhibits endotoxic shock and arthritis in an animal model. Int Immunopharmacol 5(3):485–494
33. Coimbra R, Melbostad H, Loomis W, et al. (2005) Phosphodiesterase inhibition decreases nuclear factor-kappaB activation and shifts the cytokine response toward anti-inflammatory activity in acute endotoxemia. J Trauma 59(3): 575–582
34. Col R, Keskin E, Atalay B (2005) Effect of pentoxifylline on endotoxin-induced haemostatic disturbances in rabbits. Acta Vet Hung 53(3):325–335
35. Arrieta O, Ortiz-Reyes A, Rembao D, et al. (1999) Protective effect of pentoxifylline plus thalidomide against septic shock in mice. Int J Exp Pathol 80(1):11–16
36. Haque K, Mohan P (2003) Pentoxifylline for neonatal sepsis. Cochrane Database Syst Rev 4:CD004205
37. Lauterbach R, Pawlik D, Kowalczyk D, et al. (1999) Effect of the immunomodulating agent, pentoxifylline, in the treatment of sepsis in prematurely delivered infants: a placebo-controlled, double-blind trial. Crit Care Med 27(4):807–114
38. Selim K, Huseyin C, Ibrahim KH, et al. (2004) Effect of pentoxifylline on tumor necrosis factor-alpha and interleukin-6 levels in neonatal sepsis. Med J Malaysia 59(3):391–394
39. Opal SM, Fisher CJ Jr, Dhainaut JF, et al. (1997) Confirmatory interleukin-1 receptor antagonist trial in severe sepsis: a phase III, randomized, double-blind, placebo-controlled, multicenter trial. The Interleukin-1 Receptor Antagonist Sepsis Investigator Group. Crit Care Med 25(7): 1115–1124
40. Fisher CJ Jr, Slotman GJ, Opal SM, et al. (1994) Initial evaluation of human recombinant interleukin-1 receptor antagonist in the treatment of sepsis syndrome: a randomized, open-label, placebo-controlled multicenter trial. Crit Care Med 22(1):12–21
41. Fisher CJ Jr, Dhainaut JF, Opal SM, et al. (1994) Recombinant human interleukin 1 receptor antagonist in the treatment of patients with sepsis syndrome. Results from a randomized, double-blind, placebo-controlled trial. Phase III rhIL-1ra Sepsis Syndrome Study Group. JAMA 271(23): 1836–1843
42. Haupt MT, Jastremski MS, Clemmer TP, et al. (1991) I. Effect of ibuprofen in patients with severe sepsis: a randomized, double-blind, multicenter study. The Ibuprofen Study Group. Crit Care Med 19(11):1339–1347
43. Bernard GR, Wheeler AP, Russell JA, et al. (1997) The effects of ibuprofen on the physiology and survival of patients with sepsis. The Ibuprofen in Sepsis Study Group. N Engl J Med 336(13):912–918
44. Annane D, Sebille V, Charpentier C, et al. (2002) Effect of treatment with low doses of hydrocortisone and fludrocortisone on mortality in patients with septic shock. JAMA 288(7):862–871
45. Oppert M, Schindler R, Husung C, et al. (2005) Low-dose hydrocortisone improves shock reversal and reduces cytokine levels in early hyperdynamic septic shock. Crit Care Med 33(11):2457–2464
46. Bone RC, Fisher CJ Jr, Clemmer TP, et al. (1987) A controlled clinical trial of high-dose methylprednisolone in the treatment of severe sepsis and septic shock. N Engl J Med 317(11):653–658
47. Luce JM, Montgomery AB, Marks JD, et al. (1988) Ineffectiveness of high-dose methylprednisolone in preventing parenchymal lung injury and improving mortality in patients with septic shock. Am Rev Respir Dis 138(1):62–68
48. The Veterans Administration Systemic Sepsis Cooperative Study Group (1987) Effect of high-dose glucocorticoid therapy on mortality in patients with clinical signs of systemic sepsis. N Engl J Med 317(11):659–665
49. Cronin L, Cook DJ, Carlet J, et al. (1995) Corticosteroid treatment for sepsis: a critical appraisal and meta-analysis of the literature. Crit Care Med 23(8):1430–1439
50. Confalonieri M, Urbino R, Potena A, et al. (2005) Hydrocortisone infusion for severe community-acquired pneumonia: a preliminary randomized study. Am J Respir Crit Care Med 171(3):242–248
51. Bozzette SA, Sattler FR, Chiu J, et al. (1990) A controlled trial of early adjunctive treatment with corticosteroids for *Pneumocystis carinii* pneumonia in the acquired immunodeficiency syndrome. California Collaborative Treatment Group. N Engl J Med 323(21):1451–1457
52. Gagnon S, Boota AM, Fischl MA, et al. (1990) Corticosteroids as adjunctive therapy for severe *Pneumocystis carinii* pneumonia in the acquired immunodeficiency syndrome. A double-blind, placebo-controlled trial. N Engl J Med 323(21):1444–1450
53. Mer M, Richards GA (1998) Corticosteroids in life-threatening varicella pneumonia. Chest 114(2):426–431
54. Monton C, Ewig S, Torres A, et al. (1999) Role of glucocorticoids on inflammatory response in nonimmunosuppressed patients with pneumonia: a pilot study. Eur Respir J 14(1):218–220
55. Mufson MA, Stanek RJ (1999) Bacteremic pneumococcal pneumonia in one American City: a 20-year longitudinal study, 1978–1997. Am J Med 107(1A):34S–43S
56. Waterer GW, Somes GW, Wunderink RG (2001) Monother-

apy may be suboptimal for severe bacteremic pneumococcal pneumonia. Arch Intern Med 161(15):1837 – 1842
57. Martinez JA, Horcajada JP, Almela M, et al. (2003) Addition of a macrolide to a beta-lactam-based empirical antibiotic regimen is associated with lower in-hospital mortality for patients with bacteremic pneumococcal pneumonia. Clin Infect Dis 36(4):389 – 395
58. Baddour LM, Yu VL, Klugman KP, et al. (2004) Combination antibiotic therapy lowers mortality among severely ill patients with pneumococcal bacteremia. Am J Respir Crit Care Med 170(4):440 – 444
59. Weiss K, Low DE, Cortes L, et al. (2004) Clinical characteristics at initial presentation and impact of dual therapy on the outcome of bacteremic *Streptococcus pneumoniae* pneumonia in adults. Can Respir J 11(8):589 – 593
60. Dudas V, Hopefl A, Jacobs R, Guglielmo BJ (2000) Antimicrobial selection for hospitalized patients with presumed community-acquired pneumonia: a survey of nonteaching US community hospitals. Ann Pharmacother 34(4):446 – 452
61. Brown RB, Iannini P, Gross P, Kunkel M (2003) Impact of initial antibiotic choice on clinical outcomes in community-acquired pneumonia: analysis of a hospital claims-made database. Chest 123(5):1503 – 1511
62. Houck PM, MacLehose RF, Niederman MS, Lowery JK (2001) Empiric antibiotic therapy and mortality among medicare pneumonia inpatients in 10 western states: 1993, 1995, and 1997. Chest 119(5):1420 – 1426
63. Garcia Vazquez E, Mensa J, Martinez JA, et al. (2005) Lower mortality among patients with community-acquired pneumonia treated with a macrolide plus a beta-lactam agent versus a beta-lactam agent alone. Eur J Clin Microbiol Infect Dis 24(3):190 – 195
64. Mortensen EM, Restrepo MI, Anzueto A, Pugh J (2006) The impact of empiric antimicrobial therapy with a beta-lactam and fluroquinolone on mortality for patients with severe pneumonia. Crit Care (in press)
65. Vazifeh D, Bryskier A, Labro MT (2000) Effect of proinflammatory cytokines on the interplay between roxithromycin, HMR 3647, or HMR 3004 and human polymorphonuclear neutrophils. Antimicrob Agents Chemother 44(3): 511 – 521
66. Khair OA, Devalia JL, Abdelaziz MM, et al. (1995) Effect of erythromycin on *Haemophilus influenzae* endotoxin-induced release of IL-6, IL-8 and sICAM-1 by cultured human bronchial epithelial cells. Eur Respir J 8(9):1451 – 1457
67. Kawasaki S, Takizawa H, Ohtoshi T, et al. (1998) Roxithromycin inhibits cytokine production by an neutrophil attachment to human bronchial epithelial cells in vitro. Antimicrob Agents Chemother 42(6):1499 – 1502
68. Desaki M, Takizawa H, Ohtoshi T, et al. (2000) Erythromycin suppresses nuclear factor-kappaB and activator protein-1 activation in human bronchial epithelial cells. Biochem Biophys Res Commun 267(1):124 – 128
69. Kikuchi T, Hagiwara K, Honda Y, et al. (2002) Clarithromycin suppresses lipopolysaccharide-induced interleukin-8 production by human monocytes through AP-1 and NF-kappa B transcription factors. J Antimicrob Chemother 49(5):745 – 755
70. Tamaoki J (2004) The effects of macrolides on inflammatory cells. Chest 125(2 Suppl):41S–50S; quiz 51S
71. Giamarellos-Bourboulis E, Adamis T, Sabracos L, et al. (2005) Clarithromycin: immunomodulatory therapy of experimental sepsis and acute pyelonephritis by *Escherichia coli*. Scand J Infect Dis 37(1):48 – 54
72. Giamarellos-Bourboulis EJ, Baziaka F, Antonopoulou A, et al. (2005) Clarithromycin co-administered with amikacin attenuates systemic inflammation in experimental sepsis with *Escherichia coli*. Int J Antimicrob Agents 25(2): 168 – 172
73. Giamarellos-Bourboulis EJ, Adamis T, Laoutaris G, et al. (2004) Immunomodulatory clarithromycin treatment of experimental sepsis and acute pyelonephritis caused by multidrug-resistant *Pseudomonas aeruginosa*. Antimicrob Agents Chemother 48(1):93 – 99
74. Kudoh S, Azuma A, Yamamoto M, et al. (1998) Improvement of survival in patients with diffuse panbronchiolitis treated with low-dose erythromycin. Am J Respir Crit Care Med 157(6):1829 – 1832
75. Yamamoto M, Kondo A, Tamura M, et al. (1990) [Long-term therapeutic effects of erythromycin and new quinolone antibacterial agents on diffuse panbronchiolitis]. Nihon Kyobu Shikkan Gakkai Zasshi 28(10):1305 – 1313
76. Amsden GW (2005) Anti-inflammatory effects of macrolides – an underappreciated benefit in the treatment of community-acquired respiratory tract infections and chronic inflammatory pulmonary conditions? J Antimicrob Chemother 55(1):10 – 21
77. Schultz MJ (2004) Macrolide activities beyond their antimicrobial effects: macrolides in diffuse panbronchiolitis and cystic fibrosis. J Antimicrob Chemother 54(1):21 – 28
78. Wolter JM, Seeney SL, McCormack JG (2002) Macrolides in cystic fibrosis: is there a role? Am J Respir Med 1(4):235 – 241
79. Saiman L, Marshall BC, Mayer-Hamblett N, et al. (2003) Azithromycin in patients with cystic fibrosis chronically infected with *Pseudomonas aeruginosa:* a randomized controlled trial. JAMA 290(13):1749 – 1756
80. Koh YY, Lee MH, Sun YH, et al. (1997) Effect of roxithromycin on airway responsiveness in children with bronchiectasis: a double-blind, placebo-controlled study. Eur Respir J 10(5):994 – 999
81. Gerhardt SG, McDyer JF, Girgis RE, et al. (2003) Maintenance azithromycin therapy for bronchiolitis obliterans syndrome: results of a pilot study. Am J Respir Crit Care Med 168(1):121 – 125
82. Kruger P, Fitzsimmons K, Cook D, et al. (2006) Statin therapy is associated with fewer deaths in patients with bacteraemia. Intensive Care Med 32(1):75 – 79
83. Hackam DG, Mamdani M, Li P, Redelmeier DA (2006) Statins and sepsis in patients with cardiovascular disease: a population-based cohort analysis. Lancet 367(9508):413 – 418
84. Almog Y, Shefer A, Novack V, et al. (2004) Prior statin therapy is associated with a decreased rate of severe sepsis. Circulation 110(7):880 – 885
85. Merx MW, Liehn EA, Graf J, et al. (2005) Statin treatment after onset of sepsis in a murine model improves survival. Circulation 112(1):117 – 124
86. Inoue K, Takano H, Yanagisawa R, et al. (2004) Statin, inflammation, and sepsis. Chest 125(6):2365; author reply 2365
87. Holschermann H, Schuster D, Parviz B, et al. (2005) Statins prevent NF-kappaB transactivation independently of the IKK-pathway in human endothelial cells. Atherosclerosis 185(2):240 – 245
88. Wang HR, Li JJ, Huang CX, et al. (2005) Fluvastatin inhibits the expression of tumor necrosis factor-alpha and activation of nuclear factor-kappaB in human endothelial cells stimulated by C-reactive protein. Clin Chim Acta 353 (1 – 2):53 – 60
89. Methe H, Kim JO, Kofler S, et al. (2005) Statins decrease Toll-like receptor 4 expression and downstream signaling in human CD14+ monocytes. Arterioscler Thromb Vasc Biol 25(7):1439 – 1445
90. Niessner A, Steiner S, Speidl WS, et al. (2006) Simvastatin

suppresses endotoxin-induced upregulation of toll-like receptors 4 and 2 in vivo. Atherosclerosis [Epub ahead of print]
91. Veillard NR, Braunersreuther V, Arnaud C, et al. (2005) Simvastatin modulates chemokine and chemokine receptor expression by geranylgeranyl isoprenoid pathway in human endothelial cells and macrophages. Atherosclerosis 188(1):51 - 58
92. Repine JE, Clawson CC, Goetz FC (1980) Bactericidal function of neutrophils from patients with acute bacterial infections and from diabetics. J Infect Dis 142(6):869 -875
93. Brayton RG, Stokes PE, Schwartz MS, et al. (1970) Effect of alcohol and various diseases on leukocyte mobilization, phagocytosis and intracellular bacterial killing. N Engl J Med 282(3):123 - 128
94. Welte K, Gabrilove J, Bronchud MH, et al. (1996) Filgrastim (r-metHuG-CSF): the first 10 years. Blood 88(6): 1907 - 1929
95. Dale DC, Liles WC, Llewellyn C, et al. (1998) Effects of granulocyte-macrophage colony-stimulating factor (GM-CSF) on neutrophil kinetics and function in normal human volunteers. Am J Hematol 57(1):7 - 15
96. Fujishima S, Aikawa N (1995) Neutrophil-mediated tissue injury and its modulation. Intensive Care Med 21(3): 277 - 285
97. Weiss SJ (1989) Tissue destruction by neutrophils. N Engl J Med 320(6):365 - 376
98. Fillion I, Ouellet N, Simard M, et al. (2001) Role of chemokines and formyl peptides in pneumococcal pneumonia-induced monocyte/macrophage recruitment. J Immunol 166(12):7353 - 7361
99. Karzai W, von Specht BU, Parent C, et al. (1999) G-CSF during *Escherichia coli* versus *Staphylococcus aureus* pneumonia in rats has fundamentally different and opposite effects. Am J Respir Crit Care Med 159(5):1377 - 1382
100. Bersten A, Sibbald WJ (1989) Acute lung injury in septic shock. Crit Care Clin 5(1):49 - 79
101. Quezado Z, Parent C, Karzai W, et al. (2001) Acute G-CSF therapy is not protective during lethal *E. coli* sepsis. Am J Physiol Regul Integr Comp Physiol 281(4):R1177 - 1185
102. Smith WS, Sumnicht GE, Sharpe RW, et al. (1995) Granulocyte colony-stimulating factor versus placebo in addition to penicillin G in a randomized blinded study of gram-negative pneumonia sepsis: analysis of survival and multisystem organ failure. Blood 86(4):1301 - 1309
103. Sevransky JE, Parent C, Cui X, et al. (2004) Granulocyte colony-stimulating factor has differing effects comparing intravascular versus extravascular models of sepsis. J Trauma 57(3):618 - 625
104. deBoisblanc BP, Mason CM, Andresen J, et al. (1997) Phase 1 safety trial of Filgrastim (r-metHuG-CSF) in nonneutropenic patients with severe community-acquired pneumonia. Respir Med 91(7):387 - 394
105. Nelson S, Belknap SM, Carlson RW, et al. (1998) A randomized controlled trial of filgrastim as an adjunct to antibiotics for treatment of hospitalized patients with community-acquired pneumonia. CAP Study Group. J Infect Dis 178(4):1075 - 1080
106. Nelson S, Heyder AM, Stone J, et al. (2000) A randomized controlled trial of filgrastim for the treatment of hospitalized patients with multilobar pneumonia. J Infect Dis 182(3):970 - 973
107. Root RK, Lodato RF, Patrick W, et al. (2003) Multicenter, double-blind, placebo-controlled study of the use of filgrastim in patients hospitalized with pneumonia and severe sepsis. Crit Care Med 31(2):367 - 373
108. Hartmann P, Lammertink J, Mansmann G, et al. (2005) A randomized, placebo-controlled study of the use of filgrastim in non neutropenic patients with nosocomial pneumonia. Eur J Med Res 10(1):29 - 35
109. Bauhofer A, Lorenz W, Kohlert F, et al. (2006) Granulocyte colony-stimulating factor prophylaxis improves survival and inflammation in a two-hit model of hemorrhage and sepsis. Crit Care Med 34:778 - 784
110. Karzai W, Cui X, Heinicke N, et al. (2005) Neutrophil stimulation with granulocyte colony-stimulating factor worsens ventilator-induced lung injury and mortality in rats. Anesthesiology 103(5):996 - 1005
111. Hamilton JA, Anderson GP (2004) GM-CSF biology. Growth Factors 22(4):225 - 231
112. Van Amersfoort ES, Van Berkel TJ, Kuiper J (2003) Receptors, mediators, and mechanisms involved in bacterial sepsis and septic shock. Clin Microbiol Rev 16(3):379 - 414
113. Das UN (2000) Critical advances in septicemia and septic shock. Crit Care 4(5):290 - 296
114. Haveman JW, Muller Kobold AC, Tervaert JW, et al. (1999) The central role of monocytes in the pathogenesis of sepsis: consequences for immunomonitoring and treatment. Neth J Med 55(3):132 - 141
115. Presneill JJ, Harris T, Stewart AG, et al. (2002) A randomized phase II trial of granulocyte-macrophage colony-stimulating factor therapy in severe sepsis with respiratory dysfunction. Am J Respir Crit Care Med 166(2):138 - 143
116. Rosenbloom AJ, Linden PK, Dorrance A, et al. (2005) Effect of granulocyte-monocyte colony-stimulating factor therapy on leukocyte function and clearance of serious infection in nonneutropenic patients. Chest 127(6): 2139 - 2150

Chapter 17

Antibiotic Induced Diarrhea

O.J. Pérez-Jimenez

17.1 Introduction

Antibiotic induced diarrhea is a spectrum of diseases varying from asymptomatic colonization with *Clostridium difficile* to fulminant colitis. The most common expression of this disease complex is antibiotic induced diarrhea without colitis. This chapter will cover the clinical and epidemiological manifestations of pseudomembranous colitis with special attention to the critically ill patient. Other causes of antibiotic induced diarrhea will be reviewed briefly.

Pseudomembranous colitis was initially described by Finney at the end of the nineteenth century [1]. The case was a 22-year-old female with a gastric tumor who underwent resection; the patient then developed severe diarrhea postoperatively. Postmortem examination showed the presence of a diphtheric membrane in the small bowel [1]. With the advent of antibiotics a surge in cases of nosocomial diarrhea was noted. Even with only the use of antibiotic prophylaxis there is a rate of diarrhea of 14–27% [2, 3]. Earlier microbiological studies revealed the presence of *Staphylococcus aureus* in some patients, and the fact that treatment with oral vancomycin improved the diarrhea supported the theory of *Staphylococcus aureus* as the etiologic agent.

In the 1950s the relationship of antibiotic use and the development of a syndrome of fever, diarrhea and colitis were clearly established. Anatomic studies especially in patients who received antibiotic prophylaxis prior to surgery show the presence of *Staphylococcus aureus*. These findings were based on Gram's stain and stool culture. In 1970 a group from Barnes Hospital in Saint Louis performed the first prospective study of clindamycin associated diarrhea. Ten percent of the patients showed the presence of pseudomembranes in the colon at endoscopy [4]. *Staphylococcus aureus* was not isolated in any of these patients. Further studies on stool samples in the same group showed the presence of *C. difficile* and its cytopathic toxin in patients with colitis.

Several animal studies using rodents have shown that treatment with penicillin induced fulminant colitis. In 1974, while looking at the role of viruses in a guinea pig model of antibiotic induced diarrhea, Green noted cytopathic changes in tissue cultured cells. This is probably the first report of the effect of *C. difficile* in the literature [5]. Earlier reports noted that *C. difficile* produces a toxin that was lethal to guinea pigs and rabbits and that most strains of the bacteria produce this toxin. Attention was shifted to these bacteria and in 1977 the relationship between colitis, toxin and *C. difficile* was clearly elucidated [6].

17.2 Clinical Presentation

The typical presentation for *Clostridium difficile* diarrhea is abdominal pain, profuse diarrhea, fever and leukocytosis after exposure to antibiotics. Symptoms can start 48 h after antibiotic administration, but can be seen up to 8 weeks after cessation of antibiotic therapy. The abdominal pain is crampy in nature, most frequently diffuse but can be localized to the left lower quadrant. Reports of patients with *C. difficile* colitis presenting with an acute abdomen have been noted especially in the elderly. Diarrhea is profuse, mucoid, green colored and watery with evidence of fecal leukocytes. Diarrhea can be severe with 15–30 bowel movements per day. The large volume loss can cause dehydration, electrolytic disturbances and hypotension. Bloody stools are unusual, but trace amounts of blood are frequently found. The fever is usually low grade but can be as high as 40.7°C. The leukocytosis, usually in the range of 10,000–20,000/mm^3, can reach counts greater than 40,000 cells/mm^3. Hypoalbuminemia may be present early in the disease and is attributed to a protein losing enteropathy. Polyarthritis involving large joints has been reported as an extraintestinal manifestation of pseudomembranous colitis [7].

Most of the hospitalized patients, up to 66%, will have infection with *C. difficile* as an asymptomatic carrier. These carriers are constantly shedding the organism and are reservoirs for the infection in the healthcare facility [8]. The carrier state may be due to the presence of serum IgG antibodies against toxin A, which protects against the development of diarrhea and colitis [9].

17.3 Pathophysiology

Clostridium difficile diarrhea, colitis and pseudomembranous colitis are toxin mediated mucosal inflammatory processes that are usually characterized by the presence of grossly or microscopically visible pseudomembranes consisting of nodules or large plaques containing leukocytes, fibrin, mucus and epithelial cells loosely adherent to the surface of the underlying inflamed and necrotic mucosa [7]. *Clostridium difficile* infection can manifest as asymptomatic carriage, diarrhea (secretory type), colitis with and without pseudomembranes, fulminant colitis with toxic dilatation of the colon, perforation, hypovolemia, shock and death.

Clostridium difficile associated diarrhea is caused primarily by the elaboration within the intestinal lumen of both toxin A and B. These toxins bind to the colonic mucosa inducing mucosal damage and inflammation. Most toxigenic isolates produce both toxins. Toxin A is a 308-kDa protein that is a neutrophil chemoattractant, cytotoxic to certain cell lines, and activates macrophages and mast cells. Cellular damage is induced by desegregation of actin and by the release of intracellular calcium [10]. Damage to the neuroenteric system has been reported.

Toxin B is a 270-kDa protein that causes depolymerization of filamentous actin. It is also a necrotizing enterotoxin 10 times more potent than toxin A in causing damage to the colonic mucosa in cell culture lines [11]. The diarrhea is caused by the toxins in the intestinal lumen adhering to the mucosal surface and inducing a severe inflammatory response that causes disruption of cell integrity and fluid flux into the lumen.

Newborns present a high colonization rate with *C. difficile*, up to 70% in the first 8 months but with a minimal rate of pseudomembranous colitis. Healthy adults show a prevalence of 2–3%, and when there is a recent history of antibiotic use the presence of *C. difficile* increases to 15–30% [11].

17.4 Epidemiology

Clostridium difficile is a sporulating organism that survives well in nature. Like most of the clostridia species their distribution in the environment is wide. Evaluation of epidemics includes case surveillance, stool cultures to identify carriers, typing of strains and cultures of environmental sources. These epidemiological tools have shown that *C. difficile* is the most common cause of nosocomial diarrhea. Most cases occur in hospitals, nursing homes and chronic care facilities, where cases have been reported occurring sporadically as well as in outbreaks. On the other hand, community acquired diarrhea caused by *C. difficile* is less common.

Clostridium difficile has been isolated from environmental samples in bed pans, toilets and floors of these facilities. Asymptomatic carriage of *C. difficile* has been reported in up to 30% of patients treated with antibiotics [12]. Transmission of *C. difficile* often occurs via the hands of hospital personnel and also by contact with contaminated surfaces and fomites [13, 14]. The frequency and incidence of *C. difficile* associated (CDAD) diarrhea varies widely not only geographically but within different institutions in the same geographic area. Risk factors for the development of *C. difficile* associated diarrhea other than antibiotic use are: colonic, gastric or pelvic surgery, spinal fracture, intestinal obstruction, colon carcinoma, leukemia, severe burns, uremia, heavy metal poisoning, hemolytic-uremic syndrome, ischemic vascular disease, shigellosis, severe infection, neonatal necrotizing enterocolitis, ischemic colitis and Hirschprung's disease [15]. Patients receiving postpyloric tube feeding have been noted to be at increased risk of acquiring *C. difficile* when compared to non-tube-fed patients [16].

Almost every antibiotic on the market has been implicated in cases of antibiotic induced diarrhea. The most common agents are ampicillin/amoxicillin, other penicillin derivatives, cephalosporins and clindamycin; and less frequently macrolides, fluoroquinolones and aminoglycosides. Even the drugs of choice for treatment of this condition, metronidazole and vancomycin, have been implicated in some cases of CDAD. Tetracycline, chloramphenicol and sulfonamides are now rarely implicated [17, 18]. Drugs with limited data to support a relationship are urinary antiseptics, parental aminoglycosides, parental vancomycin, antifungals, antiparasitics and antimycobacterial agents.

Antibiotics are not the only agents associated with *C. difficile* infection. Cases of patients developing *C. difficile* infection after chemotherapy have been reported [19]. Most chemotherapeutic agents also have antimicrobial activity that can alter the gut flora and cause overgrowth of *C. difficile*.

The National Nosocomial Infection Screening (NNIS) shows an increase in CDAD among ICU patients in large hospitals (>500 beds) [20]. Not only the frequency is increased but also the severity of the condition. Reports from Quebec and Pittsburg demonstrate increased mortality and more frequent colectomies in patients with CDAD. Further analysis of multiple strains revealed the presence of a variation of the tcdC segment of the genome. This mutation increases toxin production and the virulence of the strain.

17.5 Diagnostic Tests

17.5.1 Endoscopy

Endoscopy is the most rapid way to establish the diagnosis, but because of its cost and invasiveness it is usually reserved for patients who are seriously ill or in patients in whom a non-invasive test has been negative. Endoscopy is also helpful when other disease processes are being considered in the differential diagnosis. Physicians should be aware of the possibility of bowel perforation and bleeding as complications of endoscopy.

Diagnosis can be confirmed when yellowish nodules or the classic pseudomembranes are visualized. Lesions are more commonly found on the left colon, but a minority of patients will present only with right colonic lesions. Full colonoscopy should be performed especially if the left colon is unremarkable. Some patients may present with mild colonic erythema or patchy inflammation. Biopsies should be performed in cases with abnormal mucosa without the classic pseudomembranes to look for the microscopic changes suggestive of pseudomembranous colitis and to rule out other etiologies.

The histologic features of pseudomembranous colitis are not pathognomonic and can be seen in patients with ischemic colitis and other disorders.

17.5.2 Non-Invasive Tests

There is as yet no simple inexpensive, rapid, sensitive and specific test for the diagnosis of CDAD [6]. Not all laboratories provide the entire tests available on the market. Most tests target the cytotoxins produced by the pathogenic strains of *C. difficile*. The two most common tests available are: the cell culture assay for cytotoxin B and the enzyme immunoassay test for toxins A and B.

17.6 Cell Culture Assays

The cell culture assay is considered the gold standard for diagnosis of CDAD. This assay detects toxin B by its cytopathic effect in monolayer cell culture, usually in HEp-2 cells. The specificity of this assay is verified by neutralization of the cytopathic effect when antitoxin to *C. difficile* or *C. sordelli* is added. The major drawback of this test is that most laboratories do not offer tissue culture, results takes 24–48 h, and sensitivity and specificity can be affected by handling, storage of stool sample dilution and cell culture line used. On average this test is positive in more than 90% of patients with pseudomembranous colitis. The result is usually reported as detection of cytotoxin in the assay. Quantification of this response does not correlate with severity of disease.

17.7 Enzyme Immunoassays for Toxin A and B

Immunoassay is the most common and widely used test for detection of *C. difficile*. It is rapidly performed and relatively inexpensive. It provides good specificity (95–100%) and sensitivity (63–89%) [20, 21]. On average the EIA test for toxin A or B failed to detect about 10% (5–33%) of cases of *C. difficile* when compared to endoscopy or cell tissue culture assay. In cases of high clinical suspicion and a negative EIA, performing a more sensitive test like cell tissue culture assay or endoscopic evaluation should be considered to confirm the diagnosis. Sensitivity is rarely improved by sending more than one stool sample on the same day for EIA testing.

17.7.1 Other Available Tests

The latex agglutination test detects the presence of the enzyme glutamate dehydrogenase produced by *C. difficile*. This lack of specificity comes from the expression of this enzyme in non-toxigenic strains of *C. difficile*.

A test based on immunoblotting technique is commercially available (C.diffCUBE). The test detects toxin A with similar sensitivity and specificity to the EIA [22].

Culture of stool is rarely performed mostly because 30% of strains of *C. difficile* produce no toxin; it use is limited to research purposes.

17.8 Diagnostic Imaging

Plain films are usually unremarkable and should be reserved to rule out the late complications of this condition such as toxic megacolon and bowel perforation. Barium studies provide little information and can cause bowel perforation.

Computed tomography can demonstrate colonic wall thickening, colonic inflammation and ascites, but these findings can be seen in other infectious processes and also with bowel ischemia. Up to 50% of patients with CDAD have normal imaging studies. In one study CT failed to detect which patients would benefit from surgical therapy or medical therapy [23]. Nuclear medicine studies are only used on an experimental basis.

17.9 Treatment

Initial therapy includes the discontinuation of the implicated antibiotic, supportive measures and in some cases therapy with antimicrobial agents. Large volume diarrhea when present may be associated with fluid and electrolytic imbalances that need to be corrected with intravenous fluids and electrolyte replacement. Some cases may need hyperalimentation secondary to severe catabolism and the presence of protein losing enteropathy. Avoidance of antiperistaltics and opiates is encouraged to prevent prolonged mucosal exposure to toxins [24]. Selection of antibiotic used should be based on the severity of the condition. A clinical severity score was developed to help classify patients in two categories. The clinical severity score gives one point for each of the following: underlying immunosuppression/chronic medical condition, altered or depressed mental status, abdominal pain or distention, WBC >20,000 or <1,500 or bandemia >10%. Hypoalbuminemia, ascites or *Pneumatosis coli* A score >4 is considered severe [25, 35].

17.9.1 Antimicrobials

Antimicrobials are used frequently to treat pseudomembranous colitis. The most commonly used are metronidazole and vancomycin. Less frequently used are teicoplanin and bacitracin. Failure to respond to conservative treatment and a diagnostic test positive for *C. difficile* are indications for antibiotic therapy. In patients with severe symptoms empiric therapy may be started while waiting for the results of the diagnostic test.

Initial oral therapy includes vancomycin 250–500 mg four times a day or metronidazole 500 mg tid. Some advocate a combination of IV metronidazole with PO vancomycin in severe symptoms for 14–21 days followed by a slow taper of vancomycin [26, 32].

If not able to tolerate oral therapy, metronidazole 500 mg IV four times a day or vancomycin 500 mg in 100 ml normal saline via enema every 6 h are alternatives. Resistance or relapse is seen more frequently in metronidazole especially in the last 5 years [27, 36]. Adjustment in the therapeutic regimen will be necessary if this trend continues.

17.9.2 Non-Antibiotic Alternatives

Alternative ways of treating CDAD have been tried with some success. Probiotics have been tried with conflicting results. *Saccharomyces boulardii* was tried in combination with vancomycin for the prevention of recurrence; there was a decreased incidence of relapse in patients with more than two episodes but no benefit in patients with the initial episode [28]. Other probiotics used include *Lactobacillus*, non-toxigenic *C. difficile*, and *E. coli* [29, 30]. A recent review of probiotics in the treatment of CDAD showed efficacy only with S. boulardii. Limited data from Lactobacillus and commercially available bacterial combinations precluded a more definitive conclusion [31]. More radical approaches like fecal "transplant" from a donor in an attempt to repopulate the bowel with non-toxigenic flora have been attempted in limited circumstances [31]. Fecal instillation of yogurt with active cultures has been tried in the past.

Indication for surgery includes progressive severity of the colitis despite medical therapy.

Future alternatives include IVIG (normal immune globulin) and hyperimmune globulin (obtained from plasmapheresis of vaccinated donors). Monoclonal antibodies against CDA1 and CDB1 are undergoing clinical trials. Use of corticosteroids outside of a clinical trial is discouraged at this time.

New agents undergoing clinical trials include a vaccine (Acambis), a resin (Tolevamer) and multiple antibiotics (rifalaxil, ramoplanin, tinidazole, nitazoxanide, rifaximin). Preliminary reports show efficacy of 64–100%. Some of the data available on some of these agents are based on the Hamster model for colitis.

17.9.3 Treatment of Recurrence

Treatment of recurrence is a challenge because probably there is a defective immune response. There is no evidence that relates this phenomena to resistance to metronidazole or vancomycin. The probability of recurrence after a second episode is 65%. Treatment of first relapse will be retreatment with metronidazole or PO vancomycin for 10–14 days. For second relapse vancomycin should be used for 6 weeks on a slow taper: week one 125 qid, week two 125 mg bid, week three 125 mg daily, week four 125 mg qod, weeks five–six 125 mg q3d [32].

Other alternatives include a combination of vancomycin with rifampin or cholestyramine. In the pediatric population passive immunotherapy with IVIG has been successful.

17.9.4 Prevention of *C. difficile* Diarrhea

Exposure to antibiotics, hospitalization and enteral feedings are some of the risk factors for acquisition of this condition. Therefore judicious use of antibiotics has been shown to decrease the incidence of CDAD. One study restricting the use of clindamycin demonstrated a decreased incidence of antibiotic induced diarrhea [32].

Hospitalized patients are at risk of acquiring the infection nosocomially. Strict hand washing, use of gloves while manipulating patients and disinfection of objects infected with *C. difficile* with sodium hypochlorite, glutaraldehyde or ethylene oxide are effective measures to control the spread of the organism. Patients with colitis should be placed in rooms with private bathrooms at least during the diarrhea phase. Enteric isolation should be discontinued once the diarrhea resolves. Eradication of the carrier state is difficult; neither vancomycin nor metronidazole is reliably effective in eradicating the *C. difficile* carrier state.

Vaccination provides a rise in serum levels of IgG antitoxin A and this correlates with immunity [33]. (Targets for vaccination should include patients with recurrent CDAD and prevention of high risk patients. Passive immunization using hyperimmune globulin (HuMabs) can be used on recurrent CDAD patients in patients with fulminant or refractory disease and as prophylaxis in high risk hospital patients.)

The most important measure is education of the medical and nursing staff about the epidemiology and pathophysiology of this condition. The importance of hand washing between contacts with patients, the use of gloves when caring for a patient with CDAD and the judicious use of antimicrobials are simple measures that will decrease the incidence of this infection [34].

References

1. Finney JMT (1893) Gastro-enterostomy for cicatrizing ulcer of the pylorus. Bull Johns Hopkins Hosp 4:53
2. Hummel RP, Alteimer WA, Hill EQ (1964) Iatrogenic staphylococcal enterocolitis. Ann Surg 160:551
3. Wakefield RD, Sommers SC (1953) Fatal membranous staphylococcal enteritis in surgical patients. Ann Surg 138:249
4. Tedesco FJ, Barton RW, Alpers DH (1974) Clindamycin-associated colitis: A prospective study. Ann Intern Med 81:429
5. Green RH (1974) The association of viral activation with penicillin toxicity in guinea pigs and hamsters. Yale J Biol Med 47:166
6. Bartlett JG, Chang TW, Gurthwith M, et al. (1978) Antibiotic-associated pseudomembranous colitis due to toxin producing clostridia. N Engl J Med 298:531
7. Veillard E, Guggenbuhl P, Bello S, et al. (1998) Reactive oligoarthritis in a patient with *Clostridium difficile* pseudomembranous colitis, review of literature. Rev Rhum Engl Ed 65:795
8. Mcfarland LV, Mulligan ME, Kwok, et al. (1989) Nosocomial acquisition of *Clostridium difficile* infection. N Engl J Med 320:204
9. Kyne L, Warny M, Quamar A, et al. (2000) Asymptomatic carriage of *Clostridium difficile* and serum levels of IgG antibody against toxin A. N Engl J Med 342–390
10. Fekety R (1997) Guidelines for the diagnosis and management of *Clostridium difficile* diarrhea and colitis. Am J Gastroenterol 92:739
11. Riegler M, Sedivy R, Pothoulakis C, et al. (1995) *Clostridium difficile* toxin B is more potent than toxin A in damaging human colonic mucosa in vitro. J Clin Invest 95:2004
12. Johnson S, Gerding D (1996) *Clostridium difficile*. In: Mayhall CG (ed) Hospital epidemiology and infection control. Williams & Wilkins, Baltimore, p 399
13. Kim K-H, Fekety R, Batts DH, et al. (1981) Isolation of *Clostridium difficile* from the environment and contacts of patients with antibiotic induced colitis. J Infect Dis 143:42
14. Wilcox M (1996) Cleaning up *Clostridium difficile* infection. Lancet 348:767
15. Bartlett JG, Gorbach SL (1995) Pseudomembranous enterocolitis (antibiotic-related colitis). In: Stollerman GH (ed) Advances in internal medicine. Year-Book Medical Publishers, Chicago, p 445
16. Zimmaro D, Johnson S, Savik, K, et al. (1998) Acquisition of *Clostridium difficile* and *Clostridium difficile*-associated diarrhea in hospitalized patients receiving tube feeding. Ann Intern Med 129:1012
17. Kelly CP, Pothoulakis C, LaMont TT (1994) *Clostridium difficile* colitis. N Engl J Med 330:257
18. Fekety R (1996) Antibiotic-associated colitis. In: Mandell G, Bennet JE, Dolin R (eds) Principle and practices of infectious diseases, 4th edn. Churchill Livingstone, New York, p 978
19. Cudmore MA, Silva J, Feketey R, et al. (1982) *Clostridium difficile* colitis associated with cancer chemotherapy. Arch Intern Med 142:333
20. Jarvis B, Shevchuk YM (1997) Recurrent *Clostridium difficile* diarrhea associated with mitoxantrone and etoposide: a case report and review. Pharmacotherapy 17:606
21. Archibald LK, Banerjee SN, Jarvis WR (2004) Secular trends in hospital-acquired *Clostridium difficile* disease in the United States, 1987–2001. J Infect Dis 189:1585–9
22. McDonald LC, Owings M, Jernigan DB (2006) Increasing rates of *Clostridium difficile* infection among patients discharged from US short-stay hospitals, 1996–2003 CDC Emerging Infectious Diseases, Ahead of Print 12:3 March 2006
23. Merz CS, Kramer C, Forman, M, et al. (1994) Comparison of four commercially available rapid immunoassays with cytotoxin assay, and toxigenic culture for detection of *Clostridium difficile* toxin(s) from stool specimens. J Clin Microbiol 32:1142
24. Barbut F, Kajzer C, Planas N, et al. (1993) Comparison of three enzyme immunoassays, a cytotoxicity assay and toxigenic culture for diagnosis of *Clostridium difficile*-associated diarrhea. J Clin Microbiol 31:963
25. Kurzynski TA (1992) Evaluation of *C. difficile* CUBE test for detection of *Clostridium difficile*-associated diarrhea. Diagn Microbiol Infect Dis 15:493
26. Kawamoto S, Horton KM, Fishman EK (1999) Pseudomembranous colitis: can CT predict which patients will need surgical intervention? J Comput Assist Tomogr 23:79
27. Fekety R, Shah A (1993) Diagnosis and treatment of *C. difficile* colitis. JAMA 269:71
28. McFarland LV, Surawicz CM, Greenberg RN, et al. (1994) A randomized placebo control trial of *Saccharomyces boulardii* in combination with standard antibiotics for *Clostridium difficile* disease. JAMA 271:1913
29. Goerg KJ, Schorer E (1998) Probiotic therapy of pseudomembranous colitis combination of intestinal lavage and oral administration of *Escherichia coli*. Dtsch Med Wochenschr 123:1274
30. Gorbach SL (1987) Successful treatment of relapsing *Clostridium difficile* with *Lactobacillus* GG. Lancet 2:1519
31. McFarland LV (2006) Meta Analysis of probiotics for the prevention of Antibiotic Associated Diarrhea and the treatment of *Clostridium difficile* disease. Am J Gastroenterol 101:812–822
32. Tedesco FJ, Gordon D, Fortson WC (1985) Approach to pa-

tients with multiple relapses of antibiotic-associated pseudomembranous colitis. Am J Gastroenterol 80:867–868
33. Sougioultzis S, Kyne L, Drudy D, et al. (2005) *Clostridium difficile* toxoid vaccine in recurrent *Clostridium difficile*-associated diarrhea. Gastroenterology 128:764–770
34. Climo MW, Israel DS, Wong ES, et al. (1998) Hospital wide restrictions of clindamycin: effect on the incidence of *Clostridium difficile* associated diarrhea and cost. Ann Intern Med 128:989
35. Kyne L, Merry C, O'Connell B, et al. (1999) Factors associated with prolonged symptoms and severe disease due to *Clostridium difficile*. Age Aging 28:107–113
36. Aslam S, Hamill RJ, Musher DM (2005) Treatment of *Clostridium difficile* associated disease: old therapies and new strategies. Lancet Infect Dis 5:549–557

Infection Control/Epidemiology

III

Chapter 18

Fundamentals of Infection Control and Strategies for the Intensive Care Unit

18

C.E. Edmiston, Jr, P.J. Wilson, B.F. Grahn

18.1 Introduction

The mission of a hospital infection control program is to ensure continuous improvement in the delivery of patient care. This is done through a structured surveillance, which reviews, analyzes, and reports healthcare-associated infection (HAI) rates. It is the overall intent of the program to identify and reduce the risk of acquiring and transmitting infections among patients, staff, physicians, other healthcare professionals and visitors to the institution. There are in essence three specific goals of a hospital infection control program. The first goal involves the protection of the patient, which is accomplished through ensuring that a low risk exists for the acquisition of a HAI. This has become a daunting exercise in the presence of a high-risk patient population coupled with an environment that fosters the development of widespread antibiotic resistance. However, there is substantial published data demonstrating that an effective infection control program results in a reduced infection rate, increased case-specific patient survival, fewer complications and a reduction in hospitalized days [1]. Within the ICU environment there are numerous examples of opportunities where infection control interventional practices may occur. For instance, ICU patients are at high risk for acquiring a healthcare-associated urinary tract infection, ventilator-associated pneumonia (VAP), or catheter related-bloodstream infection (CR-BSI) and infection control activities, which focus upon reducing the risk of these infections, have been shown to decrease morbidity and improve patient outcome.

The second goal of an infection control program is to prevent the spread of infection from patients to healthcare workers and other individuals within the hospital environment. Many of the strategies that are used to accomplish this goal require an expertise that is above and beyond those needed for routine surveillance. By tradition, institutional based infection control programs have a broad scope of practice that encompasses a broad interdisciplinary framework (Table 18.1).

Table 18.1. Interdisciplinary responsibilities of the infection control team within the hospital environment

Scope of practice of the infection control program
• Data analysis – epidemiology and statistics
• Microbiology – clinical laboratory
• Infectious disease – surveillance
• Occupational health – policies
• Central supply – disinfection, sterilization and processing
• Administration – management and communication
• Patient care – policies and procedures
• Staff development – in-services

The infection control practitioner must be able to communicate effectively with a wide range of healthcare professions. Often this involves documenting the need for patient isolation or identifying the reasons for the use of personal protective equipment. In addition, the infection control department must work in close cooperation with employee health services when infectious exposures become an issue. Finally, employee education from top to bottom is an important function of each infection control team member and knowledge of effective teaching strategies is extremely helpful in carrying out this task.

Finally, in our current managed care environment, infection control teams represent a significant financial investment to the institution. The financial commitment associated with developing a highly trained and professional group of infection control practitioners is offset by the ability of that team to reduce the risk of HAIs within the healthcare setting. Approximately 2 million healthcare-associated infections occur each year in the United States. These infections are responsible for significant morbidity, mortality and cost. The estimated increased length of stay (LOS) associated with a healthcare-associated pneumonia is between 6 and 30 days, while the LOS associated with a CR-BSI is from 7 to 21 days. This translates into a significant monetary burden to the institution, since the cost of managing a healthcare-associated pneumonia is in the range of US $10,000 – 50,000 and treating a CR-BSI may cost as much as $50,000. This does not even begin to address the associated mortality, which is between 23% and 50% for CR-BSI and pneumonia [2 – 4]. Therefore, an effectively managed infection control program can have a positive socioeconomic impact within the institution. This is especially true in the critical care environment, where the myriad of patient risk factors can contribute to high morbidity with associated adverse clinical outcomes.

18.2 Measuring the Impact

Recently, new, innovative technologies have emerged, which claim to reduce the risk of infection within the critical care arena. It goes without saying that most of these technologies are more expensive than standard devices or practices. However, while cost may be an important factor in the current healthcare environment, it is important to determine what if any benefits may be derived by new technologies and will they have a measurable impact on reducing HAI rates within selected units or patient populations. An example of this process involves the use of antiseptic or antibiotic bonded catheters for central venous access. As discussed earlier healthcare-associated bloodstream infections, especially in the critically ill, are associated with increased LOS, higher risk of mortality and increased hospital costs. The attributed mortality associated with central lines has been reported to be 25%, with an additional LOS of 6.5 days in the SICU and an average cost of $28,690 per survivor [5]. A hypothetical comparison in shown in Table 18.2 investigating the infection control and cost effectiveness of two antiseptic/antibiotic bonded catheters versus a conventional central venous catheter (CVC).

It would appear that catheter B is superior to catheter A in preventing catheter-related bloodstream infections compared to a convention CVC. However, it should be noted that true efficacy is only apparent when sufficient statistical power is present in the study design. It is unlikely that a catheter study with less than 300 devices divided between three arms will provide that level of statistical power needed to validate clinical superiority. However, from a simple examination of the data in Table 18.1, use of catheter A reduced the number of CR-BSI by a factor of 2.6, while catheter B reduced the number of CR-BSI by a factor of 8. If the actual cost of treating a CR-BSI in the SICU is $28,690, then approximately $128,245 or $212,935 savings could in theory be realized by adopting catheters A or B compared to the conventional silastic device. It is likely that these types of comparisons will occur with greater frequency as newer innovative technologies impinge upon the critical care environment. The infection control team can and should play a central role in the development of protocols and guidelines for the evaluation of devices or technologies that as suggested reduce the HAI rate. In addition, we should recognize that the maximal benefit derived from the adoption of such innovative technology into our clinical practice is dependent entirely upon which patient populations are studied. In the case of antibiotic/antiseptic coated/bonded catheters, one approach that may be deemed most cost effective is to restrict the use of such devices to patients who are within the highest risk category for catheter-related bloodstream infections, ICU and immunosuppressed patients [6–8].

Table 18.2. Comparison of colonization and catheter related-bloodstream (CR-BSI) infections between conventional CVC and antiseptic/antibiotic coated catheters (A and B) in the SICU

Device (CVC)	N	Colonization	CR-BSI rate	Cost
Conventional device[a]	94	32%	8%	$25
Coated Catheter A	101	23%	3%	$45
Coated Catheter B	90	8%	1%	$75

[a] Silastic Hickman catheter

18.3 Responsibilities of the Infection Control Professional

An effective infection control program represents an interdisciplinary endeavor (Table 18.1) encompassing the fields of epidemiology, medicine, microbiology, pathology, nursing, and administration [9–11]. The amount of time that the infection control team spends in routine infection surveillance, prevention and control activities relates to:

- Needs of the patient population
- Risk factors of the patient population
- Complexity of the service or unit
- Adherence requirement of federal, state and local laws and regulations governing the infection control program
- Educational needs of the staff

The team is required to collect, review and analyze surveillance data and to identify current trends of HAIs. In addition, the infection control program should be viewed as an agent of change through the active participation of team members on appropriate institutional committees. This participation should result in:

- Development, review and revision of isolation guidelines as per accepted standard practice and to enforce all policies and procedures relating to isolation guidelines
- Active collaboration and consultation with all disciplines and departments to promote infection control principles into effective policies and procedures

- The development of mechanisms for evaluating the impact of new technologies and procedures as they relate to infection control (see previous section)
- The ability to utilize hospital administration as a resource for implementing infection control polices and procedures

The infection control personnel must be knowledgeable of the published literature on the epidemiology and pathogenesis of HAIs, incorporating this informational base into their current practice.

18.4 Infection Control Surveillance Criteria

The purpose of infection control surveillance whether global or unit specific is to develop and maintain a database of the institutional HAI experience. Pragmatically, surveillance attempts to define the endemic rate of infectious events within the institution. This is a dynamic process, which is in a constant state of flux, in part due to changes in patient care services, which may be impacted by new technology or changes in personnel. Surveillance will also monitor changes that occur above the endemic level. Often these changes are compared to some benchmark such as the HAI rates developed by the National Nosocomial Infection Surveillance (NNIS) program administered by the Centers for Disease control and Prevention (CDC) in Atlanta [12]. A significant component of the infection control surveillance program is the feedback or dialogue which occurs between the infection control staff and the healthcare provider. This is generally acknowledged as the interventional component, whereas the infection control personnel reviews with the clinical staff risk factors associated with care of the patient, while suggesting appropriate strategies that attempt to reduce the overall risk of infection. The measure of a successful and effective surveillance program is whether or not implementation of focused prevention and control policies results in decreasing future HAI risks.

18.5 Surveillance Strategies in the Hospital Environment

Numerous surveillance techniques have been proposed for monitoring the rates of infection within hospital and critical care environments.

- Hospital-wide or global surveillance
- Targeted or focused surveillance
- Periodic or intermittent surveillance
- Prevalence surveillance

Adoption of one or more of these techniques is dependent upon the goals and priorities of the institution. In addition, the type of surveillance performed will also be dependent upon the level of institutional resources including both monetary and personnel. The advantages and disadvantages of the three surveillance strategies are listed below:

18.5.1 Hospital-wide Surveillance

- Advantages:
  - Provide infection data from all sites within the institution
  - Establishes baseline data and identifies outbreaks early
  - Clearly identifies patterns
- Disadvantages:
  - Expensive, time consuming and labor intensive
  - Generates large amount of data often with little clinical significance
  - Reduces staff time for other important activities

18.5.2 Targeted Surveillance

- Advantages:
  - Highly flexible and mobile
  - Can focus on patients with highest risk
  - May include all hospital sites if surveillance is rotated
- Less labor intensive than hospital-wide surveillance
- Disadvantages:
  - Less opportunity for defining hospital-wide baseline rates
  - May miss initial outbreaks or clusters outside surveillance areas

18.5.3 Periodic Surveillance

- Advantages:
  - Flexible for staff, increasing opportunities for other activities
  - Allows staff to define long-term goals and objectives
- Disadvantages:
  - Possibility that infection clusters may be missed
  - Little or no consistent baseline data

18.5.4 Prevalence

- Advantages:
  - Documents trends in HAIs
  - Used to identify risk factors

  - Rapid and with relative low cost
  - Data may be used to target future areas of surveillance
- Disadvantages:
  - Unable to compare prevalence rates with incidence rates
  - Outbreaks or clusters may be missed
  - Provides information for a limited time interval

Few institutions have the available resources to provide complete hospital-wide or global surveillance. Therefore, targeted or focused surveillance has become commonplace in our healthcare institutions. At our institution we use a combination of site-specific and unit-specific surveillance to monitor HAI rates. Site-specific monitoring focuses on specific sites of infections such as respiratory tract, urinary tract, bloodstream or surgical site infections. In-hospital as well as selected postdischarge surveillance of surgical site infections are monitored in this manner. Unit-specific surveillance is designated for high-risk patient areas such as the ICUs and other units including the hematology-oncology services or the bone marrow transplant service. Studies have demonstrated that high-risk patient populations have the highest HAI rates often with significant morbidity and mortality. Therefore, it would be perceived as prudent to focus surveillance efforts on this high-risk patient population. Periodic surveillance is less time consuming than either hospital-wide or targeted; however, failure to miss sentinel clusters is a common fault of this surveillance strategy. Often this surveillance strategy may be combined with targeted surveillance so that the opportunity for missing a cluster is greatly reduced. Finally, prevalence surveillance is used to define the number of active infections within a specific time period. In this method of surveillance all new and existing infections are tabulated, which results in a rate (prevalence) that is higher than the true incidence rate. However, this strategy may be useful for studying specific risk factors, device-associated infections or the prevalence of selected antibiotic resistant pathogens within a defined patient population [9].

Frequently, several different strategies may be used within a single institution depending upon its particular goals or needs. In the end, however, the limiting factor most often is time and personnel commitments to other endeavors of the infection control program.

18.6 Data Collection, Analysis and Reporting

The process of data collection must be epidemiologically sound and driven by definable events such as CR-BSI or other device-related infections. The actual data source documents are often numerous and highly variable within a given institution (Table 18.3).

Table 18.3. Source documents for identifying healthcare-associated infections during infection control surveillance

Source documentation		
Patient	**Laboratory**	**Administration**
Physical examination	Microbiology	Admissions
Medical record	Serology	Risk assessment
Nursing Kardex	Pathology	Outpatient clinics
Clinical rounds	Antibiogram data	Employee health
Medication record		
Radiology report		
Operative report		

It is interesting to note that total chart review, Kardex screens and review of cultural results is associated with the highest level of sensitivity for detecting HAI [13, 14]. With the present widespread (inappropriate) use of antibiotics, it should come as no surprise that review of antibiotic use patterns is associated with documented infection less than 60% of the time. This is also true for fever, which as a single sentinel indicator of infection is relatively poor. In the case of surgical wound surveillance direct observation of the wound by a trained practitioner is the most accurate means of detecting a surgical site infection. Reliance upon a single source document to detect a healthcare-associated infection may often lead to underestimating the true incidence of infection. No single surveillance strategy will detect 100% of HAIs; however, in the case of ICU surveillance a focus review of positive blood cultures would likely detect most catheter-related bloodstream infections. The development of an effective surveillance program requires experience and knowledgeable infection control practitioners who recognize that in the case of surgical wound infections, direct observation is preferable to reviewing culture reports. Therefore, the most effective strategy for detecting HAIs will usually involve sifting through a combination of resources within the healthcare institution.

18.7 Comparison of Institutional Rates to National Benchmarks

In 1970, the National Nosocomial Infection Surveillance (NNIS) system was established and presently almost 300 hospitals contribute surveillance data for aggregation into a national database [12]. Data is collected using standardized protocols and encompasses Centers of Disease and Prevention (CDC) definitions that include both laboratory and clinical based criteria. For over 25 years the NNIS program included hospital-wide surveillance but has recently eliminated that component from its program. The current focus is on high-risk patient populations that include adult and pediatric ICU, high-risk nursery (HRN) and surgical site infections (SSIs). Data is collected from all sites of infection in the ICUs and HRN with an emphasis on device-related infections. A fourth component of the NNIS surveillance program is the reporting of the most common pathogens associated with bloodstream, pneumonia, and urinary tract infection in the ICU. A subset of hospitals from the NNIS system participate in a parallel program, called the Intensive Care Antimicrobial Resistance Epidemiology (ICARE) Project, which assesses antimicrobial usage and emerging patterns of resistance within the healthcare environment. While this program initially focused on the patterns of antimicrobial resistance with the critical care population, recent evaluations have also examined the emergence of antimicrobial resistance in the non-intensive care and outpatient/emergent care patient populations [15].

18.8 Strategies for the Prevention and Surveillance of Healthcare-Associated Infections in the Intensive Care Unit

18.8.1 Catheter-Related Bloodstream Infections

Catheter-related bloodstream infections (CRBSIs) have a significant impact on patient morbidity and mortality in the healthcare environment. The attributable mortality associated with a central venous access device can range from 10% to 15% [16, 17]. Table 18.4 identifies the most common microbial pathogens isolated from hospital-acquired bloodstream infections [17].

The coagulase-negative staphylococci are the most common pathogens isolated from ICU bloodstream infections. This finding is consistent with previous studies that have found the coagulase-negative staphylococci to be the most common pathogen in device-associated infections. *Staphylococcus aureus* and the enterococci are the second most common bloodstream pathogens reported in the ICU. The enterococci have vaulted from being an insignificant pathogen less than 20 years ago to their current position with many of these strains expressing multidrug resistance, including vancomycin resistance. *Candida albicans* was an organism that less than 15 years ago rarely was associated with infection in the critical care environment and now occupies the fourth position in frequency. Finally, several Gram-negative rods, including *Enterobacter* spp., *Klebsiella pneumoniae*, and *E. coli*, are shown as rounding out the top eight positions.

Table 18.5 reports the central line-associated bloodstream infection (BSI) rate for selected ICUs as tabulated by the National Nosocomial Infection Surveillance (NNIS) system [18]. The rate of catheter-related bloodstream infection ranges from a low of 2.9 per 1,000 catheter days in a cardiothoracic service to 9.7 in burn units. The variation in these rates is in part a reflection of the intrinsic risk factors that are present in this patient population. However, failure to adhere to basic principles of maximal barrier precautions at the time of line insertion and poor catheter management is also in part responsible for some CR-BSI seen in the ICU. While the pathogenesis of CR-BSI has been characterized as multifactorial, the two major mechanisms responsible for line infection involve migration of microorganisms at the site of insertion into the cutaneous tract, resulting in extraluminal colonization and contamination of catheter hub, which causes intraluminal colonization [6, 18, 19].

Surveillance and treatment strategies for catheter-related infection are dependent upon the clinical presentation. A localized infection involving a port or tunnel infection requires catheter removal, while infection localized to the exit site can usually be managed with local measures such as warm moist compresses, increasing the frequency of site care and in some cases oral antibiotics. The general treatment strategies for catheter-related infections can be characterized as follows [6, 18]:

Table 18.4. Eight most common pathogens isolated from hospital-acquired bloodstream infections [18]

Pathogen	1986–1989 (%)	1992–1999 (%)
CNS[a]	27	37
Staphylococcus aureus	16	13
Enterococcus spp.	8	13
Gram-negative rods	19	14
E. coli	6	2
Enterobacter spp.	5	5
Pseudomonas aeruginosa	4	4
Klebsiella pneumoniae	4	3
Candida spp.	8	8

[a] CNS, coagulase-negative staphylococci

Table 18.5. Central line-associated BSI rate for selected medical and surgical services reported to the National Nosocomial Infection Surveillance System, January 1992–June 2001 [18]

Type of ICU	Number of units	Central line-associated BSI rate[a]
Coronary	102	4.5
Cardiothoracic	64	2.9
Medical	135	5.9
Medical/surgical		
Major teaching	123	5.3
All others	180	3.8
Neurosurgical	47	4.7
Surgical	153	5.3
Trauma	25	7.9
Burn	18	9.7
Respiratory		

[a] Pool mean/1,000 catheter-days

- Exit site infections:
  Presents with symptoms of erythema, tenderness or purulence within 2 cm of site. Treatment is local with warm compresses, daily site care and oral antibiotics.
- Tunnel infections:
  Characterized by erythema, tenderness or purulence >2 cm from the site. This will require catheter removal.
- Pocket (implantable port) infections:
  Will present with erythema and necrosis over the port reservoir or purulent exudate in subcutaneous pocket. This requires port removal and antibiotic therapy.
- Catheter related-bloodstream infections (CR-BSI):
  Requires semiquantitative/quantitative culture with a five- to tenfold difference between central and peripheral cultures, with no other sign of infection elsewhere and associated with defervescence upon catheter removal. CNS – can be managed with in situ treatment (antibiotic lock) and systemic antibiotic. Infection due to yeast, *S. aureus* or polymicrobial recurrent infection – requires catheter removal.

Treatment of a CR-BSI is more complex than management of a localized infectious process. The fundamental question with CR-BSI is: does the line have to be removed? In situations where long-term access is required, successful treatment without removal has been reported in the literature. Removal of an infected catheter is warranted when there is a documented fungal infection, persistent bacteremia following antibiotic therapy, polymicrobial infection or infection with a highly virulent pathogen such as *Staphylococcus aureus* [6, 18–22]. Staphylococcal infections involving *Staphylococcus epidermidis* can often be managed with an antibiotic lock that utilizes a high intraluminal dose of antibiotic, which remains within the lumen of the catheter for period of up to several hours [6, 18–20].

The cornerstone of preventing CR-BSI is grounded in the basic principles of infection control, judicious handwashing and aseptic technique. Rigorous attention to aseptic principles such as maximal barrier precautions upon insertion and dedicated personnel to provide line care has repeatedly been shown to result in decreased infection. While newer technological developments in the area of wound care and the use of antiseptic/antibiotic impregnated devices has been suggested to reduce the risk of CR-BSI, there is no substitution for meticulous catheter care [6, 8, 17, 18].

To minimize the risk of contamination, all line insertions must be performed under rigorous maximal barrier precautions. This includes using sterile drapes (large), gowns, masks and gloves. Several prospective studies have demonstrated that a significant reduction in catheter colonization and bacteremia can be achieved using a rigorous aseptic protocol. While several surface antiseptics have been used to reduce skin contamination at the insertion site, cleansing with chlorhexidine has been shown to be superior to elemental iodine or an iodophor [6, 18, 21, 22]. A recent study using a 2% chlorhexidine gluconate (CHG) w/v and 70% isopropyl alcohol (IPA) skin-prepping agent demonstrate superior efficacy when compared against povidone iodine [23].Two points are worth considering: first chlorhexidine exhibits an excellent residual activity compared to other compounds and this agent is not neutralized by blood, serum or blood proteins [24].

Historically, routine guideline wire exchanges were proposed as a means to reduce the CR-BSI. However, present recommendations do not support this practice since intraluminal colonization of the previous line may serve as a source of contamination for the new line via guidewire insertion [18]. In general, central lines should only be removed when clinically expedient, while peripheral lines may be replaced at a 72-h interval [6, 18]. Routine skin asepsis and appropriate site care have been shown to be efficacious in limiting microbial growth and colonization of the catheter. At present, either gauze or transparent dressings appear to be equally effective when used appropriately [25]. It has been shown that creating a subcutaneous tract and tunneling the catheter is associated with a significant decrease in catheter-related infections [6, 18].

However, it should be pointed out that use of a dedicated IV team for care and maintenance of lines has been shown to reduce infection rates in intravascular devices [26, 27].

The consensus is now clear that the hub is an important portal for intraluminal colonization of the catheter. Catheter hub care mandates the use of aseptic technique during tubing changes and other manipulations. The hub should be cleansed with an antiseptic agent such as 70% isopropyl alcohol or 10% povidone-iodine solution before accessing the system [6]. Mechanical cleansing action alone has been found to be effective in removing most pathogens. Needleless systems have been introduced to reduce the risk of sharp injuries to healthcare workers. Because of a concern of infection with some of the needleless devices it has been recommended that additional education efforts are required that focus upon the effective maintenance of these new, innovative and at times complex devices [28, 29].

Identification of the type of catheter-related infection in a standardized manner is one key to improving patient outcomes. An understanding of the etiology and pathogenesis is also important as a basis for developing prevention and treatment guidelines. Over the past 20 years it has become evident that both the exit site and the hub can be implicated in the etiology of CR-BSI. In addition, while many innovative technologies are currently available for the prevention of infection, there is no substitution for aseptic technique and meticulous adherence to catheter care protocols.

18.8.2 Healthcare-Associated Pneumonia

Table 18.6 identifies the most common microbial pathogens associated with hospital-acquired (HAP) and ventilator-associated pneumonia (VAP) from a large US database of culture positive pneumonia [30]. Patients receiving mechanically assisted ventilation constitute the population at highest risk for infection [31].

Two organisms, *Staphylococcus aureus* (MSSA and MRSA) and *Pseudomonas aeruginosa,* stand out as the number 1 and number 2 most common pathogens associated with pneumonia in the hospital environment. *Klebsiella pneumoniae* and *Haemophilus* species ranks next in frequency followed by *Enterobacter, E. coli,* and the highly drug resistant *Acinetobacter* species. It is important to note that many of these infections are due to drug resistant bacteria, requiring the use of potent antimicrobial agents, which add significantly to the cost of managing these serious infections [32]. Diagnosis of healthcare-associated bacterial pneumonia is problematic and remains controversial, especially in the patient on mechanically assisted ventilation. A joint guideline developed by the American Thoracic Society (ATS) and Infectious Disease Society of America (IDSA) has recommended that the diagnosis of pneumonia be based on clinical samples of lower respiratory tract secretions obtained using directed methodology and not solely on clinical presentation [33]:

- Bronchoscopically acquired protective specimen brush (PSB) with quantitative culture
- Bronchoalveolar lavage (BAL)
- Protected BAL (pBAL)

Table 18.6. Most common bacterial pathogens isolated from culture positive cases of healthcare-associated pneumonia, January 2002–December 31, 2003 [30]

Pathogen	Frequency (%) Hospital-acquired	Ventilator-associated
S .aureus (MSSA)	26.2	28.5
S. aureus (MRSA)	22.9	14.6
S. pneumoniae	3.1	5.8
Other Gram-positive	8.1	8.6
Haemophilus spp.	5.6	12.2
Enterobacter spp.	4.3	5.6
Ps. aeruginosa	18.4	21.2
K. pneumoniae	7.1	8.4
E. coli	4.7	6.4
Acinetobacter spp.	2.0	3.0
Other Gram-negative	3.7	6.2

The sensitivity of these various procedures is reported to vary from 70% to 100%, with a specificity of 60–100%. The PSB is widely accepted as a reference method in diagnosing pnemonia in mechanically ventilated patients. However, false positive findings have been reported and may be related to prior antibiotic therapy. Table 18.7 reports the VAP rate for selected ICUs as tabulated by the National Nosocomial Infection Surveillance (NNIS) system [34]. Patients receiving continuous mechanical ventilation have a significantly greater risk for developing healthcare-associated pneumonia than patients not receiving mechanical support. The pathophysiology of ventilator-associated pneumonia follows a rather predictable course beginning with colonization of the airway and tracheal bronchitis, patients often presenting with acute respiratory distress or sepsis [4, 35, 36]. The attributed mortality rate hovers somewhere around 25% but a myriad of confounding variables make an accurate assessment difficult. However, mortality rates related to pneumonia have been reported to be significantly greater among patients with MRSA infection [37]. In addition, numerous risk factors have been identified that are independently associated with VAP; these include presence of intracranial pressure monitors, alteration of gastric pH, changing ventilator circuitry every 24 h, aspiration, reintubation, underlying COPD and use of ventilators for greater than 72 h [35, 36]. One approach to reducing the incidence of VAP has been directed at reducing the potential microbial contamination originating from the gastrointestinal tract. Two approaches involve the use of selective gut decontamination, which reduces the microbial burden in oropharyngeal and proximal GI tract while the other strategy involves stress ulcer prophylaxis using rimantadine.

It is unlikely that frequent, routine changes of ventilator circuitry will reduce the incidence of VAP. The current policy at our institution is to change the circuitry once a week unless the patient has an excessive production of secretions. One should not underestimate the role that hands play in cross-contamination as a mechanism for transmission of healthcare-associated

Table 18.7. Ventilator-associated pneumonia rate from selected medical/surgical units, January 1992–May 1999 [34]

Type of ICU	Number of units	Ventilator-associated pneumonia rate[a]
Medical	121	8.2
Medical/surgical		
Teaching	71	12.4
Nonteaching	138	10.3
Surgical	146	14.6
Trauma	21	16.9
Burn	17	19.9

[a] Number of ventilator-associated pneumonias/number of ventilator days × 1,000

pathogens. Cross-contamination has been well documented to occur during tracheal suctioning and manipulation of ventilator circuitry or endotracheal tubes. Therefore, aseptic technique (handwashing) is essential when caring for patients on ventilator support. In addition, it is important to note that devices associated with respiratory therapy or diagnostic examination need to be clean/sterilized/disinfected properly since they may serve as a vehicle for dissemination of healthcare-associated pathogens to at-risk patients. Finally, patient position has been proposed as a simple means for reducing the rate of VAP. A semirecumbent position (>45 degrees) is associated with a lower risk for VAP compared to patients in a supine position [4]. The use of antimicrobial prophylaxis to prevent healthcare-associated pneumonia is highly questionable and may lead to emergence of antimicrobial resistance.

18.8.3 Healthcare-Associated Urinary Tract Infections

Table 18.8 identifies the most common microbial pathogens isolated from urinary tract infections in the selected medical/surgical units [34]. Healthcare-associated urinary tract infections are the most common hospital acquired infection with the majority occurring following instrumentation. Indwelling urethral catheters that drain into an open system are associated with a higher rate of infection than closed systems.

While acute urinary tract infections may be perceived as benign and often resolve with removal of the catheter, a significant number of these patients receive antibiotic therapy. The widespread use of antibiotic in patients who may be colonized rather than truly infected contributes to antimicrobial pressure within the unit increasing the risk of emergence of antibiotic resistance, potential superinfection or the emergence of yeast (*Candida*) infections. It is interesting to note that *Candida albicans* is the number one uropathogen in both medical and surgical ICUs. At present, there has been a significant increase in the use of antifungal agents within these units. This practice has generated considerable debate, since the criteria for antifungal (*Candida*) therapy are often less than rigorous. Recovery of *Candida* from the urine (in the ICU patient) does not by itself suggest disseminated disease. While it is possible to base antifungal treatment strategies on risk factor stratification, ICU patients almost certainly express multiple risk factors in the absence of clinical disease. In addition, very few institutions perform routine susceptibility testing of *Candida* isolates, and empiric dosing is based upon "expert" opinion rather than institutional MIC data. Therefore, we are left with the premise that often colonization alone is the sole criterion for treatment and that current dosing guidelines may or may not resolve true clinical infections. There is no doubt that *Candida* has emerged as an important pathogen in the ICU and in selected patients there is an associated high morbidity and mortality. However, appropriate treatment guidelines are lacking and the current practice pattern seems to favor a "high-index of suspicion" whenever the organism is recovered in culture from a non-sterile site.

Table 18.9 reports the urinary catheter-associated UTI rate for selected ICUs as tabulated by the National Nosocomial Infection Surveillance (NNIS) system [34]. While infection can occur by a variety of mechanisms, intraluminal migration can be reduced through the use of a closed urinary drainage system. The use of surveillance cultures in catheterized patients is viewed by some practitioners as an effective strategy for the early diagnoses of urinary tract infection; however, this policy has contributed to the widespread abuse of antibiotics in the ICU. As a biomaterial, urinary catheters become rapidly colonized in asymptomatic patients and surveillance cultures should never be used as the sole criterion for therapy. It is not unusual within the ICU to see up to the third of patients whose length of stay is greater than 5 days become colonized with yeast (*Candida*). Several new urinary catheters have appeared on the market, which tout antibiotic/antiseptic coatings and suggest that use of these devices will reduce an in-

Table 18.8. Eight most common pathogens isolated from urinary tract infections in medical, surgical, trauma and burn ICUs, January 1992–May 1999 [34]

Pathogen	ICU (Percentage)			
	Medical	Surgical	Trauma	Burn
CNS[a]	2.3	1.9	3.5	2.1
Staphylococcus aureus	1.8	1.3	1.7	2.6
Enterococcus spp.	14.2	14.5	15.5	8.1
Candida albicans	20.8	16.3	10.8	8.4
Enterobacter spp.	4.1	6.2	6.5	6.7
Ps. aeruginosa	9.7	13.1	13.5	20.0
K. pneumoniae	6.3	6.1	4.5	4.7
E. coli	13.7	14.6	20.1	13.7

[a] CNS, coagulase-negative staphylococci

Table 18.9. Urinary catheter-associated UTI rate for medical, combined medical/surgical, surgical, trauma, and burn ICUs, January 1992–May 1999 [34]

Type of ICU	Number of units	Urinary catheter-associated UTI rate[a]
Medical	124	7.6
Medical/surgical		
Teaching	71	6.8
Nonteaching	140	4.5
Surgical	146	5.6
Trauma	21	7.7
Burn	17	10.1

[a] Number of urinary catheter-associated UTIs/number of urinary catheter days × 1,000

stitution's HAI rate by making the device resistant to bacterial colonization [38]. However, a recent study has suggested that silver-impregnated Foley catheters were not effective in preventing healthcare-associated urinary tract infections [39]. While there is some room for disagreement concerning the efficacy of these antiseptic devices, it is possible that these devices will have the greatest impact on those patient populations which require long-term indwelling lines. However, further studies are warranted before these devices completely replace traditional Foley catheters.

Efforts to reduce the risk of healthcare-associated UTIs in the ICU must consider the following recommendations: (a) ongoing educational efforts are required to assure that personnel are competent in catheter insertion and care, (b) attention focuses on appropriate infection control practices that emphasize aseptic technique including hand washing, and (c) insure an unobstructed urinary flow while maintaining closed sterile drainage.

18.9 Isolation Guidelines – Rationale and Practice

Isolation procedures have been developed to prevent the transmission of communicable and infectious diseases to patients, healthcare workers and visitors. The revised CDC "Isolation Precautions in Hospitals" recognizes a two tiered system of precautions, Standard Precautions and Transmission-Based Precautions [40]. Standard precautions apply to all patients and represent a standard of care that is in compliance with basic infection control practices. This standard applies to all blood, body fluids, secretions, excretions, non-intact skin surfaces and mucous membranes. Strict adherence to Standard Precautions will effectively reduce the transmission of microorganisms from both recognized and unrecognized sources of infection. In addition to the appropriate use of gloves, masks, eye/face shields, gowns and handling of patient equipment, Standard Precautions also address management/cleaning of the patient-care environment and sharp injury protection of healthcare professionals. Transmission-Based Precautions are implemented when a patient has a documented or is suspected of having being infected or colonized with a "highly transmissible or epidemiologically important pathogen." Transmission-Based Precautions are always used in addition to Standard Precautions. The CDC has recommended three specific categories of Transmission-Based Precautions: airborne, droplet and contact. In 1995, our institutional Infection Control Committee implemented a fourth category for vancomycin-resistant enterococci (VRE), Special Isolation Precautions. Recently, in response to concerns over SARS and other infectious agents that may be transmitted by a combination of contact and airborne mechanisms, a new isolation category has been proposed, Contact/Airborne Isolation Precautions, which will likely be implemented in the near future. Table 18.10 identifies the current Standard and Transmission-Based Precaution categories.

Table 18.10. Isolation precautions and microbial criteria for isolation

Precaution	Category and microbiological criteria
Standard	Formerly designated as Universal Precautions
Transmission-Based	a) Contact Multidrug-resistant bacteria Methicillin-resistant *S. aureus* (MRSA) *Cl. difficile* Infectious diarrhea Herpes zoster (immunocompromised)[a] Hemorrhagic viral infection b) Airborne[a] (prevent dissemination of particles $\leq 5\ \mu m$) Measles (rubeola) Varicella (disseminated zoster) Tuberculosis c) Droplet (prevent dissemination of particles $>5\ \mu m$) *H. influenzae* (pneumonia or meningitis) *N. meningitidis* (pneumonia or meningitis) Pertussis Influenza Rubella and mumps d) Special isolation Vancomycin-resistant enterococci (VRE)

[a] Requires that the patient be placed in a negative pressure room

18.10 Fundamental Principles of Isolation Precautions

Airborne Precautions (for known or suspected TB patients) requires patient placement in a negative pressure room (private) and all doors must be kept closed during the period of isolation. All healthcare professionals caring for known or a suspected TB patient must wear an N95 respirator mask. If the patient is to be transported within the hospital, he (she) must wear a surgical mask when outside of the negative pressure room. A patient may be removed from airborne isolation under the following conditions: (a) receiving effective therapy (TB) for at least 2 weeks and is improving clinically, (b) has had three consecutive negative sputum smears collected on different days to rule out TB, or (c) a negative BAL. Droplet Precautions requires that the patient be placed in a private room or in cohort isolation. All healthcare workers are required to wear a surgical mask when working or coming within 0.9 m of the patient. The patient must wear a surgical mask when being transported within the hospital. Patients must remain in Droplet Precaution isolation for duration of illness (viral) or following 24 h of effective antibiotic therapy (bacterial).

Contact Precautions dictate that the patient be placed in a private or cohort isolation. All personnel or visitors must wear gloves when entering the room and remove gloves upon leaving the patient's room. Hands must be washed with an antimicrobial soap immediately upon removal of the gloves. Gowns are to be worn if it is anticipated that your clothing will have substantial contact with the patient, environmental surfaces, if the patient is incontinent, has diarrhea, an ileostomy, colostomy or excessive wound drainage. Gowns are removed before leaving the patient's environment. Efforts should be made to insure that dedicated patient equipment (blood-pressure cuffs, stethoscopes, etc.) not be shared with other patients. If not disposable, these items must be thoroughly cleaned and disinfected before used on other patients. Contact precautions cannot be discontinued unless a negative culture is obtained 48 h after stopping antibiotics. Historically, patients with *Clostridium difficile* diarrhea must be symptom free or have a negative stool toxin assay before discontinuation of contact isolation. However, patients with *Clostridium difficile* diarrhea often shed the organism into the environment for several weeks after resolution of symptoms [41]. Therefore, we have implemented a policy within our institution that a negative toxin assay or resolution of symptoms does not trigger discontinuation of isolation status, but rather these patients remain in isolation until discharged. Following discharge, the patient's room undergoes a thorough terminal cleaning, which includes disposal of all patient items and privacy drapes in an effort to reduce the risk of disseminating of *C. difficile* spores to other patient rooms or units.

Because of the significant increase in vancomycin resistant enterococci (VRE) among high-risk patient populations (listed below), our institution adopted Special Isolation Precautions for VRE patients.

18.11.1 Patient Populations at Increased Risk for Acquiring Vancomycin-Resistant Enterococci (VRE)

- Receiving prolonged antimicrobials and/or vancomycin therapy
- Critically ill patients or those with severe underlying disease or immunosuppression
- ICU patients
- Oncology or transplant patients/wards
- Prolonged hospital stay
- Patients having intra-abdominal or cardiothoracic surgical procedures
- Patients with intravascular devices

Special Precautions require private or cohort isolation, dedicated patient equipment, all persons must wear gloves and gowns, and patients are restricted to their rooms and travel within the hospital only if absolutely necessary. All flat surfaces within the patient's environment must be thoroughly clean with a disinfectant cloth at least once per shift. Strict handwashing is required with an antimicrobial agent before and after leaving the patient's room. When the patient is discharged or leaves isolation the entire room is thoroughly clean with an effective disinfectant before another patient enters the room. To discontinue isolation three negative stool specimens are required (at least 1 week apart) from stool, rectal or perirectal area and from any other body site that was known to be colonized with VRE. There is a significant potential for widespread environment contamination with VRE and therefore strict enforcement of isolation policies is required to reduce transmission within the institution.

Isolation precautions should be based upon current epidemiologic information that identifies transmission patterns of infectious agents within the hospital environment. The current guidelines from the Centers from Disease Control and Prevention (CDC) are intended to recognize the importance of body fluids in the transmission of HAIs, while addressing adequate precautions for traditional routes of transmission (i.e., droplet, airborne and contact). Finally, isolation policies should always be viewed as evolutionary in nature, subject to review and updated as further data is available on the acquisition and transmission of infectious agents within the hospital environment.

18.11 Antimicrobial Use Policies and the Infection Control Practitioner

Within the critical care environment there has always been an intimate relationship between antimicrobial use policies and infection control practices. The traditional role of the infection control practitioners has been to work closely with physicians, nurses and other healthcare professional to facilitate control and prevention of transmission of infectious agents among patient, to staff and visitors within the healthcare facility. It is also appropriate for the infection control staff to maintain a close, collaborative relationship with the clinical pharmacist when tracking emerging patterns of resistance within the critical care environment. Within our institution members of the infection control team routinely participate in antimicrobial audits in high-risk patient care areas. In 1999, the infection control team was responsible for documenting a high incidence of vancomycin-resistance enterococci (VRE) among selected immunosuppressed patients on a single unit. The various isolates were collected and genotyped using pulsed-field gel electrophoresis (PFGE), which documented that several of the strains were identical, suggesting a complete breakdown in basic infection control practices within the unit. In addition, based upon an internal pharmacy audit, vancomycin usage on this unit was the highest in the institution. An alternative antibiotic use policy was presented to the attending staff physicians, resulting in a dramatic reduction (80%) in vancomycin use among patients on this unit. In addition, the infection control staff met with nursing and environmental services to heighten awareness of the problem and to review current policies and procedures relating to patient care and housekeeping practices. The impact of this comprehensive yet collegial effort has resulted in a sharp reduction in both the emergence of new cases and dissemination of existing clones over the past 12 months.

Antimicrobial resistance is a global problem; unfortunately the magnitude of the problem is not fully realized as evidenced by the continuous pattern of antimicrobial use in both the ICU and non-ICU settings. The ICU provides a daunting environment for those practitioners interested in reducing inappropriate antibiotic use. A previous study has documented that within the hospital environment, the ICU is an epicenter for antimicrobial resistance and that selected microbial populations recovered from the ICU express higher levels of resistance than non-ICU strains [15]. This is often a difficult issue to assess and current attitudes regarding appropriate antimicrobial use are steeped in ignorance, apathy or both. In the spring of 1995, the Hospital Infection Control Practice Advisory Committee (HICPAC) published in the Federal Register what amounted to a national action plan for preventing the spread of vancomycin resistance in the hospital environment. The recommendations from this committee addressed four separate areas: (1) education, (2) role of the hospital microbiology laboratory, (3) prevention and control strategies, and (4) directives for prudent vancomycin use [42]. This was in many ways a unique document that in part reflected upon an agenda for future interdisciplinary strategies aimed at reducing the acquisition and dissemination of resistant pathogens within the healthcare environment. These recommendations have stimulated other professional societies such as the Infectious Disease Society of American, Society for Healthcare Epidemiology of America, Surgical Infection Society, American Society for Microbiology and the Association for Professionals in Infection Control and Epidemiology to develop policies, procedures and indicators of appropriate antimicrobial use [43]. It is evident that antimicrobial resistance while significant in the ICU is also increasing in both Gram-positive and Gram-positive bacteria populations within all areas of the healthcare environment, adversely impacting clinical outcome and diminishing limited institutional resources [44–47].

The original HICPAC recommendations for preventing the spread of vancomycin resistance within the healthcare environment should be viewed as a blueprint for leadership in infection control, formulary restraint and microbiological support for preventing the emergence, acquisition and dissemination of all resistant healthcare-associated pathogens [48]. Therefore, the original (traditional) scope of practice (Table 18.1) for infection control professionals has been expanded to encompass the documentation of emerging trends of resistance within the hospital environment and the development of effective interventional strategies aimed at preempting future emerging patterns of resistance. Development of a judicious antimicrobial strategy for the ICU requires a close collegiality between infection control, pharmacy, microbiology and the clinical staff so that emerging patterns of antimicrobial resistance are recognized early and correlated with therapeutic efficacy.

18.12 Final Comment on Infection Control Practices Within the Critical Care Environment

Reducing the risk of healthcare-associated infection within the critical care environment requires an interdisciplinary effort, strong leadership and committed administrative (institutional) support. The foundation of this effort necessitates a commitment to basic infection control principles such as appropriate handwashing practices and adherence to isolation guidelines [40, 49]. Finally, acquisition of a healthcare-associated infection in the critical care environment is predicated on host susceptibility and other risk factors. Limiting exposure of high-risk patients to selective microbial pathogens should be viewed as the basic goal of any infection control initiative. This may require the infection control practitioner to at times "think outside of the box" or explore the clinical utility of using innovative infection control strategies, such as waterless antiseptic cloths for cleansing patients in the unit or the adoption of antibiotic or antiseptic impregnated technologies that reduce the risk of biomedical (i.e., central venous or Foley catheters) device bacterial colonization, which can lead to overt morbidity and/or mortality in susceptible high-risk patients [8, 50, 51].

References

1. Scheckler WE, Brimhall D, Buck AS, Farr BM, et al. (1998) Requirements for infrastructure and essential activities of infection control and epidemiology in hospitals: a consensus panel report. Infect Control Hosp Epidemiol 19:114–124
2. Jarvis WR (1996) Selected aspects of the socioeconomic impact of nosocomial infections. Infect Control Hosp Epidemiol 17:552–557

3. Gaynes RP (1997) Surveillance of nosocomial infections: a fundamental ingredient for quality. Infect Control Hosp Epidemiol 18:475–478
4. Flanders SA, Collard HR, Saint S (2006) Nosocomial pneumonia: state of the science. Am J Infect Control 54:84–93
5. Pittet D, Tarara D, Wenzel R (1994) Nosocomial bloodstream infections in the critically ill patients. J Am Med Assoc 271:1598–1601
6. Krzywda EA, Andris DA, Edmiston CE (1999) Catheter infections: diagnosis, etiology, treatment, and prevention. Nutr Clin Practice 14:178–190
7. Pearson ML, Abrutyn E (1997) Reducing the risk for catheter-related infection; a new strategy. Ann Intern Med 127:294–303
8. Rupp ME, Lisco SJ, Lipsett PA, Perl TM, Keating K, Civetta JM, Mermel LA, Lee D, Dellinger EP, Donahoe M, Giles D, Pfaller MA, Maki DG, Sheretz R (2005) Effect of a second-generation venous catheter impregnated with chlorhexidine and silver sulfadiazine on central catheter-related infections. Ann Internal Med 143:570–580
9. Pottinger JM, Herwaldt LA (1997) Basic surveillance – an overview. Infect Control Hosp Epidemiol 18:513–527
10. Gaynes RP, Solomon S (1996) Improving hospital-acquired infection rates: the CDC experience. Jt Comm J Qual Improv 22:457–467
11. McKibben L, Horan T, Tokars JI, Fowler G, Cardo DM, Pearson ML, Brennan ML (2005) Guidance on public reporting of healthcare-associated infections: recommendations of the healthcare infection control practices advisory committee. Am J Infect Control 33:217–226
12. Hospital Infection Program, Centers for Disease Control and Prevention (2004) National nosocomial infection surveillance (NNIS) system report, data summary from January 1992 through June 2004, issued October 2004. Am J Infect Control 32:470–485
13. Wenzel RP, Osterman CA, Hunting KJ, Gwaltney JM (1976) Hospital-acquired infection, I: surveillance in a university hospital. Am J Epidemiol 103:251–260
14. Glenister H, Taylor L, Barlett C, Cooke M, et al. (1991) An assessment of selective surveillance methods for detecting hospital acquired infection. Am J Med 91(Suppl 3B):121S–124S
15. Fridkin SK, Gaynes RP (1999) Antimicrobial resistance in intensive care units. Clin Chest Med 20:303–316
16. Wensel RP, Edmond MB (2001) Impact of hospital-acquired bloodstream infection. Emerg Infect 7:174–177
17. Lubelchek RJ, Weinstein RA (2006) Strategies for preventing catheter-related bloodstream infections: the role of new technologies. Crit Care Med 34:905–907
18. O'Grady NP, Alexander M, Dellinger EP, Gerberding JL, Heard SO, Maki DG, Masur H, McCormick RD, Mermel LA, Person ML, Raad II, Randolph A, Weinstein RA (2002) Guidelines for the prevention of intravascular catheter-related infections. MMWR 51(No.RR-10):1–36
19. Krzywda E, Andris D, Edmiston CE, Quebbeman EJ (1996) Hickman catheter sepsis: efficacy of antibiotic lock therapy. Infect Control Hosp Epidemiol 16:596–598
20. Benoit JL, Carandang G, Sitrin M, et al. (1995) Intraluminal antibiotic treatment of central venous catheter infections in patients receiving nutrition at home. Clin Infect Dis 21:1286–1288
21. Widmer AF (1997) Intravenous-related infections. In: Wenzel RP (ed) Prevention and control of nosocomial infections. Williams & Wilkins, Philadelphia, pp 771–805
22. Rubinson L, Wu AW, Haponik EF, Diette GB (2005) Why is it that internists do not follow guidelines for preventing intravascular catheter infections. Infect Control Hosp Epidemiol 26:525–533
23. Adams D, Quayum M, Worthington T, Lambert P, Elliott T (2005) Evaluation of a 2% chlorhexidine in 70 isopropyl alcohol skin disinfectant. J Hosp Infect 61:287–290
24. Chaiyakunapruk N, Veenstra DL, Lipsky BA, Saint S (2002) Chlorhexidine compared with povidone solution for vascular catheter site care: a meta analysis. Ann Intern Med 136:792–801
25. Maki DG, Rinder M (1987) Evaluation of dressing regimens for prevention of infection with peripheral venous catheters. Gauze, a transparent polyurethane dressing, and an iodophor-transparent dressing. J Am Med Assoc 258:2396–2403
26. Faubion WC, Wesley JR, Khaldi N, Silva J (1986) Total parenteral nutrition catheter sepsis: impact of the team approach. J Parenter Enteral Nutr 10:642–645
27. Tomford JW, Hershey CO, McLaren CE, Porter DK, et al. (1984) Intravenous therapy team and peripheral venous catheter-associated complications. A prospective control study. Arch Intern Med 144:1191–1194
28. Danzig LE, Short L, Collins K, et al. (1995) Bloodstream infections associated with needleless intravenous infusion systems and total parenteral nutrition. J Am Med Assoc 273:1862–1864
29. Larson EL, Cheng G, Choo JTE, Merz W (1993) In-vitro survival of skin flora in heparin locks and needleless valve infusion devices. Heart Lung 22:459–462
30. Kollef MH, Shorr A, Tabak YP, Gupta V, Liu LZ, Johannes RS (2005) Epidemiology and outcome of healthcare-associated pneumonia: results from a large US database of culture positive pneumonia. Chest 128:3854–3862
31. Edmiston CE (1999) Nosocomial infections: bacterial pneumonia, In: Atlee JL (ed) Complications in anesthesia. WB Saunders, Philadelphia, pp 208–210
32. Rello J, Ollendorf DA, Oster G, et al. (2002) Epidemiology and outcomes of ventilator-associated pneumonia in a large US database. Chest 122:2115–2121
33. Guidelines for the management of adults with hospital-acquired ventilator-associated, and healthcare-associated pneumonia (2005) Am J Respir Crit Care 171:388–416
34. Hospital Infection Control Practices Advisory Committee, Centers for Disease Control and Prevention (1999) National Nosocomial Infection Surveillance (NNIS) system report, January 1990–May 1999. Am J Infect Control 27:520–532
35. Tablan OC, Anderson LJ, Besser R, Bridges C, Hajjeh R (2004) Guidelines for preventing healthcare-associated pneumonia. MMWR 53(RR03):1–36
36. Craven DE, Kunches LM, Kilinsky V, Lichtenberg DA, et al. (1986) Risk factors for pneumonia and fatality in patients receiving continuous mechanical ventilation. Am Rev Respir Dis 133:792–796
37. Rello J, Torres A, Ricart M, Valles J, et al. (1994) Ventilator-associated pneumonia by *Staphylococcus aureus*. Am J Respir Crit Care Med 150:1545–1549
38. Darouiche RO (1999) Anti-infective efficacy of silver-coated medical prostheses. Clin Infect Dis 29:1371–1377
39. Srinivasan A, Karchmer T, Richards A, Song X, Perl TM (2006) A prospective trial of a novel, silicone-based, silver-coated Foley catheter for the prevention of nosocomial urinary tract infections. Infect Control Hosp Epidemiol 27:38–43
40. Hospital Infection Control Practices Advisory Committee, Centers for Disease Control and Prevention (1996) Guideline for isolation precautions in hospitals. Infect Control Hosp Epidemiol 17:53–80
41. Owen RC (2006) *Clostridium difficile*-associated disease: an emerging threat to patient safety. Pharmacotherapy 26:299–311

42. Hospital Infection Control Practices Advisory Committee, Centers for Disease Control and Prevention (1995) Recommendations for preventing the spread of vancomycin resistance. Infect Control Hosp Epidemiol 16:105–113
43. Shlaes DM, Gerding DN, John JF, Craig WA, et al. (1997) Society for Healthcare Epidemiology of America and Infectious Disease Society of American Joint Committee on the Prevention of Antimicrobial Resistance: Guidelines for the Prevention of Antimicrobial Resistance in Hospitals. Infect Control Hosp Epidemiol 18:275–291
44. Fridkin SK, Hill HA, Volkova NV, Edwards JR, Lawton RM, Gaynes RP, McGowan JE (2002) Temporal changes in prevalence of antimicrobial resistance in 23 US hospitals. Emerg Infect Dis 8:697–701
45. Shorr AF, Combes A, Kollef MH, Chastre J (2006) Methicillin-resistant *Staphylococcus aureus* prolongs intensive care unit stay in ventilator-associated pneumonia, despite initially appropriate antibiotic therapy. Crit Care Med 34: 700–706
46. Gaynes R, Edward JR (2005) Overview of nosocomial infections caused by Gram-negative bacilli. Clin Infect Dis 41:848–854
47. Edmiston CE, Seabrook GR, Hennen C (2001) The importance of beta-lactamase resistance in surgical infections. Surg Infect 2:1–10
48. Edmiston CE (1996) Vancomycin resistance: when failure becomes an opportunity for leadership. Ann Pharmacother 30:680–682
49. Healthcare Infection Control Practices Advisory Committee (2002) Guideline for hand hygiene in healthcare settings. MMWR 51 (No. RR-16):1–45
50. Vernon MO, Hayden MK, Trick WE, Hayes RA, Blom DW, Weinstein RA (2006) Chlorhexidine gluconate to cleanse patients in a medical intensive care unit. Arch Intern Med 166:306–312
51. Lai KK, Fontecchio SA (2002) Use of silver-hydrogel urinary catheters on the incidence of catheter-associated urinary tract infections in hospitalized patients. Am J Infect Control 30:221–225

19 Antibiotic Resistance in the Intensive Care Unit

J. Vila, F. Marco

19.1 Introduction

Nosocomial infections, especially those caused by antibacterial agent-resistant pathogens, represent an important source of morbidity and mortality for the patients in an ICU. Important antibacterial agent-resistant nosocomial pathogens include both Gram-negative (ESBL-producing Enterobacteriaceae and non-fermenting bacilli, such as *Pseudomonas aeruginosa, Acinetobacter baumannii* and *Stenotrophomonas maltophilia*) and Gram-positive (methicillin-resistant *Staphylococcus aureus* [MRSA] and vancomycin-resistant *Enterococcus* spp. [VRE]) bacteria. Overall, the prevalence of resistance is often highest in units where the most vulnerable patients are located and where antibacterial use is consequently the heaviest. For instance, ICU patients have shown twofold higher rates of MRSA, ceftazidime resistance among *Enterobacter cloacae* and *P. aeruginosa,* and vancomycin resistance among enterocci than in patients in general wards [1].

19.2 Brief Overview of the Mechanisms of Antimicrobial Resistance

Bacterial resistance to antibacterial agents may occur mainly through four mechanisms (Fig. 19.1). Altered uptake of an antibacterial agent into the bacterial cell

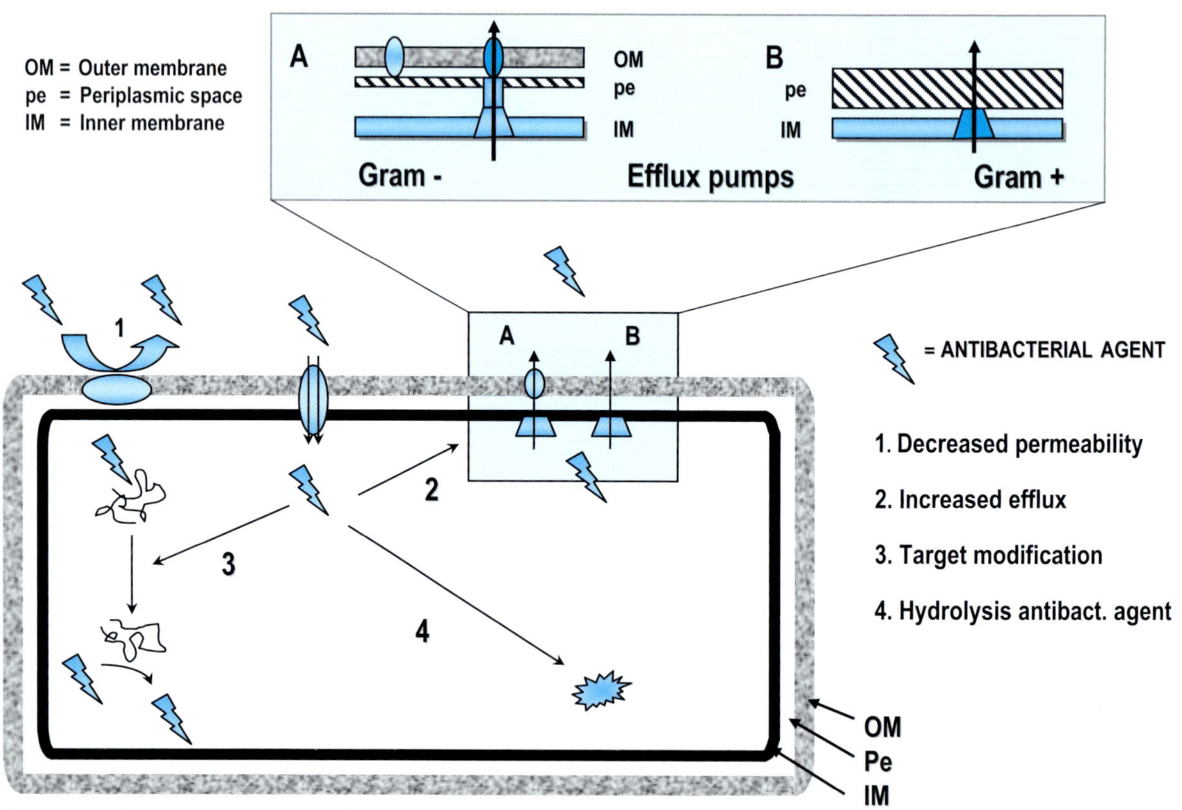

Fig. 19.1. Mechanisms of antimicrobial resistance

can be due either to a decreased permeability (entry into the cell, pathway 1 in the scheme of Fig. 19.1) or increased efflux (pumping the antibacterial agent out of the cell, pathway 2 in the scheme) or to the interplay of both mechanisms. Therefore, there is a decrease in the amount of antibacterial agent reaching its protein target. An overexpression of an efflux pump affecting one or several antibacterial agents can be found in both Gram-negative and Gram-positive bacteria, whereas a decreased permeability associated with a decrease in porin expression, the main protein which constitutes the pores used by the most hydrophobic drugs to cross the outer membrane, is exclusive of Gram-negative bacteria. The target protein for a specific antibacterial agent can be structurally modified, hence resulting in a lower affinity of this molecule for the antibacterial agent (pathway 3 in the scheme); such is the case for the penicillin-binding proteins (PBP), the protein targets for the β-lactam antibacterial agents. Finally, the most predominant mechanism of resistance is the presence of genes encoding enzymes, which hydrolyse or modify the antibacterial agent, rendering it inactive (pathway 4 in the scheme). Examples of such enzymes are the β-lactamases, aminoglycoside-modifying enzymes and chloramphenicol acetyl transferase. Bacteria often possess multiple mechanisms of antibacterial resistance for each of the antibacterial agents and some of these mechanisms can be found concomitantly, providing the bacteria with a higher level of resistance (Table 19.1). In classical cross-resistance, a single biochemical mechanism confers resistance to a single class of drugs: use of a given antibiotic can select resistance to other members of the group but not to drugs belonging to other classes. However, cross-resistance between drug classes, also called pleiotropic resistance, can occur by two mechanisms: overlapping targets and drug efflux. An example of target overlap is provided by the macrolides, lincosamides, and streptogramins (MLS), which are chemically distantly related.

Table 19.1. Main mechanisms of resistance to antibacterial agents

Antibacterial agent	Mechanism of resistance
β-Lactams	Altered penicillin-binding proteins Reduced permeability Increased efflux Synthesis of β-lactamases
Aminoglycosides	Modification of ribosomal proteins Synthesis of aminoglycoside-modifying enzymes Increased efflux
Macrolides and ketolides	Methylating enzymes Increased efflux
Glycopeptides	Altered target
Fluoroquinolones	Altered DNA gyrase and topoisomerase IV Reduced permeability Increased efflux Synthesis of peptide protecting protein targets
Tetracyclines	Ribosomal protection Increased efflux
Rifampicin	Altered RNA-polymerase
Chloramphenicol	Synthesis of chloramphenicol acetyl transferase Decreased permeability Increased efflux
Trimethoprim	Altered dihydropholate reductase Decreased permeability Increased efflux

19.3 Acquisition of Resistance

The natural (intrinsic) resistance shown by some microorganisms is normally related to specific features of these microorganisms, which prevent the arrival of the antibacterial agent to the protein target. One example of this is the constitutive expression of some efflux pumps. Moreover, this intrinsic resistance can also take place when there is a natural modification of the protein target. Although some bacteria can present an intrinsic resistance, most bacteria acquire resistance mainly by two processes. The most common mechanism of acquired resistance is the uptake of extrachromosomal DNA (plasmids, transposons or integrons) that contains antibacterial resistance genes. Conjugative plasmids and transposons are able to pass directly between bacteria through the process of conjugation in which a plasmid is transferred from the donor cell to the recipient cell. The origin of the resistance genes that can be transferred between bacteria on plasmids and transposons is unknown, but some, at least, may have originated as a self-protective mechanism in antibiotic-producing organisms. There are two other mechanisms for gene transfer in addition to conjugation: transduction and transformation. In transduction genes are transferred by bacterial viruses, called bacteriophages. In transformation, pieces of DNA in the bacteria's environment are taken into the bacteria and incorporated into the bacterial chromosome. Secondly, resistance can develop by mutation of chromosomal genes. One type of resistance that combines both mechanisms is the uptake of non-plasmid DNA fragments via transformation and recombination into the bacterial chromosome. This is exemplified by the transfer of penicillin resistance among pneumococci. Although mutations occur only rarely, prolonged exposure to antibacterial agents can select for mutations which take place during a patient's treatment.

19.4 Factors Favouring Resistance Development

The emergence, persistence and spread of resistant microorganisms in the hospital setting are associated with several factors: (1) factors dependent on the microorganism, among which is the propensity to acquire foreign genetic elements carrying resistant genes. Among these, the ability to survive in several environments and the capability to easily colonise and infect can be highlighted. (2) The existence of human and inanimate reservoirs, in which resistant bacteria can survive. Normally, these reservoirs provide a good environment for the interchange of genetic material. Finally, (3) the strategies of use of specific antibacterial agents. In addition, there are several factors which favour the spread of a resistant strain: Crowding of patients with high levels of disease acuity in a relatively small, specialised area of the hospital, reductions in nursing staff associated with economic pressure and the presence of more chronically and acutely ill patients who require prolonged hospitalisation [2–4].

Reductions in antibiotic resistance have been associated with hospital-instituted programmes aimed at combining judicious overall use of antibiotics with the use of narrow-spectrum antibiotics. The risk of acquisition of a particular infection as a function of the proportion of people colonised has been called "colonisation pressure", and has been described as a major variable affecting the spread of VRE and MRSA [5, 6]. The widespread adoption of antibiotic-control measures and promotion of strict adherence to infection-control procedures are necessary to prevent the colonisation pressure observed in hospitals, especially in ICUs. Quantitative analysis of vancomycin-resistant *Enterococcus faecalis* transmission in an ICU indicates that staffing levels have a critical role in transmission, and that a productive alliance between patients and staff is a very effective means in decreasing transmission, such that the level of adherence to hand hygiene is an inverse function of the endemic level of vancomycin-resistant *E. faecalis* colonisation [6, 7].

Prolonged length of hospital stay appears to predispose patients to infection with antibiotic-resistant bacteria. This predisposition may result, in part, from the greater likelihood over time of becoming colonised with such bacteria or the generally poorer underlying immune status of most seriously ill patients. In addition, the use of invasive devices, such as endotracheal tubes, and intravascular and urinary catheters, seems to encourage such infections. The rising presence of infections causing antibiotic resistant bacteria among patients in long-term treatment facilities can also be an important source for the entry of resistant bacteria into the ICU. Furthermore, outbreaks of multidrug resistant bacteria are also key factors promoting the spread of resistance. A reduction in the duration of mechanical ventilation could decrease the incidence of ventilator-associated pneumonia and consequently reduce the length of hospital or ICU stay. Protocols for patients requiring mechanical ventilation have been shown to reduce the duration of mechanical ventilation and the length of ICU stay.

19.5 Antimicrobial Resistance in Gram-Negative Bacteria

During the past decade, extended-spectrum β-lactamase (ESBL) producing Enterobacteriaceae, mainly *Klebsiella pneumoniae* and *Escherichia coli*, have become increasingly common nosocomial pathogens. This development is likely related to heavy use of third-generation cephalosporins [8]. The prevalence of ESBL production among the Enterobacteriaceae varies greatly from country to country and among the institutions in the country. These β-lactamases confer resistance to most β-lactam antibiotics with the exception of carbapenems. Data from the National Nosocomial Infections Surveillance (NNIS) system showed a sudden increase from 2% to 23% in ESBL-producing *K. pneumoniae* between 1989 and 1990 and this level has been maintained to date [9]. Overall, the percentage of ESBL-producing *E. coli* strains is lower than ESBL-producing *K. pneumoniae* strains (Table 19.2). Several reports have shown that the use of any β-lactam/β-lactamase inhibitor other than ceftazidime is associated with a decrease in rates of isolating ESBL-producing Enterobacteriaceae in the ICU [10]. The spread of ESBL-producing Enterobacteriaceae is worsened by their common association with other multiple resistance genes, sometimes located in the same plasmid. *Enterobacter cloacae* is another important microorganism causing ventilator-associated pneumonia. Third-generation cephalosporin treatment of infections caused by *Enterobacter* has been associated with rapid selection on AmpC cephalosporinase derepressed mutants and this scenario may limit the treatment to carbapenems. In several surveillance studies the percentage of third-generation cephalosporin-resistant *Enterobacter* strains is from 26% to 36% (Table 19.2).

Resistance to quinolones is also a growing problem. In the ICU, where changes in the prevalence of quinolone resistance can be investigated more accurately because of its closed environment, the overall quinolone resistance of Gram-negative bacilli steadily increased from 14% in 1994 to 24% in 2000 [11]. In particular, the average of quinolone-resistant *E. coli* clinical isolates in the USA is 2%, whereas in Europe it is 12% (Table 19.2).

P. aeruginosa and *A. baumannii* are the two most relevant non-fermentative Gram-negative bacteria. In

Table 19.2. Comparison of resistance rates obtained from different surveillance programs monitoring ICU infections

Microorganism	% of resistance		
	SENTRY-USA[a]	ICARE[b]	SENTRY-EU[c]
ESBL – *E. coli*	3.7	2.2	3.6
ESBL – *K. pneumoniae*	14.5	10.4	15.8
3GC[d]-resistant *Enterobacter*	26.1	33.1	36.2
FQ[e]-resistant *E. coli*	–	2.0[f]	12.1
Imipenem-resistant *P. aeruginosa*	16.1	16.4	29.0
3GC-resistant *P. aeruginosa*	–	20.6	23.3
FQ-resistant *P. aeruginosa*	24.8	23.0	30.4
Imipenem-resistant *A. baumannii*	–	–	44.6
VRE	28.4	24.7	2.9
MRSA	51.4	53.5	42

[a] Reference [13]
[b] Reference [14]
[c] Reference [15]
[d] 3GC – third generation cephalosporins
[e] FQ – fluoroquinolones
[f] Reference [16]

a surveillance study with *P. aeruginosa* and *A. baumannii* isolates from 65 laboratories in the United States collected between 1998 and 2001, Karlowsky et al. [12] found that the percentage of imipenem-resistant *P. aeruginosa* isolates was 16.7%, being 7.8% and 9.9% for cefepime and ceftazidime, respectively. In the same study it was observed that the quinolone-resistance *P. aeruginosa* strains isolated from patients in the ICU increased from 18.3% in 1998 to 25.0% in 2001. Similarly, the proportion of ciprofloxacin-resistant *A. baumannii* isolates also increased from 46.2% to 53.8%. Only 3% of the *A. baumannii* strains analysed were resistant to imipenem, in contrast with 44% of imipenem-resistant *A. baumannii* isolates found in Europe.

19.6 Antimicrobial Resistance in Gram-Positive Bacteria

Gram-positive bacteria resistant to several antibiotics have been reported as an important cause of ICU infection and in many circumstances, particularly with vancomycin-resistant *Enterococcus faecium*, few alternative antimicrobial agents remain effective.

MRSA continues to be a major nosocomial pathogen that causes severe morbidity and mortality in many hospitals worldwide. As many strategies to prevent and control the spread of MRSA microorganisms have been described [17, 18], the incidence of nosocomial MRSA in ICU patients is used to assess the quality of infection control measures. However, a continuing increase has been observed in the proportion of MRSA isolates identified from patients in the ICU with nosocomial infections. Recent data from the NNIS comparing resistance rates from January through December 2003 with those from 1998 to 2002 showed that the proportion of *Staphylococcus aureus* isolates resistant to methicillin was nearly 60% (59.5%) and the percentage increase in the rate of resistance was 11% [19]. These results underscore the continuing increase in antimicrobial resistance as surveillance programs performed previously reported lower resistance rates (Table 19.2) [13–15]. Data from the NNIS also confirm that methicillin resistance in coagulase-negative staphylococci (89.1%) is a very common feature in strains isolated from ICU patients [19].

In 1996 reduced susceptibility to vancomycin (MIC = 8 g/ml) was reported in Japan and the United States, both in association with the failure of vancomycin treatment for MRSA infection [20, 21]. The mechanism for the reduced susceptibility is not completely understood, but it appears to have developed "de novo" after antibiotic exposure [22]. It has been suggested that these strains develop independently [22] due to the different patterns of antibiotic susceptibility [23]. Recent reports of MRSA isolates resistant to vancomycin due to the acquisition of the *vanA* gene from enterococci pose a potentially serious threat to public health [24–26].

VRE have recently emerged as a significant nosocomial pathogen, especially in the ICUs. Several phenotypes of glycopeptide resistance have been described, but strains of *Enterococcus faecalis* or *E. faecium* belonging to the class VANA and VANB phenotypes are the most numerous recovered from patients. Although the first VRE isolate that harboured the *vanA* gene was identified in 1987 in Europe [27], the highest prevalence of VRE is observed in the United States [13–15]. From 1989 to 1993, a 34-fold increase in the prevalence of VRE in ICUs in the United States was observed [28]. In ICU patients, data from a recent NNIS report showed that the proportion of *Enterococcus* spp. resistant to vancomycin was 28.5% [19]. However, the rate of increase has diminished for this pathogen, which was reported as +31% in 2000 compared to +12 in 2003 [29]. In a report published by Streit et al. [30], these authors found a resistance rate of 3.9% for *E. faecalis* and 65.8% for *E. faecium* in enterococcal isolates recovered from ICU patients in North America. The emergence of vancomycin resistance among *E. faecium*, the second most frequently encountered species, is of special concern because of the high prevalence of resistance to multiple agents, including ampicillin, gentamicin and streptomycin. It is noteworthy that the spread of VRE to non-ICU wards has occurred in recent years and more than 25% of enterococci associated with bloodstream infections in hospitalised patients in the United States were resistant to vancomycin [29].

19.7 Clinical Consequences of Antimicrobial Resistance

The high frequency of antimicrobial resistant microorganisms is a major public health problem in many countries. Although it can be difficult to gather evidence on the direct relationship between antibiotic use and antimicrobial resistance, previous exposure probably exerts selective pressure favouring the emergence of resistance. Methods to reduce inappropriate or excessive antimicrobial use differ from institution to institution and deciding which is the most effective in a particular setting can be difficult [31, 32]. In addition to prudent use and scheduled rotation of antibiotics, strict compliance with infection control policies can aid in the reduction of nosocomial multidrug resistant isolates. However, several studies have shown that compliance with simple handwashing in ICUs varies from 20% to 40% [33, 34].

Antimicrobial resistance in the ICU has a clear incidence in increasing therapeutic failure, morbidity, mortality and cost [35–37]. Alvarez-Lerma et al. [38] suggested that isolation of multiresistant pathogens in critically ill patients can occur in the following circumstances: (a) detection of resistance of the original strain, particularly during treatment with cephalosporins, in relation to the development of antibacterial-induced inactivating enzymes, as in the case of Enterobacteriaceae and *P. aeruginosa*. This event is associated with failure of antimicrobial therapy and an increase in mortality; (b) isolation of one or more resistant strains of the same species in the form of an epidemic outbreak (*A. baumannii*, ESBL *K. pneumoniae*, VR *E. faecium*, MRSA). This form of presentation has an important impact on the antibiotic policy of the ICU and a major effect on the clinical course of patients with intermediate degrees of illness severity; and (c) individual isolation in a patient at risk (prolonged ICU stay, previous use of broad spectrum antimicrobial agents, high severity score). In this situation, multiresistant strains (MRSA, *P. aeruginosa*, *A. baumannii*) are frequently identified at the last phase of the clinical course of the patient. The presence of these pathogens is a marker of severity, although it has a low effect on the final outcome of the patient or on the antibiotic policy of the ICU. The infections with multidrug resistant bacteria have a significant impact on several clinical outcomes. The patients infected with multidrug-resistant microorganisms are usually treated with an effective antibacterial agent later than other patients. Several studies have demonstrated a strong association between inadequate antibiotic treatment and in-hospital mortality rates for patients with ventilator-associated pneumonia [39, 40]. In addition to higher patient mortality rates, infections caused by multidrug resistant microorganisms are associated with a significantly longer duration of hospital stay, and as a consequence greater hospital charges [41, 42].

References

1. Archivald L, Phillips L, Monnet D, et al. (1997) Antimicrobial resistance in isolates from inpatients and outpatients in the United States: increasing importance of the intensive care units. Clin Infect Dis 24:211–215
2. Haley RW, Bregman DA (1982) Role of understaffing and overcrowding in recurrent outbreaks of staphylococcal infection in a neonatal special-care unit. J Infect Dis 145: 875–885
3. McGowan JE Jr (1991) Antibiotic resistance in hospital bacteria: current patterns, modes of appearance or spread, and economic impact. Rev Med Microbiol 2:161–169
4. Kollef MH, Fraser VJ (2001) Antibiotic resistance in the Intensive Care Unit. Ann Inter Med 134:298–314
5. Merrer J, Santoli F, Appéré-De Vecchi C, et al. (2000) "Colonization pressure" and risk of acquisition of methicillin-resistant *Staphylococcus aureus* in a medical intensive care unit. Infect Control Hosp Epidemiol 21:718–723
6. Bonten MJ, Slaughter S, Ambergen AW, et al. (1998) The role of "colonization pressure" in the spread of vancomycin-resistant enterococci. Arch Inter Med 158: 1127–1132
7. Austin DJ, Bonten MJ, Weinstein RA, et al. (1999) Vancomycin-resistant enterococci in intensive-care hospital settings: transmission dynamics, persistence, and the impact of infection control programs. Proc Natl Acad Sci USA 96:6908–6913
8. Waterer GW, Wunderink RG (2001) Increasing treatment of gram-negative bacteria. Crit Care Med 29 (Suppl 4): N75–N81
9. Gaynes R, Edwards JR (2005) Overview of nosocomial infections caused by Gram-negative bacilli. Clin Infect Dis 41:848–854
10. Rice LB, Eckstein EC, DeVente J, et al. (1996) Ceftazidime-resistant *Klebsiella pneumoniae* isolates recovered at the Cleveland Department of Veterans Affairs Medical Center. Clin Infect Dis 23:118–124
11. Neuhauser MM, Weinstein RA, Rydman R, et al. (2003) Antibiotic resistance among gram-negative bacilli in US intensive care units: Implications for fluoroquinolone use. JAMA 289:885–888
12. Karlowsky JA, Draghi DC, Jones ME, et al. (2003) Surveillance for antimicrobial susceptibility among clinical isolates of *Pseudomonas aeruginosa* from hospitalised patients in the United States, 1998 to 2001. Antimicrob Agents Chemother 47:1681–1688
13. Stephen J, Mutnick A, Jones RN (2002) Assessment of pathogens and resistance patterns among intensive care unit (ICU) patients in North America: initial report from the SENTRY Antimicrobial Surveillance Program (2001). Abstract C2-297. 42nd Intersci Conf Antimicrob Agents Chemother. San Diego, 2002
14. CDC NNIS System (1999) National Nosocomial Infections Surveillance (NNIS) system report, data summary from January 1990–May 1999. Am J Infect Control 27:520–532
15. Rodriguez-Villalobos H, Struelens MJ, Jones RN, European SENTRY participants (2003) Resistance in pathogens from patients admitted to intensive care units (ICU). A report from SENTRY surveillance program Europe 2000–2002. Abstract C2-1971. 43rd Intersci Conf Antimicrob Agents Chemother, Chicago, 2003

16. Fridkin SK, Hill HA, Volkova NV, et al. (2002) Temporal changes in prevalence of antimicrobial resistance in 23 US Hospitals. Emerg Infect Dis 8:697 – 701
17. Wenzel RP, Nettelman MD, Jones RN, et al. (1991) Methicillin-resistant *Staphylococcus aureus*: implications for the 1990s and the effective control measures. Am J Med 91(Suppl 3B):221S–227S
18. Jarvis WR (1996) Preventing the emergence of multidrug-resistant microorganisms through antimicrobial use control: the complexity of the problem. Infect Control Hosp Epidemiol 17:490 – 495
19. CDC NNIS System (2004) National Nosocomial Infections Surveillance (NNIS) system report, data summary from January 1992 through June 2004, issued October 2004. Am J Infect Control 32:470 – 485
20. Hiramatsu K, Aritaka N, Hanaki H, et al. (1997) Dissemination in Japanese hospitals of strains of *Staphylococcus aureus* heterogeneously resistant to vancomycin. Lancet 350:1670 – 1673
21. Centers for Disease Control and Prevention (1997) *Staphylococcus aureus* with reduced susceptibility to vancomycin – United States. MMRW 46:765 – 766
22. Hiramatsu K (1998) The emergence of *Staphylococcus aureus* with reduced susceptibility to vancomycin in Japan. Am J Med 1004:7S–10S
23. Centers for Disease Control and Prevention (1997) Update: *Staphylococcus aureus* with reduced susceptibility to vancomycin – United States. MMRW Morb Mortal Wkly Rep 46:813 – 815
24. Centers for Disease Control and Prevention (2004) Vancomycin-resistant *Staphylococcus aureus* – New York, 2004. MMRW Morb Mortal Wkly Rep 53:322 – 323
25. Chang S, Sievert DM, Hageman JC, et al. (2003) Infection with vancomycin-resistant *Staphylococcus aureus* containing the *vanA* gene. N Engl J Med 348:1342 – 1347
26. Tenover FC, Weigel LM, Appelbaum PC, et al. (2004) Vancomycin-resistant *Staphylococcus aureus* isolate from a patient in Pennsylvania. Antimicrob Agents Chemother 48: 275 – 280
27. Leclerq R, Derlot E, Duval J, et al. (1988) Plasmid-mediated resistance to vancomycin and teicoplanin in *Enterococcus faecium*. N Engl J Med 319:157 – 161
28. Centers for Disease Control and Prevention (1995) Recommendations for Preventing the Spread of Vancomycin Resistance. Recommendations of the Hospital Infection Control Practices Advisory Committee (HICPAC). MMRW Morb Mortal Wkly Rep 44:1 – 13
29. CDC NNIS System (2001) National Nosocomial Infections Surveillance (NNIS) system report, data summary from January 1992 through June 2001, issued August 2001. Am J Infect Control 29:400 – 421
30. Streit JM, Jones RN, Sader HS, Fritsche TR (2004) Assessment of pathogen occurrences and resistance profiles among infected patients in the intensive care unit: report from the SENTRY Antimicrobial Surveillance Program (North America, 2001). Intern J Antimicrob Agents 24: 111 – 118
31. Duncan RA (1997) Controlling use of antimicrobial agents. Infect Control Hosp Epidemiol 18:260 – 266
32. Shales DM, Gerding DN, John JF, et al. (1997) Society for Healthcare Epidemiology of America and Infectious Diseases Society of America Joint Committee on the prevention of antimicrobial resistance in hospitals. Infect Control Hosp Epidemiol 18:275 – 291
33. Gould D (1994) Nurses' hand decontamination practice: results of a local study. J Hosp Infect 25:15 – 30
34. Simmons B, Bryant J, Neiman K, et al. (1990) The role of hand washing in prevention of endemic intensive care unit infections. Infect Control Hosp Epidemiol 11:589 – 594
35. Fagon JY, Chastre J, Hance AJ, et al. (1993) Nosocomial pneumonia in ventilated patients: a cohort study evaluating attributable mortality and hospital stay. Am J Med 94:281 – 288
36. Pittet D, Tarara D, Wenzel RP (1994) Nosocomial bloodstream infection in critically ill patients. Excess length of stay, extra costs and attributable mortality. JAMA 271: 1598 – 1601
37. Bueno-Cavanillas A, Delgado-Rodriguez M, Luque-Luque A, et al. (1994) Influence of nosocomial infection on mortality rate in an intensive care unit. Crit Care Med 22: 55 – 60
38. Alvarez-Lerma F, Palomar M, Grau S (2001) Management of antimicrobial use in the Intensive Care Unit. Drugs 61:763 – 775
39. Kollef MH, Ward S (1998) The influence of mini-BAL cultures on patient outcomes: implications for the antibiotic management of ventilator-associated pneumonia. Chest 113:412 – 20
40. Rello J, Gallego M, Mariscal D, et al. (1997) The value of routine microbial investigation in ventilator-associated pneumonia. Am J Respir Crit Care Med 156:196 – 200
41. Carmeli Y, Troillet N, Karchmer AW, et al. (1999) Health and economic outcomes of antibiotic resistance in *Pseudomonas aeruginosa*. Arch Intern Med 159:1127 – 32
42. Holemberg SD, Solomon SL, Blake PA (1987) Health and economic impact of antimicrobial resistance. Rev Infect Dis 9:1065 – 78

20 Epidemiology of *Pseudomonas aeruginosa* in the Intensive Care Unit

R.G. Wunderink, D.L. Mendoza

20.1 Introduction

Pseudomonas aeruginosa, a member of the family Pseudomonadaceae, is a gram-negative aerobic rod. *P. aeruginosa* can grow anaerobically if nitrates are available. Almost all strains are motile by means of a single polar flagellum. It has a predilection for growth in moist environments, probably reflecting its natural existence in soil and water. *P. aeruginosa* is tolerant of a wide variety of physical conditions, including high concentrations of salts and dyes, weak antiseptics and many commonly used antibiotics. Its growth requirements are so minimal that it can grow in distilled water and even survive in the presence of some disinfectants [1]. Optimal growth occurs in the range of 37.0–42.0 °C, but it can also grow at temperatures higher than 20.0 °C [2]. *P. aeruginosa* grows in a variety of media but does not ferment sugar. These natural properties of the bacterium contribute to its ecological success as an opportunistic pathogen.

Pseudomonas aeruginosa isolates produce three colony types. Natural isolates from soil or water typically produce a rough colony. Clinical samples, generally, yield one or another of two colony types. One type is smooth, with flat edges and an elevated appearance. The other type, frequently obtained from respiratory and urinary tract secretions, has a mucoid appearance. The smooth and mucoid phenotypes presumably play a role in colonization and virulence. This pathogen also produces two types of soluble pigments, pyoverdin and pyocyanin, which result in its characteristic green appearance in culture. The latter is relatively specific for *P. aeruginosa* and is produced by approximately half of the strains.

Pseudomonas aeruginosa is an opportunistic pathogen that is able to cause severe invasive diseases in critically ill and immunocompromised patients. Surprisingly, *P. aeruginosa* only occasionally causes serious infections in healthy persons and is infrequently identified as normal microbial flora in healthy individuals. While a common nosocomial pathogen in all departments of the hospital, *P. aeruginosa* infections are especially prevalent among intensive care unit (ICU) patients [3–5], possibly due to the severity of illness in this population as well as the high rate invasive devices or procedures. The respiratory tract is the most frequent source of *P. aeruginosa* isolates, followed by surgical wounds, urine and bloodstream [6].

The incidence of nosocomial *P. aeruginosa* infections has increased in recent decades [7]. A multicenter study placed *P. aeruginosa* as the most common gram-negative pathogen recovered in the ICU [8] and the leading cause of ventilator-associated pneumonia (VAP) [9–11]. Moreover, the high frequency of multiple resistance among *P. aeruginosa* strains makes its eradication difficult [8, 12, 13]. High mortality and morbidity rates have been observed for *P. aeruginosa* infections, especially with respiratory tract infection [14].

20.2 Environment and Nosocomial Reservoirs

Pseudomonas aeruginosa is a ubiquitous organism, both the hospital and the external environment. *P. aeruginosa* is a common inhabitant of soil, water and vegetation. These can serve as reservoirs and as agents for dissemination [15, 16]. Its ability to survive for lengthy periods as long as sufficient moisture is available may be the reason for this extensive ecologic niche. The natural and permanent reservoir of this microorganism is therefore independent of humans.

Only a small proportion of healthy individuals carry *P. aeruginosa* [17, 18]. It is found on the skin of some healthy persons and has been isolated from the throat and stool of non-hospitalized patients. The length of carriage in healthy individuals is not known. Despite abundant opportunities for exposure, community-acquired pneumonia due to *P. aeruginosa* infection is very rare in people without structural lung disease.

Hospital reservoirs for the microorganism include respiratory equipment, bronchoscopes, antiseptics, disinfectants, hand lotions, soap, sinks, artificial fingernails and physiotherapy/hydrotherapy pools [19, 20]. Many recent hospital outbreaks of *P. aeruginosa* have been reported by contamination from one of these reservoirs. The water supply in hospitals may be an important source for colonization and infection in susceptible patients [20, 21], including faucets that are contaminated during hand washing. A review of prospective studies published between 1998 and 2005 showed that between 9 % and 68 % of random tap water samples on different types of ICUs were positive for *P. aeruginosa*. Indeed, between 14 % and 50 % of infection/colonization episodes in patients were due to genotypes found in ICU water. Furthermore, this microorganism is constantly reintroduced into the hospital environment on fruits, plants, vegetables, as well as by visitors and patients transferred from other facilities.

Spread occurs by direct patient contact with contaminated reservoirs, by the ingestion of contaminated foods and water (drinking water has been associated with *P. aeruginosa* infection when used for hydrotherapy of burned patients) and from patient to patient on the hands of hospital personnel. The latter mechanism has been increasingly reported in nosocomial outbreaks [22–26] and emphasizes the role of healthcare workers as vectors and reservoirs for this pathogen.

With this degree of hospital contamination, the lower respiratory tract of mechanically ventilated patients and the skin of hospitalized patients treated with broad-spectrum antibiotics can be colonized with *P. aeruginosa* at rates exceeding 50 % [27]. The gastrointestinal carriage rates increase in hospitalized patients to 20 % within 72 h of admission.

20.3 Epidemiologic Typing of *P. aeruginosa*

Although *P. aeruginosa* was discovered more than a century ago, many aspects of its reservoirs and transmission pathways remain unknown. A possible explanation is inconsistency of epidemiologic data obtained with conventional typing methods. Phenotyping methods were widely used before molecular typing techniques substituted them. When using phenotyping techniques, establishing relationships between environmental and patient isolates was frequently impossible [28, 29].

Studies comparing the classical typing methods with genotyping confirmed that the former were of low discriminatory power and yielded variable results. The important methods of pulsed-field gel electrophoresis (PFGE), amplified fragment-length polymorphism (AFLP) analysis and random amplified polymorphic DNA polymerase chain reaction (RAPD-PCR) have successfully supplanted the phenotyping methods in terms of typeability, reproducibility and discriminatory power.

PFGE is now considered to be the most accurate method for discrimination of related and unrelated isolates of *P. aeruginosa* [30, 31] and is preferred to other typing methods for the epidemiological study of *P. aeruginosa* [32, 33]. Categories of genetic and epidemiological relatedness of isolates using PFGE can be applied for relatively small sets of isolates related to putative outbreaks of disease [34]. Thus, molecular typing is a potentially powerful screening method for continuous quality improvement. Epidemiological surveillance combined with PFGE should help to improve the targeting of preventive strategies.

The major drawbacks of PFGE are that it is time-consuming and expensive. Moreover, digitalized data management and computer analysis are required for the analysis of larger numbers of isolates, particularly for longitudinal studies on the molecular epidemiology of *P. aeruginosa*. Technical conditions must be optimized to make gel comparisons possible.

20.4 General Epidemiology of *P. aeruginosa* in the ICU

An estimated 2–13 % of individuals are colonized with *P. aeruginosa* upon admission to ICUs [17, 32, 35–37] and approximately 1 % are infected at admission [17]. These rates tend to increase during the period of hospitalization.

In the most recent National Nosocomial Infections Surveillance (NNIS) system report in the USA, *P. aeruginosa* represents the third most frequent organism associated with wound or pulmonary infections, the fourth most frequent organism causing urinary tract infection, and the fifth most frequent organism isolated from blood cultures in septicemia [38]. VAP is the main infection caused by *P. aeruginosa* in terms of frequency, morbidity and mortality [36, 37]. In primary septicemia, data from Europe and the USA show a relatively constant proportion of 4 % of cases being originated by *P. aeruginosa* [39, 40]. Both pulmonary and bloodstream infections caused by this pathogen are associated with significant morbidity and mortality rates [41, 42].

The general epidemiology of *P. aeruginosa* in the ICU suggests that colonization plays the main role and represents the true bacterial load within ICUs. An understanding of the mechanisms involved in the setting and maintenance of the endemicity of *P. aeruginosa* colonization is therefore important.

Pseudomonas aeruginosa has a remarkable capability to colonize certain subgroups of patients, with ICUs clearly established as endemic settings for this pathogen. Risk factors significantly related with the acquisition of this pathogen in ICUs include: length of stay [43], mechanical ventilation [43], widespread use of antibiotics [18, 44, 45], use of indwelling urinary catheters [18] and alcoholism [18, 43].

Even though colonization by *P. aeruginosa* frequently precedes overt infection [18], the original source of the organism and the precise mode of transmission are often unclear. Moreover, colonized patients are a source of bacteria that may colonize other patients. This may lead to *Pseudomonas* infection in patients who have none of the risk factors listed above for endogenous colonization, although endogenous is still the most frequent source of acquisition [37, 46]. Environmental sources have also been clearly demonstrated to be important in horizontal transmission and outbreaks have been reported in several ICUs [47, 48]. An understanding of the relative importance of exogenous and endogenous colonizations is vital in order to develop infection control measures and strategies to prevent infection.

Screening cultures can characterize the endemic burden in ICUs and to determine the incidence of colonization. The intestinal tract is regarded as the most important reservoir for most bacteria [35, 37]. However, the lower respiratory tract also plays an important role in the carriage of *P. aeruginosa* in ICU patients [43]. A screening program for *P. aeruginosa* carriage in ICUs must therefore include both rectal and respiratory tract specimens to identify the largest proportion of the positive patients.

20.4.1 Endemic *P. aeruginosa* Infections

Endemic infections occur with a continuous and predictable frequency, mainly from an endogenous source [49]. Molecular typing in a non-epidemic ICU setting has demonstrated in several studies that the major reservoir of *P. aeruginosa* is the endogenous flora of the patients [32, 36, 37, 50, 51]. Length of ICU stay, mechanical ventilation duration, prior antibiotic exposure and long-dwelling central venous catheters placed are risk factors for multi-drug resistant (MDR) *P. aeruginosa* infection.

Pneumonia is the main manifestation of *P. aeruginosa* infection in the ICU, being more commonly associated with late-onset VAP. *P. aeruginosa* is related with significantly worse prognosis than other pathogens [52]. Colonization of the upper respiratory tract usually precedes the onset of pneumonia. After colonization, aspiration serves as the major mode of inoculation. *P. aeruginosa* is the cause of 20% of respiratory infections in ICU patients but is also responsible for approximately 5% of bloodstream infections, 10% of urinary tract infections, and 15% of surgical infections [4, 38, 53, 54]. Bloodstream infections lead to the most significant impact on morbidity and mortality.

20.4.2 Epidemic *P. aeruginosa* Infections

A large number of nosocomial *P. aeruginosa* outbreaks have been linked to contaminated environmental sources or breakdown in infection control measures with cross-infection from colonized patients or healthcare workers [20, 35, 43, 55–59]. Endogenous infections from the intestinal tract colonization appear to play a minor role [35, 37, 46]. The majority of outbreaks reported were clonal, as identified by genomic typing systems. Because *P. aeruginosa* infection is so common in the ICU, determining whether an outbreak is caused by a single clone or by multiple isolates is important. An early hint of whether the outbreak is clonal or not and if antibiotic pressure is playing a role is whether the isolates are resistant to all available antimicrobial agents or specifically to one.

Contamination of healthcare workers hands via an environmental water source is a common cause of the outbreaks. Spread occurs mainly from patient to patient on the hands of hospital personnel and by direct patient contact with contaminated reservoirs. Transmission of *P. aeruginosa* may not only occur within an ICU but has also been reported between hospitals, spreading from one to another by transferred patients or healthcare workers working at both sites [60].

20.5 Patterns of Resistance and Virulence

Pseudomonas aeruginosa has intrinsic resistance to several β-*lactams*, commonly associated with production of high levels of a cephalosporinase (AmpC). *Pseudomonas* also exhibits acquired resistance to any antibiotic by a variety of different mechanisms. These include mutations in outer membrane porins resulting in reduced permeability, penicillin binding protein modifications, production of extended-spectrum β-*lactamases* (ESBL), acquisition of *metallo-β-lactamases* or other enzymes, and overexpression of efflux pumps systems effective against multiple antibiotics [61–66]. The higher rates of resistance in ICUs are strongly influenced by prior antibiotic use [10, 11, 67] and associated with adverse clinical outcomes [68]. Significant variability among geographic regions and hospitals must be considered [6, 10].

The main β-*lactamases* produced by *P. aeruginosa* are chromosomally encoded rather than located on plasmids. The presence of ESBLs in these bacteria has important clinical implications because they confer resistance to all penicillins and cephalosporins but are difficult to detect phenotypically by MIC testing. This problem may lead to the false susceptibility reporting and, consequently, to inappropriate therapy. Aminoglycoside resistance is usually a result of enzyme-mediated antibiotic modification [69]. Resistance to quinolones occurs principally by alterations in the binding-site structure of the DNA-gyrase enzyme, which is the site of action of quinolones. MDR strains may emerge by combinations of efflux pumps, impermeability and production of inactivating enzymes [70]. The use of combination therapy with agents that act by different mechanisms may limit the emergence of resistance but clinical data supporting this hypothesis are lacking.

The ability of *P. aeruginosa* to form biofilms greatly enhances its ability to adhere to and survive on environmental surfaces, medical devices and the airways of patients with chronic lung disease. Growth within biofilms gives rise to the potential for resistance against disinfectants and antibiotics [71].

Pseudomonas aeruginosa produces a number of substances that contribute to its pulmonary toxicity, including exotoxins, proteases, cytotoxins and hemolysins. These enzymes and toxins can cause a necrotizing pneumonia with abscess formation, limiting the antibiotic penetration [72]. Perhaps the best known and characterized of these substances is exotoxin A, produced and released by most clinical strains of this pathogen. The type III protein secretion in pneumonia caused by *P. aeruginosa* has been related with worse clinical outcome [73]. This microorganism also produces a number of pigments with biologic properties that add to its virulence. Pyocyanin is the most important. The antibiotic activity of pyocyanin favors the growth of *P. aeruginosa* rather than other bacteria in some circumstances [74, 75].

Recently, awareness of the importance of the quorum-sensing system has increased. By this mechanism, the number of bacteria of the same type remaining in a same site influences the gene transcription and protein production, generally with an alteration of the phenotype toward more invasive characteristics when adequate numbers of bacteria are present. The increased ability to incorporate new virulence and resistance genes is one aspect of the quorum-sensing system.

Interestingly, *P. aeruginosa* shares its natural habitat with free living amoebae. Amoeba host defense systems can be used to analyze the virulence of *P. aeruginosa* strains [76, 77]. Wild-type *Pseudomonas* strains are more virulent and inhibit amoebal growth. An experimental study reported that, compared to environmental isolates, *P. aeruginosa* strains causing invasive hospital-acquired infections are more virulent in amoeba assays as well as more resistant to antibiotics. These data suggest that clinical infections due to *P. aeruginosa* are, at least in part, due to increased bacterial virulence [78].

20.6 Impact of *P. aeruginosa* Infection

Pseudomonas aeruginosa infection tends to occur predominantly in patients who are severely ill and already at increased risk of dying of other causes. However, this bacterium should always be considered as a lethal pathogen, with a reported 35% attributable mortality in bacteremia [79, 80] and an overall mortality of 69% in VAP [81], with an attributable mortality of at least 10% [82]. This excess mortality represents the potential for improved outcome if prevention or better therapy of *P. aeruginosa* VAP can be developed. Unfortunately, the mortality has not improved over the last 25 years, despite the availability of increasingly potent antibiotics. This increased mortality has been attributed to the elaboration of a mucoid exopolysaccharide that offers protection from host immune factors, the production of a wide variety of enzymes and toxins responsible for tissue destruction and bacterial invasion, the immunological vulnerability of the host, and the worldwide emergence of MDR nosocomial clones [81].

Because the balance between the adequacy of host defense and the virulence of *P. aeruginosa* is often very close, the appropriateness of antibiotic treatment is extremely important. The most active agents are the carbapenems, piperacillin, cefepime, ceftazidime, quinolones and aminoglycosides [83, 84]. Nevertheless, *P. aeruginosa* is one of the predominant microorganisms associated with failure of therapy [85–87]. In the case of VAP caused by *P. aeruginosa*, the most important strategy is to change to different antibiotic combinations than the patient has received previously [85], always assuming that a resistant clone has been selected. An option unique to VAP is the addition of aerosolized antibiotics [88, 89]. No new classes of antipseudomonal antibiotics are anticipated to be available in the near future, so optimizing use of the present antibiotics remains critical.

A novel approach to *P. aeruginosa* infections may be to attack the structure of the bacterial biofilm. Although macrolides possess virtually no antipseudomonal activity per se, they have been shown to inhibit the formation of *P. aeruginosa* biofilms [90]. Possible mechanisms for such responses include inhibition of quorum-sensing system [91] and the immunomodulatory effects of macrolides.

20.7 Prevention and Infection Control Measures

Given its high mortality, prevention of *P. aeruginosa* infection is an important area for emphasis and further investigation. Preventive strategies should be designed specific to the type of ICU and surveillance should be implemented, with the availability of molecular typing to determine the diversity of the strains and identify potential exogenous outbreaks. Screening tests will document the carriage of the pathogen within the intestine and lower respiratory tract. Rectal swabs and nasal or tracheal aspirations remain the best sites for this type of screening [17].

Since *P. aeruginosa* is commonly found in tap water and other environmental sources, strict hand washing and the appropriate use of antiseptics and gloves is critical to avoid the horizontal transmission of MDR *P. aeruginosa* clones [24, 26]. Hand disinfection may be preferable to handwashing between contact with different patients [92]. In addition to hand disinfection, spread of *P. aeruginosa* can be controlled with careful attention to aseptic techniques, cleaning and monitoring all the medical devices involved in patient care, and by appropriate detection and isolation of patients colonized or infected with MDR strains. Compliance to current infection control recommendations plays a vital role in prevention.

The environment should be monitored weekly to prevent tap water from becoming colonized with *P. aeruginosa.* Techniques of water tap disinfection include mechanical cleaning of taps and aerators, chemical disinfection by hyperchlorination, and thermal disinfection [93]. Mechanical cleansing is very expensive and does not prevent retrograde recontamination. A recent study demonstrated good results with point-of-use water filtration, using disposable tap-mounted filters for 7 days [94].

Avoidance of antibiotics may be the best prevention strategy. The overwhelming majority of *P. aeruginosa* pneumonias occur in patients already exposed to antibiotics [95]. Despite its significant virulence and ubiquitous presence, *Pseudomonas* appears to require suppression of the normal host bacterial flora by antibiotics to cause infection. The eradication of normal human bacterial flora, particularly anaerobic flora, facilitates the overgrowth of *P. aeruginosa* [37, 96]. Avoidance of unnecessary antibiotic therapy may not prevent the development of pneumonia, but less antibiotic pressure may prevent *P. aeruginosa* from being the causative agent.

Active immunization with a specific vaccine appears to be too toxic for general use. Several types of vaccines are being tested, but none is currently available. Therefore, the only immunoprophylaxis demonstrated to be of benefit is the use of granulocyte-colony stimulating factor in patients with neutropenia [97].

20.8 Conclusion

Pseudomonas aeruginosa has become a dominant pathogen in most ICUs. Not only is it the most frequent pathogen in mechanically ventilated patients but mortality rates remain unacceptably high. Widespread use of broad-spectrum antimicrobials has resulted in the emergence of MDR *P. aeruginosa* strains. New resistance mechanisms are being continuously identified while few new antibacterial agents are being developed, leaving a limited number of therapeutic options available. The complex epidemiology of these MDR strains needs to be further studied in order to design measures to control their spread. Optimal management of infections with MDR strains of *P. aeruginosa* requires knowledge of local epidemiology.

Endemic infections occur with a continuous and predictable frequency, mainly from an endogenous source. *P. aeruginosa* outbreaks have been linked to contaminated environmental sources. Strains from these sources then contaminate the hands of healthcare workers and are transmitted from patient to patient. Surveillance cultures may be used in combination with molecular typing techniques to evaluate the endemicity and cross-transmission rates of *P. aeruginosa* in order to improve the targeting of preventive strategies.

Prevention and control of *P. aeruginosa* colonization and infection in ICU patients requires attention to multiple facets of pathogenesis: prudent antimicrobial use, compliance by healthcare workers with hand hygiene recommendations, identification and isolation of colonized/infected patients, prompt detection and management of outbreaks, maintenance of a clean ICU environment and appropriate cleaning and disinfection of medical equipment. Further research to further define aspects of the pathogenesis of this microorganism and to determine more effective treatments and prevention strategies is clearly needed.

References

1. Hoiby N (1974) *Pseudomonas aeruginosa* infection in cystic fibrosis. Relationship between mucoid strains of *Pseudomonas aeruginosa* and the humoral immune response. Acta Pathol Microbiol Scand [B] Microbiol Immunol 82(4): 551–558
2. Morrison AJ Jr, Wenzel RP (1984) Epidemiology of infections due to *Pseudomonas aeruginosa.* Rev Infect Dis 6(Suppl 3):S627–642
3. Jarvis WR, Martone WJ (1992) Predominant pathogens in hospital infections. J Antimicrob Chemother 29(Suppl A): 19–24
4. Richards MJ, Edwards JR, Culver DH, et al. (1999) Nosocomial infections in medical intensive care units in the United States. National Nosocomial Infections Surveillance System. Crit Care Med 27(5):887–892
5. Spencer RC (1996) Predominant pathogens found in the Eu-

ropean Prevalence of Infection in Intensive Care Study. Eur J Clin Microbiol Infect Dis 15(4):281 – 285

6. Gales AC, Jones RN, Turnidge J, et al. (2001) Characterization of *Pseudomonas aeruginosa* isolates: occurrence rates, antimicrobial susceptibility patterns, and molecular typing in the global SENTRY Antimicrobial Surveillance Program, 1997 – 1999. Clin Infect Dis 32(Suppl 2):S146 – 155
7. Cross AS (1985) Evolving epidemiology of *Pseudomonas aeruginosa* infections. Eur J Clin Microbiol 4(2):156 – 159
8. Glupczynski Y, Delmee M, Goossens H, et al. (2001) Distribution and prevalence of antimicrobial resistance among gram-negative isolates in intensive care units (ICU) in Belgian hospitals between 1996 and 1999. Acta Clin Belg 56(5):297 – 306
9. Fridkin SK, Gaynes RP (1999) Antimicrobial resistance in intensive care units. Clin Chest Med 20(2):303 – 316, viii
10. Trouillet JL, Chastre J, Vuagnat A, et al. (1998) Ventilator-associated pneumonia caused by potentially drug-resistant bacteria. Am J Respir Crit Care Med 157(2):531 – 539
11. Trouillet JL, Vuagnat A, Combes A, et al. (2002) *Pseudomonas aeruginosa* ventilator-associated pneumonia: comparison of episodes due to piperacillin-resistant versus piperacillin-susceptible organisms. Clin Infect Dis 34(8):1047 – 1054
12. Vincent JL (2000) Microbial resistance: lessons from the EPIC study. European Prevalence of Infection. Intensive Care Med 26(Suppl 1):S3 – 8
13. Vincent JL, Bihari DJ, Suter PM, et al. (1995) The prevalence of nosocomial infection in intensive care units in Europe. Results of the European Prevalence of Infection in Intensive Care (EPIC) Study. EPIC International Advisory Committee. JAMA 274(8):639 – 644
14. Fagon JY, Chastre J, Vuagnat A, et al. (1996) Nosocomial pneumonia and mortality among patients in intensive care units. JAMA 275(11):866 – 869
15. Kominos SD, Copeland CE, Grosiak B, et al. (1972) Introduction of *Pseudomonas aeruginosa* into a hospital via vegetables. Appl Microbiol 24(4):567 – 570
16. Shooter RA, Cooke EM, Faiers MC, et al. (1971) Isolation of *Escherichia coli, Pseudomonas aeruginosa*, and *Klebsiella* from food in hospitals, canteens, and schools. Lancet 2(7721):390 – 392
17. Bertrand X, Thouverez M, Talon D, et al. (2001) Endemicity, molecular diversity and colonisation routes of *Pseudomonas aeruginosa* in intensive care units. Intensive Care Med 27(8):1263 – 1268
18. Blanc DS, Petignat C, Janin B, et al. (1998) Frequency and molecular diversity of *Pseudomonas aeruginosa* upon admission and during hospitalization: a prospective epidemiologic study. Clin Microbiol Infect 4(5):242 – 247
19. Struelens MJ, Rost F, Deplano A, et al. (1993) *Pseudomonas aeruginosa* and Enterobacteriaceae bacteremia after biliary endoscopy: an outbreak investigation using DNA macrorestriction analysis. Am J Med 95(5):489 – 498
20. Trautmann M, Michalsky T, Wiedeck H, et al. (2001) Tap water colonization with *Pseudomonas aeruginosa* in a surgical intensive care unit (ICU) and relation to *Pseudomonas* infections of ICU patients. Infect Control Hosp Epidemiol 22(1):49 – 52
21. Blanc DS, Nahimana I, Petignat C, et al. (2004) Faucets as a reservoir of endemic *Pseudomonas aeruginosa* colonization/infections in intensive care units. Intensive Care Med 30(10):1964 – 1968
22. Foca M, Jacob K, Whittier S, et al. (2000) Endemic *Pseudomonas aeruginosa* infection in a neonatal intensive care unit. N Engl J Med 343(10):695 – 700
23. McNeil SA, Nordstrom-Lerner L, Malani PN, et al. (2001) Outbreak of sternal surgical site infections due to *Pseudomonas aeruginosa* traced to a scrub nurse with onychomycosis. Clin Infect Dis 33(3):317 – 323
24. Moolenaar RL, Crutcher JM, San Joaquin VH, et al. (2000) A prolonged outbreak of *Pseudomonas aeruginosa* in a neonatal intensive care unit: did staff fingernails play a role in disease transmission? Infect Control Hosp Epidemiol 21(2):80 – 85
25. Wenzel RP (1994) Healthcare workers and the incidence of nosocomial infection: can treatment of one influence the other? – a brief review. J Chemother 6(Suppl 4):33 – 37
26. Widmer AF, Wenzel RP, Trilla A, et al. (1993) Outbreak of *Pseudomonas aeruginosa* infections in a surgical intensive care unit: probable transmission via hands of a health care worker. Clin Infect Dis 16(3):372 – 376
27. Pollack M, Pier GB, Prescott RK (1984) Immunization with *Pseudomonas aeruginosa* high-molecular-weight polysaccharides prevents death from *Pseudomonas* burn infections in mice. Infect Immun 43(2):759 – 760
28. Lowbury EJ, Thom BT, Lilly HA, et al. (1970) Sources of infection with *Pseudomonas aeruginosa* in patients with tracheostomy. J Med Microbiol 3(1):39 – 56
29. Woods DE, Schaffer MS, Rabin HR, et al. (1986) Phenotypic comparison of *Pseudomonas aeruginosa* strains isolated from a variety of clinical sites. J Clin Microbiol 24(2): 260 – 264
30. Grundmann H, Schneider C, Hartung D, et al. (1995) Discriminatory power of three DNA-based typing techniques for *Pseudomonas aeruginosa.* J Clin Microbiol 33(3):528 – 534
31. Thuong M, Arvaniti K, Ruimy R, et al. (2003) Epidemiology of *Pseudomonas aeruginosa* and risk factors for carriage acquisition in an intensive care unit. J Hosp Infect 53(4):274 – 282
32. Speijer H, Savelkoul PH, Bonten MJ, et al. (1999) Application of different genotyping methods for *Pseudomonas aeruginosa* in a setting of endemicity in an intensive care unit. J Clin Microbiol 37(11):3654 – 3661
33. Tyler KD, Wang G, Tyler SD, et al. (1997) Factors affecting reliability and reproducibility of amplification-based DNA fingerprinting of representative bacterial pathogens. J Clin Microbiol 35(2):339 – 346
34. Tenover FC, Arbeit RD, Goering RV, et al. (1995) Interpreting chromosomal DNA restriction patterns produced by pulsed-field gel electrophoresis: criteria for bacterial strain typing. J Clin Microbiol 33(9):2233 – 2239
35. Bergmans DC, Bonten MJ, van Tiel FH, et al. (1998) Cross-colonisation with *Pseudomonas aeruginosa* of patients in an intensive care unit. Thorax 53(12):1053 – 1058
36. Berthelot P, Grattard F, Mahul P, et al. (2001) Prospective study of nosocomial colonization and infection due to *Pseudomonas aeruginosa* in mechanically ventilated patients. Intensive Care Med 27(3):503 – 512
37. Bonten MJ, Bergmans DC, Speijer H, et al. (1999) Characteristics of polyclonal endemicity of *Pseudomonas aeruginosa* colonization in intensive care units. Implications for infection control. Am J Respir Crit Care Med 160(4): 1212 – 1219
38. Richards MJ, Edwards JR, Culver DH, et al. (2000) Nosocomial infections in combined medical-surgical intensive care units in the United States. Infect Control Hosp Epidemiol 21(8):510 – 515
39. Panceri ML, Vegni FE, Goglio A, et al. (2004) Aetiology and prognosis of bacteraemia in Italy. Epidemiol Infect 132(4):647 – 654
40. Wisplinghoff H, Bischoff T, Tallent SM, et al. (2004) Nosocomial bloodstream infections in US hospitals: analysis of 24,179 cases from a prospective nationwide surveillance study. Clin Infect Dis 39(3):309 – 317

41. Osmon S, Ward S, Fraser VJ, et al. (2004) Hospital mortality for patients with bacteremia due to *Staphylococcus aureus* or *Pseudomonas aeruginosa*. Chest 125(2):607–616
42. Pawar M, Mehta Y, Khurana P, et al. (2003) Ventilator-associated pneumonia: Incidence, risk factors, outcome, and microbiology. J Cardiothorac Vasc Anesth 17(1):22–28
43. Talon D, Mulin B, Rouget C, et al. (1998) Risks and routes for ventilator-associated pneumonia with *Pseudomonas aeruginosa*. Am J Respir Crit Care Med 157:978–984
44. Baddour LM, Hicks DV, Tayidi MM, et al. (1995) Risk factor assessment for the acquisition of fluoroquinolone-resistant isolates of *Pseudomonas aeruginosa* in a community-based hospital. Microb Drug Resist 1(3):219–222
45. Carmeli Y, Troillet N, Eliopoulos GM, et al. (1999) Emergence of antibiotic-resistant *Pseudomonas aeruginosa*: comparison of risks associated with different antipseudomonal agents. Antimicrob Agents Chemother 43(6):1379–1382
46. Talon D, Capellier G, Boillot A, et al (1995) Use of pulsed-field gel electrophoresis as an epidemiologic tool during an outbreak of *Pseudomonas aeruginosa* lung infections in an intensive care unit. Intensive Care Med 21(12):996–1002
47. Bert F, Maubec E, Bruneau B, et al. (1998) Multi-resistant *Pseudomonas aeruginosa* outbreak associated with contaminated tap water in a neurosurgery intensive care unit. J Hosp Infect 39(1):53–62
48. Cobben NA, Drent M, Jonkers M, et al. (1996) Outbreak of severe *Pseudomonas aeruginosa* respiratory infections due to contaminated nebulizers. J Hosp Infect 33(1):63–70
49. Rutala WA, Weber DJ (1997) Water as a reservoir of nosocomial pathogens. Infect Control Hosp Epidemiol 18(9):609–616
50. Gruner E, Kropec A, Huebner J, et al. (1993) Ribotyping of *Pseudomonas aeruginosa* strains isolated from surgical intensive care patients. J Infect Dis 167(5):1216–1220
51. Kropec A, Huebner J, Riffel M, et al. (1993) Exogenous or endogenous reservoirs of nosocomial *Pseudomonas aeruginosa* and *Staphylococcus aureus* infections in a surgical intensive care unit. Intensive Care Med 19(3):161–165
52. Rello J, Jubert P, Valles J, et al. (1996) Evaluation of outcome for intubated patients with pneumonia due to *Pseudomonas aeruginosa*. Clin Infect Dis 23(5):973–978
53. National Nosocomial Infections Surveillance (NNIS) System Report, Data Summary from January 1992-June 2001 (August 2001). Am J Infect Control 29(6):404–421
54. Richards MJ, Edwards JR, Culver DH, et al. (1999) Nosocomial infections in pediatric intensive care units in the United States. National Nosocomial Infections Surveillance System. Pediatrics 103(4):39
55. Blanc DS, Parret T, Janin B, et al. (1997) Nosocomial infections and pseudoinfections from contaminated bronchoscopes: two-year follow up using molecular markers. Infect Control Hosp Epidemiol 18(2):134–136
56. Doring G, Horz M, Ortelt J, et al. (1993) Molecular epidemiology of *Pseudomonas aeruginosa* in an intensive care unit. Epidemiol Infect 110(3):427–436
57. Kollef MH (1999) The prevention of ventilator-associated pneumonia. N Engl J Med 340(8):627–634
58. Richard P, Le Floch R, Chamoux C, et al. (1994) *Pseudomonas aeruginosa* outbreak in a burn unit: role of antimicrobials in the emergence of multiply resistant strains. J Infect Dis 170(2):377–383
59. Tredget EE, Shankowsky HA, Joffe AM, et al. (1992) Epidemiology of infections with *Pseudomonas aeruginosa* in burn patients: the role of hydrotherapy. Clin Infect Dis 15(6):941–949
60. Pellegrino FL, Teixeira LM, Carvalho MD Mda G, et al. (2002) Occurrence of a multidrug-resistant *Pseudomonas aeruginosa* clone in different hospitals in Rio de Janeiro, Brazil. J Clin Microbiol 40(7):2420–2424
61. Girlich D, Poirel L, Leelaporn A, et al. (2001) Molecular epidemiology of the integron-located VEB-1 extended-spectrum beta-lactamase in nosocomial enterobacterial isolates in Bangkok, Thailand. J Clin Microbiol 39(1):175–182
62. Hocquet D, Bertrand X, Kholer T, et al. (2003) Genetic and phenotypic variations of a resistant *Pseudomonas aeruginosa* epidemic clone. Antimicrob Agents Chemother 47(6):1887–1894
63. Poirel L, Menuteau O, Agoli N, et al. (2003) Outbreak of extended-spectrum beta-lactamase VEB-1-producing isolates of *Acinetobacter baumannii* in a French hospital. J Clin Microbiol 41(8):3542–3547
64. Poirel L, Naas T, Nicolas D, et al. (2000) Characterization of VIM-2, a carbapenem-hydrolyzing metallo-beta-lactamase and its plasmid- and integron-borne gene from a *Pseudomonas aeruginosa* clinical isolate in France. Antimicrob Agents Chemother 44(4):891–897
65. Poirel L, Weldhagen GF, Naas T, et al. (2001) GES-2, a class A beta-lactamase from *Pseudomonas aeruginosa* with increased hydrolysis of imipenem. Antimicrob Agents Chemother 45(9):2598–2603
66. Poole K (2004) Efflux-mediated multiresistance in Gram-negative bacteria. Clin Microbiol Infect 10(1):12–26
67. Harris AD, Smith D, Johnson JA, et al. (2002) Risk factors for imipenem-resistant *Pseudomonas aeruginosa* among hospitalized patients. Clin Infect Dis 34(3):340–345
68. Carmeli Y, Troillet N, Karchmer AW, et al. (1999) Health and economic outcomes of antibiotic resistance in *Pseudomonas aeruginosa*. Arch Intern Med 159(10):1127–1132
69. Dever LA, Dermody TS (1991) Mechanisms of bacterial resistance to antibiotics. Arch Intern Med 151(5):886–895
70. Livermore DM (2002) Multiple mechanisms of antimicrobial resistance in *Pseudomonas aeruginosa*: our worst nightmare? Clin Infect Dis 34(5):634–640
71. Boles BR, Thoendel M, Singh PK (2004) Self-generated diversity produces "insurance effects" in biofilm communities. Proc Natl Acad Sci USA 101(47):16630–16635
72. Schulert GS, Feltman H, Rabin SD, et al. (2003) Secretion of the toxin ExoU is a marker for highly virulent *Pseudomonas aeruginosa* isolates obtained from patients with hospital-acquired pneumonia. J Infect Dis 188(11):1695–1706
73. Hauser AR, Cobb E, Bodi M, et al. (2002) Type III protein secretion is associated with poor clinical outcomes in patients with ventilator-associated pneumonia caused by *Pseudomonas aeruginosa*. Crit Care Med 30(3):521–528
74. Saiman L, Ishimoto K, Lory S, et al. (1990) The effect of piliation and exoproduct expression on the adherence of *Pseudomonas aeruginosa* to respiratory epithelial monolayers. J Infect Dis 161(3):541–548
75. Woods DE, Straus DC, Johanson WG Jr, et al. (1981) Role of salivary protease activity in adherence of gram-negative bacilli to mammalian buccal epithelial cells in vivo. J Clin Invest 68(6):1435–1440
76. Cosson P, Zulianello L, Join-Lambert O, et al. (2002) *Pseudomonas aeruginosa* virulence analyzed in a *Dictyostelium discoideum* host system. J Bacteriol 184(11):3027–3033
77. Pukatzki S, Kessin RH, Mekalanos JJ (2002) The human pathogen *Pseudomonas aeruginosa* utilizes conserved virulence pathways to infect the social amoeba *Dictyostelium discoideum*. Proc Natl Acad Sci USA 99(5):3159–3164
78. Fenner L, Richet H, Raoult D, et al. (2006) Are clinical isolates of *Pseudomonas aeruginosa* more virulent than hospital environmental isolates in amebal co-culture test?. Crit Care Med 34(3):823–828
79. Bodey GP, Jadeja L, Elting, L (1985) *Pseudomonas* bacter-

emia. Retrospective analysis of 410 episodes. Arch Intern Med 145(9):1621–1629
80. Siegman-Igra Y, Ravona R, Primerman H, et al. (1998) *Pseudomonas aeruginosa* bacteremia: an analysis of 123 episodes, with particular emphasis on the effect of antibiotic therapy. Int J Infect Dis 2(4):211–215
81. Rello J, Rue M, Jubert P, et al. (1997) Survival in patients with nosocomial pneumonia: impact of the severity of illness and the etiologic agent. Crit Care Med 25(11): 1862–1867
82. Rello J, Ausina V, Ricart M, et al. (1994) Risk factors for infection by *Pseudomonas aeruginosa* in patients with ventilator-associated pneumonia. Intensive Care Med 20(3): 193–198
83. Itokazu GS, Quinn JP, Bell-Dixon C, et al. (1996) Antimicrobial resistance rates among aerobic gram-negative bacilli recovered from patients in intensive care units: evaluation of a national postmarketing surveillance program. Clin Infect Dis 23(4):779–784
84. Troillet N, Samore MH, Carmeli Y (1997) Imipenem-resistant *Pseudomonas aeruginosa*: risk factors and antibiotic susceptibility patterns. Clin Infect Dis 25(5):1094–1098
85. Brun-Buisson C, Sollet JP, Schweich H, et al. (1998) Treatment of ventilator-associated pneumonia with piperacillin-tazobactam/amikacin versus ceftazidime/amikacin: a multicenter, randomized controlled trial. VAP Study Group. Clin Infect Dis 26(2):346–354
86. Fink MP, Snydman DR, Niederman MS, et al. (1994) Treatment of severe pneumonia in hospitalized patients: results of a multicenter, randomized, double-blind trial comparing intravenous ciprofloxacin with imipenem-cilastatin. The Severe Pneumonia Study Group. Antimicrob Agents Chemother 38(3):547–557
87. Luyt CE, Guerin V, Combes A, et al. (2005) Procalcitonin kinetics as a prognostic marker of ventilator-associated pneumonia. Am J Respir Crit Care Med 171(1):48–53
88. Ibrahim EH, Ward S, Sherman G, et al. (2001) Experience with a clinical guideline for the treatment of ventilator-associated pneumonia. Crit Care Med 29(6):1109–1115
89. Jackson BR, Thomas A, Caroll KC, et al. (2005) Use of strain typing data to estimate bacterial transmission rates in healthcare settings. Infect Control Hosp Epidemiol 26(7):638–645
90. Nagata T, Mukae H, Kadota J, et al. (2004) Effect of erythromycin on chronic respiratory infection caused by *Pseudomonas aeruginosa* with biofilm formation in an experimental murine model. Antimicrob Agents Chemother 48(6):2251–2259
91. Imamura Y, Yanagihara K, Mizuta Y, et al. (2004) Azithromycin inhibits MUC5AC production induced by the *Pseudomonas aeruginosa* autoinducer N-(3-oxododecanoyl) homoserine lactone in NCI-H292 cells. Antimicrob Agents Chemother 48(9):3457–3461
92. Pittet D, Hugonnet S, Harbarth S, et al. (2000) Effectiveness of a hospital-wide programme to improve compliance with hand hygiene. Infection Control Programme. Lancet 356(9238):1307–1312
93. Schoenen D, Stoeck B, Hienzsch S, et al. (1986) Decontamination of drinking water taps colonized with *Pseudomonas aeruginosa*. Zentralbl Bakteriol Mikrobiol Hyg[B] 182(5–6): 551–557
94. Trautmann M, Royer H, Helm E, et al. (2004) *Pseudomonas aeruginosa:* new insights into transmission pathways between hospital water and patients. Filtration 1(Suppl 1): 63–70
95. Rello J, Ausina V, Ricart M, et al. (1993) Impact of previous antimicrobial therapy on the etiology and outcome of ventilator-associated pneumonia. Chest 104(4):1230–1235
96. Vollaard EJ, Clasener HA (1994) Colonization resistance. Antimicrob Agents Chemother 38(3):409–414
97. Crawford J, Ozer H, Stoller R, et al. (1991) Reduction by granulocyte colony-stimulating factor of fever and neutropenia induced by chemotherapy in patients with small-cell lung cancer. N Engl J Med 325(3):164–170

21 How To Control MRSA Spread in the Intensive Care Unit

J.-R. Zahar, J.-F. Timsit

21.1 Epidemiology of MRSA

Staphylococcus aureus is a major human pathogen, responsible for a wide range of infections, from mild skin infections to severe wound infections and bacteremia. Since the introduction of methicillin in 1959, for the treatment of infections caused by penicillin-resistant *S. aureus*, strains of *S. aureus* resistant to methicillin have emerged. Methicillin-resistant *S. aureus* (MRSA) has evolved from methicillin-sensitive *S. aureus* (MSSA) by the acquisition of a large genetic element known as the staphylococcal cassette chromosome mec (*SCCmec*). *SCCmec* carries the *mec* gene complex and also various resistance genes against non-β-lactam antibiotics.

Usually, infections due to MRSA are acquired in hospitals, long-term care facilities or similar settings, and these strains appear to be generally resistant to multiple antibiotics and genetically closely related [1, 2].

21.1.1 Hospital and ICU Epidemiology

The spread of MRSA has been reported worldwide, with a highly variable prevalence according to the type of clinical ward (e.g., intensive care units versus outpatient departments) and the geographic area. In the US, the rate of infections due to MRSA in intensive care units (ICUs) increased from 35.9% in 1992 to 64.4% in 2003 [3]. In Europe, the overall prevalence of MRSA increased between 1999 and 2004 from 16% to 24% ($p<0.0001$) [4]. A recent survey of 3,051 *S. aureus* isolates from 25 university hospitals in 15 European countries confirmed that MRSA strains are more prevalent in southern Europe than in northern Europe, as the highest prevalence was seen in Portugal (54%) and Italy (43–58%), whereas the lowest prevalence was observed in Switzerland and the Netherlands (2%) [5]. In France, 3.7% of ICU patients have had at least one clinical sample positive with MRSA [6]. Globally, MRSA isolates accounted for 25% of all *S. aureus* isolates, and 38% of the ones from ICUs. The prevalence of methicillin resistance was the highest among *S. aureus* strains responsible for nosocomial pneumonia (34%); it was 24% among blood isolates, and the lowest among isolates associated with skin infections (22%).

21.1.2 Spread Resistance: New Features

21.1.2.1 *Emergence of Community-Acquired MRSA Strains*

Data from the Sentry Antimicrobial Surveillance Program showed an increase in methicillin resistance, not only among nosocomial *S. aureus* strains, but also among community strains [7]. Some have argued that, because of the dramatically increasing prevalence of MRSA in the hospital, the parallel epidemic in the community is attributable to individuals with MRSA from healthcare facilities and returning to the community [8]. However, findings from epidemiological and molecular typing studies suggested that community-acquired MRSA (CA-MRSA) strains are distinct from hospital-acquired MRSA (HA-MRSA). CA-MRSA have been isolated mostly from skin and soft tissue infections, and in community-dwelling patients without established risk factors for the acquisition of MRSA [9]. These CA-MRSA isolates exhibited a different chromosomal cassette *mec* element, SCCmec type IV, and have a different distribution of antibiotic resistance genes and of toxin genes [10]. The prevalence rates of CA-MRSA vary widely among studies. The pooled prevalence of CA-MRSA among MRSA isolates from hospitalized patients was 30.2% in 27 retrospective studies and 37.3% in five prospective studies, and only 0.2% among community members without healthcare contacts [9].

21.1.2.2 *Resistance to Glycopeptides*

There has been increasing concern about the possible emergence of vancomycin-resistant *S. aureus* (VRSA) strains. The concentration of vancomycin required to inhibit most strains of *S. aureus* is between 0.5 and 2 mg/l. *S. aureus* isolates with vancomycin MICs of 8–16 mg/l are currently classified as vancomycin-intermediate (VISA), and isolates with vancomycin MICs

≥32 mg/l are classified as vancomycin resistant (VRSA). Of note, the mechanisms of resistance are different. In VISA strains, cell wall is thickened by alteration of its biosynthesis, hindering glycopeptide reaching its target. In VRSA strains, the glycopeptide target itself is altered [11]. The glycopeptides – notably vancomycin – have traditionally been the mainstay of treatment of MRSA, but overuse of this antibiotic has led to the emergence of VISA and VRSA. In 1996 the world's first documented infection due to *S. aureus* with intermediate resistance to glycopeptides (GISA) was diagnosed in Japan [12], and shortly after reports from the US [13] and France [14] published cases of infections with GISA. To date only isolated cases due to VRSA isolates have been reported. The increase in the use of vancomycin to treat MRSA will increase the vancomycin selective pressure, which in turn may lead to more strains of GISA.

21.2 From Carriage to Infection

21.2.1 Risk Factors for Carriage and Infection

Humans are a natural reservoir of *S. aureus*. Both methicillin-sensitive and methicillin-resistant isolates can be persistent colonizers [15]. Ten to 20% of healthy adults are persistently colonized with *S. aureus*, and therefore are at increased risk from staphylococcal infections. Patient conditions associated with a higher risk of staphylococcal colonization are listed in Table 21.1. As ICU patients seem to be exposed simultaneously to several risk factors, they are especially prone to becoming *S. aureus* carriers.

Table 21.1. Risk factors for methicillin-resistant *Staphylococcus aureus* carriage

Risk factors for *S. aureus* carriage
Intravenous drug use
Chronic medical illness
Type I diabetes mellitus
Patients undergoing hemodialysis
Impaired immune function
AIDS
Quantitative defect in leukocyte function
Qualitative defect in leukocyte function
Risk factors for methicillin-resistant *S. aureus* carriage
Age >60 years
Previous colonization
Exposure to a patient known to be colonized or infected with MRSA
History of stay in an ICU during the last 5 years
History of surgery during the last 5 years
Prolonged hospital stay (21 days or longer)
Residence in a skilled nursing facility
Transfer from an institution with a high prevalence of MRSA
Presence of open skin lesions
Antimicrobial therapy within the last year
Surgery within the last year
Central venous catheter
Chronically poor health status

Adapted from [15]

Of note, the MRSA cross-colonization could be avoided when the overall rate of MRSA carriers is rather low. A multivariate analysis demonstrated that the colonization pressure (defined as the number of MRSA-carrier patient-days/total number of patient-days) was the only independent predictive factor for MRSA acquisition (P=0.0002) [16]. The risk of acquisition of MRSA was approximately fivefold times higher with a colonization pressure above 30% than when the colonization pressure was less than 10% [relative risk, 4.9; 95% confidence interval (95% CI), 1.2–19.9; P<0.0001]. In fact, the most important risk factor for developing an MRSA infection is MRSA carriage [17]. Workload and understaffing are also associated with MRSA infection [18].

To a lesser extent, antibiotic administration increased the risk of MRSA colonization and infection in several studies [19]. Comparison of patients colonized with MSSA and MRSA reveals that the number of antibiotics received and the duration of therapy are statistically associated with an increased risk of MRSA acquisition and infection. Although antibiotic pressure is not able to select methicillin resistance in *S. aureus* strains, many epidemiological studies suggest that MRSA is more prevalent when antimicrobials, especially the fluoroquinolones and first generation cephalosporins, are frequently used [19, 20].

21.2.2 Clinical Consequences of Infection

Infections with antibiotic-resistant organisms are thought to result in higher morbidity and mortality. However, conflicting results have been obtained with regard to the impact of methicillin resistance on outcome. A recent meta-analysis concluded that MRSA bacteremia is associated with a significantly higher mortality rate than MSSA bacteremia [21]. Indeed when data from all studies were pooled, a significant increase in mortality was associated with MRSA bacteremia as opposed to MSSA bacteremia. Recently, Combes et al. [22], and our group [23], conducted studies to analyze impact of the methicillin resistance on outcome of *S. aureus* ventilator-associated pneumonia. In these two studies and after controlling for clinical and physiologic heterogeneity between MRSA and MSSA infections, methicillin resistance did not significantly affect the 28-day mortality of patients. In vitro studies have not detected differences in virulence between MRSA and MSSA. This suggests that the discrepancies may stem from confounding factors related to differences in the populations such as duration of stay in the ICU at the time of infection, performance of invasive procedures, severity of disease at ICU admission or treatment adequacy between patients infected with MRSA and those infected with MSSA. Patients with MRSA seem to be sicker and older and will have a higher mortality because of their underlying illness.

The most important finding is that MRSA infections lead to an important increase in the use of vancomycin [17] which, in turn, increases the risk of other microorganisms such as VISA and vancomycin-resistant enterococci.

21.3 How To Control MRSA in the ICU

ICUs are particularly likely to receive patients infected or colonized with MRSA. Several studies showed that 8–10% of patients had MRSA at ICU admission [24]. These patients can form a reservoir for subsequent dissemination in the ICU unless the organism is identified through routine screening at admission and early isolation precautions are taken. Effective MRSA control has been achieved by implementing stringent infection control policies of MRSA outbreaks [25, 26]. Recent recommendations for MRSA control include two key components: identification of the MRSA reservoir using clinical and screening cultures, and contact precautions for MRSA-positive patients [27]. However, the exact modalities of the procedures to be applied then have to be adjusted to local constraints.

21.3.1 Should We Screen Everybody?

In an endemic setting, screening for MRSA on admission allows the imported cases to be identified. Identifying colonized patients early through screening is important to enable the implementation of isolation and infection control. Screening patients on admission to the ICU is recommended to establish whether the patients are colonized with MRSA, and then weekly or more frequently thereafter to identify and monitor carriage.

Recently, Lucet et al. [28] conducted a multicenter prospective study including 14 French ICUs for 6 months. Among the 2,347 admissions with MRSA screening, 7% were positive for MRSA, of whom 54.3% were detected through screening only. Carriage was detected by nasal swabs in 78% of the MRSA-positive admissions, and by nasal and skin swabs in 92%. Clinical specimens detected only 18.5% of MRSA-positive admissions. Factors associated with MRSA carriage in the multivariate analysis were age greater than 60 years, prolonged hospital stay in transferred patients, history of hospitalization or surgery, and presence of open skin lesions in directly admitted patients. However, 13% of the MRSA carriers among the transferred patients had none of the identified risk factors for MRSA carriage. Therefore, limiting screening at admission to patients with at least one risk factor would have included 70.4% of transferred patients and identified 86.8% of MRSA carriers. Limiting it to patients with at least two risk factors would have included 15.7% of transferred patients and identified 43.4% of MRSA carriers. Of the 1,443 directly admitted patients, limiting screening at admission to patients with at least one risk factor would have identified 88.4% of the MRSA carriers, and limiting it to the patients with at least two risk factors would have identified 55.8% of the MRSA carriers. The cost-benefit analysis concluded that the cost of routine MRSA screening and preventive isolation was lower than the cost of treating the MRSA infections prevented by this strategy. The sensitivity analysis indicated that universal screening and preventive isolation saved money when the prevalence of MRSA carriage varied from 2% to 20% at ICU admission. Based on similarly identified risk factors for newly detected MRSA carriage at ICU admission, a risk score was recently compiled [29]. Based on the analysis of 1,006 patients included in a case-controlled study, the probability of MRSA carriage was 8% for patients with a low risk score, as opposed to 19% for patients with an intermediate score and 46% for patients with a high score. Therefore, applying this risk score was recommended to achieve a more effective MRSA control strategy.

However, the identification of previously unknown MRSAs at ICU admission takes 2–3 days when using conventional techniques. In Geneva University Hospital, the rapid diagnostic tests such as the quick multiplex immunocapture quantitative PCR have been recently shown to reduce dramatically the delay of notification (which decreased from 87 to 21 h in the surgical ICU and from 106 to 23 h in the medical ICU), and the number of preemptive isolation days [30].

21.3.2 Hand Hygiene

The most important mode of transmission of MRSA within institutions appears to be poor hand hygiene. Once introduced into a hospital, MRSA can be spread to a large silent reservoir of colonized patients. By the time serious infections such as bacteremia draw attention to the problem, asymptomatic colonization will typically be widespread and contamination of the environment may be extensive. Hand hygiene is a fundamental aspect of infection control, with several studies showing a decline in nosocomial infection rates when compliance with hand hygiene is enhanced [31]. Despite universal acknowledgement of the pivotal role that hand hygiene plays in reducing nosocomial infection, compliance among healthcare workers remains poor, ranging from 16% to 81% [32]. Pittet et al. studied predictors of non-compliance with hand hygiene in an observational study and found that, in a multivariate analysis, physicians and nursing assistants had lower compliance rates than nurses. Worryingly, compliance was lower in ICUs, during procedures associated with a high risk of contamination and when the activity index was the highest. In a more recent cross-sectional survey of 163 physicians, the same investigators reported that adherence to hand hygiene was associated with awareness of being observed and ready availability of hand rubs [33]. A statistical model showed that the rate of carriage of resistant organisms could be reduced by a third if hand hygiene compliance increased from 40% to 70% [34]. Attempts to improve compliance have included increasing the number of accessible sinks and educating HCWs, but none of these interventions led to a marked and sustained improvement in compliance. Interventions which emphasized targeted education and frequent performance feedback were the most effective. The introduction of alcohol/chlorhexidine hand hygiene solution combined with education and motivation programs can improve hand hygiene compliance and reduce total nosocomial infections. The main reasons raised for not adhering to the recommendation to hand hygiene was the lack of time and workload in the ICU [35]. The rapid efficacy of alcohol-based solutions compared with handwashing, even with an antiseptic agent, is a major argument supporting their use in clinical practice [36]. Handrubbing also achieved a higher reduction in bacterial contamination, suggesting higher efficacy. Moreover handrubbing remained effective after a series of applications. A number of clinical studies have evaluated handwashing with plain soap versus handrubbing in everyday practice, and all showed positive results in favor of handrubbing. One randomized clinical study compared handwashing with an antiseptic soap versus handrubbing with an alcohol-based solution with the assessment of skin tolerance as the primary objective. Handrubbing was better tolerated than handwashing and achieved a comparable reduction in bacterial contamination [37].

21.3.3 Environmental Contamination

Beside the hands of HCWs as the main source of transmission for MRSA, and colonized or infected patients as the main reservoirs, the role of the environment should not be neglected. Staphylococci are able to survive for at least 1 day on five common hospital materials, with some still viable after 56 and 90 days on polyester and polyethylene plastic, respectively. Boyce et al. demonstrated that the environmental contamination of a patient's room was sufficient to contaminate the gloves of healthcare workers even without direct patient contact [38]. In a recent study, Sexton et al. assessed the degree of environmental contamination in isolation rooms with patients colonized or infected with MRSA [39]. Over half of the surface samples, including those taken from beds and mattresses, were positive, and these strains were confirmed by PFGE fingerprinting as similar to those isolated from patients.

21.3.4 Isolation and Cohorting

Most transmission of MRSA from patient to patient is thought to be mediated by transiently colonized healthcare workers (HCWs), although airborne dispersal and transmission through contacts with contaminated surfaces may also be important. Isolation measures for patients are intended to interrupt such transmission [40].

The most intensive forms of isolating patients are isolation wards (designated for the treatment of known or suspected carriers of MRSA) and nurse cohorting (the physical segregation of MRSA patients in one part of a ward, with nursing by designated staff who care exclusively for these patients). Other isolation measures include the use of single bedded rooms, cohorts of patients on general wards (without designated nursing staff), and barrier precautions (use of aprons or gowns, gloves, and, in some cases, masks by HCWs as the only physical barrier to transmission). Such control measures may place substantial burdens on hospital resources, and the value of their continued use has been questioned. National guidelines for preventing the spread of MRSA recommend mainly contact precautions and isolation of infected or colonized patients in a single room or cohort [41–43]. Although several reports have suggested a benefit from single-room isolation or cohort nursing, a systematic review pointed out the lack of well-designed studies allowing the assessment of the role of isolation measures alone. Studies were predominantly retrospective, lacking in proper statistical analysis, and generally undertaken in response to outbreaks rather than within intensive-care units of high endemicity [44]. Moreover, isolation was generally introduced within a package of measures, variably including surveillance, improved hand-washing compliance, reduction in ward activity, and addition of other treatments [45]. Despite conflicting data there is evidence that interventions including isolation can achieve major reductions in MRSA, even when endemic [40, 46, 47]. However, isolation and cohorting had to be part of a broader program to be successful. Single rooms simplify adherence to infection control guidelines by concentrating all activities on the one patient room and avoiding accidental reuse of contaminated medical devices for another patient. But such isolation of critically ill patients presents some risks. Despite higher illness severity scores, isolated patients are visited half as often as non-isolated patients (5.3 vs. 10.9 visits per hour), and are twice as likely to have adverse events (31 vs. 15 events per 1,000 patient-days) [48–50].

Lucet et al. [51], in a prospective observational cohort over 6 years assessing the effectiveness of screening strategy and contact precautions for patients with MRSA in intensive care units, concluded that MRSA control in three ICUs with a high prevalence of MRSA at admission was achieved via multiple interventions including screening, contact precautions, and use of alcohol handrub solution. Indeed, between the two compared periods, acquisition incidence of MRSA decreased from 7 % to 2.8 %. The benefits of active screening programs over a long period are still questionable; however, this is the first demonstration proving the efficacy of such a program. De Lassence et al. [52] described recently the first large outbreak of colonizations and infections with a GISA strain. This strain was associated with a high rate of infection and extensive colonization of environment. Patient isolation and barrier precautions failed when used alone. The termination of the outbreak was achieved only when a stringent policy of restricted admissions, twice daily environmental cleaning, and implementation of hand decontamination with a hydroalcoholic solution were added, associated with an increased patient/nurse ratio.

21.3.5
Eradication: What Should We Think About Mupirocin

From prospective epidemiological studies, nasal colonization with *S. aureus* is a major risk factor for infection, and suppression or eradication of this organism can help to prevent *S. aureus* infections. Many different antimicrobial agents have been used to eradicate MRSA carriage from colonized patients and HCWs. Mupirocin has emerged as the topical antibacterial agent of choice. Numerous open trials involving surgical, hemodialysis and continuous ambulatory peritoneal dialysis patients demonstrated that the use of mupirocin in patients with postoperative nasal colonization with *S. aureus* significantly reduced nosocomial *S. aureus* infections. A recent meta-analysis showed that perioperative intranasal mupirocin decreased the incidence of surgical-site infection when used as prophylaxis in non-general surgery [53]. The cost-effectiveness of this approach is still questionable, as well as the optimal regimens and strategies, and also whether infections due to other species can increase as the rate of *S. aureus* infections declines. Moreover, several investigations of outbreaks have shown that the level of resistance to mupirocin can rapidly increase, and that resistant strains can be spread from patient to patient [54]. The usefulness of mupirocin-based nasal decolonization in ICU remains a matter of debate. A recent study suggested that nasal mupirocin in ICUs can effectively prevent the occurrence of infections due to endogenous MRSA [55]. But this finding stands in contrast to double-blind randomized, placebo-controlled trials that included patients hospitalized in different types of unit [56].

21.4
Conclusion

One aspect of MRSA infections that has still not been clarified in recent years is how vigorously we should try to contain and control MRSA. It is difficult to predict the course of events when MRSA is introduced into a hospital. Rapid spread of the organism throughout the ICU and hospital could occur. Outbreaks seems to be more common following introduction of MRSA into medical or surgical intensive care units. Arguments for implementation of special control measures could be as follows:

1. MRSA can spread rapidly in hospitals and cause substantial morbidity.
2. Once MRSA strains are introduced into a facility they often become endemic and eradication could be very difficult.
3. If MRSA accounts for more than 5 % of clinical isolates, vancomycin use may increase substantially and widespread use of vancomycin increases the risk of emergence of vancomycin resistant organisms.

Despite variable outcomes of MRSA control measures, aggressive infection control measures have been shown to be cost-effective. All these studies and our own experience plead in favor of vigorous advocacy for the screening of patients at admission in the ICU and during their stay, as well as the isolation of MRSA carriers.

Acknowledgements. We thank Docteur Celine Feger for her helpful assistance in preparing the manuscript.

References

1. Agodi A, Campanile F, Basile G, Viglianisi F, Stefani S (1999) Phylogenetic analysis of macrorestriction fragments as a measure of genetic relatedness in *Staphylococcus aureus*: the epidemiological impact of methicillin resistance. Eur J Epidemiol 15:637–642
2. Van Belkum A (2000) Molecular epidemiology of methicillin-resistant *Staphylococcus aureus* strains: state of affairs and tomorrow's possibilities. Microb Drug Resist 6:173–188
3. Klevens RM, Edwards JR, Tenover FC, McDonald LC, Horan T, Gaynes R; National Nosocomial Infections Surveillance

System (2006) Changes in the epidemiology of methicillin-resistant *Staphylococcus aureus* in intensive care units in US hospitals, 1992–2003. Clin Infect Dis 42:389–391
4. The European Antimicrobial Resistance Surveillance System (EARSS). 2004 report. www.earss.rivm.nl
5. Fluit AC, Wielders CL, Verhoef J, Schmitz FJ (2001) Epidemiology and susceptibility of 3,051 *Staphylococcus aureus* isolates from 25 university hospitals participating in the European SENTRY study. J Clin Microbiol 39:3727–3732
6. The Hospital Propore II Study Group (1999) Methicillin-resistant *Staphylcoccus aureus* in French hospitals: a 2 month survey in 43 hospitals, 1995. Infect Control Hosp Epidemiol 20:478–486
7. Diekema DJ, Pfaller MA, Schmitz FJ, Smayevsky J, Bell J, Jones RN, Beach M; SENTRY Participants Group (2001) Survey of infections due to *Staphylococcus* species: frequency of occurrence and antimicrobial susceptibility of isolates collected in the United States, Canada, Latin America, Europe, and the Western Pacific region for the SENTRY Antimicrobial Surveillance Program, 1997–1999. Clin Infect Dis 32 Suppl 2:S114–132
8. Chambers HF (2001) The changing epidemiology of *Staphylococcus aureus*? Emerg Infect Dis 7:178–182
9. Fridkin SK, Hageman JC, Morrison M, Sanza LT, Como-Sabetti K, Jernigan JA, Harriman K, Harrison LH, Lynfield R, Farley MM; Active Bacterial Core Surveillance Program of the Emerging Infections Program Network (2005) Methicillin-resistant *Staphylococcus aureus* disease in three communities. N Engl J Med 352:1436–1444
10. Kluytmans-Vandenbergh MF, Kluytmans JA (2006) Community-acquired methicillin-resistant *Staphylococcus aureus:* current perspectives. Clin Microbiol Infect 12 Suppl 1:9–15
11. Ruef C (2004) Epidemiology and clinical impact of glycopeptide resistance in *Staphylococcus aureus*. Infection 32:315–327
12. Hiramatsu K, Hanaki H, Ino T, Yabuta K, Oguri T, Tenover FC (1997) Methicillin-resistant *Staphylococcus aureus* clinical strain with reduced vancomycin susceptibility. J Antimicrob Chemother 40:135–136
13. Smith TL, Pearson ML, Wilcox KR, Cruz C, Lancaster MV, Robinson-Dunn B, Tenover FC, Zervos MJ, Band JD, White E, Jarvis WR (1999) Emergence of vancomycin resistance in *Staphylococcus aureus*. Glycopeptide-intermediate *Staphylococcus aureus* Working Group. N Engl J Med 340:493–501
14. Cartolano GL, Cheron M, Benabid D, Leneveu M, Boisivon A; Association of Hospital Bacteriologists, Virologists and Hygiene Professionals (2004) Methicillin-resistant *Staphylococcus aureus* (MRSA) with reduced susceptibility to glycopeptides (GISA) in 63 French general hospitals. Clin Microbiol Infect 10:448–451
15. Sanford MD, Widmer AF, Bale MJ, Jones RN, Wenzel RP (1994) Efficient detection and long-term persistence of the carriage of methicillin-resistant *Staphylococcus aureus*. Clin Infect Dis 19:1123–1128
16. Merrer J, Santoli F, Appere de Vecchi C, Tran B, De Jonghe B, Outin H (2000) "Colonization pressure" and risk of acquisition of methicillin-resistant *Staphylococcus aureus* in a medical intensive care unit. Infect Control Hosp Epidemiol 21:718–723
17. Garrouste-Orgeas M, Timsit JF, Kallel H, Ben Ali A, Dumay MF, Paoli B, Misset B, Carlet J (2001) Colonization with methicillin-resistant *Staphylococcus aureus* in ICU patients: morbidity, mortality, and glycopeptide use. Infect Control Hosp Epidemiol 22:687–692
18. Vicca AF (1999) Nursing staff workload as a determinant of methicillin-resistant *Staphylococcus aureus* spread in an adult intensive therapy unit. J Hosp Infect 43:109–113
19. Graffunder EM, Venezia RA (2002) Risk factors associated with nosocomial methicillin-resistant *Staphylococcus aureus* (MRSA) infection including previous use of antimicrobials. J Antimicrob Chemother 49:999–1005
20. Weber SG, Gold HS, Hooper DC, Karchmer AW, Carmeli Y (2003) Fluoroquinolones and the risk for methicillin-resistant *Staphylococcus aureus* in hospitalized patients. Emerg Infect Dis 9:1415–1422
21. Cosgrove SE, Sakoulas G, Perencevich EN, Schwaber MJ, Karchmer AW, Carmeli Y (2003) Comparison of mortality associated with methicillin-resistant and methicillin-susceptible *Staphylococcus aureus* bacteremia: a meta-analysis. Clin Infect Dis 36:53–59
22. Combes A, Luyt CE, Fagon JY, Wollf M, Trouillet JL, Gibert C, Chastre J; PNEUMA Trial Group (2004) Impact of methicillin resistance on outcome of *Staphylococcus aureus* ventilator-associated pneumonia. Am J Respir Crit Care Med 170:786–792
23. Zahar JR, Clec'h C, Tafflet M, Garrouste-Orgeas M, Jamali S, Mourvillier B, De Lassence A, Descorps-Declere A, Adrie C, Costa de Beauregard MA, Azoulay E, Schwebel C, Timsit JF; Outcomerea Study Group (2005) Is methicillin resistance associated with a worse prognosis in *Staphylococcus aureus* ventilator-associated pneumonia? Clin Infect Dis 41:1224–1231
24. Talon D, Rouget C, Cailleaux V, Bailly P, Thouverez M, Barale F, Michel-Briand Y (1995) Nasal carriage of *Staphylococcus aureus* and cross-contamination in a surgical intensive care unit: efficacy of mupirocin ointment. J Hosp Infect 30:39–49
25. Boyce JM, Cookson B, Christiansen K, Hori S, Vuopio-Varkila J, Kocagoz S, Oztop AY, Vandenbroucke-Grauls CM, Harbarth S, Pittet D (2005) Methicillin-resistant *Staphylococcus aureus*. Lancet Infect Dis 5:653–663
26. Vandenbroucke-Grauls CM (1996) Methicillin-resistant *Staphylococcus aureus* control in hospitals: the Dutch experience. Infect Control Hosp Epidemiol 17:512–513
27. Muto CA, Jernigan JA, Ostrowsky BE, Richet HM, Jarvis WR, Boyce JM, Farr BM SHEA (2003) SHEA guidelines for preventing nosocomial transmission of multidrug-resistant strains of *Staphylococcus aureus* and *Enterococcus*. Infect Control Hosp Epidemiol 24:362–386
28. Lucet JC, Chevret S, Durand-Zaleski I, Chastang C, Regnier B; Multicenter Study Group (2003) Prevalence and risk factors for carriage of methicillin-resistant *Staphylococcus aureus* at admission to the intensive care unit: results of a multicenter study. Arch Intern Med 163:181–188
29. Harbarth S, Sax H, Fanfhauser-Rodriguez C, Schrenzel J, Agostinho A, Pittet D (2006) Evaluating the probability of previously unknown carriage of MRSA at hospital admission. Am J Med 119:275e15–275e23
30. Harbarth S, Masuet-Autmatell C, Schrenzel J, Francois P, Akakpo C, Renzi G, Pugin J, Ricou B, Pittet D (2006) Evaluation of rapid screening and pre-emptive contact isolation for detecting and controlling methicillin resistant *Staphylococcus aureus* in critical care: an interventional cohort study. Crit Care 10 R25
31. Pittet D, Hugonnet S, Harbarth S, Mourouga P, Sauvan V, Touveneau S, Perneger TV (2000) Effectiveness of a hospital-wide programme to improve compliance with hand hygiene. Infection Control Programme. Lancet 356:1307–1312
32. Pittet D (2001) Compliance with hand disinfection and its impact on hospital-acquired infections. J Hosp Infect 48 Suppl A:S40–46
33. Pittet D, Simon A, Hugonnet S, Pessoa-Silva CL, Sauvan V, Perneger TV (2004) Hand hygiene among physicians: performance, beliefs, and perceptions. Ann Intern Med 141: 1–148

34. Sebille V, Chevret S, Valleron AJ (1997) Modeling the spread of resistant nosocomial pathogens in an intensive-care unit. Infect Control Hosp Epidemiol 18:84–92
35. Voss A, Widmer AF (1997) No time for handwashing!? Handwashing versus alcoholic rub: can we afford 100% compliance? Infect Control Hosp Epidemiol 18:205–208
36. Girou E, Loyeau S, Legrand P, Oppein F, Brun-Buisson C (2002) Efficacy of handrubbing with alcohol based solution versus standard handwashing with antiseptic soap: randomized clinical trial. BMJ 325:362
37. Boyce JM, Kelliher S, Vallande N (2000) Skin irritation and dryness associated with two hand-hygiene regimens: soap-and-water hand washing versus hand antisepsis with an alcoholic hand gel. Infect Control Hosp Epidemiol 21:442–448
38. Rampling A, Wiseman S, Davis L, Hyett AP, Walbridge AN, Payne GC, Cornaby AJ (2001) Evidence that hospital hygiene is important in the control of methicillin-resistant *Staphylococcus aureus*. J Hosp Infect 49:109–116
39. Sexton T, Clarke P, O'Neill E, Dillane T, Humphreys H (2006) Environmental reservoirs of methicillin-resistant *Staphylococcus aureus* in isolation rooms: correlation with patient isolates and implications for hospital hygiene. J Hosp Infect 62:187–194
40. O'Connell NH, Humphreys H (2000) Intensive care unit design and environmental factors in the acquisition of infection. J Hosp Infect 45:255–262
41. Kluytmans-Vandenbergh MF, Kluytmans JA, Voss A (2005) Dutch guidelines for preventing nosocomial transmission of highly resistant microorganisms (HRMO). Infection 33:309–313
42. British Society for Antimicrobial Chemotherapy, Hospital Infection Society and the Infection Control Nurses Association (1998) Revised guidelines for the control of methicillin-resistant *Staphylococcus aureus* infection in hospitals. J Hosp Infect 39:253–290
43. Hospital Infection Control Practices Advisory Committee (1996) Guideline for isolation precautions in hospitals, part II: recommendations for isolation precautions in hospitals. Am J Infect Control 24:32–52
44. Cooper BS, Stone SP, Kibbler CC, et al. (2004) Isolation measures in the hospital management of methicillin-resistant *Staphylococcus aureus* (MRSA): systematic review of the literature. BMJ 329:533–541
45. Gastmeier P, Schwab F, Geffers C, Rilden H (2004) To isolate or not to isolate? Analysis of data from the German Nosocomial Infection Surveillance System regarding the placement of patients with methicillin-resistant *Staphylococcus aureus* in private rooms in intensive care units. Infect Control Hosp Epidemiol 25:109–113
46. Nijssen S, Bonten MJ, Weinstein RA (2005) Are active microbiological surveillance and subsequent isolation needed to prevent the spread of methicillin-resistant *Staphylococcus aureus*? Clin Infect Dis 40:405–409
47. Cepeda JA, Whitehouse T, Cooper B, et al. (2005) Isolation of patients in single rooms or cohorts to reduce spread of MRSA in intensive-care units: prospective two-centre study. Lancet 365:295–304
48. Kirkland KB, Weinstein JM (1999) Adverse effects of contact isolation. Lancet 354:1177–1178
49. Evans HL, MM Shaffer, MG Hughes, et al. (2003) Contact isolation in surgical patients: a barrier to care? Surgery 134:180–188
50. Stelfox HT, Bates DW, Redelmeier DA (2003) Safety of patients isolated for infection control. JAMA 290:1899–1905
51. Lucet JC, Paoletti X, Lolom I, Paugam-Burtz C, Trouillet JL, Timsit JF, Deblangy C, Andremont A, Regnier B (2005) Successful long-term program for controlling methicillin-resistant *Staphylococcus aureus* in intensive care units. Intensive Care Med 31:1051–1057
52. de Lassence A, Hidri N, Timsit JF, Joly-Guillou ML, Thiery G, Boyer A, Lable P, Blivet A, Kalinowski H, Martin Y, Lajonchere JP, Dreyfuss D (2006) Control and outcome of a large outbreak of colonization and infection with glycopeptide-intermediate *Staphylococcus aureus* in an intensive care unit. Clin Infect Dis 42:170–178
53. Kallen AJ, Wilson CT, Larson RJ (2005) Perioperative intranasal mupirocin for the prevention of surgical-site infections: systematic review of the literature and meta-analysis. Infect Control Hosp Epidemiol 26:916–922
54. Miller MA, Dascal A, Portnoy J, Mendelson J (1996) Development of mupirocin resistance among methicillin-resistant *Staphylococcus aureus* after widespread use of nasal mupirocin ointment. Infect Control Hosp Epidemiol 17: 811–813
55. Muller A, Talon D, Potier A, Belle E, Cappelier G, Bertrand X (2005) Use of intranasal mupirocin to prevent methicillin-resistant *Staphylococcus aureus* infection in intensive care units. Crit Care 9:246–250
56. Harbarth S, Dharan S, Liassine N, Herrault P, Auckenthaler R, Pittet D (1999) Randomized, placebo-controlled, double-blind trial to evaluate the efficacy of mupirocin for eradicating carriage of methicillin-resistant *Staphylococcus aureus*. Antimicrob Agents Chemother 43:1412–1416

Chapter 22

Epidemiology of *Acinetobacter baumannii* in the Intensive Care Unit

22

J. Garnacho-Montero, C.O. Leyba, J.A. Martín

Over the last few decades, *Acinetobacter baumannii* has become one of the main nosocomial pathogens, causing epidemics and endemics in hospitals all over the world and affecting patients in intensive care units (ICUs) in particular [1]. It is a non-fermenting Gram-negative bacillus which causes mainly nosocomial infections (it also exceptionally causes community-acquired infections) such as pneumonia, primary bacteraemia, catheter-related infections, meningitis and surgical wound infections. To date, there are eight pathogenic *Acinetobacter* species (Table 22.1); however, through DNA and 16S ribosomal DNA hybridisation studies, 21 genospecies with numerical designation have been identified [2]. The genospecies 2 (*A. baumannii*), 1 (*A. calcoaceticus*), 3 and 13 TU are of most clinical importance [3].

Table 22.1. Classification of *Acinetobacter* species

Genotypic classification	Phenotypic classification
Genospecies 1–7	*A. calcoaceticus*
Genotype 3	Biotypes 1, 2, 6 and 9
Genospecies 8/9	*A. baumannii*
Genospecies 10–12	*A. haemolyticus*
Genospecies 13–14 TU	*A. junnii*
Genotype 13 TU	*A. johnsonnii*
Genospecies BJ 14–17	*A. lwoffii*
	A. radioresistens
	A. venetianus

22.1 General Characteristics of *Acinetobacter* Outbreaks

Knowledge of the epidemiology of *Acinetobacter* spp. infections is based on traditional tools such as phenotypic and antibiotype identification, but these methods are not sufficient due to their low discrimination power, the low metabolic activity of this bacterium and its frequent multi-drug resistance pattern. It should be pointed out that microorganisms with identical antibiotic resistance patterns often belong to different genotypes [4].

The clonal identification of the isolations is firstly based on the definitive characterisation of the genospecies by means of 16S ribosomal DNA amplification of *Acinetobacter* spp. (around 1,500 base pairs) and their subsequent treatment with the restriction endonucleases *Cfo*I, *Alu*I and *Msp*I (ARDRA) [5]. Once the genospecies have been established, a molecular method such as electrophoresis in a pulsating field or the amplification of repetitive sequences and treatment using restriction endonucleases (REP-PCR) should be used for clonal identification [6].

The presence of a prevailing clone was suggested at first as the cause of nosocomial outbreaks; however, we now know that several clones often coexist in the same hospital. Hsueh et al. studied an outbreak of *A. baumannii*, which included 203 strains, and described 10 different clones although there was a predominant clone specifically located in the ICU [7]. Fernández-Cuenca et al. studied an outbreak, in the GEIH-Ab2000 project, which included 221 strains from 25 Spanish hospitals [8], and described 21 genospecies which contained a large variety of clones (79 clones) even within the same hospital. They concluded that the outbreak could be explained by the coexistence of epidemic and endemic clones. In addition, Abbo et al. [9] published a retrospective case-control study in order to understand the epidemiology of multiresistant *A. baumannii* infections. They studied 118 cases (88 of these were nosocomial infections). This outbreak had 51 clones; two of whch were predominant. They concluded that there was no temporal grouping in the cases and they appeared in multiple services, the incidence increment in an area is not due to a single clone alone and that in one clone the strains present various antibiotypes, verifying that strains with the same antibiotype may belong to various clones. Similarly, in a recent multi-centre study carried out in Spain, in the case of imipenem resistant *A. baumannii*, there was a high number of clones; a single clone was not found in any of the participating hospitals [10].

22.2 Evolution of Antimicrobial Resistance

Invariably, one of the most alarming characteristics of this Gram-negative bacillus is its ability to develop resistance to all available antibiotics, which is even higher than in other non-fermenting Gram-negative bacilli, such as *Pseudomonas aeruginosa*.

The sensitivity patterns may vary according to environmental factors, the evolution time of the outbreak and the different antimicrobial strategies. Currently, in hospitals with prolonged outbreaks or in an endemic situation, the majority of *A. baumannii* strains are resistant to aminoglycosides, ureidopenicillins, third and fourth generation cephalosporins, and fluoroquinolones; and these antibiotics are not indicated in the empirical treatment of infections in which *A. baumannii* is suspected.

One essential factor is knowledge of the resistance rates to carbapenems, the empirical treatment of choice. In fact, recently, the International Network for the Study and Prevention of Emerging Antimicrobial Resistance has defined the emergence of imipenem resistance in *Acinetobacter* spp. as a "sentinel event" which requires an urgent, coordinated response to control this multi-resistant pathogen [11]. From 1997 to 1999, SENTRY surveillance in the USA, Canada and Latin America found 8% resistance to imipenem and 10.7% resistance to meropenem, the resistance rates being greater in the isolations in the ICU. Another surveillance carried out in the United States from 1998 to 2001 showed lower rates of resistance to carbapenems; 95% of the isolations were imipenem sensitive, 90% meropenem sensitive.

At present, the situation is highly heterogeneous: there may be incidental outbreaks in hospitals or outbreaks in which 30–60% of the *A. baumannii* are imipenem resistant. These high resistance rates have been recorded all over the world, both in developed and developing countries [12–15], affecting large hospitals in particular. Figure 22.1 shows the incidence of *A. baumannii* in ICUs and the imipenem resistance rates in ICUs in Spain from 1994 to 2004.

Carbapenem resistant strains are often also resistant to the majority of antimicrobial agents, including sulbactam, a β-lactamase inhibitor which acts as a bactericide against *A. baumannii* [16]. The sole exception is colistin methanesulphonate (polymyxin E), a polypeptidic antimicrobial agent which acts as a bactericide against several Gram-negative bacterial species, including *A. baumannii* and *P. aeruginosa* [17]. It acts by means of phospholipids in the bacterial cell membrane, halting its structure. Although almost 100% of *Acinetobacter baumannii* strains are sensitive to this polypeptidic antibiotic, there are series for which in long term endemic or epidemic situations, resistance has been recorded in 1–2% of the strains [18, 19].

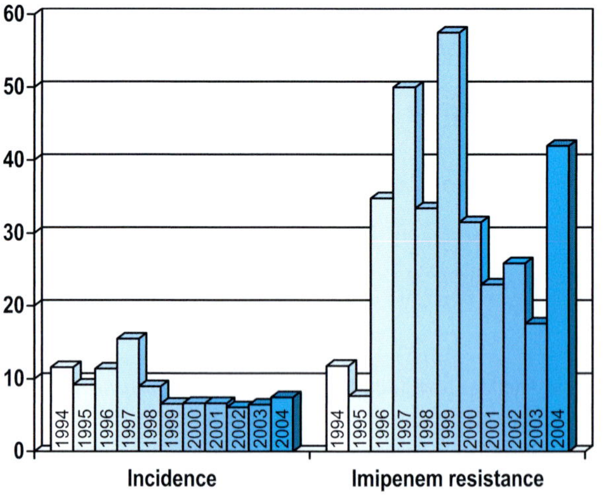

Fig. 22.1. Incidence of *A. baumannii* in Spanish ICUs and rates of imipenem resistance from 1994 to 2004 (ENVIN: National Surveillance Program for Nosocomial Infection)

Consequently, this is a very alarming situation due to the lack of therapeutic alternatives. Tigecycline, a novel glycycline derived from minocycline, should be mentioned here as the only option against multi-drug resistant *A. baumannii* that will be soon available. It has a broad antibacterial spectrum, including *A. baumannii* [20]. Clinical data are lacking in relation to the utility of tigecycline in case of multi-drug resistant *A. baumannii* infections, but it has been established that tigecycline is active in vitro against imipenem resistant strains [21].

22.3 Mechanisms of Antimicrobial Resistance

Acinetobacter baumannii has the ability to rapidly develop antimicrobial resistance. Among the factors which influence the development of resistance, the following should be considered: it is a microorganism which, throughout its phylogenetic evolution, has been exposed to antibiotic producing microorganisms from soil; its great ability to respond to antibiotics developing multiple resistance mechanisms; the wide use of antibiotics in hospitals; and its capacity to survive in any environment.

Resistance in *A. baumannii* is fundamentally carried out by conjugation, and plasmids, transposons and integrons play an important role. The encoding genes are located in both chromosomes and plasmids.

Acinetobacter baumannii has developed resistance mechanisms against the majority of antimicrobial agents. Three types of aminoglycoside-modifying enzymes have been recorded: acetylases, adenylases and phosphorylases, In addition, fluoroquinolone resistance is developed through mutations in the gyrA gene and changes in the outer membrane have not been ruled out which would contribute to the *A. baumannii* cross resistance to quinolones, aminoglycosides and all β-lactamics [22].

With respect to resistance in the latter group, the production of β-lactamases such as TEM 1 and 2, CARB-5, SHV-like (penicillinase) and ACE 1–4 (cephalosporinase) plays an important role. The carbapenems are the most efficient antibiotics in the treatment of multi-resistant *A. baumannii* infections, but the appearance of resistant strains is becoming more frequent.

In various geographic areas, there have been recordings of class B plasmids, which encode metalloenzymes that hydrolyse all β-lactamics except aztreonam and belong to the 1, 2, 4 and 5 IMP and 1 and 2 VIM families. These types of enzymes are easy to detect as they are inhibited by EDTA presence [23]. DoxA enzymes, which also inactivate carbapenems, penicillins and cephalosporins, do so less effectively than the metal β-lactamases. They are very widespread and have been involved in the development of outbreaks [24, 25], they are not inhibited by the presence of EDTA and they hydrolyse cefepime more effectively than ceftazidime, for which both antibiotics must be used to correctly identify it [26].

Other imipenem resistant mechanisms recorded in *A. baumannii* are the change in the PBP2 (penicillin binding protein), and changes in outer membrane porin due to mutations or reduced expression (Table 22.2).

Although *A. baumannii* resistance to colistin is nowadays exceptional, susceptibility breakpoints for this antimicrobial are not standardised by the Clinical and Laboratory Standards Institute. Determination of the MIC (minimum inhibitory concentration) of the strains by means of broth microdilution methods or by E test diffusion is required for the clinical use of colistin. Strains with MIC values above 4 mg/l are considered resistant [27].

Table 22.2. Mechanisms of *A. baumannii* resistance to β-lactamics

A. β-Lactamics: β-lactamase
TEM 1 and 2 (penicillin)
ACE 1–4 (cephalosporins)
AMP C
B. Carbapenems:
Carbapenemases
Metalloenzymes. Hydrolyze all β-lactamics expect aztreonam: IMP or VIM family
OXA 23 (ARI-1)-27 and 40: Hydrolyze all β lactamics
Class A: It can be inhibited by clavulanic acid
Altered PBP2: Hydrolyze carbapenems
Reduced antibiotic concentration: hydrolyze carbapenems
Absence/reduced expression of outer membrane porine
Efflux pumps

22.4 Factors Which Favour Infection/Colonisation by *Acinetobacter* spp. in the ICU

These infections usually appear in critically ill patients, with long hospital stays, in particular in ICUs, and who undergo multiple invasive procedures. It is a ubiquitous microorganism and it is estimated that there is colonisation and not a true infection in 50% of cases [28], which is very important since it implies a different therapeutic and prognostic approach. When studies of *Acinetobacter baumannii* risk factors have been carried out, prior exposure to antimicrobial agents appears constantly [29–31].

The two main infections caused by *A. baumannii* are bacteraemia and pneumonia. The most frequent origins of bacteraemia are the respiratory tract and venous catheters. Nevertheless, it should be pointed out that in a third of the cases, the clinical and microbiological criteria used to determine the origin of the bacteraemia are not exact, which is verified when genotyping the isolated strains from the blood and in the suspected focus of infection [32].

Bacteraemia due to *A. baumannii* usually affects immunodepressed patients, who have received broad spectrum antibiotherapy with long stays in the ICU and with multiple invasive procedures. This was proven in a cohort study designed to determine *A. baumannii* bacteraemia risk factors in which the invasive procedure rate (the number of invasive procedures divided by the number of days) was a predisposing factor in the multivariate analysis for the emergence of bacteraemia due to *A. baumannii* [31].

In addition, in the literature review, we found three studies designed to discover the risk factors for *A. baumannii* ventilator associated-pneumonia (VAP). The first two were carried out in an epidemic outbreak while the third was in an endemic unit due to *A. baumannii*. In a study by Baraibar et al. [33], *A. baumannii* was isolated in only 8% of the episodes. The factors independently associated with this pathogen were: neurosurgery, head trauma, acute respiratory-distress syndrome and aspiration. In contrast to other studies, it is noteworthy that the use of antimicrobial agents was not an independent determinant of *A. baumannii* VAP. The identification of the aspiration is explained by the fact that patients in ICUs are colonised with this pathogen, and aspiration is a pathogenic mechanism which causes the pulmonary infection. In addition, in a case-control study carried out in the United States, the only associated factor was prior use of ceftazidime [34].

In a third study carried out in a unit with endemic *A. baumannii*, prior use of antimicrobial agents was the only independent factor associated with VAP due to this Gram-negative bacillus [35]. It should be pointed out that reintubation was a statistically significant factor in the bivariate analysis. Undoubtedly, as with reintubation, the same occurred in a study carried out by Baraibar et al. [33] with aspiration. In both cases, colonisation occurred in the upper respiratory tract, and subsequently descended, causing pneumonia, which may be favoured by reintubation or aspiration.

Another aspect which should be analysed are risk factors linked to the isolation of *A. baumannii* strains, resistant to carbapenems, the empirical treatment of choice. Prior exposure to third generation cephalosporins and imipenem are associated independent risk factors for colonisation or infection by imipenem resistant *A. baumannii* strains [36].

The admission into units with a high number of patients colonised with carbapenem resistant strains is another factor in a study of 1,836 critically ill patients, which shows the facility with which transmission of this pathogen occurs [13].

Presentation of *A. baumannii* infections is typically slow, both in bacteriaemia and VAP. It usually affects patients with an average stay of 3 weeks and who have received antibiotics over 7 days almost without interruption [31, 37, 38]. Nevertheless, it should be pointed out that patients in endemic situations are colonised early with *A. baumannii* [39], a factor which explains the premature appearance of these patients in units in endemic situations.

22.5 Conditions Favouring *Acinetobacter* spp. Spread

Acinetobacter spp. is a ubiquitous microorganism that can survive for long periods in adverse conditions. Moreover, humans and inanimate surfaces can be easily colonised with this pathogen. In epidemic situations, *A. baumannii* may be isolated in any material or surface around the patient (bedclothes, mattresses, curtains, floors, drains, etc.), as well as in medical material (phonendoscopes, laryngoscopes, respirators, etc.) [40]. Although it is a non-spore-forming bacterium, its survival in diverse materials such as steel and dry surfaces for long periods of up to several months has been recorded, a characteristic which undoubtedly favours the transmission of this pathogen and the persistence of outbreaks [41, 42]. In addition to these environmental factors, multi-drug resistant strains have a greater capacity to spread and cause epidemics than sensitive strains, without any difference existing between them in adhesion properties, such as haemagglutination [43]. The factors which favour its spread are summarised in Table 22.3.

Table 22.3. Factors promoting *Acinetobacter* spp. transmission in the ICU

1. It can survive for long periods in inanimate surfaces
2. Heavy contamination of the environment
3. Contamination of the medical equipment
4. High rates of antibiotic resistance
5. Rapid development of resistance
6. Resistance to conventional soaps and antiseptics
7. High rates of colonised patients (especially critically ill patients)
8. Contamination of health workers' hands

Acinetobacter spp. is a normal commensal flora in the patients' and hospital staff's skin which converts them into a reservoir of infection in hospitals in epidemic and endemic situations. Many parts of the patient's body may be colonised with this Gram-negative bacillus but particularly the skin, pharynx and humid areas such as the axils, the groins or the perineum. It should be pointed out that in a critically ill patient, the digestive tract can be colonised, with *A. baumannii* becoming a reservoir in endemic situations, which is very relevant, given that *Acinetobacter* spp. is not part of the gastrointestinal flora.

The main form of *A. baumannii* transmission is through direct contact and the hospital staff are the main transmission means of this pathogen [44, 45]. In addition, it has also been recorded that it can be spread by air transmission. Thus, it has been demonstrated that *A. baumannii* can be isolated at more than 4 m away from patients with respiratory colonisation [46]. For this reason, open aspirations in patients with colonisation or respiratory infection with this pathogen can infect patients at a significant distance and therefore should be avoided.

In addition, *A. baumannii* transmission has occurred between hospitals. In Spain, this form of acquisition represents at least 3% of the cases [8]. This means of transmission should be noted by the nosocomial infection surveillance program of every hospital, and especially for the management of admissions from other hospitals in epidemic or endemic situations.

22.6 Control Measures

Given that the main transmission mechanism is by direct contact, measures such as handwashing and barrier protections should be used in order to avoid the spread of this pathogen. Strict control measures should be implemented including the use of gowns, gloves, and masks. Besides, patients colonised or infected with *A. baumannii* should be isolated from other patients in individual rooms [47].

An additional problem is that multi-drug resistant strains are almost uniformly resistant to habitual antiseptic agents such as chlorhexidine. In addition, it has been recorded that antiseptic agent dispensers may become reservoirs for *A. baumannii*, a factor favouring the spread of the pathogen [48].

The lack of strict rules with respect to washing hands favours the spread of *A. baumannii*. When coming into contact with a patient and their environment, hand hygiene with alcoholic solutions is mandatory [49, 50]. It is crucial to implement educational measures and to ensure that the alcohol-based dispensers are easily accessible to all heath workers.

Adequate cleaning of the surroundings with hypochlorite solutions is essential in order to avoid *A. baumannii* transmission, as contamination in the surroundings is an essential mechanism in the spread of this pathogen. For this reason, we must attempt to eradicate it from all the surfaces on which it survives [51]. The impact of the architectural design of the units on the spread of *A baumannii* is well known. Thus, after an ICU was transformed from an open unit to enclosed isolation rooms with handwashing facilities in each room, *A. baumannii* respiratory colonisation was reduced in patients requiring mechanical ventilation [52]. In this study, colonisation was only associated with prolonged hospital stays and not with the underlying characteristics of the patients.

22.7 Morbidity and Attributable Mortality

Crude mortality rates due to *A. baumannii* clearly depend on the focus of infection; the highest rates (approximately 50%) occurring in cases of pulmonary infections and bacteraemia, although related mortality is around 35%. The explanation is that these infections usually affect seriously ill patients and patients with long hospital stays. Therefore, this infection is considered more as a marker of the underlying severity. There is controversial data about attributable mortality resulting from *A. baumannii* bacteraemia, although it is established that this infection is associated with an increase in hospital stays and the consequent rise in costs [53].

In contrast with other Gram-negative bacilli such as *P. aeruginosa*, in which it has been shown that VAP due to this pathogen has a mortality excess [54], there are doubts about the attributable mortality of *A. baumannii* VAP. In a case-control study, it was shown that there was no attributable mortality to VAP due to this Gram-negative pathogen nor an increase in the length of hospital stays after matching cases and controls according to initial severity of illness, reason for ICU admission and hospital length of stay. In episodes caused by imipenem resistant strains, a higher mortality rate was noticed but without statistical significance, although only 25 cases were included [37].

Finally, it should be pointed out that *A. baumannii* is a ubiquitous microorganism, which explains why in almost half of the *A. baumannii* isolations it is considered as a mere coloniser, and not a true infection, which has significant prognostic consequences as mortality rates do not increase although it is associated with an increment in the length of stay and associated costs [55, 56].

22.8 Conclusions

Acinetobacter baumannii infections are a very serious problem in hospitals all over the world, occurring mainly in patients in ICUs. Undoubtedly, it remains unsolved why there are some hospitals in which the occurrence of this pathogen is high, while in others it is practically non-existent, although this problem usually affects large hospitals in which seriously ill patients are admitted.

In any case, the epidemiology of these infections is widely known. On the one hand, we are dealing with a pathogen with a high survival capacity in adverse environmental situations. As a result, colonisation may occur in inanimate surfaces, including medical material and patients, who become the main reservoir. The main transmission mechanism is through direct contact with medical staff hands although we must remember that hospital material can help in its spread as airborne transmission is possible.

Multi-drug resistant *A. baumannii* isolation requires a rapid, coordinated, multi-disciplinary response in order to avoid its spread and eliminate the reservoirs. It is clear that a correct antibiotic policy would help to mitigate this growing problem.

References

1. Bergogne-Bérézin E (2001) The increasing role of *Acinetobacter* species as nosocomial pathogens. Curr Infect Dis Rep 3:440–444
2. Ibrahim A, Gerner Smidt P, Liesack W (1997) Phylogenetic relationship of the twenty-one DNA groups of the genus *Acinetobacter* as revealed by 16S ribosomal DNA sequence analysis. Int J Sys Bacteriol 47:837–841
3. Bergogne-Bérézin E, Towner KJ (1996) *Acinetobacter* spp. as nosocomial pathogen: Microbiological, clinical, and epidemiological features. Clin Microbiol Rev 9:148–165
4. Villegas MV, Hartstein AI (2003) *Acinetobacter* outbreaks, 1977–2000. Infect Control Hosp Epidemiol 24:284–295
5. Vaneechoutee M, Dijkshoorn L, Tjenberg I, Elaichouni A, De Vos P, Caléis G, et al. (1995) Identification of *Acinetobacter* species by amplified ribosomal DNA restriction analysis. J Clin Microbiol 33:1–5
6. Martín Lozano D, Cisneros JM, Becerril B, Cuberos L, Prados T, Ortiz Leyba C, et al. (2002) Comparison of repetitive extragenic palindromic sequence-based PCR (REP-PCR) and clinical/microbiological methods in the study of nosocomial *Acinetobacter baumannii* bacteriemia sources. J Clin Microbiol 40:4571–4575
7. Hsueh PR, Teng LJ, Chen CY, Chen WH, Yu CJ, et al. (2002) Pandrug-resistant *Acinetobacter baumannii* causing noso-

comial infections in a University hospital, Taiwan. Emerg Infect Dis 8:827–831

8. Férnandez-Cuenca F, Pascual A, Vila J, Bou, Cisneros JM, Rodriguez-Baño J, et al. (2004) Diversidad clonal y sensibilidad a los antimicrobianos de *Acinetobacter baumannii* aislados en hospitales españoles. Enferm Infecc Microbiol Clin 22:267–271
9. Abbo A, Navon-Venezia S, Hammer-Muntz O, Krichali T, Siegman-Igra Y, Carmeli Y (2005) Multidrug-resistant *Acinetobacter baumannii*. Emerg Infect Dis 1122–1129
10. Cisneros JM, Rodríguez-Baño J, Fernández-Cuenca F, et al. (2005) Risk factor for the acquisition of imipenem-resistant *Acinetobacter baumannii* in Spain: A nationwide study. Clin Microbiol Infect 11:874–879
11. Richet HM, Mohammed J, McDonald LC, Jarvis WR (2001) Building communication networks: international network for the study of emerging antimicrobial resistance. Emerging Infect Dis 7:319–322
12. Go ES, Urban C, Burns J, et al. (1994) Clinical and molecular epidemiology of *Acinetobacter* infections sensitive only to polymyxon B and sulbactam. Lancet 344:1329–1332
13. Corbella X, Montero A, Pujol M, et al. (2000) Emergence and rapid spread of carbapenem resistance during a large and sustained hospital outbreak of multiresistant *Acinetobacter baumannii*. J Clin Microbiol 38:4086–4095
14. Joshi SG, Litake GM, Niphadkar KB, Ghole VS (2003) Multidrug resistant *Acinetobacter baumannii* isolates from a teaching hospital. J Infect Chemother 9:187–190
15. Landman D, Quale JM, Mayorga D, et al. (2002) Citywide clonal outbreak of multiresistant *Acinetobacter baumannii* and *Pseudomonas aeruginosa* in Brooklyn, NY. Arch Inter Med 162:1515–1520
16. Ruiz J, Núñez ML, Pérez E, et al. (1999) Evolution of resistance among clinical isolates of *Acinetobacter* over a 6-year period. Eur J Clin Microbiol Infect Dis 18:292–295
17. Garnacho-Montero J, Ortiz-Leyba C, Jiménez-Jiménez FJ, Barrero-Almodóvar AE (2003) García-Garmendia JL, Bernabeu-Wittel M, et al. Treatment of multiresistant *Acinetobacter baumannii* ventilator-associated pneumonia (VAP) with intravenous colistin: a comparison with imipenem susceptible episodes. Clin Infect Dis 36:1111–1118
18. Manikal VM, Landman D, Saurina G, et al. (2000) Endemic carbapenem-resistant *Acinetobacter* species in Brooklyn, New York: Citywide prevalence, interinstitutional spread, and relation to antibiotic usage. Clin Infect Dis 31: 101–106
19. Landman D, Quale JM, Mayorga D, et al. (2002) Citywide clonal outbreak of multiresistant *Acinetobacter baumannii* and *Pseudomonas aeruginosa* in Brooklyn, NY. Arch Inter Med 162:1515–1520
20. Milatovic D, Schmitz FJ, Verhoef J, Fluit AC (2003) Activities of the glycylcycline tigecycline (GAR-936) against 1924 recent European clinical bacterial isolates. Antimicrob Agents Chemother 47:400–404
21. Pachón-Ibáñez ME, Jiménez-Mejias ME, Pichrado C, Llanos AC, Pachón J (2004) Activity of tigecycline (GAR-936) against *Acinetobacter baumannii* strains, including those resistant to imipenem. Antimicrob Agents Chemother 48: 4479–4481
22. Urban C, Segal-Maurer S, Rahal JJ (2003) Considerations in control and treatment of nosocomial infections due to multidrug-resistant *Acinetobacter baumannii*. Clin Infect Dis 36:1268–1274
23. Walsh TR, Bolmstrom A, Qwarnstrom A, et al. (2002) Evaluation of a new E-test for detecting metallo-β lactamases in routine clinical testing. J Clin Microbiol 40:2755–2759
24. Dalle-Costa LB, Coelho JM, Souza HA, et al. (2003) Outbreak of carbapenem-resistant *Acinetobacter baumannii* producing the OXA-23 enzyme in Curiba, Brazil. J Clin Microbiol 41:3403–3406
25. Hériter C, Dubouix A, Poirel L, et al. (2005) A nosocomial outbreak of *Acinetobacter baumannii* isolates expressing the carbapenem-hydrolysing oxacillinase OXA-58. J Antimicrob Chemother 55:115–118
26. Gallego L, Canduela MJ, Sevillano E, Pujana I Calvo F, Umarán A, et al. (2004) Detección de carbapenemasas en clones de *Acinetobacter baumannii* resistentes a imipenem. Enferm Infecc Microbiol Clin 22:262–266
27. Arroyo LA, García-Curiel A, Pachón-Ibañez ME, Llanos AC, Ruiz M, Pachón J, Aznar J (2005) Reliability of the E-test method in the detection of colistin resistance in clinical isolates of *Acinetobacter baumannii*. J Clin Microbiol 43:903–905
28. Tomás MM, Cartelle M, Pertega S, et al. (2005) Hospital outbreak caused by a carbapenem-resistant strain of *Acinetobacter baumannii*: patient prognosis and risk factors for colonisation and infection. Clin Microbiol Infect 11:540–546
29. Lortholary O, Fagon JY, Buu-Hoy A, et al. (1995) Nosocomial acquisition of multiresistant *Acinetobacter baumannii*: Risk factors and prognosis. Clin Infect Dis 20:790–796
30. Levin ASS, Mendes CMF, Sinto SI, et al. (1995) An outbreak of multiresistant *Acinetobacter baumannii* in a university hospital in Sao Paulo, Brazil. Infect Control Hosp Epidemiol 16:92–97
31. García-Garmendia JL, Ortiz-Leyba C, Garnacho-Montero J, et al. (2001) Risk factors for *Acinetobacter baumannii* nosocomial bacteremia in critically ill patients: a cohort study. Clin Infect Dis 33:939–946
32. Martin-Lozano D, Cisneros JM, Becerrill B, et al. (2002) Comparison of a repetitive extragenic palindromic sequence-based PCR method and clinical and microbiological methods for determining strains sources in cases of nosocomial *Acinetobacter baumannii* bacteremia. J Clin Microbiol 23:242–247
33. Baraibar J, Correa H, Mariscal D, Gallego M, Valles J, Rello J (1997) Risk factors for infection by *Acinetobacter baumannii* in intubated patients with pneumonia. Chest 112:1050–1054
34. Husni RN, Goldstein LS, Arroliga AC, Arroliga AC, Hall GS, Fatica C, et al. (1999) Risk factors for an outbreak of multi-drug-resistant *Acinetobacter* nosocomial pneumonia among intubated patients. Chest 115:1378–1382
35. Garnacho-Montero J, Ortiz-Leyba C, Fernandez-Hinojosa E, Aldabo-Pallas T, Cayuela A, Marquez-Vacaro JA, Garcia-Curiel A, Jimenez-Jimenez FJ (2005) *Acinetobacter baumannii* ventilator-associated pneumonia: epidemiological and clinical findings. Intensive Care Med 31:649–655
36. Lee SO. Kim NJ, Choi SH, Kim TH, Chung JW, Woo JH, et al. (2004) Risk factors for acquisition of imipenem-resistant *Acinetobacter baumannii*: a case-control study. Antimicrob Agents Chemother 48:224–228
37. Garnacho-Montero J, Sole-Violan J, Sa-Borges M, Diaz-Santos E, Rello J (2003) Clinical impact of pneumonia caused by *Acinetobacter baumannii* in intubated patients: A matched cohort study. Crit Care Med 31:2478–2482
38. Wisplinghoff H, Bischoff T, Tallent SM, Seifert H, Wenzel RP, Edmond MB (2004) Nosocomial bloodstream infections in US hospitals: analysis of 24,179 cases from a prospective nationwide surveillance study. Clin Infect Dis 39:309–317
39. Corbella X, Pujol M, Ayats J, et al. (1996) Relevance of digestive tract colonisation in the epidemiology of nosocomial infections due to multiresistant *Acinetobacter baumannii*. Clin Infect Dis 23:329–334
40. Bernards AT, Harinck HI, Dijkshoorn L, et al. (2004) Per-

sistent *Acinetobacter baumannii*? Look inside your medical equipment. Infect Control Hosp Epidemiol 25:1002–1004

41. Wendt C, Dietze B, Dietz E, Ruden H (1997) Survival of *Acinetobacter baumannii* on dry surfaces. J Clin Microbiol 35:1394–1397
42. Webster C, Towner KJ, Humphreys H (2000) Survival of *Acinetobacter* on three clinically related inanimate surfaces. Infect Control Hosp Epidemiol 21:246
43. Koeleman JGM, van der Bijl MU, Stoof J, Vandenbrouche CMJE, Savelkoul PHM (2001) Antibiotic resistance is a major risk factor for epidemic behaviour of *Acinetobacter baumannii*. Infect Control Hosp Epidemiol 22:284–288
44. Wagenvoort JHT, et al. (2002) Epidemic *Acinetobacter baumanii* strain with MRSA-like behaviour carried by healthcare staff. Eur J Clin Microbiol Infect Dis 21:326–327
45. El Shafie SS, Alishaq M, Leni Garcia M (2004) Investigation of an outbreak of multidrug-resistant *Acinetobacter baumannii* in trauma intensive care unit. J Hosp Infect 56:101–105
46. Brooks SE, Walczak MA, Rizwanullah H (2000) Are we doing enough to contain *Acinetobacter* infections. Infect Control Hosp Epidemiol 21:304
47. Rello J (1999) *Acinetobacter baumannii* infections in the ICU. Customization is the key. Chest 115:1226–1229
48. Brooks SE, Walczak MA, Hameed R, Coonan P (2002) Clorhexidine resistance in antibiotic-resistant bacteria isolated from the surfaces of dispensers of soap containing clorhexidine. Infect Control Hosp Epidemiol 23:692–695
49. Cardoso CL, Pereira HH, Zequim JC, Guilhermetti M (1999) Effectiveness of hand-cleansing agents for removing *Acinetobacter baumannii* strain from contaminated hands. Am J Infect Control 27:327–331
50. Rochon-Edouard S, Pons JL, Veber B, Larkin M, Vassal S, Lemeland JF (2004) Comparative in vitro and in vivo study of nine alcohol-based handrubs. Am J Infect Control 32: 200–204
51. Denton M, Wilcox MH, Parnell P, Green D, Keer V, Hawkey PM, et al. (2004) Role of environmental cleaning in controlling an outbreak of *Acinetobacter baumannii* in a neurosurgical intensive care unit. J Hosp Infect 56:106–110
52. Mulin B, Rouget C, Clement C, et al. (1997) Association of private isolation rooms with ventilator-associated *Acinetobacter baumannii* pneumonia in a surgical intensive-care unit. Infect Control Hosp Epidemiol 18:499–503
53. Blot S, Vandewoude K, Colardyn F (2003) Nosocomial bacteremia involving *Acinetobacter baumannii* in critically ill patients: a matched cohort study. Intensive Care Med 29:471–475
54. Rello J, Jubert P, Vallés J, et al. (1996) Evaluation of outcome in intubated patients with pneumonia caused by *Pseudomonas aeruginosa*. Clin Infect Dis 23:973–978
55. García Garmendia JL, Ortiz Leyba C, Garnacho Montero J, Jiménez Jiménez FJ, Monterrubio Villar J, Gili Miner M (1999) Mortality and the increase in length of stay due to the acquisition of *Acinetobacter* in critically ill patients. Crit Care Med 27:1794–1799
56. Rodríguez-Baño J, Cisneros JM, Fernández Cuenca F, Ribera A, Vila J, Pascual A, et al. (2004) Clinical features and epidemiology of *Acinetobacter baumannii* colonization and infection in Spanish hospitals. Infect Control Hosp Epidemiol 25:819–824

Bloodstream Infections and Infection Disease Emergencies

IV

Chapter 23

Brain Abscess

23

L.M. Mundy, S.J. Bersoff-Matcha

23.1 Introduction and Historical Perspective

Brain abscess is a focal, intracerebral infection that begins as a localized area of cerebritis and develops into a collection of pus surrounded by a well-vascularized capsule [1]. Prior to the late 1800s, brain abscess was a near fatal condition with most cases diagnosed postmortem. The initial success in the treatment of brain abscess was surgical drainage or removal. This success was further enhanced during and after World War II when antibiotic therapy with penicillin and chloramphenicol became available. Over the past 25 years, there has been continued reduction in morbidity and mortality associated with brain abscesses due to advances in diagnostics and treatment strategies [1–4]. Although brain abscess is considered rare, there have been an estimated 1,500–2,500 cases diagnosed annually in the United States, with an incidence that ranges from 0.9 to 2.7 per 100,000 person-years in studied populations [5–7]. For diagnostics, neuroimaging studies, stereotactic brain biopsies, and aspiration techniques have significantly contributed to the identification of lesion(s) size, number, location, potential approaches, and evaluation over time. New antimicrobial therapies have simplified empiric- and pathogen-directed regimens. The epidemiology of this condition has evolved in recent years from a predominance of cases due to otogenic brain abscess to a rise in incidence of brain abscess among immunocompromised host populations [4, 7].

23.2 Pathophysiology and Microbiology

23.2.1 Pathophysiology

The brain is rather resistant to bacterial and fungal infection, given the frequency of overt and occult bacteremia and fungemia. This protection against seeding during bloodstream infection may be due to the abundant blood supply and relatively impermeable blood-brain barrier formed by the capillary-endothelial tight junctions. Through an experimental animal model, the natural history of brain abscess formation can be categorized into four distinct, chronological stages: early cerebritis (days 1–3), late cerebritis (days 4–9), early capsule stage (days 10–14), and late capsule stage (>14 days) [8, 9].

23.2.1.1 Source

1. Contiguous focus of infection. Organisms invade the brain parenchyma usually as a consequence of a contiguous infection of nonneural tissues such as the middle ear, mastoids, paranasal sinuses, or soft tissues of the face, orbit, or scalp.
2. Hematogenous dissemination. Bloodstream infection serves as a source of inoculum. Patients with congenital cyanotic heart disease in whom venous blood is shunted into the systemic circulation are especially prone to brain abscess formation via this mechanism.
3. Traumatic inoculation. Direct inoculation of bacteria into the brain following penetrating brain injury is common, yet unlikely to result in brain abscess formation.
4. Post-craniotomy infections. Such infections are complications of post-surgical care.
5. Other. Congenital lesions, including dermal sinuses and various forms of ruptured encephaloceles, may provide direct access from microorganisms to brain tissue. Ultimately, 20–30% of cases are cryptic and have no identified route of development.

23.2.2 Microbiology

Although most abscesses are caused by a single pathogen, mixed infections occur in up to one-third of cases and are especially common with otogenic infections. Typical intracranial brain abscess sites, likely pathogens and predisposing conditions are summarized in Table 23.1.

Most infections in immunocompetent hosts are bacterial, often polymicrobial with a combination of aero-

Predisposing conditions	Intracranial location	Usual pathogen	Initial empiric therapy[a]
Paranasal sinusitis or otitis	Frontal lobe	Aerobic streptococci, anaerobes, *Staphylococcus aureus*, *Haemophilus influenzae*	Ampilicillin-sulbactam or 3rd generation cephalosporin and metronidazole
Otogenic infection	Temporal lobe or cerebellum	Mixed infections; *Fusobacterium* spp., *Actinomyces* spp.	3rd generation cephalosporin and metronidazole
Hematogenous dissemination	MCA distribution	*S. aureus*, Enterobacteriaceae	3rd generation cephalosporin
Penetrating trauma	Site of injury	Streptococcus spp., Staphylococci spp.	3rd generation cephalosporin
HIV	Caudate nucleus	*Toxoplasma gondii*	*Pyrimethamine, sulfadiazine,* and *folinic acid*
HIV	Varies with 'soap bubble lesions'	*Cryptococcus neoformans*	Amphotericin B
Non-HIV immunosuppression	Varies	*Candida albicans* and *Aspergillus* spp.	Amphotericin B or caspofungin
Diabetes mellitus	Varies	*Mucor* or *Rhizopus*	Amphotericin B
Pyogenic lung infection	MCA distribution	Anaerobes	Penicillin G and clindamycin
Post-craniotomy	Post-surgical site		
Neonates/infants	MCA distribution	*Proteus* spp. or *Citrobacter* spp.	3rd generation cephalosporin
Post-craniotomy	Post-surgical site	Staphylococci, streptococci	Penicillin G
Cryptogenic[b]	Varies	Varies	Broad-spectrum

Table 23.1. Typical intracranial locations and pathogens of brain abscesses associated with identified predisposing conditions

MCA middle cerebral artery, *HIV* human immunodeficiency virus type-1 infection
[a] Empiric therapy: initial therapy until pathogen identified
[b] Twenty to 30% of all brain abscess cases

bic and anaerobic organisms. These occur in both adult and pediatric populations. In brain abscess associated with sinusitis, *Staphylococcus aureus*, aerobic streptococci, *Haemophilus influenzae*, and anaerobes are the most common isolates. In brain abscess associated with otogenic sources, anaerobic bacteria are the most frequent. In patients with congenital heart disease, streptococci are common. In post-craniotomy brain abscess (subdural empyema and intraparenchymal abscess), *S. aureus* and *Staphylococcus epidermidis* are most common. In post-trauma cases, *S. aureus* is the most frequent pathogen. Among persons with HIV infection, pathogens associated with brain abscess include bacteria, atypical bacteria, fungi and parasites; *Toxoplasmosis gondii* is the most frequent etiology for brain abscess with enhancing lesions noted on neuroimaging studies. In non-HIV immunosuppressed hosts, fungi such as *Candida albicans* and *Aspergillus* spp. are much more common. Diabetic patients are vulnerable to the Zygomycetes infections of *Mucor* and *Rhizopus*.

23.3 Clinical Manifestations

Although the classic triad of symptoms for patients with brain abscess is fever, headache and focal neurological deficit, less than half of patients present with all three symptoms [10]. Instead, symptoms depend more on the underlying condition of the patient, the size and location of the abscess and the organisms causing the infection. Many of the clinical manifestations of brain abscess are nonspecific, which can lead to a delay in diagnosis, although most patients (>75%) have symptoms for less than 2 weeks at the time the diagnosis is made [10, 11]. Headache, characterized by a dull, poorly localized ache, occurs in 72–92% of patients and is the most common presenting symptom in those patients who are able to report a history of present illness [1, 10–12]. Fever >100°F is seen in only 40–60% of adults and 80% of children; thus the absence of fever is not a reliable way to rule out the diagnosis [1, 11, 12]. The presence of fever is not necessarily more likely in those patients with worse initial mental status or with multiple abscesses [10, 11]. In one study, patients without fever tended to be older, had temporal lobe lesions and higher mortality [10].

Nausea and vomiting occur in about 50% of patients, probably due to increased intracranial pressure. Other central nervous system (CNS) symptoms such as papilledema, lethargy and stupor occur in 10–66% of patients; these symptoms also indicate increased intracranial pressure [1, 10, 12]. Patients with significant altered mental status tend to have a poorer prognosis [11]. Focal neurological deficits such as hemiparesis (the most common focal neurological deficit in patients with brain abscess), ataxia, or aphasia may occur in one-third to one-half of patients, and their presence depends on the location of the abscess. Nuchal rigidity also occurs in up to 50% of patients, and when it occurs with abrupt onset, may indicate intraventricular rupture of the abscess [1, 10, 12]. This is a serious complication associated with a very high (>80%) mortality [1, 11]. Seizures have been the presenting symptom in 35% of patients and occur in 25–50% of cases during initial hospitalization [10, 11].

In a 2003 study of 94 patients with bacterial brain abscess who were admitted to an intensive care unit (ICU), patients had neurological symptoms for a median of 9 days [13]. Presenting symptoms included fever in 88%, headache in 68%, neurological findings in 57%, behavioral disturbances in 50% and generalized seizures in 16%. The most common reasons for ICU transfer included neurological deterioration in 63%, respiratory insufficiency in 6% and hemodynamic failure in 6%; 21% of the patients were admitted directly to the ICU after neurosurgery. Upon admission to the ICU, the median Glasgow Coma Scale score was 11. Mechanical ventilation was required for 56% of patients for neurological reasons; median duration of mechanical ventilation was 13 days. The patients in this series spent a median duration of 22 days in the ICU and a median 32 days in the hospital [13].

23.4 Children

Children account for up to 25% of patients who develop brain abscess, often as a complication of chronic otitis media and/or mastoiditis. When frontal lobe abscess occurs in children, it is most commonly seen in male adolescents as a complication of frontal sinusitis. These patients usually present with headache, fever, and occasionally altered mental status. However, clinical findings for this condition are often subtle and routine head CT scans may initially be negative; thus a high index of suspicion is necessary. As with brain abscess in adults, both the brain abscess and sinusitis should be managed surgically and with appropriate antibiotics. In neonates, brain abscesses sometimes occur as a rare complication of meningitis from group B streptococci or *Escherichia coli* [1]. Other facultative Gram-negative organisms such as *Serratia marcescens*, *Proteus* spp., *Citrobacter* spp., and *Enterobacter* spp. are rare causes of meningitis in this age group. However, when such pathogens are cultured from the CSF, a brain abscess is present in >75% of cases [1]. Brain abscesses from these organisms are also associated with a very high mortality rate. Those who survive usually have significant long-term neurological sequelae [1]. As with any patient with brain abscess, infants and children should be managed aggressively with both surgical drainage and antimicrobial therapy.

Congenital cyanotic heart disease, particularly tetralogy of Fallot and transposition of the great vessels (and any other condition resulting in a significant right-to-left shunt), is an important predisposing factor for brain abscess in as many as 50% of children [1]. The peak incidence of brain abscess in children with this risk factor is between 4 and 7 years of age and is rare in children under 2 years [14]. Brain abscess associated with congenital cyanotic heart disease may also occur in adults. Patients who have procedures to correct the right-to-left shunt significantly reduce their risk of brain abscess, while those patients who have palliative procedures that do not completely correct the shunt do not diminish their risk [1]. Thus, the earlier and more completely the cyanotic heart disease is corrected, the lower the risk of brain abscess. The mortality from brain abscess associated with cyanotic congenital heart disease is high (30–40%) and, as with brain abscess associated with other causes, requires both aggressive surgical and antimicrobial therapy [14].

23.5 Immunocompromised Hosts

Immunocompromised hosts, including those with diabetes, as well as those receiving corticosteroids or other immunosuppressive therapies, may develop brain abscess due to a wide variety of etiologic agents, including fungi, nocardia and tuberculosis. The clinical presentation of brain abscess in these patients differs from those with pyogenic brain abscess; they are less likely to develop headache or meningismus (presumably from less inflammatory response), and are more likely to present with fever, focal neurological deficits and seizures [1]. Since the variety of etiologic agents that could potentially cause a brain abscess in these patients is so broad, choosing empiric therapy is difficult. In such cases, early surgical intervention is recommended so that cultures can be obtained and the correct antimicrobial agent(s) can be administered.

While the most common cause of brain mass in patients with acquired immune deficiency syndrome (AIDS) is toxoplasmosis, patients with AIDS may develop brain abscess from bacterial pathogens as well.

AIDS patients with radiographic evidence of space-occupying CNS lesions should be started on empiric therapy for toxoplasmosis with pyrimethamine (for adults, a loading dose of 200 mg followed by 75 – 100 mg per day), sulfadiazine (1 – 1.5 g orally every 6 h), and folinic acid (10 mg po qd) to prevent bone marrow suppression that can occur with pyrimethamine. If the patient deteriorates or fails to show clinical improvement after 2 weeks of treatment, a brain biopsy or aspiration via neurosurgical or CT-guided techniques is recommended [15]. Patients with AIDS are also more susceptible to brain abscesses due to *Salmonella* spp., *L. monocytogenes*, *Nocardia* spp., tuberculosis, and the endemic mycoses (cryptococcosis, coccidioidomycosis, blastomycosis and histoplasmosis).

23.5.1 Diagnosis

The differential diagnosis for the clinical presentation consistent with brain abscess includes brain abscess, necrotic tumor (glioblastoma), metastatic tumor, subdural abscess, sinus thrombosis, meningitis, mycotic aneurysm and encephalitis. In metastatic tumors, gadolinium-enhanced contrast studies are more likely to reveal irregular, diffuse borders. In conjunction with the history and physical examination, supportive data include:

1. Laboratory data. Laboratory findings are of minimal assistance in the diagnosis or follow-up of patients with brain abscess. As many as 40 % of patients have normal white blood cell counts with only 10 % of patients having leukocytosis that exceeds 20,000/mm^3. Higher leukocyte counts suggest a concurrent meningitis or systemic infection. The erythrocyte sedimentation rate (ESR), although not specific, is elevated in 90 % of cases; the mean ESR in patients with brain abscess is 45 – 55 mm/h [1]. C-reactive protein is also elevated. Hyponatremia may occur and in most cases indicates the syndrome of inappropriate antidiuretic hormone (SIADH) secretion. Blood cultures are most often negative, but two sets should be drawn from febrile patients because when positive can help direct antimicrobial therapy. Lumbar puncture is not recommended for patients with brain abscess due to the risk of herniation. When performed, cerebrospinal fluid (CSF) findings are non-specific among patients with brain abscess; 25 % of CSF samples reveal hypoglycorrhachia, 67 – 81 % show elevated protein, and 60 – 70 % show a mononuclear pleocytosis [10]. In many cases, CSF findings are normal, and in only 10 % of cases are CSF cultures positive. Thus, because CSF does not routinely provide useful clinical information and patients are at risk for potential 'mass effect', lumbar puncture should not be routinely performed even after neuroimaging studies have been reviewed for open cisterns and evidence of potential or existing midline intracranial shift [1, 10]. The most reliable way to make a microbiological diagnosis is to culture specimens obtained during neurosurgery or CT-guided aspiration. With appropriate handling of specimens (i.e., careful attention to anaerobic transport techniques and prompt plating of culture material), aspirate or intraopera-

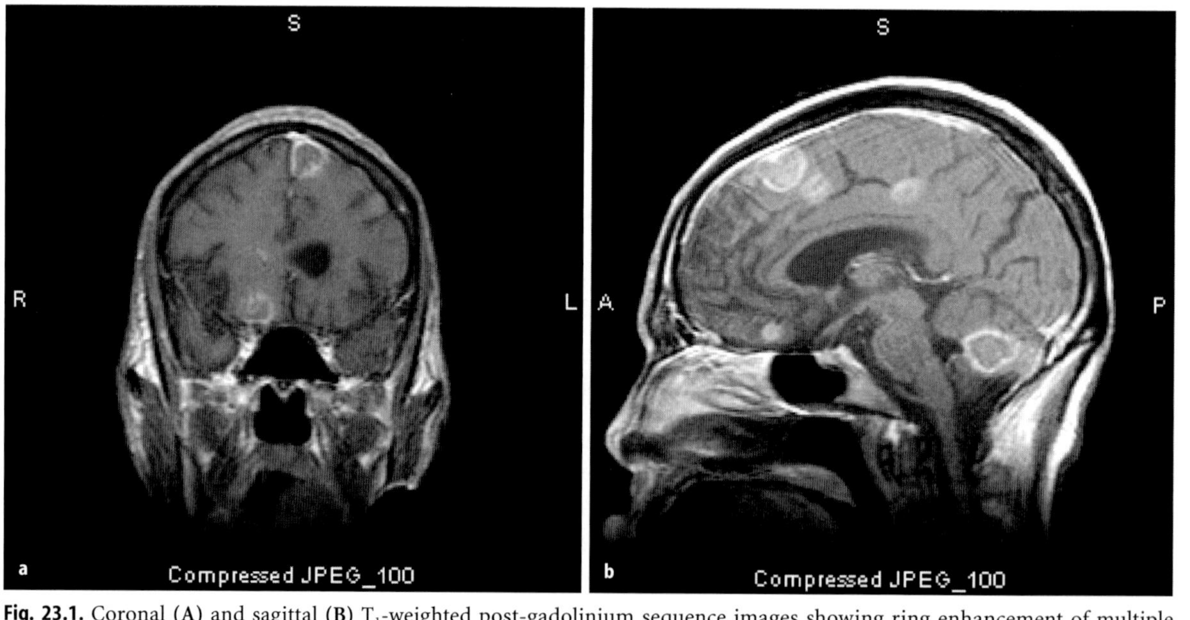

Fig. 23.1. Coronal (A) and sagittal (B) T$_1$-weighted post-gadolinium sequence images showing ring enhancement of multiple brain abscesses

tive culture yield can approximate 100% [11, 12]. In many cases, however, antimicrobial therapy has been initiated prior to surgery and in those patients cultures may be negative. While the incidence of negative cultures is greater from patients who have already begun antibiotics, material obtained during surgery should still be sent for Gram's stain and culture since findings may be helpful in guiding selection of antimicrobial agents.

2. Initial neuroimaging studies. The most important and expeditious part of the initial work-up for suspected brain abscess is a neuroimaging study with contrast, unless contraindicated. The majority of brain abscesses are ring enhancing with a thinner medial wall; intense edema is often present. Gas within the ring-enhancing lesion is highly suggestive of brain abscess. Initial neuroimaging can begin with either a head CT scan or brain magnetic radioimaging (MRI), with the selection sometimes guided by the suspected source or nidus of infection. Theoretically, based on animal models, brain MRI is better than head CT for detection of brain abscess. Head CT will enhance evaluation of bone invasion and is a quicker procedure for unstable patients. Brain MRI is best if there is involvement of a paranasal sinus or suspicion of venous sinus thrombosis. The fluid-attenuated inversion recovery (FLAIR)-weighted images are superior in depicting empyema and vasculitic CNS complications [16]. Diffusion weighted imaging (DWI) helps differentiate pyogenic abscess from ring enhancing lesions of other etiologies such as toxoplasmosis or lymphoma [16]. Pyogenic abscess has marked hyperintense signal on DWI and reduced calculated apparent diffusion coefficient which indicates restricted water diffusion [16]. In brain abscess, proton magnetic resonance spectroscopy (PMRS) reveals specific peak patterns, although this methodology is not yet routinely available [16].
   If non-contrast MRI is used, a rounded appearing lesion with edema is usually visualized. The T_1-weighted image reveals hypointensity at the central necrotic portion, surrounded by less hypointensity, representative of cerebritis and edema. The T_2-weighted images show increased or variable signal centrally surrounded by decreased signal intensity and then increased intensity (edema). After contrast the brain MRI reveals ring enhancement. If there is a brain abscess complicated by rupture of the abscess into the ventricle, there may be enhancement of the ependymal surfaces.
3. Follow-up neuroimaging studies. If non-surgical management is selected for treatment, close clinical and radiographic follow-up is necessary. Serial head CT scanning is the usual neuroimaging modality for this purpose.
   a) Radionucleotide studies. Other imaging modalities such as indium 111-labeled leukocyte scans offer little to the initial or ongoing evaluation of brain abscesses. The role of thallium-201 brain single-photon emission computed tomography (SPECT) is considered helpful in the differentiation of toxoplasmosis (low uptake) from lymphoma and tuberculoma (high uptake) [17]. The role of positron emission tomography (PET) in brain abscess remains to be determined.
   b) Cerebral angiography. This can reveal that the lesion(s) are acellular in the central bulk.
   c) Repeat head CT or brain MRI. Each of these neuroimaging studies should reveal resolution over time for persons receiving appropriate therapy. As an example, in cryptococcal meningoencephalitis, diffuse meningeal enhancement, ventriculitis, multiple punctuate lesions and "soap bubble lesions" can be visualized on MRI and resolve with targeted antifungal therapy [16].
4. Biopsy/aspiration. CT- or MRI-guided stereotactic biopsy or aspirate of the putative brain abscess can be both diagnostic and therapeutic. In cases of single lesions by MRI, stereotactic biopsy is the usual next diagnostic step [16]. Cultures and antimicrobial susceptibility data can guide pathogen-directed therapy.

23.6 Therapy

Proper management of a patient with a brain abscess includes both antimicrobial therapy and a surgical drainage procedure during which abscess material can be obtained for Gram stain and culture. Since brain abscesses are uncommon, there have been no randomized controlled trials to compare different therapies. Yet, based on the location of the abscess and previously reported experiences, some recommendations regarding therapy can be made. Bacterial brain abscesses are frequently polymicrobial and the organisms isolated depend to some extent on the source, location and predisposing condition of the patient. However, the most common agents isolated in patients from large clinical series are microaerophilic streptococci (particularly *Streptococcus milleri* and other streptococci) and anaerobic bacteria [10, 18, 19]. Other organisms such as *S. aureus* and the Enterobacteriaceae have also been seen. Thus, empiric antibiotic coverage should include antimicrobials with activity against all these organisms until material from the abscess can be obtained for culture and organism specific antimicrobial therapy can be administered.

Transplant recipients and patients who are immunocompromised from cancer chemotherapy are at risk for brain abscess from *Aspergillus* and *Candida* species. As in most patients with brain abscess, therapy for these patients should include both surgical debridement and antifungal therapy. In those patients where recovery from the immunocompromised state is possible, the likelihood of survival is greatest; however, mortality remains high. Diabetic patients, patients on chronic steroid therapy and patients with prolonged neutropenia are at risk for brain abscess due to mucormycosis. These patients frequently require extensive and disfiguring surgical debridement in addition to treatment with high-dose antifungal agents.

23.7 Surgery

Although there have been case reports documenting resolution of brain abscess using antimicrobial therapy alone [20], in most cases, both medical and surgical intervention is recommended. The two most commonly performed procedures are open craniotomy and needle aspiration. Prior to the widespread availability of intracranial radiographic imaging studies, open craniotomy under general anesthesia was the only available procedure for brain abscess drainage. Now, head CT and brain MRI scans have made it possible to more definitively localize abscesses. In addition, needle aspiration under CT guidance is less invasive and has made brain abscess drainage possible with local anesthesia. Open craniotomy is now reserved for patients with multiloculated abscesses, multiple abscesses, abscesses that fail to resolve with needle aspiration and abscesses caused by resistant pathogens. While the two procedures have not been compared in a controlled trial, retrospective analysis indicates that neither procedure has emerged as being superior in terms of outcome [11]. Because the closed needle aspiration is less invasive, most patients now initially undergo the stereotactic aspiration procedure, followed by the more invasive open procedure if deemed necessary. Patients who do undergo open craniotomy have not been shown to have a higher incidence of seizures than those who have undergone needle aspiration [1].

23.8 Antimicrobial Agents

When choosing appropriate antimicrobial therapy for brain abscesses, several issues must be considered. First, the antimicrobial agent(s) must have activity against the likely pathogen(s). Second, consideration must be given as to whether the agent will penetrate the abscess cavity. Many studies have been carried out to determine antimicrobial penetration into the CSF; yet data regarding antimicrobial penetration into brain abscess cavities is limited. The factors that predict whether an antibiotic will penetrate the CSF do not necessarily also predict penetration into a brain abscess cavity [21].

Chloramphenicol has many attractive attributes that made it one of the standard therapies for brain abscess for many years. It has a broad antimicrobial spectrum, good CNS penetration, and it has been shown to have good penetration into brain abscess cavities [10, 22]. However, because of its side effect profile, lack of available oral formulation, and because positive cultures from abscess fluid persist in many cases despite adequate drug concentrations (it is bacteriostatic against *Bacteroides fragilis* [23]), it has fallen out of favor as a first line therapy [10].

In spite of relatively poor CSF penetration, high-dose penicillin G (>24 million units daily in adults) has been found to reach therapeutic concentrations within brain abscess pus [24]. One study, however, found that after a 1-h in vitro incubation within brain abscess pus, in some cases, greater than 90% of the drug was inactivated [25]. There is limited and conflicting data regarding the penetration of the semi-synthetic penicillins (methicillin, oxacillin and nafcillin) into abscess fluid. One study showed that methicillin was detectable in brain abscess pus after standard dosing, but nafcillin was not [22]. However, there are no data to suggest that these drugs should not be used to treat brain abscess when the organisms are susceptible. In patients with staphylococci who are allergic to penicillin, or in cases when the organism is resistant to methicillin, vancomycin should be used [26].

Experiences with linezolid in the treatment of brain abscess are limited as this drug does not have an indication for CNS infections. However, it has been shown to penetrate into the brain and has been used successfully to treat brain abscess due to *Capnocytophaga* spp. [27], *Nocardia* spp. [28], and *Peptostreptococcus* spp. [29]. At the time of this writing, there have been no reports of daptomycin use for brain abscess.

First generation cephalosporins do not have good CNS penetration and should therefore not be used to treat patients with brain abscess. Third generation cephalosporins, however, have excellent CSF penetration and many of the drugs are active against most of the organisms that cause both meningitis and brain abscess. While cefotaxime, ceftizoxime, ceftriaxone and ceftazidime all have good CSF penetration, activity within a brain abscess cavity cannot be inferred. Cefotaxime has been shown to penetrate into brain abscess cavities at therapeutic levels, and it is active against many of the bacteria that cause brain abscess [30]. When used for this purpose, cefotaxime should be given at high dose (3 g IV q8), in combination with metronidazole. This regimen has been shown to be an effective combination for the treatment of brain abscess [30, 31]. Ceftazidime has been shown in one study to have good penetration into brain abscess cavities, with high enough levels for bactericidal activity against most pathogens including streptococci [32]. There are limited data for ceftriaxone and ceftizoxime, but they have been used successfully in the treatment of brain abscess in small numbers of patients [1].

Metronidazole is one of the standard drugs used in the treatment of brain abscess. It has excellent and reproducible penetration into brain abscess pus and it is bactericidal against *Bacteroides fragilis*. Metronidazole is useful only for treating strict anaerobes, and therefore must be used in combination with another agent that has activity against both aerotolerant anaerobes and microaerophilic streptococci, since these organisms are resistant to metronidazole [33]. Side effects including CNS toxicity (seizures, increased somnolence, and/or peripheral neuropathy) are more frequent in patients with hepatic insufficiency and may make it difficult to distinguish drug side effects from clinical deterioration due to the underlying infection.

Imipenem has a broad antimicrobial spectrum and has been used successfully in the treatment of brain abscess [34, 35]. However, because this drug has been known to induce seizures [36], it is usually reserved for CNS infections due to resistant pathogens [1]. Meropenem is a carbapenem with a similar antimicrobial spectrum to imipenem, but may have fewer CNS side effects.

In addition to having good CNS penetration, the quinolones have excellent activity against Gram-negative facultative anaerobes (including the Enterobacteriaceae and *Pseudomonas* spp.). However, quinolones have been shown to lower the seizure threshold.

Until recently, amphotericin B was the mainstay of therapy for brain abscess due to *Candida* spp., *Aspergillus* spp. and mucormycosis. It has poor penetration into the CNS and requires doses as high as 0.8–1.5 mg/kg/day in patients known to have brain abscess [37]. Since most patients with fungal brain abscess require 3 g or more of amphotericin, concern arises over renal toxicity. Some of the newer amphotericin B formulations may be less likely to result in renal toxicity and therefore may be preferable to traditional amphotericin in patients with fungal brain abscess. Voriconazole is a newer azole that has activity against *Aspergillus* species, CNS penetration and demonstrated superiority in invasive aspergillosis compared to amphotericin B [38]. Caspofungin is an echinocandin antifungal indicated for treatment of infections due to *Aspergillus* and *Candida* species. It is dosed at 70 mg IV on the first day as a loading dose, followed by 50 mg IV qd. It penetrates into the CNS and may be preferable to amphotericin B for long-term treatment because it does not cause renal toxicity [39]. Caspofungin does not have activity against the fungi of mucormycosis.

The definitive duration of antimicrobial therapy for brain abscess is unknown. In clinical series of bacterial brain abscess, most authors advocate a 6–8 week course of intravenous antibiotics directed at the pathogen(s) cultured from abscess pus post-drainage. Thus, if adequate surgical drainage is achieved, 6–8 weeks of intravenous therapy is likely to be sufficient. Other investigators believe that intravenous courses as short as 3 weeks may be adequate [30]. In most cases, decisions regarding duration should be individualized and based on the patient's response to therapy (both clinically and radiographically), the susceptibilities of the organism(s) to the chosen antimicrobial agent and the adequacy of surgical drainage. It is unclear whether oral antibiotics upon completion of an intravenous course are necessary; however, an additional 2–3 month course of oral antibiotics (given upon completion of the 6–8 weeks of intravenous therapy) has been suggested in order to prevent relapse [1].

Patients with fungal brain abscess may require a much longer course of therapy. As part of routine follow-up, patients should have both clinical examinations and radiographic (head CT or brain MRI) scans on a monthly or bimonthly basis, in order to document resolution of the abscess.

23.9 Adjunctive Agents

The question of whether corticosteroids are useful as adjunctive therapy in patients with brain abscess has not been evaluated by controlled clinical trials. Studies using corticosteroids in animal models of brain abscess have had conflicting results [1]. A short course of high-dose corticosteroid therapy (given po or iv at 100 mg q 6 h, which is rapidly tapered over 5–7 days) for patients with increased intracranial pressure and/or impending herniation may be beneficial [1]. However, studies indicate that prolonged use of corticosteroids should probably not be used since they have been shown in some cases to decrease penetration of antibiotics into the abscess cavity or interfere with microbial clearance [1]. In spite of these findings, clinical series with relatively large numbers of patients have shown no significant difference in outcome in those patients who received corticosteroids over those patients who did not [1, 10, 18]. While corticosteroids may be beneficial in certain circumstances, their use should be determined on a case-by-case basis.

It has been recommended that anticonvulsant medications be given to patients, even with no previous history of seizures, as prophylaxis during treatment of brain abscess and continuing for at least 3 months post-surgery [1]. After 3 months, the decision regarding whether to continue the anticonvulsants should be based on the results of a neurological evaluation. It is recommended that a few months after completion of antimicrobial therapy, patients undergo an electroencephalogram. If the result is normal, discontinuation of anticonvulsant therapy can be considered [1]. If the electro-encephalogram is abnormal, the medication should probably be continued [1].

23.10 Outcomes and Sequelae

The outcome of untreated bacterial abscess is usually death. In general, morbidity and mortality vary with location, degree of encapsulation, site of original infection, presence of complications and number of abscesses. In the literature, mortality has ranged from 35 % to 55 %, with the highest rate occurring among lesions associated with pulmonary infections [40]. In a study from Switzerland, the overall mortality rate was only 4 % [41]. This lower rate of mortality was attributed to CT-guided stereotactic aspiration and early treatment. In a study of patients with brain abscess requiring admission to the ICU that spanned from 1980 to 1999, the overall death rate was 26 % [13]. The authors did note a significant improvement in mortality with time, from more than 30 % in 1980 – 1992 falling to 8 % in 1993 – 1999 [13]. Interestingly, stereotactic brain biopsy was available as of the early 1980s and the rate of open surgical treatment did not change during the study period. The authors could pinpoint no clear reason for the improvement in prognosis seen with time [13].

Some complications of brain abscess result in worse outcomes, perhaps the most ominous of which is rupture of the brain abscess into the ventricular space. Patients typically present with sudden worsening of a preexisting headache accompanied by meningismus. This complication is usually fatal. If death is not immediate, neurosurgical intervention is warranted.

In a study by Seydoux and Francioli, sequelae of brain abscesses occurred in 44 % of patients [11]. The only factor that influenced reduction in sequelae was the clinical presentation at admission. The sequelae of brain abscess include recurrence of brain abscess, new brain abscess formation, residual focal neurological deficits and recurrent seizures. In a study of patients requiring intensive care, 36 % had long-term adverse neurological outcomes; 20 % had motor or sensory deficits, 15 % had cognitive impairment, and 7 % had seizures [13]. In this study, patients who were admitted to the ICU earlier in the hospitalization had better neurological function and better survival. Glasgow Coma scale score on admission to the ICU of ≤ 9 (indicating poor neurological function) was an independent predictor of in-hospital mortality in this series [13]. For recommendations on seizure prophylaxis and treatment see above section on treatment.

23.11 Summary

Major advances in diagnostic and therapeutic strategies have enhanced the management of brain abscess over the past 25 years. Coordinated, strategic care among neuroradiologists, neurosurgeons, infectious disease specialists and ICU physicians is recommended to optimize tailored short- and long-term care of patients with brain abscess.

Acknowledgements. The authors thank Dr. Sameer Pandit for providing the neuroimaging studies and radiographic interpretations of multiple brain abscesses.

References

1. Mathisen GE, Johnson JP (1997). Brain abscess. Clin Infect Dis 25:763
2. Tekkok IH, Erbegni A (1992) Management of brain abscess in children: review of 130 cases over a period of 21 years. Child Nerv Syst 8:411 – 6
3. Yang SY, Zhao CS (1993) Review of 140 patients with brain abscess. Surg Neurol 39:290 – 6
4. Xiao F, Tseng M, Teng L, et al. (2005) Brain abscess: clinical experience and analysis of prognostic factors. Surg Neurol 63:442 – 50
5. Mamelak AN, Mampalam TJ, Obana WG, et al. (1995) Improved management of multiple brain abscesses: a combined surgical and medical approach. Neurosurgery 36: 76 – 85
6. Nicolosi A, Hauser WA, Musicco M, et al. (1991) Incidence and prognosis of brain abscess in a defined population: Olmsted county, Minnesota, 1935 – 1981. Neuroepidemiology 10:122 – 31
7. Calfee DP, Wispelwey B (2000) Brain abscess. Semin Neurol 20:353 – 60
8. Britt RH, Enzmann DR (1983) Clinical stages of human brain abscesses on serial CT scans after contrast infusion. J Neurosurg 59:972
9. Britt RH, Enzmann DR, Yeager AS (1981) Neuropathological and computerized tomographic findings in experimental brain abscess. J Neurosurg 55:590
10. Chun CH, Johnson JD, Hofstetter M, et al. (1986) Brain abscess – a study of 45 consecutive cases. Medicine (Baltimore) 65:415
11. Seydoux C, Francioli P (1992) Bacterial brain abscesses: factors influencing mortality and sequelae. Clin Infect Dis 15:394
12. Mathiesen GE, Meyer RD, George WL, et al. (1984) Brain abscess and cerebritis. Rev Infect Dis 6(Suppl 1):S101
13. Tattevin P, Bruneel F, Clair B, et al. (2003) Bacterial brain abscesses: A retrospective study of 94 patients admitted to an intensive care unit 1980 – 1999. Am J Med (115):143 – 6
14. Kagawa M, Takeshita M, Yato S, et al. (1983) Brain abscess in congenital cyanotic heart disease. J Neurosurg 58:913
15. Chappell ET, Guthrie BL, Orenstein J (1992) The role of stereotactic biopsy in the management of HIV-related focal brain lesions. Neurosurgery 30(6):825 – 9
16. Kastrup O, Wanke I, Maschke M (2005) Neuroimaging of infections. NeuroRx 2:324 – 32
17. Skiest DJ, Erdman W, Chang WE, et al. (2000) SPECT thallium-210 combined with toxoplasma serology for the pre-

sumptive diagnosis of focal central nervous system mass lesions in patients with AIDS. J Infect 40:274–81
18. De Louvois J, Gortvai P, Hurley R (1977) Bacteriology of abscesses of the central nervous system: a multicentre prospective study. BMJ 2:981
19. Lakshmi V, Rao RR, Dinakar I (1993) Bacteriology of brain abscess – observations on 50 cases. J Med Microbiol 38:187
20. Barsoum AH, Lewis HC, Cannillo KL (1981) Non-operative treatment of multiple brain abscesses. Surg Neurol 16:283
21. Kramer PW, Griffith RS, Campbell RL (1969) Antibiotic penetration of the brain: a comparative study. J Neurosurg 31:295
22. Black P, Graybill JR, Charache P (1973) Penetration of brain abscess by systemically administered antibiotics. J Neurosurg 38:705
23. Ingham HR, Selkon JB, Roxby CM (1977) Bacteriological study of otogenic cerebral abscess: Chemotherapeutic role of metronidazole. BMJ 2:991
24. De Louvois J, Gortvai P, Hurley R (1977) Antibiotic treatment of abscesses of the central nervous system. BMJ 2:985
25. Picardi JL, Lewis HP, Tan JS, et al. (1975) Clindamycin concentrations in the central nervous system of primates before and after head trauma. J Neurosurg 43:717
26. Ogg G, Lynn WA, Peters M, et al. (1997) Cerebral nocardia abscesses in a patient with AIDS: correlation of magnetic resonance and white cell scanning images with neuropathological findings. Case Reports 311:3
27. Sabbatani S, Manfredi R, Frank G, et al. (2004) *Capnocytophaga* spp. Brain abscess in an immunocompetent host: problems in antimicrobial chemotherapy and literature review. J Chemother 16(5):497–501
28. Vigano SM, Edefonti A, Ferraresso J, et al. (2005) Successful medical treatment of multiple brain abscesses due to *Nocardia farcinica* in a paediatric renal transplant recipient. Pediatr Nephrol 20(8):1186–8
29. Salin F, Vianello F, Manara R, et al. (2006) Linezoloid in the treatment of brain abscess due to *Peptostreptococcus*. Scand J Infect Dis 38(3):203–5
30. Sjolin J, Lilja A, Eriksson N, Arneborn P, et al. (1993) Treatment of brain abscess with cefotaxime and metronidazole: prospective study on 15 consecutive patients. Clin Infect Dis 17:857
31. Gomez J, Poza M, Martinez M, et al. (1995) Use of cefotaxime and metronidazole for treating cerebral abscesses. Clin Infect Dis [letter] 21:708
32. Green HT, O'Donoghue MAT, Shaw MDM, et al. (1989) Penetration of ceftazidime into intracranial abscess. J Antimicrob Chemother 24:431
33. Ingham HR, Selkon JB (1982) Metronidazole and brain abscess. Lancet [letter] 2:613
34. Asensi V, Carton JA, Maradona JA, et al. (1996) Therapy of brain abscess with imipenem – a safe therapeutic choice? J Antimicrob Chemother 37:200
35. Asensi V, Carton JA, Maradona JA, et al. (1996) Imipenem therapy of brain abscesses. Eur J Clin Microbiol Infect Dis 15:653
36. Wong VK, Wright HT Jr, Ross LA, et al. (1991) Imipenem/cilastin treatment of bacterial meningitis in children. Pediatr Infect Dis 10:122
37. Denning DW, Stevens DA (1990) Antifungal and surgical treatment of invasive aspergillosis: Review of 2,121 published cases. Rev Inf Dis 12:1147–1201
38. Schwartz S, Thiel E (2003) CNS-aspergillosis: are there new treatment options? Mycoses 46 Suppl 2:8–14
39. Hagansee ME, Bauwens JE, Kjos B, et al. (1994) Brain abscess following marrow transplantation: experience at the Fred Hutchinson Cancer Research Center, 1984–1992. Clin Infect Dis 19:402–8
40. Loeser E Jr, Scheinberg L (1957) Brain abscesses: A review of ninety-nine cases. Neurology 7:601
41. Hasdemir MG, Ebeling U (1999) CT-guided stereotactic aspiration and treatment of brain abscesses. Acta Neurochir 125:58

24 Falciparum Malaria

C. Feldman, G.A. Richards

24.1 Introduction

Malaria is one of the most common infectious diseases in the world today, being the most important parasitic infection, and *Plasmodium falciparum* is the organism responsible for most of the mortality [1]. It has been estimated that approximately 300–500 million people contract malaria every year, with approximately 1–2 million deaths, most of these occurring in children [1–5]. *Plasmodium falciparum, Mycobacterium tuberculosis* and measles currently compete for the title of the single most important pathogen causing human morbidity and mortality [2, 3]. Infection with *Plasmodium falciparum* has a wide variety of potential clinical consequences [4, 6, 7].

Factors that may influence presentation include the age of the patient, their degree of immunity to the parasite and the duration of infection [7]. In holo- or hyperendemic areas, most adults and older children are partially immune and the disease burden is mainly in children in the first few years of life [7, 8]. The greatest mortality is between the ages of 1 and 3 years [7]. Parasitization may be almost universal in this age group and effects range from an asymptomatic infection, to a febrile illness, or even life-threatening disease [8]. In areas of low endemicity, severe malaria occurs in both adults and children and non-immune travelers and migrant workers are also vulnerable [7]. In adults infected with falciparum malaria for the first time, the range of clinical syndromes is wide and may include specific and multi-organ failure [8].

24.2 The Organism

Malaria is a protozoal disease caused by several species of *Plasmodium* which are spread by mosquitoes of the genus *Anopheles* [4]. *Plasmodium falciparum* is one of the four species of *Plasmodium* causing human infection. The period from inoculation to the appearance of parasitemia (prepatent period) is usually 9–13 days for *P. falciparum*, but may be longer, particularly in those who have been on ineffective prophylaxis [4]. During feeding the female mosquito injects saliva, within which malaria sporozoites are carried, into the skin. Within minutes the sporozoites penetrate into hepatocytes and produce tissue schizonts (also known as meronts). After 5–7 days, each tissue schizont has produced 30,000 daughter merozoites that enter the circulation, invade erythrocytes and form ring trophozoites [4]. Using hemoglobin as energy, development occurs after 48 h into late trophozoites (larger and lacier in appearance), early blood schizonts (division begins) and then mature schizonts [4]. The erythrocytes then lyse and merozoites are released into the circulation to invade other red blood cells [4]. In non-immune individuals, the process is amplified 20-fold with each cycle. When parasitemia reaches 10–15 trophozoites per microliter, it is detectable on thick blood films, ending the prepatent period [4]. After several cycles, some trophozoites differentiate into sex cells or gametocytes, which are infectious to the mosquito. The gametocyte of *P. falciparum* is characteristically banana-shaped. If male and female gametocytes are taken up by the mosquito, they mate, migrate through the midgut wall and form an oocyst which eventually leads to the release of about 1,000 sporozoites after 5–8 days [4]. These invade the salivary glands of the mosquito to complete the cycle at the next blood meal [4].

The time from first inoculation to first symptoms is the incubation period [4]. Its length depends on the patient's immune status and is usually 1–2 days longer than the prepatent period. In non-immune patients, symptoms may occur even before parasitemia is present. The other extreme is premunition where partial immunity is associated with asymptomatic parasitemia [4].

24.3 Epidemiology

Malaria persists in those parts of the world where the population of anopheline mosquitoes as well as the infected human population remain above the critical density required for sustained transmission. Approximately 40% of the world's population is at risk of acquiring malaria, resulting in those 300–500 million cases annually [4]. In Africa alone approximately 200 million cases occur every year, with a mortality of about one million. In rural Africa one in 20 children die from malaria before the age of 5 years [4]. Compounding the problem of malaria control in the developing world is the presence of drug resistance, and resistance of mosquitoes to insecticides [4].

Malaria also afflicts individuals in Southeast Asia, Latin America and South America. In 1992 approximately 75% of malarial infections were acquired in Africa, 17% in Asia, 4% in Central America and the Caribbean and 1% each in South America, North America, and Oceania [4]. In developed countries such as the United States, malaria largely occurs as a result of importation from other countries in the blood of immigrants, visitors, military personnel and occasionally also from importation of infected mosquitoes [4].

Recently there has been renewed interest in epidemiological aspects of falciparum malaria [9]. It is recognized that there are clear-cut distinctions between severe and non-severe disease and between the different forms of severe disease [10]. An important question is why *Plasmodium falciparum* causes severe infection in some, but not all, patients. This relates partly to the age of the patient, history of prior exposure to the parasite and various aspects of the hosts' immune response [7–11]. Most interestingly, it is now recognized that many of the differences in response may relate to diversity or polymorphisms in both the host and the parasite, which may impact on disease pathogenesis and be the major determinants of the outcome of a malarial infection [8–10, 12–16]. For example, in the host, possession of hemoglobin AS genotype influences the risk of both cerebral malaria and severe anemia [9], whereas possession of certain HLA genotypes (e.g., HLA-B53) may be linked to resistance to these two complications [12, 13]. Susceptibility to both these complications is linked to polymorphism in the promoter sequence for the tumor necrosis factor (TNF) gene [15, 16], whereas susceptibility to each of these complications individually is influenced by mutations at other sites [9]. Also, different strains of *P. falciparum* have been shown to vary in their ability to induce production of host TNF, and this may determine the clinical severity of the infection [14]. In addition, clonal phenotypic variation with antigenic switching is linked to, and may alter, adhesive properties of the parasite and this may be an important mechanism of immune evasion [8]. Finally, specific adhesive and linked antigenic types may be associated with severe infection [1, 8]. One of the best studied genetic markers associated with *P. falciparum* virulence is the erythrocyte membrane-protein-1 family that is responsible for antigenic variation and cytoadherence of parasitized erythrocytes to endothelial and placental syncytiotrophoblast cells. Parasites causing severe malaria express a small subset of these proteins that differ from those expressed by parasites causing uncomplicated infection [1].

24.4 Severe Malaria

The salient manifestations of severe *P. falciparum* infection are shown in Table 24.1 [5]. There has been some debate in the literature about the definition of both severe malaria and cerebral malaria. A definition of cerebral malaria proposed by the World Health Organization (WHO) reads as follows "A clinical syndrome characterized by coma (inability to localize a painful stimulus) at least one hour after termination of a seizure or correction of hypoglycemia, detection of asexual forms of *P. falciparum* malaria parasites on peripheral blood smears, and exclusion of other causes of encephalopathy" [17, 18]. More recently, severe malaria has been recognized to be a complex multi-system disorder and to have many of the features in common with severe sepsis or a severe inflammatory response syndrome [19, 20]. Studies of outcome of patients with falciparum malaria in the intensive care unit (ICU) commonly report that markers of severity of illness (such as the SAPS or APACHE II score), shock, acidosis, coma, pulmonary edema and coagulation disorders are indicators of poor outcome [21]. The level of parasitemia has not consistently been shown to be a good predictor of outcome. Metabolic acidosis has long been recognized as a major predictor of, as well as a significant contributor to, death [6, 20]. Whereas lactate has been considered to be the major contributor to the acidosis, unidentified anions other than lactate have been shown, more recently, to be even more important [22]. Attempts to assess severity of infection objectively have included other markers, such as the procalcitonin level, which has shown some promise [23].

One other consideration with regard to severe infection, at least in certain areas of the world, is the potential interaction between malaria and human immunodeficiency virus (HIV) infection in those patients who

Table 24.1. Manifestations of severe *Plasmodium falciparum* infection

Cerebral malaria
Severe anemia
Acute renal failure
Pulmonary edema
Metabolic acidosis
Coagulation disturbances
Hypoglycemia
Hypotension
High severity of illness score (e.g., APACHE II, SAPS)

are co-infected [24–26]. On the one hand it has been suggested that this may be associated with increased HIV viral replication, viral genotypic heterogeneity and CD4 T-lymphocyte loss leading to accelerated decline in immune function, reduced survival and increased HIV transmission [25]. On the other hand studies have suggested that HIV infection may be significantly associated with the development of severe and complicated malaria [24], being associated with a high parasite burden with the associated risk that this may potentially lead to poor malaria control and a greater chance for the development of resistance to anti-malarial agents [26].

24.5 Pathogenesis of Severe Disease and Cerebral Malaria

The adhesive properties that the parasite confers on the host's erythrocytes appear to play a central role in malaria pathogenicity [27–29]. As the parasite grows in the red blood cells it induces the expression of surface ligands, as well as various endothelial receptors, that mediate adhesion to the endothelium of post-capillary venules, which results in sequestration of the parasite within the peripheral circulation [27, 28]. In addition, some isolates induce expression of receptors on non-infected red cells, leading to rosette formation, and still others induce expression of adhesion molecules on other parasitized cells causing auto-agglutination [27]. These phenomena can lead to reduced microcirculatory flow or even obstruction to local blood flow and/or cause local metabolic disturbances, such as the production of lactic acid, which may manifest as organ-specific dysfunction [27–30]. Multiple endothelial receptors have been recognized (reviewed elsewhere [30, 31]), and it has now been demonstrated that endothelial activation and leukocyte sequestration in the brain appear to be a feature of fatal malaria [27, 32].

A number of theories have been forwarded to more fully explain the mechanisms of cerebral malaria [3, 27–29, 33–40]. Initially it was assumed that it was simply a mechanical effect related to sludging of parasitized red blood cells within the vasculature, causing decreased cerebral perfusion with hypoxia [28]. Other theories have included altered microvascular permeability, secondary to malarial "toxins" or mediators such as kinins, causing cerebral edema, but this has largely been discounted [35]. Immunological mechanisms were considered following the detection of immune complexes and complement in affected brains [7, 34] and still others have investigated the possibility that disseminated intravascular coagulation (DIC) [34] or endotoxemia [36] may be involved.

Clarke and co-workers proposed the cytokine theory of human cerebral malaria [38–40]. They recognized that cytokines such as TNF and interleukin (IL)-l when overproduced could themselves cause clinical syndromes such as those seen in human malaria [38–40].

Many of these may simply be manifestations of a severe systemic inflammatory response syndrome. Products of schizogony have been shown to trigger release of TNF and IL-l and serum levels of these cytokines correlate with the severity of malaria infection, including the presence of cerebral symptoms [38–40]. The cytokine theory is also consistent with the concept of sequestration of parasites in the cerebral circulation in that schizogony could cause higher local levels of cytokines and their products [40].

Sequestration, however, may not be essential to the development of cerebral dysfunction according to the cytokine theory [40]. Cytokines themselves may alter cerebral function through the local generation of nitric oxide (NO), which may act as a vasodilator to increase intracranial pressure and which may also function as a false neurotransmitter [39, 40]. Cytokines, especially IFNγ, TNF, and lymphotoxins, and chemokine receptors are also said to be responsible for both blood-brain barrier alterations and biochemical changes that may also lead to parenchymal brain lesions [41]. It is also important to consider that septic encephalopathy may be a feature of any severe critical illness and may be indistinguishable clinically from cerebral malaria [42].

24.6 Laboratory Diagnosis of Malaria

For the laboratory diagnosis of malaria, thick and thin blood smears should be made according to standard procedures [4, 43]. Thick smears are 20–40 times more sensitive and should be used for screening. Thin smears fixed with methanol, to preserve erythrocyte morphology, and Giemsa stained allow speciation as well as determination of the level of parasitemia [4, 43]. Various clues to distinguish falciparum malaria on thin smear include the finding of small tight rings, appliqué forms and banana-shaped gametocytes.

Parasitemia should be quantified and counted on thin smears as parasites per 1,000 red blood cells corrected to percentage [4, 43]. After initiation of treatment, parasitemia should be followed regularly until resolution to confirm therapeutic efficacy. The time from initiation of treatment until thick smears are repeatedly negative is called the parasite clearance time. A number of newer techniques have been developed for the diagnosis of malaria including quantitative buffy coat methods, antigen detection, enzyme linked immunosorbent assay, polymerase chain reaction (PCR), including real time PCR, and indirect fluorescent antibody tests [4, 43–46].

24.7 Treatment of Severe and Complicated Malaria

If possible, patients with severe or cerebral malaria should be treated in an intensive care Unit (ICU) [6]. Treatment should be initiated as rapidly as possible, and should not necessarily await parasitological confirmation of the diagnosis if this is likely to be delayed [6]. Patients should be weighed in order to determine drug dosages accurately [6]. Careful fluid management is essential and may be aided by the placement of a central venous catheter and a urinary catheter. The importance of hypovolemia in severe malaria is well recognized, particularly in children, and early recognition and treatment may be associated with an improved outcome [47, 48]. However, care should be taken to avoid fluid overload with the possibility of precipitating pulmonary edema. In patients with severe hemodynamic instability, non-invasive cardiac output monitoring may be of value. A recent meta-analysis of exchange transfusion as adjunctive management of severe malaria concluded that there was no evidence of an increase in survival with its use [49]. However, the authors indicated that there were substantial problems with the comparability of the two treatment groups and suggested that only a randomized controlled trial would give definitive answers. Hyperpyrexia >38.5 °C should be treated with tepid sponging, fanning and a cooling blanket [6].

The drug treatment of severe or complicated malaria is shown in Table 24.2 [1, 4–7, 50, 51].

Chloroquine is only used in areas where the infection is definitively known to be sensitive to this agent. Parenteral antimalarial drugs are recommended initially in most cases, at least until there is clear evidence of clinical improvement and oral medication is able to be tolerated [4, 6, 7, 51].

Parenteral quinine is the drug of choice in most of the tropical world. In some countries, such as in the United States, quinidine may be the drug of choice. An intravenous loading dose of either agent is recommended to achieve therapeutic levels rapidly since most deaths occur within the first 48 h [4, 6, 7, 50–52]. A total of 7 days medication is required, which may be completed with oral quinine or quinidine.

Artemisinin and its derivatives, although not yet licensed in many areas, appear to be exciting new agents for the treatment of severe and multidrug-resistant malaria [53–71]. This group of drugs is being used more commonly and it has been suggested that these agents may be the drugs of choice for severe malaria because of their efficacy and safety [53–71]. Artesunate is water soluble and may be given intravenously or intramuscularly, while artemeter is oil-based and is given intramuscularly [61]. Both preparations come in suppository form and may be given rectally, which has also been shown to be effective in the treatment even of severe malaria [59–62]. However, there is growing concern about the development of resistance to these agents, which is already beginning to emerge [72–74]. This, together with the fact that these agents have a short half-life, has led to the recommendation that they always be

Table 24.2. The parenteral treatment of severe and complicated falciparum malaria

Drug	Regimen
Chloroquine[a]	Chloroquine 10 mg base/kg by constant infusion over 8 h followed by 15 mg base/kg over 24 h
Quinine (intravenous)	Quinine dihydrochloride salt 20 mg/kg intravenously in 200 ml 5% dextrose and/or saline over 4 h (loading dose) followed by quinine dihydrochloride salt 10 mg/kg infusion over 4 h every 8 h (maintenance dose) beginning 8 h after start of the loading dose, until patient can take oral medication
	ALTERNATIVE[b] Quinine dihydrochloride salt 7 mg/kg intravenously over 30 min (loading dose) followed immediately by 10 mg/kg infusion over 4 h repeated 8 hourly (maintenance dose) until patient can take oral medication
Quinidine (intravenous)	Quinidine base 15 mg/kg intravenously over 4 h (loading dose) followed by quinidine base 7.5 mg/kg over 4 h (maintenance dose) every 8 h beginning 8 h after start of loading dose, until patient can take oral medication
	ALTERNATIVE[b] Quinidine base 10 mg/kg intravenously over 1–2 h (loading dose) followed immediately by 0.02 mg/kg/min by infusion (maintenance dose) for 72 h or until patient can take oral medication[c]
Artemesinin derivatives	
Artesunate	2.4 mg/kg IVI or IM bolus initially followed by 1.2 mg/kg at 12 h and 24 h then 1.2 mg/kg daily for 5–7 days OR
Artemether	3.2 mg/kg IM initially followed by 1.6 mg/kg IM daily for 5–7 days

[a] For the parenteral treatment of severe malaria in cases of drug-sensitive infections; if any doubt treat as for resistant infections

[b] Alternative regimens suggested particularly in the ICU setting

[c] The same dosing regimen has also been reported for the quinidine salt [5]

given with another agent such as mefloquine, doxycycline or clindamycin, which may be associated not only with a better and/or more rapid cure of the infection, but also limit the development of resistance [5, 53, 63, 75].

Combination therapy with various drugs with different modes of action is increasingly being recommended for the treatment of malaria and a number of new combinations are at different stages of development [1, 75]. Additional drugs that are sometimes recommended as combination therapy with quinine include antibiotics such as the macrolides (e.g., azithromycin), doxycycline or clindamycin, which should be added particularly in areas of intense quinine resistance or where prolonged treatment with quinine would otherwise be necessary [50, 75]. Tetracyclines are contraindicated in pregnancy and childhood. Where initial response to therapy is poor, halofantrine or mefloquine have been recommended [6, 7]. Other agents that have been used in treatment of malaria, but which are now no longer recommended, include dexamethasone, mannitol, heparin and dextran [3, 6, 76, 77].

24.8 Cerebral Malaria

In many parts of the world cerebral malaria is said to be the most common clinical presentation of severe malaria in man, with a mortality in the region of 20%, or greater, and accounting for 80% of deaths [6, 7]. However, in some parts of Africa, anemia is a more common severe manifestation particularly in children. Patients fulfilling the criteria for cerebral malaria [3, 6, 17, 18] manifest features of a diffuse symmetrical encephalopathy.

In adults cerebral malaria tends to develop after several days of fever and other non-specific symptoms [3, 7]. In children it tends to be more acute in onset, usually after less than 2 days [3, 7]. It may start dramatically with a generalized convulsion followed by persistent unconsciousness. Post-ictal coma should resolve within 30 min, but coma due to cerebral malaria usually persists more than 24–72 h. The most common neurological picture of cerebral malaria is that of a bilateral symmetrical upper motor neuron lesion with increased muscle tone and reflexes [7].

Various forms of posturing may be observed, including decerebrate and decorticate rigidity [6, 7]. These may occur in hypoglycemic and normoglycemic patients. While neck rigidity and photophobia do not tend to occur, mild neck stiffness is not uncommon [3, 6, 7]. Neck retraction and opisthotonus may, however, occur in both adults and children [7]. Corneal and eyelash reflexes and papillary responses are usually normal in adults, but disorders of conjugate gaze are common [6, 7]. The gag reflex is usually maintained but abdominal reflexes are invariably absent. This latter may be a valuable clinical sign [6, 7]. Papilledema is not a feature of cerebral malaria, probably reflecting the fact that raised intracranial pressure is not found in the majority of patients early in the course of the illness [6, 7, 78]. Forcible jaw closure and bruxism are common [6, 7].

Studies in children recovering from cerebral malaria have shown neurological sequelae in approximately 10% or more of cases and these occur especially with infections that were complicated by hypoglycemia [3, 7]. Hemiplegia, cortical blindness, behavior disturbances, cranial nerve lesions, extrapyramidal tremor, polyneuropathy, mononeuritis multiplex, Guillain-Barre syndrome, and prolonged coma have all been described as neurological sequelae of patients with cerebral malaria [3, 7].

The APACHE II severity of illness scoring index has been used to predict the mortality of patients with cerebral malaria. In one study, a cut-off of 24 stratified patient mortality with an accuracy of >95%. In that study, high APACHE II score, deep unconsciousness, acute renal failure and acidemia were identified as poor prognostic factors [79].

24.9 Convulsions

Convulsions may occur in as many as 50% of cases of cerebral malaria and are more common in children [6]. In children it may be difficult to differentiate febrile convulsions from those due to cerebral malaria and the possibility that they may be related to hypoglycemia should also always be considered [6]. Convulsions are usually generalized, but other types, including focal seizures, may occur [6]. Generalized convulsions appear to impact negatively on the outcome.

The role of prophylactic anticonvulsants in patients with cerebral malaria is under investigation. Once seizures occur they should be managed in the usual way [6, 80]. Treatment is initially with lorazepam 0.1 mg/kg or midazolam 0.2 mg/kg intravenously, together with maintenance of the airway and appropriate cooling of the patient [6, 80]. Studies of generalized convulsive status epilepticus have suggested that 0.1 mg/kg lorazepam, or 15 mg/kg phenobarbital, or diazepam 0.15 mg/kg followed by 18 mg/kg phenytoin, are all acceptable initial treatment regimens; however most people would treat status with lorazepam initially followed by midazolam (0.2 mg/kg then infusion at 0.1 mg/kg/h) or propofol (5 mg/kg then infusion at 30 μg/kg/min) if not successful [80].

24.10 Severe Anemia

The occurrence of anemia is invariable in patients with severe falciparum malaria [6, 7].

It is due to hemolysis of parasitized red blood cells, shortened survival of unparasitized cells and bone marrow dysfunction [6]. Certain red cell enzyme defects, such as G6PD deficiency, may increase susceptibility to antimalarial induced oxidant-mediated hemolysis. Coombs positive hemolytic anemia and microangiopathic hemolytic anemia also occur [6]. It is recommended that patients should be transfused if the hematocrit falls below 20% [6]. Specific clotting factors should be administered as needed [6]. Transfusions should be carefully monitored to prevent fluid overload with its associated complications and in some patients low dose loop diuretics (e.g., furosemide 20 mg) may be administered during the transfusion to prevent its occurrence [6].

24.11 Blackwater Fever

This was previously described as the occurrence of unusually severe intravascular hemolysis with other severe manifestations of falciparum malaria, including renal failure, hypotension and coma, despite relatively low levels of parasitemia [6, 7]. The condition was attributed to some form of immunological response to quinine or one of the other anti-malarial agents, but it is also possible that it may have represented unrecognized G6PD deficiency [6, 7]. No special treatment of hemoglobinuria is currently recommended, although alkalinization of the urine may be desirable [6].

24.12 Renal Failure

Some degree of renal dysfunction, as manifested by a raised serum creatinine, is common in patients with severe falciparum malaria [81, 82]. This may be related to hypovolemia and blackwater fever, but more commonly occurs in association with severe malaria in which the mechanism is said to be a reduction in renal capillary blood flow [6].

A variety of glomerular lesions have been described; however the clinical course of all three forms of renal failure is usually that of acute tubular necrosis [6, 7, 82]. The management is similar to that of renal failure in other critical care settings [83, 84]. Attention should be given to fluid status, electrolytes and acid-base balance. If there is anuria or oliguria after fluid replacement, increasing intravenous doses of furosemide should be given in an attempt to increase urine output [6]. Whereas the absolute indications for dialysis are similar to those of other situations and include severe hyperkalemia, fluid overload, metabolic acidosis and uremia, continuous dialysis should be initiated early, prior to the development of fluid overload, and not be dictated by an arbitrary metabolic parameter such as creatinine [6, 83, 84].

It has been recommended that the doses of antimalarials should be reduced in patients with renal failure [6]. This was based on the observation of high plasma concentrations of quinine in patients with renal failure. However, this was probably due to impaired hepatic clearance as a consequence of severe infection, rather than impaired renal clearance, which has not been documented to occur even in patients with moderately elevated serum creatinine levels [6]. A suggested dosing regimen is as follows: initial dose 20 mg/kg of intravenous quinine dihydrochloride (salt) over 4 h followed by 10 mg/kg every 8 h [6]. The infusion volume may be reduced to 50–100 ml of 5% dextrose. After the second day the dose should be reduced to 5 mg/kg eight hourly [6].

Hemodialysis removes quinine and in this situation the dose should remain 10 mg/kg every 8 h [6]. There does not appear to be a need to alter the dose of chloroquine in patients in renal failure, even in those on hemodialysis [6].

24.13 Pulmonary Edema

This is a particularly serious consequence of severe falciparum malaria and is often fatal [6, 7]. It is similar in most respects to the acute respiratory distress syndrome (ARDS), and hyperparasitemia (>10%) and pregnancy are important predisposing factors [6]. The pathogenesis is not entirely clear, but as it is associated with a normal/low pulmonary capillary wedge pressure it is most likely due to an increase in pulmonary capillary permeability, as occurs with ARDS [6, 7]. The first indication of the onset of this condition is an increase in the respiratory rate, which precedes the development of any of the other chest signs [6, 7]. Careful fluid management is the cornerstone of the prevention and management [6]. Hemodynamic monitoring by means of a central venous catheter or a non-invasive cardiac output monitor may aid in management of fluid status.

24.14 Metabolic Acidosis

Metabolic acidosis is common in patients with pulmonary edema, although it may also occur in its absence [6]. The mechanism is not entirely certain and it may occur even in the absence of significant hypoxia or hypoperfusion [6]. It appears to be due to tissue hypoxia as a consequence of stagnant flow of parasitized red blood cells through capillary beds [6]. Other factors may include impaired hepatic blood flow (a site of lactate disposal) and high cytokine levels (TNF leads to lactate production) [6]. In addition, the malaria parasite itself produces large amounts of lactate as a by-product of glycolysis. The possible important role of unidentified anions other than lactate has been described above [22]. The acidosis of severe bacterial sepsis appears to involve peroxynitrite induced mitochondrial dysfunction and it is possible that a similar mechanism is involved with severe malaria [85]. Therapy should include correction of hypotension and hypoxemia, if present [6]. Whether correction of an acidosis improves outcome is not known. It should only be corrected if the pH falls below 7.15, if at all, since infusion may worsen pulmonary edema due to the large sodium load [6]. The prognosis of patients with severe lactic acidosis is poor [6].

24.15 Hyperthermia

Progressively increasing body temperature may be associated with convulsions, delirium and coma [6]. High fever increases metabolic demand, which may further compromise tissues damaged by stagnant capillary blood flow [6]. Heat stroke may be associated with permanent neurological sequelae [6]. Patients with cerebral malaria often improve with a decrease in the temperature, which may be achieved by tepid sponging, fanning and cooling blankets [6].

24.16 Coagulation Disturbances

While thrombocytopenia is very common in severe falciparum malaria, in most cases it does not appear to be an indicator of disseminated intravascular coagulation as it usually occurs in the setting of normal coagulation and without evidence of bleeding [6, 7]. It appears that the previous concerns of an important pathogenic role for DIC in severe falciparum malaria were exaggerated and that full blown DIC with bleeding probably only occurs in 5% or less of patients with severe malaria [6, 7].

24.17 Hyperparasitemia

Patients with a blood parasitemia of > 10% were previously said to be at increased risk for the complications of severe malaria, which was said to be proportionate to the degree of parasitemia [6]. It was further recommended that patients with hyperparasitemia should have an exchange blood transfusion [6, 86]. This recommendation was not based on large prospective randomized studies, but followed individual case reports and is confounded in some cases by patients with malaria with higher levels of parasitemia who recover without transfusion and in others by the fact that total parasite burden may not be reflected in the peripheral smear [4, 6, 86]. In addition, as described above, a recent meta-analysis of exchange transfusion in the literature, while acknowledging problems with the studies reviewed, concluded that there was no evidence, in general, of its benefit [49]. It has also been noted that facilities for full exchange transfusions (6–8 units of blood) are often not widely available, although in these situations it was previously suggested that partial exchange transfusion (e.g., 4 units) could be undertaken [3, 6].

24.18 Hepatic Dysfunction

While abnormalities in "liver function tests" are quite common in patients with severe malaria, true hepatic dysfunction is uncommon and if present is mild [6]. Raised bilirubin levels are often noted and are mostly due to hemolysis [6]. Raised serum levels of aspartate aminotransaminase may also be associated with hemolysis. Occasional patients with severe falciparum malaria do, however, have marked jaundice with raised serum levels of both aspartate and alanine aminotransferases in addition to prolonged prothrombin time [6]. These patients may have true hepatic dysfunction contributed to by hemolysis and DIC [6].

24.19 Hypoglycemia

Hypoglycemia is a commonly reported complication in severe malaria [6, 7]. It occurs in two situations in particular [6, 7, 87]. Firstly it may occur in pregnant women, where in addition to neurological sequelae it may also cause fetal distress [6, 7]. Unless it has been prolonged and very severe it is associated with a good prognosis and responds well to glucose administration. Secondly, hypoglycemia may occur in severely ill patients and be associated with severe anemia, jaundice, hyperparasitemia, lactic acidosis and coma [6, 7]. Quinine-induced stimulation of insulin release may be an important mechanism, but other factors, including glucose consumption by the parasite, may be contributory [6, 7, 87]. Other mechanisms that have been considered as possible causes of hypoglycemia include depleted hepatic glycogen stores and inhibition of hepatic gluconeogenesis [7]. Many of the usual clinical features of hypoglycemia are absent, or are masked by, or interpreted as the symptoms of malaria, but whenever the level of consciousness deteriorates in patients with malaria, hypoglycemia should be suspected [6, 7, 87]. Glucose requirements may be high and infusions of 50% glucose followed by 10–20% glucose, preferably through a central venous catheter, may be required to maintain adequate blood levels [6].

24.20 Bacteremia/Septicemia

Gram-negative microorganisms are frequently cultured from the blood of patients with severe malaria [6, 7]. While there is often no apparent source for these organisms it is possible that they may arise via translocation through ischemic bowel. In addition these patients often have central venous and urinary catheters in place [6, 7]. The manifestations of bacteremia vary from asymptomatic to severe sepsis with shock [6]. One study has shown a high incidence of bacterial infection in patients with falciparum malaria presenting in shock [88]. The previously described "algid malaria" is very reminiscent of Gram-negative sepsis and it has been suggested that they may represent one and the same condition [6, 7]. Many authorities recommend both conventional antibiotics and antimalarial agents in the initial therapy of patients with severe malaria [6].

24.21 Gastrointestinal Bleeding

This complication has been noted particularly in patients who have been given high-dose corticosteroids, and is thought to be due to gastric erosion [3, 6, 76]. It should be treated in the usual way together with the infusion of fresh blood [6].

24.22 Aspiration Pneumonia

This complication may occur in any patient with a decreased level of consciousness and is particularly common in severe malaria since these patients often vomit [6]. The latter may be associated with convulsions or be due to anti-malarial agents. Antiemetics may be given but their efficacy has not been consistently demonstrated [6].

24.23 Special Considerations in Pregnancy

Falciparum malaria is a particularly dangerous disease in pregnancy, especially during the second and third trimester [6]. The mortality of cerebral malaria is approximately 40% in pregnant women and both mother and fetus may die despite aggressive treatment [4, 6]. Pregnant women are at particular risk of hypoglycemia and pulmonary edema [4, 6]. The exact mechanism by which pregnancy enhances the susceptibility to, and the risk of, complicated disease is not certain. However, red cells containing mature forms of the asexual parasites are found in the placenta, being a key feature of maternal infection with *P. falciparum*, and are associated with significant compromise of placental function [6, 89]. Placental parasites express different surface ligands that facilitate immune evasion and their adhesion to specific placental molecules [89]. Treatment should start immediately and the potential teratogenic or abortifacient properties of quinine and chloroquine in this severe situation should be ignored and in any case are considered by many authorities to have been largely exaggerated [4, 6, 7, 90]. Blood glucose levels should be measured frequently and, where possible, fetal monitoring should be undertaken [6]. Some clinicians favor cesarian section or induction of labor if the fetus is viable [6].

24.24 Special Considerations in Children

Children tend to have a shorter disease course and progress much more rapidly than adults to severe malaria [4]. Hypoglycemia, seizures, severe anemia and sudden death are more common, whereas renal failure, pulmonary edema and jaundice are less likely than in adults [4, 6, 7]. Although respiratory distress does not appear in the original WHO definition of severe malaria, it is recognized by clinicians treating children with malaria as an important sign which is not usually due to pulmonary edema or ARDS [91–93]. It has also been termed the malaria hyperpneic syndrome [91]. Possible causes include cardiac failure, coexistent pneumonia, direct sequestration of parasites in the lungs, or a sign of cerebral malaria [93]. It is important to remember that the clinical features of pneumonia and malaria, both common causes of childhood morbidity and mortality in the developing world, overlap considerably and many children fulfilling the WHO criteria for pneumonia may actually have malaria [9, 94]. The majority of cases of respiratory distress in children are associated with lactic acidosis and this is well documented as a poor prognostic factor [93, 95]. After cerebral malaria, 9–26% of children may have neurologic sequelae of which half will resolve completely [3, 4, 96]. Hypoglycemic children are at greater risk of neurologic sequelae and/or death [4]. It is important to remember in the treatment of children with malaria that drug dosages need to be modified [4].

24.25 Conclusions

The enormous cost in lives, as well as the cost of treatment, makes malaria a considerable socioeconomic burden. Control of the disease through control of parasite and insect vectors has become largely ineffective due to mosquito and parasite mutation with subsequent development of resistance, together with a change in the social behavior of the host [97]. The need for effective control measures has never been greater [97–99]. Measures to achieve this should include prevention, such as insecticide impregnated bednets and mosquito repellents as well as targeted chemoprophylaxis, and provision of easy access to early treatment once infection occurs [97, 98, 100].

Measures for the future include the possibility of a vaccine which could be anti-parasite or even anti-disease, a variety of which are currently being tested [101–109]. However, a recent Cochrane meta-analysis [110] of some of the studies of currently available vaccine candidates suggested that they were not yet optimal. The possible substantial socioeconomic savings that would occur with effective vaccine use underlies the need for emphasis on immunoprophylaxis.

References

1. Greenwood BM, Bojang K, Whitty CJM, Targett GAT (2005) Malaria. Lancet 365:1487–1498
2. Murray CJL, Lopez AD (1997) Mortality by cause for eight regions of the world: global burden of disease study. Lancet 349:1269–1276
3. Warrell DA (1997) Cerebral malaria: clinical features, pathophysiology and treatment. Ann Trop Med Parasitol 91:875–884
4. Murphy GS, Oldfield EC III (1996) Falciparum malaria. Infect Dis Clin North Am 10:747–775
5. Trampuz A, Jereb M, Muzlovic I, Prabhu RM (2003) Clinical review: Severe malaria. Critical Care 7:315–323
6. White NJ, Warrel DA (1988) The management of severe malaria. In: Wernsdorfer WH, McGregor I (eds) Principles and practice of malariology. Churchill Livingstone, Edinburgh, pp 865–888
7. World Health Organization (1990) Severe and complicated malaria. Trans R Soc Trop Med Hyg 84:1–65
8. Roberts DJ, Biggs B-A, Brown G, Newbold CI (1993) Protection, pathogenesis and phenotypic plasticity in *Plasmodium falciparum* malaria. Parasitol Today 9:281–286
9. Greenwood BM (1997) The epidemiology of malaria. Ann Trop Med Parasitol 91:763–769
10. Molineaux L (1996) *Plasmodium falciparum* malaria: some epidemiological implications of parasite and host diversity. Ann Trop Med Parasitol 90:379–393
11. Urquhart AD (1994) Putative pathophysiological interactions of cytokines and phagocytic cells in severe human falciparum malaria. Clin Infect Dis 19:117–131
12. Hill AV, Allsopp CEM, Kwiatkowski D, Anstey NM, Twumasi P, et al. (1991) Common West African HLA antigens are associated with protection from severe malaria. Nature 352:595
13. Hill AV, Elvin J, Willis AC, Aidoo M, Allsopp CEM, et al. (1992) Molecular analysis of the association of HLA B 53 and resistance to severe malaria. Nature 360:434–439
14. Allan RJ, Rowe A. Kwiatkowski D (1993) *Plasmodium falciparum* varies in its ability to induce tumor necrosis factor. Infect Immun 61:4772–4776
15. McGuire W, Knight JC, Hill AVS, Allsopp CEM, Greenwood BM, et al. (1999) Severe malarial anemia and cerebral malaria are associated with different tumor necrosis factor promoter alleles. J Infect Dis 179:287–290
16. McGuire W, Hill AVS, Allsopp CEM, Greenwood BM, Kwiatkowski D (1994) Variation in the TNF-α promoter region associated with susceptibility to cerebral malaria. Nature 371:508–510
17. Idro R, Jenkins NE, Newton CRJC (2005) Pathogenesis, clinical features, and neurological outcome of cerebral malaria. Lancet Neurol:827–840
18. WHO (2000) Severe falciparum malaria. Trans R Soc Trop Med Hyg 94(Suppl 1):1–90
19. Clark IA, Alleva LM, Mills AC, Cowden WB (2004) Pathogenesis of malaria and clinically similar conditions. Clin Microbiol Rev 17:509–539
20. Mackintosh CL, Beeson JG, Marsh K (2004) Clinical features and pathogenesis of severe malaria. Trends Parasitol 20:597–603
21. Bruneel F, Hocqueloux L, Alberti C, Wolff M, Chevret S, Bedos J-P, Durand R, Le Bras J, Regnier B, Vachon F (2003) The clinical spectrum of severe imported falciparum malaria in the intensive care unit. Report of 188 cases in adults. Am J Respir Crit Care Med 167:684–689
22. Dondorp AM, Chau TTH, Phu NH, Mai NTH, Loc PP, Chuong LV, Sinh DX, Taylor A, Hien TT, White NJ, Day NPJ (2004) Unidentified acids of strong prognostic significance in severe malaria. Crit Care Med 32:1683–1688
23. Chiwakata CB, Manegold C, Bonicke L, Waase I, Julch C, Dietrich M (2001) Procalcitonin as a parameter of disease severity and risk of mortality in patients with *Plasmodium falciparum* malaria. J Infect Dis 183:1161–1164
24. Chirenda J, Siziya S, Tshimanga M (2000) Association of HIV infection with the development of severe and complicated malaria cases at a rural hospital in Zimbabwe. Cent Afr J Med 46:5–9
25. Lawn SD (2004) AIDS in Africa: the impact of coinfections on the pathogenesis of HIV-1 infection. J Infect 48:1–12
26. White NJ (2004) Antimalarial drug resistance. J Clin Invest 113:1084–1092
27. Pasloske BL, Howard RJ (1994) Malaria, the red cell, and the endothelium. Annu Rev Med 45:283–295
28. Berendt AR, Turner GDH, Newbold CI (1994) Cerebral malaria: the sequestration hypothesis. Parasitol Today 10:412–414
29. MacPherson GG, Warrell MJ, White NJ, Looareesuwan S, Warrell DA (1985) Human cerebral malaria. A quantitative ultrastructural analysis of parasitized erythrocyte sequestration. Am J Pathol 119:385–401
30. Dondorp AM, Pongponratn E, White NJ (2004) Reduced microcirculatory flow in severe falciparum malaria: pathophysiology and electron-microscopic pathology. Acta Tropica 89:309–317

31. Kirchgatter K, Del Portillo HA (2005) Clinical and molecular aspects of severe malaria. An Acad Bras Cienc 77: 455–475
32. Armah H, Dodoo AK, Wiredu EK, Stiles JK, Adjei AA, Gyasi RK, Tettey Y (2005) High-level cerebellar expression of cytokines and adhesion molecules in fatal, paediatric, cerebral malaria. Ann Trop Med Parasitol 99:629–647
33. Miller LH, Good MF, Milon G (1994) Malaria pathogenesis. Science 264:1878–1883
34. Phillips RE, Warrell DA (1986) The pathophysiology of severe falciparum malaria. Parasitol Today 2:271–282
35. Warrell DA, Looareeuwan S, Phillips RE, White NJ, Warrel MJ, et al. (1986) Function of the blood-cerebrospinal fluid barrier in human cerebral malaria: rejection of the permeability hypothesis. Am J Trop Med Hyg 35:882–889
36. Usawattanakul W, Tharavanij S, Warrell DA, Looareesuwan W, White NJ, et al. (1985) Factors contributing to the development of cerebral malaria II. Endotoxin. Clin Exp Immunol 61:562–568
37. Grau GE, de Kossodo S (1994) Cerebral malaria: mediators, mechanical obstruction or more? Parasitol Today 10:408–409
38. Clark IA, Chaudhri G, Cowden WB (1989) Roles of tumour necrosis factor in the illness and pathology of malaria. Trans R Soc Trop Med Hyg 83:436–440
39. Clark IA, Rockett KA, Cowden WB (1991) Proposed link between cytokines, nitric oxide and human cerebral malaria. Parasitol Today 7:205–207
40. Clark IA, Rockett KA (1994) The cytokine theory of human cerebral malaria. Parasitol Today 10:410–412
41. Coltel N, Combes V, Hunt NH, Grau GE (2004) Cerebral malaria – a neurovascular pathology with many riddles still to be solved. Curr Neurovasc Res 1:91–110
42. Vespa P (1998) Neurological complications of critical medical illnesses and transplantation. Curr Opin Crit Care 4:69
43. Bain BJ, Chiodini PL, England JM, Bailey JW (1997) The laboratory diagnosis of malaria. Clin Lab Haem 19:165–170
44. Perandin F, Manca N, Calderaro A, Piccolo G, Galati L, Ricci L, Medici MC, Arcangeletti MC, Snounou G, Dettori G, Chezzi C (2004) Development of a real-time PCR assay for detection of *Plasmodium falciparum*, *Plasmodium vivax*, and *Plasmodium ovale* for routine clinical diagnosis. J Clin Microbiol 42:1214–1219
45. Farcas GA, Zhong KJ, Lovegrove FE, Graham CM, Kain KC (2003) Evaluation of the Binax NOW ICT test versus polymerase chain reaction and microscopy for the detection of malaria in returned travelers. Am J Trop Med Hyg 69: 589–592
46. Durand F, Crassous B, Fricker-Hidalgo H, Carpentier F, Brion JP, Grillot R, Pelloux H (2005) Performance of the Now Malaria rapid diagnostic test with returned travellers: a 2-year retrospective study in a French teaching hospital. Clin Microbiol Infect 11:903–907
47. Pamba A, Maitland K (2004) Fluid management of severe falciparum malaria in African children. Tropical Doctor 34:67–70
48. Maitland K, Pamba A, English M, Peshu N, Levin M Marsh K, Newton CRJC (2005) Pre-transfusion management of children with severe malarial anaemia: a randomized controlled trial of intravascular volume expansion. Br J Haematol 128:393–400
49. Riddle MS, Jackson JL, Sanders JW, Blazes DL (2002) Exchange transfusion as an adjunct therapy in severe *Plasmodium falciparum* malaria: A meta-analysis. Clin Infect Dis 34:1192–1198
50. Molyneux M, Fox R (1993) Diagnosis and treatment of malaria in Britain. Br Med J 306:1175–1180
51. White NJ (1996) Current concepts: the treatment of malaria. N Engl J Med 335:800–806
52. Lesi A, Meremikwu M (2004) High first dose quinine regimen for treating severe malaria. The Cochrane database of systematic reviews, Issue 3. John Wiley, Chichester, UK
53. White NJ, Nosten F, Looareeuwan S, Watkins WM, Marsh K, et al. (1999) Averting a malaria disaster. Lancet 353: 1965–1967
54. Hoffman SL (1996) Artemether in severe malaria – still too many deaths. N Engl J Med 335:124–126
55. Tran TH, Day NP, Nguyen HP, Nguyen TH, Tran TH, Pham PL, Dinh XS, Ly VC, Ha V, Waller D, Peto TE, White NJ (1996) A controlled trial of artemether or quinine in Vietnamese adults with severe falciparum malaria. N Engl J Med 335:76–83
56. Mohanty S, Mishara SK, Satpathy SK, Dash S, Patnaik J (1997) α, β-Arteether for the treatment of complicated falciparum malaria. Trans R Soc Trop Med Hyg 91:328–330
57. van Hensbroek MB, Onyiorah E, Jaffar S, Schneider G, Palmer A, et al. (1996) A trial of artemether or quinine in children with cerebral malaria. N Engl J Med 335:69–75
58. van Vugt M, Brockman A, Gemperli B, Luxemburger C, Gathmann I, et al. (1998) Randomized comparison of artemether-benflumetol and artesunate-mefloquine in treatment of multidrug-resistant falciparum malaria. Antimicrob Agents Chemother 42:135–139
59. Awad MI, Alkadru AMY, Behrens RH, Baraka OZ, Eltayeb IB (2003) Descriptive study on the efficacy and safety of artesunate suppository in combination with other antimalarials in the treatment of severe malaria in Sudan. Am J Trop Med Hyg 68:153–158
60. Aceng JR, Byarugaba JS, Tumwine JK (2005) Rectal artemether versus intravenous quinine for the treatment of cerebral malaria in children in Uganda: randomized clinical trial. BMJ 330:334–338
61. Ashley EA, White NJ (2005) Artemisinin-based combinations. Curr Opin Infect Dis 18:531–536
62. Whitty CJM, Ansah E, Reyburn H (2005) Treating severe malaria. BMJ 330:317–318
63. South East Asian Quinine Artesunate Malaria Trial (SEAQUAMAT) Group (2005) Artesunate versus quinine for treatment of severe falciparum malaria: a randomized trial. Lancet 366:717–725
64. McIntosh HM, Olliaro P (2000) Artemisinin derivatives for treating severe malaria. The Cochrane database of systematic reviews, Issue 2. John Wiley, Chichester, UK
65. Huda SN, Shahab T, Ali SM, Afzal K, Khan HM (2003) A comparative clinical trial of artemether and quinine in children with severe malaria. Indian Pediatr 40:939–945
66. Adam I, Idris HM, Mohamed-Ali AA, Aelbasit IA, Elbashir MI (2002) Comparison of intramuscular artemether and intravenous quinine in the treatment of Sudanese children with severe falciparum malaria. East Afr Med J 79:621–625
67. Haynes RK, Krishna S (2004) Artemisinins: activities and actions. Microbes Infection 6:1339–1346
68. Newton PN, Angus BJ, Chierakul W, Dondorp A, Ruangveerayuth R, Silamut K, Teerapong P, Suputtamongkol Y, Looareesuwan S, White NJ (2003) Randomized comparison of artesunate and quinine in the treatment of severe falciparum malaria. Clin Infect Dis 37:7–16
69. Krudsood S, Wilairatana P, Vannaphan S, Treeprasertsuk S, Silachamroon U, Phomrattanaprapin W, Gourdeuk VR, Brittenham GM, Looareesuwan S (2003) Clinical experience with intravenous quinine, intramuscular artemeter and intravenous artesunate for the treatment of severe malaria in Thailand. Southeast Asian J Trop Med Public Health 34:54–61

70. Mohanty AK, Rath BK, Mohanty R, Samal AK, Mishra K (2004) Randomized control trial of quinine and artesunate in complicated malaria. Indian J Pediatr 71:291–295
71. Woodrow CJ, Haynes RK, Krishna S (2005) Artemisinins. Postgrad Med J 81:71–78
72. Menard D, Matsika-Claquin MD, Djalle D, Yapou F, Manirakiza A, Dolmazon V, Sarda J, Talarmin A (2005) Association of failures of seven-day courses of artesunate in a non-immune population in Bangui, central African Republic with decreased sensitivity of *Plasmodium falciparum*. Am J Trop Med Hyg 73:616–621
73. Jambou R, Legrand E, Niang M, Khim N, Lim P, Volney B, Ekala MT, Bouchier C, Esterre P, Fandeur T, Mercereau-Puijalan O (2005) Resistance of *Plasmodium falciparum* field isolates to in-vitro artemether and point mutations of the SERCA-type PfATPase6. Lancet 366:1960–1963
74. Duffy PE, Sibley CH (2005) Are we losing artemisinin combination therapy already? Lancet 366:1908–1909
75. Maitland K, Makanga M, Williams TN (2004) Falciparum malaria: current therapeutic challenges. Curr Opin Infect Dis 17:405–412
76. Warrell DA, Looareesuwan S, Warrell M, Kasemsarn P, Intaraprasert R, et al. (1982) Dexamethasone proves deleterious in cerebral malaria. A double-blind trial in 100 comatose patients. N Engl J Med 306:313–319
77. Hoffman SL, Rustama D, Punjabi NH, Surampaet B, Sanjaya B, et al. (1988) High dose dexamethasone in quinine-treated patients with cerebral malaria: A double-blind, placebo-controlled trial. J Infect Dis 158:325–331
78. Looareesuwan S, Warrell DA, White NJ, Sutharasamai P, Chanthavanich, et al. (1983) Do patients with cerebral malaria have cerebral oedema? A computed tomography study. Lancet i:434–437
79. Wilairatana P, Looareesuwan S (1995) APACHE II scoring for predicting outcome in cerebral malaria. J Trop Med Hyg 98:256–260
80. Marik P, Varon J (2004) The management of status epilepticus. Chest 126:582–591
81. Trang TTM, Phu NH, Vinh H, Hien TT, Cuong BM, et al. (1992) Acute renal failure in patients with severe falciparum malaria. Clin Infect Dis 15:874–880
82. Wilairatana P, Westerlund EK, Ausudkij B, Vannaphan S, Krudsood S, et al. (1999) Treatment of malarial acute renal failure by hemodialysis. Am J Trop Med Hyg 60:233–237
83. Bunchman TE (2004) Fluid overload in multiple organ dysfunction syndrome: prediction of survival. Crit Care Med 32:1805–1806
84. Ronco C, Bellomo R, Homel P, Brendolan A, Dan M, Piccinni P, LaGreca G (2000) Effects of different doses in continuous veno-venous hemofiltration on outcomes of acute renal failure: a prospective randomized trial. Lancet 356: 26–30
85. Brealey D, Brand M, Hargreaves I, Heales S, Land J, Smolenski R, Davies NA, Cooper CE, Singer M (2002) Association between mitochondrial dysfunction and severity and outcome of septic shock. Lancet 360:219–223
86. Panosian CB (1998) Editorial response: Exchange blood transfusion in severe falciparum malaria – the debate goes on. Clin Infect Dis 26:853–854
87. White NJ, Warrell DA, Chanthavanigh P, Looareesuwan S, Warrell MJ, et al. (1983) Severe hypoglycemia and hyperinsulinemia in falciparum malaria. N Engl J Med 309:61–66
88. Bruneel F, Gachot B, Timsit JF, Wolff M, Bedos JP, et al. (1997) Shock complicating severe falciparum malaria in European adults. Intensive Care Med 23:698–701
89. Beeson JG, Duffy PE (2005) The immunology and pathogenesis of malaria during pregnancy. Curr Top Microbiol Immunol 297:187–227
90. Adam I, Mirghani OA, Saed OK, Ahmed SM, Mohamadani AA, Ahmed HM, Mackenzie CD, Homeida MM, Elbashir MI (2004) Quinine therapy in severe *Plasmodium falciparum* malaria during pregnancy in Sudan. East Mediterr Health J 10:159–166
91. Newton CRJC, Taylor TE, Whitten RO (1998) Pathophysiology of fatal falciparum malaria in African children. Am J Trop Med Hyg 58:673–683
92. Marsh K, Forster D, Waruiru C, Mwangi I, Winstanley M, et al. (1995) Indicators of life-threatening malaria in African children. N Engl J Med 332:1399–1404
93. Marsh K, English M, Crawley J (1996) The pathogenesis of severe malaria in African children. Ann Trop Med Parasitol 90:395–402
94. O'Dempsey TJ, McArdle TF, Laurence BE, Lamont AC, Todd JE, et al. (1993) Overlap in the clinical features of pneumonia and malaria in African children. Trans R Soc Trop Med Hyg 87:662–665
95. Allen SJ, O'Donnell A, Alexander NDE, Clegg JB (1996) Severe malaria in children in Papua New Guinea. QJ Med 89:779–788
96. Brewster DR, Kwiatkowski D, White NJ (1990) Neurological sequelae of cerebral malaria in children. Lancet 336:1039–1043
97. Greenwood BM (1997) What's new in malaria control? Ann Trop Med Parasitol 91:523–531
98. WHO Malaria Unit (1993) Global malaria control. Bull World Health Organ 71:281–284
99. Tripathi RP, Mishra RC, Dwivedi N, Tewari N, Verma SS (2005) Current status of malaria control. Curr Med Chem 12:2643–2659
100. Brown GV (1993) Chemoprophylaxis of malaria. Med J Aust 159:187–196
101. Playfair JHL, Taverne J, Bate CAW, de Souza JB (1990) The malaria vaccine: anti-parasite or anti-disease? Immunol Today 11:25–27
102. Clark IA, Rockett KA (1994) Immunizing against toxic malarial antigens. Parasitol Today 10:6
103. Amador R, Patarroyo M (1996) Malaria vaccines. J Clin Immunol 16:183–189
104. Kwiatkowski D, Marsh K (1997) Development of a malaria vaccine. Lancet 350:1696–1701
105. Urdaneta M, Prata A, Stuchiner CJ, Tosta CE, Tauil P, et al. (1998) Evaluation of SPf66 malaria vaccine efficacy in Brazil. Am J Trop Med Hyg 58:378–385
106. Stoute JA, Slaoui M, Heppner DG, Momin P, Kester KE, et al. for the RTS, S Malaria Vaccine Evaluation Group (1997) A preliminary evaluation of a recombinant circumsporozoite protein vaccine against *Plasmodium falciparum* malaria. N Engl J Med 336:86–91
107. Greenwood B (2005) Malaria vaccines evaluation and implementation. Acta Tropica 95:298–304
108. Shibui A, Shiibashi T, Nogami S, Sugano S, Watanabe J (2005) A novel method for development of malaria vaccines using full-length cDNA libraries. Vaccine 23:4359–4366
109. Moorthy VS, Good MF, Hill AVS (2004) Malaria vaccine developments. Lancet 363:150–156
110. Graves P, Gelband H (2003) Vaccines for preventing malaria. The Cochrane database of systematic reviews, Issue 1. John Wiley, Chichester, UK

Chapter 25

Toxic Shock Syndromes

K.B. Laupland, H. Dele Davies

25.1 Introduction

Staphylococcal toxic shock syndrome (TSS) was first described in seven children aged 8–17 years by Todd et al. in 1978 [1]. It shortly thereafter became well known as an illness of menstruating women who used tampons [2, 3]. The syndrome is characterized by rapid onset of fever, hypotension, and multisystem failure with desquamating rash occurring in convalescence [4]. The majority of early cases reported were menstrually associated (MTSS) but this has been changing with an increasing proportion of cases non-menstrually associated (NMTSS) [5].

In the late 1980s, cases of severe invasive group A streptococcal (GAS) infections associated with a similar clinical presentation to staphylococcal TSS began to appear in the literature [6–8]. This streptococcal toxic shock-like or streptococcal toxic shock syndrome (STSS) shares in common features of fever, shock, and multisystem organ failure with staphylococcal TSS [4, 9]. In contrast, STSS has no menstrual association, is more common at extremes of age and is a much more lethal condition compared to TSS with case fatality rates of approximately 50% as compared to 5–10% respectively [5, 10–14]. STSS is occasionally associated with the severe soft tissue infection necrotizing fasciitis, which has been popularly called "flesh eating disease" by the media [15].

25.2 Epidemiology

25.2.1 Staphylococcal Toxic Shock Syndrome

There have been significant changes in the rates of TSS since its first description nearly three decades ago. In the early 1980s the incidence peaked and there was much public awareness [14]. Case-control studies identified white race, young women (under 20 years), barrier contraceptives, and use of tampons, particularly the superabsorbent variety Rely brand, as risk factors for acquiring TSS [2, 16–18]. The Rely brand tampon was withdrawn from the market in 1980 and there was a temporally associated decrease in TSS incidence from rates of approximately 10 per 100,000 young women in 1980 to 1 per 100,000 in 1986 [2, 14, 19–21].

Following the initial identification of MTSS cases, there were increasing numbers of NMTSS cases reported. The majority of NMTSS cases are nosocomially acquired and the sources of infection may be either genital, such as with postpartum or contraceptive diaphragm associated illness, or non-genital such as with postoperative wound infection, burns, cellulitis, and rarely necrotizing fasciitis [5, 22, 23]. Since the mid 1980s rates of NMTSS have been similar to those for MTSS. The overall incidence of TSS has been less well documented since the late 1980s but rates did not evidently increase for years after until just recently when an increase in cases was noted in the Minneapolis-St. Paul (Twin Cities) area in the United States [24, 25]. The case fatality rate for TSS is lowest for vaginally associated disease in young females under 15 years old (2%) and highest in men (17%) and non-vaginally associated cases in women (13%) over 45 years old [26].

25.2.2 Streptococcal Toxic Shock Syndrome

Invasive GAS infections, defined as the isolation of *Streptococcus pyogenes* from normally sterile sites such as blood or cerebrospinal, pleural, or deep tissue aspirate fluid, have re-emerged in recent decades as significant causes of severe infections. These infections were common until the middle of the twentieth century but then decreased in incidence for poorly defined reasons. The global burden of invasive GAS disease is estimated at more than 600,000 cases yearly with rates dramatically higher in less developed countries [27]. Population-based studies have shown that invasive GAS disease in Europe and North America occurs at an incidence of 2–5 per 100,000 [10, 13, 28, 29]. Among cases of invasive GAS infection, STSS occurs in approximately 5–15% (incidence of 0.2–0.7 per 100,000 population) and necrotizing fasciitis in 3–6% [12, 13, 29, 30].

Although early studies suggested that STSS was more common among healthy young individuals, prospective population based studies have demonstrated that this is not the case [8, 10, 11, 13]. The risk for development of STSS is highest in the elderly and those with chronic underlying illnesses [10, 13]. Important risk factors for development of invasive GAS infection and STSS determined by population-based studies include extremes of age, black as compared to white race, and coexistent HIV infection, malignancy, heart disease, diabetes, lung disease, and alcohol abuse [10, 12, 28]. Skin trauma or breakdown is observed as a preceding event to invasive GAS disease in approximately one-third of cases but the relative risk associated with this is unknown. In children, varicella is the most important documented risk factor for acquisition of invasive GAS disease and necrotizing fasciitis [10, 12, 13].

Approximately one-half of patients with necrotizing fasciitis have concomitant STSS, although only one-quarter of cases of STSS have necrotizing fasciitis [10, 12, 15]. The most common foci of infection associated with STSS include soft tissue infection, pneumonia, bacteremia with no focus, and septic arthritis [10]. The case fatality rate of invasive GAS infection is markedly increased when associated with STSS, with rates of 45–81% identified in population based studies [10, 12, 28, 29]. Necrotizing fasciitis in the absence of criteria for STSS does not increase the case fatality rate above that for invasive GAS infections alone.

25.3 Etiology and Pathogenesis

25.3.1 Staphylococcal Toxic Shock Syndrome

TSS is caused by toxigenic strains of *Staphylococcus aureus*. The evidence supporting a toxic pathogenesis in TSS includes the clinical findings of multisystem involvement in the absence of systemic infection (positive blood cultures in less than 10% of cases) and the ability to reproduce a TSS-like illness in rabbits using purified *S. aureus* toxins [5, 31, 32]. There is strong evidence implicating toxic shock syndrome toxin-1 (TSST-1) and the staphylococcal enterotoxins as the etiologic agents of TSS [33]. TSST-1 was identified independently by Bergdoll et al. and Schlievert et al. in 1981 and its role in TSS is widely accepted [34, 35]. This protein is produced by over 90% of MTSS isolates and the majority of NMTSS isolates [33, 35]. The staphylococcal enterotoxins are commonly co-produced with TSST-1 and are likely responsible for the syndrome in non-TSST-1 producing isolates from TSS cases [33, 36]. Staphylococcal enterotoxin B is produced by the majority of NMTSS isolates in which TSST-1 is not produced and is likely the cause of the disease in these cases [5, 36–38]. TSST-1 negative TSS has a higher case-fatality rate which may reflect the higher rate of co-morbid medical conditions typical of NMTSS patients or the different toxins mediating the illness [33].

It is not clear why TSS emerged as a "new" complication of *S. aureus* infections in the late 1970s. Retrospective studies have identified that *S. aureus* has had the ability to produce TSST-1 since at least the 1950s [39]. The onset of MTSS in the 1980s appears to be closely related to the use of superabsorbent tampons, as these products probably increase the risk of MTSS by altering the vaginal milieu to encourage *S. aureus* colonization and promote toxin production. In vitro studies of TSST-1 expression by *S. aureus* have identified that production is highly variable according to the environment and that an aerobic, pH neutral, low magnesium environment optimizes toxin production [40]. Tampons may increase the risk of TSS by promoting these conditions. A recent study conducted in North America found that colonization by TSST-1 producing *S. aureus* strains was common in young women and that most had neutralizing titers of antibodies [41]. It is less clear which factors have been involved in the development of NMTSS. It is possible that this condition has been present at a low baseline rate for many years but not widely identified until surveillance for MTSS brought it to attention. MTSS and NMTSS appear to be distinct microbiologically as one clone appears to be responsible for the majority of cases of MTSS whereas isolates from NMTSS are heterogeneous [42].

TSST-1 and the staphylococcal enterotoxins are superantigens which induce widespread immune activation and subsequent shock [43–45]. In the usual cell mediated immune response, T cells recognize antigen presented by the major histocompatibility complex II positive antigen presenting cells with high specificity. The population of T cells that respond are selected based on the specificity of their T cell receptor, which is determined by the combination of the variable gene segments Vα, Vβ, Jα, Jβ, and Dβ [43]. However, superantigens bypass the usual antigen presenting process and activate T cells based on Vβ specificity alone [43, 46]. This leads to a relatively non-specific activation of large populations of T cells. For instance, TSST-1 is Vβ2 restricted and may stimulate up to 50% of all T cells [47]. The result of this activation is the release of potent mediators of inflammation including interleukins 1 and 6 and tumor necrosis factor, which ultimately lead to the clinical manifestations of TSS.

25.3.2 Streptococcal Toxic Shock Syndrome

The pathogenesis of STSS is less well defined than TSS and it appears to be related to both the invasiveness of the organism as well as to the systemic toxins it produces. Identification of virulence determinants is further complicated by the fact that the same strains that cause severe invasive disease are commonly non-disease associated, and that there is considerable heterogeneity among isolates from different cases of STSS [48]. Unlike in TSS where systemic effects are observed typically in association with a localized infection, STSS is characterized by severe bacteremic infection typically in with a rapidly progressive local focus of disease. No single factor has been identified that enables *S. pyogenes* to aggressively invade tissue but potential virulence determinants include M proteins and enzymes such as streptokinase, hyaluronidase, deoxyribonucleases, and proteinases [49]. Although there is a broad range of M protein types observed with severe GAS disease, M1 and M3 have been observed to occur at higher rates with invasive infection [28, 50]. However, the association of M-type with severe disease is modest and these proteins may be markers for other yet identified invasive factors.

There are a number of exotoxins that may potentially mediate STSS although a single one has not been identified as the cause. The streptococcal pyrogenic exotoxins (SPE) function as superantigens and are structurally related to the staphylococcal enterotoxins [43–45]. Strains of GAS producing SPE A in North America and SPE B and SPE C in Europe have been associated with STSS [51, 52]. Mitogenic factor and streptococcal superantigen have been identified from STSS isolates but their role is unclear [53, 54]. Watanabe-Ohnishi et al. showed that characteristic Vβ restricted T cell population changes occurred in cases of STSS that were not related to SPE and suggested that an unidentified superantigen may be involved [55].

25.4 Diagnosis

The diagnosis of TSS or STSS is based on identifying a syndrome of shock, fever, and multisystem failure with the fulfillment of criteria for one of these conditions. The Centers for Disease Control and Prevention case definition for TSS is shown in Table 25.1 and the criteria for STSS as defined by the Working Group on Severe Streptococcal Infections are shown in Table 25.2 [4, 9]. The diagnosis of TSS requires a high index of suspicion because it is a clinical diagnosis having no single diagnostic test and the infection source is often mild or clinically not readily evident. The diagnosis of TSS does not necessarily require isolation of *S. aureus* although most cases will have evidence of this infection. STSS is usually easier to diagnose than TSS because of the usually fulminant illness and high rate of blood culture positivity (>90%) in this condition [10]. However, the early presentation of patients who later develop STSS is often non-specific and delays in diagnosis and treatment are not uncommon. Unlike in TSS where the causative agent

Table 25.1. Staphylococcal toxic shock syndrome: case definition[4]

All of:
1. Fever: temperature ≥38.9 °C
2. Rash: diffuse macular erythroderma
3. Desquamation: 1–2 weeks after onset of illness, particularly of palms, soles, fingers, and toes
4. Hypotension: systolic blood pressure <90 mmHg for adults or <5th percentile by age for children or orthostatic syncope

And

Involvement of three or more of the following organ systems:
- A. Gastrointestinal: vomiting or diarrhea at onset of illness
- B. Muscular: severe myalgia or creatinine phosphokinase level greater than twice the upper limit of normal
- C. Mucous membranes: vaginal, oropharyngeal, or conjunctival hyperemia
- D. Renal: BUN or serum creatinine greater than twice the upper limit of normal; or ≥5 white blood cells per high power field in the absence of a urinary tract infection
- E. Hepatic: total bilirubin, or transaminase greater than twice the upper limit of normal
- F. Hematology: platelets <100,000/mm^3
- G. Central nervous system: disorientation or alterations in consciousness without focal neurologic signs when fever and hypotension are absent

And

Negative results on the following tests if obtained:
- A. Blood, throat or cerebrospinal fluid cultures; blood cultures may be positive for *S. aureus*
- B. Serologic tests for Rocky Mountain spotted fever, leptospirosis, or measles

Table 25.2. Streptococcal toxic shock, case definition [9]

I. Isolation of group A streptococcus (*S. pyogenes*)
- A. From a normally sterile site (e.g., blood, CSF, pleural or peritoneal fluid, tissue biopsy, surgical wound)
- B. From a non-sterile site (e.g., throat, sputum, vagina, superficial skin lesion)

II. Clinical signs of severity
- A. Hypotension: systolic blood pressure ≤90 mmHg in adults or <5th percentile for age in children

And
- B. ≥2 of the following:
  1. Renal impairment (creatinine >177 μmol/l for adults or twice upper limit of normal for age or baseline level in chronic renal insufficiency)
  2. Coagulopathy (platelets ≤100,000 or disseminated intravascular coagulation)
  3. Liver involvement (transaminases or bilirubin ≥ twice upper limit normal or baseline in pre-existing liver impairment)
  4. Adult respiratory distress syndrome (pulmonary infiltrates and hypoxemia without heart failure) or evidence of diffuse capillary leak (generalized edema or pleural or peritoneal effusions with hypoalbuminemia)
  5. Generalized erythematous macular rash that may desquamate
  6. Soft tissue necrosis (necrotizing fasciitis, myositis, or gangrene)

Illness with:
IA and II (A and B) – definite case
IB and II (A and B) – probable case, if no other etiology defined for illness

does not need to be isolated, the definition of STSS requires the isolation of GAS from the patient [4, 9].

TSS and STSS share many clinical features in common which may be the result of the shock state or more specifically related to individual toxin effects. In these syndromes, shock is multi-factorial and may be due to vasodilatation, non-hydrostatic protein leakage with subsequent intravascular volume depletion, hypovolemia from diarrhea, vomiting, and fever, and myocardial depression [56–58]. The myocardial dysfunction when it occurs demonstrates the picture of a reversible toxic cardiomyopathy or myocarditis. The shock state commonly leads to renal impairment from pre-renal failure or acute tubular necrosis [59]. Electrolyte abnormalities are non-specific and may include low serum calcium, magnesium, sodium, potassium, and phosphate. The elevated transaminase and bilirubin levels commonly observed are most likely related to shock liver. Adult respiratory distress syndrome (ARDS) is more common in STSS but may also occur in TSS. Pleural effusions are common in severe cases of toxic shock and may be complicated by empyema [60].

Toxin manifestations that may be independent of the shock state occur commonly especially in TSS. In TSS the rash is typically a diffuse macular erythroderma with desquamation most pronounced in the hands and soles at approximately 1–3 weeks after illness onset. The rash in STSS is similar but desquamation occurs less commonly. TSS may be associated with mental status changes ranging from headache to encephalopathy, which may lead to persistent cognitive impairment [61]. Vomiting and inflammatory diarrhea are common in TSS, as is sterile pyuria, and may be a result of severe illness or secondary to toxin(s).

Necrotizing fasciitis occurs commonly in association with STSS and is diagnosed if histopathological examination reveals necrosis of fascia with edema and polymorphonuclear infiltrate [15]. This diagnosis may also be made if tissue necrosis is evident clinically or at surgical exploration. Necrotizing fasciitis is a rapidly progressive infection that is often difficult to diagnose clinically. In the early stages there may be necrosis of the underlying fascia despite normal overlying skin. Clues to the diagnosis include pain out of proportion to physical findings, edema, and/or erythema in the setting of symptoms and signs of infection including fever, arthralgias, and myalgias [62]. Rapid changes in clinical findings are particularly worrisome for this diagnosis. Creatine kinase levels are often elevated but this test is both insensitive and non-specific and therefore inadequate to rule out necrotizing fasciitis. Soft tissue radiograms rarely show air in tissue in necrotizing fasciitis due to GAS and are unhelpful to exclude this diagnosis. Magnetic resonance imaging has been proposed as a test to diagnose necrotizing fasciitis but performance of this test should not delay definitive diagnosis by surgical exploration and biopsy which is the standard of care [62]. Since no symptom, sign, or non-invasive investigation reliably rules out a diagnosis of potentially limb or life-threatening necrotizing fasciitis, surgical exploration should be performed in all cases for which the diagnosis is entertained. The procedure has minimal morbidity but a missed or delayed diagnosis of necrotizing fasciitis has very serious and often lethal consequences.

In both TSS and STSS the differential diagnosis includes a broad range of inflammatory conditions. Rocky Mountain spotted fever caused by *Rickettsia rikkettsii*, typhus, meningococcemia, Lyme disease, and leptospirosis are all infections associated with rash that may mimic TSS. Toxic epidermal necrolysis, erythema multiforme, and Stevens-Johnson syndrome all present with rash and fever. Septic shock due to other bacterial organisms may also be difficult to differentiate from toxic shock. Kawasaki disease is an acute illness of children characterized by fever, rash, lymphadenopathy, oral involvement and peripheral extremity changes that must be differentiated from TSS because this condition is complicated by coronary artery aneurysms in approximately 25% of untreated cases [63].

25.5 Treatment

The general principles of treatment of TSS and STSS are similar to other causes of severe sepsis and septic shock and may involve supportive care, anti-microbials, source investigation and control, and adjunctive therapies [64]. There have been no large randomized trials in the specific treatment of TSS or STSS and management is based primarily on expert opinion and from experience in related conditions. The spectrum of TSS ranges from relatively mild to severe disease whereas STSS is nearly always severe. For example, in one prospective study, 80% of cases of STSS required ICU care, 60% needed mechanical ventilation and 52% vasopressor support [12]. In all cases of STSS and TSS, if ICU care is not initially deemed to be necessary, close monitoring on the hospital ward is required with a low threshold to transfer to ICU care in the event of clinical deterioration.

The general principles of supportive care for patients with TSS and STSS are shared in common with other etiologies of severe sepsis and septic shock and should reflect current widely accepted guidelines [64]. These may include, but are not limited to, early recognition and prompt and aggressive hemodynamic support [65], endotracheal intubation and mechanical ventilation using a lung protective low tidal volume strategy [66], appropriate use of sedative medications and paralytic agents [67], renal replacement therapy

[68], aggressive glucose and electrolyte management [69], activated protein C infusion in severe cases [70, 71], and low-dose adrenocorticoid replacement therapy [72].

Antibiotic therapy is essential in the treatment of TSS and STSS. Antibiotics for TSS are most important for preventing relapse in MTSS but are usually also needed to treat the local infection in NMTSS [73]. Prompt use of antibiotics in STSS is critical because this is nearly always a systemic infection. *S. aureus* is usually resistant to penicillin and in some regions it is commonly methicillin resistant. *S. pyogenes* is universally susceptible to penicillin. However, even if in vitro susceptible, in TSS and STSS beta-lactam antibiotics may be limited in treatment because of the "inoculum effect" [74]. This occurs when the bacteria are present in high concentrations and are in stationary phase with the subsequent reduced production of penicillin binding proteins, the target of beta-lactam antibiotics. Clindamycin is a protein synthesis inhibitor antibiotic that has in vitro activity against both *S. aureus* and *S. pyogenes*. It is not affected by the inoculum effect and also may treat toxic shock by inhibiting toxin production [75]. Clindamycin has been shown to be more effective than penicillin in mouse models of GAS myositis and in case-control studies in humans with STSS [76]. Our recommendations are that high doses of clindamycin should be used with a penicillinase resistant penicillin in TSS, and with penicillin in STSS unless susceptibility testing demonstrates resistance. Since in many cases it is difficult to differentiate among TSS, STSS, and Gram-negative septic shock in the initial presentation, clindamycin should be used with a broad spectrum, β-lactamase resistant agent until microbiologic diagnosis is achieved. In regions where MRSA is a concern, vancomycin or linezolid should be added to this empiric regimen.

Source control is commonly required in TSS and STSS. Any localized infection source requires intervention such as removal of tampons or wound packing, or surgical drainage of infected wounds, abscesses, or empyemas. Necrotizing fasciitis must be investigated and treated surgically without delay because this condition is typically fulminant. Adequate drainage and excision of necrotic tissue is mandatory and repeated surgical procedures or repeated exploration are needed in the treatment of this condition. Wounds should generally be packed open until the infection has been cured, at which time closure or grafting may be performed as appropriate.

There are many proponents of intravenous immunoglobulin (IVIG) therapy as an adjunctive treatment for TSS and STSS and in many regions it is viewed as a standard of care [77, 78]. Intravenous immunoglobulin contains neutralizing antibodies to staphylococcal and streptococcal superantigens and has anti-cytokine activity [15, 79, 80]. Although there is rationale for IVIG use in these syndromes based in theory, several lines of laboratory investigation, and retrospective clinical series, no definitive clinical trial has been conducted and there remains clinical equipoise as to whether IVIG should be used in the treatment of TSS and STSS [81]. One prospective, randomized control comparing IVIG and placebo in the treatment of STSS has been reported [82]. However, this study was ended prematurely after enrolling only 21 patients and as a result was underpowered to detect any significant mortality difference. We recommend the use of IVIG as an adjunctive therapy for STSS and TSS where the disease presentation is particularly severe or rapidly progressive despite prompt institution of other recommended therapies. In children with TSS or STSS it is important to exclude Kawasaki disease as this condition shares many features with toxic shock and may be diagnosed simultaneously [63]. If there are clinical criteria for Kawasaki disease or evidence of coronary involvement then IVIG is clearly indicated based on its proven efficacy in reducing the risk of developing coronary aneurysms from 23% to 2% [83]. Echocardiography is the screening procedure of choice to detect coronary aneurysms and it is our recommendation that this test is performed on all children with TSS or STSS.

Preventive measures may play a role in the management of TSS and STSS. In MTSS it is prudent to recommend against the use of superabsorbent tampons. If these products are used then the absorbency and amount of time they are left in place may best be minimized [25]. Risks for NMTSS may be reduced by careful wound care and prompt treatment of infection in surgical cases. Recurrence is common in TSS and there may be a role for eliminating *S. aureus* asymptomatic carriage in the nares using topical mupirocin [2, 84]. Invasive GAS disease has an estimated household contact transmission risk of 3 per 1,000 that is comparable to rates observed for meningococcal disease [10]. Antibiotic prophylaxis for close contacts of patients with STSS may be beneficial but the best way to approach this issue remains to be defined [85, 86]. In children, 16% of all cases of invasive GAS disease are complications of varicella infection and it has been estimated that 10% of all invasive GAS in children would be prevented by routine vaccination for varicella at 1 year of age [13].

References

1. Todd J, Fishaut M, Kapral F, Welch T (1978) Toxic-shock syndrome associated with phage-group-I Staphylococci. Lancet 2(8100):1116–1118
2. Davis JP, Chesney PJ, Wand PJ, LaVenture M (1980) Toxic-shock syndrome: epidemiologic features, recurrence, risk factors, and prevention. N Engl J Med 303(25):1429–1435
3. Shands KN, Schmid GP, Dan BB, Blum D, Guidotti RJ, Har-

grett NT, Anderson RL, Hill DL, Broome CV, Band JD, et al. (1980) Toxic-shock syndrome in menstruating women: association with tampon use and *Staphylococcus aureus* and clinical features in 52 cases. N Engl J Med 303(25): 1436–1442
4. Wharton M, Chorba TL, Vogt RL, Morse DL, Buehler JW (1990) Case definitions for public health surveillance. MMWR Recomm Rep 39(RR-13):1–43
5. Kain KC, Schulzer M, Chow AW (1993) Clinical spectrum of nonmenstrual toxic shock syndrome (TSS): comparison with menstrual TSS by multivariate discriminant analyses. Clin Infect Dis 16(1):100–106
6. Cone LA, Woodard DR, Schlievert PM, Tomory GS (1987) Clinical and bacteriologic observations of a toxic shock-like syndrome due to *Streptococcus pyogenes*. N Engl J Med 317(3):146–149
7. Bartter T, Dascal A, Carroll K, Curley FJ (1988) 'Toxic strep syndrome'. A manifestation of group A streptococcal infection. Arch Intern Med 148(6):1421–1424
8. Stevens DL, Tanner MH, Winship J, Swarts R, Ries KM, Schlievert PM, Kaplan E (1989) Severe group A streptococcal infections associated with a toxic shock-like syndrome and scarlet fever toxin A. N Engl J Med 321(1):1–7
9. The Working Group on Severe Streptococcal Infections (1993) Defining the group A streptococcal toxic shock syndrome. Rationale and consensus definition. JAMA 269(3): 390–391
10. Davies HD, McGeer A, Schwartz B, Green K, Cann D, Simor AE, Low DE (1996) Invasive group A streptococcal infections in Ontario, Canada. Ontario Group A Streptococcal Study Group. N Engl J Med 335(8):547–554
11. Hoge CW, Schwartz B, Talkington DF, Breiman RF, MacNeill EM, Englender SJ (1993) The changing epidemiology of invasive group A streptococcal infections and the emergence of streptococcal toxic shock-like syndrome. A retrospective population-based study. JAMA 269(3):384–389
12. Zurawski CA, Bardsley M, Beall B, Elliott JA, Facklam R, Schwartz B, Farley MM (1998) Invasive group A streptococcal disease in metropolitan Atlanta: a population-based assessment. Clin Infect Dis 27(1):150–157
13. Laupland KB, Davies HD, Low DE, Schwartz B, Green K, McGeer A (2000) Invasive group A streptococcal disease in children and association with varicella-zoster virus infection. Ontario Group A Streptococcal Study Group. Pediatrics 105(5):E60
14. Schuchat A, Broome CV (1991) Toxic shock syndrome and tampons. Epidemiol Rev 13:99–112
15. Kaul R, McGeer A, Low DE, Green K, Schwartz B (1997) Population-based surveillance for group A streptococcal necrotizing fasciitis: Clinical features, prognostic indicators, and microbiologic analysis of seventy-seven cases. Ontario Group A Streptococcal Study. Am J Med 103(1): 18–24
16. Schlech WF, 3rd, Shands KN, Reingold AL, Dan BB, Schmid GP, Hargrett NT, Hightower A, Herwaldt LA, Neill MA, Band JD, et al. (1982) Risk factors for development of toxic shock syndrome. Association with a tampon brand. JAMA 248(7):835–839
17. Osterholm MT, Davis JP, Gibson RW, Mandel JS, Wintermeyer LA, Helms CM, Forfang JC, Rondeau J, Vergeront JM (1982) Tri-state toxic-state syndrome study. I. Epidemiologic findings. J Infect Dis 145(4):431–440
18. Schwartz B, Gaventa S, Broome CV, Reingold AL, Hightower AW, Perlman JA, Wolf PH (1989) Nonmenstrual toxic shock syndrome associated with barrier contraceptives: report of a case-control study. Rev Infect Dis 11 Suppl 1:S43–48; discussion S48–49
19. Gaventa S, Reingold AL, Hightower AW, Broome CV, Schwartz B, Hoppe C, Harwell J, Lefkowitz LK, Makintubee S, Cundiff DR, et al. (1989) Active surveillance for toxic shock syndrome in the United States, 1986. Rev Infect Dis 11 Suppl 1:S28–34
20. Osterholm MT, Forfang JC (1982) Toxic-shock syndrome in Minnesota: results of an active-passive surveillance system. J Infect Dis 145(4):458–464
21. Latham RH, Kehrberg MW, Jacobson JA, Smith CB (1982) Toxic shock syndrome in Utah: a case-control and surveillance study. Ann Intern Med 96(6):906–908
22. Davis JP, Osterholm MT, Helms CM, Vergeront JM, Wintermeyer LA, Forfang JC, Judy LA, Rondeau J, Schell WL (1982) Tri-state toxic-shock syndrome study. II. Clinical and laboratory findings. J Infect Dis 145(4):441–448
23. Chesney PJ, Davis JP, Purdy WK, Wand PJ, Chesney RW (1981) Clinical manifestations of toxic shock syndrome. JAMA 246(7):741–748
24. Schlievert PM, Tripp TJ, Peterson ML (2004) Reemergence of staphylococcal toxic shock syndrome in Minneapolis-St. Paul, Minnesota, during the 2000–2003 surveillance period. J Clin Microbiol 42(6):2875–2876
25. Tierno PM, Jr (2005) Reemergence of staphylococcal toxic shock syndrome in the United States since 2000. J Clin Microbiol 43(4):2032; author reply 2032–2033
26. Broome CV (1989) Epidemiology of toxic shock syndrome in the United States: overview. Rev Infect Dis 11 Suppl 1:S14–21
27. Carapetis JR, Steer AC, Mulholland EK, Weber M (2005) The global burden of group A streptococcal diseases. Lancet Infect Dis 5(11):685–694
28. O'Brien KL, Beall B, Barrett NL, Cieslak PR, Reingold A, Farley MM, Danila R, Zell ER, Facklam R, Schwartz B, et al. (2002) Epidemiology of invasive group a streptococcus disease in the United States, 1995–1999. Clin Infect Dis 35(3):268–276
29. Eriksson BK, Andersson J, Holm SE, Norgren M (1998) Epidemiological and clinical aspects of invasive group A streptococcal infections and the streptococcal toxic shock syndrome. Clin Infect Dis 27(6):1428–1436
30. Ekelund K, Skinhoj P, Madsen J, Konradsen HB (2005) Invasive group A, B, C and G streptococcal infections in Denmark 1999–2002: epidemiological and clinical aspects. Clin Microbiol Infect 11(7):569–576
31. Kum WW, Laupland KB, See RH, Chow AW (1993) Improved purification and biologic activities of staphylococcal toxic shock syndrome toxin 1. J Clin Microbiol 31(10): 2654–2660
32. Parsonnet J, Gillis ZA, Richter AG, Pier GB (1987) A rabbit model of toxic shock syndrome that uses a constant, subcutaneous infusion of toxic shock syndrome toxin 1. Infect Immun 55(5):1070–1076
33. Garbe PL, Arko RJ, Reingold AL, Graves LM, Hayes PS, Hightower AW, Chandler FW, Broome CV (1985) *Staphylococcus aureus* isolates from patients with nonmenstrual toxic shock syndrome. Evidence for additional toxins. JAMA 253(17):2538–2542
34. Bergdoll MS, Crass BA, Reiser RF, Robbins RN, Davis JP (1981) A new staphylococcal enterotoxin, enterotoxin F, associated with toxic-shock-syndrome *Staphylococcus aureus* isolates. Lancet 1(8228):1017–1021
35. Schlievert PM, Shands KN, Dan BB, Schmid GP, Nishimura RD (1981) Identification and characterization of an exotoxin from *Staphylococcus aureus* associated with toxic-shock syndrome. J Infect Dis 143(4):509–516
36. Crass BA, Bergdoll MS (1986) Involvement of staphylococcal enterotoxins in nonmenstrual toxic shock syndrome. J Clin Microbiol 23(6):1138–1139
37. Lee VT, Chang AH, Chow AW (1992) Detection of staphy-

lococcal enterotoxin B among toxic shock syndrome (TSS)- and non-TSS-associated *Staphylococcus aureus* isolates. J Infect Dis 166(4):911–915
38. Schlievert PM (1986) Staphylococcal enterotoxin B and toxic-shock syndrome toxin-1 are significantly associated with non-menstrual TSS. Lancet 1(8490):1149–1150
39. Hayes PS, Graves LM, Feeley JC, Hancock GA, Cohen ML, Reingold AL, Broome CV, Hightower AW (1984) Production of toxic-shock-associated protein(s) in *Staphylococcus aureus* strains isolated from 1956 through 1982. J Clin Microbiol 20(1):43–46
40. Schlievert PM, Blomster DA (1983) Production of staphylococcal pyrogenic exotoxin type C: influence of physical and chemical factors. J Infect Dis 147(2):236–242
41. Parsonnet J, Hansmann MA, Delaney ML, Modern PA, Dubois AM, Wieland-Alter W, Wissemann KW, Wild JE, Jones MB, Seymour JL, et al. (2005) Prevalence of toxic shock syndrome toxin 1-producing *Staphylococcus aureus* and the presence of antibodies to this superantigen in menstruating women. J Clin Microbiol 43(9):4628–4634
42. Musser JM, Schlievert PM, Chow AW, Ewan P, Kreiswirth BN, Rosdahl VT, Naidu AS, Witte W, Selander RK (1990) A single clone of *Staphylococcus aureus* causes the majority of cases of toxic shock syndrome. Proc Natl Acad Sci U S A 87(1):225–229
43. Marrack P, Kappler J (1990) The staphylococcal enterotoxins and their relatives. Science 248(4959):1066
44. Proft T, Fraser JD (2003) Bacterial superantigens. Clin Exp Immunol 133(3):299–306
45. Llewelyn M, Cohen J (2002) Superantigens: microbial agents that corrupt immunity. Lancet Infect Dis 2(3):156–162
46. Kum WW, Laupland KB, Chow AW (2000) Defining a novel domain of staphylococcal toxic shock syndrome toxin-1 critical for major histocompatibility complex class II binding, superantigenic activity, and lethality. Can J Microbiol 46(2):171–179
47. Choi Y, Lafferty JA, Clements JR, Todd JK, Gelfand EW, Kappler J, Marrack P, Kotzin BL (1990) Selective expansion of T cells expressing V beta 2 in toxic shock syndrome. J Exp Med 172(3):981–984
48. Cockerill FR, 3rd, MacDonald KL, Thompson RL, Roberson F, Kohner PC, Besser-Wiek J, Manahan JM, Musser JM, Schlievert PM, Talbot J, et al. (1997) An outbreak of invasive group A streptococcal disease associated with high carriage rates of the invasive clone among school-aged children. JAMA 277(1):38–43
49. Bisno AL, Brito MO, Collins CM (2003) Molecular basis of group A streptococcal virulence. Lancet Infect Dis 3(4):191–200
50. Talkington DF, Schwartz B, Black CM, Todd JK, Elliott J, Breiman RF, Facklam RR (1993) Association of phenotypic and genotypic characteristics of invasive *Streptococcus pyogenes* isolates with clinical components of streptococcal toxic shock syndrome. Infect Immun 61(8):3369–3374
51. Hauser AR, Stevens DL, Kaplan EL, Schlievert PM (1991) Molecular analysis of pyrogenic exotoxins from *Streptococcus pyogenes* isolates associated with toxic shock-like syndrome. J Clin Microbiol 29(8):1562–1567
52. Musser JM, Hauser AR, Kim MH, Schlievert PM, Nelson K, Selander RK (1991) *Streptococcus pyogenes* causing toxic-shock-like syndrome and other invasive diseases: clonal diversity and pyrogenic exotoxin expression. Proc Natl Acad Sci U S A 88(7):2668–2672
53. Yutsudo T, Murai H, Gonzalez J, Takao T, Shimonishi Y, Takeda Y, Igarashi H, Hinuma Y (1992) A new type of mitogenic factor produced by *Streptococcus pyogenes*. FEBS Lett 308(1):30–34
54. Mollick JA, Miller GG, Musser JM, Cook RG, Grossman D, Rich RR (1993) A novel superantigen isolated from pathogenic strains of *Streptococcus pyogenes* with aminoterminal homology to staphylococcal enterotoxins B and C. J Clin Invest 92(2):710–719
55. Watanabe-Ohnishi R, Low DE, McGeer A, Stevens DL, Schlievert PM, Newton D, Schwartz B, Kreiswirth B, Kotb M (1995) Selective depletion of V beta-bearing T cells in patients with severe invasive group A streptococcal infections and streptococcal toxic shock syndrome. Ontario Streptococcal Study Project. J Infect Dis 171(1):74–84
56. Paris AL, Herwaldt LA, Blum D, Schmid GP, Shands KN, Broome CV (1982) Pathologic findings in twelve fatal cases of toxic shock syndrome. Ann Intern Med 96(6):852–857
57. Larkin SM, Williams DN, Osterholm MT, Tofte RW, Posalaky Z (1982) Toxic shock syndrome: clinical, laboratory, and pathologic findings in nine fatal cases. Ann Intern Med 96(6):858–864
58. Forni AL, Kaplan EL, Schlievert PM, Roberts RB (1995) Clinical and microbiological characteristics of severe group A streptococcus infections and streptococcal toxic shock syndrome. Clin Infect Dis 21(2):333–340
59. Chesney RW, Chesney PJ, Davis JP, Segar WE (1981) Renal manifestations of the staphylococcal toxic-shock syndrome. Am J Med 71(4):583–588
60. Demeter SL, Fuenning C, Klein JJ (1982) Pleural effusion in toxic shock syndrome. Ann Intern Med 97(1):148–149
61. Rosene KA, Copass MK, Kastner LS, Nolan CM, Eschenbach DA (1982) Persistent neuropsychological sequelae of toxic shock syndrome. Ann Intern Med 96(6):865–870
62. Stamenkovic I, Lew PD (1984) Early recognition of potentially fatal necrotizing fasciitis. The use of frozen-section biopsy. N Engl J Med 310(26):1689–1693
63. Laupland KB, Dele Davies H (1999) Epidemiology, etiology, and management of Kawasaki disease: state of the art. Pediatr Cardiol 20(3):177–183
64. Dellinger RP, Carlet JM, Masur H, Gerlach H, Calandra T, Cohen J, Gea-Banacloche J, Keh D, Marshall JC, Parker MM, et al. (2004) Surviving Sepsis Campaign guidelines for management of severe sepsis and septic shock. Intensive Care Med 30(4):536–555
65. Rivers E, Nguyen B, Havstad S, Ressler J, Muzzin A, Knoblich B, Peterson E, Tomlanovich M (2001) Early goal-directed therapy in the treatment of severe sepsis and septic shock. N Engl J Med 345(19):1368–1377
66. Ventilation with lower tidal volumes as compared with traditional tidal volumes for acute lung injury and the acute respiratory distress syndrome. The Acute Respiratory Distress Syndrome Network. N Engl J Med 342(18):1301–1308
67. Kress JP, Pohlman AS, O'Connor MF, Hall JB (2000) Daily interruption of sedative infusions in critically ill patients undergoing mechanical ventilation. N Engl J Med 342(20):1471–1477
68. Schiffl H, Lang SM, Fischer R (2002) Daily hemodialysis and the outcome of acute renal failure. N Engl J Med 346(5):305–310
69. van den Berghe G, Wouters P, Weekers F, Verwaest C, Bruyninckx F, Schetz M, Vlasselaers D, Ferdinande P, Lauwers P, Bouillon R (2001) Intensive insulin therapy in the critically ill patients. N Engl J Med 345(19):1359–1367
70. Bernard GR, Vincent JL, Laterre PF, LaRosa SP, Dhainaut JF, Lopez-Rodriguez A, Steingrub JS, Garber GE, Helterbrand JD, Ely EW, et al. (2001) Efficacy and safety of recombinant human activated protein C for severe sepsis. N Engl J Med 344(10):699–709
71. Doig CJ, Laupland KB, Zygun DA, Manns BJ (2003) The epidemiology of severe sepsis syndrome and its treatment

with recombinant human activated protein C. Expert Opin Pharmacother 4(10):1789–1799

72. Annane D, Sebille V, Charpentier C, Bollaert PE, Francois B, Korach JM, Capellier G, Cohen Y, Azoulay E, Troche G, et al. (2002) Effect of treatment with low doses of hydrocortisone and fludrocortisone on mortality in patients with septic shock. JAMA 288(7):862–871
73. Chesney PJ, Crass BA, Polyak MB, Wand PJ, Warner TF, Vergeront JM, Davis JP, Tofte RW, Chesney RW, Bergdoll MS (1982) Toxic shock syndrome: management and long-term sequelae. Ann Intern Med 96(6):847–851
74. Eagle H (1952) Experimental approach to the problem of treatment failure with penicillin. I. Group A streptococcal infection in mice. Am J Med 13(4):389–399
75. Tanaka M, Hasegawa T, Okamoto A, Torii K, Ohta M (2005) Effect of antibiotics on group A *Streptococcus* exoprotein production analyzed by two-dimensional gel electrophoresis. Antimicrob Agents Chemother 49(1):88–96
76. Stevens DL, Gibbons AE, Bergstrom R, Winn V (1988) The Eagle effect revisited: efficacy of clindamycin, erythromycin, and penicillin in the treatment of streptococcal myositis. J Infect Dis 158(1):23–28
77. Laupland KB, Boucher P, Rotstein C, Cook DJ, Doig CJ (2004) Intravenous immunoglobulin for severe infections: a survey of Canadian specialists. J Crit Care 19(2):75–81
78. Norrby-Teglund A, Ihendyane N, Darenberg J (2003) Intravenous immunoglobulin adjunctive therapy in sepsis, with special emphasis on severe invasive group A streptococcal infections. Scand J Infect Dis 35(9):683–689
79. Takei S, Arora YK, Walker SM (1993) Intravenous immunoglobulin contains specific antibodies inhibitory to activation of T cells by staphylococcal toxin superantigens [see comment]. J Clin Invest 91(2):602–607
80. Skansen-Saphir U, Andersson J, Bjork L, Andersson U (1994) Lymphokine production induced by streptococcal pyrogenic exotoxin-A is selectively down-regulated by pooled human IgG. Eur J Immunol 24(4):916–922
81. Kaul R, McGeer A, Norrby-Teglund A, Kotb M, Schwartz B, O'Rourke K, Talbot J, Low DE (1999) Intravenous immunoglobulin therapy for streptococcal toxic shock syndrome – a comparative observational study. The Canadian Streptococcal Study Group. Clin Infect Dis 28(4):800–807
82. Darenberg J, Ihendyane N, Sjolin J, Aufwerber E, Haidl S, Follin P, Andersson J, Norrby-Teglund A (2003) Intravenous immunoglobulin G therapy in streptococcal toxic shock syndrome: a European randomized, double-blind, placebo-controlled trial. Clin Infect Dis 37(3):333–340
83. Durongpisitkul K, Gururaj VJ, Park JM, Martin CF (1995) The prevention of coronary artery aneurysm in Kawasaki disease: a meta-analysis on the efficacy of aspirin and immunoglobulin treatment. Pediatrics 96(6):1057–1061
84. Laupland KB, Conly JM (2003) Treatment of *Staphylococcus aureus* colonization and prophylaxis for infection with topical intranasal mupirocin: an evidence-based review. Clin Infect Dis 37(7):933–938
85. Centers for Disease Control and Prevention (2002) Prevention of invasive group A streptococcal disease among household contacts of case patients and among postpartum and postsurgical patients: recommendations from the Centers for Disease Control and Prevention. Clin Infect Dis 35(8):950–959
86. Smith A, Lamagni TL, Oliver I, Efstratiou A, George RC, Stuart JM (2005) Invasive group A streptococcal disease: should close contacts routinely receive antibiotic prophylaxis? Lancet Infect Dis 5(8):494–500

Chapter 26

Acute Infective Endocarditis

C.N. Gentry, J.R. McDonald

26.1 Introduction

Infective endocarditis (IE), an infection of the endocardial lining of the heart, accounts for about 1 in 1,000 admissions to hospital. Because IE often occurs in patients with multiple co-morbid illnesses and those who have undergone recent invasive procedures, it is commonly diagnosed and treated in the intensive care unit (ICU) [1, 2]. IE is the cause of 0.8–3.0% of admissions to ICUs, with mortality exceeding 50% in some reported series of ICU patients [3, 4].

Infective endocarditis has traditionally been classified as acute, subacute, or chronic. Acute disease is characterized by sudden clinical onset with a fulminant course. In the pre-antibiotic era, it usually led to death in less than 6 weeks. Acute IE has historically been associated with *Staphylococcus aureus*, *Streptococcus pyogenes*, or *Streptococcus pneumoniae* [2]. In contrast, subacute and chronic IE have more indolent courses and are usually accompanied by more subtle clinical signs and symptoms. In the pre-antibiotic era, subacute and chronic IE typically led to death in greater than 6 weeks.

Several epidemiologic trends support the observation that acute IE is increasing in frequency relative to subacute and chronic IE, including the increasing use of invasive procedures and intravascular prosthetic devices, the increasing role of *S. aureus* in IE, and rising rates of nosocomial IE [5, 6]. In this chapter, when possible, discussion of endocarditis will focus on acute endocarditis, though much of the relevant literature includes all classifications of IE without distinguishing between acute, subacute, or chronic endocarditis.

26.2 Pathophysiology

Several events must take place in order for an episode of IE to occur: endocardial injury, sterile thrombus formation, bacteremia, microbial adherence, and formation of a mature vegetation.

Endocardial injury may occur by many mechanisms. Most commonly, an acquired or congenital cardiac condition causes turbulent blood flow leading to injury to the valve surface or the mural endocardium. Alternatively, the endocardium may be damaged by an intravascular catheter or other device that directly abrades the inner surface of the heart. In injection drug users, endocardial damage to the tricuspid valve may occur due to the direct injection of contaminating debris. The damaged endothelial surface triggers platelet and fibrin deposition, and the formation of a sterile thrombus.

In some animal models, endocarditis can be induced without preexisting endocardial trauma [7]. Physiologic stresses including high cardiac output, hypersensitivity states, hormonal manipulation, cold exposure, and high altitude have been shown to induce sterile endocardial thrombosis in experimental settings [7]. Clinical states associated with sterile endocardial thrombosis include malignancy, rheumatic diseases, and uremia.

Transient bacteremia plays a key role in the pathogenesis of IE. Bacteria are introduced into the bloodstream when a body surface that is heavily colonized by bacteria (oral cavity, gut lumen, genitourinary mucosa) is traumatized. The trauma and subsequent bacteremia often go unrecognized [8].

In the setting of endocardial injury and/or sterile thrombus, bloodborne bacteria may adhere to the endocardial surface. Bacteria differ in their likelihood of adherence. In animal models of endocarditis, when pathogens are injected into the bloodstream, pathogens which commonly cause endocarditis (*S. aureus*, viridans streptococci, and enterococci) are more likely to adhere to an experimentally damaged heart valve than pathogens which less commonly cause IE [9]. These differences can be explained by adhesion factors that vary between types of bacteria. For example, the amount of dextran present in the streptococcal cell wall has been linked to that strain's likelihood of adhesion [10], and variations in *S. aureus* strains' ability to bind to fibronectin appear to play a role in adhesion to damaged endocardium [11].

Once bacteria have attached to the endocardium, additional deposition of fibrin occurs on the surface of the vegetation, and bacterial proliferation continues within. Because vegetations are typically avascular, penetration of phagocytic cells is minimal, resulting in relative protection from host immune defenses. The avascular nature of most vegetations also results in poor penetration of antimicrobial agents.

26.3 Epidemiology

26.3.1 Demographics and Risk Factors

Approximately 10,000–15,000 new cases of IE are diagnosed annually in the United States [12]. Although some studies have reported that the rate of IE has been stable over time [6, 13], changes in both diagnostic tools and diagnostic criteria make such comparisons difficult. In addition, rates of several major endocarditis risk factors have changed over time, including increases in invasive medical procedures and intravenous drug use, and decreases in rheumatic heart disease.

Infective endocarditis is diagnosed more frequently in men than in women, in approximately a 2:1 ratio [12]. The mean age of patients at the time of diagnosis has been steadily increasing over time, from less than 30 years in the pre-antibiotic era [14] to nearly 60 years in a recent multicenter, international cohort [15]. IE most commonly affects the left-sided heart valves. In a large international cohort, 40 % of patients had mitral valve IE, while 36 % had aortic valve IE [15, 16]. Tricuspid valve IE is common among intravenous drug users but is otherwise rare. The pulmonic valve is least likely to be involved in IE.

Prior episodes of IE, invasive medical procedures, and intravenous drug use are risk factors for IE [1]. Underlying structural heart disease is present in about 75 % of patients who develop IE [13]. Historically, rheumatic heart disease, and specifically mitral stenosis, was the major underlying valvular defect in patients with IE, but the incidence of rheumatic heart disease has decreased dramatically. More recently, the most common predisposing valvular lesions are mitral regurgitation, aortic valve disease (stenosis and regurgitation), and congenital heart disease [17]. Mitral valve prolapse without regurgitation is associated with only a slightly increased risk of IE [18]. Patients with prosthetic cardiac valves are at a high risk for IE. One to 4 % of prosthetic valve recipients develop IE in the first year after surgery, and an additional 1 % are diagnosed per year thereafter [12]. Some comorbid medical conditions such as diabetes mellitus and kidney disease have been shown to be risk factors for IE in some studies as well [1].

26.3.2 Nosocomial IE

Nosocomial IE is a relatively new category of IE that has emerged in recent decades. Recent case series show that between 14 % and 31 % of all IE is nosocomial in origin [19–21]. In an analysis of IE occurring at a single institution in Spain, the proportion of IE that was nosocomial increased from 3.4 % in the mid-1980s to 31 % in the late 1990s. Mortality among nosocomial IE was significantly higher than in community-acquired IE. Nosocomial IE was more commonly caused by *S. aureus*, coagulase-negative staphylococci, and enterococci, and rarely by streptococci [20].

Nosocomial IE can usually be attributed to a hospital acquired infection at a primary site, most commonly an intravenous catheter insertion site, surgical wound site, or as a result of an invasive procedure. Of 31 nosocomial cases of IE described by Mourvillier et al., 21 were related to intravenous catheter infection, 4 to an infected arteriovenous fistula, 3 to surgical site infection, 2 to pneumonia, and 1 to a digestive procedure [4]. Of 22 nosocomial IE cases in an ICU, Gouello et al. found that 11 were related to an intravascular device (5 central venous catheters, 3 peripheral venous catheters, and 3 arteriovenous fistulas), 8 to a surgical site infection, 1 to endotracheal intubation, 1 to a skin infection, and 1 had no identifiable source [22].

26.3.3 Infective Endocarditis in Critical Care

Few studies have described the occurrence of IE in critical care settings. Karth et al. described 33 cases of IE occurring in 4 medical ICUs in Vienna, Austria, between 1994 and 1999 [3]. IE was identified in 0.8 % of all ICU patients. In 55 % of patients with IE in this study, IE was diagnosed prior to ICU admission; in the remaining 45 % it was diagnosed in the ICU. The most common reasons for ICU admission in patients with known IE were congestive heart failure (CHF) (64 % of cases), septic shock (21 %) and neurologic deterioration (15 %). Mechanical ventilation was required by 79 % of IE patients, inotropes and/or vasoconstrictors by 73 %, and acute renal failure occurred in 39 %. The majority (79 %) had native valve IE. *S. aureus* was the leading pathogen, causing 36 % of IE. Cardiac surgery was performed for IE in 60 % of cases, and 54 % of patients died during their hospital stay. The leading causes of death were cardiogenic shock and septic shock. Acute renal failure on ICU admission was the only independent predictor of mortality [3].

Mourvillier et al. described a large cohort of 228 cases of IE occurring in 2 medical ICUs in France between 1993 and 2000 [4]. IE was diagnosed in 3 % of ICU patients during this time period. IE occurred on a native valve in 64 % of cases. *S. aureus* was the causative agent in half of all cases. Of the native valve cases, 21% were nosocomial. Neurological events occurred in nearly 40% of patients, CHF complicated 29% of cases, and septic shock occurred in 26%. In-hospital mortality was 45%. Several factors independently predicted in-hospital mortality, including septic shock, neurological complications, and immunocompromised state [4].

A study by Gouello et al. focused only on nosocomial IE in patients admitted to the ICU [22]. Among more than 4,000 patients admitted to an ICU in a single French hospital between 1992 and 1997, the incidence of nosocomial IE was 0.5%. The majority (68%) of these patients had no predisposing cardiac lesion. *S. aureus* was the causative pathogen in 68% of cases. Overall mortality was 68% [22].

One study examined prosthetic valve IE only in the ICU setting [23]. Between 1978 and 1992, 122 cases of prosthetic valve IE occurred in a French ICU. *S. aureus* was the most frequent pathogen in early disease, accounting for 61% of isolates, while streptococci and *S. aureus* were most common among cases of late disease. Heart failure complicated 50% of cases, non-neurologic emboli 35%, prosthesis instability 32%, and neurologic emboli 27%. Mortality was 34% at 4 months. Predictors of mortality among *S. aureus* cases were septic shock, heart failure, mediastinitis, and prothrombin time <30%; predictors among non-*S. aureus* cases were renal failure, heart failure, and prothrombin time <30% [23].

In summary, these studies show that the incidence of IE in ICUs ranges from 0.8% to 3%. *S. aureus* is the most frequent pathogen. Complication rates, including heart failure, sepsis, and neurologic events, are higher than typical rates seen among IE in non-ICU populations. The incidence of nosocomial IE is high in this population, and the mortality rates are high compared to other IE populations.

26.4 Diagnosis

26.4.1 History and Physical Examination

The spectrum of clinical presentation of IE is broad, and clinical features are often non-specific. IE can affect virtually any organ, but certain elements of the history and physical examination should raise suspicion of IE. Unlike patients with subacute bacterial endocarditis who often report nonspecific constitutional symptoms, patients with acute endocarditis typically describe the abrupt onset of fever and rigors. The presence of known risk factors for IE, such as invasive procedures, dental work, intravenous drug use, structural heart disease, or prior endocarditis, suggest the possibility of IE. The clinical history may indicate a potential source of bacteremia. History should also include inquiry into complications of IE, including the sequelae of embolization to the brain, lungs, spleen, gut, kidneys, bones and joints, and skin.

Physical examination in patients with suspected or confirmed IE should be comprehensive, with special attention to examination of the heart, skin and mucosal surfaces, ocular fundi, central nervous system, spleen, dentition, and all current or recent sites of invasive devices and procedures. Although heart murmur is present in 85% of patients diagnosed with IE, a changing murmur is identified in only 5–10% of cases. Approximately 50% of patients with IE have evidence of embolic phenomena on physical examination. Clinical sequelae of embolization include skin manifestations in 18–50% of patients, splenomegaly in 20–57%, and retinal lesions in 2–10% [2]. An absence of clinical findings should not rule out the diagnosis of IE in the presence of clinical suspicion.

26.4.2 Diagnostic Criteria

The Duke Criteria are commonly used in making the diagnosis of IE. Originally proposed in 1994 [24], they have since been modified [25], and have been shown to be superior to the previously used criteria [26, 27]. Diagnosis is classified as "definite," "probable," or "rejected" based on the presence of major and minor criteria including information from blood cultures, echocardiography, pathology, serology, history, and clinical examination. The modified Duke Criteria are shown in Table 26.1.

Table 26.1. Modified Duke criteria for diagnosis of infective endocarditis (IE)[a]. Adapted with permission from Li et al. [25]

Major criteria
Microbiologic: typical organisms cultured from two separate blood cultures, OR persistently positive blood cultures, OR single culture (or phase 1 IgG >1:800) for *Coxiella burnetii*
Evidence of endocardial involvement: echocardiogram showing oscillating intracardiac mass, abscess, or partial dehiscence of prosthetic valve; OR new valvular regurgitation
Minor criteria
Predisposition to IE: previous IE, intravenous drug use, prosthetic heart valve, cyanotic congenital heart disease, mitral valve prolapse, or other cardiac lesion causing turbulent blood flow within the heart
Fever >38 °C
Vascular phenomena: major arterial emboli, septic pulmonary infarcts, mycotic aneurysm, intracranial hemorrhage, conjunctival hemorrhages, or Janeway's lesions
Immunologic phenomena: glomerulonephritis, Osler's nodes, Roth's spots, or rheumatoid factor
Microbiologic findings not meeting major criteria

[a] Definite endocarditis requires two major criteria, or one major and three minor criteria, or five minor criteria. Possible endocarditis requires one major and one minor criterion, or three minor criteria

26.4.3 Echocardiography

Echocardiographic findings which are suggestive of IE include vegetation, abscess, aneurysm, fistula, leaflet perforation, or, in the case of prosthetic valves, valvular dehiscence [28]. Both transthoracic echocardiography (TTE) and transesophageal echocardiography (TEE) can be useful in the diagnosis and evaluation of IE. The sensitivity of TTE is low (46%) compared to TEE (93%), though the specificities are similar (95–96%) [29]. Obesity, hyperinflation of the lungs (as occurs in mechanically ventilated patients), and the presence of a prosthetic heart valve all reduce the sensitivity of TTE.

In patients with a negative TTE but "possible" IE by modified Duke Criteria, TEE has been shown to improve the ability to diagnose IE. In one study, both TTE and TEE were performed on 114 patients with IE. Three patients who were classified as "rejected" cases by TTE became "possible" cases of IE with TEE, and 22 patients who were "possible" cases became "definite" [30]. In another study of 103 patients with *S. aureus* bacteremia, TTE was positive in 7% of patients and indeterminate in 18%. Subsequent TEE identified vegetations in 19% of those who initially had negative TTE, and in 21% of those with an indeterminate TTE [31]. In addition to its superior diagnostic ability, TEE can better identify complications of IE, such as perivalvular abscess and fistula, which may alter clinical management. TEE is now considered by many experts to be the initial echocardiographic modality of choice for IE, except in patients with low clinical suspicion of IE [32].

26.4.4 Additional Tests

In addition to a history and physical examination, when IE is suspected, several additional tests should be considered. A minimum of three blood cultures should be drawn, with the first and last drawn at least 1 h apart. The microbiology lab should be alerted to the possible diagnosis of IE so that culture techniques may be altered if isolation of more fastidious organisms is required. Electrocardiogram should be obtained to evaluate for new conduction disturbance. Additional testing which may be useful includes chest radiograph to evaluate for the presence of embolism or heart failure, urinalysis to evaluate for possible glomerulonephritis, and rheumatoid factor. Glomerulonephritis and positive rheumatoid factor are minor diagnostic criteria in the modified Duke criteria.

26.5 Specific Pathogens

26.5.1 *Staphylococcus aureus*

Over the last 15 years, the incidence of *S. aureus* IE has increased, overtaking viridans streptococci as the predominant organism in many reports [32–36]. Several researchers have postulated that medical advances and increasing use of technology including intravenous catheters and implanted prosthetic devices have resulted in a higher incidence of nosocomial or healthcare-associated staphylococcal bacteremia, placing more patients at risk for endocarditis [33].

Staphylococcus aureus commonly causes acute IE and is associated with higher mortality than other organisms [15, 37, 38]. It involves the mitral valve more often than the aortic valve and is a frequent cause of right-sided IE among intravenous drug users [15]. *S. aureus* IE is frequently complicated by embolic events. In one large international cohort study, embolization occurred in 60% of cases of *S. aureus* IE versus 31% of cases caused by other organisms. Embolic events to the central nervous system are also more frequent in *S. aureus* IE than in IE caused by other organisms (20% vs. 13%) [15].

In general, antibiotic treatment of *S. aureus* IE should include a minimum of 6 weeks of nafcillin or oxacillin for oxacillin-susceptible strains, or 6 weeks of vancomycin for oxacillin-resistant strains. Vancomycin should not be used for treatment of oxacillin-susceptible strains unless a serious β-lactam allergy is documented [32]. Most experts also endorse the addition of gentamicin for 3–5 days at the beginning of treatment for oxacillin-susceptible strains. The addition of an aminoglycoside has been associated with more rapid clearance of bacteremia, but has not resulted in improvements in morbidity or mortality [39]. Short-course therapy (2 weeks) using a β-lactam plus aminoglycoside has been shown to be effective in selected cases of right-sided *S. aureus* IE in intravenous drug users [32]. When treating prosthetic valve endocarditis (PVE) caused by *S. aureus*, rifampin should be added to the treatment regimen for the duration of therapy, and gentamicin should be added for the first 2 weeks of therapy for both oxacillin-susceptible and oxacillin-resistant strains [32]. Please see Tables 26.2 and 26.3 for further treatment recommendations.

26.5.2 Coagulase-Negative Staphylococci

A recent study estimated that 6% of native valve endocarditis (NVE) is caused by coagulase-negative staphylococci [40]. Most of these cases are caused by *S. epidermidis*, though many facilities do not identify coagulase-

Table 26.2. Selected native valve endocarditis treatment regimens. Adapted with permission from Baddour et al. [32]

Organism	Drug	Duration	Alternative/comments
Oxacillin-sensitive *Staphylococcus*	Oxacillin/nafcillin 2 g q4 h **with or without** Gentamicin 1 mg/kg q8 h	6 weeks 3–5 days	For non-anaphylactoid penicillin allergy, substitute cefazolin 2 g IV q8 h for oxacillin/nafcillin. For anaphylactoid penicillin allergy, vancomycin 15 mg/kg q12 h[a]
Oxacillin-resistant *Staphylococcus*	Vancomycin 15 mg/kg q12 h[a]	6 weeks	
Viridans streptococci/*S. bovis* Highly penicillin-susceptible (PCN MIC ≤ 0.12 μg/ml)	Penicillin G 12–18 million U/24 h[b] or Ceftriaxone 2 g IV/IM q24 h	4 weeks 4 weeks	For penicillin allergy, vancomycin 15 mg/kg q12 h[a]
Viridans streptococci/*S. bovis* Relatively penicillin-resistant (PCN MIC > 0.12–0.5 μg/ml)	Penicillin G 24 million U/24 h[b] **plus** Gentamicin 3 mg/kg q24 h **or** Ceftriaxone 2 g IV/IM q24 h **plus** Gentamicin 3 mg/kg q24 h	4 weeks 2 weeks 4 weeks 2 weeks	For penicillin allergy, vancomycin 15 mg/kg IV q12 h[a]
Viridans streptococci/*S. bovis* or Nutritionally variant streptococci Penicillin-resistant (PCN MIC > 0.5 μg/ml)	See treatment regimen for penicillin/ampicillin-resistant enterococcal endocarditis	–	–
Enterococcus spp. Pan-sensitive	Ampicillin 2 g IV q4 h **plus** Gentamicin 1 mg/kg q8 h[c] **or** Penicillin G 18–30 million U/24 h[b] **plus** Gentamicin 1 mg/kg q8 h[c]	4–6 weeks 4–6 weeks 4–6 weeks 4–6 weeks	For penicillin allergy, vancomycin 15 mg/kg IV q12 h[a] **plus** Gentamicin 1 mg/kg IV/IM q8 h[c] for 6 weeks
Enterococcus spp. Penicillin/ampicillin-resistant	Vancomycin 15 mg/kg q12 h[a] **plus** Gentamicin 1 mg/kg q8 h[c]	6 weeks 6 weeks	If β-lactamase production, ampicillin-sulbactam 3 g q6 h **plus** Gentamicin 1 mg/kg q8 h[c] for 6 weeks
Enterococcus spp. Aminoglycoside resistant[d]	Ampicillin 2 g IV q4 h **or** Penicillin G 24 million U IV/24 h[b]	4–6 weeks[g]	For penicillin allergy, vancomycin 15 mg/kg IV q12 h[a] for 6 weeks
HACEK organisms	Ceftriaxone 2 g IV/IM q24 h **or** Ampicillin-sulbactam 3 g q6 h	4 weeks 4 weeks	For penicillin allergy, ciprofloxacin 400 mg IV q12 h

[a] Goal Vancomycin through 10–15 μg/mL
[b] Penicillin G dosing can be continuous infusion or given q4h
[c] Both gentamicin and streptomycin susceptibilities should be obtained. High-level aminoglycoside resistance is defined as gentamicin MIC > 500 to 2000 μg/mL or streptomycin MIC > 2000 μg/mL
[d] Isolates resistant to gentamicin should be tested for streptomycin sensitivity. If streptomycin-susceptible, streptomycin should be substituted for gentamicin at a dose of 7.5 mg/kg q12h

negative staphylococci to the species level. Coagulase-negative staphylococcal IE is associated with fewer embolic events but more frequent intracardiac abscesses than *S. aureus* IE. Mortality rates are similar between the two organisms [40]. IE caused by coagulase-negative staphylococci is typically more indolent in onset than IE caused by other organisms, making coagulase-negative staphylococci a less frequent cause of acute IE. One notable exception to this is the species *S. lugdunensis*, a coagulase-negative staphylococcus that has been described as causing acute IE with an aggressive clinical course [41].

Coagulase-negative staphylococci are a common cause of PVE, particularly in the first year after prosthetic valve implantation [32, 33, 42]. Because most coagulase-negative staphylococci readily form biofilm, they are well adapted to cause infections of prosthetic materials. Please refer to Tables 26.2 and 26.3 for treatment recommendations.

26.5.3 Streptococci

The proportion of IE caused by streptococci appears to be decreasing, but these organisms are still common pathogens, identified in almost 30 % of definite IE cases in one recent study [15]. The most common streptococ-

Table 26.3. Selected prosthetic valve endocarditis treatment regimens. Adapted with permission from Baddour et al. [32]

Organism	Drug	Duration	Alternative/comments
Oxacillin-sensitive *Staphylococcus*	Oxacillin/nafcillin 2 g IV q4 h **plus** Rifampin 300 mg IV/po q8 h **plus** Gentamicin 1 mg/kg IV/IM q8 h	≥6 weeks ≥6 weeks 2 weeks	For non-anaphylactoid penicillin allergy, substitute cefazolin 2 g IV q8 h for oxacillin/nafcillin For anaphylactoid penicillin allergy, vancomycin 15 mg/kg q12 h[a] for 6 weeks
Oxacillin-resistant *Staphylococcus*	Vancomycin 15 mg/kg IV q12 h[a] **plus** Rifampin 300 mg IV/po q8 h **plus** Gentamicin 1 mg/kg IV/IM q8 h	≥6 weeks ≥6 weeks 2 weeks	For penicillin allergy, vancomycin 15 mg/kg q12 h[a] for 6 weeks
Viridans streptococci/*S. bovis*[c] Highly penicillin-susceptible (PCN MIC ≤ 0.12 μg/ml)	Penicillin G 24 million U/24 h[b] **or** Gentamicin 3 mg/kg q24 h **or** Ceftriaxone 2 g IV/IM q24 h **with or without** Gentamicin 3 mg/kg q24 h	6 weeks 2 weeks 6 weeks 2 weeks	For penicillin allergy, vancomycin 15 mg/kg q12 h[a] for 6 weeks
Viridans streptococci/*S. bovis*	Penicillin G 24 million U/24 h[b] **plus** Gentamicin 3 mg/kg q24 h OR Ceftriaxone 2 g IV/IM q24 h **plus** Gentamicin 3 mg/kg q24 h	6 weeks 6 weeks 6 weeks 6 weeks	Relatively or fully penicillin-resistant (PCN MIC >0.12)
Enterococcus spp.	PVE treatment regimens identical to NVE treatment regimens. See Table 26.2	–	–
HACEK organisms	PVE treatment regimens identical to NVE treatment regimens. See Table 26.2	–	–

[a] Goal: vancomycin trough 10–15 μg/ml, [b] Penicillin G dosing can be continuous infusion or given q4 h, [c] Optional addition of gentamicin 3 mg/kg q24 h for 2 weeks

cal species causing IE are found in the viridans streptococcus group. Viridans streptococci are α-hemolytic oral flora, and include the following species: *S. mitis*, *S. mutans*, *S. salivarius*, *S. sanguis*, and the *S. milleri* group (also known as the *S. anginosus* or *S. intermedius* group, which includes *S. intermedius*, *S. anginosus*, and *S. constellatus*) [12, 32]. Nutritionally variant streptococci including *Abiotropha* and *Granulicatella* species are also classified as viridans streptococci.

Streptococcus bovis is a group D streptococcal species distinct from viridans streptococci. *S. bovis* is found in enteric flora, and bacteremia with this organism is associated with colon polyps, colon cancer and liver disease [43]. *S. bovis* accounts for 5–15% of cases of IE in the United States, is associated with involvement of multiple valves, and is typically diagnosed in older patients with more comorbid diseases [43, 44]. Treatment of IE caused by viridans streptococci or by *S. bovis* is determined by the MIC of the infecting organism to penicillin. Aminoglycosides are sometimes required for synergistic effects. Please refer to Tables 26.2 and 26.3 for treatment recommendations.

Other streptococci (including *S. pneumoniae* and streptococci in Groups A, B, C and G) account for less than 5% of cases of definite IE [15]. Of these organisms, group B streptococci (*S. agalactiae*) are the most commonly identified pathogens in IE [35]. Like *S. bovis*-associated IE, IE due to *S. agalactiae* is commonly seen in older patients with multiple co-morbid diseases. Group B streptococcal IE is often an aggressive clinical entity characterized by large vegetations, frequent embolic events, and high mortality [45]. Treatment of IE caused by these streptococcal species should include a β-lactam or other cell wall-active agent and, in some cases, an aminoglycoside [12, 32].

26.5.4 Enterococci

Enterococci are the third most common etiology of IE, causing approximately 10% of all cases [16, 33]. Endocarditis caused by enterococcal species is commonly diagnosed in older men and is associated with lower mortality rates than IE caused by other organisms [16, 46]. A gastrointestinal or urinary source of enterococcal bacteremia can often be identified. Enterococcal NVE frequently involves the aortic valve and causes symptoms of heart failure. Compared to other organisms, it is less commonly associated with embolic events [16]. PVE caused by enterococcal species is associated with intracardiac abscess formation [46].

Treatment of enterococcal IE is complex. Enterococcal isolates from patients with IE should be tested for susceptibility to penicillin, ampicillin, and vancomycin as well as for high-level resistance to both gentamicin and streptomycin. In general, successful therapy requires two antimicrobial agents with a typical regimen consisting of a cell wall-active agent (penicillin, ampicillin or vancomycin) plus an aminoglycoside for synergistic effect. Aminoglycosides are typically given for the duration of therapy (4–6 weeks) though recent data suggest that shorter courses may be adequate [47]. Please refer to Tables 26.2 and 26.3 for treatment recommendations.

26.5.5 Gram-Negative Bacilli

Gram-negative bacilli account for approximately 5% of IE diagnoses, and are typically divided into HACEK and non-HACEK organisms [33]. The HACEK group includes organisms from the following genera: *Haemophilus*, *Actinobacillus*, *Cardiobacterium*, *Eikenella*, and *Kingella*. Though these fastidious organisms traditionally have required prolonged incubation periods to grow on culture media, many HACEK organisms grow within 5 days using modern culture techniques [48]. Because β-lactamase production in the HACEK organisms is becoming more frequent, ceftriaxone is now the recommended empiric therapy [32].

Enterobacteriaceae and other non-HACEK gram-negative bacilli are unusual causes of IE, and are often associated with intravenous drug use or underlying valvular abnormalities. These cases are characterized by frequent heart failure and high mortality rates. *Pseudomonas* IE has been strongly associated with intravenous drug use [12, 32].

26.5.6 *Candida* Species

Candida is an uncommon cause of IE, accounting for approximately 2% of cases [33, 49]. In one recent series, candidal endocarditis was much more frequently observed in patients with prosthetic valves [49]. Although previous studies have reported mortality rates of almost 80%, others have found the mortality rate to be comparable to that of *S. aureus* IE at approximately 40% [12, 49]. Because candidal endocarditis is rare, treatment guidelines have not been clearly established. Many experts recommend surgical intervention in conjunction with antifungal therapy with amphotericin B [12, 32].

26.5.7 Culture-Negative IE

Between 5% and 10% of IE cases are diagnosed in the setting of negative blood cultures [33, 50, 51]. Because the diagnostic criteria for IE are less accurate in this situation, some experts estimate that culture-negative IE may actually account for more than 20% of true cases [32, 52]. Reasons for negative blood cultures among patients with IE include: prior antibiotic therapy, inadequate culture techniques, fastidious or unexpected pathogens, or non-infectious endocarditis [32, 51, 52]. A recent review of culture-negative IE suggested that up to 50% of cases are caused by *Coxiella burnetii*, and almost 25% are caused by *Bartonella* species [51]. Serologic studies are instrumental in diagnosing both Q fever and *Bartonella* endocarditis. PCR of valve tissue or of serum has also increased detection rates of *Bartonella* species in IE [53]. Recent studies have shown mortality rates in culture-negative IE of less than 10%, much lower than previously reported [51, 52].

26.6 Complications

26.6.1 Congestive Heart Failure

Over half of patients with IE suffer at least one complication from the disease [54]. CHF is one of the most common complications of IE in both native and prosthetic valves, and is usually due to infection-induced valvular dysfunction [55]. In retrospective studies of IE patients with CHF, medical management alone is associated with higher mortality than surgical and medical management combined (60% vs. 29%) [56]. Patients with aortic valve IE are more likely to develop severe CHF than those with mitral valve IE [32, 56, 57]. CHF is an important indication for surgical intervention, particularly in the setting of aortic valve IE [12, 32, 55–57].

26.6.2 Perivalvular/Intracardiac Abscess

Perivalvular or intracardiac abscesses complicate approximately 20–40% of cases of IE [58–60]. Periannular extension of infection is more common in IE of the aortic valve [56, 59] and occurs more frequently in PVE than in NVE [55, 56, 59, 60]. Intracardiac infection extending to the conduction system and causing heart block is more common in aortic valve IE [55, 56, 59]. Patients with perivalvular or intracardiac abscesses have increased rates of embolization and higher mortality [56, 58, 59]. Staphylococcal IE has been associated with an increased incidence of perivalvular abscess

[58–60]. Periannular infection is best diagnosed using TEE and usually requires surgical intervention [55, 58].

26.6.3 Embolization

Twenty to 50% of patients with IE experience at least one embolic event during the course of illness [32, 54, 61]. Embolization to the central nervous system accounts for 40–65% of embolic events, and the middle cerebral artery is the most commonly affected vascular distribution [32, 54, 62]. Other common sites of embolization include the spleen, kidneys, lungs, and liver [54, 57]. Many studies have shown rates of embolic events to be highest in the first 2 weeks after diagnosis, with decreasing risk once antibiotic therapy is begun [62, 63]. Several echocardiographic characteristics have been correlated with increased risk of embolization including vegetation size greater than 10 mm and vegetation on the mitral valve, particularly on the anterior mitral valve leaflet [32, 57]. Overall, embolic events during the course of IE have been associated with a two- to fourfold increase in mortality [57].

26.7 Management Issues

26.7.1 Antibiotic Therapy

The complexity of antibiotic selection and the long-term nature of treatment of IE make consultation with an infectious diseases specialist advisable in most cases. Over 50% of IE cases are managed with antibiotic therapy alone [32]. Parenteral therapy is preferred because of consistently higher antibiotic levels as compared to oral regimens, which often yield inconsistent drug levels due to variable GI absorption [12]. Long durations of therapy are necessary because of both poor penetration of antibiotics into valvular vegetations and high concentrations of microorganisms within those vegetations [12].

Combination regimens with a cell wall-active agent (β-lactam or vancomycin) and an aminoglycoside are used for synergistic effects in the treatment of many cases of gram-positive IE. Because cell wall-active agents increase aminoglycoside entry into susceptible bacteria, these agents should be dosed in close temporal proximity to one another to maximize synergistic effects. Though in vitro and animal studies provide the rationale for this combination therapy, clinical data are scarce. The combination of a β-lactam and aminoglycoside for *S. aureus* IE reduced the duration of bacteremia in one study but did not improve clinical outcomes [39]. A recent meta-analysis examining the addition of an aminoglycoside to a cell wall-active agent in treatment of *S. aureus* and viridans streptococci showed no clinical benefit of combination therapy [64]. When using aminoglycosides for synergy in treatment of gram-positive IE, doses and resultant peak and trough levels are generally lower than those recommended for primary treatment of gram-negative infections [12, 32].

Once antibiotic therapy has been initiated, blood cultures should be drawn at least every 48 h until clearance of bacteremia has been documented. Treatment duration should be counted from the time of the first negative blood cultures. If an aminoglycoside or vancomycin is used, levels should be monitored intermittently to prevent toxicity [12, 32].

26.7.2 Surgical Intervention

Because decisions regarding surgery for patients with IE are complex, and because the need for surgical intervention is often sudden, it is often advisable to include a surgeon in the management of patients with IE. Current guidelines for surgical treatment of IE are based primarily on observational data rather than prospective randomized trials [12, 65]. Limitations in the quality of evidence should be taken into account when considering existing recommendations for surgical intervention.

The presence of CHF is a strong indication for surgical treatment [55, 57]. Mortality among patients with moderate to severe CHF is greater than 50% in those managed medically, but decreases to only 10–35% in those managed both surgically and medically [57]. Severe valvular dysfunction or dehiscence is also considered an indication for surgery because of the potential for the development of CHF with sudden clinical deterioration [55, 56]. This risk appears to be higher for patients with aortic valve IE than for those with mitral valve IE [56, 66].

Patients with perivalvular or intracardiac abscess should be strongly considered for surgery. Abscess formation results in decreased penetration of antibiotics to the site of infection, making medical treatment alone less likely to be successful [59]. In addition, abscesses often cause heart block and valvular insufficiency with resultant CHF [55, 56, 59].

In general, IE of a prosthetic valve is considered an indication for surgery based on data showing higher mortality in patients who receive medical management alone [57, 67]. Some studies suggest that certain patients with late PVE may be adequately managed with medical therapy alone [68, 69]. Patients with PVE but without clinically significant heart failure, those who improve on antibiotic therapy, and those who have IE caused by less virulent organisms such as viridans streptococci may be considered for initial non-surgical management [68].

Patients with organisms that have been historically refractory to medical management, such as *Pseudomo-*

nas, *Brucella*, *Coxiella*, and *Candida*, may benefit from surgical management [32, 55, 57]. In addition, patients with IE caused by organisms resistant to multiple bactericidal agents should be considered for surgery.

Surgical interventions based on echocardiographic predictors of embolism, or on a history of an embolic event, have not been associated with decreased mortality [32, 57]. Specific echocardiographic criteria can predict risk of embolization [61, 63], but this risk of embolization must be weighed against surgical risk for each individual patient. If surgical treatment is undertaken to minimize embolization risk, this intervention is most useful when performed early after the initial diagnosis of IE is made [32, 57].

Forty to 45% of patients with IE undergo surgery, and recent data suggest that the rates of surgical intervention are essentially the same in NVE and PVE [67, 70]. Surgical intervention is more common in younger patients with CHF, perivalvular abscess, and coagulase-negative staphylococcal IE. In selected patients, surgical treatment has been associated with lower mortality. In-hospital mortality is marginally decreased in patients with PVE who undergo surgery, but decreases dramatically in patients receiving surgery for NVE [67, 70]. Longitudinal outcome studies show continued survival benefit after surgical intervention in patients with multiple indications for surgery. In cases of PVE, long-term survival at 10 years has been predicted at 28% with medical therapy and 58% with surgery [70]. Analysis of 6-month mortality in a cohort of patients with NVE showed a sustained mortality benefit in patients managed surgically (14%) compared to patients receiving medical therapy (51%) [73]. Overall, surgery is associated with lower mortality in selected patients with either NVE or PVE.

26.7.3 Right-Sided IE

Approximately 10% of IE cases involve the right side of the heart, almost always affecting the tricuspid valve [32, 72]. Right-sided IE is primarily a disease of intravenous drug users and has different clinical characteristics than left-sided IE [73]. Patients with right-sided IE are younger and have less underlying valve disease than patients with left-sided IE [32, 73]. Clinical manifestations of right-sided IE are often the result of septic pulmonary emboli and include pleuritic chest pain, dyspnea and hemoptysis. More than two-thirds of patients with right-sided IE have abnormal chest X-rays [32]. Echocardiography often reveals large vegetations (> 20 mm), and valvular destruction may be severe [73]. Right-sided IE can present with symptoms of right-sided heart failure caused by tricuspid valve damage.

Staphylococcus aureus is the most commonly isolated organism in right-sided IE. In contrast to the recommended 6-week course of antibiotic therapy for left-sided *S. aureus* IE, select cases of tricuspid valve *S. aureus* IE may be managed with shorter courses of parenteral antibiotics or with oral regimens [32, 73–75]. Patients with concurrent left-sided IE, evidence of metastatic infection, CHF, prosthetic valves, vegetations larger than 10 mm, immunocompromised status, or infection with methicillin-resistant *S. aureus* are not considered candidates for shorter course therapy or oral regimens [73]. Overall, the prognosis for right-sided IE is good with mortality rates less than 10% [72, 73].

26.7.4 Prosthetic Valve Endocarditis

The risk of prosthetic valve endocarditis (PVE) is highest in the initial postoperative period, and is estimated at 1–5% in the first 12 months [57, 76, 77]. Overall, the risk of PVE is similar for mechanical and bioprosthetic valves and does not appear to differ between the aortic and mitral positions [77–79]. Early-onset PVE, occurring within the first 12 months after surgery, is usually nosocomial in origin and is most often caused by coagulase-negative staphylococci or *S. aureus* [78]. Late-onset PVE, diagnosed more than 12 months after surgery, has similar microbiology to NVE [42, 79].

The antibiotics used for treatment of PVE are similar to NVE, but longer courses of therapy are typically required. One notable exception to this rule is the addition of rifampin to the treatment regimen for PVE caused by *S. aureus*. Please see Table 26.3 for treatment recommendations. Surgical intervention should be considered in patients with PVE, particularly those at high risk for treatment failure.

26.7.5 Mortality

In recent studies, in-hospital mortality among patients with IE has been estimated at 15–20%, with subsequent 12-month mortality rates of 20–30% [16, 61, 80–82]. Mortality is similar in NVE and PVE [57]. While there does not appear to be a significant difference in survival between mitral and aortic valve IE, patients with right-sided IE have significantly lower mortality rates when compared to those with left-sided IE [57]. Mortality has been shown to vary by causative organism as well. Viridans streptococci and enterococci are associated with lower mortality in native valve IE while *S. aureus* IE is associated with higher mortality [16]. IE caused by gram-negative bacilli or by fungi is associated with greater than 50% mortality [57].

Many of the complications of IE are also independent risk factors for mortality. CHF [15, 61], periannular abscess [15], embolic events [4, 82, 83], and large mobile vegetations on echocardiogram [61, 82, 84] have all been associated with mortality. Patient factors such as nosocomial acquisition of infection [83], older age [61], immunocompromised status [4], diabetes [80], severity of illness such as APACHE II score [80], hemodynamic instability [4], altered mental status [4, 82, 83] and renal failure [61, 82, 83] are significant predictors of mortality.

Table 26.4. Cardiac conditions associated with endocarditis. Adapted with permission from Dajani et al. [8]

Endocarditis prophylaxis recommended
High-risk category
Prosthetic cardiac valves, including bioprosthetic and homograft valves
Previous bacterial endocarditis
Complex cyanotic congenital heart disease (e.g., single ventricle states, transposition of the great arteries, tetralogy of Fallot)
Surgically constructed systemic pulmonary shunts or conduits
Moderate-risk category
Most other congenital cardiac malformations (other than above and below)
Acquired valve dysfunction (e.g., rheumatic heart disease)
Hypertrophic cardiomyopathy
Mitral valve prolapse with valve regurgitation and/or thickened leaflets
Endocarditis prophylaxis not recommended
Negligible-risk category (no greater risk than the general population)
Isolated secundum atrial septal defect
Surgical repair of atrial septal defect, ventricular septal defect, or patent ductus arteriosus (without residual abnormality, greater than 6 months after repair)
Previous coronary artery bypass graft surgery
Mitral valve prolapse without valve regurgitation
Physiologic, functional, or innocent heart murmurs
Previous Kawasaki disease without valve dysfunction
Previous rheumatic fever without valve dysfunction
Cardiac pacemakers (intravascular and epicardial) and implanted defibrillators

26.8 Antimicrobial Prophylaxis

Many procedures that cause mucosal or cutaneous trauma cause transient bacteremia. Patients with certain cardiac defects are more likely to develop IE after bacteremia. This is the rationale for antimicrobial prophylaxis to prevent IE at the time of certain procedures. There have been no randomized controlled trials in at-risk patients to prove definitively that prophylaxis works, but nevertheless it is common practice [8]. The AHA Practice Guideline for the Prevention of Bacterial Endocarditis is an excellent source of information regarding antimicrobial prophylaxis [8].

Table 26.5. Selected procedures and antimicrobial prophylaxis. Adapted with permission from Dajani et al. [8]

Endocarditis prophylaxis recommended
Surgical operations that involve respiratory, intestinal, or biliary mucosa
Bronchoscopy with a rigid bronchoscope
Sclerotherapy for esophageal varices
Esophageal stricture dilation
Endoscopic retrograde cholangiography with biliary obstruction
Cystoscopy
Urethral dilation
Endocarditis prophylaxis not recommended
Endotracheal intubation
Bronchoscopy with a flexible bronchoscope, with or without biopsy[a]
Transesophageal echocardiography[a]
Esophagogastroduodenoscopy (EGD) with or without gastrointestinal biopsy[a]
Urethral catheterization
Cardiac catheterization, including balloon angioplasty
Implantation of cardiac pacemakers, defibrillators, or coronary stents
Incision or biopsy of surgically scrubbed skin

[a] Prophylaxis is optional for high-risk patients

Table 26.6. Prophylactic antibiotic regimens for prevention of endocarditis in adults. Adapted with permission from Dajani et al. [8]

Procedure	Recommended regimen	Alternatives
Respiratory/esophageal	Amoxicillin 2 g PO 1 h before procedure	Penicillin allergy: clindamycin 600 mg PO, or cephalexin[a] or cefadroxil[a] 2 g PO, or azithromycin or clarithromycin 500 mg PO 1 h before procedure Unable to take oral medications: ampicillin 2 g IM/IV or cefazolin[a] 1 g IM/IV or clindamycin 600 mg IV within 30 min before procedure
Genitourinary/gastrointestinal (other than esophageal), patient with high-risk cardiac condition	Ampicillin 2 g IM/IV plus gentamicin 1.5 mg/kg IV/IM (not to exceed 120 mg) within 30 min of starting procedure; 6 h later, ampicillin 1 g IM/IV or amoxicillin 1 g orally	Penicillin allergy: vancomycin 1 g IV over 1–2 h plus gentamicin 1.5 mg/kg IV/IM (not to exceed 120 mg); complete injection/infusion within 30 min of starting procedure
Genitourinary/gastrointestinal (other than esophageal), patient with moderate-risk cardiac condition	Amoxicillin 2 g PO 1 h before procedure, or ampicillin 2 g IM/IV within 30 min of starting procedure	Penicillin allergy: vancomycin 1 g IV over 1–2 h; complete infusion within 30 min of starting procedure

[a] Cephalosporins should not be used in individuals with immediate-type hypersensitivity reaction (urticaria, angioedema, or anaphylaxis) to penicillins

Prophylaxis is recommended when a patient with a moderate- or high-risk cardiac lesion undergoes a procedure for which prophylaxis is recommended. The cardiac lesion classification is presented in Table 26.4, and a partial list of procedures is shown in Table 26.5. In general, if prophylaxis is indicated, oral regimens should be given 1 h prior to the procedure, and intravenous regimens should be completed 30 min prior to the procedure. Prophylactic antibiotic recommendations are shown in Table 26.6.

References

1. Strom BL, Abrutyn E, Berlin JA, Kinman JL, Feldman RS, Stolley PD, Levison ME, Korzeniowski OM, Kaye D (2000) Risk factors for infective endocarditis: oral hygiene and nondental exposures. Circulation 102:2842–8
2. Bayer AS (1993) Infective endocarditis. Clin Infect Dis 17:313–320
3. Karth GD, Koreny M, Binder T, Knapp S, Zauner C, Valentin A, Honninger R, Heinz G, Siostrzonek C (2002) Complicated infective endocarditis necessitating ICU admission: clinical course and prognosis. Crit Care 6:149–154
4. Mourvillier B, Trouillet J, Timsit J, Baudot J, Chastre J, Regnier B, Gibert C, Wolff M (2004) Infective endocarditis in the intensive care unit: clinical spectrum and prognostic factors in 228 consecutive patients. Intensive Care Med 30:2046–2052
5. Harris SL (1992) Definitions and demographic characteristics. In: Kaye D (ed) Infective endocarditis. Raven Press, New York, pp 1–30
6. Durack DT, Petersdorf RG (1977) Changes in the epidemiology of endocarditis. In: Kaplan EL, Taranta AV (eds) Infective endocarditis. An American Heart Association Symposium. American Heart Association, Dallas, pp 3–23
7. Tunkel AR, Scheld WM (1992) Experimental models of endocarditis. In: Kaye D (ed) Infective endocarditis. Raven Press, New York, pp 37–61
8. Dajani AS, Taubert KA, Wilson W, Bolger AF, Bayer A, Ferrieri P, Gewitz MH, Shulman ST, Nouri S, Newburger JW, Hutto C, Pallasch TJ, Gage TW, Levison ME, Peter G, Zuccaro G (1997) Prevention of bacterial endocarditis: Recommendations by the American Heart Association. Circulation 96:358–66
9. Gould K, Ramirez-Ronda CH, Holmes RK, Sanford JP (1978) Adherence of bacteria to heart valves in vitro. J Clin Invest 56:1314–1325
10. Scheld WM, Valvone JA, Sande MA (1978) Bacterial adherence in the pathogenesis of endocarditis. Interaction of bacterial dextran, platelets, and fibrin. J Clin Invest 61: 1394–1403
11. Kuypers JM, Proctor RA (1989) Reduced adherence to traumatized rat heart valves by a low-fibronectin-binding mutant of *Staphylococcus aureus*. Infect Immun 57:2306–2312
12. Fowler VG, Scheld WM, Bayer AS (2005) Endocarditis and intravascular infections. In: Mandell GL, Bennett JE, Dolin R (eds) Mandell, Douglas and Bennett's principles and practice of infectious diseases, 6th edn. Churchill Livingstone, Philadelphia, pp 975–1021
13. Griffin MR, Wilson WR, Edwards WD, O'Fallon WM, Kurland LT (1985) Infective endocarditis. Olmsted County, Minnesota, 1950 through 1981. JAMA 254:1199–1202
14. Thayer WS (1926) Studies on bacterial (infective) endocarditis. Johns Hopkins Hosp Rep 22:1–8
15. Miro JM, Anguera I, Cabell CH, Chen AY, Stafford JA, Corey GR, Olaison L, Eykyn S, Hoen B, Abrutyn E, Raoult D, Bayer A, Fowler VG, and the International Collaboration on Endocarditis Merged Database Study Group (2005) *Staphylococcus aureus* native valve infective endocarditis: Report of 566 episodes from the International Collaboration on Endocarditis Merged Database. Clin Infect Dis 41:507–514
16. McDonald JR, Olaison L, Anderson DJ, Hoen B, Miro JM, Eykyn S, Abrutyn E, Fowler VG Jr, Habib G, Selton-Suty C, Pappas PA, Cabell CH, Corey GR, Marco R, Sexton DJ (2005) Enterococcal native valve endocarditis: Report of 107 episodes from the International Collaboration on Endocarditis Merged Database. Am J Med 11:759–766
17. Michel PL, Acar J (1995) Native cardiac disease predisposing to infective endocarditis. Eur Heart J 16 Suppl B:2–9
18. Clemens JD, Horwitz RI, Jaffe CC, Feinstein AR, Stanton BF (1982) A controlled evaluation of the risk of bacterial endocarditis in persons with mitral-valve prolapse. N Engl J Med 307:776–780
19. Pelletier LL, Petersdorf RG (1977) Infective endocarditis: A review of 125 cases from the University of Washington Hospitals, 1963–72. Medicine (Baltimore) 56:287–299
20. Martín-Dávila P, Fortún J, Navas E, Cobo J, Jiménez-Mena M, Moya JL, Moreno S (2005) Nosocomial endocarditis in a tertiary hospital: An increasing trend in native valve cases. Chest 128:772–779
21. Terpenning MS, Buggy BP, Kaufmann CA (1988) Hospital-acquired infective endocarditis. Arch Intern Med 148: 1601–03
22. Gouello JP, Asfar P, Brenet O, Kouatchet A, Berhelot G, Alquier P (2000) Nosocomial endocarditis in the intensive care unit: an analysis of 22 cases. Crit Care Med 28: 377–382
23. Wolff M, Witchitz S, Chastang C, Regnier B, Vachon F (1995) Prosthetic valve endocarditis in the ICU. Prognostic factors of overall survival in a series of 122 cases and consequences for treatment decision. Chest 108:688–694
24. Durack DT, Lukes AS, Bright DK (1994) New criteria for diagnosis of infective endocarditis: utilization of specific echocardiographic findings. Duke Endocarditis Service. Am J Med 96:200–207
25. Li JS, Sexton DJ, Mick N, Nettles R, Fowler VG Jr, Ryan T, Bashore T, Corey GR (2002) Proposed modifications to the Duke criteria for the diagnosis of infective endocarditis. Clin Infect Dis 30:633–638
26. Bayer AS, Ward JL, Ginzton LE, Shapiro SM (1994) Evaluation of new clinical criteria for the diagnosis of infective endocarditis. Am J Med 96:211–215
27. Hoen B, Selton-Suty G, Danchin N, Weber M, Villemot JP, Mathieu P, Floquet J, Canton P (1995) Evaluation of the Duke criteria versus the Beth Israel criteria for the diagnosis of infective endocarditis. Clin Infect Dis 21:905–911
28. Sachdev M, Peterson GE, Jollis JG (2002) Imaging techniques for diagnosis of infective endocarditis. Infect Dis Clin North Am 16:319–37
29. Bashore TM, Cabell C, Fowler VJ Jr (2006) Update on infective endocarditis. Curr Probl Cardiol 4:274–352
30. Roe MT, Abramson MA, Li J, Heinle SK, Kisslo J, Corey GR, Sexton DJ (2000) Clinical information determines the impact of transesophageal echocardiography on the diagnosis of infective endocarditis by the Duke criteria. Am Heart J 139:945–51
31. Fowler VG, Li J, Corey GR, Boley J, Marr KA, Gopal AK, Kong LK, Gottlieb G, Donovan CL, Sexton DJ, Ryan T (1997) Role of echocardiography in evaluation of patients with *Staphylococcus aureus* bacteremia: experience in 103 patients. J Am Coll Cardiol 30:1072–8

32. Baddour LM, Wilson WR, Bayer AS, Fowler VG Jr, Bolger AF, Levison ME, Ferrieri P, Gerber MA, Tani LY, Gewitz MH, Tong DC, Steckelberg JM, Baltimore RS, Shulman ST, Burns JC, Falace DA, Newburger JW, Pallasch TJ, Takahashi M, Taubert KA (2005) Infective endocarditis: Diagnosis, antimicrobial therapy, and management of complications. A statement for healthcare professionals from the Committee on Rheumatic Fever, Endocarditis, and Kawasaki Disease, Council of Cardiovascular Disease in the Young, and the Councils on Clinical Cardiology, Stroke, and Cardiovascular Surgery and Anesthesia, American Heart Association. Circulation 6:e394–e434
33. Fowler VG, Miro JM, Hoen B, Cabell CH, Abrutyn E, Rubinstein E, Corey GR, Spelman D, Bradley SF, Barsic B, Pappas PA, Anstrom KJ, Wray D, Fortes CQ, Anguera I, Athan E, Jones P, van der Meer JTM, Elliott TSJ, Levine DP, Bayer AS (2005) *Staphylococcus aureus* endocarditis: A consequence of medical progress. JAMA 293:3012 – 3021
34. Brusch JL (1998) Infective endocarditis in critical care. In: Cunha BA (ed) Infectious diseases in critical care medicine, 1st edn. Marcel Dekker, New York, pp 387 – 434
35. Sanchez JL, Little R (2001) Acute infective endocarditis. In: Rello J, Valles J, Kollef MH (eds) Critical care infectious diseases, 1st edn. Kluwer Academic, Norwell, MA, pp 435 – 445
36. Tleyjeh IM, Steckelberg JM, Murad HS, Anavekar NS, Ghomrawi HM, Mirzoyev Z, Moustafa SE, Hoskin TL, Mandrekar JN, Wilson WR, Baddour LM (2005) Temporal trends in infective endocarditis: a population-based study in Olmsted County, Minnesota. JAMA 293:3061 – 2
37. Cabell CH, Jollis JG, Peterson GE, Corey GR, Anderson DJ, Sexton DJ, Woods CW, Reller LB, Ryan T, Fowler VG Jr (2002) Changing patient characteristics and the effect on mortality in endocarditis. Arch Intern Med 162:90 – 97
38. Chirouze C, Cabell CH, Fowler VG, Khayat N, Olaison L, Miro JM, Habib G, Abrutyn E, Eykyn S, Corey GR, Selton-Suty C, Hoen B, and the International Collaboration on Endocarditis Study Group (2004) Prognostic factors in 61 cases of *Staphylococcus aureus* prosthetic valve infective endocarditis from the International Collaboration on Endocarditis Merged Database. Clin Infect Dis 38:1323 – 1327
39. Korzeniowski O, Sande MA (1982) Combination antimicrobial therapy for *Staphylococcus aureus* endocarditis in patients addicted to parenteral drugs and in nonaddicts: A prospective study. Ann Intern Med 97:496 – 503
40. Chu VH, Cabell CH, Abrutyn E, Corey GR, Hoen B, Miro JM, Olaison L, Stryjewski ME, Pappas P, Anstrom KJ, Eykyn S, Habib G, Benito N, Fowler VG, and the International Collaboration on Endocarditis Merged Database Study Group (2004) Native valve endocarditis due to coagulase-negative staphylococci: Report of 99 episodes from the International Collaboration on Endocarditis Merged Database. Clin Infect Dis 39:1527 – 1530
41. Anguera I, Del Rio A, Miró JM, Matínez-Lacasa X, Marco F, Gumá JR, Quaglio G, Claramonte X, Moreno A, Mestres CA, Mauri E, Azqueta M, Benito N, García-de la Maria C, Almela M, Jiménez-Expósito M-J, Sued O, De Lazzari E, Gatell JM, and the Hospital Clinic Endocarditis Study Group (2005) *Staphylococcus lugdunensis* infective endocarditis: description of 10 cases and analysis of native valve, prosthetic valve, and pacemaker lead endocarditis clinical profiles. Heart 91:e10
42. Baddour LM, Wilson WR (2005) Prosthetic valve endocarditis and cardiovascular device-related infections. In: Mandell GL, Bennett JE, Dolin R (eds) Mandell, Douglas and Bennett's principles and practice of infectious diseases, 6th edn. Churchill Livingstone, Philadelphia, pp 1022 – 1044
43. Tripodi MF, Adinolfi LE, Ragone E, Durante Mangoni E, Fortunato R, Iarussi D, Ruggiero G, Utili R (2004) *Streptococcus bovis* endocarditis and its association with chronic liver disease: An underestimated risk factor. Clin Infect Dis 38:1394 – 1400
44. Hoen B, Chirouze C, Cabell CH, Selton-Suty C, Duchêne F, Olaison L, Miro JM, Habib G, Abrutyn E, Eykyn S, Bernard Y, Marco F, Corey GR, and the International Collaboration on Endocarditis Study Group (2005) Emergence of endocarditis due to group D streptococci: Findings derived from the merged database of the International Collaboration on Endocarditis. Eur J Clin Microbiol Infect Dis 24: 12 – 16
45. Sambola A, Miro JM, Tornos MP, Almirante B, Moreno-Torrico A, Gurgui M, Martinez E, Del Rio A, Azqueta M, Marco F, Gatell JM, and the *Streptococcus agalactiae* Endocarditis Study Group (2002) *Streptococcus agalactiae* infective endocarditis: Analysis of 30 cases and review of the literature, 1962 – 1998. Clin Infect Dis 34:1576 – 1584
46. Anderson DJ, Olaison L, McDonald JR, Miro JM, Hoen B, Selton-Suty C, Doco-Lecompte T, Abrutyn E, Habib G, Eykyn S, Pappas PA, Fowler VG, Sexton DJ, Almela M, Corey GR, Cabell CH (2005) Enterococcal prosthetic valve infective endocarditis: Report of 45 episodes from the International Collaboration on Endocarditis Merged Database. Eur J Clin Microbiol Infect Dis 24:665 – 670
47. Olaison L, Schadewitz K (2002) Enterococcal endocarditis in Sweden, 1995 – 1999: Can shorter therapy with aminoglycosides be used? Clin Infect Dis 34:159 – 166
48. Baron EJ, Scott JD, Tompkins LS (2005) Prolonged incubation and extensive subculturing do not increase recovery of clinically significant microorganisms from standard automated blood cultures. Clin Infect Dis 41:1677 – 80
49. Benjamin DK, Miro JM, Hoen B, Steinbach WJ, Fowler VG, Olaison L, Habib G, Abrutyn E, Perfect J, Zaas A, Corey GR, Eykyn S, Thuny F, Jiménez-Expósito MJ, Cabell CH, and the ICE-MD Study Group (2004) Candida endocarditis: contemporary cases from the International Collaboration of Infectious Endocarditis Merged Database (ICE-MD). Scand J Infect Dis 36:453 – 455
50. Tunkel BR, Kaye D (1992) Endocarditis with negative blood cultures. N Engl J Med 326:1215 – 17
51. Houpikian P, Raoult D (2005) Blood culture-negative endocarditis in a reference center: Etiologic diagnosis of 348 cases. Medicine 84:162 – 173
52. Werner M, Anderson R, Olaison L, Hogevik H (2003) A clinical study of culture-negative endocarditis. Medicine 82:263 – 273
53. Zeaiter Z, Fournier PE, Greub G, Raoult D (2003) Diagnosis of *Bartonella* endocarditis by a real-time nested PCR assay using serum. J Clin Microbiol 41:919 – 25
54. Mouly S, Ruimy R, Launay O, Arnoult F, Brochet E, Trouillet JL, Leport C, Wolff M (2002) The changing clinical aspects of infective endocarditis: Descriptive review of 90 episodes in a French teaching hospital and risk factors for death. J Infect 45:246 – 256
55. Sexton DJ, Spelman D (2003) Current best practices and guidelines: Assessment and management of complications in infective endocarditis. Cardiol Clin 21:273 – 282
56. Moon MR, Stinson EB, Miller DC (1997) Surgical treatment of endocarditis. Prog Cardiovasc Surg 40:239 – 264
57. Mylonakis E, Calderwood SB (2001) Infective endocarditis in adults. N Engl J Med 345:1318 – 1330
58. Daniel WG, Mugge A, Martin RP, Lindert O, Hausmann D, Nonnast-Daniel B, Laas J, Lichtlen PR (1991) Improvement in the diagnosis of abscesses associated with endocarditis by transesophageal echocardiography. N Engl J Med 324:795 – 800

59. Graupner C, Vilacosta I, San Román JA, Ronderos R, Sarriá C, Fernández C, Mújica R, Sanz O, Sanmartín JV, Pinto AG (2002) Periannular extension of infective endocarditis. J Am Coll Cardiol 39:1204 - 1211
60. Anguera I, Mire JM, Cabell CH, Abrutyn E, Fowler VG, Hoen B, Olaison L, Pappas PA, de Lazzari E, Eykyn S, Habib G, Pare C, Wang A, Corey R, and the ICE-MD Investigators (2005) Clinical characteristics and outcome of aortic endocarditis with periannular abscess in the International Collaboration on Endocarditis Merged Database. Am J Cardiol 96:976 - 981
61. Thuny F, Disalvo G, Belliard O, Avierinos JF, Pergola V, Rosenberg V, Casalta JP, Gouvernet J, Derumeaux G, Iarussi D, Ambrosi P, Calabro R, Riberi A, Collart F, Metras D, Lepidi H, Raoult D, Harle JR, Weiller PJ, Cohen A, Habib G (2005) Risk of embolism and death in infective endocarditis: Prognostic value of echocardiography, a prospective multicenter study. Circulation 112:69 - 75
62. Heiro M, Nikoskelainen J, Engblom E, Kotilainen E, Marttila R, Kotilainen P (2000) Neurologic manifestations of infective endocarditis: A 17-year experience in a teaching hospital in Finland. Arch Intern Med 160:2781 - 2787
63. Steckelberg JM, Murphy JG, Ballard D, Bailey K, Tajik AJ, Taliercio CP, Giuliani ER, Wilson WR (1991) Emboli in infective endocarditis: The prognostic value of echocardiography. Ann Inter Med 114:635 - 640
64. Falagas ME, Matthaiou DK, Bliziotis IA (2006) The role of aminoglycosides in combination with a beta-lactam for the treatment of bacterial endocarditis: a meta-analysis of comparative trials. J Antimicrob Chemother 57:639 - 47
65. Cabell CH, Abrutyn E, Fowler VG, Hoen B, Miro JM, Corey GR, Olaison L, Pappas P, Anstrom KJ, Stafford JA, Eykyn S, Habib G, Mestres CA, Wang A, and ICE-MD Investigators (2005) Use of surgery in patients with native valve infective endocarditis: Results from the International Collaboration on Endocarditis Merged Database. Am Heart J 150:1092 - 1098
66. Mills J, Utley J, Abbott J (1974) Heart failure in infective endocarditis: Predisposing factors, course, and treatment. Chest 66:151 - 157
67. Vlessis AA, Hovaguimian H, Jaggers J, Ahmad A, Starr A (1996) Infective endocarditis: Ten-year review of medical and surgical therapy. Ann Thorac Surg 61:1217 - 1222
68. Akowuah EF, Davies W, Oliver S, Stephens J, Riaz I, Zadik P, Cooper G (2003) Prosthetic valve endocarditis: Early and late outcome following medical or surgical treatment. Heart 89:269 - 272
69. Habib G, Tribouilloy C, Thuny F, Giorgi R, Brahim A, Amazouz M, Remadi JP, Nadji G, Casalta JP, Coviaux F, Avierinos JF, Lescure X, Riberi A, Weiller PJ, Metras D, Raoult D (2005) Prosthetic valve endocarditis: who needs surgery? A multicentre study of 104 cases. Heart 91:954 - 959
70. Wang A, Pappas P, Anstrom KJ, Abrutyn E, Fowler VG, Hoen B, Miro JM, Corey GR, Olaison L, Stafford JA, Mestres CA, Cabell CH, and the International Collaboration on Endocarditis Investigators (2005) The use and effect of surgical therapy for prosthetic valve infective endocarditis: A propensity analysis of a multicenter, international cohort. Am J Heart 150:1086 - 1091
71. Vikram HR, Buenconsejo J, Hasbun R, Quagliarello VJ (2003) Impact of valve surgery on 6-month mortality in adults with complicated, left-sided native valve endocarditis. JAMA 290:3207 - 3214
72. Hoen B, Alla F, Selton-Suty C, Béguinot I, Bouvet A, Briançon S, Casalta JP, Danchin N, Delahaye F, Etienne J, Moing VL, Leport C, Mainardi JL, Ruimy R, Vandenesch F for the Association pour l'Etude et la Prévention de l'Endocardite Infectieuse (AEPEI) Study Group (2002) Changing profile of infective endocarditis: Results of a 1-year survey in France. JAMA 288:75 - 81
73. Moss R, Munt B (2003) Injection drug use and right sided endocarditis. Heart 89:577 - 581
74. DiNubile MJ (1994) Short-course antibiotic therapy for right-sided endocarditis caused by *Staphylococcus aureus* in injection drug users. Ann Intern Med 121:873 - 876
75. Heldman AW, Hartert TV, Ray SC, Daoud EG, Kowalski TE, Pompili VJ, Sisson SD, Tidmore WC, vom Eigen KA, Goodman SN, Lietman PS, Petty BG, Flexner C (1996) Oral antibiotic treatment of right-sided staphylococcal endocarditis in injection drug users: Prospective randomized comparison with parenteral therapy. Am J Med 101:68 - 76
76. Mahesh B, Angelini G, Caputo M, Jin XY, Bryan A (2005) Prosthetic valve endocarditis. Ann Thorac Surg 80:1151 - 1158
77. Stanbridge TN, Isalska BJ (1997) Aspects of prosthetic valve endocarditis. J Infect 35:1 - 6
78. Piper C, Körfer R, Horstkotte D (2001) Prosthetic valve endocarditis. Heart 85:590 - 593
79. Karchmer AW, Longworth DL (2003) Infections of intracardiac devices. Cardiol Clin 21:253 - 271
80. Chu VH, Cabell CH, Benjamin DK Jr, Kuniholm EF, Fowler VG Jr, Engemann J, Sexton DJ, Corey GR, Wang A (2004) Early predictors of in-hospital death in infective endocarditis. Circulation 110:1745 - 9
81. Wallace SM, Walton BI, Kharbanda RK, Hardy R, Wilson AP, Swanton RH (2002) Mortality from infective endocarditis: clinical predictors of outcome. Heart 88:53 - 60
82. Leblebicioglu H, Yilmaz H, Tasova Y, Alp E, Saba R, Caylan R, Bakir M, Akbulut A, Arda B, Esen S (2006) Characteristics and analysis of risk factors for mortality in infective endocarditis. Eur J Epidemiol 21:25 - 31
83. Hsu CN, Wang JY, Tseng CD, Hwang JJ, Hsueh PR, Liau CS (2006) Clinical features and predictors for mortality in patients with infective endocarditis at a university hospital in Taiwan from 1995 to 2003. Epidemiol Infect 134:589 - 97
84. Martin-Davila P, Navas E, Forun J, Moya JL, Cobo J, Pintado V, Quereda C, Jimenez-Mena M, Moreno S (2005) Analysis of mortality and risk factors associated with native valve endocarditis in drug users: the importance of vegetation size. Am Heart J 150:1099 - 106

27 Influenza

P.R. Brookmeyer, K.F. Woeltje

27.1 Introduction

Influenza infections account for significant morbidity and mortality both in the United States and worldwide. Approximately 5 – 15 % of the world's population develops the disease annually. In the United States, 114,000 hospitalizations and 36,000 deaths are thought to occur annually [1], with an estimated annual economic impact of 3 – 5 billion dollars [2]. Complications of influenza include primary and secondary pneumonias, respiratory failure and rarely myositis and neurologic failures. These complications often lead to ICU admission, especially in the elderly or immunocompromised population.

Superimposed on these annual epidemics are periodic pandemics, the most famous being the "Spanish Influenza" of 1918 – 1919, in which at least 20 million and perhaps as many as 100 million persons succumbed worldwide [3]. Based on conservative attack and mortality rates, it is estimated that in the United States alone the next influenza pandemic may result in 314,000 – 734,000 hospitalizations, and claim between 89,000 and 207,000 lives, with an economic impact of 70 – 170 billion dollars [4]. In the new pandemic, it is projected that the ICU capacity in the United States will be overwhelmed, requiring the painful decision to withhold care from patients unlikely to survive, focusing on patients most likely to respond to ventilatory and other therapy.

27.2 History

The influenza virus has likely been causing annual epidemics and periodic pandemics since antiquity. One of the first references to influenza in the "modern literature" appears to be Sydenham's account in 1679 [5]. In a classic review of historical pathology by Hirsch, 299 outbreaks of influenza occurring at an average interval of 2.4 years were calculated between 1173 and 1875 [6]. Industrialization and the increased pace of transportation resulted in increasingly rapid spread of severe pandemic influenza. This culminated in the 1918 – 1919 "Spanish Influenza." This famous pandemic was notable for its surprisingly heavy toll on young adults, with mortality rates in some areas reaching 5 – 10 %. In the United States, draconian infection control measures included closing public schools, creating quarantines, and travel passes. At least three additional somewhat milder pandemics occurred throughout the remainder of the 20th century (Fig. 27.1).

27.3 Virology

The influenza virus is a member of the Orthomyxoviridae family, a family which includes influenza A, B, C, Thogoto virus, and the infectious salmon anemia virus. This family is characterized by a host derived envelope, a negative sense single stranded, segmented RNA genome, and envelope glycoproteins important in viral entry and exit from cells. The morphology of the three

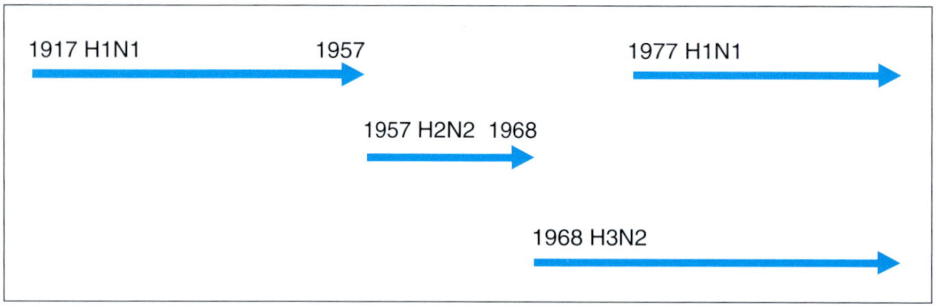

Fig. 27.1. Influenza A antigenic shifts

subtypes of influenza is similar, with an 80–120 nm viron size, 9–12 structural proteins, and 7–8 gene segments. On the surface of the influenza virus are spike-like projections of glycoproteins that possess either hemagglutinin or neuraminidase activity, both of which are critical to viral replication. The hemagglutinin facilitates entry of the virus into host cells by attachment to sialic-acid receptors. A major function of the neuraminidase is to catalyze the cleavage of glycosidic linkages to sialic acid, which allows the completed virion to be released from infected cells [7]. There are at least 16 antigenetically diverse hemagglutinins and 9 distinct neuraminidases in influenza A, the majority of which exist in non-human hosts [8]. Influenza A viruses are typically designated HxNy where the x and y represent which hemagglutinin and neuraminidase, respectively, the virus carries. Thus influenza A H3N2 possesses a type 3 hemagglutinin and a type 2 neuraminidase. The numbering scheme is arbitrary and carries no intrinsic meaning; the numbers only represent a way to distinguish between types of the molecules. In contrast, influenza B has only one known hemagglutinin and only one neuraminidase. Other viral proteins include the Matrix (M) protein, which controls nuclear transport, the Nucleoprotein (NP), a regulator of transcription, and Matrix 2 (M2) protein, an ion channel required for uncoating.

Influenza is classified into types A, B and C based on differences in viral proteins. Influenza C is somewhat morphologically distinct, and is classified in a different genus from influenza A and B. It infects both humans and swine, but tends to cause only mild disease without season variation [9]. In contrast, both influenza A and B are major causes of disease. Influenza B infects only humans, typically causing severe disease in the elderly or high risk patients. It rarely causes epidemics, and does not cause pandemics. Influenza A infects many hosts, including humans, birds, swine, horses, and marine mammals. It is a common cause of both annual epidemics and periodic pandemics.

27.3.1 Antigenic Variation

While infection with influenza results in the development of both humoral and cell mediated protective immunity, individuals may be re-infected periodically. This is secondary to changes in influenza antigens resulting in virus subtypes to which humans have little or no resistance. Through these changes, influenza has remained a significant pathogen over the ages despite the advent of vaccines. The changes occur via changes in the surface glycoproteins of the virus, neuraminidase and hemagglutinin. Two types of antigenic change are described, known as antigenic drift and antigenic shift.

27.3.1.1 Antigenic Drift

Antigenic drift refers to the minor antigenic changes which occur in the hemagglutinin and neuraminidase proteins. The mechanism of antigenic drift is the gradual accumulation of amino acid substitutions due to point mutations in the hemagglutinin and neuraminidase genes [10, 11]. As mutations accumulate, antibodies generated by exposure to previous strains do not neutralize current strains to the same extent, resulting in only limited or partial immunity to the new strains. It is felt that decreased recognition of the new strains acts as a type of natural selection; new strains with less immune recognition become the predominant strain in annual epidemics. Antigenic drift is present in both the influenza A and B subtypes.

27.3.1.2 Antigenic Shift

Antigenic shift occurs only in influenza A. Compared with previous strains, the predominant circulating virus possesses a different hemagglutinin, neuraminidase, or both. There is little or no antibody recognition of these new stains, thereby creating strains that may become a source of epidemic and pandemic influenza. There is a strong association between antigenic shifts with the occurrence of pandemics. The severe pandemics of 1918–1919 (shift to H1N1) and 1957 (shift to H2N2) were associated with shifts of both the hemagglutinin and neuraminidase [12, 13]. The less extensive pandemic of 1968 was associated with only a shift to a new hemagglutinin (shift to H3N2) [14]. Interestingly, the "pseudo-pandemic" of 1977, which involved an influenza A virus which had shifted back to H1N1, affected primarily younger individuals, born after the H1N1 virus had last circulated [15].

Antigenic shift can occur through a variety of mechanisms. Non-human influenza is selective in its tropism, and cannot easily replicate in humans [16]. However, avian influenza viruses may replicate in non-avian, non-human reservoirs (like swine). A pig that was co-infected with both avian and human strains of influenza might result in a genetic reassortment that produces a novel virus capable of replication in and transmission between humans [17]. This reassortment process may happen frequently, but may result in viruses with decreased pathogenicity or limited tropism in humans, and therefore severe pandemics do not begin.

Alternatively, mutations may occur directly in a non-human virus, such as an avian virus, that allow the virus to readily spread from person to person [18]. This process may occur partially, so that spread from animals to humans is possible, but human-to-human spread does not occur. An example is H5N1 avian influenza. Beginning in late 2003 an epizootic developed in Southeast Asia, which by the spring of 2006 had become a panzootic in wild birds and domestic poultry involving parts of Europe and Africa as well. Between December 2003 and March 2006, a total of 186 persons had cases of H5N1 influenza confirmed by the World Health Organization, of whom 105 (56%) died. Almost all patients who developed the infection appear to have acquired it directly from sick birds, presumably because the virus had restricted tropism and was not able to spread readily from person to person [19]. At the time this chapter was written the H5N1 avian influenza panzootic was still spreading.

27.4 Epidemiology

In temperate regions influenza spread occurs annually with the peak epidemic during winter months. Conversely, in tropical regions outbreaks of influenza may occur year round. In annual influenza epidemics between 5% and 15% of the population may develop disease. While attack rates are greatest in the young, influenza-associated mortality is highest in the elderly and immunocompromised. Risk factors for influenza-associated complications include chronic lung, heart and renal disease [20, 21]. The entire epidemic appears to take approximately 5–6 weeks to circulate through the community. How influenza persists between the annual epidemics is poorly understood.

Epidemic influenza occurs annually. However, an influenza pandemic occurs every several decades and involves the entire world. Influenza strains causing pandemic influenza are usually the result of antigenic shift, with little immunity in the populace. While past pandemics such as the 1918 pandemic took many months to spread throughout the world, the rapid pace of modern travel would likely allow a new pandemic to spread much more rapidly, allowing little time for initially unaffected regions to prepare.

27.5 Transmission and Pathophysiology

Influenza spreads rapidly in communities. The mechanism of spread from person to person is primarily droplet via small particle sized aerosols [22]. Once the virus is deposited on the respiratory epithelium, the influenza virus attaches to ciliated columnar epithelial cells via the hemagglutinin molecule. The cells are then invaded and viral replication occurs. Released viruses then infect large numbers of adjacent epithelial cells, and therefore within a few replication cycles large numbers of cells may be infected. The incubation period from exposure to the onset of illness appears to range from 1 to 3 days, with the average period 2 days. Adults can be infectious from the day before symptoms begin through approximately 5 days after illness onset. Children can be infectious for 10 days or more, and young children can shed virus for several days before their illness onset. Severely immunocompromised persons can shed virus for weeks or months [23]. Immune responses to influenza infection include both nonspecific and specific immunity. Nonspecific defenses include nonspecific mucoproteins which bind virus and the mechanical apparatus of the muco-ciliary apparatus. Patients with defective muco-ciliary apparatuses, such as smokers, tend to have higher attack rates and more severe complications of influenza infection. Specific defenses include both humeral and cell mediated responses. Infection with influenza results in long-lived resistance to re-infection with the same virus subtype. However, because of antigenic shift and drift, there is only limited protection against new subtypes. A good illustration of the long lived immunity to specific viruses is the 1977 reemergence of the H1N1 subtype, where people alive during the 1918 pandemic were largely immune and not affected.

Antibody responses to the influenza virus are typically directed against the hemagglutinin, neuraminidase, structural proteins M and NP, and to some degree to the M2 protein. Antibodies responses have variable cross protection within viral subtypes depending on the amount of change of the antigen resulting from antigenic shift or drift. Antibodies to hemagglutinin appear most important in protecting against disease and future infection with the same subtype. Antibodies to neuraminidase reduce efficient release of virus and decreases plaque size in in-vitro assays. Peak antibodies are formed approximately 4–7 weeks after infection, then slowly decline. There appears to be a significant mucosal response to the hemagglutinin antigen, with nasal secretions containing IgG and IgA.

27.6 Clinical Disease

The clinical features of an uncomplicated influenza are nondescript, and virtually indistinguishable from other respiratory viral infections. Influenza is characterized by an abrupt onset of headache, fevers, often high grade, dry cough, myalgia, malaise and anorexia. The cough is variable, often initially nonproductive, then productive of small amounts of mucous, usually nonpurulent. Duration of fevers average 3 days, with a range of 4–8 days. Cough and weakness ("post-influenza asthenia") may persist for weeks after fever and upper respiratory tract symptoms have resolved. Physical exam usually reveals flushing, tachycardia, and occasionally tachypnea. The pulmonary exam is generally unremarkable in uncomplicated cases. Early in the illness even otherwise healthy people may appear quite ill, and during times of epidemic both physician practices and emergency rooms are often swamped with influenza patients, which potentiates the spread to noninfected patients.

27.6.1 Complications

The most common complication of influenza is pneumonia. Pneumonia can either be primary influenza pneumonia or a secondary bacterial pneumonia. Primary influenza pneumonia was first well documented in the influenza pandemic of 1957–1958 [24]. It is thought to be a major cause of death during the earlier pandemic of 1918–1919. Symptoms include high fever, dyspnea, hypoxemia, and respiratory distress. Chest radiographs are similar to other viral pneumonias, revealing scant bilateral interstitial infiltrates. Primary influenza pneumonia has become increasingly rare in the current interpandemic era.

Secondary bacteria pneumonias are similar to non-influenza associated pneumonias. Up to 25% of all mortality from influenza and a large proportion of ICU admission secondary to influenza are due to secondary bacterial pneumonias [25]. *S. pneumonia* is the most common pathogen associated with post-influenza pneumonia, accounting for up to 48% in some series. *S. aureus*, an otherwise uncommon cause of community-acquired pneumonia, is the second most common organism isolated in this setting (19%). Other more typical pneumonia pathogens, such as *Haemophilus influenza*, are common as well [26]. Secondary pneumonias often develop as the patient is improving from the primary influenza infection, with the patient improving briefly, then becoming again febrile, now with worsening respiratory status and purulent secretion. Some patients may have features of both viral and bacterial pneumonia. While influenza usually does not require ICU care, high risk patients with severe pneumonia may require intubation and ICU level care.

Non-pneumonia complications of influenza have also been reported. An important complication of influenza is myositis with elevated muscle enzymes. This must be differentiated from the myalgias, which are very common with the influenza syndrome. Other complications include pericarditis, myocarditis, and CNS complications, the most common of which appears to be a Guillain-Barre type syndrome [27]. Finally, Reye's syndrome has been reported in children infected with influenza B and receiving aspirin [28].

27.6.2 Diagnosis

In times of a confirmed epidemic, when influenza is widespread in the community, a clinical definition based on fever greater than 37.8 °C, and two of four symptoms: cough, myalgia, sore throat and headache, was found to have a sensitivity of 77.6% and specificity of 55%, for the diagnosis of influenza [29, 30]. However, at the beginning of epidemics, with sporadic cases, and with atypical presentation, the clinical laboratory must be utilized to differentiate influenza from other respiratory viruses. Available tests include viral culture, a rapid diagnosis using viral antigens, and the investigational PCR tests.

Viral culture is the gold standard for laboratory diagnosis. Virus can be easily isolated by nasal swabs, throat cultures, and sputum or bronchoalveolar lavage samples. One study concluded that sputum and nasal aspirates had the highest positive predictive value, and throat swabs the worst; however, this study did not include bronchoalveolar lavage specimens [31]. After collection and transport in viral transport medium, the specimens are inoculated into specific cell cultures, where virus is detected by cytopathic effect [32]. Less commonly, embryonated eggs can be used for virus propagation, followed by characterization of the virus by hemagglutination inhibition. Unfortunately, viral culture takes up to 72 h to see a cytopathic effect, but has the benefit of allowing for sub-typing of viral strains, which is critical in the assessment of the current year's vaccine and development of the next.

As rapid diagnosis of influenza is very important for treatment and infection control, a number of commercial rapid diagnostic tests have recently been developed. These tests can yield results in as little as 30 min. They differ in the types of influenza viruses they can detect and whether they can distinguish between influenza types. Different tests can detect: (1) only influenza A viruses; (2) both influenza A and B viruses, but not distinguish between the two types; or (3) both influenza A and B and differentiation between the two [33]. These tests are based on the immunologic detection of viral antigens via immunofluorescence or enzyme immunoassays. The reported sensitivities of these rapid diagnostic methods range from 40% to 80% [34].

PCR has also been used for diagnosis, though usually in a research setting. Some authors have suggested that PCR may be more sensitive than viral culture, as it can detect virons which have lost replicative viability [35]. Unfortunately, PCR is expensive, and labor intensive, and currently tends to be confined to research institutions.

Serological diagnosis of influenza is possible, but can be difficult to interpret as most people have been previously infected. Acute and convalescent specimens, which reveal a fourfold rise in titers, are considered diagnostic.

27.6.3 Treatment

While prevention of influenza is by the far the best measure to combat influenza, four antiviral drugs in two mechanistic classes are currently available and FDA approved for the treatment of influenza. These drugs, when used in the first 24–48 h of illness, appear to shorten duration of symptoms for between 1 and 2 days [36, 37]. The M2 inhibitors amantidine and rimantidine have been used since the 1960s, but are only active against influenza A. The M2 inhibitors target the M2 ion channel, which is important in replication of the viron. The major side effects of amantidine are central nervous system symptoms such insomnia, impaired thinking, dizziness and lightheadedness, resulting in discontinuation rates of up to 13%. Ramantidine appears to have far fewer symptoms, and discontinuation rates of about 6% have been reported [38]. In recent years an increasing M2 channel inhibitor resistance has surfaced. During the 2005–2006 influenza year, CDC testing of 120 influenza A (H3N2) viruses isolated from patients in 23 states revealed resistance rates of 91%. Therefore, during this season, the CDC has recommended against the use of M2 inhibitors in the treatment or prevention of influenza A [39]. Continuation of this resistance trend appears likely in the future.

Neuraminidase inhibitors, including inhaled zanamivir and oral oseltamivir, are newer potent agents, active and approved against both influenza A and B. The neuraminidase inhibitors inhibit the functioning of the viral neuraminidase, which cleaves sialic acid containing receptors, allowing release of completed viron from the infected cell. Oseltamivir is generally well tolerated, and major side effects are limited to nausea and vomiting, which typically do not require drug cessation. Zanamivir is supplied as a dry powder for inhalation, and has been linked to bronchospasm and decrease in peak flows in asthmatics [40], as well as gastrointestinal upset. The manufacturer has released a warning advising patients with COPD or asthma to have a fast acting inhaler available prior to administration.

27.7 Prevention

27.7.1 Vaccination

Vaccination is by far the best method for prevention of influenza. Influenza is unique among vaccine preventable illnesses because its high rate of mutation requires development and implementation of a new vaccine annually. Worldwide surveillance and a degree of luck are required to select the proper antigenic variants of influenza to include in the vaccine months before the start of the annual flu season [41]. In the United States there are currently two licensed vaccines, a trivalent inactivated vaccine (TIV), and a trivalent live-attenuated influenza vaccine (LAIV).

The inactivated vaccine was first licensed in 1943, and now usually contains three influenza antigenic strains – two type A, and one type B. After the likely predominant strains are identified, the viruses are grown in embryonated chicken eggs. They are then inactivated, purified, split into viral fragments, and finally combined into vaccine. Nearly 6 months after identification of target strains is required for vaccine production. Therefore if the educated guesses regarding the dominant strains are incorrect there is no time to develop alternative vaccines. When there is a good match between vaccine and epidemic virus, levels of protection from influenza infection range from 70% to 90% [42], although it is typically less in elderly and chronically ill patients. Patients who do get infected with influenza despite having been vaccinated tend to have less severe disease, and have lower mortality rates. The inactivated vaccine is well tolerated; contraindications are limited to allergies to eggs and a history of a severe adverse reaction. Individuals with a febrile infection should not be vaccinated until its resolution, since they may have a decreased immune response to the vaccine.

The live attenuated influenza vaccine was licensed in 2003. Although it is a live viral vaccine, the virus is cold adapted, so that it only replicates at the lower temperatures found in the anterior nares [43]. While both the inactivated and live vaccines induce systemic antibody responses, the cold adapted vaccine additionally confers a significant specific mucosal antibody response (IgA). The cold adapted vaccine is currently only FDA approved for those between 5 and 49 years of age. Contraindications include immunosuppression, HIV infection, malignancy, leukemia, or lymphoma, and those between age 5 and 17 receiving aspirin products, because of the association of Reye syndrome with aspirin and wild-type influenza infection [44]. The live attenuated vaccine can be given to healthcare workers. Work restrictions are not necessary after this vaccine except for those caring for immunocompromised patients who require a protective environment (e.g., bone-marrow transplant patients) [45].

Influenza vaccine is recommended for patients at increased risk for complications, including those older than 50, and those with chronic pulmonary or cardiac disease, diabetes, renal disfunction, or immunosuppression (see Table 27.1). Vaccination is also strongly recommended for all healthcare workers.

During the 2004–2005 influenza season, manufacture problems resulted in large shortages of the killed vaccine, resulting in rationing of vaccine. The CDC has recommended a triage system to identify those at highest risk who should receive vaccination priority in

Table 27.1. Priority groups for the inactivated influenza vaccine in case of shortages (adapted from [54])

Tier	Priority group
1 A	Persons aged ≥65 years with comorbid conditions Residents of long-term-care facilities
1 B	Persons aged 2–64 years with comorbid conditions Persons aged >65 years without comorbid conditions Children aged 6–23 months Pregnant women
1 C	Healthcare personnel Household contacts and out-of-home caregivers of children aged <6 months
2	Household contacts of children and adults at increased risk for influenza-related complications Healthy persons aged 50–64 years
3	Persons aged 2–49 years without high-risk conditions

Table 27.2. CDC recommendations for influenza vaccination (adapted from [54])

Persons at increased risk for complications
Persons aged ≥65 years
Residents of nursing homes and other chronic care
Adults and children who have chronic pulmonary or cardiovascular system diseases, including asthma (hypertension is excluded)
Adults and children with chronic metabolic diseases (including diabetes mellitus), renal dysfunction, hemoglobinopathies, or immunosuppression
Adults and children who have any condition (e.g., cognitive dysfunction, spinal cord injuries, seizure disorders, or other neuromuscular disorders) that can compromise respiratory function or the handling of respiratory secretion
Children and adolescents (aged 6 months–18 years) who are receiving long-term aspirin
Women who will be pregnant during the influenza season
Children aged 6–23 months
Persons aged 50–64 years
Vaccination is recommended for all persons aged 50–64 years
Persons who can transmit influenza to those at high risk
Healthcare workers including physicians, nurses, and other personnel
Employees of assisted living and other residences for persons in groups at high risk
Persons who provide home care to persons in groups at high risk; and household contacts (including children) of persons in groups at high risk
Household contacts of children aged 0–23 months

times of shortages (see Table 27.2). New vaccine development and production techniques, such as acellular vaccines, that allow for rapid production and deployment need to be developed in order to avoid future shortages. These methods would also allow rapid vaccine development during the influenza seasons when antigen matches are poor. In the setting of a vaccine shortage, consideration could also be given to using the LAIV in an expanded patient population (although this would be an off-label use) [46].

27.7.2 Antiviral Prophylaxis

All of the antiviral medicines used for therapy have also been used as post-exposure prophylaxis during times when influenza is circulating in the community. However, because of the rapid development of resistance in the H_3N_2 influenza virus noted during the 2005–2006 influenza season, the M2 inhibitors amantadine and rimantadine are no longer recommended for prophylaxis. Among neuraminidase inhibitors, zanamivir has not been FDA approved for prophylaxis. As antiviral prophylaxis is expensive, and not without side effects, prophylaxis must not be used in place of vaccination. Additionally, all individuals who are initiated on antiviral prophylaxis should also receive the influenza vaccine. The Advisory Committee on Immunization Practices recommends consideration of antiviral prophylaxis for patients at high risk of complications who have not received vaccination, those who are unlikely to respond to vaccination and healthcare workers who have not received vaccination, during times when influenza is active in the community [47]. Duration of prophylaxis is controversial and depends of the aim. As a bridge to vaccination, antiviral drugs should be continued for 2 weeks after vaccination. In "seasonal prophylaxis," where the individual cannot receive or is not expected to amount an immune response to the vaccination, prophylaxis should be initiated upon widespread reports of influenza in the community and should continue for 4–6 weeks [48]. Antiviral drugs can also be used as post-exposure prophylaxis, where drugs are given for 7–10 days after contact with an infected person [49]. This will not protect against influenza contracted from outside the contact after the prophylactic period, and may be best suited to times of sporadic cases. Many anecdotal reports also support the use of antiviral drugs in aborting epidemics in nursing homes, and could be extrapolated to outbreaks in intensive care units [50].

27.8 Infection Control

Patients with influenza should be placed in isolation to prevent nosocomial spread of the disease. There have also been several well documented cases of intra-ICU spread of influenza [51]. The Centers for Disease Control and Prevention (CDC) recommend that patients with known **or suspected** influenza be placed in "Droplet Precautions." [52]. Patients should be placed in a private room if possible; otherwise cohorting of influenza patients is acceptable. Healthcare workers should wear a surgical or procedure mask when entering the room (or working within 0.9 m of the patient). The mask should be removed upon leaving the room, and hand hygiene should be implemented. Patients should stay in their rooms to the extent possible. If a patient with known or suspected influenza must travel to a procedure, a surgical or procedure mask should be placed on the patient prior to leaving the room. Negative pressure rooms and N-95 respirators are not recommended for routine influenza patients. ICUs should have policies to exclude visitors who have febrile respiratory symptoms. Healthcare workers with febrile respiratory illnesses should likewise not come to work, thereby avoiding the risk of spreading influenza to patients and coworkers.

If there is suspicion of nosocomial acquisition of influenza in an ICU, an investigation should be conducted by the hospital's infection control program. Surveillance for possible additional patients with influenza who may have gone unrecognized should be conducted. ICU personnel should also be surveyed to determine who might have served as a source. Good infection control practices should be reinforced, especially the prompt isolation of patients (using droplet precautions) as soon as influenza is even suspected. Patients and HCW in the ICU who have not been vaccinated should be offered the flu vaccine. If additional nosocomial cases of influenza occur despite infection control measures, or if the outbreak is due to a strain of influenza that is a poor match to the current vaccine, strong consideration should be given to administering chemoprophylaxis to non-infected ICU patients for at least 2 weeks [53]. Active surveillance for additional cases of influenza should continue for at least 2 weeks after the last diagnosed case.

References

1. Thompson WW, Shay D, Weintraub E, et al. (2003) Mortality associated with influenza and respiratory syncytial virus in the United States. JAMA 289(2):179–186
2. Schoenbaum SC (1987) Economic impact of influenza. The individual's perspective. Am J Med 82(6A):26–30
3. Johnson NP, Mueller J (2002) Updating the accounts: global mortality of the 1918–20 "Spanish" influenza pandemic. Bull Hist Med 76(1):105–115
4. Meltzer MI, Cox NJ, Fukuda K (1999) The economic impact of pandemic influenza in the United States: priorities for intervention. Emerg Infect Dis 5(5):659–671
5. Treanor JJ (2005) Influenza virus. In: Mandell GL, Bennett JE, Dolin R (eds) Principles and practice of infectious diseases. Churchill Livingstone, Philadelphia, PA, p 2060
6. Hirsch A (1883) Handbook of geographical and historical pathology, 2nd edn. New Sydenham Society, London
7. Gubareva LV, Kaiser L, Hayden FG (2000) Influenza virus neuraminidase inhibitors. Lancet 355(9206):827–835
8. Nicholson KG, Wood JM, Zambon M (2003) Influenza. Lancet 362(9397):1733–1745
9. Zambon MC (1999) Epidemiology and pathogenesis of influenza. J Antimicrob Chemother 44 Suppl B:3–9
10. Luther P, Bergmann KC, Oxford JS (1984) An investigation of antigenic drift of neuraminidases of influenza A (H1N1) viruses. J Hyg (Lond) 92(2):223–229
11. Webster RG, Kendal AP, Gerhard W (1979) Analysis of antigenic drift in recently isolated influenza A (H1N1) viruses using monoclonal antibody preparations. Virology 96(1):258–264
12. Taubenberger JK, Reid AH, Lourens RM, et al. (2005) Characterization of the 1918 influenza virus polymerase genes. Nature 437(7060):889–893
13. Kilbourne ED (1959) Studies on influenza in the pandemic of 1957–58. III. Isolation of influenza A (Asian strain) viruses from influenza patients with pulmonary complications. Details of virus isolation and characterization of isolates, with quantitative comparison of isolation methods. J Clin Invest 38:266–274
14. Schulman JL, Kilbourne ED (1969) Independent variation in nature of the hemagglutinin and neuraminidase antigens of influenza virus: distinctiveness of the hemagglutinin antigen of Hong Kong-68 virus. Proc Natl Acad Sci U S A 63(2):326–333
15. Kilbourne ED (2006) Influenza pandemics of the 20th century. Emerg Infect Dis 12(1):9–14
16. Beare AS, Webster RG (1991) Replication of avian influenza viruses in humans. Arch Virol 119(1–2):37–42
17. Scholtissek C, Rohde W, Von Hoyningen V, Rott R (1978) On the origin of the human influenza virus subtypes H2N2 and H3N2. Virology 87(1):13–20
18. Belshe RB (2005) The origins of pandemic influenza – lessons from the 1918 virus. N Engl J Med 353(21):2209–2211
19. Beigel JH, Farrar J, Han AM, et al. (2005) Avian influenza A (H5N1) infection in humans. N Engl J Med 353(13): 1374–1385
20. Glezen WP, Keitel WA, Taber LH, et al. (1991) Age distribution of patients with medically-attended illnesses caused by sequential variants of influenza A/H1N1: comparison to age-specific infection rates, 1978–1989. Am J Epidemiol 133(3):296–304
21. Baker WH, Mullooly JP (1980) Impact of epidemic type A influenza in a defined adult population. Am J Epidemiol 112(6):798–811
22. Alford RH, Kasel JA, Gerone PJ (1966) Human influenza from aerosol inhalation. Proc Soc Exp Biol Med 122(3): 800–804
23. http://www.cdc.gov/flu/professionals/diagnosis/, accessed 3/27/2006
24. Louria DB, Blumenfeld HL, Ellis JT, et al. (1959) Studies on influenza in the pandemic of 1957–1958. II. Pulmonary complications of influenza. J Clin Invest 38(1 Part 2):213–265
25. Simonsen L (1999) The global impact of influenza on morbidity and mortality. Vaccine 17(Suppl 1):3–10
26. Oliveira EC, Marik PE, Colice G (2001) Influenza pneumonia: a descriptive study. Chest 119(6):1717–1723
27. Hayase Y, Tobita K (1997) Influenza virus and neurological diseases. Psychiatry Clin Neurosci 51(4):181–184
28. Nishida N, Chiba T, Ohtani M, Yoshioka N (2005) Sudden unexpected death of a 17-year-old male infected with the influenza virus. Leg Med (Tokyo) 7(1):51–57
29. Boivin G, Hardy I, Tellier G, Maziade J (2000) Predicting influenza infections during epidemics with use of a clinical case definition. Clin Infect Dis 31(5):1166–1169
30. Zambon M, Hays J, Webster A, et al. Relationship of clinical diagnosis to confirmed virological, serologic or molecular detection of influenza. Arch Intern Med 161(17): 2116–2122
31. Covalciuc KA, Webb KH, Carlson CA (1999) Comparison of four clinical specimen types for detection of influenza A and B viruses by optical immunoassay (FLU OIA Test) and cell culture methods. J Clin Microbiol 37(12):3971–3974
32. Treanor JJ (2005) Influenza virus. In: Mandell GL, Bennett

JE, Dolin R (eds) Principles and practice of infectious diseases. Churchill Livingstone, Philadelphia, PA, p 2071
33. http://www.cdc.gov/flu/professionals/labdiagnosis.htm, accessed on 3/7/2006
34. Treanor JJ (2005) Influenza virus. In: Mandell GL, Bennett JE, Dolin R (eds) Principles and practice of infectious diseases. Churchill Livingstone, Philadelphia, PA, pp 2070–2071
35. Newton DW, Mellen CF, Baxter BD, et al. (2002) Practical and sensitive screening strategy for detection of influenza virus. J Clin Microbiol 40(11):4353–4356
36. Nicholson KG, Aoki FY, Osterhaus AD, et al. (2000) Efficacy and safety of oseltamivir in treatment of acute influenza: a randomised controlled trial. Lancet 355(9218):1845–1850
37. Hayden FG, Osterhaus ADME, Treanor JJ, et al. (1997) Efficacy and safety of the neuraminidase inhibitor zanamivir in the treatment of influenza virus infections. N Engl J Med 337(13):927–928
38. Dolin R, Reichman RC, Madore HP, et al. (1982) A controlled trial of amantadine and rimantadine in the prophylaxis of influenza A infection. N Engl J Med 307(10):580–584
39. http://www.cdc.gov/flu/han011406.htm, accessed on 3/7/2006
40. Neuraminidase inhibitors for treatment of influenza A and B infections. MMWR Morb Mortal Wkly Rep 48(49):1139
41. Treanor J (2004) Weathering the influenza vaccine crises. N Engl J Med 351(20):2037–2040
42. Boyce TG, Gruber WC, Coleman-Dockery SD, et al. (1999) Mucosal immune response to trivalent live attenuated intranasal influenza vaccine in children. Vaccine 18(1–2):82–88
43. Maassab HF, DeBorde DC (1985) Development and characterization of cold-adapted viruses for use as live virus vaccines Vaccine 3(5):355–69
44. Prescribing Information for FluMist™, Influenza Virus Vaccine Live, Intranasal, 2004–2005 Formula. MedImmune Vaccines, Inc. Gaithersburg, MD
45. Talbot TT, Bradley SF, Cosgrove SE (2005) Influenza vaccination of healthcare workers and vaccine allocation for healthcare workers during vaccine shortages. Infect Control Hosp Epidemiol 26(11):882–890
46. Advisory Committee on Immunization Practices (ACIP) (2004) Prevention and control of influenza. Recommendations of the Advisory Committee on Immunization Practices (ACIP). MMWR Recomm Rep 53(RR06):1
47. Cosgrove SE, Fishman NO, Talbot TR, Woeltje KF, Schaffner W, Fraser VJ, McMillan JA, Perl TM (2005) Strategies for use of a limited influenza vaccine supply. JAMA 293(2):229–232
48. Hayden FG, Atmar RL, Schilling M, et al. (1999) Use of the selective oral neuraminidase inhibitor oseltamivir to prevent influenza. N Engl J Med 341(18):1336–1343
49. Welliver R, Monto AS, Carewicz O, et al. (2001) Effectiveness of oseltamivir in preventing influenza in household contacts: a randomized controlled trial. JAMA 285(6):748–754
50. Schilling M, Povinelli L, Krause P, et al. (1998) Efficacy of zanamivir for chemoprophylaxis of nursing home influenza outbreaks. Vaccine 16(18):1771–1774
51. Oliveira EC, Lee B, Colice GL (2003) Influenza in the intensive care unit. J Intensive Care Med 18(2):80–91
52. Garner JS, Hospital Infection Control Practices Advisory Committee (1996) Guideline for isolation precautions in hospitals. Infect Control Hosp Epidemiol 17:53–80
53. Centers for Disease Control and Prevention. Prevention and control of influenza: recommendations of the Advisory Committee on Immunization Practices (ACIP). MMWR 53(RR-6):1–40
54. Centers for Disease Control and Prevention (CDC) Tiered use of inactivated influenza vaccine in the event of a vaccine shortage. MMWR Morb Mortal Wkly Rep 54(30):749–750

28 Bloodstream Infection in the Intensive Care Unit

J. VALLES

28.1 Introduction

Nosocomial infections occur in 5–10% of patients admitted to hospitals in the United States [1]. The endemic rates of nosocomial infections vary markedly between hospitals and between areas of the same hospital. Patients in intensive care units (ICUs), representing 8–15% of hospital admissions, suffer a disproportionately high percentage of nosocomial infections compared with patients in non-critical care areas [2–7]. Wenzel et al. [3] reported that patients admitted to ICUs account for 45% of all nosocomial pneumonias and bloodstream infections, although critical care units comprise only 5–10% of all hospital beds. Severity of underlying disease, invasive diagnostic and therapeutic procedures, contaminated life-support equipment, and the prevalence of resistant microorganisms are critical factors in the high rate of infection in ICUs [8].

Donowitz et al. [5] reported a threefold increase in the risk of nosocomial infection for ICU patients when compared with ward patients (18% vs. 6%; $p<0.001$); and bloodstream infections were 7.4 times as likely to occur in ICU patients as in ward patients, with an infection rate in the ICU of 5.2 episodes per 100 admissions compared with 0.7 episodes per 100 admissions in a general ward ($p<0.001$). Trilla et al. [9], in a study of the risk factors for nosocomial bloodstream infection in a large Spanish university hospital, found that among other variables, the admission to an ICU was linked with a marked increase in the risk of nosocomial bloodstream infection (OR=2.37; CI 95%: 1.67–3.38; $p=0.02$).

On the other hand, 40% of patients admitted to the ICU present infections acquired in the community, and 17% of them present bacteremia [10]. The incidence rate of patients with community-acquired bacteremia admitted in a general ICU is about 9–10 episodes per 1,000 admissions [11, 12], representing 30–40% of all episodes of bacteremia in the ICU (Fig. 28.1).

The aim of this chapter is to discuss the clinical importance of bloodstream infection in the ICU, including nosocomial and community-acquired episodes.

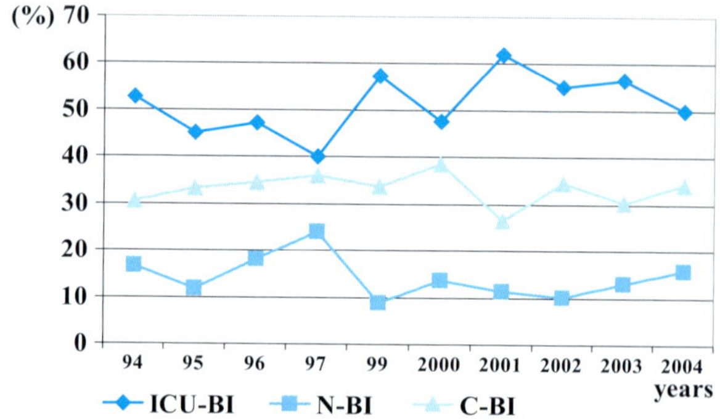

Fig. 28.1. Distribution of bacteremias in the medical-surgical ICU of Hospital Sabadell (period 1994–2004). *ICU-BI* intensive care unit-acquired bloodstream infection, *N-BI* nosocomial (outside ICU)-acquired bloodstream infection, *C-BI* community-acquired bloodstream infection

28.2 Pathophysiology of Bloodstream Infection

Invasion of the blood by microorganisms usually occurs via one of two mechanisms: drainage from the primary focus of infection via the lymphatic system to the vascular system, or direct entry from needles (e.g., in intravenous drug users) or other contaminated intravascular devices such as catheters or graft material. The presence of bloodstream infection represents either the failure of an individual's host defenses to localize an infection at its primary site or the failure of a physician to remove, drain, or otherwise sterilize that focus. Ordinarily, host defenses respond promptly to a sudden influx of microorganisms, particularly by efficient phagocytosis by macrophages or the mononuclear phagocytic system that helps clear the blood within minutes to hours. Clearance may be less efficient when microorganisms are encapsulated, or it may be enhanced if the host has antibodies specific for the infecting organism. Clearance of the bloodstream is not always successful. Examples of this problem are bloodstream infections associated with intravascular foci and endovascular infections and episodes that occur in individuals whose host defense mechanisms either are too impaired to respond efficiently or are simply overwhelmed [13].

For that reason, the presence of living microorganisms in blood is of substantial clinical importance; it is an indicator of disseminated infection and, as such, generally indicates a poorer prognosis than that associated with localized disease.

28.3 Definitions

Nosocomial bloodstream infection in the ICU is defined in a patient with a clinically significant blood culture positive for a bacterium or fungus that is obtained more than 72 h after admission to the ICU or previously, if it is directly related to a invasive manipulation on admission to the ICU (e.g., urinary catheterization or insertion of intravenous line). By contrast, a community-acquired bacteremia is defined when the infection develops in a patient prior to hospital and ICU admission, or if this episode of bacteremia develops within the first 48 h of hospital and ICU admission, and it is not associated with any procedure performed after hospital or ICU admission. These definitions from the Centers for Disease Control and Prevention (CDC) consider that infections that are not nosocomial infections are community-acquired by default [14]. However, there are patients residing in the community, who are receiving care at home, living in nursing homes and rehabilitation centers, receiving chronic dialysis, and receiving chemotherapy in physicians' offices who may present bloodstream infections. These infections have traditionally been categorized as community-acquired infections. For this reason, recently a new classification scheme for bloodstream infection has been proposed that distinguishes among patients with community-acquired, healthcare-associated, and nosocomial infections. Healthcare-associated bloodstream infection has been defined when a positive blood culture is obtained from a patient at the time of hospital admission or within 48 h of admission if the patient fulfilled any of the following criteria: (1) received intravenous therapy at home, received wound care or specialized nursing care or had self-administered intravenous medical therapy; (2) attended a hospital hemodialysis clinic or received intravenous chemotherapy; (3) was hospitalized in an acute care hospital for 2 or more days in the 90 days before the bloodstream infection; or (4) resided in a nursing home or long-term care facility [15].

Bloodstream infections may be classified as primary or secondary according to the source of the infection [14]. Primary bloodstream infection occurs without any recognizable focus of infection with the same organism at another site at the time of positive blood culture, and secondary bloodstream infections are infections that developed subsequent to a documented infection with the same microorganism at another site. Episodes secondary to intravenous or arterial lines have traditionally been classified as primary bacteremias; however, if local infection (defined as redness, tenderness, and pus) is present at the site of an intravascular line, and if the semiquantitative (yielding >15 colonies) or quantitative culture of a segment catheter is positive to the same strain as in the blood cultures, they may be classified as secondary bacteremias. According to this definition, in the absence of an identified source, primary bacteremias should be designated bacteremias of unknown origin [16–19].

According to clinical patterns of bacteremia, it may also be useful to categorize bloodstream infection as transient, intermittent, or continuous [13]. Transient bacteremia, lasting minutes to hours, is the most common and occurs after manipulation of infected tissues (e.g., abscesses); during certain surgical procedures; when procedures are undertaken that involve contaminated or colonized mucosal surfaces (e.g., gastrointestinal endoscopy); and, predictably, at the onset of acute bacterial infections such as pneumonia, meningitis, and complicated urinary infections. Intermittent bacteremia is that which occurs, clears, and then recurs in the same patient due to the same microorganism. Classically, this type of bacteremia is associated with undrained closed space infections, such as intra-abdominal abscesses. Continuous bacteremia is characteristic of infective endocarditis as well as other endovascular infections such as arterial graft infections, and suppurative thrombophlebitis associated with intravenous line infections commonly seen in critically ill patients.

Bloodstream infections may also be categorized as unimicrobial or polymicrobial depending on the number of microorganisms isolated during a single bacteremic episode.

Blood cultures which are found to be positive in the laboratory but which do not truly reflect bloodstream infection in the patient have been termed contaminant bloodstream infections or, more recently, pseudobloodstream infections [16]. Several techniques are available to assist the clinician and microbiologist in interpreting the clinical importance of a positive blood culture. The categorical decision to consider the bloodstream infection as true infection or a contaminant should take into account, at least: the patient's clinical history, physical findings, body temperature at the time of the blood culture, leukocyte count and differential cell counts, the identity of microorganism isolated and the result of cultures of specimens from other sites. Indeed, the type of microorganism isolated may have some predictive value: common blood isolates that always or nearly always (>90%) represent true infection include *S. aureus*, *E. coli* and other members of the Enterobacteriaceae, *Pseudomonas aeruginosa*, *Streptococcus pneumoniae*, and *Candida albicans*. Other microorganisms such as *Corynebacterium* spp., *Bacillus* spp., and *Propionibacterium acnes* rarely (<5%) represent true bloodstream infection. More problematic are the viridans group streptococci which represent true bloodstream infection in 28% of cases, enterococci in 78%, and coagulase-negative staphylococci (CNS) in 15% [20, 21].

The number of positive blood cultures out of the total number performed is frequently used to determine the clinical significance of the isolate, but recent data suggest that this technique is flawed. Mirret and colleagues [22] examined the significance of CNS in blood cultures. For conventional two-bottle culture sets, 49% of those classified as significant infections and 68% classified as contaminants grew in one bottle, whereas 51% of pathogens and 68% of contaminants grew in both bottles. The degree of overlap is so great that it is difficult to predict the clinical significance based on the number of positive bottles. It is important to note that although coagulase-negative staphylococci have frequently been considered as contaminants in the past, recent studies have shown that even a single blood-culture positive for these microorganisms is frequently associated with clinically relevant episodes of bloodstream infections [23–25].

When a culture is unexpectedly positive (in the absence of signs or symptoms) or when only one of several cultures is positive for a microorganism, it can often be dismissed as a contaminant. Every positive blood culture, however, should be carefully evaluated before being dismissed as insignificant [16].

28.4 Epidemiology

Nosocomial infection in ICU patients is a frequent event with potentially lethal consequences. Because patients in ICUs are severely ill and undergo invasive procedures, they suffer a disproportionate percentage of nosocomial infections [5, 7, 26–28]. Compared with patients in general medical/surgical wards, who have been found to have an overall risk of 6% of acquiring an infection during their hospital stay, the risk in critically ill patients in the ICU is around 18% [5]. The nosocomial infection rates among ICU patients are as much as 5–10 times higher than those recorded for patients admitted to other wards, meaning that nearly 25% of all hospital-acquired infections occur in ICU patients [29]. Nosocomial infections are more common in ICUs because of the severity of the underlying disease, the duration of hospital stay, the use of invasive procedures, contaminated life-support equipment, and the prevalence of multiply resistant microorganisms. Data from the European Prevalence of Infection in Intensive Care study (EPIC) collected in 1992 shown that on the day of study a total of 21% of patients admitted to the ICU had an infection acquired in the ICU [30].

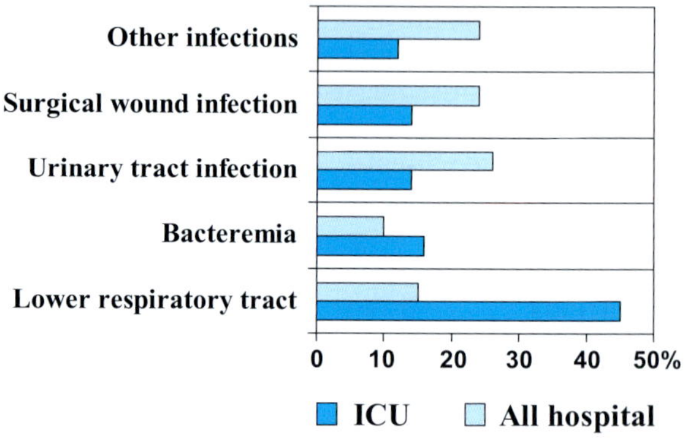

Fig. 28.2. Distribution of nosocomial infections in the ICU versus the whole hospital (NNIS) (from ref. [29], with permission)

Patients in the ICU not only have higher endemic rates of nosocomial infection than patients in general wards, but the distribution of their nosocomial infections also differs. The two most important nosocomial infections in general wards are urinary tract infections and surgical wound infections, whereas in the ICU lower respiratory tract and bloodstream infections are the most frequent [29] (Fig. 28.2). This distribution is related to the widespread use of mechanical ventilation and intravenous catheters. Data compiled through the National Nosocomial Infections Surveillance System (NNIS) of the Centers for Disease Control and Prevention in the USA revealed that bloodstream infections accounted for almost 20% of nosocomial infections in ICU patients, 87% of which were associated with a central line [31].

Despite the higher incidence of nosocomial bloodstream infection in ICUs, few studies have adequately analyzed this infection in this selected population. The studies conducted in critically ill patients in recent years show that the incidence rate of nosocomial bloodstream infection in the ICU ranges from 27 to 67 episodes per 1,000 admissions [18, 19, 32, 33] (Table 28.1), depending on the type of ICU (surgical or medical or coronary care unit), the severity of patients, the use of invasive devices and the length of ICU stay. These infection rates among ICU patients are as much as 5–10 times higher than those recorded for patients admitted to general wards.

Table 28.1. Rates of nosocomial bloodstream infection in the ICU

Year	Type of ICU	ENBI/1000[a]	Reference
1994	Medical-surgical ICU	67.2	Rello [18]
1994	Surgical ICU	26.7	Pittet [32]
1996	Adult ICUs Multicenter study	41	Brun-Buisson [33]
1997	Adult ICUs Multicenter study	36	Vallés [19]

[a] Episodes of nosocomial bloodstream infection per 1,000 admissions

A few epidemiologic studies focusing solely on community-acquired BSI on admission to the ICU are available. Data from a recent multicenter study reported a community-acquired bloodstream infections rate of 10.2 episodes per 1,000 ICU admissions [34].

28.5 Microbiology

28.5.1 Nosocomial Bloodstream Infection

The spectrum of microorganisms that invade the bloodstream in patients with nosocomial infections during their stay in the ICU has been evaluated in several recent studies. Although almost any microorganism can produce bloodstream infection, staphylococci and gram-negative bacilli account for the vast majority of cases. However, among the staphylococci, coagulase-negative staphylococci (CNS) have recently become a clinically significant agent of bloodstream infection in the ICU [18–21]. The ascendance of this group of staphylococci has increased the interpretative difficulties for clinicians, since a high number of CNS isolations represent contamination rather than true bloodstream infection. The increased importance of CNS bloodstream infection seems to be related to the high incidence of utilization of multiple invasive devices in critically ill patients and to the multiple antimicrobial therapy used for gram-negative infections in ICU patients, which results in selection of gram-positive microorganisms. The change in the spectrum of organisms causing nosocomial bloodstream infection in an adult ICU is confirmed in the recent study by Edgeworth and colleagues [35], which analyzed the evolution of nosocomial bloodstream infection over 25 years in the same ICU. Between 1971 and 1990, the frequency of isolation of individual organisms changed little, with *S. aureus*, *P. aeruginosa*, *E. coli*, and *K. pneumoniae* species predominating. However, between 1991 and 1995, the number of bloodstream infections doubled, largely due to the increased isolation of CNS, *Enterococus* spp., and intrinsically antibiotic-resistant gram-negative organisms, particularly *P. aeruginosa* and *Candida* spp.

Currently, the leading pathogens among cases of nosocomial bloodstream infection in the ICU are gram-positive microorganisms, representing nearly half of the organisms isolated [18, 19, 32, 36] (Table 28.2). Coagulase-negative staphylococci (CNS), *S. aureus* and enterococci are the most frequent gram-positive bacteria in all studies, and CNS is isolated in 20–30% of all episodes of bloodstream infection. Gram-negative bacilli are responsible for 30–40% of bloodstream infection episodes, and the remaining cases are mostly due to *Candida* spp. Polymicrobial episodes are relatively common, representing about 10%. Anaerobic bacteria are isolated in fewer than 5% of cases.

Among gram-positive bloodstream infections, the incidence of the pathogens is similar in the different ICUs, CNS being the most frequently isolated organism, and *S. aureus* the second commonest pathogen in all studies. Only the incidence of strains with antibiotic resistance such as methicillin-resistant *Staphylococcus aureus* (MRSA) or vancomycin-resistant enterococci (VRE) differs substantially according to the characteristics of individual institutions, and depending on whether they become established as endemic nosocomial pathogens in the ICU. On the other hand, the gram-negative species isolated from nosocomial bloodstream infections in the ICUs of different institutions show marked variability. The relative contribution of each gram-negative species to the total number of isolates from blood varies from hospital to hospital and over time. The antibiotic policy of the institution may induce the appearance of highly resistant microorganisms and the emergence of endemic nosocomial pathogens, in particular *Pseudomonas* spp, *Acinetobacter* spp., and Enterobacteriaceae with extended-spectrum beta-lactamase (ESBL).

Table 28.2. Microorganisms causing nosocomial bloodstream infection in adult ICUs

Reference	Gram-positive microorganisms	Gram-negative microorganisms	Fungi	Polymicrobial episodes
Rello [18]	44.1% CNS *S. aureus* Enterococci	40.5% *P. aeruginosa* *E. coli* *Enterobacter* spp.	5.4% *Candida* spp.	9.9%
Pittet [32]	51.0% CNS *S. aureus* *Enterococci*	39.0% *Enterobacter* spp. *Klebsiella* spp. *S. marcescens*	4.8% *Candida* spp.	21%
Vallés [19]	49.8% CNS *S. aureus* Enterococci	32.6% *P. aeruginosa* *A. baumannii* *K. pneumoniae*	4.4% *Candida* spp.	12.7%
Jamal [36]	46.8% CNS *S. aureus* Enterococci	36.6% *Enterobacter* spp. *S. marcescens* *K. pneumoniae*	17.6% *Candida* spp	9.8%

CNS coagulase-negative staphylococci

Table 28.3. Microorganisms and sources of community-acquired bacteremias admitted in the ICU

Reference	Sources		Microorganisms	
Forgacs [11]	Pulmonary	38.5%	*S. pneumoniae*	32.3%
	Genitourinary	23.0%	*E. coli*	27.2%
	Endocarditis	8.0%	*S. aureus*	13.5%
	Biliary tract	5.9%	Other GNB	14.2%
	Other	11.1%	Other GPC	8.2%
	Unknown origin	20.0%	Other	14.2%
Vallés [12]	Pulmonary	20.0%	*E. coli*	28.1%
	Abdominal	20.1%	*S. pneumoniae*	17.9%
	Genitourinary	19.8%	*S. aureus*	14.9%
	Other	10.3%	Other GNB	18.6%
	Unknown origin	29.2%	Other GPC	9.5%
			Other	11.07%

The incidence of polymicrobial and anaerobic bloodstream infections depends on the incidence of surgical patients in each ICU, because in two-thirds of these bacteremic episodes the origin is an intra-abdominal infection.

28.5.2 Community-Acquired Bloodstream Infection

In the bacteremic episodes acquired in the community and admitted in the ICU, the incidence of gram-positive is similar to that of gram-negative microorganisms and near to 10% are polymicrobial episodes. *E. coli*, *S. pneumoniae* and *S. aureus* are the leading pathogens, and the prevalence of these microorganisms is related to the main sources of bacteremia found in these patients, such as urinary, pulmonary tract, and unknown origin [11, 12, 34] (Table 28.3).

28.6 Sources

According to a more recent analysis, the vast majority (70%) of nosocomial bloodstream infections in the ICU are secondary bacteremias, including the bloodstream infections related to an intravascular catheter-infection, and the remaining 30% are bacteremias of unknown origin. Table 28.4 summarizes the sources of nosocomial bacteremias in the ICU in several recent series [18, 19, 32, 35]. As shown, intravascular catheter-related infections and respiratory tract infections are the leading sources of secondary episodes.

The source of nosocomial bloodstream infections varies according to microorganism. Coagulase-negative staphylococci and *Staphylococcus aureus* commonly complicate intravenous-related infections, whereas gram-negative bacilli are the main etiology for secondary bloodstream infections following respiratory tract, intra-abdominal and urinary tract infections. Among

Table 28.4. Major sources of nosocomial bloodstream infection in the ICUs

Type of infection	Rello [18] (%)	Pittet [32] (%)	Vallés [19] (%)	Edgeworth [35] (%)
Intravenous catheter	35	18	37.1	62
Respiratory tract	10	28	17.5	3
Intra-abdominal infection	9	NA	6.1	6.9
Genitourinary tract	3.6	5.4	5.9	2.4
Surgical wound or soft tissue	8	8	2.4	3
Other	7	14.5	2.9	–
Unknown origin	27	20	28.1	22.4

bacteremias of unknown origin, most are caused by gram-positive microorganisms, mainly CNS, and they may originate in device-related infections not diagnosed at the time of the development of the bloodstream infection.

Among community-acquired bloodstream infections, lower respiratory tract, intra-abdominal and genitourinary infections represent more than 80% of episodes of bacteremia admitted in the ICU (Table 28.3). Near to 30% of episodes are of unknown origin including mainly meningococcal and staphylococcal infections [11, 12, 34].

28.7 Systemic Response to Bloodstream Infection

The host reaction to invading microbes involves a rapidly amplifying polyphony of signals and responses that may spread beyond the invaded tissue. Fever or hypothermia, chills, tachypnea, and tachycardia often herald the onset of the systemic inflammatory response to microbial invasion, also called sepsis. However, the interchangeable use of terms such as "bloodstream infection," "sepsis," and "septicemia" has led to confusion.

A recent definition of bloodstream infection classifies patients with severe infection and its sequelae [37]. Bloodstream infection and fungemia have been simply defined as the presence of bacteria or fungi in blood cultures, and four stages of increasing severity of systemic response have been described: the systemic inflammatory response syndrome (SIRS), which is identified by a combination of simple and readily available clinical signs and symptoms (i.e., fever or hypothermia, tachycardia, tachypnea, and changes in blood leukocyte count); sepsis, in patients in whom the SIRS is caused by documented infection; severe sepsis when patients have a dysfunction of the major organs; and septic shock, which describes patients with hypotension and organ dysfunction in addition to sepsis. As sepsis progresses to septic shock, the risk of death increases substantially. Early sepsis is usually reversible, whereas many patients with septic shock succumb despite aggressive therapy.

The presence of organisms in the blood is one of the most reliable criteria for characterizing a patient presenting with SIRS as having sepsis or one of its more severe presentations, such as severe sepsis or septic shock.

In a recent multicenter study, Brun-Buisson and colleagues [33] analyzed the relationship between bloodstream infection and severe sepsis in adults in ICUs and general wards in 24 hospitals in France. In this study, of the 842 episodes of clinically significant bloodstream infection recorded, 162 (19%) occurred in patients hospitalized in ICUs. Three hundred and seventy-seven episodes (45%) of bloodstream infection were nosocomial, and their incidence was 12 times greater in ICUs than in wards. The frequency of severe sepsis during bloodstream infection differed markedly between wards and ICUs (17% vs. 65%, $p<0.001$). The nosocomial episodes acquired in the ICU represented an incidence rate of 41 episodes per 1,000 admissions and the incidence rate of severe sepsis among patients with nosocomial bloodstream infection in the ICU was 24 episodes per 1,000 admissions.

Another recent multicenter study reported by our group [19] analyzed exclusively nosocomial bloodstream infections acquired in adult ICUs of 30 hospitals in Spain, and classified their systemic response according to new definitions as sepsis, severe sepsis and septic shock. Among 590 episodes of nosocomial bloodstream, the host reaction was classified as sepsis in 371 episodes (62.8%), severe sepsis in 109 episodes (18.5%), and septic shock in the remaining 110 (18.6%). The systemic response differed markedly according to source of bloodstream infection (Table 28.5). The episodes of bloodstream infection associated with intravascular catheters showed the lowest rate of septic shock (12.8%), whereas the episodes of bloodstream infection secondary to lower respiratory tract, intra-abdominal or genitourinary tract infections showed the highest incidence of severe sepsis and septic shock. In the study by Brun-Buisson et al. [33], in patients hospitalized in ICUs, intravascular catheter-related bloodstream infection was also associated with a lower risk of severe sepsis (OR=0.2; 95% CI: 0.1 – 0.5; $p<0.01$).

The systemic response may differ according to the microorganism causing the episode of bloodstream infection. Gram-negative and *Candida* spp. have been associated with a higher incidence of severe sepsis and septic shock in our multicenter study [19], whereas CNS was the microorganism causing the lowest incidence of septic shock. The multicenter study of Brun-Buisson et al. [33] analyzed ICU bloodstream infections separately and found the episodes caused by CNS to be also associated with a reduced risk of severe sepsis (OR = 0.2; $p=0.02$) relative to other organisms.

These results suggest that the source of infection and probably the type of microorganism causing the episode of bloodstream infection, especially if a species other than CNS is involved, may be important in the development of severe sepsis and septic shock.

Among community-acquired episodes the incidence of severe sepsis and septic shock is higher than in nosocomial episodes, in part because the severity of systemic response is the motive for ICU admission. In the multicenter French study, a 74% of community-acquired episodes presented severe sepsis or septic shock at admission in the ICU [33]. In a multicenter Spanish study carried out in 30 ICUs, the incidence of severe sepsis and septic shock was also 75%. In this study, gram-negative microorganisms and the urinary and intra-abdominal infections were associated more frequently with septic shock [34].

28.8 Risk Factors for Nosocomial Bloodstream Infection in the ICU

The conditions that predispose an individual to bloodstream infection include not only host underlying conditions but therapeutic, microbial and environmental factors as well. The illnesses that have been associated with an increased risk of bloodstream infection include hematologic and nonhematologic malignancies, diabetes mellitus, renal failure requiring dialysis, chronic hepatic failure, immune deficiency syndromes, and conditions associated with the loss of normal skin barriers such as serious burns and decubitus ulcers. In the ICU, therapeutic maneuvers associated with an increased

Table 28.5. Distribution of systemic response according to source of 590 episodes of ICU nosocomial bloodstream infection

Source	Number (%) of episodes			
	Sepsis	Severe sepsis	Septic shock	Total
Intravenous catheter	158 (68.5)	41 (18.7)	28 (12.8)	219 (37.1)
Lower respiratory tract	53 (51.5)	27 (26.2)	23 (22.3)	103 (17.5)
Intra-abdominal infection	12 (33.3)	9 (25)	15 (41.7)	36 (6.1)
Urinary tract	23 (65.7)	5 (14.3)	7 (20)	35 (5.9)
Surgical wound and soft tissue	7 (50)	2 (14.3)	5 (35.7)	14 (2.4)
Other	11 (64.7)	4 (23.5)	2 (11.8)	17 (2.9)
Unknown	115 (69.3)	21 (12.6)	30 (18.1)	166 (28.1)
Total	371 (62.8)	109 (18.5)	110 (18.6)	590 (100)

risk of nosocomial bloodstream infection include procedures such as placement of intravascular and urinary catheters, endoscopic procedures, and drainage of intra-abdominal infections.

Several risk factors have been associated with the acquisition of bloodstream infection by specific pathogens. Coagulase-negative staphylococci are mainly associated with central venous line infection and with the use of intravenous lipid emulsions. *Candida* spp. infections are related to the exposure to multiple antibiotics, hemodialysis, isolation of *Candida* species from sites other than the blood, azotemia, and the use of indwelling catheters [38]. In a recent analysis of risk factors for nosocomial candidemia in ICU patients with nosocomial bloodstream infections, we found that exposure to more than four antibiotics during the ICU stay (OR: 4.10), parenteral nutrition (OR: 3.37), previous surgery (OR: 2.60) and the presence of solid malignancy (OR: 1.57) were the variables that were independently associated with the development of *Candida* spp. infection [39].

28.9 Prognosis

28.9.1 Nosocomial Bacteremia

The crude mortality associated with bacteremic sepsis averages 35% (range 20–50% [17, 40, 41]. The mortality directly attributable to the nosocomial bloodstream infection averaged 27% (range 14–38%) [42]. Although one-third of the deaths occur within the first 48 h after the onset of symptoms, mortality can occur 14 or more days later. Late deaths are often due to poorly controlled infection, complications during the stay in the ICU, or failure of multiple organs [43]. Nosocomial bloodstream infection is associated with higher crude mortality rates than community-acquired infection [16, 41]. In a study, Bueno-Cavanillas et al. [44] analyzed the impact of nosocomial infection on the mortality rate in an ICU. In that study, overall crude relative risk of mortality was 2.48 (95% CI=1.47–4.16) in patients with a nosocomial infection compared with non-infected patients. When the type of infection was evaluated, the risk of mortality for patients with bloodstream infection was 4.13 (95% IC=2.11–8.11).

The risk of dying is influenced by the prior clinical condition of the patient and the rate at which complications develop. Analysis using prognostic stratification systems (such as the APACHE scoring system) indicate that factoring in the patients' age and certain physiologic variables results in more accurate estimates of the risk of dying. Variables associated with the high care-fatality rates include acute respiratory distress syndrome (ARDS), disseminated intravascular coagulation (DIC), renal insufficiency, and multiple organ dysfunction (MOD). Microbial variables are less important, although high care-fatality rates have been observed for patients with bloodstream infection due to *Pseudomonas aeruginosa*, *Candida* spp. and for patients with polymicrobial bloodstream infection.

In another study of bloodstream infection in an adult ICU of a teaching hospital in the UK over a 12-year period, Crowe and colleagues [45] analyzed 315 episodes of bloodstream infection, of which 82% were hospital-acquired, and found an overall mortality related to bloodstream infection of 44.4%. They also observed that ICU stay was longer in bacteremic patients (12 days) than non-bacteremic patients (3 days).

The crude mortality from bloodstream infection is often 35–60%, ranging from 12% to 80%. The attributable mortality defines the mortality directly associated with the episode of bloodstream infection, and excludes the mortality attributable to underlying conditions. It averages 26%, but varies according to the specific microorganisms involved: CNS averaged 13.6%; enterococci, 31%; and *Candida* spp. 38% [23, 46, 47].

Pittet et al. in 1994 [32] analyzed the attributable mortality, excess length of stay and extra costs due to nosocomial bloodstream infection in a surgical ICU. In this case-control study, the crude mortality rate was 50%, differing significantly from that of the matched controls (15%, $p<0.01$). In consequence, the attributable mortality associated with nosocomial bloodstream infection was 35%. These authors also observed that median length of hospital stay for cases was 14 days longer than for controls. Furthermore, nosocomial bloodstream infection was associated with a doubling of time of SICU stays, and consequently with a significant economic burden.

This study demonstrates that nosocomial bloodstream infections cause excess mortality and significantly prolong ICU and hospital stay among critically ill patients.

In another study of nosocomial bloodstream infection in a medical-surgical ICU reported by Rello et al. [18], the overall mortality was 31.5%, and 65.7% of all deaths were directly attributable to infection. Bloodstream infections from intra-abdominal, lower respiratory tract or unknown origin were associated with a poor prognosis. A logistic regression analysis defined intra-abdominal origin ($p=0.01$, OR:15.7) and presence of shock ($p<0.004$, OR: 3.3) as independently influencing the risk of death.

In a more recent study, Pittet et al. [48] analyzed the importance of preexisting co-morbidities for the prognosis of bloodstream infection in critically ill patients. The study was performed in a surgical ICU, and the authors analyzed 176 patients with bloodstream infection, of whom 125 (71%) were nosocomially acquired. The mean total length of ICU stay of bacteremic pa-

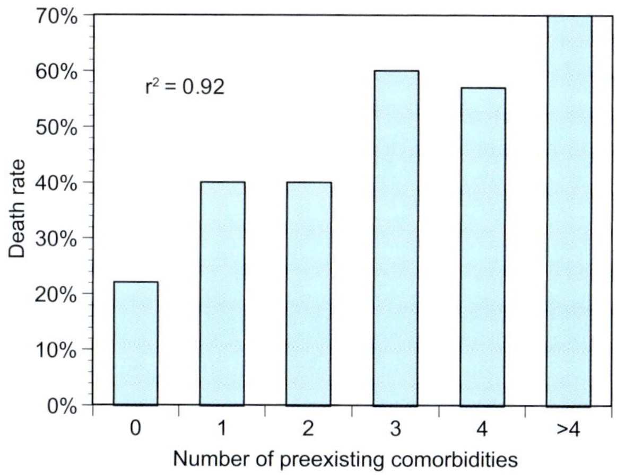

Fig. 28.3. Importance of preexisting co-morbidities for prognosis of septicemia in critically ill patients (from ref. [48], with permission)

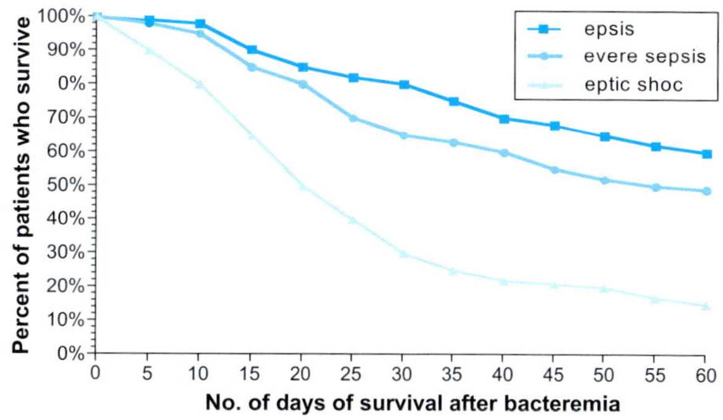

Fig. 28.4. Survival after nosocomial bloodstream infection according to systemic response

tients was also four times longer than that of non-bacteremic patients (17.6 days vs. 4.3 days). The overall mortality rate of non-bacteremic was 8.8%, whereas that of bacteremic patients was 44.3%. Thus, bacteremic patients had a fivefold increased risk of dying when compared with non-bacteremic patients (RR = 5.03, CI 95% 4.17–6.07, $p < 0.0001$). In this study they found a close correlation between the number of co-morbidities and fatality rates (Fig. 28.3). In addition, APACHE II ≥ 20 was also identified as an independent predictor of mortality.

A number of factors have been suspected as being associated with mortality in bloodstream infection. The most widely recognized prognostic factors are age, severity of the patient's underlying disease, and the appropriateness of antimicrobial therapy. Among other factors potentially related to the outcome of bloodstream infection, a multiple source of infection, secondary infection, bloodstream infection caused by some difficult-to-treat organisms such as *Pseudomonas* or *Serratia* spp., polymicrobial bloodstream infection, and factors related to host response such as the occurrence of hypotension, shock, or organ failure have all been described as prognostically important. In a French multicenter study of bloodstream infection and severe sepsis in ICUs and wards of 24 hospitals, Brun-Buisson et al. [33] reported that bloodstream infection due to *E. coli* or CNS was associated with a lower risk of severe sepsis and death, whereas *S. aureus* and gram-positive organisms other than CNS were associated with an increased risk of death. The results of that study emphasize the impact of end-organ dysfunction (i.e., severe sepsis and septic shock) on prognosis in bloodstream infection.

In the multicenter study on nosocomial bloodstream infection carried out by our group [19] in 30 Spanish ICUs, crude mortality was 41.6%, and 56% of all deaths were directly attributable to the bloodstream infection. The crude mortality was correlated to the severity of systemic response; it was as high as 80% among patients with septic shock, compared with 26% among patients whose bacteremic episodes were manifested exclusively as sepsis. The cumulative probability of survival stratified according to the grade of systemic response is shown in Fig. 28.4. In addition, bloodstream infections originating in the abdomen or respiratory tract were associated with the highest mortality ($p = 0.04$).

Because crude mortality cannot differentiate between mortality directly related to bloodstream infection and mortality attributable to underlying conditions, we were aware that different factors may influence the prognosis if we considered directly related mortality or crude mortality. For this reason we performed a double multivariate analysis with different dependent variables: one, related mortality, and the other, crude mortality. In the related mortality analysis, in addition to the level of systemic response and associated complications, we found that the type of microorganisms involved and the source of bloodstream infection played an important role in the prognosis. In the crude mortality analysis, we found that in addition to the systemic response and associated complications, mechanical ventilation at the time of development of bloodstream infection, chronic hepatic failure, and APACHE II > 15 at the time of diagnosis of bloodstream infection were chosen as factors by the statistical model; this seems to indicate that underlying diseases and the severity of patient's conditions markedly influence crude mortality among ICU patients with nosocomial bloodstream infection. On the other hand, the immediate prognosis after an episode of nosocomial bloodstream infection (related mortality) correlated with level of systemic response, type of microorganism involved and the different sources of bloodstream infection.

Pittet et al. [49] recently conducted a large cohort study to determine prognostic factors of mortality in

ICU patients with positive blood cultures. They analyzed 173 patients with bacteremia, of whom 53.1% were nosocomially acquired. Among patients with bacteremic sepsis, 75 died (43%); in 81% of them, the cause of death was considered to be directly or indirectly related to the infection. In this study, the best two independent prognostic factors were the APACHE II score at the onset of sepsis (OR, 1.13; CI 95% 1.08–1.17; $p<0.001$) and the number of organ dysfunctions developing thereafter (OR, 2.39; CI 95% 2.02–2.82; $p<0.001$). This study suggests that in ICU patients with positive blood cultures outcome can be predicted by the severity of illness at onset of sepsis and the number of vital organ dysfunctions developing subsequently.

28.9.2 Community-Acquired Bacteremia

Patients admitted in the ICU with community-acquired bacteremia present a crude mortality near to 40%, compared with a mortality of 18% in bacteremic patients admitted in general wards [12, 34, 50]. This elevated mortality in part is due to the severity of systemic response that presents in these patients and that is the cause of admission in the ICU [12, 34]. In addition to the severity of systemic response (severe sepsis and septic shock) and associated complications, the appropriateness of empiric antimicrobial treatment is the most important variable influencing the outcome of these patients [12, 34]. The incidence of inappropriate antibiotic treatment community-acquired bacteremias admitted in the ICU in two studies range between 15% and 20% and the mortality among patients with empiric inappropriate antibiotic treatment was more than 70% [12, 34, 51]. The correlation between survival time, systemic response to community-acquired bloodstream infection, and delayed antibiotic treatment is shown as Kaplan-Meier curves in Fig. 28.5.

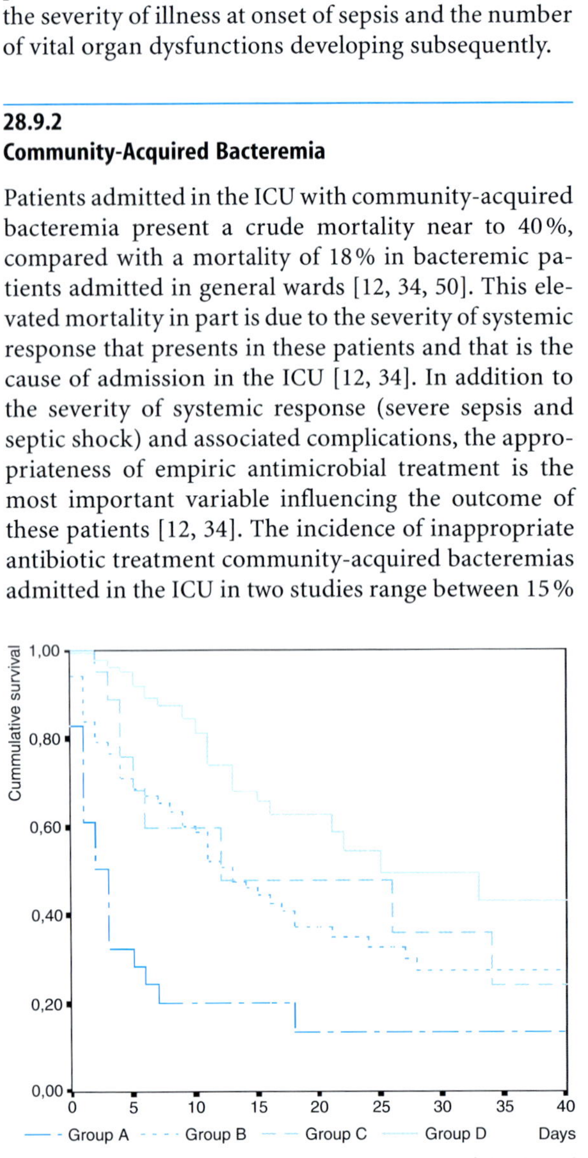

Fig. 28.5. Survival rate according to the presence of shock and initial antibiotic treatment. Log-rank test: $p<0.001$. *Group A* septic shock + delayed antibiotic treatment; *Group B* septic shock + appropriate antibiotic treatment; *Group C* no septic shock + delayed antibiotic treatment; *Group D* no septic shock + appropriate antibiotic treatment. (From ref. [34], with permission)

28.10 Conclusions

1. Nosocomial bloodstream infections occur two to seven times more often in intensive care unit (ICU) patients than in ward patients. Recent studies have shown that the incidence rate ranges between 26 and 67 episodes per 1,000 ICU admissions, depending on the type of ICU.
2. Patients with nosocomial ICU bloodstream infection have a higher prevalence of intravenous lines and respiratory sources of infection than ward patients in whom urinary tract infection is the most prevalent source of bloodstream infection.
3. Gram-positive microorganisms are the most prevalent cause of nosocomial bloodstream infection in ICU patients. This high incidence is related to the high prevalence of bloodstream infection associated with intravascular catheters in critically ill patients, and to the multiple antibiotic therapy used for gram-negative infections in ICU patients, which results in the selection of gram-positive microorganisms.
4. Currently, gram-negative microorganisms cause between 30% and 40% of ICU-acquired bloodstream infections, and multiresistant organisms, such as *P. aeruginosa*, *Serratia* spp, or *A. baumannii*, are the most frequently isolated pathogens.
5. Approximately 40% of ICU patients with nosocomial bloodstream infection show a severe systemic response, such as severe sepsis or septic shock, associated with high mortality.
6. The attributable mortality from nosocomial bloodstream infections is high in critically ill patients, and the infection is associated with excessively long ICU and hospital stays, and a significant economic burden.
7. The incidence rate of community-acquired bacteremia in adult ICUs is 10 episodes/1,000 admissions. *S. pneumoniae, S. aureus and E. coli* represent more than 80% of microorganisms causing community-acquired bacteremia in the critically ill patients. Most episodes are associated with severe sepsis or septic shock, and they are associated with a high mortality, and in the majority of cases directly related with the infection. The severity of systemic response and the appropriateness of empiric antibiotic treatment significantly influence the prognosis of these patients.

References

1. Wenzel RP (1990) Organization for infection control. In: Mandell GL, Douglas RG Jr, Bennett JE (eds) Principles and practice of infectious diseases, 3rd edn. Churchill Livingstone, New York, pp 2176–2180
2. Weinstein RA (1991) Epidemiology and control of nosocomial infections in adult intensive care units. Am J Med 91(Suppl 3B):179S–184S
3. Wenzel RP, Thompson RL, Landry SM, et al. (1983) Hospital-acquired infections in intensive care unit patients: an overview with emphasis on epidemics. Infect Control 4: 371–5
4. Maki DG (1989) Risk factors for nosocomial infection in intensive care: "devices vs nature" and goals for the next decade. Arch Intern Med 149:30–35
5. Donowitz LG, Wenzel RP, Hoyt JW (1982) High risk of hospital-acquired infection in the ICU patient. Crit Care Med 10:355–7
6. Brown RB, Hosmer D, Chen HC, et al. (1985) A comparison of infections in the different ICUs within the same hospital. Crit Care Med 13:472–476
7. Daschner F (1985) Nosocomial infections in intensive care units. Intensive Care Med 11:284–287
8. Massanari RM, Hierholzer WJ Jr (1986) The intensive care unit. In: Bennett JV, Brachman PS (eds) Hospital infections, 2nd edn. Little, Brown and Company, Boston, pp 285–298
9. Trilla A, Gatell JM, Mensa J, et al. (1991) Risk factors for nosocomial bacteremia in a large Spanish teaching hospital: A case-control study. Infect Control Hosp Epidemiol 12:150–156
10. Ponce de León-Rosales S, Molinar-Ramos F, Domínguez-Cherit G, Rangel-Frausto S, Vázquez-Ramos V (2000) Prevalence of infections in intensive care units in Mexico: A multicenter study. Crit Care Med 28:1316–1321
11. Forgacs IC, Eykyn SJ, Bradley RD (1986) Serious infection in the intensive therapy unit: a 15-year study of bacteraemia. Q J Med 60:773–779
12. Vallés J, Ochagavía A, Rué M, Díaz E, et al. (2000) Critically ill patients with community-acquired bacteremia: Characteristics and prognosis. Intensive Care Med 26(Suppl.3): S222
13. Reimer LG, Wilson ML, Weinstein MP (1997) Update on detection of bacteremia and fungemia. Clin Microbiol Rev 10:444–465
14. Garner JS, Jarvis WR, Emori TG, et al. (1988) CDC definitions for nosocomial infections. Am J Infect Control 16: 128–140
15. Friedman ND, Kaye KS, Stout JE, et al. (2002) Health care-associated bloodstream infections in adults: A reason to change the accepted definition of community-acquired infections. Ann Intern Med 137:791–797
16. Pittet D (1993) Nosocomial bloodstream infections. In: Wenzel RP (ed) Prevention and control of nosocomial infections, 2nd edn. Williams & Wilkins, Baltimore, MD, pp 512–555
17. Gatell JM, Trilla A, Latorre X, et al. (1988) Nosocomial bacteremia in a large Spanish teaching hospital: analysis of factors influencing prognosis. Rev Infect Dis 10:203–210
18. Rello J, Ricart M, Mirelis B, et al. (1994) Nosocomial bacteremia in a medical-surgical intensive care unit: epidemiologic characteristics and factors influencing mortality in 111 episodes. Intensive Care Med 20:94–98
19. Vallés J, León C, Alvarez-Lerma F, et al. (1997) Nosocomial bacteremia in critically ill patients: a multicenter study evaluating epidemiology and prognosis. Clin Infect Dis 24:387–395
20. Towns ML, Quartey SM, Weinstein MP, et al. (1993) The clinical significance of positive blood cultures: a prospective, multicenter evaluation, abstr. C-232. In: Abstracts of the 93rd General Meeting of the American Society for Microbiology 1993. American Society for Microbiology, Washington, DC
21. Weinstein MP, Towns ML, Quartey SM, et al. (1997) The clinical significance of positive blood cultures in the 1990s: a prospective comprehensive evaluation of the microbiology, epidemiology, and outcome of bacteremia and fungemia in adults. Clin Infect Dis 24:584–602
22. Mirret S, Weinstein MP, Reimer LG, et al. (1994) Interpretation of coagulase-negative staphylococci in blood cultures: does the number of positive bottles help? Abstr. C-69. In: Abstracts of the 93rd General Meeting of the American Society for Microbiology 1994. American Society for Microbiology, Washington, DC
23. Martin MA, Pfaller MA, Wenzel RP (1989) Coagulase-negative staphylococci bacteremia. Mortality and hospital stay. Ann Intern Med 110:9–16
24. Ponce de León S, Wenzel RP (1984) Hospital-acquired bloodstream infections with *Staphylococcus epidermidis*. Am J Med 77:639–644
25. Domínguez-de Villota E, Algora-Weber A, Millan I, et al. (1987) Early evaluation of coagulase-negative staphylococci in blood samples of intensive care unit patients. A clinically uncertain judgement. Intensive Care Med 13: 390–394
26. Craven DE, Kunches LM, Lichtenberg DA, et al. (1988) Nosocomial infections and fatality in medical and surgical intensive care unit patients. Arch Intern Med 148:1161–1168
27. Constantini M, Donisi PM, Turrin MG, et al. (1987) Hospital-acquired infections surveillance and control in intensive care services. Results of an incidence study. Eur J Epidemiol 3:347–355
28. Daschner FD, Frey P, Wolff G, et al. (1982) Nosocomial infections in intensive care wards: A multicenter prospective study. Intensive Care Med 8:5–9
29. Trilla A (1994) Epidemiology of nosocomial infections in adult intensive care units. Intensive Care Med 20:S1–S4
30. Vincent JL, Bihari DJ, Suter PM, et al. (1995) The prevalence of nosocomial infection in intensive care units in Europe. JAMA 274:634–644
31. Richards MJ, Edwards JR, Culver DH, et al. (1999) Nosocomial infections in medical intensive care units in the United States. Crit Care Med 27:887–892
32. Pittet D, Tarara D, Wenzel RP (1994) Nosocomial bloodstream infection in critically ill patients. Excess length of stay, extra costs, and attributable mortality. JAMA 271: 1598–1601
33. Brun-Buisson C, Doyon F, Carlet J, et al. (1996) Bacteremia and severe sepsis in adults: A multicenter prospective survey in ICUs and wards of 24 hospitals. Am J Respir Crit Care Med 154:617–624
34. Vallés J, Rello J, Ochagavía A, Garnacho J, Alcalá MA, and Spanish Collaborative Group for Infections in Intensive Care Units of Sociedad Española de Medicina Intensiva, Crítica y Unidades Coronarias (2003) Community-acquired bloodstream infection in critically ill adult patients: Impact of shock and inappropriate antibiotic therapy on survival. Chest 123:1615–1624
35. Edgeworth JD, Treacher DF, Eykyn SJ (1999) A 25-year study of nosocomial bacteremia in an adult intensive care unit. Crit Care Med 27:1421–1428
36. Jamal WY, El-Din K, Rotimi VO, et al. (1999) An analysis of hospital-acquired bacteraemia in intensive care unit patients in a university hospital in Kuwait. J Hosp Infect 43:49–56

37. Bone RC, Balk RA, Cerra FB, et al. (1992) Definitions for sepsis and organ failure and guidelines for the use of innovative therapies in sepsis. Chest 101:1644 - 1655
38. Wenzel RP (1995) Isolation of *Candida* species from sites other than the blood. Clin Infect Dis 20:1531 - 1534
39. Díaz E, Villagrá A, Martínez M, et al. (1998) Nosocomial candidemia risk factors. Intensive Care Med 24 (Suppl 1): S143
40. Leibovici L, Konisberger H, Pitlik SD (1992) Bacteremia and fungemia of unknown origin in adults. Clin Infect Dis 14:436 - 439
41. Weinstein MP, Reller LB, Murphy JR, et al. (1983) The clinical significance of positive blood cultures: a comprehensive analysis of 500 episodes of bloodstream infection and fungemia in adults. I. Laboratory and epidemiologic observations. Rev Infect Dis 5:35 - 53
42. Wenzel RP (1988) The mortality of hospital-acquired bloodstream infections: need for a new vital statistic? Int J Epidemiol 17:225 - 227
43. Munford RS (1994) Sepsis and septic shock. In: Isselbacher KJ, Braunwald E, Wilson JD, Martin JB, Fauci AS, Kasper DL (eds) Harrison's principles of internal medicine, 13rd edn. McGraw-Hill, New York, pp 511 - 515
44. Bueno-Cavanillas A, Delgado-Rodríguez M, López-Luque A, et al. (1994) Influence of nosocomial infection on mortality rate in an intensive care unit. Crit Care Med 22: 55 - 60
45. Crowe M, Ispahani P, Humphreys H, et al. (1998) Bacteraemia in the adult intensive care unit of a teaching hospital in Nottingham, UK, 1985 - 1996. Eur J Clin Microbiol Dis 17:377 - 384
46. Landry SL, Kaiser DL, Wenzel RP (1989) Hospital stay and mortality attributed to nosocomial enterococcal bacteremia: a controlled study. Am J Infect Control 17:323 - 329
47. Wey SB, Motomi M, Pfaller MA, et al. (1988) Hospital-acquired candidemia: the attributable mortality and excess length of stay. Arch Intern Med 148:2642 - 2645
48. Pittet D, Thiévent B, Wenzel RP, et al. (1993) Importance of pre-existing co-morbidities for prognosis of septicemia in critically ill patients. Intensive Care Med 19:265 - 272
49. Pittet D, Thiévent B, Wenzel RP, et al. (1996) Bedside prediction of mortality from bacteremic sepsis. A dynamic analysis of ICU patients. Am J Respir Crit Care Med 153:684 - 693
50. Cartón JA, García-Velasco G, Maradona JA, Pérez F, Asensi V, Arribas JM (1988) Bacteriemia extrahospitalaria en adultos. Análisis prospectivo de 333 episodios. Med Clin (Barc) 90:525 - 530
51. Ibrahim EH, Sherman G, Ward S, Fraser VJ, Kollef MH (2000) The influence of inadequate antimicrobial treatment of bloodstream infections on patient outcomes in the ICU setting. Chest 118:146 - 155

Chapter 29

Bloodstream Infections in Patients with Total Parenteral Nutrition Catheters

R. SIERRA, A. RAMÍREZ

29.1 Introduction

Vascular access is an essential procedure in the management of critically ill patients, especially the insertion of central venous catheters (CVCs). The most commonly used CVCs are noncuffed percutaneously inserted catheters placed in the femoral, internal jugular or subclavian veins [1–3]. Unfortunately, these intravascular devices are associated with the risk of complications. Potential CVC-related complications include chiefly arterial puncture, pneumothorax, hemothorax, thrombosis, hematoma, and infectious complications. Among the most important life-threatening complications of intravascular devices are catheter-related bloodstream infections (CRBSIs) [2–7], which represent a major cause of nosocomial infection in intensive care units (ICUs) [8–10]. The National Nosocomial Infections Surveillance (NNIS) System reported in 2004 [11] a CRBSI mean rate in United States ICUs of 4.85 CRBSI cases per 1,000 central line-days (mean value of pooled means from different types of surveyed ICU). Mean rates of the other two main sources of nosocomial infection in US ICUs were 4.9 urinary catheter-associated urinary tract infections per 1,000 urinary-catheter-days, and 11.1 ventilator-associated pneumonias per 1,000 ventilator-days. Twenty-five percent of bloodstream infections that occur in the ICU are secondary to catheter-related infections (CRIs). In addition, up to 80% of primary bacteremia may be linked to CRIs [9, 12, 13].

Attributable mortality from CRIs in critically ill patients has been found high in some studies [14–16], though this finding is controversial [8]. Between 2,400 and 20,000 deaths are estimated to be produced by CRIs yearly in the USA [1, 17, 18], giving mortality rates ranging from 14% to 28% [6, 10, 14, 19–24]. Nevertheless, mortality rates from CRBSI are relatively low, if they are compared with the mortality from other infectious foci [9]. CRBSI is also associated with an excess of length of stay both in ICUs and hospital, further increasing cost [8, 9, 14, 17, 22, 24–29].

29.2 Definitions

29.2.1 CVCs

CVCs may be classified according to the insertion length, e.g., (1) short-term catheters, in place < 10 days, and (2) long-term catheters, in place > 10 days [6]. However, other researchers have defined short-term catheters as those with placement duration < 7 days, and long-term catheters as those in place > 7 days [30].

29.2.2 Exit Site Infection

Exit site infection is considered when local signs occur, such as tenderness, skin erythema, induration within 2 cm of the catheter exit site (with or without fever), or cellulitis along the subcutaneous tract, in the absence of pus at the exit site. Except for the presence of pus, these signs lack specificity and may be caused by host immune response against the CVC, or by the administered fluid as well. The presence of pus is usually a diagnostic sign of infection, even when a culture from the catheter tip is not available [30–35].

29.2.3 Colonization

Colonization occurs when a positive culture from either catheter tip, subcutaneous segment of the catheter, or catheter hub is obtained with a result of ≥ 15 colony-forming units (cfu)/ml [6, 30, 36].

29.2.4 Catheter-Related Bloodstream Infection

Catheter-related bloodstream infection is defined when signs of systemic infection (i.e., sepsis) are associated with positive blood cultures which have been obtained by any diagnostic method. Matched microorganisms should be isolated in the catheter tip, and in blood cultures from the peripheral vein. Furthermore, other apparent sources of infection should not occur [30].

Diagnosing CRBSI by coagulase-negative staphylococci requires microbial growth to be obtained in at least two peripheral-blood samples [37].

29.2.5 Infusate-Related Infection

Infusate-related infection is present when there are signs of systemic infection, in the absence of other apparent infectious sources. In addition, the same microorganism should grow in both peripheral-blood samples, and in the fluids administered. Cultures of the catheter tip are not required to be positive [30].

29.3 Etiology

Catheter-related infection is caused mainly by microorganisms from the skin flora. However, in the hospital setting, a normal flora is usually replaced by pathogenic bacteria. Patients who are receiving antimicrobial therapy are often colonized by gram-negative bacilli, *Staphylococcus aureus* or fungi. Besides, microorganisms from the airways are frequently isolated in patients with tracheostomy. Microorganism types which are isolated from catheters appear to be related to insertion sites. Aerobic gram-negative bacilli, *Candida* species, and anaerobes are isolated in the inguinal region more frequently.

The most frequent pathogens related to the etiology of CRBSI are coagulase-negative staphylococci, *Staphylococcus aureus*, enterococci, aerobic gram-negative bacilli, and *Candida* spp. (especially *C. albicans*). The microorganism most commonly isolated in catheter-related sepsis is *Staphylococcus epidermidis*, which seems to be associated with a lower mortality rate than other pathogens. A higher rate of mortality has been found associated with *Staphylococcus aureus* CRI. Antimicrobial treatment of these pathogens may be difficult because many isolates are increasingly becoming resistant to oxacillin and other antibiotics [1, 38, 39].

29.4 Risk Factors

Multilumen central venous catheters are associated with a greater risk of CRI when compared with the risk from single-lumen catheters, since multilumen catheters are more frequently manipulated so increasing the chance of a breakdown in protective barriers [40–46].

Heavy cutaneous colonization is also a major risk factor for CRI [6]. CRI rate was decreased in patients who received chlorhexidine gluconate for insertion-site skin disinfection, compared with those who received povidone-iodine. Such a practice constitutes a simple measure for reducing the occurrence of CRI [47].

Femoral vein insertion site is considered to be associated with the highest rate of microbial colonization, since this skin zone usually has a heavier cutaneous colonization. Colonization risk is lower for the jugular site [6, 48]. Infection occurs more frequently in the jugular vein than in the subclavian vein. It may be favored by neck movements, which make dressing care of catheters difficult. Infection risk is lower for subclavian vein insertion sites [49–51].

The longer the catheter is in place the higher the probability of CRI occurrence [34]. CRI is also more frequent in patients in whom two or more catheters have been inserted [9].

Recent studies carried out on hematology-oncological patients have shown an association between fibrin deposition, catheter-related thrombosis and infection [52–56], but these findings have not been confirmed in other studies [3, 56].

Administration of blood products through CVCs is another risk factor for CRBI, although thrombocytopenia during catheterization may provide some protection against CRBI [57, 58].

Parenteral nutrition (PN) was identified as an independent risk factor for CRI in hospitalized patients, particularly those in the ICU, which is probably explained by hyperglycemia. The pathogenic role of hyperglycemia in other patients groups is uncertain [35, 59–63].

ICU admission when nursing staff are less available has also been identified as a risk factor for CRI.

Unstable clinical status has not been demonstrated to be a risk factor for CRI [35].

Malnutrition appears not to be a risk factor for CRI but influences clinical outcome, and is associated with more complications, increased mortality rates, and increased hospital length of stay and costs [64, 65].

29.5 Pathogenesis

CRBSI principally occurs by two routes, extraluminally and intraluminally. The extraluminal route occurs when there is concordance among isolates from catheter segments, skin, and blood cultures. The intraluminal route occurs when isolates from a hub, or infusate fluids, and blood cultures are concordant. The route of infection is considered as being indeterminate when both routes are possible [6].

CRBSI often occurs following catheter colonization [1, 20]. Pathogens firstly have to gain access to the intraluminal or extraluminal surface of the catheter [6]. Intravascular devices cause a local inflammatory response in the site of insertion, and then several proteins covering the catheter [66–71] favor the adherence of microorganisms by diverse mechanisms [66, 67].

Microorganisms gain access into the body through one of the three following mechanisms:

1. At the time of insertion or later, the skin flora invades the percutaneous tract through the insertion site, involving initially the external surface of the catheter (extraluminal colonization). This mechanism is regarded to be the major mechanism in short-term nontunneled catheter-associated infections.
2. Microorganisms contaminate the catheter hub and lumen (intraluminal colonization). This mechanism results from frequent manipulations, or when the catheter is inserted over a percutaneous guidewire. When epidemic CRBSI occurs, a contaminated infusion should also be considered.
3. Microorganisms may occasionally be carried hematogenously to the intravascular device from a remote source of infection. This mechanism is not frequent [1, 6, 48, 72–76].

Most infections associated with short-term catheters are caused by skin flora surrounding the insertion site which gains access via an extraluminal route, and occasionally intraluminally. With long-term catheters, there is a predomination of intraluminal colonization with contamination of the hub and afterwards of the lumen. The intraluminal route commonly predominates when the placement is longer than 1–2 weeks [6]. The mechanism of infection that is attributed to CVCs inserted in old sites over a guidewire appears to be no different from that of catheters inserted in de novo sites [6, 48].

After microorganisms gain access to the intravascular device, they can adhere to it, and produce extracellular polymer substances ("slime"), which facilitate further adhesion to CVC surfaces. These polymers develop into a matrix which leads to biofilm formation. Infection is derived from the microbes' ability to adhere, proliferate, and elaborate biofilm. These actions allow sustained infection, and hematogenous dissemination [1, 6, 48].

The microorganisms commonly associated with biofilm formation in catheters are: coagulase-negative staphylococci, *Staphylococcus aureus*, *Enterococcus faecalis*, *Klebsiella pneumonia*, *Pseudomonas aeruginosa*, and *Candida albicans* [1, 77].

All catheters develop biofilms in vivo. Initially, this effect is not significant; however, when the catheter has been in place for a long time, biofilms can become a persistent source of infection, and may oppose host defenses by decreasing the effect of antibiotics [1, 78]. In addition there is decreased diffusion of antibiotics in biofilms, and other mechanisms which favor resistance occurrence. Biofilm-associated pathogens require a greater concentration of antibiotics to be eliminated since they have decreased antimicrobial susceptibility [1, 77, 79].

29.6 Diagnosis

The diagnosis of CRI is often based on the exclusion of the presence of other inflammatory sources [34]. CRBSI diagnostic methods may be categorized into two groups, those with catheter removal, and those without catheter removal. The most common methods are those with catheter removal and catheter-tip culturing when CRBSI is suspected (Table 29.1). Nevertheless, most of the catheters are not usually infected and replacement may increase the risk of complications and cost [76, 80–83]. The methods for diagnosing CRI without catheter removal are listed in Table 29.2.

Subcutaneous segment cultures appear not to be useful for diagnosing CRBSI [84].

Table 29.1. Diagnostic methods with catheter removal [1, 2, 34]

	Description	Diagnostic cut-off value	Pooled sensitivity (95% CI)	Pooled specificity (95% CI)
Qualitative catheter segment culture	Catheter segment is immersed in a broth media, and then incubated for 24–72 h. This method is not recommended since it has a poor specificity	Any growth	0.87 (0.79–0.96)	0.75 (0.72–0.78)
Semiquantitative catheter segment culture (Maki method)	The most used method to diagnose CRBSI. The catheter tip is rolled 4 times across an agar plate, then incubated, and observed after an overnight period	≥15 cfu/ml	0.83 (0.79–0.87)	0.86 (0.85–0.87)
Quantitative catheter segment culture	It requires vortex or sonicating catheter samples in broth, or flushing the broth through the catheter, and then plating on blood agar serial dilutions	≥ 10^3 cfu/ml	0.82 (0.78–0.86)	0.89 (0.87–0.91)

Table 29.2. Diagnostic methods without catheter removal [1, 2, 34]

	Description	Diagnostic cut-off value	Pooled sensitivity (95% CI)	Pooled specificity (95% CI)
Qualitative blood culture through catheter	≥1 blood samples for cultures are drawn from the catheter	Any growth	0.91 (0.84–0.98)	0.86 (0.83–0.89)
Quantitative blood culture through catheter	A blood sample for culture is drawn from the catheter, and processed by pour-plate or lysis-centrifugation technique	≥100 cfu	0.84 (0.80–0.89)	0.90 (0.88–0.92)
Paired qualitative blood cultures	Concomitant blood samples for cultures are both drawn through the catheter, and percutaneously	Microorganisms are ≥5-fold greater in central blood sample	0.79 (0.74–0.84)	0.99 (0.98–1.0)
Differential time to positivity	Concomitant blood samples for cultures are both drawn through the catheter, and percutaneously, and then are monitored continuously	Central blood sample turns positive 120 min before	0.89 (0.86–0.92)	0.83 (0.79–0.87)
Acridine orange leukocyte cytospin (AOLC)	1 ml of blood is aspirated from the catheter, then the cells are lysed with sterile water, centrifuged, stained with acridine orange, and observed. Simple and rapid test. It allows an early targeted antimicrobial therapy, and is recommended as the first line investigation of CRBSI [76, 85]	Any microorganism is visualized	0.87 (0.80–0.94)	0.93 (0.89–0.97)

29.7 Management

Catheter removal whenever a CRI is suspected is the common approach to managing these frequent nosocomial infections. However, many catheters are removed unnecessarily, since in many cases they are not associated with infection. Besides, CVC reinsertion may be further associated with complications [1].

Antibiotic therapy is empirically initiated by the intravenous route. The choice of a given antibiotic regime usually depends on illness severity, patient risk factors, and likely pathogens associated with the intravascular device.

Vancomycin is recommended in hospitals where there are frequently methicillin-resistant *Staphylococci* (MRSA). Oxacillin should be used in the absence of epidemic, or endemic, MRSA flora.

In addition, empiric treatment with an antipseudomonal beta-lactamic agent should be considered in immunocompromised, or seriously ill, patients, to cover enteric gram-negative bacteria and *Pseudomonas* spp. When fungemia is suspected, then amphotericin B or intravenous fluconazole should be used. Caspofungin or voriconazole are alternative therapies when candidiasis is suspected in an unstable patient. If the clinical status of the patient has been stabilized, switching to oral agents can be considered [30].

Catheters may not have to be removed initially, particularly if the microorganism isolated is coagulase-negative staphylococci [30, 86].

If severe sepsis is not in evidence (i.e., the presence of hypotension, hypoperfusion, or organ failure) and no infection signs are observed at the insertion site, the catheter should be removed only when either: (a) cultures of blood drawn from the catheter yield positive results, (b) there is persistent fever, or (c) the results of peripheral blood cultures are negative because the catheter was not cultured.

Whenever patients exhibit a serious illness, sepsis, or signs of infection at the exit site, the catheter should be removed.

For treatment purposes, patients with non-tunneled catheters and CRBSI may be distributed into two groups: complicated CRBSI (with septic thrombosis, endocarditis, osteomyelitis, or emboli) or non-complicated CRBSI.

In the case of a peripheral blood culture negative result, and the catheter culture reveals significant growth of *S. aureus* or *C. albicans* (either febrile patients with valvular heart disease or neutropenic patients), then the patient should be observed and peripheral blood cultures repeated. Some authors advise the delivery of a short course (5–7 days) of antibiotic therapy [1, 30].

CRI caused by coagulase-negative staphylococcus must receive a 5–7 day course of antimicrobial therapy, combined with catheter removal. A course of 10–14 days of local antibiotic lock (ABL) may be applied if the catheter is not removed. The catheter should be removed for pathogens other than coagulase-negative staphylococci, and patients should receive 10–14 days of antimicrobial therapy. A course of 4–6 weeks should be considered in the case of persistent bacteremia or fungemia after catheter removal, or if there is evidence of complicated infection (except in cases of osteomyelitis, which requires 6–8 weeks of therapy). The antimicrobial treatment for

Candida spp. should last up to 14 days after the last positive blood culture.

Streptokinase in combination with antimicrobial therapy has not been demonstrated to be beneficial for the treatment of CRI [30].

In the case of persistent bacteremia, fungemia, or when clinical improvement after 3 days of appropriate antibiotic therapy and catheter withdrawal is lacking, endocarditis should be ruled out with transesophageal echocardiography. If the results of such a test are negative, then aggressive workup for septic thrombosis or for another metastasic infection should ensue [1, 30].

In cases of tunneled CVCs or implantable devices it is important to confirm that a related infection has occurred. Catheters must be removed in cases of complicated infections, CRI by *Candida* spp., tunnel infection, port abscess, and when following an initially maintained catheter there is clinical deterioration or persistent bacteremia.

The treatment regime is similar to that of non-tunneled catheters, in the case of pathogens other than *Candida* spp., and those mentioned above. However, if the catheter has to be retained, systemic antibiotic therapy should be combined with ABL for 10–14 days (Table 29.3) [30]. ABL has been used to decrease the duration of systemic antibiotic treatment, and to maintain a high antibiotic concentration within the CVC. ABL comprises a mixture of 0.3 ml (40 mg) of teicoplanin (400 mg per 3 ml) and 0.2 ml of sodium heparin at 500 IU per 5 ml, although other antibiotics or antifungal agents can be also used. When CRBSI is confirmed, this 0.5-ml lock is injected into the catheter, and left for 12 h. Later, this small volume is aspirated before initiating PN. ABL is administered for 12–15 days, in combination with short-duration systemic antibiotherapy (usually a glycopeptide plus an aminoglycoside). Systemic antiobiotherapy is administered in general for the first 5 days [39].

Table 29.3. Management of tunneled CVCs [30]

	Evidence level
Ensure that the CVC is really the source of infection	IIIB
The CVC should be removed in case of complicated infections	IIB
For salvage of the CVC in patients with uncomplicated infections, ABL should be used for 2 weeks with standard systemic antibiotic therapy in the absence of tunnel or pocket infection	IIB
Tunneled catheter pocket infections or port abscess require removal of catheter and usually 7–10 days of appropriate antibiotic therapy	IIIC
Antibiotic lock therapy is recommended for treatment when the catheter is retained	IIIB

ABL success depends on antibiotic concentrations within the catheter [87]. High antibiotic concentrations augment antimicrobial efficacy and lessen the secondary effects of systemic antibiotic treatment.

The ABL method is recommended and supported by findings from in vitro models which have shown reductions in staphylococcal, gram-negative and fungal colonization rates. Some trials have also demonstrated clinical efficacy for CRBSI, especially for non-tunneled catheters [39]. However, ABL is not recommended in long-term PN, because ABL appears not to prevent a second or third episode of CRI by the same bacterial strain but with an increase in teicoplanin resistance [38, 88, 89].

29.8 Bloodstream Infections in Patients with Total Parenteral Nutrition Catheters

Parenteral nutrition is indicated when gut function is altered, and enteral nutrition is not suitable. PN serves to prevent the adverse effects of malnutrition, and its use is not exclusive to hospitalized patients. Delivery of PN to outpatients is known as home PN (HPN). PN is not indicated for unstable patients. The impact of PN on mortality and morbidity is a controversial issue, because of the occurrence of frequent complications related to PN use. CRI constitutes a major complication derived from PN, and represents the main cause for readmission to hospital in HPN patients [39, 90–96].

Subclavian vein access is a common approach for delivering PN, whether subcutaneously or not [97]. Subclavian vein access is preferred for infection control purposes. Frequency of mechanical complications may be decreased by using bedside ultrasound for catheter placement [31].

Peripherally inserted central catheters (PICCs) can also be used for delivering PN. PICCs are small-size catheters inserted into the subclavian vein through the basilic or cephalic vein. PICCs are associated with fewer mechanical complications during the insertion procedure than other venous access, but are long-term catheters in HPN patients. The use of such catheters appears to be more associated with increased risk of phlebitis, thrombosis or sepsis when compared with that of CVCs [98–103]. A higher frequency of CRI cases related to PICCs used for HPN may be related to a higher exposure of the arms to microbes than the chest wall surface. It is crucial not only to use a sterile technique during insertion, but also to deliver proper catheter care [97]. HPN patients should report to their healthcare provider any changes in their catheter site, and any new discomfort, and as well as avoiding submerging the catheter under water. Showering can be allowed whenever the catheter and connecting device are protected with an impermeable cover during the shower [31].

By tunneling CVC appears to reduce the CRI risk. This measure should be considered when circumstances make it not feasible to cannulate a subclavian vein [6]. For patients requiring frequent or continuous venous access, a PICC or tunneled CVC is usually employed. However, a totally implantable access device is the recommended approach for patients who require long-term, intermittent vascular access [31].

Candida spp. and *Malassetia* spp. are more frequently isolated in PN patients with CRI than in patients with CVCs not used to PN. Certain *Candida* spp., in the presence of glucose-containing fluids, may also produce slime, which may explain the elevated rate of CRBSI caused by fungal pathogens found among patients receiving PN [31].

Increased blood glucose levels have been related to higher infection rates in hospitalized patients [104], especially in critically ill patients [105]. Hyperglycemia in PN patients can be explained by the intense activation of contraregulatory hormones, and cytokine responses, which are both associated with circumstances such as severe disease, and excessive administration of glucose. Patients with PN exhibit frequently sustained hyperglycemia, and often receive insulin. Hyperglycemia impairs immune response as well, reducing neutrophil chemotaxis and phagocytosis, which can increase risk of infection onset [59, 105, 106]. Tight control of glycemia may reduce mortality rates significantly in surgical ICU patients [105]; however, such intensive insulin therapy has been demonstrated to reduce only morbidity, but not mortality, rates, in patients in the medical ICU [107].

Possibly the contamination by particulates, such as undetected trace elements, could also favor CRI occurrence [108, 109].

A high CRI incidence rate occurring in PN patients could favor the use of antiseptic- or antibiotic-impregnated catheters [50, 110–113]. The use of antibiotic-impregnated catheters is associated with lower colonization rates. However, such CRBSI incidence rates appear to be no different when they are compared with those of non-impregnated catheters [114–124]. Antimicrobial-impregnated catheters have been demonstrated to reduce the risk of CRBSI only among patients whose catheters were used for delivering total PN [116, 125]. Minocycline plus rifampin-impregnated catheters were demonstrated to be effective only against staphylococci strains (*S. aureus* and *S. epidermidis*). However, colonization frequency by *Candida* spp. is higher than in non-impregnated catheters [116, 121, 126]. Utilization of miconazole plus rifampin-impregnated catheters is associated with lower rates of CRI when compared to standard catheters. These special catheters may be effective on prevention of CRI by *Candida* spp., although it has not yet been demonstrated [10].

Tubing used for administering total PN, or lipid emulsions, should be replaced within 24 h after initiating the infusion.

For infection control purposes, all CVCs must have the least number of ports or lumens needed for the management of the patient, and should be removed as soon as their use is no longer essential [31]. Catheter colonization risk in PN patients is decreased when single-lumen catheters are inserted through the subclavian vein, are used exclusively for PN, and are cared for by and under the control of a multidisciplinary team [97, 127].

References

1. Lane RK, Matthay MA (2002) Central line infections. Curr Opin Crit Care 8:441–8
2. Safdar N, Fine JP, Maki DG (2005) Meta-analysis: methods for diagnosing intravascular device-related bloodstream infection. Ann Intern Med 142:451–466. Erratum in: Ann Intern Med 142:803
3. Abdelkefi A, Torjman L, Ladeb S, et al. (2005) Randomized trial of prevention of catheter-related bloodstream infection by continuous infusion of low-dose unfractionated heparin in patients with hematologic and oncologic disease. J Clin Oncol 23:7864–7870
4. Maki DG (1989) Pathogenesis, prevention and management of infections due to intravascular devices used for infusion therapy. In: Waldwogel F (ed) Infections associated with indwelling medical devices. American Society for Microbiology, Washington, DC, pp 161–177
5. Maki DG, Goldman DA, Rhame FS (1973) Infection control in intravenous therapy. Ann Intern Med 79:867–887
6. Safdar N, Maki DG (2004) The pathogenesis of catheter-related bloodstream infection with noncuffed short-term central venous catheters. Intensive Care Med 30:62–67
7. Valles J, Leon C, Alvarez-Lerma F (1997) Nosocomial bacteremia in critically ill patients: a multicenter study evaluating epidemiology and prognosis. Clin Infect Dis 24: 387–395
8. Rello J, Ochagavia A, Sabanes E, et al. (2002) Evaluation of outcome of intravenous catheter-related infections in critically ill patients. Am J Respir Crit Care Med 162:1027–1030
9. Brun-Buisson C, Doyon F, Sollet JP, et al. (2004) Prevention of intravascular catheter-related infection with newer chlorhexidine-silver sulfadiazine-coated catheters: a randomized controlled trial. Intensive Care Med 30:837–843
10. Yucel N, Lefering R, Maegele M, et al. (2004) Reduced colonization and infection with miconazole-rifampicin modified central venous catheters: a randomized controlled clinical trial. J Antimicrob Chemother 54:1109–1115
11. National Nosocomial Infections Surveillance System (2004) National Nosocomial Infections Surveillance (NNIS) System Report, data summary from January 1992 through June 2004, issued October 2004. Am J Infect Control 32:470–485
12. Maki DG (1981) Nosocomial bacteremia. An epidemiologic overview. Am J Med 70:719–732
13. Richards MJ, Edwards JR, Culver DH, et al. (2000) Nosocomial infections in combined medical-surgical intensive care units in the United States. Infect Control Hosp Epidemiol 21:510–515
14. Pittet D, Tarara D, Wenzel RP (1994) Nosocomial bloodstream infection in critically ill patients. Excess length of

stay, extra costs, and attributable mortality. JAMA 271: 1598–1601
15. Gastmeier P, Weist K, Ruden H (1999) Catheter-associated primary bloodstream infections: epidemiology and preventive methods. Injection 27(Suppl 1):S1–6
16. Pittet D, Wenzel RP (1995) Nosocomial bloodstream infections. Secular trends in rates, mortality, and contribution to total hospital deaths. Arch Intern Med 155:1177–1184
17. Hu KK, Veenstra DL, Lipsky BA, et al. (2004) Use of maximal sterile barriers during central venous catheter insertion: clinical and economic outcomes. Clin Infect Dis 39: 1441–1445
18. Saint S, Savel RH, Matthay MA (2002) Enhancing the safety of critically ill patients by reducing urinary and central venous catheter-related infections. Am J Respir Crit Care Med 165:1475–1479
19. Russell LM, Weinstein RA (1998) Antimicrobial-coated central venous catheters – icing on the cake or the staff of life? Crit Care Med 26:195–196
20. Polderman KH, Girbes AR (2002) Central venous catheter use. Part 2: infectious complications. Intensive Care Med 28:18–28
21. Smith RL, Meixler SM, Simberkoff MS (1991) Excess mortality in critically ill patients with nosocomial bloodstream infections. Chest 100:164–167
22. Arnow PM, Quimosing EM, Beach M (1993) Consequences of intravascular catheter sepsis. Clin Infect Dis 16:778–784
23. Collignon PJ (1994) Intravascular catheter associated sepsis: a common problem. The Australian Study on Intravascular Catheter Associated Sepsis. Med J Aust 161:374–378
24. Sherertz RJ, Ely EW, Westbrook DM, et al. (2000) Education of physicians-in-training can decrease the risk for vascular catheter infection. Ann Intern Med 132:641–648
25. McConnell SA, Gubbins PO, Anaissie EJ (2003) Do antimicrobial-impregnated central venous catheters prevent catheter-related bloodstream infection? Clin Infect Dis 37:65–72
26. O'Grady NP, Alexander M, Dellinger EP, et al. (2002) Healthcare Infection Control Practices Advisory Committee. Guidelines for the prevention of intravascular catheter-related infections. Am J Infect Control 30:476–489
27. Mermel LA (2000) Prevention of intravascular catheter-related infections. Ann Intern Med 132:391–402
28. National Nosocomial Infections Surveillance (NNIS) System (1998) National Nosocomial Infections Surveillance (NNIS) System report, data summary from October 1986–April 1998, issued June 1998. Am J Infect Control 26:522–533
29. Renaud B, Brun-Buisson C; ICU-Bacteremia Study Group (2001) Outcomes of primary and catheter-related bacteremia. A cohort and case-control study in critically ill patients. Am J Respir Crit Care Med 163:1584–1590
30. Mermel LA, Farr BM, Sherertz RJ, et al. (2001) Infectious Diseases Society of America; American College of Critical Care Medicine; Society for Healthcare Epidemiology of America. Guidelines for the management of intravascular catheter-related infections. Clin Infect Dis 32:1249–1272
31. Guidelines for prevention of intravascular catheter-related infections (2002) MMWR Morb Mortal Wkly Rep 51:1–32
32. Pearson ML (1996) Guideline for prevention of intravascular device-related infections. Hospital Infection Control Practices Advisory Committee. Infect Control Hosp Epidemiol 17:438–473
33. Lugauer S, Regenfus A, Boswald M, et al. (1999) A new scoring system for the clinical diagnosis of catheter-related infections. Infection 27(Suppl 1):S49–53
34. Calandra T, Cohen J (2005) International Sepsis Forum Definition of Infection in the ICU Consensus Conference. The international sepsis forum consensus conference on definitions of infection in the intensive care unit. Crit Care Med 33:1538–1548
35. Beghetto MG, Victorino J, Teixeira L, et al. (2005) Parenteral nutrition as a risk factor for central venous catheter-related infection. JPEN J Parenter Enteral Nutr 29:367–373
36. Maki DG, Weise CE, Sarafin HW (1977) A semiquantitative culture method for identifying intravenous-catheter-related infection. N Engl J Med 296:1305–1309
37. Leon C, Ariza J (2004) SEIMC; SEMICYUC. Guidelines for the treatment of short-term intravascular catheter-related infections in adults; SEIMC-SEMICYUC Consensus Conference. Enferm Infecc Microbiol Clin 22:92–101
38. Guedon C, Nouvellon M, Lalaude O, et al. (2002) Efficacy of antibiotic-lock technique with teicoplanin in *Staphylococcus epidermidis* catheter-related sepsis during long-term parenteral nutrition. JPEN J Parenter Enteral Nutr 26:109–113
39. Cuntz D, Michaud L, Guimber D, et al. (2002) Local antibiotic lock for the treatment of infections related to central catheters in parenteral nutrition in children. JPEN J Parenter Enteral Nutr 26:104–108
40. Dezfulian C, Lavelle J, Nallamothu BK, et al. (2003) Rates of infection for single-lumen versus multilumen central venous catheters: a meta-analysis. Crit Care Med 31:2385–2390
41. Hilton E, Haslett TM, Borenstein MT, et al. (1988) Central catheter infections: single- versus triple-lumen catheters. Influence of guide wires on infection rates when used for replacement of catheters. Am J Med 84:667–672
42. Yeung C, May J, Hughes R (1988) Infection rate for single lumen v triple lumen subclavian catheters. Infect Control Hosp Epidemiol 9:154–158
43. Kemp L, Burge J, Choban P, et al. (1994) The effect of catheter type and site on infection rates in total parenteral nutrition patients. JPEN J Parenter Enteral Nutr 18:71–74
44. Gil RT, Kruse JA, Thill-Baharozian MC, et al. (1989) Triple- vs single-lumen central venous catheters. A prospective study in a critically ill population. Arch Intern Med 149: 1139–1143
45. Gowardman JR, Montgomery C, Thirlwell S, et al. (1998) Central venous catheter-related bloodstream infections: an analysis of incidence and risk factors in a cohort of 400 patients. Intensive Care Med 24:1034–1039
46. Farkas JC, Liu N, Bleriot JP, et al. (1992) Single- versus triple-lumen central catheter-related sepsis: a prospective randomized study in a critically ill population. Am J Med 93:277–282
47. Chaiyakunapruk N, Veenstra DL, Lipsky BA, et al. (2002) Chlorhexidine compared with povidone-iodine solution for vascular catheter-site care: a meta-analysis. Ann Intern Med 136:792–801
48. Rupp ME, Lisco SJ, Lipsett PA, et al. (2005) Effect of a second-generation venous catheter impregnated with chlorhexidine and silver sulfadiazine on central catheter-related infections: a randomized, controlled trial. Ann Intern Med 143:570–580
49. Still JM, Law E, Thiruvaiyaru D, Belcher K, et al. (1998) Central line-related sepsis in acute burn patients. Am Surg 64:165–170
50. Darouiche RO, Raad II, Heard SO, et al. (1999) A comparison of two antimicrobial-impregnated central venous catheters. Catheter Study Group. N Engl J Med 340:1–8
51. Merrer J, De Jonghe B, Golliot F, et al. (2001) French Catheter Study Group in Intensive Care. Complications of femoral and subclavian venous catheterization in critically ill patients: a randomized controlled trial. JAMA 286:700–707

52. Darouiche RO (2001) Device-associated infections: a macroproblem that starts with microadherence. Clin Infect Dis 33:1567–1572
53. Musher D, Goldsmith E, Dunbar S, et al. (2002) Association of hypercoagulable states and increased platelet adhesion and aggregation with bacterial colonization of intravenous catheters. J Infect Dis 186:769–773
54. Mehall JR, Saltzman DA, Jackson RJ, et al. (2002) Fibrin sheath enhances central venous catheter infection. Crit Care Med 30:908–912
55. Lordick F, Hentrich M, Decker T, et al. (2003) Ultrasound screening for internal jugular vein thrombosis aids the detection of central venous catheter-related infections in patients with haemato-oncological diseases: a prospective observational study. Br J Haematol 120:1073–8
56. van Rooden CJ, Schippers EF, Barge RM, et al. (2005) Infectious complications of central venous catheters increase the risk of catheter-related thrombosis in hematology patients: a prospective study. J Clin Oncol 23:2655–2660
57. Hanna HA, Raad I (2001) Blood products: a significant risk factor for long-term catheter related bloodstream infections in cancer patients. Infect Control Hosp Epidemiol 22:165–166
58. Mermel LA (1996) Bacteriology, safety and prevention of infection associated with continuous intravenous infusions. Blood Coagul Fibrinolysis 7(Suppl 1):S45–S51
59. Braunschweig CL, Levy P, Sheean PM, et al. (2001) Enteral compared with parenteral nutrition: a meta-analysis. Am J Clin Nutr 74:534–542
60. Borzotta AP, Beardsley K (1999) *Candida* infection in critically ill trauma patients: a retrospective case-control study. Arch Surg 134:657–665
61. Robert J, Fridkin SK, Blumberg HM, et al. (2000) The influence of the composition of the nursing staff on primary bloodstream infection rates in a surgical intensive care unit. Infect Control Hosp Epidemiol 21:12–17
62. Kudsk KA, Croce MA, Fabian TC, et al. (1992) Enteral versus parenteral feeding. Effects on septic morbidity after blunt and penetrating abdominal trauma. Ann Surg 215:503–511
63. Moore FA, Moore EE, Jones TN, et al. (1989) TEN versus TPN following major abdominal trauma – reduced septic morbidity. J Trauma 29:916–922
64. Correia MI, Waitzberg DL (2003) The impact of malnutrition on morbidity, mortality, length of hospital stay and costs evaluated through a multivariate model analysis. Clin Nutr 22:235–239
65. Naber TH, Schermer T, de Bree A, et al. (1997) Prevalence of malnutrition in nonsurgical hospitalized patients and its association with disease complications. Am J Clin Nutr 66:1232–1239
66. Franson TR, Sheth NK, Rose HD, et al. (1984) Scanning electron microscopy of bacteria adherent to intravascular catheters. J Clin Microbiol 20:500–505
67. Marrie TJ, Costerton JW (1984) Scanning and transmission electron microscopy of in situ bacterial colonization of intravenous and intraarterial catheters. J Clin Microbiol 19:687–693
68. Anaissie E, Samonis G, Kontoyiannis D, et al. (1995) Role of catheter colonization and infrequent hematogenous seeding in catheter-related infections. Eur J Clin Microbiol Infect Dis 14:134–13
69. Raad II, Luna M, Khalil SA, et al. (1994) The relationship between the thrombotic and infectious complications of central venous catheters. JAMA 271:1014–1016
70. Francois P, Vaudaux P, Foster TJ, et al. (1996) Host-bacteria interactions in foreign body infections. Infect Control Hosp Epidemiol 17:514–520
71. Reid G (1999) Biofilms in infectious disease and on medical devices. Int J Antimicrob Agents 11:223–226
72. Sitges-Serra A, Jaurrieta E, Linares J, et al. (1983) Bacteria in total parenteral nutrition catheters: where do they come from? Lancet 1:531
73. Sitges-Serra A, Puig P, Linares J, et al. (1984) Hub colonization as the initial step in an outbreak of catheter-related sepsis due to coagulase negative staphylococci during parenteral nutrition. JPEN J Parenter Enteral Nutr 8:668–672
74. Sitges-Serra A, Linares J, Garau J (1985) Catheter sepsis: the clue is the hub. Surgery 97:355–357
75. Blot F, Nitenberg G, Chachaty E, et al. (1999) Diagnosis of catheter-related bacteraemia: a prospective comparison of the time to positivity of hub-blood versus peripheral-blood cultures. Lancet 354:1071–1077
76. Kite P, Dobbins BM, Wilcox MH, McMahon MJ (1999) Rapid diagnosis of central-venous-catheter-related bloodstream infection without catheter removal. Lancet 354:1504–1507
77. Donlan RM (2001) Biofilm formation: a clinically relevant microbiological process. Clin Infect Dis 33:1387–1392
78. Raad I, Costerton W, Sabharwal U, Sacilowski M, Anaissie E, Bodey GP (1993) Ultrastructural analysis of indwelling vascular catheters: a quantitative relationship between luminal colonization and duration of placement. J Infect Dis 168:400–407
79. Ceri H, Olson ME, Stremick C, Read RR, Morck D, Buret A (1999) The Calgary Biofilm Device: new technology for rapid determination of antibiotic susceptibilities of bacterial biofilms. J Clin Microbiol 37:1771–1776
80. Ryan JA Jr, Abel RM, Abbott WM, Hopkins CC, Chesney TM, Colley R, Phillips K, Fischer JE (1974) Catheter complications in total parenteral nutrition. A prospective study of 200 consecutive patients. N Engl J Med 290:757–761
81. Kite P, Dobbins BM, Wilcox MH, Fawley WN, Kindon AJ, Thomas D, Tighe MJ, McMahon MJ (1997) Evaluation of a novel endoluminal brush method for in situ diagnosis of catheter related sepsis. J Clin Pathol 50:278–282
82. American College of Chest Physicians/Society of Critical Care Medicine Consensus Conference (1992) Definitions for sepsis and organ failure and guidelines for the use of innovative therapies in sepsis. Crit Care Med 20:864–874
83. Widmer AF, Nettleman M, Flint K, Wenzel RP (1992) The clinical impact of culturing central venous catheters. A prospective study. Arch Intern Med 152:1299–1302
84. Raad II, Hanna HA, Darouiche RO (2001) Diagnosis of catheter-related bloodstream infections: is it necessary to culture the subcutaneous catheter segment? Eur J Clin Microbiol Infect Dis 20:566–568
85. Bong JJ, Kite P, Ammori BJ, Wilcox MH, McMahon MJ (2003) The use of a rapid in situ test in the detection of central venous catheter-related bloodstream infection: a prospective study. JPEN J Parenter Enteral Nutr 27:146–150
86. Flynn PM, Shenep JL, Stokes DC, Barrett FF (1987) In situ management of confirmed central venous catheter-related bacteremia. Pediatr Infect Dis J 6:729–734
87. McCarthy A, Byrne M, Breathnach F, O'Meara A (1995) "In-situ" Teicoplanin for central venous catheter infection. Ir J Med Sci 164:125–127
88. Krzywda EA, Andris DA, Edmiston CE Jr, Quebbeman EJ (1995) Treatment of Hickman catheter sepsis using antibiotic lock technique. Infect Control Hosp Epidemiol 16:596–598
89. Faintuch J, Waitzburg DL, Bertevello PL, Silva ML, Borges VC, Pereira SS, Gama-Rodrigues JJ, Pinotti HW (1995) Conservative management of septic parenteral nutrition catheters. JPEN J Parenter Enteral Nutr 19:428–429

90. Savage AP, Picard M, Hopkins CC, Malt RA (1993) Complications and survival of multilumen central venous catheters used for total parenteral nutrition. Br J Surg 80:1287–1290
91. Freund HR, Rimon B (1990) Sepsis during total parenteral nutrition. JPEN J Parenter Enteral Nutr 14:39–41
92. Mitchell A, Atkins S, Royle GT, Kettlewell MG (1982) Reduced catheter sepsis and prolonged catheter life using a tunnelled silicone rubber catheter for total parenteral nutrition. Br J Surg 69:420–422
93. Nehme AE (1980) Nutritional support of the hospitalized patient. The team concept. JAMA 243:1906–1908
94. Yeung CY, Lee HC, Huang FY, Wang CS (1998) Sepsis during total parenteral nutrition: exploration of risk factors and determination of the effectiveness of peripherally inserted central venous catheters. Pediatr Infect Dis J 17:135–142
95. Chan S, McCowen KC, Blackburn GL (1999) Nutrition management in the ICU. Chest 115(5 Suppl):145S–148S
96. August DA, Thorn D, Fisher RL, Welchek CM (1991) Home parenteral nutrition for patients with inoperable malignant bowel obstruction. JPEN J Parenter Enteral Nutr 15:323–327
97. DeLegge MH, Borak G, Moore N (2005) Central venous access in the home parenteral nutrition population-you PICC. JPEN J Parenter Enteral Nutr 29:425–428
98. Alhimyary A, Fernandez C, Picard M, Tierno K, Pignatone N, Chan HS, Malt R, Souba W (1996) Safety and efficacy of total parenteral nutrition delivered via a peripherally inserted central venous catheter. Nutr Clin Pract 11:199–203
99. Goodwin ML, Carlson I (1993) The peripherally inserted central catheter: a retrospective look at three years of insertions. J Intraven Nurs 16:92–103
100. Merrell SW, Peatross BG, Grossman MD, Sullivan JJ, Harker WG (1994) Peripherally inserted central venous catheters. Low-risk alternatives for ongoing venous access. West J Med 160:25–30
101. Rutherford C (1988) A study of single lumen peripherally inserted central line catheter dwelling time and complications. J Intraven Nurs 11:169–173
102. Cowl CT, Weinstock JV, Al-Jurf A, Ephgrave K, Murray JA, Dillon K (2000) Complications and cost associated with parenteral nutrition delivered to hospitalized patients through either subclavian or peripherally-inserted central catheters. Clin Nutr 19:237–243
103. Duerksen DR, Papineau N, Siemens J, Yaffe C (1999) Peripherally inserted central catheters for parenteral nutrition: a comparison with centrally inserted catheters. JPEN J Parenter Enteral Nutr 23:85–89
104. McCowen KC, Friel C, Sternberg J, Chan S, Forse RA, Burke PA, Bistrian BR (2000) Hypocaloric total parenteral nutrition: effectiveness in prevention of hyperglycemia and infectious complications – a randomized clinical trial. Crit Care Med 28:3606–3611
105. van den Berghe G, Wouters P, Weekers F, Verwaest C, Bruyninckx F, Schetz M, Vlasselaers D, Ferdinande P, Lauwers P, Bouillon R (2001) Intensive insulin therapy in the critically ill patients. N Engl J Med 345:1359–1367
106. van den Berghe G, Wouters PJ, Bouillon R, Weekers F, Verwaest C, Schetz M, Vlasselaers D, Ferdinande P, Lauwers P (2003) Outcome benefit of intensive insulin therapy in the critically ill: Insulin dose versus glycemic control. Crit Care Med 31:359–366
107. van den Berghe G, Wilmer A, Hermans G, Meersseman W, Wouters PJ, Milants I, van Wijngaerden E, Bobbaers H, Bouillon R (2006) Intensive insulin therapy in the medical ICU. N Engl J Med 354:449–461
108. Ball PA, Bethune K, Fox J, Ledger R, Barnett M (2001) Particulate contamination in parenteral nutrition solutions: still a cause for concern? Nutrition 17:926–929
109. Failla ML, Benedict CD, Weinberg ED (1975) Bacterial and fungal growth in total parenteral nutrition solutions. Antonie Van Leeuwenhoek 41:319–328
110. Maki DG, Mermel LA, Klugar D, et al. (2000) The efficacy of a chlorhexidine impregnated sponge (Biopatch) for the prevention of intravascular catheter-related infection – a prospective randomized controlled multicenter study. Presented at the Interscience Conference on Antimicrobial Agents and Chemotherapy. American Society for Microbiology, Toronto, Ontario, Canada
111. Marin MG, Lee JC, Skurnick JH (2000) Prevention of nosocomial bloodstream infections: effectiveness of antimicrobial-impregnated and heparin-bonded central venous catheters. Crit Care Med 28:3332–3338
112. Pluhator-Murton MM, Fedorak RN, Audette RJ, Marriage BJ, Yatscoff RW, Gramlich LM (1999) Trace element contamination of total parenteral nutrition. 1. Contribution of component solutions. JPEN J Parenter Enteral Nutr 23:222–227
113. O'Grady NP, Gerberding JL, Weinstein RA, Masur H (2003) Patient safety and the science of prevention: the time for implementing the Guidelines for the prevention of intravascular catheter-related infections is now. Crit Care Med 31:291–292
114. Crnich CJ, Maki DG (2002) The promise of novel technology for the prevention of intravascular device-related bloodstream infection. I. Pathogenesis and short-term devices. Clin Infect Dis 34:1232–1242
115. Maki DG, Stolz SM, Wheeler S, Mermel LA (1997) Prevention of central venous catheter-related bloodstream infection by use of an antiseptic-impregnated catheter. A randomized, controlled trial. Ann Intern Med 127: 257–266
116. Leon C, Ruiz-Santana S, Rello J, de la Torre MV, Valles J, Alvarez-Lerma F, Sierra R, Saavedra P, Alvarez-Salgado F; Cabana Study Group (2004) Benefits of minocycline and rifampin-impregnated central venous catheters. A prospective, randomized, double-blind, controlled, multicenter trial. Intensive Care Med 30:1891–1899
117. Bach A, Bohrer H, Motsch J, Martin E, Geiss HK, Sonntag HG (1994) Prevention of bacterial colonization of intravenous catheters by antiseptic impregnation of polyurethane polymers. J Antimicrob Chemother 33:969–978
118. Greenfeld JI, Sampath L, Popilskis SJ, Brunnert SR, Stylianos S, Modak S (1995) Decreased bacterial adherence and biofilm formation on chlorhexidine and silver sulfadiazine-impregnated central venous catheters implanted in swine. Crit Care Med 23:894–900
119. Maki DG, Cobb L, Garman JK, Shapiro JM, Ringer M, Helgerson RB (1988) An attachable silver-impregnated cuff for prevention of infection with central venous catheters: a prospective randomized multicenter trial. Am J Med 85:307–314
120. Kamal GD, Pfaller MA, Rempe LE, Jebson PJ (1991) Reduced intravascular catheter infection by antibiotic bonding. A prospective, randomized, controlled trial. JAMA 265:2364–2368
121. Raad I, Darouiche R, Dupuis J, Abi-Said D, Gabrielli A, Hachem R, Wall M, Harris R, Jones J, Buzaid A, Robertson C, Shenaq S, Curling P, Burke T, Ericsson C (1997) Central venous catheters coated with minocycline and rifampin for the prevention of catheter-related colonization and bloodstream infections. A randomized, double-blind trial. The Texas Medical Center Catheter Study Group. Ann Intern Med 127:267–274

122. Raad II, Hanna HA (2002) Intravascular catheter-related infections: new horizons and recent advances. Arch Intern Med 162:871–878
123. Coopersmith CM, Rebmann TL, Zack JE, Ward MR, Corcoran RM, Schallom ME, Sona CS, Buchman TG, Boyle WA, Polish LB, Fraser VJ (2002) Effect of an education program on decreasing catheter-related bloodstream infections in the surgical intensive care unit. Crit Care Med 30:59–64
124. Raad II, Darouiche RO, Hachem R, Abi-Said D, Safar H, Darnule T, Mansouri M, Morck D (1998) Antimicrobial durability and rare ultrastructural colonization of indwelling central catheters coated with minocycline and rifampin. Crit Care Med 26:219–224
125. Alonso-Echanove J, Edwards JR, Richards MJ, Brennan P, Venezia RA, Keen J, Ashline V, Kirkland K, Chou E, Hupert M, Veeder AV, Speas J, Kaye J, Sharma K, Martin A, Moroz VD, Gaynes RP (2003) Effect of nurse staffing and antimicrobial-impregnated central venous catheters on the risk for bloodstream infections in intensive care units. Infect Control Hosp Epidemiol 24:916–925
126. Gaonkar TA, Modak SM (2003) Comparison of microbial adherence to antiseptic and antibiotic central venous catheters using a novel agar subcutaneous infection model. J Antimicrob Chemother 52:389–396
127. Dimick JB, Swoboda S, Talamini MA, Pelz RK, Hendrix CW, Lipsett PA (2003) Risk of colonization of central venous catheters: catheters for total parenteral nutrition vs other catheters. Am J Crit Care 12:328–335

Chapter 30

Hemodialysis Catheter-Related Infections

R. Lombardi

30.1 Introduction

End-stage renal disease (ESRD) patients are more susceptible to infection due to defects in the immune system, particularly at the skin barrier and in cellular immunity [1]. On the other hand, the dialysis procedure itself, which requires repeated access to the bloodstream and exposed blood to the extracorporeal circuit, acts as a relevant associated risk factor [2]. Malnutrition and old age are supplementary risk factors.

Bacteremia is one of the most serious complications in dialysis patients and is mainly related to the vascular access, being caused more often by temporary or permanent catheters than by the arteriovenous fistula or the graft [3, 4]. On the other hand, vascular access related infection represents the most common cause of bacteremia in the patient undergoing dialysis [3–7]. A comprehensive study carried out in Denmark showed that out of 14,387 cases of *Staphylococcus aureus* bacteremia, 5.5 % occurred in hemodialysis patients and 80 % of the cases were catheter-related [8].

The most effective measure to reduce the incidence of catheter-related infections (CRI) is to lessen the number of patients using a catheter for hemodialysis. Approximately 17 % of prevalent hemodialysis patients in the USA and 8 % in Europe have a catheter as vascular access (VA) [9]. According to the Uruguayan Registry of Dialysis, which includes the whole population of patients with ESRD in the country, 7 % of prevalent patients and 4.8 % of incident patients in 2004 had a central venous catheter as VA [10].

30.2 Definitions

30.2.1 Catheter Colonization

Growth of ≥ 15 colony-forming units by semiquantitative culture of the extraluminal segment of the catheter tip [11] or > 10^3 by quantitative culture of the intraluminal surface [12, 13] in the absence of clinical symptoms is taken as the definition of catheter colonization, which can be considered as a localized infection. A lower count corresponds to *contamination of the catheter.* Some studies have suggested that a combination of different catheter-segment cultures increase sensitivity and specificity for the diagnosis of colonization. Rello et al. [14] found that a combination of the semiquantitative culture of the external surface of the tip with the quantitative culture of the intraluminal surface of the subcutaneous segment has had the best performance in detecting catheter colonization.

30.2.2 Exit Site Infection

Erythema, tenderness, edema and suppuration within 2 cm from the exit site are signs of exit site infection.

30.2.3 Tunnel Infection

Inflammation or suppuration along the catheter subcutaneous tunnel, more than 2 cm from the exit site.

30.2.4 Catheter-Related Bloodstream Infection (CR-BSI)

1. *Definitive:* isolation of the same microorganism from the catheter and from blood drawn through a peripheral vein, in the absence of another evident source of infection
2. *Probable:* isolation of a microorganism in only blood culture or catheter tip in a symptomatic patient with no other apparent source of infection
3. *Possible:* blood and tip culture negative and defervescence of the clinical picture after the catheter removal in a symptomatic patient with no other apparent source of infection [15]

30.2.5 Catheter-Related Sepsis

Catheter-related sepsis is defined by the association of one or more organ dysfunctions with colonization of the catheter and corresponds to so-called severe sepsis, in accordance with the definitions of the Consensus Conference of the American College of Chest Physicians/Society of Critical Care Medicine 1992 [16].

30.3 Epidemiology

The number of ESRD patients is increasing all over the world. In addition, survival in dialysis has increased, which leads to more frequent problems with definitive vascular access and therefore to an increase in the use of catheters for temporary or prolonged vascular access.

The available information about the incidence of hemodialysis catheter-related infections is diverse, and there are few controlled trials. In general, publications show a frequency of infections that exceeds those reported in other settings [17, 18]. Variations in the type of catheter used (tunneled, non-tunneled, cuffed or non-cuffed), the material from which they are made (polyethylene, polyurethane, silicone), the duration of placement (temporary, prolonged), as well as the insertion site could be some reasons for the differences found in the literature.

Incidence of bacteremia ranges between 1.6 and 13.5 episodes per 1,000 catheter-days, using non-tunneled, non-cuffed devices. Tunneled, cuffed catheters are associated with a lower risk of infection, which ranges between 0.2 and 0.8 episodes per 1,000 catheter-days [15] (Table 30.1). According to data from the Epidemiological Surveillance System from four Dialysis Units in Montevideo directed by the author, frequency of CR-BSI was 2.31 and 0.72 episodes/1,000 catheter-days, in non-tunneled and tunneled catheters, respectively [19].

Exit-site infection is another frequent and potentially severe complication. The incidence ranges between 0.4 and 4.5 episodes per 1,000 catheter-days [20]. The frequency of episodes per patient-year has been estimated to be between 0.36 [21] and 0.57 [22]. Exit site infection represents a potential risk for the colonization of the intravascular segment of the catheter and bacteremia. Likewise, it may determine the loss of the access, unless controlled by treatment.

30.4 Pathogenesis

The development of catheter-related infection depends on the presence of three conditions: *invasion, adherence* and *multiplication* of microorganisms in the catheter. Infective organisms can migrate into the endovascular segment of the catheter through the insertion site (*periluminal*); through the catheter hub during its manipulation (*endoluminal*) or from a distant focus of infection that leads to bacteremia and subsequent colonization of the tip (*hematogenous*). The type of catheter and the setting in which it is inserted could determine the mechanism of colonization. In short-term catheters (less than 1 month) the periluminal route is the more likely mechanism of colonization [23]. In long-term catheters, particularly when they are used for parenteral nutrition, colonization is more frequent through the catheter hub [24].

Staphylococcus aureus and coagulase-negative *Staphylococcus* are the prevailing microorganisms, so it is reasonable to think of a mucocutaneous origin of catheter-related infections. Hemodialysis patients are more frequently *S. aureus* nasal carriers than the general population. The frequency has been estimated to be 50–60% [25, 26], and therefore periluminal colonization is likely to take place. Likewise, the high frequency of *S. aureus* carriage in these patients endures the risk of autocontamination at the time of connection unless appropriate preventive measures are applied (use of surgical mask by the patients). In one study [27], the same strain of *S. aureus* was identified simultaneously in the nares and in the blood of patients in 50% of cases. Such studies demonstrate the predictive value of colonization of the insertion site by *S. aureus* for the development of bacteremia. Finally, staff members' hands might be a vehicle for transmission during catheter connection and disconnection, especially coagulase-negative *Staphylococcus*.

There is little and contradictory information available about the mechanism of colonization of hemodialysis catheters [17, 18, 28, 29]. According to Almirall et al. [18], the prevailing mechanism would seem to be periluminal, from migration of skin flora to the tip

Table 30.1. Epidemiology of catheter related-bloodstream infection (references in text)

Author	Date	Number of catheters	Type of catheter	Incidence (CR-BSI/ 1,000 catheter-days)
Vanherweghem	1986	200	Non-tunneled	6/1,000 catheter-days
Almirall	1989	53	Non-tunneled	10/1,000 catheter-days
Capello	1989	107	Hickman	0.8/1,000 catheter-days
Kinnaert	1990	19	Hickman	07/1,000 catheter-days
Marr	1997	102	Cuffed-tunneled	3.9/1,000 catheter-days
Lombardi	2003	80	Non-tunneled	2.31/1,000 catheter-days
			Tunneled	0.72/1,000 catheter-days
Betjes	2004	76	Non-tunneled	2.61/1,000 catheter-days
			Tunneled	1.7/1,000 catheter-days

(correspondence skin/tip: 58.6%; hub/tip: 17.2%). Cheesbrough et al. [17] found a greater relationship between the hub cultures (57%) and the tip than the skin (36%). Studying a group of patients with weekly quantitative cultures taken through the catheter, Dittmer et al. [28] found a high incidence of endoluminal catheter colonization (68%) and bacteremia (35%). Other investigators assume that skin colonization plays a very important role, since they found a relation between the condition of the skin in the exit site and the frequency of catheter colonization and bacteremia [29]. Typing organisms by phage, Nielson et al. [27] also found evidence favoring the periluminal route.

ESRD patients are prone to infection due to defense mechanism dysfunction caused by uremia, as well as to the specific risk associated with renal replacement therapies.

Uremia affects the barrier function of skin and mucosa, as well as the humoral immunity, even though the typical disorder is the cellular immunity impairment. Lymphopenia, decrease of delayed hypersensitivity, lymphoid system and thymus atrophy are the characteristic disorders in ESRD, and experimental data suggests the existence of immune inhibitor factors in the serum of uremic patients [1, 30]. It has not been possible to establish which are the substances responsible for such disorders, but they are very likely not to be related to the well known markers of uremia (urea, creatinine), but to other factors such as phosphate, potassium, indoles, phenols, PTH, and others [1]. Deficiencies in vitamins E and C and folic acid, as well as the increase in serum levels of trace elements (copper, cadmium) and zinc depletion, have been related to immune disorders in uremic patients [31]. Malnutrition, which also develops in end-stage renal disease patients, has been proven to be a risk factor for infection [32].

Iron overload, caused by excessive iron replacement or repeated blood transfusions, leads to granulocyte malfunction and infection [4, 6, 33], increasing the risk of bacteremia by up to three times [34].

Nasal carriage of *S. aureus* is another risk factor for infection in this group of patients, as already mentioned. Approximately 15% of healthy individuals are nasal carriers of *S. aureus* but this percentage could rise to more than 60% in dialysis patients [25].

The contact of blood with the dialysis circuit triggers an inflammatory-anti-inflammatory response mediated by cytokines, complement and other mediators of the inflammatory cascade which leads to a decrease in the granulocyte function and the release of oxygen-free radicals. These disturbances have been associated with a higher risk of bacterial infection, as well as catabolic stress and β_2-microglobulin amyloidosis, particularly if cellulosic membranes are used [2, 35].

30.5 Microbiology

Hemodialysis catheter-related infections are caused mainly by gram-positive cocci, especially *Staphylococcus* spp. (Table 30.2). Coagulase-negative *Staphylococcus* is a prevalent organism as in other settings, but the incidence of *S. aureus* is comparatively higher due to the frequent skin and nasal colonization with this agent among dialysis patients. Both represent approximately 70% of total catheter colonization. Bacteremia is caused by coagulase-negative *Staphylococcus* in 14–76% of cases, while *S. aureus* has been isolated in 12–44% of cases according to different authors [5, 18, 19, 36–38]. However, in a large series of 63 CR-BSIs, *S. aureus* was prevalent (43%) compared to *S. epidermidis* (14%) [5].

Enterococcus is the second most frequent gram-positive coccus after *Staphylococcus* (5–13%) and, finally, gram-negative aerobic bacilli (11–24%), among which *Pseudomonas* species prevail since they frequently contaminate dialysis water. Other bacteremia-causing agents less frequently isolated are fungi and diphtheroids. In our unit we have had eight catheter-related bacteremia episodes due to *Bacillus* spp., which have also been reported by other authors [39].

30.6 Diagnosis

The diagnosis criteria for the different forms of catheter-related infections are mentioned elsewhere in this section. Diagnosis of catheter-related infection by

Table 30.2. Organisms isolated in blood cultures (references in text)

Author	Date	Number of bacteremias	*S. aureus* (%)	Coagulase-negative staphylococcus (%)	Enterococcus (%)	Gram negative bacilli (%)
Marr	1997	63	43	14	5	24
Robinson	1998	23	35	22	13	13
Capdevilla	1993	13	16	3		38
Almirall	1989	9	44	33	11	11
Schaffer	1995	8	12	62	12	12
Lombardi	1998	7	57	14		14

semiquantitative or quantitative methods requires removal of the device. However, if catheter removal is undesirable, quantitative blood culture is an alternative diagnostic method. Blood is drawn through the device and from a peripheral vein simultaneously. Capdevilla and colleagues [40] demonstrated that a count fourfold greater or more in the catheter blood culture than in the peripheral blood one has a sensitivity of 94% and a specificity of 100% for the diagnosis of catheter-related infection. Likewise, a count of > 100 cfu/ml in the catheter blood with the same organism in peripheral blood also has a high predictive value. Other authors suggest a cutoff of sevenfold greater [41]. The quantitative culture methods are safer but less practical, so they are not recommended for clinical practice. Recently, the differential time to positivity for central versus peripheral blood cultures for the diagnosis of CR-BSI has been proposed [42]. Using automated culture systems, positive results from CVC at least 2 h earlier than peripheral blood samples could be considered as definitive CR-BSI.

Exhaustion of peripheral vein in hemodialysis patients can be a serious limitation to diagnosis. Poole et al. [43] in a recent study found that in 39% of suspected CR-BSIs, a peripheral vein could not be used. Efforts to obtain peripheral blood samples must be made in an attempt to improve diagnosis performance.

30.7 Morbidity and Mortality Associated with Catheters for Hemodialysis

Infection is the second most frequent cause of death in ESRD patients [44]. In the Uruguayan Dialysis Registry, which includes the entire population of ESRD patients in Uruguay, infection represents 23% of all-cause mortality [10].

Placement of a catheter as vascular access is a well known risk factor for bacteremia and sepsis. Nevertheless, only recently has a link between type of vascular access and outcome [45, 46] been demonstrated in observational and retrospective studies in large series of patients. Randomized controlled trials cannot be performed to demonstrate this fact for ethical reasons. However, Polkinghorne et al. [47], using the propensity score analysis, a statistical tool that minimizes bias due to non-randomization, demonstrated a significantly higher risk of death in patients with catheter or arteriovenous graft (AVG) compared to arteriovenous fistula (AVF). The risk of all-cause mortality and infection mortality increased from 1.5- to three-fold when patients with catheter were compared with those with AVF.

Timing of creation of vascular access is also related to the risk of infection and outcome. In a recently published study by Oliver et al. [48], early creation of VA (at least 4 months before starting hemodialysis) was associated with lower risk of infection when compared with late created VA (within 1 month prior to starting dialysis or after). Catheter use increased the risk of infection by 1.41 (CI 95% 1.14 – 18.1).

The use of catheter as VA for hemodialysis is also related to anemia and cardiovascular disease. Roberts et al. [49] in a cohort of 186348 prevalent and incident ESRD patients found that the extent of catheter use as well as VA infection was associated with anemia and a higher requirement for rHuEPO.

Assuming the hypothesis that inflammatory state predisposes to cardiovascular disease, Ishani et al. [50] showed that septicemia or bacteremia was associated with death, myocardial infarction, heart failure, peripheral vascular disease and stroke, particularly in patients without a previous history of cardiovascular disease. In this study, the higher rates of septicemia or bacteremia were observed in patients with catheter as VA. So, the authors concluded that septicemia is a potentially preventable cardiovascular risk factor in this setting.

Catheter-related infections may become complicated with metastatic localizations, especially when there is persistent bacteremia or it is associated with thrombophlebitis. The most frequent complications among others are infective endocarditis, osteomyelitis, suppurative arthritis, spinal epidural abscess and pulmonary septic emboli.

Osteomyelitis and osteoarthritis are frequent localizations and are observed in 5 – 15% of all hemodialysis catheter-related bacteremias [5, 8, 27, 33, 51]. Vertebral, clavicular, and pelvic involvement are the most common. Pain is the most frequent symptom, while fever is only seen in 30% of cases [51]. The most reliable methods for the diagnosis are bone scintigraphy and CT scan. Recently, the use of labeled human polyclonal IgG has been suggested and preliminary studies have shown promising results [52].

Infective endocarditis is a serious complication that is associated with high rates of morbimortality. The real incidence of endocarditis is not yet known with certainty, because there are no well designed epidemiological studies and the criteria for diagnosis have been modified since the introduction of Duke's diagnosis criteria [53]. According to the scarce literature available, the incidence ranges between 3% and 4.4% [8, 54]. Diagnosis may be difficult due to the low frequency of classical symptoms of endocarditis, and the high frequency of preexisting cardiac murmur in these patients. Infective endocarditis may be suspected in all dialysis patients who have fever or bacteremia of unexplained origin. The most sensitive and specific diagnosis procedure is the transesophageal echocardiography. According to Robinson and coworkers [54], catheter in-

Table 30.3. Infective endocarditis in a series of ESRD patients (non-published)

Number of cases	20
Age	53.8 ± 12.4 years
Source of infection	
Catheter	8
Fistula	3
Other	6
Unknown	3
Microbiology	
S. aureus	6
Enteroccocus	5
Gram-negative bacilli	5
Enteroccocus + GN bacilli	1
Negative	3
Valve affected	
Aortic	9
Mitral	5
Aortic + mitral	5
Tricuspid	1
Surgery	2 (10%)
Mortality rate	7 (35%)

fection was the cause in 55% of patients. Fever and cardiac murmur were the most frequent manifestations, and the mitral valve was the most frequently affected. The prevalent germ was *S. aureus*, followed by *S. epidermidis*. Only five patients underwent valve replacement and the mortality rate was 30%. The above data is very similar to that from an unpublished series studied by the author in 1993, the results of which are shown in Table 30.3 [55].

Recently, Fernandez-Cean and coworkers [56] have proposed a strategy based on the removal of vascular access and the transient switch from hemodialysis to peritoneal dialysis in patients with infective endocarditis, because of a better outcome in a series of 21 patients.

Spinal epidural abscess is a rare and serious infection. However, its frequency has been increasing due to the more extensive use of hemodialysis catheters, especially when catheter salvage has been used [57]. The main symptom is persistent and intense back pain [57, 58]. Fever and leukocytosis are not constant. In some cases, neurological manifestations due to medullar compression (paresis, hypoesthesia or paresthesia) could be observed. The prevailing organism is *S. aureus*, which is isolated in 60% of cases. The diagnostic test of choice is magnetic resonance imaging. Treatment consists of a prolonged course of antibiotics for 4–6 weeks, the antibiotic being selected according to the susceptibility of the causative organism and its bone tissue penetration. Surgery for drainage of the epidural space is indicated when symptoms of medullar compression are observed. Diagnosis and treatment must be made without delay, to minimize the risk of neurological sequelae, which are in fact frequent.

30.8 Prevention

Universal precautions and adhesion to aseptic technique in the placement and management of the catheter are the cornerstones in the prevention of catheter-related infections. Selection of the site of insertion, dressing technique, type of catheter, replacement of catheter, prophylactic use of antimicrobial and other strategies are complementary issues to be considered.

Several studies have shown that infection rate is less frequent when the subclavian vein is used as the placement site [15], and that is the reason why it has been the insertion site of choice. However, the frequency with which subclavian vein stenosis and thrombosis occur [59–61] has determined the preference for the internal jugular vein. There is controversy about the femoral vein, traditionally considered to be more risky and used for just a few days. However, some studies show that it can be used as a prolonged access without major infection risks. Montagnac et al. [62] found a colonization rate of 21.8% in a group of 55 patients with silicone-rubber femoral catheters that on average stayed in for 41 days. In another study [63], carried out with polyurethane double-lumen catheters in hospitalized patients, the rate of infection found was not higher than the usual one, even though the duration of placement was 7 days. Recently, Oliver et al. [64] proposed to remove non-tunneled femoral catheters after 1 week, because of a higher relative risk of bacteremia when compared with devices inserted in the internal jugular vein. If the femoral vein needs to be used because of exhausted vein access, a tunneled catheter could be as safe as an internal jugular vein one [65].

Catheter site dressing regimens are controversial and a very active topic of research. Levin and associates [66] have demonstrated that the use of povidone-iodine ointment and sterile gauze on the catheter exit site has significantly decreased the frequency of catheter-related infection. Exit site infection falls from 5 to 1.23 episodes/1,000 catheter-days, tip colonization from 11.26 to 5.33/1,000 catheter-days, and bacteremia from 4.59 to 0.41 episodes/1,000 catheter-days. Decrease of the relative risk was 72%, 52%, and 93%, respectively. On the other hand, they proved the reduction to be more evident in *S. aureus* nasal carriers. Other authors have studied the effect of mupirocin, an active anti-staphylococcal topical antibiotic, in the form of an ointment at the exit site level, for the prevention of infections caused by *S. aureus*. Sesso and associates [67] randomized 136 ESRD patients with non-tunneled non-cuffed catheters to disinfect their skin with povidone-iodine versus 2% mupirocin ointment after catheter placement and in every hemodialysis. They found significantly less catheter colonization (1.76 vs. 14.27 episodes/1,000 catheter-days) and bacteremia (0.71 vs.

8.92 episodes/1,000 catheter-days) with the use of mupirocin.

Similar results were found recently by Johnson et al. [68] in a group of dialysis patients with tunneled-cuffed catheters. Using an ointment with three antibiotics (bacitracin, gramicidin and polymixin B), Lok and coworkers [69] in a well designed study demonstrated a dramatic reduction of CR-BSI from 2.48 to 0.63 episodes/1,000 catheter-days. Our own experience is in accordance with these results: after the implementation of the routine use of mupirocin in July 2001, the historical incidence of CR-BSI dropped from 2.1 to 0 episodes/1,000 catheter-days.

There is growing evidence that tunneled, cuffed catheters are associated with less risk of infection when compared to non-tunneled, non-cuffed ones. In a non-controlled study [70] using Hickman catheters, the authors found a lower rate of CR-BSI (0.8 episodes/1,000 catheter-days) than that previously reported by the same group. In another paper [71], 80 tunneled, cuffed catheters were compared prospectively to standard double-lumen catheters. Incidence of bacteremia was significantly lower in the tunneled device group (1.3% vs. 3.6%), but exit site infection was higher (29% vs. 9%). The device composed of two separated single lumen catheters introduced by Canaud [72] has been used increasingly largely because it provides good dialysis adequacy with an acceptable catheter survival and a relatively low risk of infection [73]. However, implementation of measures tending to select AVF as the preferred vascular access should be stressed and the use of central venous catheters as permanent access should be discouraged [74].

Likewise, there is not enough information to sustain the use of antiseptic or antimicrobial-impregnated catheters (silver, chlorhexidine, cefazolin, etc.). Even though there are studies that show beneficial effects in other kinds of patients [75], there is no evidence to prove the results are similar in a hemodialysis setting. A randomized study carried out on 100 patients using silver-impregnated catheters could not demonstrate any preventive effect of this type of catheter on colonization rate, and they are also more expensive [76]. Finally, a small series of four patients with silver-impregnated cuffed catheters was compared to another four patients with regular catheters. The latter had less infectious complications than the study group [77]. Since the activity of coated antibiotics and antiseptic declines with time, the efficacy of this approach could be limited in long-term central venous-catheters.

Replacement of the catheter over a guidewire, which is common practice and is safe in critically ill patients [78], has not been studied enough in hemodialysis patients. Uldall [79] compared the weekly replacement over a guidewire with clinically indicated replacement, and did not find differences in the infection rates between the two groups.

Table 30.4. Antibiotic-anticoagulant lock solutions

Antibiotic	Anticoagulant
Gentamicin 40 mg/ml	Tri-sodium citrate 3.13%
Vancomycin 2.5 mg/ml	Heparin 2,500 units/ml
Vancomycin 2.5 + gentamicin 1 mg/ml	Heparin 2,500 units/ml
Cefazolin 5 mg/ml	Heparin 2,500 units/ml
Cefazolin 5 mg/ml + gentamicin 1 mg/ml	Heparin 2,500 units/ml
Taurolidine 1.35%	Sodium citrate 4%

There are no data about the effect of prophylactic antibiotics in hemodialysis catheters, but if we take into account the results in other settings [15], such practice is not recommendable.

New strategies for the prevention of catheter related infection were proposed recently. Antibiotic-locking of catheter, a well known therapeutic approach for the treatment of CR-BSI, was tested with the aim of preventing infection (Table 30.4). When gentamicin [80, 81], cephazolin [82], and taurolidine [83] with citrate or heparin were compared to heparin alone, a lower rate of CRI and greater CRI-free catheter survival was observed. A supplementary beneficial effect of locking catheters with antibiotics on epoietin requirement was also observed in one study [81]. However, there is concern about the consequences of systemic exposure to gentamicin (ototoxicity) and citrate (hypocalcemia), as well as the risk of development of bacterial resistance. Further studies are required to establish the efficacy and safety of the antibiotic-lock technique.

In 2001, the National Kidney Foundation updated the guidelines for improving the dialysis patient quality of life and life expectancy [74]. The K/DOQI recommendations formulated regarding the prevention of infections related to catheters are:

1. Trained dialysis staff should only perform hemodialysis-catheter dressing changes and catheter manipulations (evidence/opinion).
2. Catheter exit site should be examined at each hemodialysis treatment for signs of infection (opinion).
3. Catheter exit site dressings should be changed at each hemodialysis treatment (opinion).
4. Use of sterile gauze and povidone-iodine or mupirocin ointment at the catheter exit site at the end of each dialysis session is recommended (evidence).
5. During catheter connection and disconnection procedures, nurses and patients should wear a surgical mask. Nurses should also wear sterile gloves (opinion).
6. Manipulating a catheter and accessing the patient's bloodstream should be performed in a manner that minimizes contamination. Hubs should be disinfected with povidone-iodine for 3–5 min. Hubs should be covered in order to prevent exposure.

30.9 Treatment

Removing the catheter and the use of systemic antibiotics, followed by delayed placement of another catheter in a new site, is the most effective and safe strategy for the treatment of catheter-related bacteremia. However, this modality of treatment implies the loss of venous access, which is critical in ESRD because of the need for preservation of the vascular bed.

There is general agreement that non-tunneled CR-BSI should be treated promptly with systemic antibiotics and the removal of the device [78]. On the contrary, in tunneled catheters the decision to remove the device is based mainly on the severity of the infection (severe sepsis, metastasic seeding, endocarditis, etc.) and salvage strategies could be attempted [84, 85].

30.9.1 Antibiotic Therapy

When a catheter-related infection is suspected, systemic empiric antibiotic therapy must be started, based upon the prevailing organism and its sensitivity pattern. As previously mentioned, in 70–80% of cases, the causative organisms are *Staphylococcus,* which is frequently resistant to methicillin, and *Enterococcus.* For that reason, the empiric antibiotic of choice is vancomycin, which has the additional advantage of a low dosage requirement (1 g weekly) for pharmacokinetic reasons [86]. An aminoglycoside must be added in order to cover gram-negative aerobic bacilli; dosage must also be adapted to renal function and body mass (amikacin: 7 mg/kg body weight, postdialysis). Seric levels of vancomycin and aminoglycoside must be monitored to avoid toxicity. Third-generation cephalosporin could be used instead of aminoglycosides to prevent ototoxicity [85]. Once the agent has been identified and susceptibility data are available, therapy should be adjusted accordingly. The widespread use of vancomycin must be discouraged because of its relatively lower antimicrobial activity with regard to antistaphyloccal beta-lactamines and the risk of vancomycin-resistant enterococcus selection [87, 88], which is emerging as a frequent pathogen in this population. Cefazolin, in a schedule of 1–2 g postdialysis, has shown satisfactory results in the case of methicillin-sensitive *S. aureus* [89, 90]. Recommended duration of treatment is 2–3 weeks.

30.9.2 Catheter Management

As was stated, non-tunneled catheters should be removed immediately, which implies the elimination of the source of infection and enhances the chances of cure.

On the contrary, when prolonged, tunneled-cuffed, double-lumen or twin catheters are used, salvage of the catheter or the venous site should be attempted. Three alternatives have been suggested: (1) maintenance of the catheter in place, (2) replacement over a guidewire using the same venous access, and (3) instillation of antibiotics in the lumen of the device. In spite of the fact that some authors [36, 91, 92] have obtained satisfactory results with catheter maintenance and systemic antibiotics, the majority of investigators did not obtain satisfactory results [21, 93, 94]. Therefore, this practice could be considered as a suboptimal and non-recommended approach. Catheter replacement over a guidewire keeping the same venous access has been suggested as an alternative. This procedure may be rehearsed if the access is not severely infected (sepsis, endocarditis or other metastatic colonizations) and if the tunnel or the exit site is not infected. If this is the case, the catheter may be placed in the same vein through a new tunnel [95]. In a series of 21 catheters, replacement over a guidewire failed in the four cases in which the exit site was infected [96]. Robinson et al. [37] achieved a resolution rate of 92% in a series of 23 cases of CR-BSI without infection on the exit site, treated with replacement over a guidewire and 3 weeks of systemic antibiotics. In a short series of 13 episodes of persistent bacteremia in spite of the systemic antibiotic and in which the tunnel was not infected, Schaffer [38] achieved cure of infection in all the cases by combining the replacement over a guidewire with a new tunnel and a short systemic antibiotic course (1–2 weeks), even in those cases of mycotic infection. In a recent work, Beathard [95] prospectively studied a series of CR-BSIs in hemodialysis patients that he divided into three categories: (1) minimal symptoms without skin infection, in which he replaced the catheter over a guidewire after a 48-h treatment with systemic antibiotics; (2) minimal symptoms with tunnel or exit site infection, in which he replaced the catheter over a guidewire and created a new tunnel; and (3) severe clinical symptoms, which were treated by removing and delayed replacement. In all cases systemic antibiotics were used for 3 weeks. With these practices, cure rates were 87.8%, 75%, and 86.5%, respectively.

Finally, instillation of an antibiotic-anticoagulant solution in the catheter lumen has been used successfully in some recent studies. Krishnasami et al. [97], using vancomycin plus gentamicin plus heparin as a lock solution in addition to systemic vancomycin/gentamicin, achieved a cure rate of 65% and an infection-free catheter survival of about 65% at 45 days. The same group, in another study using ceftazidime instead of gentamicin, obtained a 70% cure of catheter-related bacteremia. The type of causative microorganism makes a difference in the likelihood of cure, being higher in gram-negative bacilli, intermediate in

Table 30.5. Guidelines for the treatment of CR-BSI

Type of catheter	Management of catheter	Antibiotics
Non-tunneled	Remove	Systemic antibiotic for 2 weeks
Tunneled-cuffed	1. Remove	Systemic antibiotic for 2 weeks
	2. Non-remove (salvage)	Systemic antibiotic for 2–3 weeks plus antibiotic lock
	3. Change over guidewire a) Same tunnel (non-infected) b) New tunnel (if infected)	Systemic antibiotic for 2–3 weeks

negative-coagulase staphylococcus and lower in *S. aureus.*

Infection of the exit site without systemic infection is treated topically. If it persists, systemic antibiotics are prescribed. Tunnel suppuration is treated with systemic antibiotics.

To summarize (Table 30.5):

1. CR-BSI in non-tunneled catheter: catheter removal, with replacement in another venous site, associated with systemic antibiotics for 2 weeks
2. CR-BSI in tunneled catheter:
   a) Catheter removal with replacement of a new non-tunneled catheter and systemic antibiotics. Criteria for the removal are severe infection (sepsis, endocarditis, osteoarthritis, spinal epidural abscess); persistent bacteremia beyond 48–72 h of antibiotic therapy or worsening of clinical status; blood cultures positive to fungi; exit tunnel suppuration
   b) Non-removal of catheter
      i) Salvage of catheter with systemic antibiotics and antibiotic-lock
      ii) Replacement over a guidewire and insertion of a new tunneled catheter in the same venous site. If there is tunnel suppuration, maintaining the venous site and replacing the catheter through a new tunnel can be tried. In all cases, systemic antibiotic therapy selected according to susceptibility of the offending organism must be performed for 2–3 weeks.
3. Exit site infection. Antiseptic or local antibiotic treatment (mupirocin, iodo-povidone, chlorhexidine)
4. Tunnel infection. It is recommended to remove the catheter and administrate systemic antibiotics, but replacement over a guidewire with a new tunnel could be attempted.

References

1. Vanholder R, Van Loo A, Dhondt AM, De Smet R, Ringoir S (1996) Influence of uremia and haemodialysis on host defense and infection. Nephrol Dial Transplant 11:593–598
2. Hakim RM (1993) Clinical implications of hemodialysis membrane bioincompatibility. Kidney Int 44:484–494
3. Powe NR, Jaar B, Furth SL, Hermann J, Briggs W (1999) Septicemia in dialysis patients: incidence, risk factors, and prognosis. Kidney Int 55:1081–1090
4. Hoen B, Paul-Dauphin A, Hestin D, Kessler M (1998) EPIBACDIAL: A multicenter prospective study of risk factors for bacteremia in chronic hemodialysis patients. J Am Soc Nephrol 9:869–876
5. Marr KA, Kong LK, Fowler VG, Gopal A, Sexton DJ, Conlon PJ, Corey GR (1998) Incidence and outcome of *Staphylococcus aureus* bacteremia in hemodialysis patients. Kidney Int 54:1684–1689
6. Hoen B, Kessler M, Hestin D, Mayeux D (1995) Risk factors for bacterial infections in chronic hemodialysis adult patients: a multicenter prospective survey. Nephrol Dial Transplant 10:377–381
7. Tokars JI, Miller ER, Alter MJ, Arduino MJ (2000) National surveillance of dialysis-associated diseases in the United States. Semin Dial 15:162–171
8. Nielsen J, Kolmos HJJ, Espersen F (1998) *Staphyloccocus aureus* bacteraemia among patients undergoing dialysis – focus on dialysis catheter-related cases. Nephrol Dial Transplant 13:139–145
9. Pisoni RL, Young EW, Dykstra DM, Greenwood RN, Hekking E, Gillespie B, Wolfe RA, Goodkin DA, Held PJ (2002) Vascular access use in Europe and the United States: results from the DOPPS. Kidney Int 61:305–316
10. Uruguayan Registry of Dialysis. http://fp.chasque.apc.org:8081/sun/REGISTRO.HTM
11. Maki DG, Weise CE, Sarafin HW (1977) Semiquantitative culture method for identifying intravenous catheter-related infections. N Engl J Med 296:1305–1309
12. Cleri DJ, Corrado ML, Seligman SJ (1980) Quantitative culture of intravenous catheters and other intravascular inserts. J Infect Dis 141:781–786
13. Brun-Buisson C, Abroug F, Legrand P, Huet Y, Larabe S, Rapin M (1987) Diagnostic of central venous catheter-related sepsis. Critical level of quantitative tip cultures. Arch Intern Med 47:83–877
14. Rello J, Gatell JM, Almirall J, Campistol JM, González J, Puig de la Bellacasa J (1989) Evaluation of culture techniques for identification of catheter-related infection in hemodialysis patients. Eur J Clin Microbiol Infect Dis 8:620–622
15. Pearson ML and the Hospital Infection Control Practices Advisory Committee (1996) Guidelines for prevention of intravascular device-related infections. Am J Infect Control 24:262–293
16. American College of Chest Physicians, Society of Critical Care Medicine Consensus Conference (1992) Definitions for sepsis and organ failure and guidelines for the use of innovative therapies in sepsis. Crit Care Med 20:864–874
17. Cheesbrough JS, Finch RG, Burden RP (1986) A prospective study of the mechanisms of infection associated with hemodialysis catheters. J Infect Dis 154:579–589
18. Almirall J, Gonzalez J, Rello J, Campistol JM, Montoliu J, Puig de la Bellacasa J, Revert L, Gatell JM (1989) Infection of hemodialysis catheters: incidence and mechanisms. Am J Nephrol 9:454–459
19. Lombardi R, Gómez T, Pacheco G, Giménez M, Bogio M, De los Santos M (2006) Programa de Vigilancia Epidemiológica de 4 Centros de Diálisis en Montevideo. Rev Med Uruguay (submitted)

20. Dryden MS, Samson A, Ludlam HA, Wing AJ, Phillips I (1991) Infective complications associated with the use of Quinton Permcath for long-term central vascular access for hemodialysis patients. J Hosp Infect 19:257–262
21. Moss AH, Vasilakis C, Holley JL, Foulks CJ, Pillai K, McDowell DE (1990) Use of a silicone dual-lumen catheter with a Dacron cuff as a long-term vascular access for hemodialysis patients. Am J Kidney Dis 16:211–215
22. Prabhu PN, Kems SR, Sabatelli FW, Hawkins IF, Ross EA (1997) Long-term performance and complications of the Tesio twin catheter system for hemodialysis access. Am J Kidney Dis 30:213–218
23. Raad I, Costerton W, Sabharwal U, Sacilowski M, Anaissie E, Bodey GP (1993) Ultrastructural analysis of indwelling vascular catheters: a quantitative relationship between luminal colonization and duration of placement. J Infect Dis 168:400–407
24. Sitges-Serra A, Puig P, Liñares J, Pérez JL, Farreró N, Jaurrieta E, Garau J (1984) Hub colonization as the initial step in an outbreak of catheter-related sepsis due to coagulase negative staphylococci during parenteral nutrition. J Parent Enter Nutrit 8:668–672
25. Bargman JM (1995) Nasal carriage of *Staphyloccocus aureus* in dialysis patients. Semin Dialysis 8:220–225
26. Wanten GJA, Schneeberger PM, Bevers A, van Ginneken E, Koolen MI (1998) Optimizing screening procedures for *Staphyloccocus aureus* nasal carriage in patients on hemodialysis. Nephrol Dial Transplant 13:1256–1258
27. Nielsen J, Daustrand Ladefoged S, Kolmos HJJ (1998) Dialysis catheter-related septicaemia – focus on *Staphyloccocus aureus* septicaemia. Nephrol Dial Transplant 13:2847–2852
28. Dittmer ID, Sharp D, McNulty CAM, Williams AJ, Banks RA (1999) A prospective study of central venous hemodialysis catheter colonization and peripheral bacteremia. Clin Nephrol 51:34–39
29. Hung K-Y, Tsai T-J, Yen C-J, Yen T-S (1995) Infection associated with double lumen catheterization for temporary haemodialysis: experience of 168 cases. Nephrol Dial Transplant 10:247–251
30. Goldblum SE, Reed WP (1980) Host defenses and immunologic alterations associated with chronic hemodialysis. Ann Intern Med 93:597–613
31. Briggs WA, Pedersen MM, Mahajan SK, Sillix DH, Prasad AS, McDonald FD (1982) Lymphocyte and granulocyte function in zinc-treated and zinc-deficient hemodialysis patients. Kidney Int 21:827–832
32. Churchill DN, Taylor W, Cook RJ, LaPlante P, Barre P, Cartier P, Fay WP, Goldstein MB, Jindal K, Mandin H, McKenzie JK, Muirhead N, Parfrey PS, Posen GA, Slaughter D, Ulan RA, Werb R (1992) Canadian hemodialysis morbidity study. Am J Kidney Dis 19:214–234
33. Kessler M, Hoen B, Mayeux D, Hestin D, Fontenaille C (1993) Bacteremia in patients on chronic hemodialysis. Nephron 64:95–100
34. Boelaert JR, Daneels RF, Schugers ML, Matthys EG, Goedts BZ, Van Landuyt HW (1990) Iron overload in hemodialysis patients increases the risk of bacteremia: a prospective study. Nephrol Dial Transplant 5:130–134
35. Bonomini V, Coli Ren, Scolari MP, Stefoni S (1995) Structure of dialysis membranes and long-term clinical outcome. Am J Nephrol 15:455–462
36. Capdevila JA, Segarra A, Planes AM, Ramirez-Arellano M, Pahissa A, Piera L, Martínez-Vázquez JM (1993) Successful treatment of hemodialysis catheter-related sepsis without catheter removal. Nephrol Dial Transplant 8:231–234
37. Robinson D, Suhocki P, Schwab SJ (1998) Treatment of infected tunneled venous access hemodialysis catheters with guidewire exchange. Kidney Int 53:1792–1794
38. Shaffer D (1995) Catheter-related sepsis complicating long-term, tunneled central venous dialysis catheters: management by guidewire exchange. Am J Kidney Dis 25:593–596
39. Curtis JR, Wing AJ, Coleman JC (1967) *Bacillus cereus* bacteraemia. A complication of intermittent haemodialysis. Lancet i:136–138
40. Capdevila JA, Planes AM, Palomar M, Gasser I, Almirante B, Pahissa A, Crespo E, Martínez-Vázquez JM (1992) Value of differential quantitative blood culture in the diagnosis of catheter-related sepsis. Eur J Clin Microbiol Infect Dis 11:403–407
41. Fan ST, Teoh-Chan CH, Lau KF (1989) Evaluation of central venous catheter sepsis by differential quantitative blood culture. Eur J Clin Microbiol Infect Dis 8:142–144
42. Blot F, Nitenberg G, Chachaty E, Raynard B, Germann N, Antoun S, Laplanche A, Brun-Buisson C, Tancrede C (1999) Diagnosis of catheter-related bacteremia: a prospective comparison of the time to positivity of hub-blood versus peripheral-blood cultures. Lancet 354:1071–1077
43. Poole CV, Carlton D, Bimbo L, Allon M (2004) Treatment of catheter-related bacteremia with an antibiotic lock protocol: effect of bacterial pathogen. Nephrol Dial Transplant 19:1237–1244
44. U.S Renal Data System (2005) USRDS 2005 Annual Data Report. National Institutes of Health. NIDDK, Bethesda
45. Dhingra RK, Young EW, Hulbert-Shearon TE, Leavey SF, Port FK (2001) Type of vascular access and mortality in US hemodialysis patients. Kidney Int 60:1443–1451
46. Pastan S, Soucie M, McClellan W (2002) Vascular access and increased risk of death among hemodialysis patients. Kidney Int 62:620–626
47. Polkinghorne KR, McDonald SP, Atkins RC, Kerr PG (2004) Vascular access and all-cause mortality: a propensity score analysis. J Am Soc Nephrol 15:477–486
48. Oliver MJ, Rothwell DM, Fung K, Hux JE, Lok CE (2004) Late creation of vascular access for hemodialysis and increased risk of sepsis. J Am Soc Nephrol 15:1936–1942
49. Roberts TL, Obrador GT, St Peter WL, Pereira BJG, Collins AJ (2004) Relationship among catheter insertions, vascular access infection, and anemia management in hemodialysis patients. Kidney Int 66:2429–2436
50. Ishani A, Collins AJ, Herzog CA, Foley RN (2005) Septicemia, access and cardiovascular disease in dialysis patients: the USRDS wave 2 study. Kidney Int 68:311–318
51. Torda AJ, Gottlieb T, Bradbury R (1995) Pyogenic vertebral osteomyelitis: analysis of 20 cases and review. Clin Infect Dis 20:320–328
52. Palermo F, Boccaletto, Paolin A, Carniato A, Zoli P, Giusto F, Turra S (1998) Comparison of technetium-99m-MDP, technetium-99m-WBC and technetium-99m-HIG in musculoskeletal inflammation. J Nucl Med 39:516–521
53. Durack DT, Lukes AS, Bright DK (1994) New criteria for diagnosis of infective endocarditis: utilization of specific echocardiographic findings. Duke Endocarditis Service. Am J Med 96:200–209
54. Robinson DL, Fowler VG, Sexton DJ, Corey RG, Conlon PJ (1997) Bacterial endocarditis in hemodialysis patients. Am J Kidney Dis 30:521–524
55. Lombardi R, Mautone M, Rodríguez O, Alvarez A, Kuster F, Zinno E (1993) 2° Congreso Uruguayo de Nefrología, Montevideo
56. Fernandez-Cean J, Alvarez A, Burguez S, Baldovinos G, Larre-Borges P, Cha M (2002) Infective endocarditis in chronic hemodialysis: two treatment strategies. Nephrol Dial Transplant 17:2226–2230
57. Kovalik EC, Raymond JR, Albers FJ, Berkoben M, Butterly DW, Montella B, Conlon PJ (1996) A clustering of epidural

abscesses in chronic hemodialysis patients: risk of salvaging access catheters in cases of infection. J Am Soc Nephrol 7:2264–2267
58. Obrador GT, Levenson DJ (1996) Spinal epidural abscess in hemodialysis patients: report of three cases and review of the literature. Am J Kidney Dis 27:75–83
59. Clark DD, Albina JE, Chazan JA (1990) Subclavian vein stenosis and thrombosis: a potential serious complication in chronic hemodialysis patients. Am J Kidney Dis 15:265–268
60. Cimochowski GE, Worley E, Rutherford WE, Sartain JA, Blondin J, Harter H (1990) Superiority of the internal jugular over the subclavian access for temporary dialysis. Nephron 54:154–161
61. Hernandez, D, Díaz F, Suria S, Machado M, Lorenzo V, Losada M, González-Posada JM, De Bonis E, Domínguez ML, Rodríguez AP, Torres A (1993) Subclavian catheter-related infection is a major risk factor for the late development of subclavian vein stenosis. Nephrol Dial Transplant 8:227–230
62. Montagnac R, Bernard C, Gullaumie J, Hanhart P, Clavel P, Yazji J, Martínez LM, Schillinger F (1997) Indwelling silicone femoral catheters: experience of three hemodialysis centers. Nephrol Dial Transplant 12:772–775
63. Kirkpatrick WG, Culpepper RM, Sirmon MD (1996) Frequency of complications with prolonged femoral vein catheterization for hemodialysis access. Nephron 73:58–62
64. Oliver MJ, Callery SM, Thorpe KE, Schab SJ, Churchill DN (2000) Risk of bacteremia from temporary hemodialysis catheters by site of insertion and duration of use: a prospective study. Kidney Int 58:2543–2545
65. Maya ID, Allon M (2005) Outcomes of tunneled femoral hemodialysis catheters: comparison with internal jugular vein catheters. Kidney Int 68:2886–2889
66. Levin A, Mason AJ, Jindal KK, Fong IW, Goldstein MB (1991) Prevention of hemodialysis subclavian vein catheter infections by topical povidone-iodine. Kidney Int 40: 934–938
67. Sesso R, Barbosa D, Leme IL, Sader H, Canzani ME, Manfredi S, Draibe S, Pignatari AC (1998) *Staphyloccocus aureus* prophylaxis in hemodialysis patients using central venous catheter: effect of mupirocin ointment. J Am Soc Nephrol 9:1085–1092
68. Johnson DW, MacGinley R, Kay TD, Hawley CM, Campbell SB, Isbel NM, Hollett P (2002) A randomized controlled trial of topical exit site mupirocin application in patients with tunneled, cuffed hemodialysis catheters. Nephrol Dial Transplant 17:1802–1807
69. Lok CE, Stanle KE, Hux JE, Richardson R, Tobe SW, Conly J (2003) Haemodialysis infection prevention with polysporin ointment. J Am Soc Nephrol 13:169–179
70. Capello M, De Pauw L, Bastin G, Prospert F, Delcour C, Thaysse C, Dhaene M, Vanherweghem JL, Kinnaert P (1989) Central venous access for hemodialysis using the Hickman catheter. Nephrol Dial Transplant 4:988–992
71. Schwab SJ, Buller GL, McCann RL, Bollinger RR, Stickel DL (1988) Prospective evaluation of a Dacron cuffed hemodialysis catheter for prolonged use. Am J Kidney Dis 11:166–169
72. Canaud B, Beraud JJ, Joyeux H, Mion C (1986) Internal jugular vein cannulation with two silicone rubber catheters: A new and safe temporary vascular access for hemodialysis. Thirty month's experience. Artif Organs 10:397–403
73. Lee T, Barker J, Allon M (2005) Tunneled catheters in hemodialysis patients: reasons and subsequent outcomes. Am J Kidney Dis 46:501–508
74. National Kidney Foundation (2001) K/DOQI Clinical Practice Guidelines for Vascular Access. Am J Kidney Dis 37(Suppl 1):S137–S181
75. Maki DG, Stolz SM, Wheeler S, Mermel LA (1997) Prevention of central venous catheter-related bloodstream infection by use of an antiseptic-impregnated catheter. Ann Int Med 127:257–266
76. Trerotola SO, Kraus M, Johnson MS, Harris VJ, Snidow JJ, Shah H, McKusky M (1996) Randomized study of silver coating (Silvergard) for prevention of infection in tunneled hemodialysis catheters. J Am Soc Nephrol 7:1422
77. Diskin CJ, Stokes TJ (1995) Efficacy of an attachable silver impregnated subcutaneous cuff for the prevention of catheter-associated infections in patients on chronic maintenance hemodialysis. Nephron 69:357–359
78. Hagley MT, Martin B, Gast P, Traeger SM (1992) Infectious and mechanical complications of central venous catheters placed by percutaneous venipuncture and over guidewires. Crit Care Med 20:1426–1430
79. Uldall PR (1981) Subclavian cannulation for hemodialysis. Int Artif Org 4:213–214
80. Dogra GK, Herson H, Hutchinson B, Irish AB, Heath CH, Golledge C, Luxton G, Moody H (2002) Prevention of tunneled hemodialysis catheter-related infections using catheter-restricted filling with gentamicin and citrate: a randomized controlled study. J Am Soc Nephrol 13:2133–2139
81. McIntyre CW, Hulme LJ, Taal M, Fluck RJ (2004) Locking of tunneled hemodialysis catheters with gentamicin and heparin. Kidney Int 66:801–80
82. Kim SH, Song KI, Chang JW, Kim SB, Sung SA, Jo SK, Cho WY, Kim HK (2006) Prevention of uncuffed hemodialysis catheter-related bacteremia using an antibiotic lock technique: a prospective, randomized clinical trial. Kidney Int 69:161–164
83. Betjes MG, van Agteren M (2004) Prevention of dialysis catheter-related sepsis with a citrate-taurolidine-containing lock solution. Nephrol Dial Transplant 19:1546–1551
84. Schwab SJ, Beathard G (1999) The hemodialysis catheter conundrum: hate living with them, but can't live without them. Kidney Int 56:1–17
85. Allon M (2004) Dialysis catheter-related bacteremia: treatment and prophylaxis. Am J Kidney Dis 44:779–791
86. DeSoi CA, Sahm DF, Umans JG (1992) Vancomycin elimination during high-flux hemodialysis: kinetic model and comparison of four membranes. Am J Kidney Dis 20: 354–360
87. Brady JP, Snyder JW, Hasbargen JA (1998) Vancomycin-resistant enterococcus in end-stage renal disease. Am J Kidney Dis 32:415–418
88. Tokars JI (1998) Vancomycin use and antimicrobial resistance in hemodialysis centers. Am J Kidney Dis 32:521–523
89. Marx MA, Frye RF, Matzke GR, Golper TA (1998) Cefazolin as empiric therapy in hemodialysis-related infections: efficacy and blood concentrations. Am J Kidney Dis 32: 410–414
90. Fogel MA, Nussbaum PB, Feintzeig ID, Hunt WA, Gavin JP, Kim RC (1998) Cefazolin in chronic hemodialysis patients: a safe, effective alternative to vancomycin. Am J Kidney Dis 32:401–409
91. Domoto DT, Kennedy DJ (1987) Antibiotic treatment of chronic central venous hemodialysis catheter infection without catheter removal. Int J Artif Org 10:239–240
92. Donnelly PK, Hoenich NA, Lennard TWJ, Proud G, Taylos RMR (1988) Surgical management of long-term central venous access in uraemic patients. Nephrol Dial Transplant 3:57–65
93. Marr KA, Sexton DJ, Conlon PJ, Corey GR, Schwab SJ, Kirkland KB (1997) Catheter-related bacteremia and out-

come of attempted catheter salvage in patients undergoing hemodialysis. Ann Intern Med 127:275 – 280

94. Swartz RD, Messana JM, Boyer CJ, Lunde NM, Weitzel WF (1994) Successful use of cuffed central venous hemodialysis catheters inserted percutaneously. J Am Soc Nephrol 4:1719 – 1725
95. Beathard GA (1999) Management of bacteremia associated with tunneled-cuffed hemodialysis catheters. J Am Soc Nephrol 10:1045 – 1049
96. Carlisle EJ, Blake P, McCarthy F, Vas S, Uldall R (1991) Septicemia in long-term jugular hemodialysis catheters; eradicating infection by changing the catheter over a guidewire. Int J Artif Organs 14:150 – 153
97. Krishnasami Z, Carlton D, Bimbo L, Taylor ME, Balkovetz DF, Barker J, Allon M (2002) Management of hemodialysis catheter-related bacteremia with an adjunctive lock solution. Kidney Int 61:1136 – 1142

31 Infection of Pulmonary Arterial and Peripheral Arterial Catheters

A. Rodríguez, J. Rello

31.1 Background

The pulmonary arterial catheter (PAC) and the peripheral arterial catheter (AC) are used frequently in the management of critically ill patients, but not without risk. The use of the catheter has been associated with complications such as infection of catheter insertion site and catheter-related infection with and without subsequent catheter-related bacteremia (CRB) [1].

Current information about infections associated with the central venous catheter (CVC) is extensive. However, less information is available about arterial catheters used temporarily in specific hospital areas like the intensive care unit (ICU). Insertion complications may occur during central venous catheterization, while infectious complications have occurred with catheter maintenance. In1998, Raad [2] estimated that in the USA at least 400,000 episodes of vascular catheter-related bloodstream infection occur every year. The Center of Disease Control (CDC) guidelines [3] indicate the rate of AC-related bloodstream infection is comparable to that of temporary CVCs (2.9/1,000 catheter-days). The attributable cost of treating one episode for a patient in the ICU increased from US $28,000 in 1994 to more than US $56,000 [4, 5] in 2000.

In 1979, Band and Maki [6] reported a 4 % incidence of catheter-related bloodstream infection (CRBSI) associated with an arterial catheter that had remained in place for over 96 h. Myres et al. [7] reported a catheter-related infection (CRI) rate of 5.8 % when the mean duration of catheterization was 4.2 days, while Hudson-Civetta et al. [1] reported a 10 % rate of positive catheter segment cultures at 3 days in a large group of patients with sepsis. At the same time, Pinilla et al. [8] reported that the rate of infectious complications associated with the internal jugular site (29 %) and the antecubital site (20 %) was higher than with the subclavian approach (7 %). The rates of PAC-related infection and CRB reportedly range from 1.7 % to 35 % [1–10], which may reflect differences in the patient population and the methods used to recognize infection.

While the most frequently selected arteries for peripheral arterial catheterization are the radial and femoral arteries, there are currently no specific guidelines on the type of catheter (venous/arterial) to use to prevent a catheter-associated infection. Few studies have evaluated the incidence and pathogenesis of colonization and bloodstream infection secondary to the placement of AC.

In this chapter, we summarize current knowledge of infectious complications associated with these catheters and focus on laboratory diagnosis and clinical approach.

31.2 Pulmonary Arterial Catheter

The benefits of arterial catheterization in critically ill patients must be balanced by the potential technical and septic risks. The risk of CRBSI from PAC has been difficult to assess due to the reported variable incidence of catheter colonization (ranging from 5.8 [4] to 40 % [8]) and bloodstream infection (ranging from 0 % [7, 12–14] to 10 % [15]). The characteristics of pulmonary arterial catheter colonization and bloodstream infection are shown in Table 31.1. As Rello et al. [16] state, these results are heterogeneous and cannot be compared since they have used different methods of diagnosis, incomplete data or too few cases. Also, they have different populations and risk factors.

The cumulative incidence of bloodstream infection associated with PAC is generally low, i.e. <5 % in most reports (Table 31.1). The risk of developing catheter-related sepsis has been shown to vary from 0.3 % to 0.5 % per day per catheter [17]. In contrast, the cumulative incidence of colonization is generally high, ranging from 5.8 % to 40 %. Given that in most series the period of catheterization is short, the incidence of colonization ranged from 1.3 to 15.5 episodes per 100 catheterization days [7, 11] or from 0.9 to 12.2 episodes per 1,000 catheterization days [18, 19]. The CDC [3] recommends that the rate of CRBSI be expressed as the number of catheter associated bloodstream infections (BSIs) per 1,000 catheter days. This parameter is more adequate than the rate expressed as the number of CRBSIs per 100 catheters (or percentage), because it ac-

Table 31.1. Characteristics of pulmonary arterial colonization or bloodstream infection. Adapted from [16]

Ref., year	ICU[a]	Design[b]	Culture[c]	No. cases	Days[d]	Bacteremia (%)	Colonization (%)	Colonization (× 100 d)	Colonization (× 1,000 d)
[21], 1978	Q	P	Qual.	57	3.2	0	25	7.81	–
[22], 1978	C	R	Qual.	152	2.5	0	30	12.00	–
[23], 1980	G	P	–	71	2.8	2.8	–	–	–
[26], 1981	G	P	Semi.	31	2.9	–	6.4	2.2	–
[24], 1982	M	P	Qual.	153	–	0	19	–	–
[20], 1982	G	P	Semi.	37	3.5	–	8.1	2.31	–
[25], 1983	G	P	Semi.	133	2.6	2	10	3.84	–
[8], 1983	Q	P	Semi.	37	–	2.7	16	–	–
[15], 1984	G	P	Quan.	10	–	10	20	–	–
[27], 1985	G	P	Semi.	12	6.0	0	33.3	5.55	–
[7], 1985	Q	P	Semi.	170	4.4	0	5.8	1.31	–
[28], 1987	Q	P	Semi.	63	3.0	0	6.1	2.03	–
[11],1987	G	P	Quan.	20	2.6	–	40	15.83	–
[1], 1987	Q	P	Semi.	49	3.0	0	10.2	3.4	–
[29], 1988	G	P	Semi.	272	–	5	12	–	–
[12],1988	Q	P	Semi.	102	3.5	0	5.9	1.68	–
[13], 1988	Q	P	Semi.	60	2.5	0	6	2.4	–
[10], 1993	G	P	Semi.	69	4.5	2.9	21.7	4.98	–
[30], 1994	Q	P	Semi.	297	3.0	0.7	21.9	–	–
[31], 1994	Q	P	Semi.	442	3.1	1.1	21.7	6.8	–
[14], 1996	G	P	Semi.	66	5.0	0	28.7	5.6	–
[19], 2001	C	P	Semi	157	6.6	0.6	11.5	–	0.93
[32], 2001	Ca	P	Semi.	77	3.0	0	8.9	–	15.5
[18], 2003	G	P	Semi.	98	4.8	0	4.5	–	7.0
				85	6.5	0.8	9.6	–	12.2

[a] Intensive Care Unit: *Q* surgical, *C* coronary, *G* general, *M* medical, *Ca* cancer center
[b] Design: *P* prospective, *R* retrospective
[c] Culture: *Qual.* qualitative, *Semi.* semiquantitative, *Quan.* quantitative
[d] Mean days of catheterization

counts for BSIs over time and therefore adjusts risk for the number of days the catheter is in use. Local inflammation at the insertion site (erythema, cellulites, etc.) occurs in 0.9–16% of patients [16, 19, 20] and is usually resolved by withdrawing the catheter.

In CRI, bacteria may gain access to the bloodstream in two ways: they may migrate from the catheter-skin interface over the external surface or down the internal surface of the catheter to the catheter trip. Widmer [33] thinks that the physician should adhere strictly to the recommendation that the PAC should be replaced after 5 days, because the risk of CRI or CRB after 5 days is substantial, i.e., up to 80% after 14 days of catheterization.

There are several potential sources of microorganism contamination for catheter colonization and bloodstream infection. Maki et al. [34] believe that the external surface is the most important source of infection because [33]:

1. The colonization of the catheter is mainly detected by microorganisms on the external surface.
2. Bacteria have been shown to move along the other surface, possibly by capillary action.
3. There is a strong link between the semiquantitative culture (SQC) of the external surface of CRB.
4. Colonization of the skin is a strong predictor of CRI and CRB.
5. Topical disinfectants reduce the rate of infection.
6. Maximal barrier precautions taken at the time of catheter insertion prevent infection.

The catheter may be colonized internally secondary to contamination of the hub or infusate derivate from skin or infusate. Nevertheless, cutaneous colonization of the device at the insertion site is the main source of microorganism contamination. Hubs are frequently colonized, and their contribution as a primary source of infection is well established [30, 31]. Liñares et al. [35] have highlighted the importance of hubs as a source of microorganism contamination in parenteral nutrition catheters. Similarly, PAC hubs are frequently manipulated by caregivers, usually without optimal aseptic technique. Moreover, repeatedly injecting a frozen saline solution to monitor cardiac output, drawing multiple blood samples for biochemical tests, measuring oxygen pressure in mixed venous blood and repeatedly manipulating the catheter to administer drugs to critically ill patients increases the risk of bloodstream infection from hubs [16]. Bacteria can migrate from the hub to the tip of the catheter while protected from any host-defense mechanism. This hypothesis is also supported in animal models [36] and clinical studies [37].

Important pathogenic determinants of CRI are: (a) the material from which the device is made and (b) the intrinsic virulence factors of the infecting microorganisms. Catheters made of Teflon, silicone or polyurethane are likely to be more resistant to the adherence of microorganisms than catheters made of polyvinylchoride or polyethylene [38]. Furthermore, higher rates of CRI have been reported with triple-lumen catheters (three hubs) than with single-lumen catheters (one hub) [39].

Finally, as Widmer [33] states, contamination of the skin at the insertion site may be the most important variable in short-term catheterization, whereas the hub becomes more important as a source of infection as the duration of catheterization increases.

The microorganisms involved in both catheter colonization and bloodstream infection include: coagulase-negative staphylococci, *Staphylococcus aureus*, *Streptococcus* sp., Gram-negative bacilli (such as *Pseudomonas* sp., *Proteus* sp., *Escherichia coli*, or *Klebsiella* sp.) and *Candida albicans* [11, 24]. In a prospective study, Rello et al. [10] analyzed 69 PACs that remained in situ over 24 h in a general ICU. Eighteen strains of microorganisms were isolated from 15 catheters. In 13 (72.2%) cases, the pathogens identified were coagulase-negative staphylococci, which were simultaneously recovered from the skin around the insertion site in 10 cases. The remaining five pathogens isolated were Gram-negative bacilli, which were isolated from the hubs but not from the insertion site. These findings suggest the need to culture hubs when pulmonary arterial catheter-related bloodstream infection is suspected.

Henderson [40] grouped risk factors for CRI and CRB into patient-related factors and hospital-related factors. Age, altered host-defense mechanism, the severity of the underlying disease, remote infections and sepsis are all considered patient-related risk factors and cannot usually be altered but should be considered when developing catheter maintenance protocols [41].

Hospital-related factors include catheter type and material, insertion sites, type of placement (percutaneous vs. cutdown), duration of site use, emergency vs. selective placement, the skill of the individual who places the catheter and alterations in skin microflora [41].

In particular, several risk factors have been considered regarding PAC infection, but the most frequently analyzed variable is probably the length of catheterization. This may be a co-factor in the severity of the underlying illness; septic patients are at a much higher risk than nonseptic patients. The length of hospitalization prior to catheter insertion may also be a risk factor, but this is difficult to distinguish from the severity of illness [41].

The CDC recommended in its guidelines for preventing intravascular infections "the proper and frequent changing of central venous cannulas that are used for pressure monitoring" [42]. Several studies have demonstrated a significant increase in the rate of positive PAC aspirate cultures [21], catheter-related infection [43] and intra-arterial catheter-related infection [6] after 72 h in situ. In their study, Hudson-Civetta et al. [1] evaluated the risk of PAC infection in septic surgical patients but found no cases of bloodstream infection after 72 h of catheterization and no relationship between the percentage of positive catheter-aspirate cultures and the duration of catheterization. However, all subjects received antibodies to treat their primary infection. On the other hand, Sise et al. [44], using a qualitative culture method, found that local and other septic complications are infrequent within the first 72 h but rise significantly thereafter. Another study [45] used a protocol to determine whether PAC sites (and those of other types of catheters) could be used for longer periods to avoid the risk of repeating central venopunctures. The rate of CRI increased in nonseptic patients when catheter use was extended from 4 days to 6 (33% vs. 12%, $p<0.05$). There was also a strong relationship between number of days of catheter placement in the ICU and the likelihood of subsequent CRI, e.g., catheters placed at ≤ 6 days versus those placed after 7 days ($p<0.05$).

Infections are probably more frequent when catheters are exposed to bloodstream infections from other sites [1, 21], or where there are local signs of inflammation at the insertion site [21]. Senagore et al. [28] prospectively studied the infection rate by evaluating two different vascular accesses (subclavian vein vs. jugular vein) and whether they were replaced by new puncture or through a guide wire; they found no significant differences. An earlier randomized trial [46] to evaluate scheduled replacement was carried out on 112 patients and 460 catheters. It compared the changes performed every 7 days either with guide assistance or new puncture sites with the changes performed with new puncture sites when indicated clinically. There were no significant differences in the complication rates between the three groups, but infections and mechanical complications were slightly more frequent in patients in the scheduled-change group than in the group whose catheters were changed when indicated clinically. Recently, in another randomization trial, Cobb et al. [47] compared four methods of catheter exchange. These were: replacement every 3 days either by insertion at a new site (group 1), exchange over a guide wire (group 2), replacement when clinically indicated by insertion at a new site (group 3) or exchange over a guide wire (group 4). The incidence rates (per 100 days of catheter use) of bloodstream infection were: 3 in group 1, 6 in group 2, 2 in group 3 and 3 in group 4. The incidence rates of mechanical complications were 14%, 4%, 8% and 3% for groups 1, 2, 3, and 4, respectively, and the patients randomly assigned to guide-wire-assisted exchange were more likely to have bloodstream infection after the first 3 days of catheterization (6% vs. 0%, $p<0.05$).

Table 31.2. Risk factors for colonization of pulmonary-artery catheter. Adapted from [16]

Ref.	Risk factor	Odds ratio
12	Children	–
	Long catheterization	–
	Inotropic use	–
47	Skin colonization	5.5
	Jugular access	4.3
	>3 days	3.1
	Antisepsis violation	2.1
10	>5 days	2.1
	Antibiotic use	0.2

The authors concluded that routinely replacing central vascular catheters every 3 days does not prevent infection, but exchanging catheters with a guide wire increased the risk of bloodstream infection. Recently, Chen et al. [18] reported no statistically significant difference for PAC colonization and CRBSI rate when intervals of 4 or 7 days between insertion and replacement were compared. The catheter colonization rate was 7.0 episodes/1,000 catheter days in the 4-days group versus 12.2 episodes/1,000 catheter day (OR 1.7, 95% CI 0.6–5.1) and the CRBSI was 0.0 vs. 1.0 episodes/1,000 catheter day, respectively.

Since most of the clinical and epidemiologic variables often cited affect the risk of CRI and RCBSI, a multivariate statistical analysis such as multiple logistic regressions is the only way to identify which variables independently influence the risk after adjustment has been made for all others. Table 31.2 summarizes the results of three reports [10, 12, 48] that evaluated potential risk factors by multivariate analysis. In the study by Rello et al. [10], 20 potential risk factors were analyzed. Only seven variables had an odds ratio (OR) >2. These were: (1) the duration of catheterization over 5 days, (2) jugular access, (3) insertion technique, (4) complications, (5) diurnal insertion, (6) absence of microbial use, and (7) cardiorespiratory arrest. However, when these variables were included in the logistic regression analysis, only the duration of catheterization (>5 days) was statistically linked to a greater risk of PAC colonization. In contrast, antimicrobial use was associated with negative cultures.

It is difficult to diagnose CRI and CRB. Clinical criteria alone, such as fever or inflammation at the catheter insert site, are nonspecific and usually of little help [49, 50]. When CRI is suspected it is common practice to remove the catheter and replace it at a new site. However, 80–90% of new febrile episodes in patients in intensive care are not caused by catheter infection. It has therefore been estimated that 75–85% of catheters are removed unnecessarily during a new fever episode [47, 49, 51]. So the increased risks of infection or traumatic complications secondary to unnecessary catheter replacement should also be considered.

Table 31.3. Definitions on catheter infection

Term	Definition
Catheter-related infection (CRI)	Catheter segment culture with presence of = or >15 colonies on a blood agar by semiquantitative culture[a]
Catheter-related bloodstream infection (CRBSI)	Isolated from the same organism from a catheter segment quantitative or semiquantitative culture and from a peripheral blood culture in a patient with sepsis syndrome
Catheter contamination	Presence in a specimen taken for culture, of organisms introduced by the person collecting the specimen during the course of obtaining the sample
Catheter colonization	Catheter segment culture with presence of <15 colonies on blood agar by semiquantitative culture

[a] The Centers of Disease Control and Prevention (CDC) definition includes necessary signs of infection, fever or elevated white blood cell count, and local signs of inflammation such as erythema

"Catheter-related infection" is an imprecise term. Erroneous delineation of contamination, colonization and true catheter-related infection can lead to confusion and an incorrect interpretation of this paper. Table 31.3 shows, therefore, which definitions of catheter infection are now generally accepted [33, 41]. Clinical markers show a poor correlation with infection associated with PAC or central-venous lines. Laboratory tests are therefore needed to confirm a clinically suspected diagnosis of CRI. Interpretation of the laboratory results depends on the culture method and the gold standard used. Diagnostic methods can be classified as:

1. *Qualitative broth culture*, when colonies are not counted. This method is highly sensitive but not very specific and does not help to distinguish contamination from infection.
2. *Semi-quantitative culture*, when the specimen is cultured directly and the colonies are counted on agar plates to allow an enumeration just within a limited range. This technique has several important limitations: only the external surface of the catheter is explored, so endoluminal infections may be undetected. Sensitivity is optimal (almost 100%) but specificity is low (20–50%) [50].
3. *Quantitative culture*, when the serial dilutions of the original specimen are used for culture. This technique only explores the internal part of the catheter. The quantitative culture technique has been simplified with catheter vortexing in sterile water by Brun-Bruisson et al. [52]. Both specificity (88%) and sensitivity (97%) are high.

In 1979, Wing et al. [53] had the idea of performing cultures of blood withdrawn from the catheter and a peripheral vein. More recently, Hudson-Civetta et al. [1] evaluated multiple samples from 49 patients with PAC to confirm the hypothesis that bloodstream infection could be diagnosed on the basis of qualitative catheter-drawn cultures. However, neither blood cultures from peripheral veins, arterial blood, or catheter-drawn blood were found to be useful. This study concluded that pulmonary arterial catheter-related bloodstream infection should only be evaluated with segment-catheter cultures and blood samples drawn by direct venipuncture. Several authors [2, 50, 54], however, state that paired quantitative blood cultures should be used to diagnose CRI. These techniques are based on the premise that, when a bacteremia is linked to a CRI, the number of microorganisms retrieved by the blood culture drawn from the catheter is higher than in the blood peripheral culture. A diagnosis is proposed when the number of colonies isolated from the cultures of blood taken through the vascular catheter is at least five times the number in the culture of a concurrent peripheral blood sample. The predictive value of this method has been studied using a threshold for positive of between 15 and 10^3 CFU/ml with a specificity of 99% but a sensitivity of just 20% for diagnosing CRI in cancer patients [55]. Fan et al. [56] found that differential blood cultures correctly identified seven out of nine infected catheters. In this study, sensitivity was 77.8% and specificity was 100%, with no false-positive results. Similarly, Douard et al. [57] found that differential blood cultures had a specificity and positive predictive value of 100%, while their sensitivity (38%) and negative predictive values (78%) were slightly lower. Despite their accuracy, paired cultures are not routinely used in clinical practice, mainly because of their relative complexity and cost.

Passerini et al. [11] used electron microscopy and the quantitative culture method in the CRI. They showed that the extent of catheter colonization in internal and external surfaces is different. Even more important is the fact that colonization is not uniform along the length of the catheter surface. This method has no clinical interest, but it questions the real value of using a single segment of the catheter to diagnose colonization. Rello et al. [58] evaluated the usefulness of semiquantitative cultures of distal, intradermal and atrial segments (3 cm around the proximal orifice) for diagnosing PAC colonization. In this study, the semiquantitative culture of the tip detected 66% of colonized catheters. Results were similar when the other segment was considered independently. Rello et al. therefore concluded that a combination of both intradermal and distal segment cultures is the most practical and reliable method for identifying colonized PAC. In another study, the same authors [59] showed the need to culture both the catheter tip and the introducer segment to obtain an accurate diagnosis of PAC colonization when an indwelling introducer is present. A further meta-analysis [51] confirmed the superiority of quantitative techniques for catheter segment culture. This method had a higher pooled sensitivity and specificity (above 90%) than semiquantitative or quantitative cultures.

In summary, the optimal way to diagnose CRI and replace PAC is unknown. If temperature inexplicably increases more than 48 h after catheter insertion and there is evidence of local signs of infection with or without positive blood culture, the catheter and introducer can be exchanged and treated according to the results of the semiquantitative culture. However, because of the particularly high colonization rate of the PAC and the introducers, it is recommended that Swan-Ganz catheters be removed before the 5th day of placement.

Infection of short-term catheters is mainly prevented by avoiding contamination of the catheter by the skin flora at the catheter insertion site. As Rello [60] indicated in a recent editorial, the best strategy for protecting against colonization from the hub or the skin depends on the conservative affinities (skin hypothesis) or otherwise (hub hypothesis) of the physician. However, the pathogenesis of colonization is probably different in each type of catheter and the results cannot be extrapolated. The full barrier precautions during central-venous catheter insertion significantly reduce the risk of intravenous CRI and CRB [30, 33, 48]. These precautions have been linked to a fourfold decrease in the rate of CRB to PAC [48] and a more than sixfold decrease in the rate of sepsis related to central-venous catheters [61]. Table 31.4 shows preventive strategies for catheter-related infections. All these preventive strategies should be evaluated at the time of selection. They should never be considered as a substitute for the traditional practice of adhering to an aseptic and careful technique during insertion and maintenance of the catheters [60].

Table 31.4. Preventive strategies for catheter-related infections

- Maximum sterile barriers
- Cutaneous antimicrobials and antiseptic
- Tunneling
- Ionic silver cuffs
- Infusion therapy team
- Intraluminal antibiotic locks
- Antiseptic hubs
- Antimicrobial coating of catheter

31.3 Peripheral Arterial Catheter

The peripheral arterial catheter (AC) for measuring intra-arterial pressure and monitoring arterial gases is one of the most common devices in an ICU setting. The maximal sterile barrier precautions are not normally used during AC insertion, yet the majority of patients in the ICU are monitored with ACs. The risk of colonization and infection of ACs might approach that for central venous catheters (2.9 vs. 2.3 episodes/1,000 catheter-days [3]). However, few studies have evaluated the true incidence and pathogenesis of colonization and infection secondary to the placement of an AC. The incidence of AC colonization and infection reported in the literature varies depending on the catheter-tip culture technique used. The incidence of colonization is reported to range from 0% to 36% and from 1.1 to 8.8 episodes/100 catheter-days (Table 31.5). Catheter-related bloodstream infection (CRBSI) is uncommon and its incidence ranges from 0 to 0.95 episodes/100 catheter-days [8, 66]. In the study by Pinilla et al. [8], ACs showed a very low rate of catheter infection and were not associated with bacteremia. This infection rate is low possibly because: (a) most of the catheters were removed within 4 days, (b) the vessel is deeply situated, (c) the catheter shaft is short, (d) the catheter is secured and inserted more easily (especially in a radial site), (e) the staff are more familiar with the maintenance, or (f) high-pressure conditions in the artery may be effective in flushing out potential pathogens and a fast arterial flow may help to prevent bacterial adherence [33].

The skin is probably the most common source of microorganisms that cause peripheral arterial bloodstream infection [62, 65]. Many clinical and microbiologic data indicate that most CRBSIs are caused by microorganisms that invade the intracutaneous area surrounding the catheter. Several studies [62, 63, 65] have shown a strong correlation between organisms present on the skin surrounding the catheter wound and microorganisms recovered from a catheter that has been linked to bacteremia.

The microorganisms responsible are usually coagulase-negative staphylococci and *Staphylococcus aureus* [49]. When rare microorganisms such as *Candida parapsilosis, Serratia marcescens, Klebsiella oxytoca, Pseudomonas cepacia, Acinetobacter baumannii* or *Flavobacterium* spp. are isolated, contamination of the fluid should be considered, especially inside the transducer assembly [64]. The risk of developing bloodstream infection from infusate contamination is reported to be low and generally occurs in epidemics, especially during summer time [33, 64]. Using normal saline solution in intra-arterial infusion, which does not support the growth of most microbial pathogens, probably provides protection against contamination in hemodynamic monitoring [16]. Table 31.6 details the CDC official recommendations [3] for the administration sets and parenteral fluid replacement. For instance, Shinozaki et al. [71] reported no increase of bacterial fluid contamination in relation to the duration of catheterization. Ducharme et al. [62] reported that manipulating the system as little as possible probably reduces the risk of contamination of both the infusate and insertion site significantly. Good aseptic technique with standard sterile barrier precautions during insertion is therefore much more important than any systematic change [69].

Table 31.5. Summary of studies on peripheral arterial catheter. Adapted from [16]

Ref., year	ICU[a]	Design[b]	Culture[c]	No. cases	Days[d]	Bacteremia (%)	Colonization (%)	Colonization (×100 d)	Colonization (×1,000 d)
[6], 1979	G	P	Semi.	130	4.4	3.8	18.0	4.4	–
[20], 1982	–	P	Semi.	52	3.3	–	11.1	2.6	–
[8], 1983	Q	P	Semi.	172	3.0	0	4.0	1.2	–
[62], 1988	P	P	Qual./Semi.	70	2.9	0	0	0	–
[63], 1988	Q	P	Semi.	75	4.0	0	9.5	1.19	–
[64], 1989	G	P	Semi.	164	6.4	0	22.5	3.49	–
[65], 1991	C	P	Semi.	340	2.7	0	2.3	8.8	–
[66], 1993	O	P	Semi.	71	–	5.6	16.0	–	–
[67], 1993	G	P	Semi.	71	10.6	7.0	36.0	3.4	–
[68], 2001	G	P	Semi.	132	13.3	0	9.3	–	–
[69], 2003	G	P	Semi.	129[e]	8.8	1.5	17.8	–	20.2
				143[f]	8.4	1.4	13.3	–	15.8
[73], 2004	G	P	Semi.	817	7.1	0.2	1.4	–	–
[70], 2005	G	P	Semi.	212	8.2		7.7	–	9.3

[a] Intensive care unit: *G* polyvalent, *Q* surgical, *P* pediatric, *C* coronary, *O* oncologic
[b] Design: *P* prospective
[c] Culture: *Semi.* semiquantitative, *Qual.* qualitative
[d] Mean period of catheterization
[e] Includes patients with maximal sterile barrier precautions use
[f] Includes patients with standard-of-care

Table 31.6. CDC recommendations for replacement of administration sets and parenteral fluids. (Adapted from [3])

Administration sets	Parenteral fluids
1. Replace administration sets, including secondary sets and add-on devices, no more frequently than at 72-h intervals	1. Complete the infusion of lipid-containing solutions within 24 h of hanging the solution
2. Replace tubing used to administered blood, blood products, or lipid emulsions within 24 h of initiating the in fusion	2. Complete the infusion of lipid emulsions alone within 12 h of hanging the emulsion. If volume considerations require more time, the infusion should be completed within 24 h
3. Replace tubing used to administer propofol infusion every 6 or 12 h, depending on its use	3. Complete infusion of blood or other blood products within 4 h of hanging the blood

As with PAC, few studies have attempted to identify the risk factors associated with AC colonization and bloodstream infection. Several studies [6, 62, 64, 66] agreed that systemic antimicrobial therapy does not protect against arterial catheter-related infection. In fact, most episodes of bloodstream infections in these studies occurred in patients receiving antibiotics. In 1979 Band and Maki [6] studied CRBSI from AC and determined that three factors were associated with a significant increase in both local and bloodstream catheter-related infections: (1) insertion of the catheter by surgical cutdown (ninefold increase in catheter-related bacteremia), (2) cannulation that exceeded 4 days, and (3) inflammation of the insertion site. The incidence of catheter-related infection was 18 %, while 70 % of infections occurred in catheters that had been used for more than 96 h. All CRBSIs in this study occurred in patients whose catheter sites were used for over 96 h.

Most ICU policies recommend the radial artery as first choice, but there are no guidelines that relate site selection to the prevention of CRI. The femoral artery access is frequently selected in patients with multiorgan dysfunction or shock. Some advantages of this site are: the catheters are easy to place, blood specimens can be taken and the incidence of thromboembolism is low. However, this site is frequently avoided because of the increased possibility of bacterial contamination from the perineal area [20, 72, 73]. Thomas et al. [72] conducted a study to evaluate the risk of infection related to radial versus femoral sites for arterial catheterization. They found that the incidence of local infection was similar for both insertion sites. Frezza et al. [74] compared the complications rate of AC in a medical ICU to those in a surgical ICU. They found that the infection rate was similar in both ICUs and between radial and femoral sites.

Several researchers have studied the duration of cannulation. Some found that long period catheterization increased the cumulative incidence of colonization (%) but did not increase the incidence rate when the days of catheterization were considered [20, 64, 72]. Band and Maki [6] reported that the duration of the arterial catheterization was the major determinant for the infection, but Thomas et al. [72] found no correlation between the incidence of CRI and days of catheterization. In the opinion of Ducharme et al. [62], the risk of CRI in children is very low and does not demand systemic replacement. Consequently, the efficacy of periodically changing the arterial catheters as a measure of prevention is still unconfirmed. In this way, no specific recommendations were made regarding replacement of peripheral arterial catheter in newer CDC guidelines [3]. However, AC and the entire administration sets must be changed if there is: (a) ischemia of the distal extremity, (b) evidence of microembolization, (c) signs of inflammation at the insertion site, (d) an unsafe location, (e) unexplained fever, or (f) positive blood cultures without an obvious source of infection [16, 41].

As with PAC, the semiquantitative culture technique reported by Maki et al. [43] seems to be the best method for diagnosing AC colonization. Bloodstream infection is found almost exclusively among patients with positive semiquantitative AC culture. Finally, we should keep in mind that fever without other sources of infection is the most frequent picture of presentation of AC bloodstream infection.

References

1. Hudson-Civetta J, Civetta JM, et al. (1987) Risk and detection of pulmonary artery catheter-related infection in septic surgical patients. Crit Care Med 15:29 – 32
2. Raad I (1998) Intravascular-catheter-related infections. Lancet 351:893 – 95
3. Centers for Disease Control and Prevention (2002) Guidelines for the prevention of intravascular catheter-related infections. MMWR Morb Mortal Wkly Rep 51(RR-10)
4. Soufir L, Timsit JF, Mahe C, et al. (1999) Attributable morbidity and mortality of catheter-related septicaemia in critically ill patients: a matched, risk-adjusted, cohort study. Infect Control Hosp Epidemiol 20:396 – 401
5. Rello J, Ochagavia A, Sabanes E, et al. (2000) Evaluation of outcome of intravenous catheter-related infection in critically ill patients. Am J Respir Crit Care Med 162:1027 – 30
6. Band JD, Maki DG (1979) Infection caused by arterial catheters used for hemodynamic monitoring. Am J Med 67:735 – 38
7. Myres ML, Austin TW, Sibbald WJ (1985) Pulmonary artery catheter infections. Ann Surg 201:237 – 40
8. Pinilla JC, Ross DF, Martin T, et al. (1983) Study of the incidence of intravascular catheter infection and associated septicemia in critically ill patients. Crit Care Med 11:21 – 24
9. Elliot CG, Zimmerman GA, Clemmer TP (1979) Complications of pulmonary artery catheterization in the care of critically ill patients. Chest 76:647 – 50
10. Rello J, Coll P, Net A, Prats G (1993) Infection of pulmonary artery catheters. Chest 103:132 – 36

11. Passerini L, Phang PT, Jackson FL, et al. (1987) Biofilms on right heart flow-directed catheters. Chest 92:440–42
12. Damen J (1988) The microbiologic risk of invasive haemodynamic monitoring in open-heart patients requiring prolonged ICU treatment. Intensive Care Med 14:156–58
13. Levy JH, Nagle DM, Curling PE, et al. (1988) Contamination reduction during central venous catheterization. Crit Care Med 16:165–69
14. Vallés J, Rello J, Matas L, et al. (1996) Pulmonary artery catheter colonization: influence of using an indwelling introducer. Eur J Clin Microbiol Infect Dis 15:71–75
15. Miller JJ, Venus B, Mathru M (1984) Comparison of the sterility of long-term central venous catheterization using single lumen, triple lumen and pulmonary artery catheters. Crit Care Med 12:634–36
16. Rello J, Jubert P, Esandi M, et al. (1997) Specific problems of arterial, Swan-Ganz, and hemodialysis catheters. Nutrition 13(Suppl):36S–39S
17. Jarvis WR, Edwards JR, Culver DH, et al. (1991) Nosocomial infection rates in adult and pediatric ICVs in the United States. NNIS System. Am J Med 91:1855–1915
18. Chen YY, Yen DHS, Yang YG, et al. (2003) Comparison between replacement at 4 days and 7 days of the infection rate for pulmonary artery catheters in an intensive care unit. Crit Care Med 31:1353–58
19. Kac G, Durain E, Amrein C, et al. (2001) Colonization and infection of pulmonary artery catheter in cardiac surgery patients: epidemiology and multivariate analysis of risk factors. Crit Care Med 29:971–75
20. Singh S, Nelson N, Acosta I, et al. (1982) Catheter colonization and bacteremia with pulmonary and arterial catheters. Crit Care Med 10:736–40
21. Applefeld JJ, Caruthers RE, Reno DJ, et al. (1978) Assessment of the sterility of long-term cardiac catheterization using the thermodilution Swan-Ganz catheter. Chest 74:377–81
22. Prachar H, Dittel M, Jobst CH, et al. (1978) Bacterial contamination of central venous catheter. Intensive Care Med 4:79–82
23. Puri V, Carlson R, Bamder J, et al. (1980) Complications of vascular catheterization in critically ill. Crit Care Med 8:495–97
24. Michel L, Marsh M, McMichan JC, et al. (1981) Infection of pulmonary artery catheters in critically ill patients. JAMA 245:1032–36
25. Kaye W, Wheaton M, Potter-Bynoe G (1983) Radial and pulmonary artery catheter-related sepsis (abstract). Crit Care Med 11:249
26. Nelson N, Singh S, Check F, et al. (1981) Colonization and catheter-related sepsis with pulmonary and arterial sepsis (abstract). Crit Care Med 11:144
27. Samsoondar W, Freeman J, Coultish I, et al. (1985) Colonization of intravascular catheter in the intensive care unit. Am J Surg 145:730–33
28. Senagore A, Waller J, Bonnel B, et al. (1987) Pulmonary artery catheterization: a prospective study of internal jugular and subclavian approach. Crit Care Med 15:35–38
29. Hilton E, Haslett T, Borenstein M, et al. (1988) Central catheter infections: single versus triple-lumen catheters. Am J Med 84:662–65
30. Mermel LA, Maki DG (1994) Infectious complications of Swan-Ganz pulmonary artery catheters. Pathogenesis, epidemiology, prevention and management. Am J Respir Crit Care Med 149:1020–24
31. Maki DG, Stolz SS, Wheeler S, et al. (1994) A prospective randomized trial of gauze and two polyurethane dressings for site care of pulmonary artery catheters: implications for catheter management. Crit Care Med 15:1729–32
32. Blot F, Chachaty E, Raynard B, et al. (2001) Mechanisms and risk factors for infection of pulmonary artery catheter and introducer sheaths in cancer patients admitted to intensive care units. J Hosp Infect 48:289–297
33. Widmer AF (1997) Intravenous-related infections. In: Wenzel RP (ed) Prevention and control of nosocomial infections. Williams and Wilkins, Baltimore, MD, pp 556–79
34. Maki DG, Goldman DA, Rhame FS (1973) Infection control in intravenous therapy. Ann Intern Med 79:867–90
35. Liñares J, Sitges-Serra A, Garau J, et al. (1985) Pathogenesis of catheter sepsis: a prospective study with quantitative and semiquantitative cultures of catheter hub and segment. J Clin Microbiol 21:357–60
36. Segura M, Alia C, Valverde J, et al. (1990) Assessment of a new hub design and the semiquantitative catheter culture method using an in vivo experimental model of catheter sepsis. J Clin Microbiol 28:2551–55
37. Segura M, Alvarez-Lerma F, Tellado JM, et al. (1995) Clinical trial of the effect of a new catheter hub on the prevention of central venous catheter-related sepsis. Interscience Conference on Antimicrobial Agents and Chemotherapy, San Francisco, p 258 (Abstract)
38. Ashkenazi S, Weiss E, Drucker MM, et al. (1986) Bacterial adherence to intravenous catheters and needles and its influence by cannula type and bacterial surface hydrophobicity. J Lab Clin Med 107:136–140
39. Yeung AC, May J, Hughes R (1988) Infection rate for single lumen versus triple lumen subclavian catheter. Infect Control Hosp Epidemiol 9:154–59
40. Henderson DK (1988) Intravascular device-associated infection: current concepts and controversies. Infect Surg 7:365–69
41. Norwood S, Ruby A, Civetta J, et al. (1991) Catheter-related infections and associated septicemia. Chest 99:968–70
42. Simmons BP, Hooton TM, Wong ES, et al. (1982) Guidelines for prevention of intravascular infections. National Technical Information Service, Springfield, VA
43. Maki DG, Weise CE, Sarafin HW (1977) A semiquantitative method for identified intravenous-catheter-related infection. N Engl J Med 296:1305–08
44. Sise MJ, Hollinsworth P, Brimm JE (1981) Complications of the flow-directed pulmonary artery catheter: a prospective analysis in 219 patients. Crit Care Med 9:315–18
45. Civetta JM, Hudson-Civetta JA, Dion L (1998) Duration of illness affects catheter-related infection and bacteremia (abstract). In: Program and abstracts of the 27th interscience conference on antimicrobial agents and chemotherapy. Atlanta, October 11–12, 1998
46. Eyer S, Brummitt C, Crossley K, et al. (1990) Catheter related-sepsis: prospective, randomized study of three methods of long-term catheter maintenance. Crit Care Med 18: 1073–76
47. Cobb D, High K, Sawyer RG, et al. (1992) A controlled trial of scheduled replacement of central venous and pulmonary-artery catheters. N Engl J Med 327:1062–66
48. Mermel L, Stolz S, Maki DG (1991) Epidemiology of infection with PA/Swan-Ganz catheter: a prospective study using molecular epidemiology. Am J Med 91 (31B):197S
49. Raad II, Bodey GP (1992) Infectious complications of indwelling vascular catheters. Clin Infect Dis 15:197
50. Blot F, Brun-Buisson C (1999) Current approaches to the diagnosis and prevention of catheter-related infections. Curr Opin Crit Care 5:341–46
51. Siegman-Igra Y, Anglim AM, Shapiro DE, et al. (1997) Diagnosis of vascular catheter-related bloodstream infection: a meta-analysis. J Clin Microbiol 35:928–32
52. Brun-Buisson C, Abroug F, Legrand P, et al. (1987) Diagno-

sis of central venous catheter-related sepsis: critical level of quantitative tip cultures. Arch Intern Med 147:873–76
53. Wing EJ, Norden CW, Shadduck RK, et al. (1979) Use of quantitative bacteriologic techniques to diagnose catheter-related sepsis. Arch Intern Med 139:482–85
54. Moyer MA, Edwards LD, Farley L (1983) Comparative culture methods on 101 intravenous catheters: routine, semiquantitative and blood cultures. Arch Intern Med 143:66–69
55. Andremont A, Paulet R, Nitenberg G, et al. (1988) Value of semi-quantitative cultures of blood drawn through catheter hubs for estimating the risk of catheter tip colonization in cancer patients. J Clin Microbiol 26:2297–2301
56. Fan ST, Teoh-Chan CH, Lau KF (1989) Evaluation of central venous catheter sepsis by differential quantitative blood culture. Eur J Clin Microbiol Infect Dis 8:142–45
57. Douard MC, Arlet G, Leverger G, et al. (1991) Quantitative blood cultures for diagnosis and management of catheter-related sepsis in pediatric hematology and oncology patients. Intensive Care Med 17:30–34
58. Rello J, Coll P, Net A, et al. (1991) Evaluation of different catheter parts for identification of pulmonary artery catheter colonization. Scand J Infect Dis 23:655–69
59. Vallés J, Rello J, Matas L, et al. (1996) Pulmonary artery catheter colonization: influence of using an indwelling introducer. Eur J Clin Microbiol Infect Dis 15:71–75
60. Rello J (1998) Prevención de las infecciones por catéter: ha llegado la hora del cambio? Enferm Infecc Microbiol Clin 16:53–4
61. Raad II, Honh DC, Gilbreath BJ, et al. (1994) Prevention of central venous catheter-related infection by using maximal sterile barrier precautions during insertion. Infect Control Hosp Epidemiol 15:231–35
62. Ducharme F, Gauthier M, Lacroix J, et al. (1988) Incidence of infection related to arterial catheterization in children: a prospective study. Crit Care Med 16:272–75
63. Norwood S, Cormier B, McMahon N, et al. (1988) Prospective study of catheter-related infection during prolonged arterial catheterization. Crit Care Med 16:836–89
64. Leroy O, Billiau V, Beuscart C, et al. (1989) Nosocomial infections associated with long-term radial artery cannulation. Intensive Care Med 15:241–45
65. Furfaro S, Gauthier M, Lacroix J, et al. (1991) Arterial catheter-related infections in children. Am J Dis Child 145: 1037–42
66. Raad I, Umphrey J, Khan A, et al. (1993) The duration of placement as a predictor of peripheral and pulmonary arterial catheter infection. J Hosp Infect 23:17–22
67. León MA, León C, Mateu A, et al. (1993) Infecciones relacionadas con catéteres intravasculares en el paciente crítico. Estudio multicéntrico. Med Intensiva 17:531–35
68. Martin C, Saux P, Papazian L, et al. (2001) Long-term arterial cannulation in the ICU patients using the radial artery or dorsalis pedis artery. Chest 119:901–906
69. Rijnders BAJ, Van Wijngaerden E, Wilmer A, et al. (2003) Use of full sterile barrier precautions during insertion of arterial catheters: A randomized trail. Clin Infect Dis 36: 743–48
70. Traoré O, Liotier J, Souweine B (2005) Prospective study of arterial and central venous catheter colonization and of arterial and central venous catheter-related bacteremia in intensive care units. Crit Care Med 33:1276–80
71. Shinozaki T, Deane RS, Mazuzan JE, et al. (1983) Bacterial contamination of arterial lines. JAMA 249:223–25
72. Thomas F, Burke JP, Parker J, et al. (1983) The risk of infection related to radial vs femoral sites for arterial catheterization. Crit Care Med 11:807–11
73. Lorente L, Villegas J, Martin M, et al. (2004) Catheter-related infection in critically ill patients. Intensive Care Med 30:1681–84
74. Frezza EE, Mezghebe H (1998) Indications and complications of arterial catheter use in surgical or medical intensive care units: analysis of 4932 patients. Am Surg 64: 127–31

Chapter 32

Prevention of Catheter-Related Bloodstream Infections in Critical Care Patients

P. Muñoz, E. Bouza

32.1 Introduction

Catheter-related bloodstream infections (CR-BSIs) are one of the most frequent causes of sepsis in intensive care units. They are associated with a high morbidity and considerable mortality and economic burden [1, 2]. In ICUs the main type of catheters inserted and used are short-term central vascular catheters (CVCs), meaning those inserted percutaneously either peripherally (basilic or cephalic veins) or centrally (jugular, subclavian or femoral). These catheters are usually intended to stay "in situ" for less than 30 days. Incidence of CR-BSI in ICUs ranges habitually from 2 to 10 episodes per 1,000 days on IV catheterization, depending on type of population, type of catheter inserted, point of entry of insertion and other variables [3–5]. In most polyvalent ICUs figures of less than 5 episodes of CR-BSI/1,000 days of catheterization are considered a good standard of care [6].

The real impact of CR-BSIs in overall mortality in the ICU is difficult to assess but attributable mortality is usually less than 10%, considerably inferior to bacteremic sepsis of other origins [7, 8]. Nevertheless, CR-BSIs prolong the ICU stay by between 5 and 8 days and have an associated cost calculated as approximately $30,000 in 1993 [9].

CR-BSIs are one of the infectious diseases more amenable to preventive interventions with different measures, which have been well summarized in the guidelines issued by the international societies [2, 10–13]. In this review we will address some of these preventive measures particularly applicable to adults admitted to ICUs on which scientific information has been produced in the last 5 years.

32.2 Value of Continuous Medical Education

Educational strategies targeting specific problems after observing CVC care practices have been demonstrated to be effective in decreasing the rates of CR-BSI and in our opinion should always be included in infection control schemes [4, 13–18]. Education-based programs are now recommended as a first-line strategy in the recently revised guidelines for the prevention of these infections [19].

Programs targeted specifically to medical intensive care units highlighting correct practices have demonstrated significant reductions in the incidence of CR-BSI, but some of them were performed on populations that had very high basal rates of CR-BSI [20, 21]. More data are required on the efficacy of such programs for units that begin the education process with a basal rate of CR-BSI of under 5 episodes of CR-BSI/1,000 days of catheter use.

In the work of Warren et al. [22], the intervention program in an ICU consisted of a 10-page self-study module on risk factors and practice modifications involved in CR-BSI; fact sheets and posters reinforced the information in the study module. Following the implementation of the intervention, the rate of CR-BSI decreased from 9.4 to 5.5 per 1,000 catheter-days ($p=0.019$), with estimated cost savings of between $103,600 and $1,573,000.

32.3 Measures To Take Before or During Catheter Insertion

It is possible to intervene using different targets and steps.

32.3.1 Multi-Lumen or Single-Lumen Catheters

The influence of the number of catheter lumens in the risk of infection has received much discussion since the introduction of multi-lumen central venous catheters more than 2 decades ago. A recent meta-analysis has compared the risk of CR-BSI and catheter colonization in multi-lumen, short-term catheters, compared to single-lumen catheters. The study selected a total of 15 studies for review and concluded that although CR-BSI was more common in multi-lumen catheters, catheter colonization was not so, but the studies were heterogeneous. When only studies of higher quality were included, multi-lumen catheters were found to be associated with a slight increase in CR-BSI. The authors concluded that the slight increase in infectious risk when using multi-lumen catheters is likely offset by their improved convenience, thereby justifying the continued use of multi-lumen vascular catheters when required [23]. We fully agree with this statement.

In another systematic review, including five randomized trials with data on 255 single-lumen and 275 multi-lumen catheters, CR-BSI occurred in 23 patients (8.4%) with multi-lumen and in 8 patients (3.1%) with single-lumen catheters (OR 2.58, 95% CI 1.24–5.37, NNT 19, 95% CI 11–75). For every 20 single-lumen catheters inserted, one bloodstream infection will be avoided that would have occurred had multi-lumen catheters been used [24].

32.3.2 Antimicrobial-Coated Catheters

The issue of antibiotic impregnated catheters continues to be debated. Despite data showing a reduction of catheter colonization and even slight reductions in CR-BSI, the significant cost difference with uncoated catheters, the potential toxicity of the coating substances and the risk of selection of antimicrobial resistant microorganisms precludes their introduction as a standard of care.

Several papers show that the use of catheters impregnated with antiseptic or antibiotic agents decrease the risk for catheter colonization and CR-BSIs in comparison with non-impregnated catheters [2, 25–36, 30, 38–47]. Coating substances include a combination of chlorhexidine and silver sulfadiazine (C-SS) [27, 28, 30, 31, 37] or minocycline and rifampin (R-M) [26, 32, 34, 38–42]. Catheters coated with C-SS have been shown to decrease colonization and CR-BSI by at least fourfold compared with uncoated catheters [26, 29] in short term CVCs, but failed to reduce the risk for CR-BSI in long-term catheters [31].

A new generation of chlorhexidine-silver sulfadiazine coated catheters with a higher concentration of antiseptics and better bonding to both the internal and external surface of the catheter has been associated with a reduction of colonization but not with a clear reduction of CR-BSI [35, 43, 44]. In a study comparing standard, un-impregnated central venous catheters with silver-coated and chlorhexidine-silver-sulfadiazine impregnated CVCs, antiseptic-impregnated CVCs could not prevent catheter colonization when compared with standard polyurethane catheters in a critical care setting with infrequent catheter colonization rates and CVCs left in place for >10 days [45].

In hematology-oncology patients, a prospective double-blind, randomized, controlled trial showed that second generation chlorhexidine and silver sulfadiazine (CHSS) catheters were effective in reducing the rate of catheter colonization (12% coated vs. 33% uncoated) but there was no significant difference in the incidence of CR-BSI (3% coated vs. 7% uncoated) [44].

Catheters coated with M-R have been associated with a lower rate of infection than uncoated catheters in patients with long-term catheters [40, 41], but a multicenter randomized trial carried out in Spain by Leon et al. in ICU patients showed no reduction in CR-BSI and an increase in *Candida* spp. colonization with no change in 30-day survival or reduced length of hospital stay [34].

A prospective and randomized study compared the infection rate of silver-platinum-carbon (SPC)-impregnated catheters with rifampin-minocycline (RM)-coated catheters in a single center in Australia. Colonization rates were lower for the RM catheters but no significant differences could be achieved in CR-BSI [38]. The same results were obtained in former studies [46, 47].

In our opinion, antimicrobial coated catheters still have to demonstrate a real cost-benefit to be incorporated as a standard of care in intensive care units. Issues like the potential selection of antimicrobial resistant pathogens also have to be clarified.

32.3.3 Selection of Insertion Point

The potential relationship between the location of CVC placement and the risk of infection is still controversial. Available evidence suggests that subclavian catheterization is less likely to result in catheter-related infection than internal jugular catheterization, and both have a lower risk than the femoral insertion [5, 48–57].

In a recent epidemiologic, prospective, observational study, the site of insertion in an intensive care unit population (subclavian, internal jugular, and femoral sites) was studied. The optimal insertion site for each individual patient was selected by intensive care physicians and a uniform protocol stressing strict sterile insertion was enforced. A total of 831 central venous catheters and 4,735 catheter days in 657 patients were studied. The incidence of catheter infection (4.01/1,000 catheter days, 2.29% catheters) and colonization (5.07/1,000 catheter days, 2.89% catheters) was low overall. There was no statistically significant difference in the incidence of infection and colonization or duration of catheters ($p=0.89$) [58]. Despite these encouraging results, femoral access should remain as an alternative but not a first choice for catheter placement in adult intensive care units [59].

Regarding the technique of tunneling, the current evidence does not support the routine use of tunneling in CVCs in patients in ICUs because there is no evidence of an associated reduction of CR-BSI [60–62].

Randolph et al. [62] in a meta-analysis evaluated the efficacy of tunneling short-term central venous catheters to prevent catheter-related infections. They included seven trials in the analysis and the conclusion was that current evidence does not support routine tunneling until its efficacy is evaluated at different placement sites and relative to other interventions.

32.3.4 Skin Preparation and Aseptic Insertion Technique

Povidone iodine 10% and alcohol 70% are effective for the skin preparation, but aqueous chlorhexidine 2% has been shown to be superior in preventing central venous catheter colonization and is the recommended practice nowadays. In a recent meta-analysis [63], evaluating the skin disinfection with chlorhexidine gluconate compared with povidone-iodine solution in preventing CR-BSI, the authors selected 8 studies involving a total of 4,143 catheters and concluded that the incidence of CR-BSI is significantly reduced in patients with central vascular lines who receive chlorhexidine gluconate versus povidone-iodine for insertion-site skin disinfection.

A more recent study compares povidone-iodine 10% (PVP-iodine), chlorhexidine 0.5%/propanol 70%, or chlorhexidine 0.5%/propanol 70% followed by PVP-iodine 10%. Bacteria were isolated from 30.8% of the catheters placed after skin disinfection with povidone-iodine, from 24.4% after disinfection with propanol/chlorhexidine and from 4.7% after disinfection with propanol/chlorhexidine followed by povidone-iodine ($p=0.006$) [64].

Use of maximum sterile barriers lowered costs (from $621 to $369 per catheter insertion), decreased the incidence of catheter-related bloodstream infections (from 5.3% to 2.8%) and improved patient safety in a prospective and comparative trial [65].

Skin preparation should include hair-cutting rather than shaving [66] and maximal sterile barrier precautions during insertion. Using fenestrated drapes, sterile gloves, gown, cap, mask, and a large drape can minimize catheter colonization and subsequent catheter related infection [15, 67, 68]. The use of full sterile barriers, however, has not been demonstrated to reduce the risk of infection for arterial catheters, but is a standard of care for central venous catheters [69].

32.3.5 Antimicrobial Prophylaxis at Insertion

Antibiotic prophylaxis at the time of catheter insertion is not recommended at the present time [70]. In routine cardiothoracic surgery patients, extending routine perioperative antibiotic prophylaxis until all IVCs have been removed does not influence rates of IVC colonization [71]. There is no evidence from randomized trials to support or refute the use of prophylactic antibiotics when umbilical artery catheters are inserted in newborn infants, or to support or refute continuing antibiotics once initial cultures rule out infection in newborn infants with umbilical artery catheters [72].

Cutdowns to insert either venous or arterial catheters are not recommended [2, 73].

32.4 Prevention of Infection After Catheter Insertion

32.4.1 Surveillance Cultures of the Skin and Hubs as a Way to Anticipate "At Risk" Populations for CR-BSI

In a prospective cohort study, carried out in an 11-bed heart surgery intensive care unit, all catheters were surveyed. Cultures were obtained from the skin insertion site and all hubs (surface cultures) every 72 h and on catheter removal. All samples were processed semiquantitatively. Over the study period, 561 catheters were inserted in 130 patients, and there were 15 episodes of CR-BSI. Validity indexes for the capacity of surface cultures to predict catheter colonization and CR-BSI were as follows: accuracy, 71.4, 65.6; sensitivity, 83.5%, 100%; specificity, 67.1%, 64.7%; positive predictive value, 47.6%, 7.2%; negative predictive value, 91.9%, 100%; positive likelihood ratio, 2.5, 2.83; and negative likelihood ratio, 0.2, 0, respectively. The process is time-consuming and expensive and is recommended only for the selection of a subpopulation prone to preventive interventions [74]. Otherwise, systematic surveillance cultures of catheters are not recommended at the present time [75–77].

32.4.2 Periodic Flush and Lock with Antimicrobial Agents

The antibiotic lock technique is a controversial method for sterilizing the catheter lumen and involves instilling high concentrations of antibiotics with or without heparin into the catheter lumen for extended periods of time. The lock technique with high concentration of antibiotics has been mainly used for the treatment of CR-BSI [78] but less frequently in the prevention of CR-BSI [79–81].

The lock technique has been successful in numerous small uncontrolled studies, suggesting that an antibiotic lock may be effective in salvaging infected central venous access devices. Currently, the Centers for Disease Control and Prevention Guidelines on the management of central venous access device infections support the use of this technique only for patients requiring long-term access who repeatedly experience catheter-related bloodstream infections despite stringent catheter care, but not for primary prophylaxis [82, 83].

In vitro studies demonstrate that many antibiotic combinations are stable and maintain high drug concentrations for prolonged periods of time. In vivo studies report the success of multiple combinations for both prevention and treatment with antibiotic lock technique in salvaging these catheters [79].

Prophylactic use of a vancomycin-heparin lock solution markedly reduced the incidence of CRBSI in high-risk neonates with long-term central catheters and did not promote vancomycin resistance, but was associated with asymptomatic hypoglycemia [84].

In patients receiving hemodialysis, locking prophylaxis with the use of gentamicin and heparin (5 mg/ml) was compared with standard heparin (5,000 IU/ml) alone. The gentamicin-locked group suffered only one infective episode (0.3/1,000 catheter days) compared to ten episodes in six patients in the heparin alone group (4/1,000 catheter days, $p=0.02$) [85].

Prophylactic monthly catheter flushes with 5,000 IU urokinase did not significantly decrease the number of documented bacteremic events in children with cancer who have CVCs [86].

32.4.3 Alcohol, Taurolidine and Other Non-Antibiotic Flushes

The ethanol-lock technique has been developed in recent years as a means to treat central venous line infections. In a study carried out by Dannenberg et al. [87] in children and adolescents with CR-BSI from Broviac catheters, 18 patients were treated with ethanol locks and the remaining 15 only with systemic antibiotic treatment. In the ethanol group 67% had no infectious relapse within 4 weeks of treatment compared with 47% treated with systemic antibiotics alone. No severe clinical side effects of ethanol flush were observed. Exposure to a 70% ethanol lock solution does not appreciably alter the integrity of selected commercial polyetherurethane and silicone catheters [88]. A good prospective and comparative study on the value of ethanol flushes in the prophylaxis of CR-BSI is badly lacking.

Taurolidine is an antiseptic substance developed more than 30 years ago, active in vitro against Gram positive and Gram negative bacteria and also with antifungal activity. It is available as a 2% solution that can be administered intraperitoneally and also intravenously. Taurolidine is metabolized to taurine, CO_2 and water. In a pilot study, taurolidine solution was used as an intravenous (i.v.) lock in the totally implantable intravascular devices of 11 consecutive oncological patients with CR-BSI not responding to systemic antimicrobial chemotherapy. All patients recovered completely from the infection and no adverse drug effects were seen [89].

A solution containing both taurolidine and citrate (Neutrolin; Biolink Corporation, Norwell, MA) has been shown to be very active in an "in vitro" model on biofilm containing bacteria and *Candida* [90].

In a group of patients on hemodialysis, catheters were randomly selected for lock prevention with either heparin or a citrate-taurolidine-containing solution. In the heparin group, four cases of catheter-related sepsis occurred as opposed to no sepsis episodes in the patients with catheters locked with the citrate-taurolidine-containing solution ($p<0.5$), and no side effects with the use of citrate-taurolidine catheter lock solution were noted [91].

Taurolidine can also be used as a daily flush solution in the reduction of CR-BSI in patients on home TPN [92], but the final role of taurolidine requires the realization of well designed prospective and comparative clinical trials.

32.4.4 Topical Antimicrobial Agents at the Portal of Entry

Topical polysporin (a triple antibiotic ointment) applied to the central venous catheter insertion site could reduce the incidence of catheter-related infections in patients receiving hemodialysis. In a randomized, double-blind study, infections were observed in more patients in the placebo group than in the polysporin group (34 vs. 12%; relative risk 0.35, 95% CI 0.18–0.68, $p=0.0013$). The number of infections per 1,000 catheter days (4.10 vs. 1.02, $p<0.0001$) and the number of bacteremias per 1,000 catheter days (2.48 vs. 0.63, $p=0.0004$) were also greater in the placebo group. Within the 6-month study period, there were 13 deaths in the placebo group as compared with 3 deaths in the polysporin triple group ($p=0.0041$). The prophylactic application of topical polysporin triple antibiotic ointment to the central venous catheter insertion site reduced the rate of infections and was associated with improved survival in hemodialysis patients [93].

Regarding the use of povidone solutions at the exit site of the catheter, povidone-iodine applied at the insertion site reduces the incidence of catheter-related infections when compared with no ointment in hemodialysis catheters. The alcoholic solution of iodine was better than the aqueous one in patients in adult intensive care units [94].

In a prospective and randomized trial, 119 patients scheduled electively to receive 140 CVCs were divided into 3 groups for different skin disinfection techniques: One group received povidone-iodine 10% (PVP-iodine); the second received chlorhexidine 0.5%/propanol 70%. A final group received chlorhexidine 0.5%/propanol 70% followed by PVP-iodine 10%. Prior to disinfection, a swab from the site of insertion was taken for culture. All catheters were cultured quantitatively after removal. Bacterial growth was found in 30.8% of the catheters placed after skin disinfection with povidone-iodine, in 24.4% after disinfection with propanol/chlorhexidine and in 4.7% after disinfection with propanol/chlorhexidine followed by povidone-iodine ($p=0.006$). The authors conclude that skin disinfection with propanol/chlorhexidine followed by PVP-iodine was superior in the prevention of microbial CVC colonization compared to either of the regimens alone [64].

In patients receiving hemodialysis, mupirocin applied thrice-weekly at the exit site is superior to no ointment on infection rates and catheter survival. Compared with controls, mupirocin-treated patients experienced significantly fewer catheter-related bacteremias (7 vs. 35%, $p<0.01$) and a longer time to first episode of bacteremia. Mupirocin use was not associated with any adverse patient effects or the induction of antimicrobial resistance [95].
In another study, mupirocin was compared with the topical application of a standardized antibacterial honey (Medihoney) in a randomized trial. A total of 101 patients undergoing hemodialysis were enrolled. The incidences of catheter-associated bacteremias in honey-treated ($n=51$) and mupirocin-treated ($n=50$) patients were comparable (0.97 vs. 0.85 episodes per 1,000 catheter days, respectively; NS). Thrice-weekly application of standardized antibacterial honey to hemodialysis catheter exit sites was safe, cheap, and effective and resulted in a comparable rate of catheter-associated infection to that obtained with mupirocin. The effectiveness of honey against antibiotic-resistant microorganisms and its low likelihood of selecting for further resistant strains suggests that this agent may represent a satisfactory alternative means of chemoprophylaxis in patients with central venous catheters [96].

Disinfection with a skin antiseptic that contains octenidine hydrochloride is also highly active and well tolerated, leads to a decrease in skin colonization over time and may be a new option for CVC care [97].

Application of chlorhexidine at the portal of entry is nowadays the recommended practice in the most recent guidelines and recommendations and is cost effective [63, 98–102]. A chlorhexidine gluconate-impregnated dressing (Biopatch) reduces the rate of CVCs in infants and children after cardiac surgery when compared with a standard polyurethane dressing (study group) but not the rate of CR-BSI [103].

In a prospective randomized clinical trial in a hematology unit, tunneled intravascular catheters were randomized to receive a standard dressing regimen, or a sustained-release chlorhexidine dressing. Of the 112 catheters which were randomized, exit-site or combined exit-site/tunnel infections occurred in 23 (43%) of 54 catheters in the control group, and five (9%) of 58 catheters in the intervention group (CI 0.04–0.37, $p<0.001$). Chlorhexidine dressings reduced the incidence of exit-site/tunnel infections of indwelling tunneled intravascular catheters without prolonging catheter survival in neutropenic patients [104].

32.4.5 Needleless Devices To Protect and Seal Hubs

Catheter hubs are a common source of contamination, especially during prolonged catheterization. A new hub model (Segur-Lock) that incorporates an antiseptic chamber filled with 3% iodinated alcohol has been compared with standard Luer-lock connectors. Rates of catheter colonization and CR-BSI are lower with the new hub model [105–107]; however, this new system is not needle-free.

New disinfectable, needle-free connectors have been compared with conventional open systems. These systems decrease catheter colonization and CR-BSI in prospective and comparative trials [108, 109].

References

1. Richards MJ, Edwards JR, Culver DH, et al. (2000) Nosocomial infections in combined medical-surgical intensive care units in the United States. Infect Control Hosp Epidemiol 21(8):510–5
2. O'Grady NP, Alexander M, Dellinger EP, et al. (2002) Guidelines for the prevention of intravascular catheter-related infections. Infect Control Hosp Epidemiol 23(12):759–69
3. Saint S, Veenstra DL, Lipsky BA (2000) The clinical and economic consequences of nosocomial central venous catheter-related infection: are antimicrobial catheters useful? Infect Control Hosp Epidemiol 21(6):375–80
4. Sherertz RJ, Ely EW, Westbrook DM, et al. (2000) Education of physicians-in-training can decrease the risk for vascular catheter infection. Ann Intern Med 132(8):641–8
5. Merrer J, De Jonghe B, Golliot F, et al. (2001) Complications of femoral and subclavian venous catheterization in critically ill patients: a randomized controlled trial. JAMA 286(6):700–7
6. Leon C, Ariza J (2004) Guías para el tratamiento de las infecciones relacionadas con catéteres intravasculares de corta permanencia en adultos: conferencia de consesnso SEIMC-SEMICYUC. Enferm Infecc Microbiol Clin 22(2):92–101
7. Rello J, Ochagavia A, Sabanes E, et al. (2000) Evaluation of outcome of intravenous catheter-related infections in critically ill patients. Am J Respir Crit Care Med 162(3):1027–30
8. Valles J, Leon C, Alvarez-Lerma F (1997) Nosocomial bacteremia in critically ill patients: a multicenter study evaluating epidemiology and prognosis. Spanish Collaborative Group for Infections in Intensive Care Units of Sociedad Espanola de Medicina Intensiva y Unidades Coronarias (SEMIUC). Clin Infect Dis 24(3):387–95
9. Pittet D, Tarara D, Wenzel RP (1994) Nosocomial bloodstream infection in critically ill patients. Excess length of stay, extra costs, and attributable mortality. JAMA 271(20):1598–601
10. Schiel X, Hebart H, Kern WV, et al. (2003) Sepsis in neutropenia – guidelines of the Infectious Diseases Working Party (AGIHO) of the German Society of Hematology and Oncology (DGHO). Ann Hematol 82(Suppl 2):S158–66

11. Miller DL, O'Grady NP (2003) Guidelines for the prevention of intravascular catheter-related infections: recommendations relevant to interventional radiology. J Vasc Interv Radiol 14(2):133–6
12. Fatkenheuer G, Buchheidt D, Cornely OA, et al. (2003) Central venous catheter (CVC)-related infections in neutropenic patients – guidelines of the Infectious Diseases Working Party (AGIHO) of the German Society of Hematology and Oncology (DGHO). Ann Hematol 82(Suppl 2):S149–57
13. Mermel LA, Farr BM, Sherertz RJ, et al. (2001) Guidelines for the management of intravascular catheter-related infections. J Intraven Nurs 24(3):180–205
14. Eggimann P, Hugonnet S, Harbarth S, et al. (2001) Reduction of bloodstream infections 2 years following a global prevention strategy targeted at vascular access in ICU [abstract]. Abstracts of the 41th Interscience Conference on Antimicrobial Agents and Chemotherapy. American Society for Microbiology, Chicago, IL, p 2050
15. Coopersmith CM, Rebmann TL, Zack JE, et al. (2002) Effect of an education program on decreasing catheter-related bloodstream infections in the surgical intensive care unit. Crit Care Med 30(1):59–64
16. Warren DK, Zack JE, Cox MJ, et al. (2003) An educational intervention to prevent catheter-associated bloodstream infections in a nonteaching, community medical center. Crit Care Med 31(7):1959–63
17. Warren DK, Zack JE, Mayfield JL, et al. (2004) The effect of an education program on the incidence of central venous catheter-associated bloodstream infection in a medical ICU. Chest 126(5):1612–8
18. Mermel LA (2000) Prevention of intravascular catheter-related infections. Ann Intern Med 132(5):391–402
19. O'Grady NP, Alexander M, Dellinger EP, et al. (2002) Guidelines for the prevention of intravascular catheter-related infections. Centers for Disease Control and Prevention. MMWR Recomm Rep 51(RR-10):1–29
20. Lobo RD, Levin AS, Gomes LM, et al. (2005) Impact of an educational program and policy changes on decreasing catheter-associated bloodstream infections in a medical intensive care unit in Brazil. Am J Infect Control 33(2): 83–7
21. Higuera F, Rosenthal VD, Duarte P, et al. (2005) The effect of process control on the incidence of central venous catheter-associated bloodstream infections and mortality in intensive care units in Mexico. Crit Care Med 33(9):2022–7
22. Warren DK, Yokoe DS, Climo MW, et al. (2006) Preventing catheter-associated bloodstream infections: a survey of policies for insertion and care of central venous catheters from hospitals in the prevention epicenter program. Infect Control Hosp Epidemiol 27(1):8–13
23. Dezfulian C, Lavelle J, Nallamothu BK, et al. (2003) Rates of infection for single-lumen versus multilumen central venous catheters: a meta-analysis. Crit Care Med 31(9): 2385–90
24. Zurcher M, Tramer MR, Walder B (2004) Colonization and bloodstream infection with single- versus multi-lumen central venous catheters: a quantitative systematic review. Anesth Analg 99(1):177–82
25. Cicalini S, Palmieri F, Petrosillo N (2004) Clinical review: new technologies for prevention of intravascular catheter-related infections. Crit Care 8(3):157–62
26. Raad I, Darouiche R, Dupuis J, et al. (1997) Central venous catheters coated with minocycline and rifampin for the prevention of catheter-related colonization and bloodstream infections. A randomized, double-blind trial. The Texas Medical Center Catheter Study Group. Ann Intern Med 127(4):267–74
27. Maki DG, Stolz SM, Wheeler S, et al. (1997) Prevention of central venous catheter-related bloodstream infection by use of an antiseptic-impregnated catheter. A randomized, controlled trial. Ann Intern Med 127(4):257–66
28. Kamal GD, Pfaller MA, Rempe LE, et al. (1991) Reduced intravascular catheter infection by antibiotic bonding. A prospective, randomized, controlled trial. JAMA 265(18): 2364–8
29. Veenstra DL, Saint S, Sullivan SD (1999) Cost-effectiveness of antiseptic-impregnated central venous catheters for the prevention of catheter-related bloodstream infection. JAMA 282(6):554–60
30. Veenstra DL, Saint S, Saha S, et al. (1999) Efficacy of antiseptic-impregnated central venous catheters in preventing catheter-related bloodstream infection: a meta-analysis. JAMA 281(3):261–7
31. Logghe C, Van Ossel C, D'Hoore W, et al. (1997) Evaluation of chlorhexidine and silver-sulfadiazine impregnated central venous catheters for the prevention of bloodstream infection in leukaemic patients: a randomized controlled trial. J Hosp Infect 37(2):145–56
32. Darouiche RO, Raad II, Heard SO, et al. (1999) A comparison of two antimicrobial-impregnated central venous catheters. Catheter Study Group. N Engl J Med 340(1):1–8
33. Crnich CJ, Maki DG (2002) The promise of novel technology for the prevention of intravascular device-related bloodstream infection. I. Pathogenesis and short-term devices. Clin Infect Dis 34(9):1232–42
34. Leon C, Ruiz-Santana S, Rello J, et al. (2004) Benefits of minocycline and rifampin-impregnated central venous catheters. A prospective, randomized, double-blind, controlled, multicenter trial. Intensive Care Med 30(10): 1891–9
35. Brun-Buisson C, Doyon F, Sollet JP, et al. (2004) Prevention of intravascular catheter-related infection with newer chlorhexidine-silver sulfadiazine-coated catheters: a randomized controlled trial. Intensive Care Med 30(5): 837–43
36. Walder B, Pittet D, Tramer MR (2002) Prevention of bloodstream infections with central venous catheters treated with anti-infective agents depends on catheter type and insertion time: evidence from a meta-analysis. Infect Control Hosp Epidemiol 23(12):748–56
37. Greenfeld JI, Sampath L, Popilskis SJ, et al. (1995) Decreased bacterial adherence and biofilm formation on chlorhexidine and silver sulfadiazine-impregnated central venous catheters implanted in swine. Crit Care Med 23(5): 894–900
38. Fraenkel D, Rickard C, Thomas P, et al. (2006) A prospective, randomized trial of rifampicin-minocycline-coated and silver-platinum-carbon-impregnated central venous catheters. Crit Care Med 34(3):668–75
39. Darouiche RO, Berger DH, Khardori N, et al. (2005) Comparison of antimicrobial impregnation with tunneling of long-term central venous catheters: a randomized controlled trial. Ann Surg 242(2):193–200
40. Hanna H, Benjamin R, Chatzinikolaou I, et al. (2004) Long-term silicone central venous catheters impregnated with minocycline and rifampin decrease rates of catheter-related bloodstream infection in cancer patients: a prospective randomized clinical trial. J Clin Oncol 22(15): 3163–71
41. Chatzinikolaou I, Hanna H, Graviss L, et al. (2003) Clinical experience with minocycline and rifampin-impregnated central venous catheters in bone marrow transplantation recipients: efficacy and low risk of developing staphylococcal resistance. Infect Control Hosp Epidemiol 24(12): 961–3

42. Crnich CJ, Maki DG (2002) The promise of novel technology for the prevention of intravascular device-related bloodstream infection. II. Long-term devices. Clin Infect Dis 34(10):1362–8
43. Rupp ME, Lisco SJ, Lipsett PA, et al. (2005) Effect of a second-generation venous catheter impregnated with chlorhexidine and silver sulfadiazine on central catheter-related infections: a randomized, controlled trial. Ann Intern Med 143(8):570–80
44. Ostendorf T, Meinhold A, Harter C, et al. (2005) Chlorhexidine and silver-sulfadiazine coated central venous catheters in haematological patients – a double-blind, randomised, prospective, controlled trial. Support Care Cancer 13(12):993–1000
45. Dunser MW, Mayr AJ, Hinterberger G, et al. (2005) Central venous catheter colonization in critically ill patients: a prospective, randomized, controlled study comparing standard with two antiseptic-impregnated catheters. Anesth Analg 101(6):1778–84
46. Corral L, Nolla-Salas M, Ibanez-Nolla J, et al. (2003) A prospective, randomized study in critically ill patients using the Oligon Vantex catheter. J Hosp Infect 55(3):212–9
47. Ranucci M, Isgro G, Giomarelli PP, et al. (2003) Impact of oligon central venous catheters on catheter colonization and catheter-related bloodstream infection. Crit Care Med 31(1):52–9
48. Lee SH, Hahn ST (2005) Comparison of complications between transjugular and axillosubclavian approach for placement of tunneled, central venous catheters in patients with hematological malignancy: a prospective study. Eur Radiol 15(6):1100–4
49. Sadoyama G, Gontijo Filho PP (2003) Comparison between the jugular and subclavian vein as insertion site for central venous catheters: microbiological aspects and risk factors for colonization and infection. Braz J Infect Dis 7(2):142–8
50. Vinod KP (2002) Jugular versus subclavian central venous catheter insertion: search for the better approach. Crit Care Med 30(2):486–7
51. Ruesch S, Walder B, Tramer MR (2002) Complications of central venous catheters: internal jugular versus subclavian access – a systematic review. Crit Care Med 30(2): 454–60
52. Gutierrez JA, Bagatell R, Samson MP, et al. (2003) Femoral central venous catheter-associated deep venous thrombosis in children with diabetic ketoacidosis. Crit Care Med 31(1):80–3
53. Murai DT (2002) Are femoral Broviac catheters effective and safe? A prospective comparison of femoral and jugular venous Broviac catheters in newborn infants. Chest 121(5):1527–30
54. Goldstein AM, Weber JM, Sheridan RL (1997) Femoral venous access is safe in burned children: an analysis of 224 catheters. J Pediatr 130(3):442–6
55. Durbec O, Viviand X, Potie F, et al. (1997) A prospective evaluation of the use of femoral venous catheters in critically ill adults. Crit Care Med 25(12):1986–9
56. Trottier SJ, Veremakis C, O'Brien J, et al. (1995) Femoral deep vein thrombosis associated with central venous catheterization: results from a prospective, randomized trial. Crit Care Med 23(1):52–9
57. Murr MM, Rosenquist MD, Lewis RW, et al. (1991) A prospective safety study of femoral vein versus nonfemoral vein catheterization in patients with burns. J Burn Care Rehabil 12(6):576–8
58. Deshpande KS, Hatem C, Ulrich HL, et al. (2005) The incidence of infectious complications of central venous catheters at the subclavian, internal jugular, and femoral sites in an intensive care unit population. Crit Care Med 33(1):13–20; discussion 234–5
59. O'Grady NP, Dezfulian C (2005) The femoral site as first choice for central venous access? Not so fast. Crit Care Med 33(1):234–5
60. Foo R, Fujii A, Harris JA, et al. (2001) Complications in tunneled CVL versus PICC lines in very low birth weight infants. J Perinatol 21(8):525–30
61. Nahum E, Levy I, Katz J, et al. (2002) Efficacy of subcutaneous tunneling for prevention of bacterial colonization of femoral central venous catheters in critically ill children. Pediatr Infect Dis J 21(11):1000–4
62. Randolph AG, Cook DJ, Gonzales CA, et al. (1998) Tunneling short-term central venous catheters to prevent catheter-related infection: a meta-analysis of randomized, controlled trials. Crit Care Med 26(8):1452–7
63. Chaiyakunapruk N, Veenstra DL, Lipsky BA, et al. (2002) Chlorhexidine compared with povidone-iodine solution for vascular catheter-site care: a meta-analysis. Ann Intern Med 136(11):792–801
64. Langgartner J, Linde HJ, Lehn N, et al. (2004) Combined skin disinfection with chlorhexidine/propanol and aqueous povidone-iodine reduces bacterial colonisation of central venous catheters. Intensive Care Med 30(6):1081–8
65. Hu KK, Veenstra DL, Lipsky BA, et al. (2004) Use of maximal sterile barriers during central venous catheter insertion: clinical and economic outcomes. Clin Infect Dis 39(10):1441–5
66. Eggimann P, Harbarth S, Constantin MN, et al. (2000) Impact of a prevention strategy targeted at vascular-access care on incidence of infections acquired in intensive care. Lancet 355(9218):1864–8
67. Raad, II, Hohn DC, Gilbreath BJ, et al. (1994) Prevention of central venous catheter-related infections by using maximal sterile barrier precautions during insertion. Infect Control Hosp Epidemiol 15(4):231–8
68. Mermel LA, McCormick RD, Springman SR, et al. (1991) The pathogenesis and epidemiology of catheter-related infection with pulmonary artery Swan-Ganz catheters: a prospective study utilizing molecular subtyping. Am J Med 91(3B):197S–205S
69. Rijnders BJ, Van Wijngaerden E, Wilmer A, et al. (2003) Use of full sterile barrier precautions during insertion of arterial catheters: a randomized trial. Clin Infect Dis 36(6):743–8
70. van de Wetering MD, van Woensel JB (2003) Prophylactic antibiotics for preventing early central venous catheter Gram positive infections in oncology patients. Cochrane Database Syst Rev (2):CD003295
71. Sandoe JA, Kumar B, Stoddart B, et al. (2003) Effect of extended perioperative antibiotic prophylaxis on intravascular catheter colonization and infection in cardiothoracic surgery patients. J Antimicrob Chemother 52(5):877–9
72. Inglis GD, Davies MW (2004) Prophylactic antibiotics to reduce morbidity and mortality in neonates with umbilical artery catheters. Cochrane Database Syst Rev (3):CD004697
73. Povoski SP (2000) A prospective analysis of the cephalic vein cutdown approach for chronic indwelling central venous access in 100 consecutive cancer patients. Ann Surg Oncol 7(7):496–502
74. Bouza E, Muñoz P, Burillo A, et al. (2005) The challenge of anticipating catheter tip colonization in major heart surgery patients in the intensive care unit: Are surface cultures useful? Crit Care Med 33(9):1953–1960
75. Raad, II, Baba M, Bodey GP (1995) Diagnosis of catheter-related infections: the role of surveillance and targeted quantitative skin cultures. Clin Infect Dis 20(3):593–7
76. Atela I, Coll P, Rello J, et al. (1997) Serial surveillance cultures of skin and catheter hub specimens from critically ill

patients with central venous catheters: molecular epidemiology of infection and implications for clinical management and research. J Clin Microbiol 35(7):1784–90
77. Nielsen J, Kolmos HJ, Rosdahl VT (1998) Poor value of surveillance cultures for prediction of septicaemia caused by coagulase-negative staphylococci in patients undergoing haemodialysis with central venous catheters. Scand J Infect Dis 30(6):569–72
78. Rijnders BJ, Van Wijngaerden E, Vandecasteele SJ, et al. (2005) Treatment of long-term intravascular catheter-related bacteraemia with antibiotic lock: randomized, placebo-controlled trial. J Antimicrob Chemother 55(1):90–4
79. Bestul MB, Vandenbussche HL (2005) Antibiotic lock technique: review of the literature. Pharmacotherapy 25(2): 211–27
80. Oncu S, Ozturk B, Kurt I, et al. (2004) Elimination of intraluminal colonization by antibiotic lock in catheters. Tohoku J Exp Med 203(1):1–8
81. Metcalf SC, Chambers ST, Pithie AD (2004) Use of ethanol locks to prevent recurrent central line sepsis. J Infect 49(1):20–2
82. Bagnall-Reeb H (2004) Evidence for the use of the antibiotic lock technique. J Infus Nurs 27(2):118–22
83. De Sio L, Jenkner A, Milano GM, et al. (2004) Antibiotic lock with vancomycin and urokinase can successfully treat colonized central venous catheters in pediatric cancer patients. Pediatr Infect Dis J 23(10):963–5
84. Garland JS, Alex CP, Henrickson KJ, et al. (2005) A vancomycin-heparin lock solution for prevention of nosocomial bloodstream infection in critically ill neonates with peripherally inserted central venous catheters: a prospective, randomized trial. Pediatrics 116(2):e198–205
85. McIntyre CW, Hulme LJ, Taal M, et al. (2004) Locking of tunneled hemodialysis catheters with gentamicin and heparin. Kidney Int 66(2):801–5
86. Aquino VM, Sandler ES, Mustafa MM, et al. (2002) A prospective double-blind randomized trial of urokinase flushes to prevent bacteremia resulting from luminal colonization of subcutaneous central venous catheters. J Pediatr Hematol Oncol 24(9):710–3
87. Dannenberg C, Bierbach U, Rothe A, et al. (2003) Ethanol-lock technique in the treatment of bloodstream infections in pediatric oncology patients with broviac catheter. J Pediatr Hematol Oncol 25(8):616–21
88. Crnich CJ, Halfmann JA, Crone WC, et al. (2005) The effects of prolonged ethanol exposure on the mechanical properties of polyurethane and silicone catheters used for intravascular access. Infect Control Hosp Epidemiol 26(8):708–14
89. Koldehoff M, Zakrzewski JL (2004) Taurolidine is effective in the treatment of central venous catheter-related bloodstream infections in cancer patients. Int J Antimicrob Agents 24(5):491–5
90. Shah CB, Mittelman MW, Costerton JW, et al. (2002) Antimicrobial activity of a novel catheter lock solution. Antimicrob Agents Chemother 46(6):1674–9
91. Betjes MG, van Agteren M (2004) Prevention of dialysis catheter-related sepsis with a citrate-taurolidine-containing lock solution. Nephrol Dial Transplant 19(6):1546–51
92. Jurewitsch B, Jeejeebhoy KN (2005) Taurolidine lock: the key to prevention of recurrent catheter-related bloodstream infections. Clin Nutr 24(3):462–5
93. Lok CE, Stanley KE, Hux JE, et al. (2003) Hemodialysis infection prevention with polysporin ointment. J Am Soc Nephrol 14(1):169–79
94. Parienti JJ, du Cheyron D, Ramakers M, et al. (2004) Alcoholic povidone-iodine to prevent central venous catheter colonization: A randomized unit-crossover study. Crit Care Med 32(3):708–13
95. Johnson DW, MacGinley R, Kay TD, et al. (2002) A randomized controlled trial of topical exit site mupirocin application in patients with tunnelled, cuffed haemodialysis catheters. Nephrol Dial Transplant 17(10):1802–7
96. Johnson DW, van Eps C, Mudge DW, et al. (2005) Randomized, controlled trial of topical exit-site application of honey (Medihoney) versus mupirocin for the prevention of catheter-associated infections in hemodialysis patients. J Am Soc Nephrol 16(5):1456–62
97. Tietz A, Frei R, Dangel M, et al. (2005) Octenidine hydrochloride for the care of central venous catheter insertion sites in severely immunocompromised patients. Infect Control Hosp Epidemiol 26(8):703–7
98. Krau SD (2003) Review: chlorhexidine gluconate is more effective than povidone-iodine for preventing vascular catheter related bloodstream infection. Evid Based Nurs 6(1):18
99. Crawford AG, Fuhr JP, Jr, Rao B (2004) Cost-benefit analysis of chlorhexidine gluconate dressing in the prevention of catheter-related bloodstream infections. Infect Control Hosp Epidemiol 25(8):668–74
100. Carson SM (2004) Chlorhexidine versus povidone-iodine for central venous catheter site care in children. J Pediatr Nurs 19(1):74–80
101. Chaiyakunapruk N, Veenstra DL, Lipsky BA, et al. (2003) Vascular catheter site care: the clinical and economic benefits of chlorhexidine gluconate compared with povidone iodine. Clin Infect Dis 37(6):764–71
102. Maki DG, Ringer M, Alvarado CJ (1991) Prospective randomised trial of povidone-iodine, alcohol, and chlorhexidine for prevention of infection associated with central venous and arterial catheters. Lancet 338(8763):339–43
103. Levy I, Katz J, Solter E, et al. (2005) Chlorhexidine-impregnated dressing for prevention of colonization of central venous catheters in infants and children: a randomized controlled study. Pediatr Infect Dis J 24(8):676–9
104. Chambers ST, Sanders J, Patton WN, et al. (2005) Reduction of exit-site infections of tunnelled intravascular catheters among neutropenic patients by sustained-release chlorhexidine dressings: results from a prospective randomized controlled trial. J Hosp Infect 61(1):53–61
105. Segura M, Alvarez-Lerma F, Tellado JM, et al. (1996) A clinical trial on the prevention of catheter-related sepsis using a new hub model. Ann Surg 223(4):363–9
106. Leon C, Alvarez-Lerma F, Ruiz-Santana S, et al. (2003) Antiseptic chamber-containing hub reduces central venous catheter-related infection: a prospective, randomized study. Crit Care Med 31(5):1318–24
107. Segura M, Alia C, Valverde J, et al. (1990) Assessment of a new hub design and the semiquantitative catheter culture method using an in vivo experimental model of catheter sepsis. J Clin Microbiol 28(11):2551–4
108. Bouza E, Muñoz P, Lopez-Rodriguez J, et al. (2003) A needleless closed system device (CLAVE) protects from intravascular catheter tip and hub colonization: a prospective randomized study. J Hosp Infect 54(4):279–87
109. Yebenes JC, Vidaur L, Serra-Prat M, et al. (2004) Prevention of catheter-related bloodstream infection in critically ill patients using a disinfectable, needle-free connector: a randomized controlled trial. Am J Infect Control 32(5):291–5

Chapter 33

Meningococcemia

P. Domingo, N. Barquet

"No microbe can kill more quickly"
Harry A. Feldman, 1979

33.1 Definition

Meningococcemia literally means the presence and isolation of *Neisseria meningitidis* in the blood of a patient. Although it is an invariable phenomenon in the pathogenesis of meningococcal disease, it may in itself dominate the clinical picture. The clinical spectrum of meningococcemia ranges from a clinically inapparent, mostly oligo-symptomatic bacteremia as in benign or inapparent meningococcemia to overwhelming cases with early multiple-organ failure as in fulminant meningococcemia [1].

There are few diseases which cause as much social alarm, even among healthcare staff, as that triggered by meningococcal disease when a case is detected in the community. The reasons for this alarm are: (1) its high death rate (6–13% and rising to 44–70% in fulminant meningococcemia); (2) the speed with which it can kill. A case has been described with a start of symptoms-death interval of just 3 h 20 min in a previously healthy child; (3) the seriousness of the sequelae among survivors (e.g., amputations in meningococcemia); (4) the impossibility of reducing the death rate in fulminant meningococcemia despite the early establishment of antibiotic therapy, life support measures for patients in critical condition and aggressive treatments; (5) the impossibility of predicting the appearance of epidemic outbreaks; (6) the high risk of contagion among family members (300 times more risk than the general population); and (7) the lack of an effective vaccine against *N. meningitidis* serogroup B.

33.2 The Meningococcus

Neisseria meningitidis is a Gram-negative diplococcus which typically appears with the adjacent sites flattened to produce a biscuit shape. It is an exclusively human pathogen. This bacterium is considered fastidious in its growth conditions, and tends to readily undergo autolysis. Optimal growth conditions include moist environment at 35–37°C with an atmosphere of 5–10% carbon dioxide. The organism grows well on a number of medium bases including blood agar base, trypticase soy agar, supplemented chocolate agar, and Mueller-Hinton agar. *N. meningitidis* is identified by acid production tests or by chromogenic enzyme substrate tests [2].

An outer membrane composed of lipids, lipo-oligosaccharides and outer membrane proteins surrounds the meningococcus. Between the outer membrane and the cytoplasmic membrane lies a peptidoglycan cell wall. A polysaccharide capsule produced by the bacteria and attached to this outer membrane envelops pathogenic meningococci. At least 13 meningococcal serogroups have been defined according to the immunologic reactivity of their capsular polysaccharide antigens: A, B, C, D, H, I, K, L, X, Y, Z, Z' (29E), and W-135; meningococcal disease usually being caused by serogroups A, B, C, L, X, Y, and W-135 [1]. Based on the class 2/3 or 1 outer membrane proteins, at least 20 meningococcal serotypes and 10 serosubtypes have been identified [3]. Endemic meningococcal disease is caused by a broad number of serotypes in contrast with epidemic disease that is caused by a single serotype [4]. There are other classification systems, based on differential antigenic properties of lipo-oligosaccharide with at least 13 immunotypes [5–8]. It is possible to use the antigenic properties of immunoglobulin A1 proteases and pili for additional typing [9].

Serogrouping and serotyping are used to characterize the *N. meningitidis* strains and are very important in the development of vaccines, but cannot be used to determine the origin of epidemic and resistant clones [10]. Multilocus enzyme electrophoresis, pulsed-fields gel electrophoresis, DNA fingerprinting and protein chain reaction provide a better insight into the epidemiology and clonal expansion of *N. meningitidis* strains [11–14].

Neisseria meningitidis has the capacity to exchange the genetic material responsible for capsule production and thereby switch from serogroup B to C or vice versa [15, 16]. A similar event with W-135 isolates has been described [17]. This process occurs on exchanging at random the gene encoding for the capsular polysaccharide in such a way that the new recombinant strain will express a different capsular polysaccharide to the one that it expressed before. Thus, all the serogroups should be capable of changing to any other. Capsule-switching may become an important mechanism of virulence with the widespread use of vaccines that provide serogroup-specific protection [18]. The existence of a capsule-switching genetic mechanism and the lack of vaccine against *N. meningitidis* serogroup B have led to the identification of a new noncapsular candidate for vaccine.

33.3 Epidemiology

Meningococcemia obviously shares epidemiological characteristics with other forms of meningococcal disease, especially meningococcal meningitis. It may occur worldwide as sporadic, endemic or epidemic disease [19]. There are marked differences in the epidemiology of meningococcal disease in different countries and geographic locations.

In developed countries, such as the United States and western Europe, meningococcal disease usually causes sporadic or endemic disease with a peak in late winter and early spring. The annual incidence rates range from 1 to 3 cases per 100,000 inhabitants and are caused by strains of serogroups B and C [20, 21].

In developing countries, such as sub-Saharan Africa, meningococcal disease causes endemic or epidemic disease. During the endemic period the annual incidence rate is approximately 10 times higher (10–25/100,000/year) than developed countries. Meningococcal disease is caused by serogroup A and occurs in seasonal annual cycles, with the attack rate rising at the end of the dry season and declining after the beginning of the rainy season [22]. For more than one century serogroup A and C strains have been responsible for recurrent epidemics in sub-Saharan Africa, which extends from Ethiopia in the East, to Senegal in the West, mainly within the range of 300 mm to 1,000 mm annual rainfall [23]. The large-scale epidemics occur at wider intervals with irregular patterns every 5–12 years and last for two to three dry seasons, dying out during the intervening rainy seasons [24]. During epidemics, the incidence is as high as 400–800 per 100,000 inhabitants (even 1,000/100,000). In 1996, in the largest epidemic ever recorded, there were more than 200,000 cases and 20,000 deaths [25].

The differences in incidence rates between developed and developing countries reflect the different pathogenic properties of *N. meningitidis* strains and socioeconomic, environmental, and climatological differences [26].

Epidemics of meningococcal disease can be caused by clonal *N. meningitidis* strains migrating across continents [27]. The clonal serogroup A meningococcus originated in China and spread to Nepal and India between 1983 and 1987 [10, 28], reaching Saudi Arabia in 1987, and causing an epidemic among pilgrims during the Hajj in Mecca. The organism was then transported with the Hajjis, leading to epidemics in 1988 in central Africa and in later years in eastern Africa [29]. The epidemic spread to South Africa in 1996 [30]. The transfer of strains of the same clonal complex by Hajjis to the United States and Europe did not give rise to epidemics there [31]. It is not known why potential pathogenic strains cause major epidemics in some areas while others are not affected [22]. The occurrence of meningococcal disease would not appear to be determined solely by the introduction of a new virulent *N. meningitidis* strain but also by other factors that enhance transmission and by the susceptibility of the local population [32].

In Spain, there have been four epidemic waves of meningococcal disease in the last 35 years with interepidemic periods of variable duration (Fig. 33.1). The first three epidemic waves (1979, 1981 and 1983) were caused by strains of *N. meningitidis* serogroup B while the last one (1996–1997) was provoked by a serogroup C strain.

Since 1988, incidence of meningococcal disease in Spain caused by serogroup B meningococci has declined, and incidence due to serogroup C meningococci has increased. This change of pattern led to the carrying out of a mass vaccination campaign against serogroup C with polysaccharide A+C vaccine in Spain during 1996–97. The campaign succeeded in reducing the rate of incidence of serogroup C meningococcal disease in 1998 and 1999. However, there was an upturn in this incidence in the year 2000 attributable to the ineffectiveness of the polysaccharide vaccine to protect children under the age of 2.

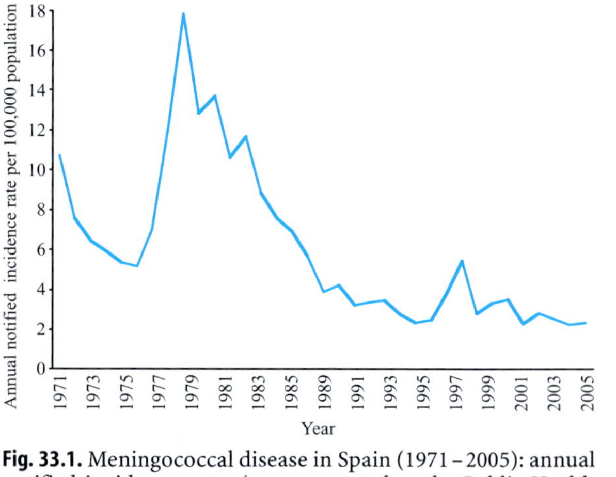

Fig. 33.1. Meningococcal disease in Spain (1971–2005): annual notified incidence rates (cases reported to the Public Health Service)

Serogroup C meningococcal polysaccharide-protein conjugate vaccines were introduced into the Spanish pediatric vaccine calendar in the autumn of 2000, immediately after their commercialization, and this has led to a spectacular decrease in the incidence of serogroup C meningococcal disease in those vaccinated. The greatest reduction among those vaccinated was observed in children under 1 year old, an age group in which the incidence has gone from 12.6/100,000 in the first 20 weeks of the season 1999–2000, before the introduction of serogroup C meningococcal polysaccharide-protein conjugate vaccines, to 1.4/100,000 during the same period of the season 2001–2002. In non-vaccinated groups, the incidence rate for serogroup C remains high.

In Spain, the annual notified incidence rates of meningococcal disease over recent years have been around 2–3 cases per 100,000 inhabitants (Fig. 33.1), with an annual average of 800–1,000 cases. The case-fatality rate is still stagnant, at around 10%. The incidence rates and case-fatality rates in other western European countries were similar in recent years, with a trend to increase in the late 1990s [33].

With the aim of knowing the population groups at greatest risk of acquiring meningococcal disease, among other objectives, and consequently the main candidates for preventive interventions, an epidemiological study was carried out in Barcelona with detection of cases using two active epidemiologic surveillance systems for 6 years (1987–1992) [34]. The intention was to detect all the cases of meningococcal disease diagnosed in people resident in this big city and on knowing the population census to be able to calculate the average annual incidence rate by age group. This would provide highly reliable incidence data not influenced by the population pyramid. The estimated incidence using passive epidemiological surveillance systems is not reliable as it is not known whether or not there is under-notification.

No meningococcal vaccination campaign was carried out during the 6 years of the study, which helped it to reflect the epidemiology of meningococcal disease in the most natural conditions possible. Epidemiological studies on meningococcal disease had never been carried out previously in a large urban community, such as a big city like Barcelona, using active epidemiologic surveillance systems for a long period of time.

In the study mentioned, patient detection was carried out using two active epidemiologic surveillance systems. The main case detection system consisted of a member of the Barcelona Meningococcal Disease Surveillance Group (an ad hoc group created and made up of 107 doctors from the 24 acute care hospitals in the metropolitan area of Barcelona) that reviewed, on a daily basis, the diagnostic orientations written in the blood culture or cerebrospinal fluid (CSF) culture request sheets that had been sent to the microbiology laboratories serving all the acute care hospitals ($n=24$) in the area of the city of Barcelona, together with the pertinent sample, to search for a presumptive diagnosis consistent with meningococcal disease. Patients with diagnostic orientations suggesting meningococcal disease were monitored and an epidemiological survey was carried out. The main system also included the monitoring of the cultures and the rapid notification when a strain of *N. meningitidis* was isolated and identified.

The complementary case detection system involved reviewing, on a daily basis, the diagnoses on admission and discharge of all the patients attended on at the 24 acute care hospitals in the area of the city of Barcelona. When a diagnosis consistent with meningococcal disease was detected, for example meningitis of unknown cause, the patient was evaluated by a member of the Barcelona Meningococcal Disease Surveillance Group. The complementary system was established to assess the reliability of the main system [34].

The study revealed that, in Barcelona during the period 1987–1992, of every three cases of meningococcal disease diagnosed, one was not notified to the health authorities (under-notification of 30%), despite being a notifiable disease [34]. It also demonstrated that meningococcal disease has the highest incidence rate in children under 10 years old, especially among those aged 1 year or less in whom the incidence rate approaches 100 cases per 100,000 inhabitants per annum (Fig. 33.2). This is true for meningococcemia as well as for other clinical forms of meningococcal disease. The risk of contracting meningococcal disease is inversely related to age. After childhood, the incidence rate shows a sharp decline with a second incidence peak during adolescence (age group 15–19 years) and a slight upturn in old persons (age group 70 years) (Fig. 33.2) [34]. Meningococcal disease is more frequently seen in patients living in the inner city, where other risk factors for infectious diseases, such as overcrowded homes, poor nutrition and hygiene, low levels of education and low family income, are also prevalent [35].

Several risk factors, which we have grouped in Table 33.1, have classically been identified for the acquisition of meningococcal disease, the most serious being exposure to a pathogenic strain of *N. meningitidis* contained in nasopharyngeal secretions of a healthy carrier or patient. Most meningococcal cases acquire the invading strain from a healthy carrier, and secondary cases, i.e., those who acquire the bacterium from another case, constitute no more than 5% of the total number of cases [34]. Unexpectedly, as Osler pointed out as early as 1915, physicians, nurses and other healthcare workers rarely acquire *N. meningitidis* from a patient [36].

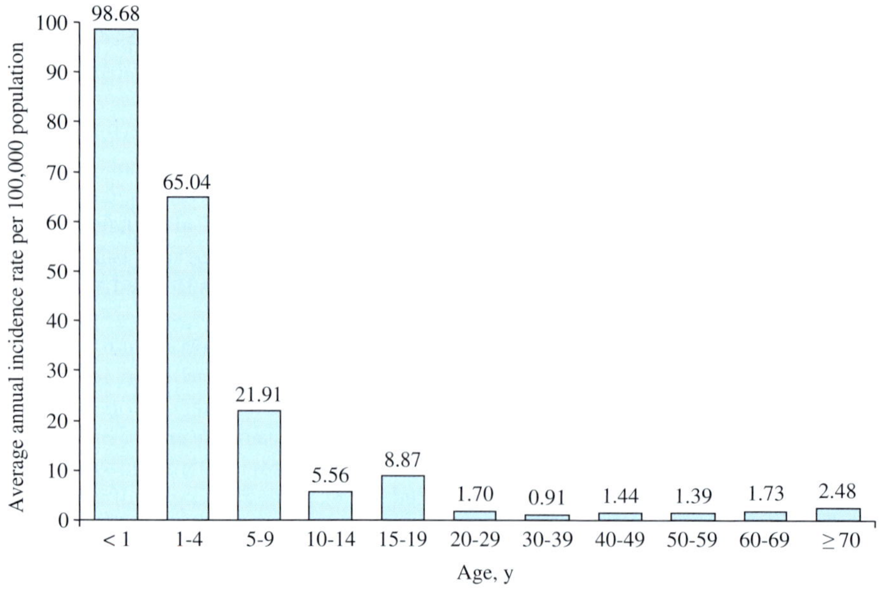

Fig. 33.2. Meningococcal disease in Barcelona (1987–1992): average annual incidence rate by age group (cases detected by active epidemiologic surveillance systems). (From ref. [34])

Table 33.1. Principal factors predisposing to the acquisition of meningococcal disease

Host dependent factors

- Absence of bactericidal antibodies against antigens of the invasive strain
- Age (maximum incidence between 6 months and 5 years)
- Congenital or acquired deficits of complement factors (C2, C3, inactivator of C3b, C5, C6, C7, C8, C9)
- Properdin deficiency
- Immunoglobulin deficiency
- Anatomic or functional asplenia
- FcRIIA polymorphism

***Neisseria meningitidis* dependent factors**

- Presence of capsule
- Certain serogroups and serotypes
- Production and release of endotoxin
- Ability to capture and use iron
- Production of hyaluronidase
- Production of specific IgA1 proteases

Environment dependent factors

- Exposure to a pathogenic strain of *Neisseria meningitidis* contained in nasopharyngeal secretions of a healthy carrier or patient with meningococcal disease
- Crowding (household, day-care centers, schools, universities, barracks, army, closed communities)
- Climatic factors (winter and spring, windy weather in sub-Saharan Africa)
- Recent viral respiratory illness, especially influenza
- Active or passive smoking
- Poor socioeconomic status
- Travel to areas with a high incidence of meningococcal disease

Other risk factors for acquiring meningococcal disease include the immune status of the patient, preceding or concomitant *Mycoplasma pneumoniae* or viral respiratory tract infections, climatological and social conditions and bacterial properties. The formation of protective antibodies against homologous strains was induced by nasopharyngeal carriage of *N. meningitidis*, but, on some occasions, this also produced cross-reacting antibodies to heterologous strains of pathogenic meningococci [37]. Approximately 10% of the population harbors meningococci in the nasopharynx during endemic periods. Nine out of ten strains isolated from carriers are, however, nonpathogenic *Neisseria lactamica* or nonpathogenic *N. meningitidis*, as they are not associated with the clones isolated from patients with meningococcal disease [38].

The carriage rate of meningococci in children younger than 4 years was below 3%. This rate increases with age to a maximum of 24–37% at 15–24 years, and decreases to below 10% in older age groups [38–41]. The carriage rate is higher in lower socioeconomic classes, probably because of crowding, and under conditions where people from different regions are brought together, for example military recruits, prisoners, boarding-school students, or pilgrims [37, 42–44]. Virulent clones have a higher transmission rate, with invasive disease often occurring within the first week after acquisition [45, 46], whereas some people may carry pathogenic meningococci for many months or years without falling ill [47, 48]. A randomly sampled population study performed in an endemic period suggests that acquisition of the pathogenic *N. meningitidis* strains induced illness in only 1% of persons harboring these strains [40].

Vaccination with serogroup C meningococcal polysaccharide-protein conjugate vaccines may reduce nasopharyngeal carriage [49] and could alter the pattern of disease in the unvaccinated [50].

Certain strains of enteric bacteria, such as *Escherichia coli* 07:K1(L):NM and *Bacillus pumilus*, produce capsular polysaccharides that are immunologically identical to the capsular polysaccharides of *N. meningitidis* serogroups A, B, and C, and contribute to the defense against meningococci by the induction of cross-reacting antibodies. This is another potential source of immunization against meningococcal disease [51, 52].

It was suggested that the polymorphism in the neutrophilic receptor for the Fc portion of the immunoglobulins IgG (FcγRIIA) may play a role in the development of meningococcal disease, since neutrophils from patients with low affinity allotypes are less efficient in removing meningococci from the bloodstream [53, 54]. Patients with deficits of the terminal factors of the complement are also colonized more frequently with virulent meningococcal strains that, as serum meningococcidal capacity is diminished, may more frequently cause invasive disease [55].

33.4 Pathogenesis and Pathophysiology

The development of full-blown meningococcal disease necessarily involves three steps, although sometimes only two are necessary to cause clinically apparent disease (Fig. 33.3). First, *N. meningitidis* must colonize the nasopharyngeal mucosa of the patient and must also survive and eventually multiply there. Second, the meningococcus must be able to pass through that mucosa and reach the bloodstream and successfully evade the host defense mechanisms, basically complement-mediated lysis and phagocytosis of immunoglobulin-opsonized meningococci by neutrophils [56]. Finally, if *N. meningitidis* has managed to survive in the bloodstream, it may reach the blood-brain barrier, crossing it only to obtain a sanctuary, the subarachnoid space, where it will virtually have no real limitation to multiply and eventually cause a severe surbarachnoidal inflammatory response [57]. All these steps are modulat-

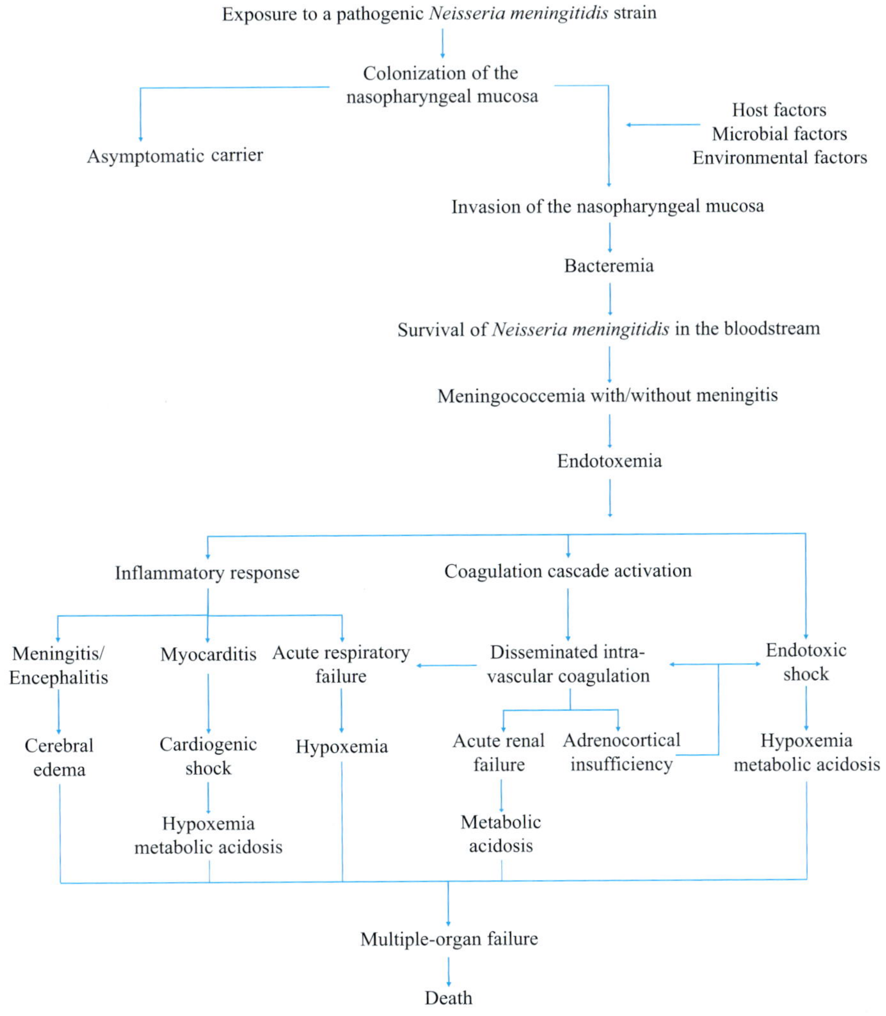

Fig. 33.3. Algorithm of pathogenesis and pathophysiology of meningococcemia

ed in a definite manner by the dynamic interaction established between the microorganism properties, the host and environmental conditions. The main factors are listed in Table 33.1.

Colonization of the human nasopharynx is the first event in the development of human meningococcal disease. The human nasopharyngeal mucosa is the only natural reservoir of *N. meningitidis* [58]. Transmission of meningococcus always occurs from one person to another, by direct contact or via droplets, and the newly infected person is at the greatest risk of developing meningococcal disease [48]. The survival of bacteria in these droplets would appear to be influenced by climatological conditions, such as temperature and humidity. Multiple factors have been identified as favoring meningococcal nasopharyngeal carriage, such as being a close contact of a patient with meningococcal disease, for example household members, healthcare workers, and day-care center workers [59, 60]. Physical damage of nasopharyngeal mucosa by active or passive smoking increases the risk of *N. meningitidis* carriage and meningococcal disease [61–64], as do stressful events and preceding or concomitant *Mycoplasma pneumoniae* or viral upper respiratory tract infections which either alter the integrity of the mucosal surface or influence local or systemic immunity [65–69]. Pili contribute to the attachment to nasopharyngeal mucosal cells [56]. The mechanisms for nasopharyngeal colonization and survival of *N. meningitidis* are not well understood, but since IgA and ciliary activity constitute the cornerstone of mucosal defense, the meningococcus is able to diminish the ciliary activity and to produce an IgA protease [70].

Meningococcus can survive and proliferate in the bloodstream when intravascular killing is impaired, either because of specific virulence factors of the meningococcus itself or because of a naive or defective immune system of the host. The polysaccharide capsule is the most important bacterial virulence factor for survival of the meningococcus in the bloodstream. This protects against complement-mediated bacteriolysis and phagocytosis by neutrophils, and hepatic and spleen macrophages [71]. The capacity to acquire iron from human transferrin by using transferrin binding proteins is another factor involved [72, 73].

Defense against meningococcus within the bloodstream is based on the presence of serum bactericidal antibodies against *N. meningitidis*, a functioning complement system, and its cornerstone is antibody-mediated lysis of meningococci via classical activation. The incidence of meningococcal disease in normal individuals is reciprocally related to the serum concentration of specific antibodies, with the highest incidence occurring from 6 to 24 months of age, when maternal antibodies have disappeared and own antibodies have not yet been generated [34, 37, 42]. Specific antibodies are induced throughout life by the continuously repeated and intermittent carriage of meningococci and *N. lactamica* [74, 75]. As already mentioned, certain strains of enteric bacteria with capsular polysaccharides immunologically identical to certain capsular polysaccharides of *N. meningitidis* induce the production of cross-reacting antibodies [51, 52].

After *N. meningitidis* invades the bloodstream, three main cascade pathways are activated. The first cascade is the complement system that induces the inflammatory reaction via C3a and C5a. The second is the coagulation and fibrinolysis pathway which results in a prothrombotic stage. The third is the inflammatory response mediated by cytokines and chemokines. Genetic polymorphisms among components of these cascade pathways have been involved in the susceptibility, severity, and outcome of meningococcal disease [76].

Effective removal of encapsulated bacteria requires phagocytosis of opsonized bacteria, a process that depends on efficient interaction between antibodies and Fc receptors and between complement and complement receptors [77]. The IgG receptors (FcγRs) are of crucial importance in directing the uptake and destruction of encapsulated bacteria, since FcγRs on phagocytes detect IgG-opsonized microorganisms [78, 79]. The naturally occurring polymorphism of the FcγRIIA may influence neutrophil phagocytic capacity, thus predisposing a patient to handling more or less efficiently the presence of meningococci within the bloodstream [80]. The presence of adequate concentrations of complement, especially terminal factors, is of paramount importance for killing meningococci, since they not only directly damage the bacterial membrane but also improve opsonization and phagocytosis [81]. Patients who have deficits of the terminal factors of the complement exemplify how important it is, and usually present recurrent episodes of meningococcal disease. The possibility of acquiring meningococcal disease increases by up to 6,000-fold due to deficiency of one of the terminal complement factors [55]. Only a few cases can be explained by terminal complement factors or properdin deficiency, due to their rarity. Only 5 cases (1.0%) of 643 patients living in Barcelona diagnosed as having meningococcal disease during 1987–1992 had a complement deficit, this being C7 in 3 cases and C8 in 2 others [34].

Once *N. meningitidis* has been able to survive and eventually multiply within the bloodstream, it may reach the blood-brain barrier and cross it. However, the pathogenic events underlying the development of meningococcal meningitis are beyond the scope of this chapter and will be discussed in the chapter devoted to bacterial meningitis.

Common complications of meningococcemia are vascular collapse and shock and coagulation disorders ranging from laboratory abnormalities to disseminat-

Table 33.2. Meningococcal disease in Barcelona (1987–1992): clinical manifestations by bacteriological form (cases detected by active epidemiologic surveillance systems). (From ref. [34])

Clinical feature	No. (%) of patients				
	Meningococcemia ($n=152$)	Meningitis ($n=165$)	Meningococcemia with meningitis ($n=150$)	Meningococcal disease not microbiologically proved ($n=176$)	All cases ($n=643$)
Fever	148 (97.4)	165 (100)	148 (98.7)	176 (100)	637 (99.1)
Petechiae	112 (73.7)	94 (57.0)	121 (80.7)	176 (100)	503 (78.2)
Headache	25 (16.4)	123 (74.5)	105 (70.0)	101 (57.4)	354 (55.1)
Nausea/vomiting	51 (33.6)	92 (55.8)	73 (48.7)	85 (48.3)	301 (46.8)
Meningeal signs	12 (7.9)	129 (78.2)	83 (55.3)	59 (33.5)	283 (44.0)
Pharyngeal erythema	46 (30.3)	70 (42.4)	58 (38.7)	65 (36.9)	239 (37.2)
Chills[a]	67 (44.1)	36 (21.8)	33 (22.0)	29 (16.5)	165 (25.7)
Abnormal level of consciousness (excluding coma)	11 (7.2)	55 (33.3)	49 (32.7)	40 (22.7)	155 (24.1)
Maculopapular rash	32 (21.1)	20 (12.1)	26 (17.3)	23 (13.1)	101 (15.7)
Ecchymosis	20 (13.2)	12 (7.3)	17 (11.3)	24 (13.6)	73 (11.4)
Myalgia[a]	22 (14.5)	9 (5.5)	15 (10.0)	21 (11.9)	67 (10.4)
Abdominal pain[a]	12 (7.9)	3 (1.8)	9 (6.0)	12 (6.8)	36 (5.6)
Coma	3 (2.0)	17 (10.3)	5 (3.3)	6 (3.4)	31 (4.8)
Arthralgia[a]	6 (3.9)	9 (5.5)	6 (4.0)	6 (3.4)	27 (4.2)
Hemorrhagic diathesis	9 (5.9)	3 (1.8)	8 (5.3)	5 (2.8)	25 (3.9)
Seizures	2 (1.3)	6 (3.6)	6 (4.0)	8 (4.5)	22 (3.4)
Cranial nerve palsies	1 (0.7)	10 (6.1)	3 (2.0)	1 (0.6)	15 (2.3)
Other focal neurologic signs	0 (0)	5 (3.0)	3 (2.0)	3 (1.7)	11 (1.7)

[a] Only patients aged ≥6 years were considered

ed intravascular coagulation (DIC) [82]. Both complications are primarily due to the effects of meningococcal lipo-oligosaccharide, which is a potent endotoxin [83]. There are common causal mechanisms for shock and DIC, two interrelated processes which reinforce each other. For example, microvascular thrombosis leads to hypoperfusion (i.e., shock) and shock induces endothelial damage and DIC [26]. Capillary leakage, inappropriate vascular tone, intravascular microthrombi, and myocardial dysfunction cause shock. DIC and myocardial depression further aggravate the state of shock. Its effects are mediated by TNF-α, IL-1 and IL-6 and by an extensive complement activation, and all these mediators may contribute to the multiple-organ failure and death occurring in the most severe cases [84, 85]. Cytokines also play a pivotal role in the activation and regulation of the coagulation cascade, which in its most severe form causes overwhelming DIC with the formation of microvascular thrombi in various organs [82].

It has been demonstrated that factors intrinsic to the host, such as genetic influences on cytokine production, may contribute to a severe or fatal outcome of meningococcal disease. Among them, death associated with meningococcal disease has been related to a TNF-α gene promoter polymorphism [86], to a low level of TNF production and a high level of IL-10 production [87], and to a functional insertion/deletion (4G/5G) polymorphism in the promoter region of the plasminogen activator inhibitor (PAI)-1 gene [88, 89]. These findings may constitute a genetic background that modulates the host response to meningococcal infection, and eventually its clinical manifestations and outcome.

The major mechanism of death in meningococcemia is circulatory collapse resulting from a combination of capillary leak, intravascular volume depletion, vasodilation and myocardial failure.

33.5 Clinical Features and Forms of Meningococcemia

Meningococcal disease is a protean disease, i.e., its clinical manifestations can be quite varied, ranging from transient fever and bacteremia to fulminant disease with death ensuing within hours of the onset of clinically apparent disease [90]. Despite the fact that variations in the clinical manifestations of meningococcal disease can occur, the trained physician has little doubt when facing a case of full-blown meningococcemia, but diagnosis of sporadic cases requires a high index of suspicion and a careful search for clues of the disease. This is particularly true for patients of extreme ages, where subtle symptoms and signs may be the prodrome of overt disease.

Despite the variety of clinical presentations of meningococcal disease, fever and petechiae are usually present. Petechiae are present in 78.2% of patients, independently of the clinical form of the disease [34]. They usually appear as discrete lesions, 1–2 mm in diameter, most frequently on the trunk and lower portions of the body (Figs. 33.4–33.7). However, in patients with scarce lesions, the mucous surfaces such as the conjunctiva may be the only site affected. Petechiae commonly cluster in areas where pressure may be applied to the skin by elastic underwear or stockings, thus demonstrating the importance of completely disrobing the patient for an adequate examination [1]. The initial number and progression of petechiae is important and a simple means to monitor both the evolution of the disease and the effectiveness of therapy. A common practice is to circle areas with petechiae, count those within the circle, and document the number of petechial lesions present per a given unit of time. The counts should be performed hourly early in the disease or until the patient clinically stabilizes.

Petechiae are a common harbinger of meningococcal disease, but occasionally if the patient is not completely undressed when examined or if examination of mucous surfaces such as the palpebral conjunctiva is omitted, important telltale lesions can be missed [1]. The finding of petechiae or purpura in a febrile patient should increase the index of suspicion for meningococcemia.

Petechial rash is not the only cutaneous manifestation of meningococcal disease, and a maculopapular eruption that can resemble a viral exanthem, particularly rubella, has also been described [91]. This rash is neither purpuric nor pruritic and is usually transient, generally not lasting more than 2 days, and most frequently disappears hours after the first observation. In cases of fulminant meningococcal disease, the skin lesions dominate the clinical appearance and may evidence coalescence of increasing petechiae, septic vas-

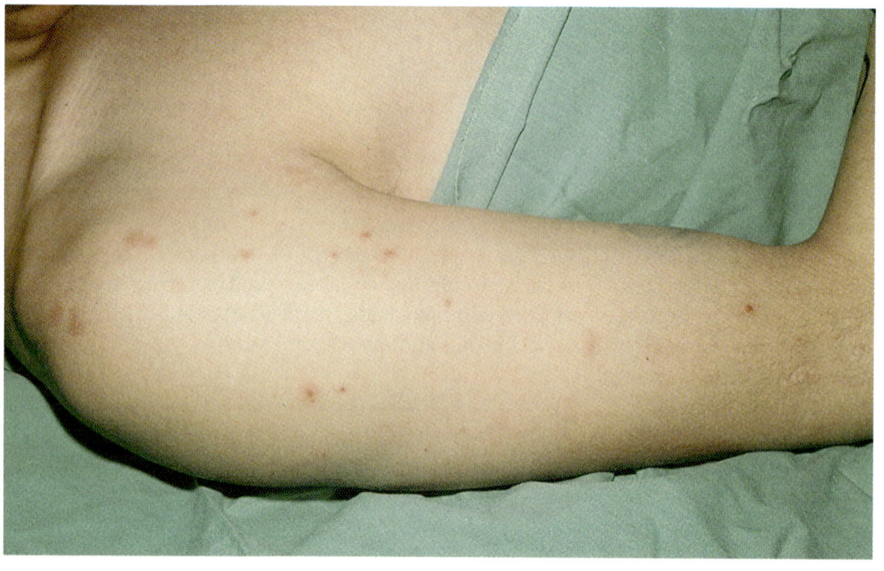

Fig. 33.4. Petechiae in the arm of a patient with meningococcemia

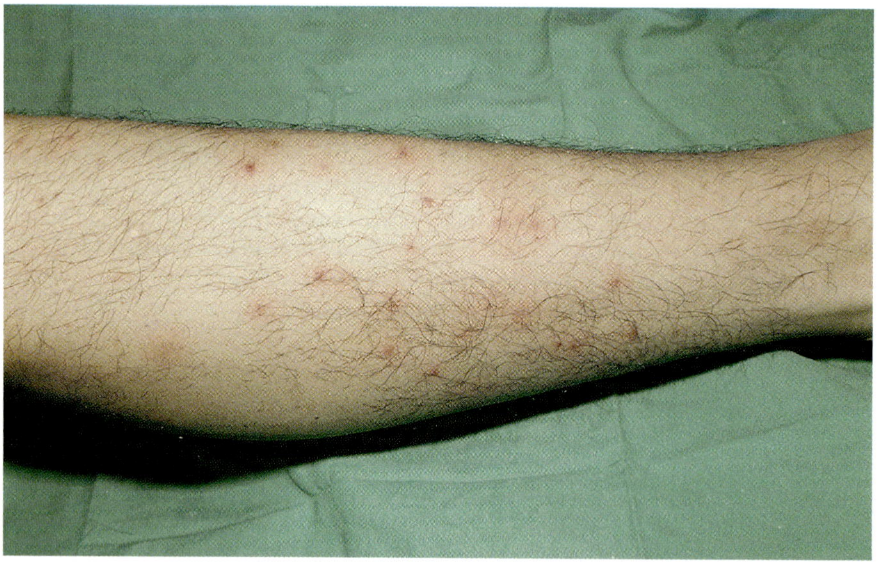

Fig. 33.5. Petechiae in the leg of a patient with meningococcemia

culitis, together with ecchymoses, purpura, subcutaneous hematoma, and hemorrhagic bullae covering a majority of the body surface [92]. Skin hemorrhages are the distinguishing feature par excellence of meningococcal disease and are usually the visual manifestations of DIC (Figs. 33.8, 33.9). These cutaneous signs frequently coexist with other signs of DIC, such as spontaneous clinically apparent bleeding, including bleeding from wounds, hematuria, spontaneous gingival bleeding, epistaxis, gastrointestinal or gynecological bleeding, and peripuncture bruises or puncture bleeding at the time of establishing venous or arterial access, intramuscular injection, lumbar puncture, or others.

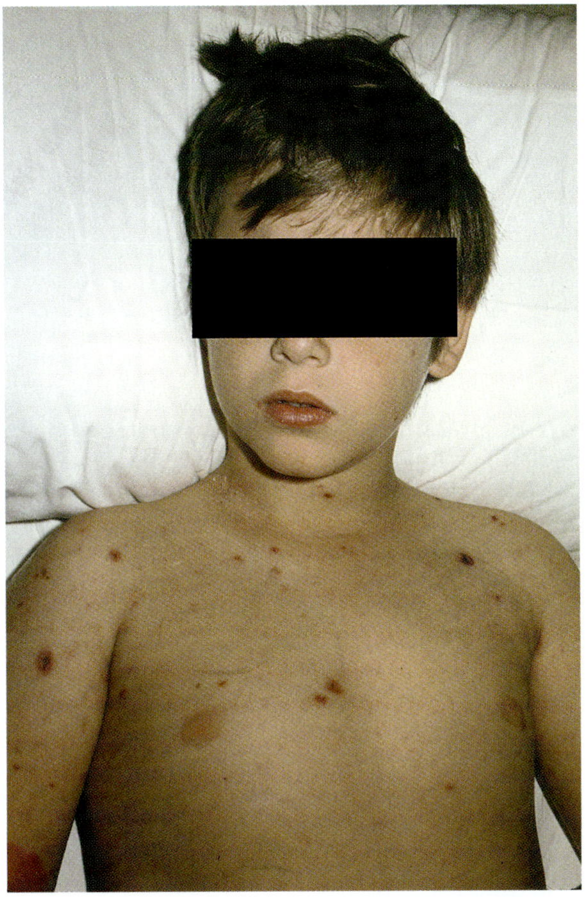

Fig. 33.6. Purpuric lesions in a young child with meningococcemia

All of these are signs of ominous prognosis [34, 93] and are present characteristically in the fulminant form of meningococcemia, together with a profound endotoxic shock with hemorrhagic destruction of adrenal glands (Waterhouse-Friderichsen syndrome) or peripheral symmetric gangrene (*purpura fulminans*) (Fig. 33.10). DIC is a generalized phenomenon which affects all organs, but the adrenals are especially vulnerable [94]. Adrenal hemorrhages can cause adrenal insufficiency [95]. However, the intracerebral vessels are spared during fulminant meningococcemia [26].

The fulminant form of meningococcal disease, defined as interval of symptoms to therapy lower than 7 h and shock on hospital admission, affects 3.9–5.3% of patients [34, 93]. When present, shock dominates the clinical picture, with a poorly responsive patient, intense peripheral vasoconstriction and cyanotic and poorly perfused extremities. Blood analyses demonstrate metabolic acidosis and usually hypoxia. Fulminant meningococcemia is characterized by shock and DIC, two interrelated processes. Shock and DIC have a rapid onset and characteristic skin hemorrhages that allow bedside diagnosis. Shock and DIC have common causal mechanisms and reinforce each other. For example, microvascular thrombosis leads to hypoperfusion and shock leads to endothelial damage and DIC [26]. To quote Hardaway, "Shock is both cause and effect of DIC" [96].

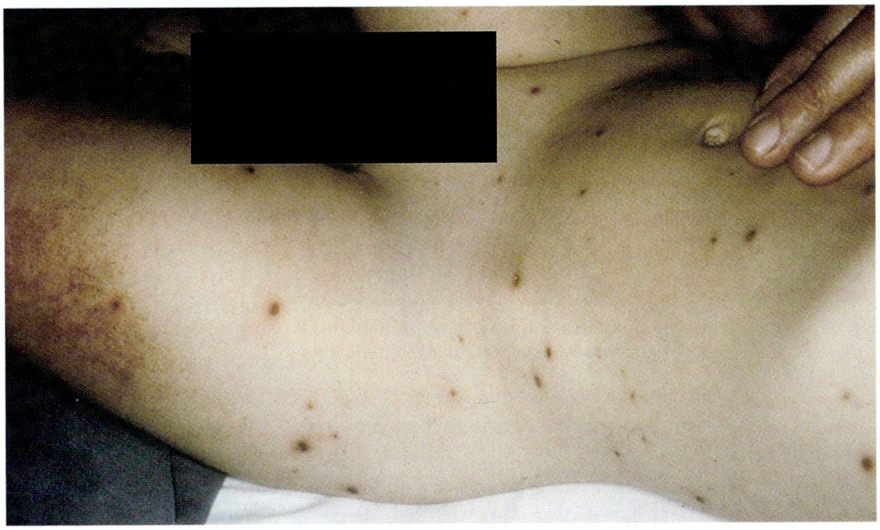

Fig. 33.7. Septic vasculitis in a patient with meningococcemia

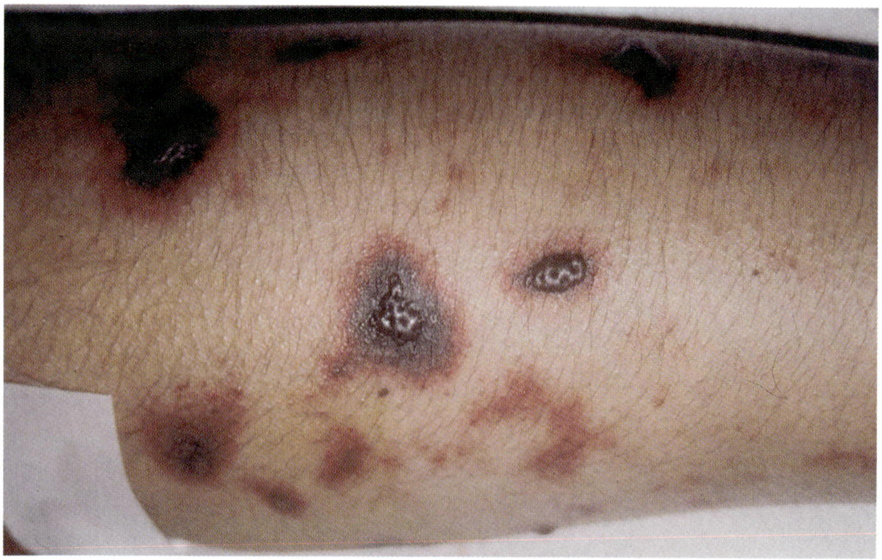

Fig. 33.8. Subcutaneous ecchymosis in a patient with fulminant meningococcemia

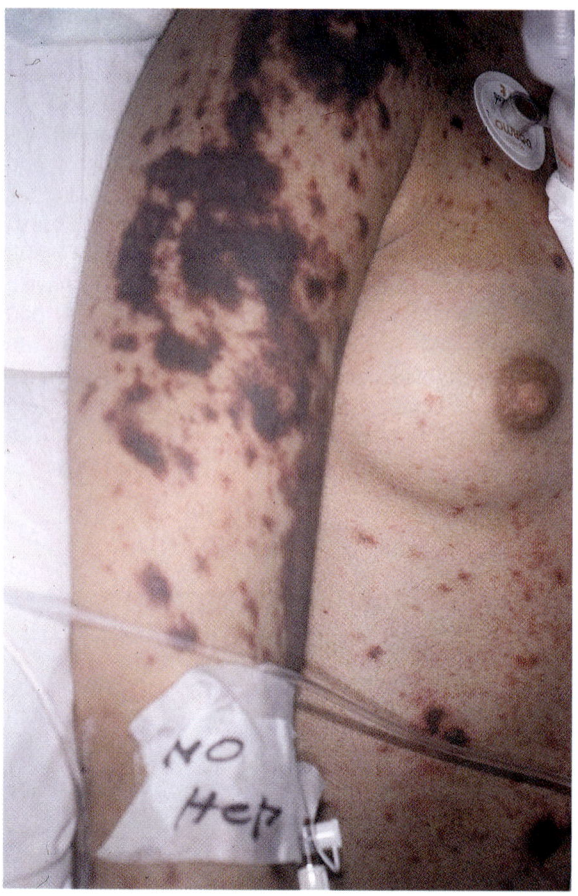

Fig. 33.9. Extensive ecchymosis in a patient with fulminant meningococcemia and disseminated intravascular coagulation

A very important prognostic sign is myocardial involvement that manifests itself by the presence of gallop rhythm, congestive cardiac failure with pulmonary edema and poor peripheral perfusion [97]. Some degree of myocarditis has been demonstrated in more than half of the patients who die of meningococcal disease [98, 99]. Another frequent complaint in meningococcemia is generalized muscle tenderness, sometimes with very intense pain, that can be an important differential sign [90].

Wolfe and Birbara have distinguished four clinical situations in meningococcal disease: bacteremia without sepsis, meningococcemia without meningitis, meningitis with or without meningococcemia, and the meningoencephalitic presentation [100]. The latter two clinical forms will be discussed in the chapter devoted to bacterial meningitis. Benign, occult or inapparent meningococcemia is caused by a low-degree bacteremia, ranging from 22 to 325 organisms per milliliter, from a primary upper respiratory source [101]. In fact, the patient or parent seeks medical attention because of an upper respiratory illness or rash of presumed viral origin [34]. After recovery, or more frequently after discharge from the hospital without specific antimicrobial therapy, the results of blood cultures are reported positive for *N. meningitidis*. This form of meningococcal disease accounts for 2% of the total number of cases [34].

When isolated meningococcemia or meningococcemia without meningitis is present, the patient looks septic, usually with a skin rash, generalized malaise, weakness, headache, and muscle tenderness. Frequently hypotension appears on admission or shortly thereafter. Isolated meningococcemias represents around 23.6% of the total cases of meningococcal disease [34]. When meningococcemia occurs in the setting of meningococcal meningitis, symptoms and signs attributable to meningitis usually dominate the clinical picture. Finally, variations of manifestations may occur, and the patient can progress from one to the other form during the course of the disease [102].

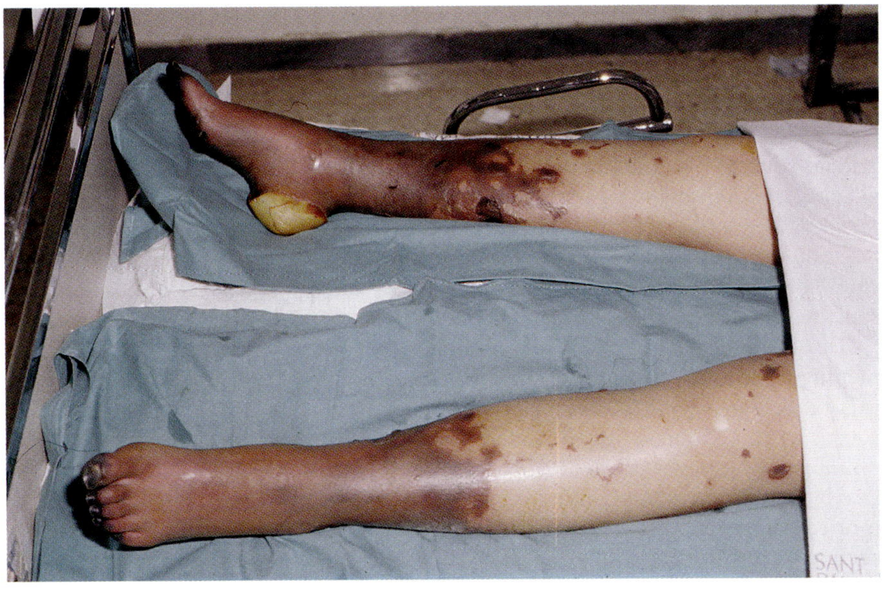

Fig. 33.10. Symmetric peripheral gangrene in *purpura fulminans*

A specific and infrequent form of meningococcal disease called chronic meningococcemia, that is characterized by low-grade fever, rash, and arthritis, is also known [103–107]. Chronic meningococcemia is defined as meningococcal septicemia without meningeal symptoms in which fever has persisted for at least 1 week before initiation of any antibiotic therapy [108]. From a clinical point of view, the cutaneous lesions are identical to those seen in chronic gonococcemia, and *N. meningitidis* is thought to be increasing as a cause of the arthritis-dermatitis syndrome [109].

In patients with repeated flares of meningococcemia, complement deficiencies must be ruled out [55]. Although a primary focus for meningococcemia is seldom found, a portal of entry can sometimes be identified. The most frequent are the conjunctiva, and the lung [110, 111].

33.6 Diagnosis

Early diagnosis and immediate recognition of deterioration are of crucial importance because meningococcal disease can be fatal within a few hours. The clinical diagnosis of meningococcal disease does not usually pose many problems for an experienced physician from an endemic area when faced with a characteristic case. However, in some cases, early diagnosis of meningococcemia is extremely difficult and requires a high degree of suspicion [112, 113].

The hallmarks for the clinical diagnosis of meningococcal disease are the presence of fever and petechiae, and they form the basis for the criteria of the Meningococcal Disease Surveillance Group to establish a clinical diagnosis of meningococcal disease [114]. Following its criteria, a patient can be diagnosed as having meningococcal disease when having an illness with fever and petechiae, diagnosed as meningococcal disease by the local physician, even if there is no blood or CSF isolate of *N. meningitidis*. In our epidemiological environment (western Europe), there are only a few diseases that may resemble meningococcal disease. Among them, viral illnesses, bacteremia caused by *Haemophilus influenzae*, *Streptococcus pneumoniae* and other Gram-positive cocci, rickettsiosis, and autoimmune purpuras may cause a rash that can simulate meningococcal disease. In North America, rickettsiosis of the Rocky Mountain spotted fever group may pose a greater diagnostic dilemma. Furthermore, only 78 % of the patients with meningococcal disease will present an identifiable rash, and in those cases in which there are no cutaneous signs, the clinical presentation is entirely indistinguishable from other bacteremic diseases, and these patients are more prone not to be identified when they first seek medical attention [34].

Twelve percent of patients diagnosed as having meningococcal disease in Barcelona from 1987 to 1992 had been seen by a hospital physician but were sent home from the emergency service with an erroneous diagnosis of upper respiratory tract infection or viral illness. Meningococcal disease was only diagnosed in a subsequent visit [34].

The gold standard for diagnosis of meningococcal disease (a definite diagnosis) is based on recovering *N. meningitidis* from a usually sterile body fluid such as blood, CSF, or rarely synovial, pleural or pericardial fluids. Obviously, the CSF and blood are the most fruitful sources of positive cultures. In our experience, blood cultures were positive in 47.0 % of cases [34], whereas in the experience of others they were positive in 51.4% of cases [115]. However, even in patients who do not have clinical meningitis, *N. meningitidis* can be recovered from a CSF culture, and CSF is otherwise normal in terms of protein and glucose contents and cellular count [116]. Another possible source of meningococci, although with a variable ability to isolate *N. meningitidis*, is the petechial skin or mucosal lesions. Some authors have reported isolation in 69.8% of petechial smears, but once again interpretation of these specimens may be difficult [115].

Throat swabs play a limited role in the diagnosis of meningococcal disease, since a third of young adults carry meningococci, and thus isolation of a meningococcus from a young adult with meningococcemia is uninformative. However, meningococci are rarely carried by infants and young children (1–4%), and therefore isolation of a well-capsulated meningococcus from such a patient with meningococcemia must be valid [117]. Rapid methods for microbiologic diagnosis, such as Gram stain, detection of meningococcal antigens by means of counterimmunoelectrophoresis, latex agglutination, and coagglutination, and the polymerase chain reaction, have been useful for the diagnosis of meningococcal meningitis, but their use in an environment of meningococcemia has yet to be determined. Polymerase chain reaction analysis offers the advantages of detecting serogroup-specific *N. meningitidis* DNA and of not requiring live organisms for a positive result.

From 35.2% to 43.7% of patients with meningococcal disease have received antibiotics prior to hospital admission [34, 93]. These patients, who can still be diagnosed as having meningococcal disease if they fulfill the criteria established by the Meningococcal Disease Surveillance Group [114], will have in a greater proportion no positive microbiologic data to support the diagnosis. Meningococcal disease not microbiologically proved represents 27.4% of the total number of patients with the disease [34]. In these patients, methods such as those that look for bacterial antigens or bacterial DNA may play a diagnostic role.

33.7 Management of Meningococcemia

Although significant advances in the treatment of meningococcal disease were made early in the twentieth century by means of serum therapy from immunized horses [118, 119], the introduction of sulfonamides by Schwentker [120] in 1937, and penicillin by Rosenberg and Arling [121] in 1944, dramatically altered the previously ominous prognosis of meningococcal disease. However, sulfonamides play a very limited role in the treatment of meningococcal disease since meningococci became widely resistant to sulfonamides early in the 1960s [122].

Antibiotics are the cornerstone of treatment. It is necessary to begin antibiotic therapy as soon as possible, and this should never be delayed by diagnostic procedures (Fig. 33.11). A gold standard of therapeutics is to establish antibiotic treatment before 30 min following patient admission to the hospital emergency unit. Therapy should be extended to include immediate fluid resuscitation, a prompt beginning of mechanical ventilation, and transfer to a suitably equipped ICU in patients with poor prognostic signs or imminent shock [26]. The usual doses of the most common antibiotics used in the treatment of meningococcal disease are given in Table 33.3.

Penicillin has for decades been the treatment of choice for meningococcal disease. However, since the mid-1980s, there has been an increasing frequency of isolation of meningococcal strains with decreased susceptibility to penicillin, mainly from Spain [123], the United Kingdom [124], and South Africa [125]. In Spain, the prevalence of meningococcal strains relatively resistant to penicillin rose from the mid-1980s to a maximum of 70.0% in 1997 and 75.2% in 2002 (Fig. 33.12) [123]. Since then, these figures have stabilized at around 50–60% of strains. This reduced sensitivity is due to a reduced affinity to penicillin binding protein type 2 [123]. Penicillin resistance due to plasmid-related β-lactamase production occasionally occurs [126]. Although the present rate of partially resistant strains has potential implications for empiric therapy of bacterial meningitis, it probably should not affect penicillin-based therapeutic strategies of meningococcemia. Standard doses of penicillin (i.e., 250,000 units/kg/day) will provide an adequate serum level that usually surpasses the MIC for partially resistant isolates by many times [127]. Thus, penicillin can still be used safely in the treatment of meningococcemia. The usual recommended dose of penicillin is 300,000 units/kg/day with an upper limit of 24 million units/day as 2 million units q2 h.

Notwithstanding the fact that penicillin or chloramphenicol therapy may be successful, it does not eradicate the meningococcus from the nasopharynx [128], as bactericidal concentrations are not reached in the nasopharyngeal and respiratory secretions, and thus patients treated with penicillin or chloramphenicol should be given rifampin chemoprophylaxis before discharge from the hospital to prevent reentry of the pathogenic *N. meningitidis* strain into the household or another group of which the patient forms part [129, 130]. It has, however, been shown that on discharge from hospital only 1% of patients were nasopharyngeal carriers of pathogenic meningococci [128, 131, 132]. It is not necessary to establish chemoprophylaxis if the meningococcal disease has been treated with ceftriaxone or cefotaxime.

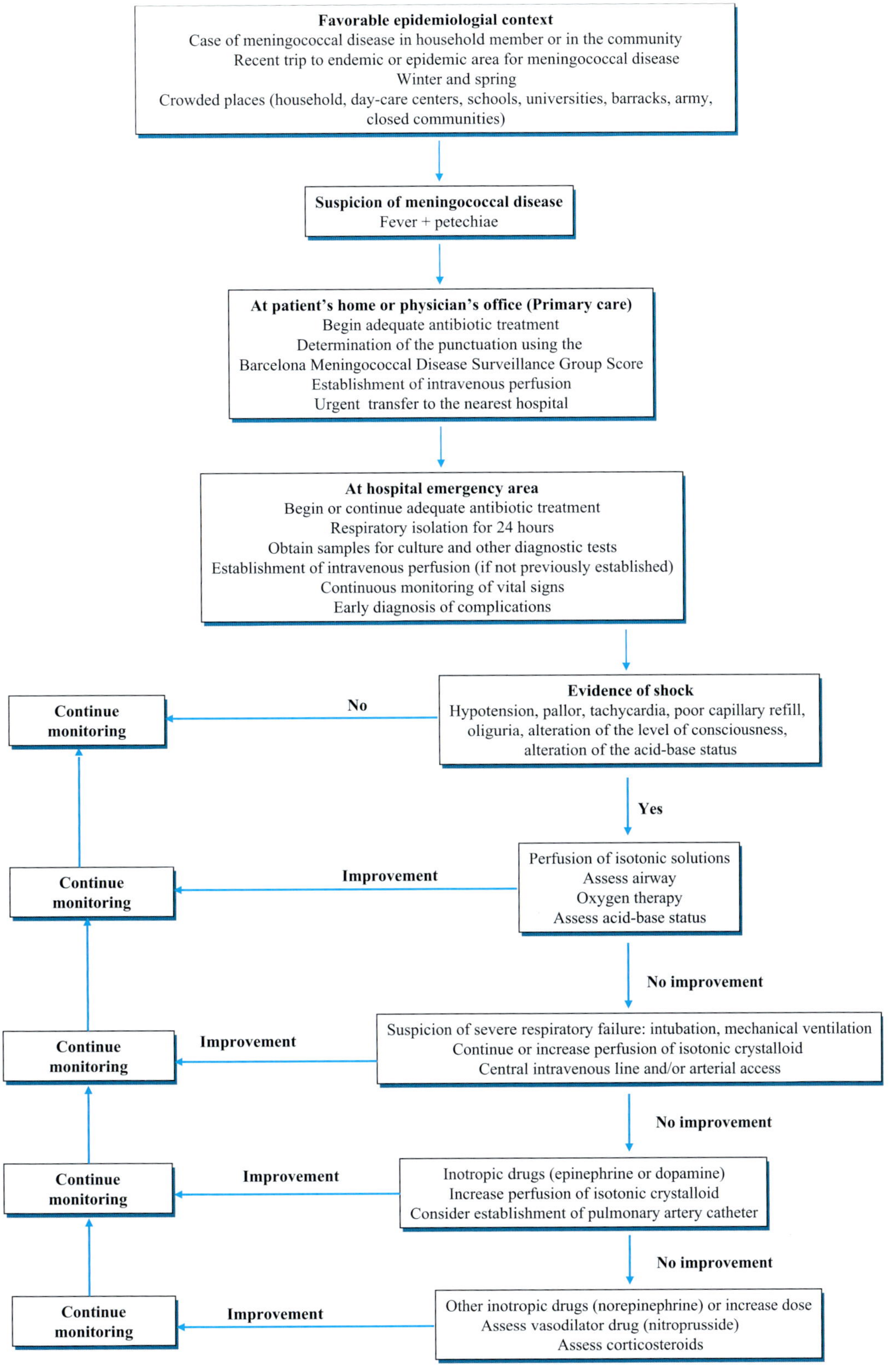

Fig. 33.11a. Algorithm of management for meningococcemia

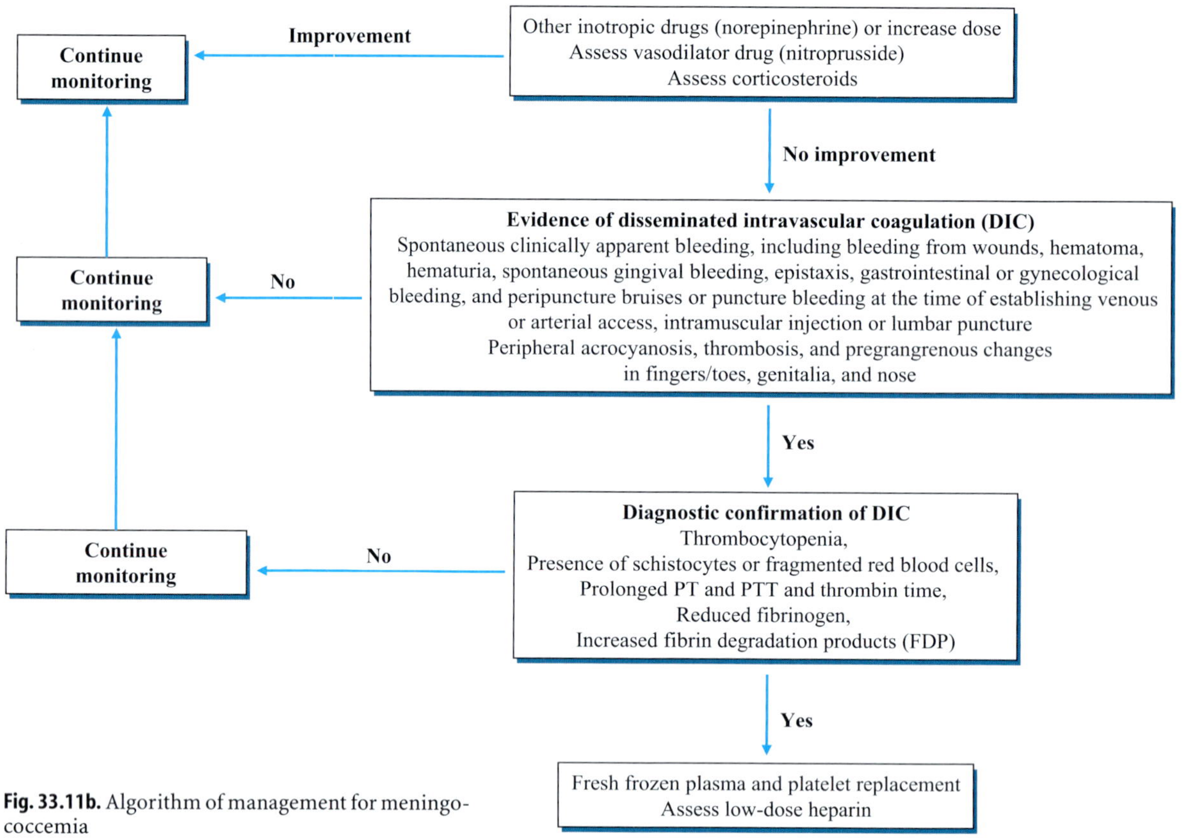

Fig. 33.11b. Algorithm of management for meningococcemia

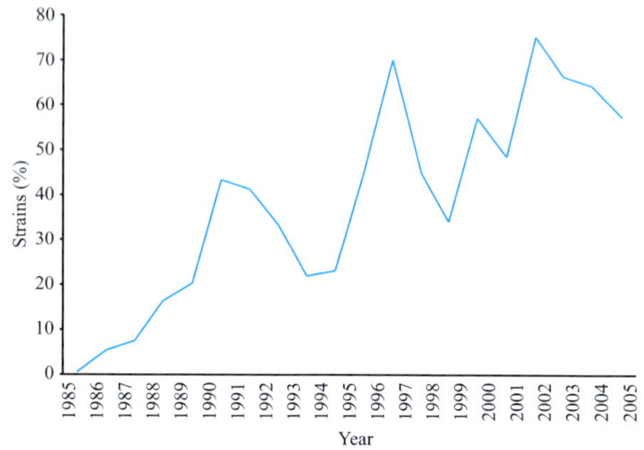

Fig. 33.12. Prevalence of decreased susceptibility to penicillin *Neisseria meningitidis* strains isolated in Spain (1985–2005)

With indiscriminate chemoprophylaxis it is possible to sterilize the nasopharynx in the absence of pathogenic strains of meningococcus and to eliminate the nonpathogenic strains of *Neisseria* or other nonpathogenic germs which compete with *N. meningitidis* for the colonization of the nasopharynx. Nonselective chemoprophylaxis prevents the protective immunological response by means of crossed reactivity and allows the colonization de novo of pathogenic *N. meningitidis* strains. It is therefore recommended to proceed with selective chemoprophylaxis which consists in carrying out a nasopharyngeal exudate culture, having obtained the sample by smear, and only carrying out chemoprophylaxis in the event of detecting the presence of pathogenic meningococci strains.

Third-generation cephalosporins are increasingly used in the empirical treatment of bacterial meningitis and meningococcal disease due to a better coverage of all possible etiologies of bacterial meningitis and because of the fear of resistance. Third-generation cephalosporins, including cefotaxime, ceftriaxone, ceftizoxime, and ceftazidime and the second-generation cefuroxime have been successfully used for the treatment of meningococcal meningitis [133–135]. For patients who are allergic to penicillin, aztreonam may be a safe alternative. Also, for patients allergic to penicillin, chloramphenicol at a dose of 100 mg/kg/day up to a maximum of 4 g/day administered intravenously may be an effective substitute for penicillin and in Third World countries it can be administered in its depot formulation by the intramuscular route. The duration of antibiotic therapy will vary, but usually 7 days is enough when the meningococcus is sensitive to the antibiotic used.

The epidemiological study on meningococcal disease carried out in Barcelona during 1987–1992 dem-

Table 33.3. Antibiotics used in the treatment and chemoprophylaxis of meningococcal disease

Meningococcemia treatment

Non-penicillin-allergic
Penicillin G Na
Adults: 300,000 units/kg/day IV (in divided doses every 4 h), up to 24 million units/day
Ceftriaxone
Adults: 100 mg/kg/day IV (in divided doses every 12 h), up to 4 g/day
Children: 50 mg/kg/day IV (in divided doses every 12 h), up to 2 g/day
Cefotaxime
Adults: 200 mg/kg/day IV (in divided doses every 6 h), up to 12 g/day
Meropenem
Adults: 3.0 g/day IV (in divided doses every 8 h)

Penicillin-allergic
Chloramphenicol
Adults: 100 mg/kg/day IV (in divided doses every 6 h), up to 4 g/day
Aztreonam
Adults: 150 mg/kg/day IV (in divided doses every 8 h), up to 12 g/day

Chemoprophylaxis
Rifampin
Adults: 600 mg/12 h PO, for 2 days (4 doses)
Children > 1 month: 10 mg/kg/12 h PO, up to 600 mg/12 h, for 2 days (4 doses)
Children ≤ 1 month: 5 mg/kg/12 h PO, for 2 days (4 doses)
Ceftriaxone
Adults: 250 mg IM, single dose
Children > 12 years: 250 mg IM, single dose
Children ≤ 12 years: 125 mg IM, single dose
Ciprofloxacin
Adults: 500 mg PO, single dose
Levofloxacin
Adults: 500 mg PO, single dose
Ofloxacin
Adults: 400 mg PO, single dose
Minocycline
Adults: 100 mg/12 h PO, for 5 days
Spiramycin
Adults: 500 mg/6 h PO, for 5 days
Children: 10 mg/kg/6 h PO, for 5 days
Azithromycin
Adults: 500 mg PO, single dose

[a] Ciprofloxacin, ofloxacin, and minocycline are contraindicated in children, pregnant woman or lactating women

onstrated that pre-admission antibiotic therapy was an independent predictor of a better outcome, reducing mortality and the incidence of sequelae in surviving patients [34, 93]. On the basis of this result, the administration of adequate antibiotic prior to hospitalization is recommended as soon as meningococcal disease is suspected, as this is the only way that the physician has, at a non-hospital level (at patient's home or physician's office), to improve the patient's prognosis. This measure should be carried out provided that it does not represent an important delay in the

Table 33.4. Prognostic factors for patients with meningococcal disease: bedside clinical parameters for prediction of outcome. (From ref. [93])

Barcelona Meningococcal Disease Surveillance Group Score Parameter	Points
Preadmission antibiotic therapy	−1
Age ≥ 60 years	1
Focal neurologic signs[a]	1
Hemorrhagic diathesis[b]	2

Probability of death according to observed score Prediction score	Case-fatality rate (%)
−1	0
0	2.3
1	27.3
2	73.3
≥ 3	100

[a] Motor, sensory, or cranial nerve disturbances of central origin
[b] Spontaneous clinically apparent bleeding, including bleeding from wounds, hematoma, hematuria, spontaneous gingival bleeding, epistaxis, gastrointestinal or gynecological bleeding, and peripuncture bruises or puncture bleeding at the time of establishing venous or arterial access, intramuscular injection or lumbar puncture

transfer of the patient to hospital. Before carrying out this study, microbiologists advised against administering antibiotics before obtaining the blood and/or CSF samples for culture, as this significantly reduces the likelihood of recovering *N. meningitidis*. At present, with methods such as PCR which do not require live bacteria to obtain a positive result, this inconvenience is no longer relevant. Studies in the United Kingdom have suggested that early administration of parenteral penicillin by general practitioners, as soon as the diagnosis was entertained, significantly improved the prognosis of patients pre-treated in this way [136–141].

The clinical management of a patient with meningococcal disease, whether meningococcemia or meningococcal meningitis, should always be treated as a medical emergency. The initial management of meningococcemia includes the rapid administration of antibiotic therapy and the continuous monitoring of the patient's vital signs for early detection of the appearance of complications (Fig. 33.11). Respiratory isolation is indicated until 24 h after the first dose of antibiotics. The infectivity of the patient disappears quickly once the first doses of antibiotic have been administered. The measures aimed at preventing contagion in the initial hours, apart from respiratory isolation, are the use by healthcare staff of masks, eye protection, white coat, gloves and hand-washing.

The most common and important manifestation requiring urgent intervention in meningococcal disease is vascular collapse and shock. This occurs in 12.1% of all the cases of meningococcal disease and is far more frequent in isolated meningococcemia than when there is concomitant meningitis [34]. For the first few hours, it is necessary to monitor patients closely as shock can develop after starting antibiotic therapy [142]. It should be taken into account that monitoring the systolic blood pressure in children is not sufficient to trace the development of shock. Low diastolic blood pressure, delayed capillary refill, cold extremities, and tachycardia are better indicators [26]. Good clinical surveillance and frequent laboratory monitoring are crucial. For example, on observing an increase in the number and size of skin hemorrhages and a decrease in the platelet count, it is easy to monitor the progression of DIC [26, 143].

Patients with the fulminant form of meningococcal disease characteristically have a severe capillary leak syndrome together with myocardial dysfunction. Thus, supportive care should include optimizing preload, decreasing afterload, and improving myocardial contractility. All of this is best accomplished in the ICU setting. Intravenous fluid administration should be implemented, together with inotropic and vasopressive support with dobutamine or dopamine, tailored to the needs of each patient on the basis of clinical assessment and of monitoring of systemic arterial pressure and central venous pressure or pulmonary wedge pressure [144–147]. During the first 24 h, administration of 8–10 l of intravenous fluid may be necessary. The severity of shock has been correlated by various studies with serum levels of TNF-α, IL-1, IL-6, and lipo-oligosaccharide [84, 148, 149]. These findings and the encouraging results obtained in animal models have suggested that treatment with monoclonal antibodies against some of the cytokines or the endotoxin could be of use in humans [150–153].

Some therapeutic successes were initially published with the humanized anti-lipid A IgM antibody HA-1A and with protein C concentrate infusions [154]. However, in human controlled trials *E. coli* J5 antibodies, humanized anti-lipid A IgM antibody HA-1A, and recombinant bactericidal/permeability-increasing protein (rBPI) failed to show protection [155–158]. The negative results of the antiendotoxin therapies can be explained by the poor neutralizing potency of the antibodies or by the timing of administration [26].

The use of glucocorticoids in the treatment of meningococcemia in patients with evidence of *purpura fulminans* and adrenal hemorrhagic necrosis (Waterhouse-Friderichsen syndrome) is still controversial [159, 160]. Several controlled studies of patients with shock have demonstrated no benefit of high-dose glucocorticoid treatment. However, in many acute care hospitals glucocorticoids belong to the standard treatment protocol of fulminant meningococcemia with extensive DIC and shock or suspicion of Waterhouse-Friderichsen syndrome [26]. Some patients with meningococcemia have a profound respiratory failure, and in this case and in those who have received high amounts of intravenous fluid and those in which profound shock has occurred, mechanical ventilation should be started immediately [161].

The problem of DIC is particularly ominous and its presence is an independent predictor of death [34, 93]. As shock and DIC are interrelated processes, the only successful treatment of DIC is the therapy against shock. The routine use of heparin has not improved the prognosis of DIC. Endovascular thrombosis, ischemia, and imminent autoamputation may, however, lead to additional treatment. Heparin therapy has been suggested for this purpose [162, 163]. Patients with impending peripheral gangrene (Fig. 33.10) and severe coagulopathy should be treated with low-dose heparin (10 units/kg/h) together with fresh frozen plasma with the aim of restoring depleted levels of antithrombin III, protein C, and protein S [164–166].

Antithrombin III infusion [167], topical nitroglycerin [168, 169], extracorporeal membrane oxygenation [170, 171], hemofiltration [163, 172], and plasma or whole-blood exchange with or without leukapheresis [173–176] have been tried in a few cases of fulminant and refractory meningococcemia with variable results. Continuous caudal block has been used to restore lower extremity perfusion in a child with meningococcemia [177]. In order to restore perfusion to pregangrenous limbs, thrombolytic therapy offers the best hope, and there are anecdotal reports of the beneficial effects of recombinant tissue plasminogen activator [146, 178–181].

Metabolic acidosis as a result of poor tissue perfusion in shock may appear, and serum electrolytes and acid-base balance may be monitored closely and abnormalities corrected immediately. Correction is often hampered by acute renal failure, and thus continuous plasma filtration or dialysis may be necessary in anuria due to acute tubular necrosis or cortical necrosis associated with meningococcal septic shock [182]. Alkalinization is recommended in patients with severe rhabdomyolysis in order to prevent myoglobin-induced renal failure [26].

33.8 Outcome and Prognosis

Despite adequate antibiotic therapy and supportive care, meningococcal disease causes an overall mortality of 6–15% of patients [21, 34, 183, 184]. Still today meningococcal disease is the third cause of death in children, only surpassed by casual injuries and malignant diseases. In Barcelona, over 6 years meningococcal disease caused the loss of 1,842 potential years of life (average annual, 18 per 100,000 inhabitants) [34]. In this study, performed in Barcelona by active epidemiologic surveillance systems from 1987 to 1992, the average annual mortality rate was 0.40 per 100,000 and among children under 10 years it was 2.23 per 100,000 (Fig. 33.13) [34]. Multiple-organ failure is the most frequent cause of death (65.0–76.5% of deaths), followed by cerebral edema (13.7–25.0%), and myocarditis (9.8–10.0%) [34, 93].

Meningococcemia is the clinical form of meningococcal disease with the highest case-fatality rate (11.2%), and with fulminant meningococcemia this is 43.8–44.0% of patients [34, 93]. There is rapid clinical deterioration, and approximately half of the patients who die will do so within 24 h of the appearance of the first symptoms. A third of the patients with fatal meningococcal disease die within 6 h of hospital admission and another third die between 6 and 18 h [26, 185, 186]. Death at a later stage is still determined by the course in the early hours, as shown by the fact that the main cause of death after 24 h is withdrawal of treatment because of poor neurological prognosis after prolonged cerebral hypoperfusion in the early hours [187].

The ability to define the outcome of meningococcal disease based on a number of indicators has been extensively studied and several scoring systems, with clinical and laboratory parameters, may be applied to patients in order to identify severity [186, 188–200]. The Barcelona Meningococcal Disease Surveillance Group designed and validated a very simple scoring system that is based entirely on clinical parameters very easy to determine at the patient's bedside [93].

The Barcelona Meningococcal Disease Surveillance Group Score was prospectively developed (624 patients in the derivation set) and validated (283 patients in the validation set) in all age groups and in all clinical forms of microbiologically proved meningococcal disease (meningococcaemia and/or meningococcal meningitis) [93]. The score was also validated in microbiologically unproved meningococcal disease [34]. Hemorrhagic diathesis was scored with 2 points, presence of focal neurologic signs with 1 point, age of 60 years or older with 1 point, and preadmission antibiotic therapy was scored as −1. The clinical scores of −1, 0, 1, 2, and 3 or more points were associated with a probability of death of 0%, 2.3%, 27.3%, 73.3%, and 100%, respectively (Table 33.4). Prospective validation of this score has shown a score >1 to best identify patients at high risk of dying and a score equal to −1 accurately identifying patients with no mortality. It is one of the more accurate scoring systems and was predictive of death in 82.4% of the patients [93].

The main attraction of the Barcelona Meningococcal Disease Surveillance Group Score is its simplicity, and therefore its speed, as it includes only four easily available clinical parameters obtained at the bedside by the physician or another well-trained health professional and not just in the hospital emergency area or intensive care unit, but even in the physician's office or the patient's home.

The Barcelona Meningococcal Disease Surveillance Group Score is a widely used score, in many hospital emergency areas and intensive care units, and has been used to select the patients for which speed of transfer to hospital (ambulance vs. helicopter), admission to an intensive care unit, and establishment of more aggressive treatments is a priority or to stratify the patients according to their prognosis for clinical trials. It also provides a useful tool for evaluating the impact on survival of new therapeutic strategies.

The probability of death in meningococcal disease related to the presence or absence of predictors of death is shown in Fig. 33.13. Patients with the highest probability of dying were those with hemorrhagic diathesis, whereas those with no predictor of death and who had received preadmission adequate antibiotics had the best prognosis.

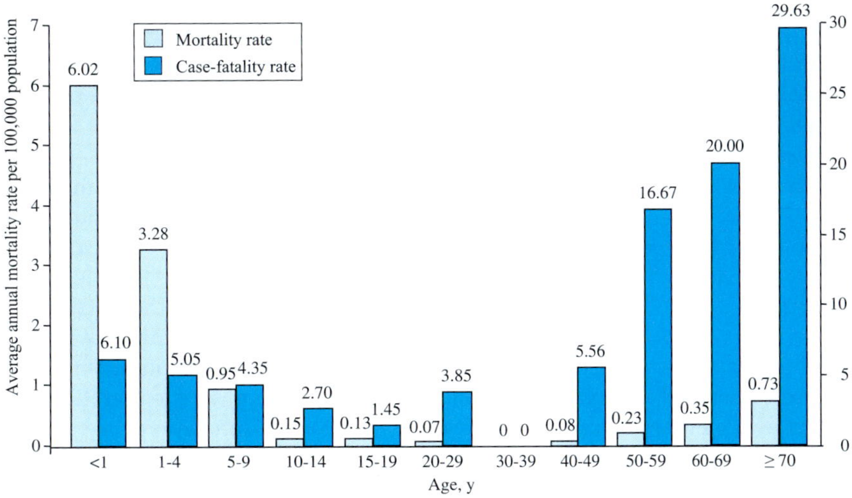

Fig. 33.13. Meningococcal disease in Barcelona (1987–1992): average annual mortality rate and case-fatality rate by age group (cases detected by active epidemiologic surveillance systems). (From ref. [34])

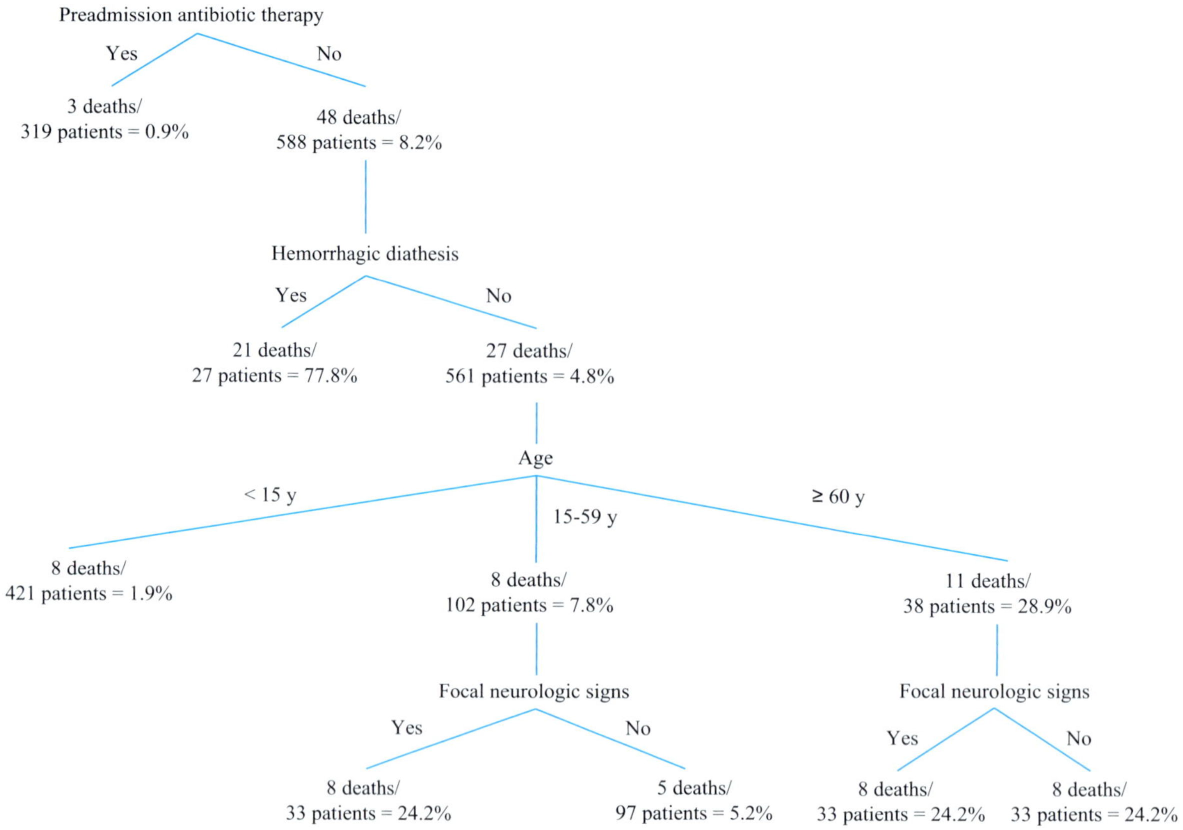

Fig. 33.14. Algorithm of probability of death in meningococcal disease related to the presence or absence of predictors of death. The fraction expresses the number of deaths/the number of patients with the condition, equal to the case-fatality rate. (From ref. [93])

The rate of permanent and disabling sequelae in meningococcemia is 2.6–11% of patients [26, 34, 201]. When they occur they are usually severe, with limb, finger-toe or extremity amputation being the most prevalent. Approximately 15% of cases require extensive skin and peripheral limb necrosis requiring amputation or reconstructive skin surgery [202–204]. Independent predictors of sequelae in patients with meningococcal disease are age over 60 years, the presence of focal neurologic signs on admission to the hospital and the presence of hemorrhagic diathesis, whereas preadmission antibiotic therapy plays a protective role [34]. The clinical factors which independently allow the appearance of sequelae to be predicted are the same as those which allow death to be predicted.

33.9 Prevention

It has long been known that household members and day-care center and schoolchildren contacts of index patients with meningococcal disease have a 50–1,000-fold higher chance of acquiring invasive disease than do members of the general population [129, 205, 206]. A reason for this increased risk is that the household members share some factors predisposing to the acquisition of meningococcal disease such as the genetic factors and the occurrence of recent viral respiratory illness. Since these factors are not shared with the healthcare workers or laboratory personnel, secondary cases acquired in the hospital [207–217] or in the laboratory are uncommon [218–227].

Chemoprophylaxis can protect susceptible persons from acquiring meningococcal disease by eliminating meningococci colonization (eradication of the carrier status) in close contacts. To quote Feldman "If there are no carriers, there are no cases" [228]. Chemoprophylaxis eradicates *N. meningitidis* from the nasopharynx and should be administered, as soon as possible, to intimate contacts such as household members or roommates, day-care center contacts, childcare contacts, frequent playmates of young children, and persons exposed to the patient's oral secretions in the 7 days before the onset of illness (kissing, sharing eating utensils or toothbrushes, mouth-to-mouth resuscitation, exposure to secretions aerosolized during endotracheal intubation), preferably within 24 h of diagnosis of the index case [77, 229, 230]. Healthcare workers do not have an increased risk if the latter circumstances are excluded and should not be routinely offered chemoprophylaxis.

The antibiotics that are highly effective in eradicating meningococcus from the nasopharynx and the recommended chemoprophylaxis regime are listed in Table 33.3 [231–234]. Rifampin, which achieves high concentrations in nasopharyngeal and respiratory secretions, is one of the most effective antibiotics for eliminating meningococci from the nasopharynx. Rifampin is contraindicated in pregnant women (teratogenicity in laboratory animals) and is generally well tolerated although it has various side effects, including orange urine and sweat, orange staining of contact lenses, stimulation of liver microsomal enzymes, and reduction in levels of other concurrent medications (i.e., oral contraceptives, anticoagulants, digoxin, phenytoin). Rifampin may reduce efficacy of oral contraceptives; therefore alternative contraceptive measures should be used during and for the month after rifampin administration. Ciprofloxacin, ofloxacin, and minocycline are contraindicated in children, pregnant woman or lactating women. Ceftriaxone is probably the drug of choice for a pregnant contact. Ciprofloxacin is contraindicated in individuals younger than 18 years of age because of evidence of cartilage damage in juvenile beagles [235].

Chemoprophylaxis should be instituted as soon as possible because the risk of secondary cases is greatest during the first days after onset of disease in the index case. Chemoprophylaxis usually fails if given too late, to the inadequate person, because of meningococci resistant to the antibiotic administered or due to the incorrect dose or interval [206, 230, 236–239].

Physicians should not obtain nasopharyngeal cultures to determine whether or not to administer prophylaxis; this only delays prompt chemoprophylaxis. Selective chemoprophylaxis is only indicated in patients with meningococcal disease treated with penicillin or chloramphenicol.

Chemoprophylaxis is further limited as it does not prevent reintroduction of the pathogenic *N. meningitidis* strain from a carrier outside the group, and late secondary cases still therefore occur [240].

Immunization of contacts may be useful in order to prevent secondary cases as a supplement to chemoprophylaxis of household members, and day-care centers, schoolchildren and other contacts of index cases of meningococcal disease caused by the serogroups carried by vaccine [241]. About 40% of secondary cases may occur 5 or more days after presentation of the index cases.

Due to the fact that half of secondary cases in household members develop within 24 h in children under 15 years, the Norwegian health authorities advise treating these possible coprimary cases with phenoxymethyl-penicillin for 1 week [242–244]. The preventive treatment with penicillin has considerably reduced the number of coprimary fatalities in families [245]. However, this strategy is criticized because it can favor the development of meningococcal strains resistant to penicillin [246, 247].

Respiratory isolation of patients with meningococcal disease is recommended for the first 24 h of admission to hospital. In all situations in which there is potential for secondary cases, this risk must be explained to families and it is absolutely essential to educate contacts in relation to the need to seek immediate medical attention if they develop signs or symptoms of a febrile illness. No prophylactic strategy is 100% effective, and ill contacts should therefore be evaluated with a high suspicion of meningococcal disease [235].

In view of the fact that the protection offered by vaccination is not immediate, and the limited value of chemoprophylaxis in the prevention of secondary cases, immediate medical attention if signs or symptoms of a febrile illness develop, early diagnosis and prompt appropriate treatment are still the only ways to reduce morbidity and mortality [235].

Meningococcal disease only occurs in patients devoid of specific bactericidal or opsonizing antibodies. The best way to prevent meningococcal disease is therefore to use vaccination to induce these antibodies [26]. Primary prevention is crucial for many reasons. The presentation of the meningococcal disease may be fulminant, with no opportunity for antibiotics to influence the evolution of the disease. Antibiotic-resistant strains have been discovered, and chemoprophylaxis of contacts is a difficult and often ineffective public health measure. Mass immunization is essential to help prevent both endemic and epidemic meningococcal disease worldwide [235].

Pathogenic meningococci are encapsulated in polysaccharide, which has a different structural biochemistry defining the serogroup of the microorganism. The polysaccharide capsules of meningococci are important determinants of virulence. Mutants of *N. meningitidis* without capsular expression are non-pathogenic. Serum antibody to capsule polysaccharide protects against meningococcal disease by activating complement-mediated bacteriolysis and/or opsonization [25].

The primary successful approach to the development of meningococcal vaccines has been to purify capsular polysaccharides from the cell surface of *N. meningitidis* and obtain a product free of contaminating endotoxin. The first unconjugated capsular polysaccharide vaccines against *N. meningitidis* serogroup A and C were developed in the 1960s, in response to epidemics of meningococcal disease among United States military recruits [248–250]. Large trials demonstrated that these vaccines were safe and effective in adults and older children [251–254] and are able to control community outbreaks of meningococcal disease caused by serogroups A and C, epidemics in United States military centers, and large epidemics in sub-Saharan Africa and Brazil [255–263].

The currently available A/C bivalent and A/C/Y/W135 tetravalent meningococcal unconjugate vaccines contain purified preparations of the specific capsular polysaccharide antigens of these two or four serogroups [248, 264]. These meningococcal unconjugated polysaccharide vaccines induce a T-cell-independent immune response which is age dependent, this being its main limitation: scarce immune response in children under 18 months old and, consequently, deficient protection in the age group at most risk of acquiring meningococcal disease; non-lasting protection, and a scarce antibody response to booster doses of serogroup C meningococcal vaccine [265, 266]. Administration of these "thymus-independent" vaccines does not therefore tend to be recommended for children under 18 months old.

The administration of A/C or A/C/Y/W135 meningococcal unconjugated polysaccharide vaccines is indicated in the following situations: epidemics and outbreaks of meningococcal disease caused by the serogroups carried by vaccine; groups at high risk of acquiring meningococcal disease (individuals with functional or anatomic asplenia and persons with complement or properdin deficiencies); travelers who are visiting areas or countries with a high incidence of meningococcal disease; day-care center contacts, schoolchildren contacts and household members of an index case of meningococcal disease as an adjunct to antibiotic chemoprophylaxis; and military training camps [267].

Polysaccharides are T-cell-independent antigens and consequently induce an immune response through the direct presentation of the antigen and the activation of the B cells without the intervention of the T cells. In children under 18 months old this produces a response predominantly of IgM antibodies of little intensity and scarce duration and does not establish immune memory. The B cells of this age group are in an insufficient stage of maturity to trigger an adequate immune response without the collaboration of the T cells [268].

Experience with *Haemophilus influenzae* type b and pneumococcal conjugate vaccines showed that the immunogenicity of capsular polysaccharides can be improved by chemical conjugation to a protein carrier [269, 270]. To obtain an effective response in children under 18 months old it is necessary to combine the capsular polysaccharides with a conveying protein, which grants them the characteristics of a T-cell-dependent antigen. The immune response then involves the stimulation of the T cells which activate the B cells by means of soluble factors. This allows an early production of long-lasting IgG antibodies, and the establishment of immune memory which is demonstrated by a marked strengthening effect after revaccination [267].

In order to overcome the lack of adequate immunogenicity of meningococcal unconjugated polysaccharide vaccines in infants, several C and A/C meningococcal protein-polysaccharide conjugate vaccines were developed through the 1980s [271, 272], and the first human trials were conducted in 1991 [273]. These vaccines have demonstrated their ability to induce immunological memory and greater effectiveness in children under 18 months old, thus offering protection to the age group most in need of protection against meningococcal disease [274, 275]. The A/C meningococcal protein-polysaccharide conjugate vaccines are differentiated by the conveying protein (e.g., tetanic toxoid, bovine albumin, diphtheric toxoid CRM197), by the structure and length of the polysaccharide, by the method linking the protein to the polysaccharide which can be in a direct covalent manner or with an additional molecule and by the protein/polysaccharide ratio [267].

In November 1999, serogroup C meningococcal polysaccharide-protein conjugate vaccine was introduced into routine immunization in the United Kingdom in an attempt to control hyperendemic serogroup C meningococcal disease. The United Kingdom became the first country to introduce routine serogroup C meningococcal immunization [276]. Ireland and Spain, in 2000, were the next countries to introduce the serogroup C meningococcal polysaccharide-protein conjugate vaccine into their routine immunization schedule. The United Kingdom campaign was followed by an 81 % reduction in the numbers of serogroup C meningococcal disease in the immunized group (from 537 in July 1998 to April 1999 to 103 in the equivalent period from 2001 to 2002) [277]. Vaccine efficacy has been estimated at 92–97 % for teenagers [278–280], 92 % for toddlers [280], and 91 % for infants [279], and deaths due to serogroup C meningococcal disease fell from 67 in 1999 to 5 in 2001 [281]. In Ireland the incidence from 1999 to 2002 has fallen by 96 % from 3.7 to 0.13/100,000 persons/year. In Spain the incidence from 1999 to 2001 has fallen by 58 % from 0.93 to 0.39/100,000 persons/year, despite low vaccine coverage in teenagers.

In January 2005, the Food and Drug Administration approved serogroup A, C, Y, W-135 meningococcal polysaccharide-protein (diphtheria toxoid) conjugate vaccine indicated for active immunization of adolescents and adults between 11 and 55 years old to prevent meningococcal disease due to serogroups contained by the vaccine. The employment of this vaccine in older high school or college students will reduce the meningococcus transmission and decrease the risk of meningococcal disease in this age group without the concern of inducing immune hyporesponsiveness, which is observed after serogroup C meningococcal polysaccharide immunization [267].

The serogroup A, C, Y, W-135 meningococcal polysaccharide-protein conjugate vaccine will be extraordinarily useful for controlling epidemic meningococcal disease in sub-Saharan Africa caused by serogroups A, C and W-135 [282], outbreaks of serogroup W-135 strains related to Hajj pilgrims [283–285], and frequent outbreaks of serogroup Y detected in North America and Latin America. This vaccine will also be useful in developed countries with a low incidence of serogroup A, C, Y, and W-135 meningococcal disease, administered either as a travel vaccine or as a booster vaccine after primary immunization with serogroup C meningococcal polysaccharide-protein conjugate vaccine [276].

The lack of activity against serogroup B meningococci is the main disadvantage of the vaccines currently available in western Europe. It has not been possible to develop serogroup B polysaccharide vaccines, even when polysaccharide was conjugated to a carrier protein, because the specific capsular polysaccharide of serogroup B induces a weak immune response [268]. This polysaccharide is a 200-residue $\alpha(2\rightarrow8)$ homopolymer of *N*-acetylneuraminic acid and bears an extraordinary resemblance to the human neuronal cell adhesion molecule [286]. It is considered that this resemblance could be responsible for the scarce immunogenicity, due to a phenomenon of immunological tolerance caused by developmental exposure of the fetus to cross-reactive polysialated glycoproteins, expressed in several host tissues. Cross-reactive, long chain polysialated glycoproteins are particularly plentiful in the fetal brain, where they can be observed on the neural cell adhesion molecule [286, 287]. Expression of this cross-reactive polysialic acid diminishes in almost all adult tissues [25].

The disappointing immunogenic behavior of the specific capsular polysaccharide of serogroup B has not only been demonstrated in those vaccinated but also in patients surviving a recent episode of serogroup B meningococcal disease and in the nasopharyngeal carriers of strains of meningococcus of this serogroup. In all of them it is not possible to find plasmatic concentrations of antibodies aimed at the specific capsular polysaccharide of serogroup B.

One approach is to use a conjugated chemically modified serogroup B polysaccharide capsule where the native *N*-acetyl group has been replaced by the *N*-propionyl group and conjugated to a protein carrier [288]. Given that the attempts to increase the tolerance for own antigens entail the risk of inducing autoimmunity, most research aimed at obtaining a vaccine against serogroup B concentrates on non-capsular antigens [267].

Promising alternative vaccines against serogroup B meningococcal disease include the detoxified lipo-oligosaccharides, surface-exposed outer membrane protein vesicles, iron regulating proteins (transferrin binding protein B), neisserial surface protein A, and commensal *Neisseria* species. Vaccines not based on capsular polysaccharide have the advantage of avoiding the potential risk of capsule-switching.

A B/C meningococcal vaccine, consisting of a mixture mainly of outer membrane proteins from serogroup B meningococci noncovalently complexed with capsular polysaccharide from serogroup C, was developed in Cuba. Different success rates were obtained from large-scale trials in Chile, Cuba, and Brazil [289–292]. The vaccine effectiveness varied extraordinarily with age, being scarcely effective in children under 4 years old and ineffective under 2 years old. A similar outer membrane protein vesicle without serogroup C polysaccharide vaccine is also being developed in Cuba [267].

The Walter Reed Army Institute of Research prepared an experimental vaccine based on outer membrane proteins from serogroup B meningococci strain (responsible for an epidemic in Iquique, Chile) noncovalently complexed with capsular polysaccharide from serogroup C, with low concentration of lipopolysaccharide. The effectiveness of the mass vaccination campaign carried out in Iquique was 51% (ineffective in children under 4 years old; effectiveness of 70% in the group 5–21 years old) and the protection granted was of short duration [293].

A vaccine based on outer membrane proteins of a strain of serogroup B *N. meningitidis* was elaborated by the National Institute of Public Health in Norway, in response to serogroup B meningococcal outbreaks in this country. The results of the clinical trial were so discouraging that it was concluded that the protection was insufficient to justify its inclusion in a systematic vaccination program [294]. This Norwegian institute prepared a vaccine designed to combat the epidemic of meningococcal disease due to the strain B:4:P1.7b,4 suffered by New Zealand for more than a decade. The clinical trials began in May 2002.

A nasal vaccine, consisting of outer membrane vesicles from serogroup B *N. meningitidis*, may induce systemic and local mucosal immune responses and offers protection against meningococcal disease in humans [295–297].

A hexavalent recombinant PorA meningococcal vaccine was developed in the Netherlands at Rijksinstituut voor Volksgezondheid en Milieu with outer membrane proteins prepared from two strains that each express three different PorA proteins. A trial in the United Kingdom and the Netherlands with a Dutch outer membrane protein vaccine (without capsular polysaccharide) offered promising results [298, 299].

The protective immunity offered by outer membrane protein vaccines is mainly directed at the highly variable, immunodominant outer membrane proteins [300]. Consequently, these vaccines do not elicit serum bactericidal antibody against many heterologous meningococcal strains. As outer membrane protein vaccines do not afford good protection in children under the age of 4 years either [25], the applicability of these vaccines for routine immunization programs to decrease endemic serogroup B meningococcal disease provoked by antigenically diverse meningococci is brought into question. It is, however, possible that these vaccines are important as an intervention to disrupt outbreaks of disease caused by a single meningococcal clone [296].

All the meningococcal vaccines described above were obtained using conventional vaccine development methodology. The vaccines developed with the conventional methodology are based on attenuated live or killed whole microorganisms, subunit microorganisms and toxins detoxified by chemical treatment. They are characterized by their high immunogenicity and scarce purity. This inconvenience has been solved in the last few decades using recombinant DNA technology to produce subunit vaccines based on specific very purified antigens [301].

With the conventional vaccine development methodology, the identification of the antigen candidate to be transformed into a future vaccine is based on the cultivation of a certain microorganism and subsequent dissection into its components using biochemical, immunological and microbiological means. Once its individual components have been identified and produced in a pure form, either directly from the microorganism or through recombinant DNA technology, the immunogenicity of each component is then determined to assess whether it is a candidate to be transformed into a vaccine. This methodology requires the growth of the pathogen in vitro (not all pathogens can be cultivated in vitro) and only identifies those antigens that can be obtained in the large quantities necessary to prove their immunogenicity. Moreover, not all the antigens expressed during in vivo infection are expressed during the in vitro culture. Therefore, the conventional methodology requires much time and can fail to identify protective antigens [302].

Technologies such as genome sequencing, *in silico* analysis, proteomics technologies (two-dimensional gel electrophoresis and mass spectrometry), DNA microarrays, in vivo expression technology and signature tagged mutagenesis have revolutionized the approach to vaccine design [303].

The recent genome sequencing of certain microorganisms has permitted a new methodological approach to vaccine development, in a reverse way, called reverse vaccinology [304]. The availability of complete genome sequences allows the identification of all proteic antigens and the prediction *in silico* of their ability to induce a protective immune response, independently of their abundance and without the need to grow the microorganism in vitro [303].

Once the genome sequences are known, a computer analysis is performed with the aim of predicting those segments of DNA that code for novel antigens. Then, using *in silico* analysis, the genes that code for outer membrane or surface exposed proteins are selected. Later, these genes are expressed by DNA recombinant technology. Finally, by immunogenicity testing in animal models, those proteins that have induced a better immune response of bactericidal antibodies are selected [303].

Vaccine candidates are identified using computer predictions. It is not necessary to culture the microorganism, and the method can therefore also be applied to microorganisms that cannot be cultured. The process is carried out in a computer room rather than a laboratory. The analysis of the vaccine candidates begins with the virtual catalogue of all the protein antigens that the microorganism can express either in vivo or in vitro and irrespective of whether it can be obtained in large quantities. Every single proteic antigen of a pathogen can be tested for its ability to induce a protective immune response. For this reason, the number of candidate antigens for new vaccines, identified by reverse vaccinology, will increase considerably in the near future [303]. The main limitation of this genome-based approach to vaccine development is the inability to identify non-protein antigens, such as polysaccharides, lipopolysaccharides, glycolipids, and other CD1-restricted antigens [304].

Complete genome sequencing of *N. meningitidis* serogroup B strain MC58 was obtained in 2000 by the random shotgun strategy [305]. Using reverse vaccinology, fragments of DNA were screened by computer analysis in order to select putative open reading frames (ORFs) that potentially encoded novel surface-exposed or secreted proteins while the nucleotide sequence was being determined [306]. The 2,272,351-base pair genome of this strain contained 2,158 ORFs, 600 of which coded for surface-exposed or secreted proteins. These antigens included different classes of proteins, according to their predicted localization on the bacterial surface such as outer membrane or secreted proteins, lipoproteins, inner membrane proteins, periplasmic proteins, and proteins with homologies to bacterial factors involved in virulence and pathogenesis [307].

The selected 600 ORFs were amplified from meningococcus by PCR, and cloned into *Escherichia coli* in order to express each gene. A total of 350 of them were successfully expressed recombinant proteins, purified, and used to immunize mice. The sera allowed the identification of proteins that are surface exposed and that are conserved in sequence across a range of strains. Finally, sera were tested in bactericidal assay for the ability to induce complement mediated in vitro killing of bacteria, an assay which correlates with vaccine efficacy in humans [307]. Ninety-one proteins were found to be surface exposed, and 29 of them were able to induce bactericidal antibodies by immunogenicity testing in animal models [303]. Fifteen very promising antigens are under investigation and are likely to enter into vaccine development.

The use of reverse vaccinology allows the discovery of previously unknown and undescribed proteins as vaccine candidates and an understanding of their role and function. Many of the novel outer membrane or surface exposed proteins share homologies to known virulence factors. Among these the newly identified antigens are GNA33 (genome derived *Neisseria* antigen), NadA (*Neisseria* adhesin A, NMB1994), GNA992, and App (Adhesin penetration protein; GNA1985). In only a few years reverse vaccinology has resulted in the identification of more vaccine candidates as compared to those discovered during the previous 4 decades of research [303]. What is surprising is not just the high number of new vaccine candidates identified but also the quality of the new proteins, which provides an optimal basis for the development of an effective vaccine against *N. meningitidis* serogroup B [304].

Current research into meningococcal vaccines is aimed at improving the immunogenicity of the capsular polysaccharides by conjugation with different types of proteins or using other components of the bacterial surface as antigens identified by reverse vaccinology. The final objective is to obtain a polyvalent meningococcal vaccine, preferably for intranasal administration, which is highly effective and safe in all age groups, and which offers protection against all the serogroups of *N. meningitidis* which cause meningococcal disease.

References

1. Apicella MA (2005) *Neisseria meningitidis.* In: Mandell GL, Bennett JE, Dolin R (eds) Mandell, Douglas, and Bennett's principles and practice of infectious diseases, 6th edn, vol. 2. Elsevier-Churchill Livingstone, Philadelphia, pp 2498–2513
2. Janda WM, Knapp JS (2003) *Neisseria* and *Moraxella catarrhalis.* In: Murray PR, Baron EJ, Jorgensen JH, Pfaller MA, Yolken RH (eds) Manual of clinical microbiology, 8th edn, vol. 1. American Society for Microbiology Press, Washington, DC, pp 585–608
3. Frasch CE, Zollinger WD, Poolman JT (1985) Serotype antigens of *Neisseria meningitidis* and a proposed scheme for designation of serotypes. Rev Infect Dis 7:504–510
4. Broud DD, Griffiss JM, Baker CJ (1979) Heterogeneity of serotypes of *Neisseria meningitidis* that cause endemic disease. J Infect Dis 140:465–470
5. Mandrell RE, Zollinger WD (1977) Lipopolysaccharide serotyping of *Neisseria meningitidis* by hemagglutination inhibition. Infect Immun 16:471–475
6. Jennings HL, Johnson KG, Kenne L (1983) The structure of the R-type oligosaccharide core obtained from some lipopolysaccharides of *Neisseria meningitidis.* Carbohydrate Res 121:233–241
7. Gamian A, Beurret M, Michon F, Brisson JR, Jennings HJ (1992) Structure of the L2 lipopolysaccharide core oligosaccharides of *Neisseria meningitidis.* J Biol Chem 267: 922–925
8. Scholten RJ, Kuipers B, Vankenburg A, Dankert J, Zollinger WD, Poolman JT (1994) Lipo-oligosaccharide immunotyping of *Neisseria meningitidis* by a whole-cell ELISA with monoclonal antibodies. J Med Microbiol 41:236–243
9. Stephens DS, Whitney AM, Rothbard J, Schoolnik GK (1985) Pili of *Neisseria meningitidis*: analysis of structure and investigation of structural and antigenic relationships to gonococcal pili. J Exp Med 161:1539–1553
10. Caugant DA (1998) Population genetics and molecular epidemiology of *Neisseria meningitidis.* APMIS 106:505–525
11. Selander RK, Caugant DA, Ochman H, Musser JM, Gilmour MN, Whittam TS (1986) Methods of multilocus enzyme electrophoresis for bacterial population genetics and systematics. Appl Environ Microbiol 51:873–884
12. Fox AJ, Jones DM, Gray SJ, Caugant DA, Saunders NA (1991) An epidemiologically valuable typing method for *Neisseria meningitidis* by analysis of restriction fragment length polymorphisms. J Med Microbiol 34:265–270
13. Bjorvatn B, Hassan-King B, Greenwood B, Haimanot RT, Fekade D, Sperber G (1992) DNA fingerprinting in the epidemiology of African serogroup A *Neisseria meningitidis.* Scand J Infect Dis 24:323–332
14. Woods JP, Kersulyte D, Tolan RW Jr, Berg CM, Berg DE (1994) Use of arbitrarily primed polymerase chain reaction analysis to type disease and carrier strains of *Neisseria meningitidis* isolated during a university outbreak. J Infect Dis 169:1384–1389
15. Swartley JS, Marfin AA, Edupuganti S, Liu LJ, Cieslak P, Perkins B, et al. (1997) Capsule switching of *Neisseria meningitidis.* Proc Natl Acad Sci USA 94:271–276
16. Kertesz DA, Coulthart MB, Ryan JA, Johnson WM, Ashton FE (1998) Serogroup B, electrophoretic type 15 *Neisseria meningitidis* in Canada. J Infect Dis 177:1754–1757
17. Kriz P, Giorgini D, Musilek M, Larribe M, Taha MK (1999) Microevolution through DNA exchange among strains of *Neisseria meningitidis* isolated during an outbreak in the Czech Republic. Res Microbiol 150:273–280
18. Rosenstein NE, Perkins BA, Stephens DS, Popovic T, Hughes JM (2001) Meningococcal disease. N Engl J Med 344:1378–1388
19. Diaz PS (1999) The epidemiology and control of invasive meningococcal disease. Pediatr Infect Dis J 18:633–634
20. Centers for Disease Control and Prevention (2005) Prevention and control of meningococcal disease recommendations of the Advisory Committee on Immunization Practices (ACIP). MMWR Morb Mortal Wkly Rep 54(RR-7): 1–21
21. Peltola H (1983) Meningococcal disease: still with us. Rev Infect Dis 5:71–91
22. Achtman M (1995) Global epidemiology of meningococcal disease. In: Cartwright K (ed) Meningococcal disease. John Wiley & Sons, Chichester, pp 159–175
23. Lapeyssonnie L (1963) La méningite cerebro-spinale en Afrique. Bull World Health Organ 28 (Suppl):1–114
24. Moore PS (1992) Meningococcal meningitis in sub-Saharan Africa: a model for epidemic process. Clin Infect Dis 14:515–525
25. Jódar L, Feavers IM, Salisbury D, Granoff DM (2002) Development of vaccines against meningococcal disease. Lancet 359:1499–1508
26. van Deuren M, Brandtzaeg P, van der Meer JW (2000) Update on meningococcal disease with emphasis on pathogenesis and clinical management. Clin Microbiol Rev 13:144–166
27. Moore PS, Reeves MW, Schwartz B, Gellin BG, Broome CV (1989) Intercontinental spread of an epidemic group A *Neisseria meningitidis* strain. Lancet ii:260–263
28. Zhu P, Hu X, Xu L (1995) Typing *Neisseria meningitidis* by analysis of restriction fragment length polymorphisms in the gene encoding the class 1 outer membrane protein: ap-

plication to assessment of epidemics throughout the last 4 decades in China. J Clin Microbiol 33:458–462
29. Guibourdenche M, Høiby EA, Riou JY, Varaine F, Joguet C, Caugant DA (1996) Epidemics of serogroup A *Neisseria meningitidis* of subgroup III in Africa, 1989–94. Epidemiol Infect 116:115–120
30. McGee L, Koornhof HJ, Caugant DA (1998) Epidemic spread of subgroup III of *Neisseria meningitidis* serogroup A to South Africa in 1996. Clin Infect Dis 27:1214–1220
31. Moore PS, Harrison LH, Telzak EE, Ajello GW, Broome CV (1988) Group A meningococcal carriage in travelers returning from Saudi Arabia. JAMA 260:2686–2689
32. Stephens DS (1999) Uncloaking the meningococcus: dynamics of carriage and disease. Lancet 353:941–942
33. Jones D (1995) Epidemiology of meningococcal disease in Europe and the USA. In: Cartwright K (ed) Meningococcal disease. John Wiley & Sons, Chichester, pp 147–157
34. Barquet N, Domingo P, Caylà JA, González J, Rodrigo C, Fernández-Viladrich P, et al. (1999) Meningococcal disease in a large urban population (Barcelona, 1987–1992): predictors of dismal prognosis. Arch Intern Med 159: 2329–2340
35. Schwartz B, Moore PS, Broome CV (1989) Global epidemiology of meningococcal disease. Clin Microbiol Rev 2 (Suppl):S118–S124
36. Osler W (1915) Special discussion on the epidemiology of cerebrospinal meningitis. Proc Roy Soc Med 8:41–64
37. Goldschneider I, Gotschlich EC, Artenstein MS (1969) Human immunity to the meningococcus: I. The role of humoral antibodies. J Exp Med 129:1307-1326
38. Bevanger L, Bergh K, Gisnås G, Caugant DA, Frøholm LO (1998) Identification of nasopharyngeal carriage of an outbreak strain of *Neisseria meningitidis* by pulsed-field gel electrophoresis *versus* phenotypic methods. J Med Microbiol 47:993–998
39. Cartwright KA, Stuart JM, Jones DM, Noah ND (1987) The Stonehouse survey: nasopharyngeal carriage of meningococci and *Neisseria lactamica*. Epidemiol Infect 99:591–601
40. Caugant DA, Høiby EA, Magnus P, Scheel O, Hoel T, Bjune G, et al. (1994) Asymptomatic carriage of *Neisseria meningitidis* in a randomly sampled population. J Clin Microbiol 32:323–330
41. Caugant DA, Kristiansen BE, Frøholm LO, Bøvre K, Selander RK (1988) Clonal diversity of *Neisseria meningitidis* from a population of asymptomatic carriers. Infect Immun 56:2060–2068
42. Goldschneider I, Gotschlich EC, Artenstein MS (1969) Human immunity to the meningococcus: II. Development of natural immunity. J Exp Med 129:1327–1348
43. Pether JV, Lightfood NF, Scott RJ, Morgan J, Steele-Perkins AP, Sheard SC (1988) Carriage of *Neisseria meningitidis*: investigations in a military establishment. Epidemiol Infect 101:21–42
44. Tappero JW, Reporter R, Wenger JD, Ward BA, Reeves MW, Missbach TS, et al. (1996) Meningococcal disease in Los Angeles County, California, and among men in the county jails. N Engl J Med 335:833–840
45. Edwards EA, Devine LF, Sengbusch GH, Ward HW (1977) Immunological investigations of meningococcal disease: III. Brevity of group C acquisition prior to disease occurrence. Scand J Infect Dis 9:105–110
46. Marks MI, Frasch CE, Shapera RM (1979) Meningococcal colonization and infection in children and their household contacts. Am J Epidemiol 109:563–571
47. Broome CV (1986) The carrier state: *Neisseria meningitidis*. J Antimicrob Chemother 18 (Suppl A):25–34
48. Cartwright K (1995) Meningococcal carriage and disease. In: Cartwright K (ed) Meningococcal disease. John Wiley & Sons, Chichester, pp 115–146
49. Takala AK, Santosham M, Almeido-Hill J, Wolff M, Newcomer W, Reid R, et al. (1993) Vaccination with *Haemophilus influenzae* type b meningococcal protein conjugate vaccine reduces oropharyngeal carriage of *Haemophilus influenzae* type b among American Indian children. Pediatr Infect Dis J 12:593–599
50. Pollard AJ, Levin M (2000) Vaccines for prevention of meningococcal disease. Pediatr Infect Dis J 19:333–345
51. Kasper DL, Winkelhake JL, Zollinger WD, Brandt BL, Artenstein MS (1973) Immunochemical similarity between polysaccharide antigens of *Escherichia coli* 07:K1(L):NM and group B *Neisseria meningitidis*. J Immunol 110: 262–268
52. Vann WF, Liu TY, Robbins JB (1976) *Bacillus pumilus* polysaccharide cross-reactive with meningococcal group A polysaccharide. Infect Immun 13:1654–1662
53. Platonov AE, Shipulin GA, Vershinina IV, Dankert J, van de Winkel JGJ, Kuijper EJ (1998) Association of human Fc gamma RIIa (CD32) polymorphism with susceptibility to and severity of meningococcal disease. Clin Infect Dis 27:746–750
54. Domingo P, Muñiz-Díaz E, Baraldés MA, Arilla M, Barquet N, Pericas R, et al. (2002) Associations between Fc gamma receptor IIA polymorphisms and the risk and prognosis of meningococcal disease. Am J Med 112:19–25
55. Ross SC, Densen P (1984) Complement deficiency states and infection: epidemiology, pathogenesis and consequences of neisserial and other infections in an immune deficiency. Medicine (Baltimore) 63:243–273
56. de Voe IW (1982) The meningococcus and mechanisms of pathogenicity. Microbiol Rev 46:162–190
57. Quagliarello V, Scheld WM (1992) Bacterial meningitis: pathogenesis, pathophysiology, and progress. N Engl J Med 327:862–872
58. Stephens D, Hoffman L, McGee Z (1983) Interaction of *Neisseria meningitidis* with human nasopharyngeal mucosa: attachment and entry into columnar epithelial cells. J Infect Dis 148:369–376
59. Andersen J, Berthelsen L, Bech-Jensen B, Lind I (1998) Dynamics of the meningococcal carrier state and characteristics of the carrier strains: a longitudinal study within three cohorts of military recruits. Epidemiol Infect 121: 85–94
60. Griffiss JMcL, Brandt BL, Jarvis GA (1987) Natural immunity to *Neisseria meningitidis*. In: Vedros NA (ed) Evolution of meningococcal disease, vol. 2. CRC Press, Boca Raton, pp 99–119
61. Haneberg B, Tønjum T, Rodahl K, Gedde-Dahl TW (1983) Factors preceding the onset of meningococcal disease, with special emphasis on passive smoking, stressful events, physical fitness and general symptoms of ill health. NIPH Ann 6:169–173
62. Stuart JM, Cartwright KAV, Robinson PM, Noah ND (1989) Effect of smoking on meningococcal carriage. Lancet ii:723–725
63. Stanwell-Smith RE, Stuart JM, Hughes AO, Robinson P, Griffin MB, Cartwright K (1994) Smoking, the environment and meningococcal disease: a case control study. Epidemiol Infect 112:315–328
64. Fischer M, Hedberg K, Cardosi P, Plikaytis BD, Hoesly FC, Steingart KR, et al. (1997) Tobacco smoke as a risk factor for meningococcal disease. Pediatr Infect Dis J 16:979–983
65. Levitt LP, Bond JO, Hall IE Jr, Dame GM, Buff EE, Marston C, et al. (1970) Meningococcal and ECHO-9 meningitis: report of an outbreak. Neurology 20:45–51
66. Young LS, LaForce FM, Head JJ, Feeley JC, Bennett JV (1972) A simultaneous outbreak of meningococcal and influenza infections. N Engl J Med 287:5–9

67. Moore PS, Hierholzer J, de Witt W, Gouan K, Djore D, Lippeveld T, et al. (1990) Respiratory viruses and mycoplasma as cofactors for epidemic group A meningococcal meningitis. JAMA 264:1271 - 1275
68. Cartwright KAV, Jones DM, Smith AJ, Stuart JM, Kaczmarski EB, Palmer SR (1991) Influenza A and meningococcal disease. Lancet 338:554 - 557
69. Raza MW, El-Ahmer OR, Ogilvie MM, Blackwell CC, Saadi AT, Elton RA, et al. (1999) Infection with respiratory syncytial virus enhances expression of native receptors for non-pilate *Neisseria meningitidis* on HEp-2 cells. FEMS Immunol Med Microbiol 23:115 - 124
70. Plaut A (1989) Microbial subversion of host defenses. In: Schaechter M, Medoff G, Schlessinger D (eds) Mechanisms on microbial diseases. Williams & Wilkins, Baltimore, pp 139 - 146
71. Klein NJ, Ison CA, Peakman M, Levin M, Hammerschmidt S, Frosch M, et al. (1996) The influence of capsulation and lipooligosaccharide structure on neutrophil adhesion molecule expression and endothelial injury by *Neisseria meningitidis*. J Infect Dis 173:172 - 179
72. Schryvers AB, Gonzalez GC (1990) Receptors for transferrin in pathogenic bacteria are specific for the host's protein. Can J Microbiol 36:145 - 157
73. Pettersson A, Poolman JT, van der Ley P, Tommassen J (1997) Response of *Neisseria meningitidis* to iron limitation. Antonie van Leeuwenhoek 71:129 - 136
74. Gold R, Goldschneider I, Lepow ML, Draper TF, Randolph M (1978) Carriage of *Neisseria meningitidis* and *Neisseria lactamica* in infants and children. J Infect Dis 137:112 - 121
75. Jones GR, Christodoulides M, Brooks JL, Miller AR, Cartwright KA, Heckels JE (1998) Dynamics of carriage of *Neisseria meningitidis* in a group of military recruits: subtype stability and specificity of the immune response following colonization. J Infect Dis 178:451 - 459
76. Emonts M, Hazelzet JA, de Groot R, Hermans PWM (2003) Host genetic determinants of *Neisseria meningitidis* infections. Lancet Infect Dis 3:565 - 577
77. van de Winkel JGJ, Anderson CL (1991) Biology of human immunoglobulin G Fc receptors. J Leukocyte Biol 49: 511 - 524
78. van de Winkel JGJ, Capel PJA (1993) Human IgG Fc receptor heterogeneity molecular aspects and clinical implication. Immunol Today 14:215 - 221
79. Gessner JE, Heiken H, Tamm A, Schmidt RE (1998) The IgG Fc receptor family. Ann Hematol 76:231 - 248
80. Salmon JE, Edberg JC, Brogie NL, Kimberly RP (1992) Allelic polymorphisms of human Fcγ receptor IIA and Fcγ receptor IIIB: independent mechanisms for differences in human phagocyte function. J Clin Invest 89:1274 - 1281
81. de Kleijn ED, Hazelzet JA, Kornelisse RF, de Groot R (1998) Pathophysiology of meningococcal sepsis in children. Eur J Pediatr 157:869 - 880
82. van Gorp EC, Suharti C, ten Cate H, Domans WM, van der Meer JM, ten Cate JW, et al. (1999) Infectious diseases and coagulation disorders. J Infect Dis 180:176 - 186
83. Brandtzaeg P, Kierulf P, Gaustad P, Skulberg A, Bruun JN, Halvorsen S, et al. (1989) Plasma endotoxin as a predictor of multiple organ failure and death in systemic meningococcal disease. J Infect Dis 159:195 - 204
84. Girardin E, Grau GE, Dayer JM, Roux-Lombard P, Lambert PH (1988) Tumor necrosis factor and interleukin-1 in the serum of children with severe infectious purpura. N Engl J Med 319:397 - 400
85. Brandtzaeg P, Mollnes TE, Kierulf P (1989) Complement activation and endotoxin levels in systemic meningococcal disease. J Infect Dis 160:58 - 65
86. Nadel S, Newport MJ, Booy R, Levin M (1996) Variation in the tumor necrosis factor-α promoter region may be associated with death from meningococcal disease. J Infect Dis 174:878 - 880
87. Westendorp RG, Langermans JA, Huizinga TW, Elouali AH, Verweij CL, Boomsma DI, et al. (1997) Genetic influence on cytokine production and fatal meningococcal disease. Lancet 349:170 - 173
88. Hermans PW, Hibberd ML, Booy R, Daramola O, Hazelzet JA, de Groot R, et al. (1999) 4G/5G promoter polymorphism in the plasminogen-activator-inhibitor-1 gene and outcome of meningococcal disease. Lancet 354: 556 - 560
89. Westendorp RGJ, Hottenga JJ, Slagboom PE (1999) Variation in plasminogen-activator-inhibitor-1 gene and risk of meningococcal septic shock. Lancet 354:561 - 563
90. Gold R (1987) Clinical aspects of meningococcal disease. In: Vedros NA (ed) Evolution of meningococcal disease, vol. 2. CRC Press, Boca Raton, pp 69 - 97
91. Kingston ME, Mackey D (1986) Skin clues in the diagnosis of life-threatening infections. Rev Infect Dis 8:1 - 11
92. Steven N, Wood M (1995) The clinical spectrum of meningococcal disease. In: Cartwright K (ed) Meningococcal disease. John Wiley & Sons, Chichester, pp 177 - 205
93. Barquet N, Domingo P, Caylà JA, González J, Rodrigo C, Fernández-Viladrich P, et al. (1997) Prognostic factors in meningococcal disease: development of a bedside predictive model and scoring system. JAMA 278:491 - 496
94. Böhm N (1982) Adrenal, cutaneous and myocardial lesions in fulminating endotoxinemia (Waterhouse-Friderichsen syndrome). Pathol Res Pract 174:92 - 105
95. Hardman JM, Earle KM (1967) Meningococcal infections: a review of 200 fatal cases. J Neuropathol Exp Neurol 26:119
96. Hardaway RM (1982) Pathology and pathophysiology of disseminated intravascular coagulation. In: Cowley RA, Trump BF (eds) Pathophysiology of shock, anoxia and ischaemia. Williams & Wilkins, Baltimore, pp 186 - 197
97. Levin S, Painter MB (1966) The treatment of acute meningococcal infection in adults. Ann Intern Med 64:1049 - 1056
98. Gore I, Saphir Q (1947) Myocarditis, a classification of 1402 cases. Am Heart J 34:827 - 831
99. Hardman JM (1968) Fatal meningococcal infections: the changing pathologic picture in the '60's. Milit Med 133:951 - 964
100. Wolfe RE, Birbara CA (1968) Meningococcal infections at an army training center. Am J Med 44:243 - 255
101. Sullivan TD, LaScolea LJ (1987) *Neisseria meningitidis* bacteremia in children: quantitation of bacteremia and spontaneous clinical recovery without antibiotic therapy. Pediatrics 80:63 - 87
102. Casado-Flores J, Osona B, Domingo P, Barquet N (1997) Meningococcal meningitis during penicillin therapy for meningococcemia. Clin Infect Dis 25:1479
103. Dock W (1924) Intermittent fever of seven months duration due to meningococcemia. JAMA 83:399 - 400
104. Saslaw S (1962) Chronic meningococcemia: report of a case. N Engl J Med 266:605 - 607
105. Benoit F (1963) Chronic meningococcemia: case report and review of the literature. Am J Med 35:103 - 112
106. Frank ST, Gómez RM (1968) Chronic meningococcemia. Milit Med 133:918 - 920
107. Leibel R, Fangman J, Ostrovsky M (1974) Chronic meningococcemia in childhood. Am J Dis Child 127:94 - 98
108. Ognibene A, Dito W (1964) Chronic meningococcemia. Arch Intern Med 114:29 - 32
109. Rompalo AM, Hook EW III, Roberts PL, Ramsey PG, Handsfield HH, Holmes KK, et al. (1987) The acute ar-

thritis-dermatitis syndrome: the changing importance of *Neisseria gonorrhoeae* and *Neisseria meningitidis*. Arch Intern Med 147:281–283
110. Barquet N, Gasser I, Domingo P, Moraga FA, Macaya A, Elcuaz R (1990) Primary meningococcal conjunctivitis: report of 21 patients and review. Rev Infect Dis 12: 838–847
111. Koppes GM, Ellenbogen C, Gebhart RJ (1977) Group Y meningococcal disease in United States Air Force recruits. Am J Med 62:661–666
112. Riordan FAI, Thomson APJ, Sills JA, Hart CA (1996) Who spots the spots? Diagnosis and treatment of early meningococcal disease in children. BMJ 313:1255–1256
113. Granier S, Owen P, Pill R, Jacobson L (1998) Recognising meningococcal disease in primary care: qualitative study of how general practitioners process clinical and contextual information. BMJ 316:276–279
114. Meningococcal Disease Surveillance Group (1976) Analysis of endemic meningococcal disease by serogroup and evaluation of chemoprophylaxis. J Infect Dis 134:201–204
115. Hoyne AL, Brown RH (1948) 727 meningococcic cases: an analysis. Ann Intern Med 28:248–259
116. Domingo P, Mancebo J, Blanch L, Coll P, Net A, Nolla J (1990) Bacterial meningitis with "normal" cerebrospinal fluid in adults: a report of five cases. Scand J Infect Dis 22:115–116
117. Cartwright KAV (1999) Early management of meningococcal disease. Infect Dis Clin North Am 13:661–684
118. Jochmann G (1906) Versuche zur Serodiagnostik und Serotherapie der epidemischen Genickstarre. Dtsch Med Wochenschr 32:788–793
119. Flexner S, Jobling JW (1908) An analysis of four hundred cases of epidemic meningitis treated with the anti-meningitis serum. J Exp Med 10:690–710
120. Schwentker FF, Gelman S, Long PH (1937) The treatment of meningococcic meningitis with sulfanilamide: preliminary report. JAMA 108:1407–1408
121. Rosenberg DH, Arling PA (1944) Penicillin in the treatment of meningitis. JAMA 125:1011–1017
122. Scheld WM, Mandell GL (1984) Sulfonamides and meningitis. JAMA 251:791–794
123. Sáez-Nieto JA, Lujan R, Berrón S, Campos J, Viñas M, Fusté C, et al. (1992) Epidemiology and molecular basis of penicillin-resistant *Neisseria meningitidis* in Spain: a 5-year history (1985–1989). Clin Infect Dis 14:394–402
124. Sutcliffe EM, Jones DM, El-Sheikh S, Percival A (1988) Penicillin-insensitive meningococci in the UK. Lancet i:657–658
125. Botha P (1988) Penicillin-resistant *Neisseria meningitidis* in Southern Africa. Lancet i:54
126. Dillon JR, Paizé M, Yeung KH (1983) Spread of penicillinase-producing and transfer plasmids from the gonococcus to *Neisseria meningitidis*. Lancet i:779–781
127. Hieber JP, Nelson JD (1977) A pharmacologic evaluation of penicillin in children with purulent meningitis. N Engl J Med 297:410–413
128. Abramson JS, Spika JS (1985) Persistence of *Neisseria meningitidis* in the upper respiratory tract after intravenous antibiotic therapy for systemic meningococcal disease. J Infect Dis 151:370–371
129. Meningococcal Disease Surveillance Group (1976) Meningococcal disease: secondary attack rate and chemoprophylaxis in the United States, 1974. JAMA 235:261–265
130. Voss L, Lennon D (1994) Epidemiology, management, and prevention of meningococcal infections. Curr Opin Pediatr 6:23–28
131. Álvarez F, Aguilera A, García-Gago M (1991) Effect of chemoprophylaxis on the meningococcal carrier state after infection. Pediatr Infect Dis J 10:700
132. Weis N, Lind I (1994) Pharyngeal carriage of *Neisseria meningitidis* before and after treatment of meningococcal disease. J Med Microbiol 41:339–342
133. Grubbauer HM, Dornbusch HJ, Dittrich P, Weippl G, Mutz I, Zobel G, et al. (1990) Ceftriaxone monotherapy for bacterial meningitis in children. Chemotherapy 36:441–447
134. Neu HC (1987) Cephalosporins in the treatment of meningitis. Drugs 34 (Suppl 2):135–153
135. Shaad UB, Krucko J, Pfenninger J (1984) An extended experience with cefuroxime therapy of childhood bacterial meningitis. Pediatr Infect Dis 3:410–415
136. Begg N (1992) Reducing mortality from meningococcal disease. BMJ 305:133–134
137. Strang JR, Pugh EJ (1992) Meningococcal infections: reducing the case fatality rate by giving penicillin before admission to hospital. BMJ 305:141–143
138. Cartwright K, Reilly S, White D, Stuart J (1992) Early treatment with parenteral penicillin in meningococcal diseases. BMJ 305:143–147
139. Palmer SR, Corson J, Hall R, Payne S, Ludlow J, Deere B, et al. (1992) Meningococcal disease in Wales: clinical features, outcome and public health management. J Infect 25:321–328
140. Woodward CM, Jessop EG, Wale MC (1995) Early management of meningococcal disease. Commun Dis Rep Rev 5:R135–R137
141. Wilks D, Lever AMM (1996) Reasons for delay in administration of antibiotics to patients with meningitis and meningococcaemia. J Infect 32:49–51
142. Jacobs RF, Sowell MK, Moss MM, Fiser DH (1990) Septic shock in children: bacterial etiologies and temporal relationships. Pediatr Infect Dis J 9:196–200
143. van Deuren M, Neeleman C, van't Hek LGFM, van der Meer JWM (1998) A normal platelet count at admission in acute meningococcal disease does not exclude a fulminant course. Intensive Care Med 24:157–161
144. Mercier JC, Beaufils F, Hartmann JF, Azema D (1988) Hemodynamic patterns of meningococcal shock in children. Crit Care Med 16:27–33
145. Kennedy NJ, Duncan AW (1996) Acute meningococcaemia: recent advances in management (with particular reference to children). Anaesth Intensive Care 24:197–216
146. Kirsch EA, Barton RP, Kitchen L, Giroir BP (1996) Pathophysiology, treatment and outcome of meningococcemia: a review and recent experience. Pediatr Infect Dis J 15:967–978
147. Hodgetts TJ, Brett A, Castle N (1998) The early management of meningococcal disease. J Accid Emerg Med 15: 72–76
148. Waage A, Brandtzaeg P, Halstensen A, Kierulf P, Espevik T (1989) The complex pattern of cytokines in serum from patients with meningococcal septic shock: association between interleukin 6, interleukin 1, and fatal outcome. J Exp Med 169:333–338
149. Prins JM, Lauw FN, Derkx BH, Speelman P, Kuijper ES, Dankert J, et al. (1998) Endotoxin release and cytokine production in acute and chronic meningococcaemia. Clin Exp Immunol 114:215–219
150. Nassif X, Mathison JC, Wolfson E, Koziol JA, Ulevitch RJ, So M (1992) Tumour necrosis factor alpha antibody protects against lethal meningococcaemia. Mol Microbiol 6:591–597
151. Wester JP, Breumelhof R, Geers AB (1992) Monoclonal antibodies in the treatment of adult fulminant meningococcaemia. Eur J Med 1:372–373
152. Villard J, Roux-Lombard P, Hugli A, Dayer JM (1993)

Could natural inhibitors of tumor necrosis factor-α modify the clinical course of fulminant meningococcemia? Crit Care Med 21:1396–1400
153. Nadel S, Macintosh I, Levin M (2001) Evaluation of new treatments for meningococcal disease. In: Pollard AJ, Maiden MCJ (eds) Meningococcal disease: methods and protocols. Serie: Methods in molecular medicine n0 67 (JM Walker, series ed.). Humana Press, Totowa, NJ, pp 549–586
154. Syed SDA, Taylor RH, Crean PM, Stewart RJ (1992) Successful use of monoclonal anti-lipid-A IgM in infant with meningococcal sepsis. Lancet 339:496
155. J5 Study Group (1992) Treatment of severe infectious purpura in children with human plasma from donors immunized with *Escherichia coli* J5: a prospective double-blind study. J Infect Dis 165:695–701
156. Giroir BP, Quint PA, Barton P, Kirsch EA, Kitchen L, Goldstein B, et al. (1997) Preliminary evaluation of recombinant amino-terminal fragment of human bactericidal/permeability-increasing protein in children with severe meningococcal sepsis. Lancet 350:1439–1443
157. Derkx B, Wittes J, McCloskey R (1999) Randomized placebo-controlled trial of HA-1A, a human monoclonal antibody to endotoxin, in children with meningococcal septic shock. Clin Infect Dis 28:770–777
158. Levin M, Quint P, Goldstein B, Barton P, Bradley P, Bradley JS, et al. (2000) Recombinant bactericidal/permeability-increasing protein (rBPI21) as adjunctive treatment for children with severe meningococcal sepsis: a randomized trial. Lancet 356:961–967
159. Riordan FA, Thomson AP, Ratcliffe JM, Sills JA, Diver MJ, Hart CA (1999) Admission cortisol and adrenocorticotrophic hormone levels in children with meningococcal disease: evidence of adrenal insufficiency? Crit Care Med 27:2257–2261
160. Pollard AJ, Britto J, Nadel S, de Munter C, Habibi P, Levin M (1999) Emergency management of meningococcal disease. Arch Dis Child 80:290–296
161. Wajchenberg B, Leme CE, Tambascia M, Boulos M, Okada H, Cesar FP, et al. (1978) The adrenal response to exogenous adrenocorticotropin in patients with infections due to *Neisseria meningitidis*. J Infect Dis 138:387–391
162. Corrigan JJ Jr, Jordan CM (1970) Heparin therapy in septicemia with disseminated intravascular coagulation: effect on mortality and on correction of hemostatic defects. N Engl J Med 283:778–782
163. Smith OP, White B, Vaughan D, Rafferty M, Claffey L, Lyons B, et al. (1997) Use of protein-C concentrate, heparin, and haemodiafiltration in meningococcus-induced *purpura fulminans*. Lancet 350:1590–1593
164. Wilson F, Morse S (1972) Therapy of acute meningococcal infections: early volume expansion and prophylactic low dose heparin. Am J Med Sci 264:445–455
165. Gerard P, Moriau M, Bachy A, Malvaux P, de Meyer R (1973) Meningococcal purpura: report of 19 patients treated with heparin. J Pediatr 82:780–786
166. Kuppermann N, Inkelis S, Saladino R (1994) The role of heparin in the prevention of extremity and digit necrosis in meningococcal *purpura fulminans*. Pediatr Infect Dis J 13:867–873
167. Cobroft R, Henderson A (1994) Meningococcal *purpura fulminans* treated with antithrombin III concentrate: what is the optimal replacement therapy? Aust N Z J Med 24:575–576
168. Irazuzta J, McManus ML (1990) Use of topically applied nitroglycerin in the treatment of *purpura fulminans*. J Pediatr 117:993–995
169. Meyer M, Irazuzta J, Tozibikian H (1999) Topical nitroglycerin and pain in *purpura fulminans*. J Pediatr 134:639–641
170. Goldman AP, Kerr SJ, Butt W, Marsh MJ, Murdoch IA, Paul T, et al. (1997) Extracorporeal support for intractable cardiorespiratory failure due to meningococcal disease. Lancet 349:466–469
171. Leclerc F, Martinot A, Cremer R, Fourier C (1997) ECMO for refractory cardiorespiratory failure due to meningococcal disease. Lancet 349:1397–1398
172. Kumar A, Kanagasundaram NS, Collyns TA, Davison AM (1998) Plasma exchange and haemodiafiltration in fulminant meningococcal sepsis. Nephrol Dial Transplant 13:484–487
173. Bjorvatn B, Bjertnaes L, Fadnes HO, Flaegstad T, Gutteberg TJ, Kristiansen BE, et al. (1984) Meningococcal septicaemia treated with combined plasmapheresis and leucapheresis or with blood exchange. BMJ 288:439–441
174. Drapkin MS, Wisch JS, Gelfand JA, Cannon JG, Dinarello CA (1989) Plasmapheresis for fulminant meningococcemia. Pediatr Infect Dis J 8:399–400
175. van Deuren M, Santman FW, van Dalen R, Sauerwein RW, Span LF, van der Meer JW (1992) Plasma and whole blood exchange in meningococcal sepsis. Clin Infect Dis 15: 424–430
176. Churchwell KB, McManus ML, Kent P, Gorlin J, Galacki D, Humphreys D, et al. (1995) Intensive blood and plasma exchange for treatment of coagulopathy in meningococcemia. J Clin Apher 10:171–177
177. Tobias JD, Haun SE, Helfaer M, Nichols DG (1989) Use of continuous caudal block to relieve lower-extremity ischaemia caused by vasculitis in a child with meningococcemia. J Pediatr 115:1019–1021
178. Keeley SR, Matthews NT, Buist M (1991) Tissue plasminogen activator for gangrene in fulminant meningococcaemia. Lancet 337:1359
179. Zenz W, Muntean W (1998) New therapies for severe meningococcal disease. Lancet 351:528
180. Aiuto LT, Barone SR, Cohen PS, Boxer RA (1997) Recombinant tissue plasminogen activator restores perfusion in meningococcal *purpura fulminans*. Crit Care Med 25:1079–1082
181. Nadel S, de Munter C, Britto J, Habibi P, Levin M (1998) Recombinant tissue plasminogen activator restores perfusion in meningococcal *purpura fulminans*. Crit Care Med 26:971–972
182. Marotto MS, Marotto PC, Sztajnbok J, Seguro AC (1997) Outcome of acute renal failure in meningococcemia. Renal Failure 19:807–810
183. Havens PL, Garland JS, Brook MM, Dewitz BA, Stremski ES, Troshynski TJ (1989) Trends in mortality in children hospitalized with meningococcal infections, 1957 to 1987. Pediatr Infect Dis J 8:8–11
184. Hart CA, Rogers TRF (1993) Meningococcal disease. J Med Microbiol 39:3–25
185. Cahalane SF, Waters M (1975) Fulminant meningococcal septicaemia: a hospital experience. Lancet ii:120–121
186. Emparanza JI, Aldamiz-Echevarría L, Pérez-Yarza EG, Larranaga P, Jímenez JL, Labiano M, et al. (1988) Prognostic score in acute meningococcemia. Crit Care Med 16:168–169
187. Mok Q, Butt W (1996) The outcome of children admitted to intensive care with meningococcal septicaemia. Intensive Care Med 22:259–263
188. Stiehm ER, Damrosch DS (1966) Factors in the prognosis of meningococcal infection. J Pediatr 68:457–467
189. Niklasson PM, Lundbergh P, Strandell T (1971) Prognostic factors in meningococcal disease. Scand J Infect Dis 3:17–25

190. Kahn A, Blum D (1978) Factors for poor prognosis in fulminating meningococcemia: conclusions from observations of 67 childhood cases. Clin Pediatr (Phila) 17:680–687
191. Vik-Mo H, Lote K, Nordøy A (1978) Disseminated intravascular coagulation in patients with meningococcal infection: laboratory diagnosis and prognostic factors. Scand J Infect Dis 10:187–191
192. Lewis LS (1979) Prognostic factors in acute meningococcemia. Arch Dis Child 54:44–48
193. Gårdlund B (1986) Prognostic evaluation in meningococcal disease. Intensive Care Med 12:302–307
194. Sinclair JF, Skeoch CH, Hallworth D (1987) Prognosis of meningococcal septicaemia. Lancet ii:38
195. Gedde-Dahl TW, Bjark P, Høiby EA, Høst JH, Bruun JN (1990) Severity of meningococcal disease: assessment by factors and scores and implications for patient management. Rev Infect Dis 12:973–992
196. Giraud T, Dhainaut JF, Schremmer B, Regnier B, Desjars P, Loirat P, et al. (1991) Adult overwhelming meningococcal purpura: a study of 35 cases, 1977–1989. Arch Intern Med 151:310–316
197. Thomson APJ, Sills JA, Hart CA (1991) Validation of the Glasgow Meningococcal Septicemia Prognostic Score: a 10-year retrospective survey. Crit Care Med 19:26–30
198. Busund R, Starume B, Revhaug A (1993) Fatal course in severe meningococcemia: clinical predictors and effect of transfusion therapy. Crit Care Med 21:1699–1705
199. Domingo P, Muñíz-Díaz E, Baraldés MA, Arilla M, Barquet N, Pericas R, et al. (2004) Relevance of genetically determined host factors to the prognosis of meningococcal disease. Eur J Clin Microbiol Infect Dis 23:634–637
200. Festa M, Derkx B (2001) Clinical scoring systems in meningococcal disease. In: Pollard AJ, Maiden MCJ (eds) Meningococcal disease: methods and protocols. Serie: Methods in molecular medicine n0 67 (JM Walker, series ed). Humana Press, Totowa, NJ, pp 411–425
201. Edwards MS, Baker CJ (1981) Complications and sequelae of meningococcal infections in children. J Pediatr 99:540–545
202. Genoff MC, Hoffer MM, Achauer B, Formosa P (1992) Extremity amputations in meningococcemia-induced *purpura fulminans*. Plast Reconstr Surg 89:878–881
203. Harris NJ, Gosh M (1994) Skin and extremity loss in meningococcal septicaemia treated in a burn unit. Burns 20:471–472
204. Huang S, Clarke JA (1997) Severe skin loss after meningococcal septicaemia: complications in treatment. Acta Pediatr 86:1263–1266
205. de Wals P, Hertoghe L, Borlée-Grimée I, de Maeyer-Cleempoel S, Reginster-Haneuse G, Dachy A, et al. (1981) Meningococcal disease in Belgium: secondary attack rate among household, day-care nursery and pre-elementary school contacts. J Infec 3 (Suppl 1):53–61
206. Cooke RPD, Riordan T, Jones DM, Painter MJ (1989) Secondary cases of meningococcal infection among close family and household contacts in England and Wales, 1984–7. BMJ 298:555–558
207. Fairley NH, Stewart CA (1916) Cerebro-spinal fever. Quarantine Service Publication, No. 9. Commonwealth of Australia, Melbourne, pp 13, 15, 16, 21, 22
208. Feldman HA (1966) Recent developments in the therapy and control of meningococcal infections. Disease-a-Month (Chicago) February:19–20
209. Center for Disease Control (1972) Methods of prevention and control of nosocomial infections. In: Center for Disease Control (eds) National Nosocomial Infections Study: fourth quarter 1971. Center for Disease Control, Atlanta, pp 19–23
210. Center for Disease Control (1978) Nosocomial meningococcemia – Wisconsin. MMWR Morb Mortal Wkly Rep 27:358, 363
211. Cohen MS, Steere AC, Baltimore R, von Graevenitz A, Pantelick E, Camp B, et al. (1979) Possible nosocomial transmission of group Y *Neisseria meningitidis* among oncology patients. Ann Intern Med 91:7–12
212. Riewerts-Eriksen NHR, Espersen F, Laursen L, Skinhøj P, Høiby N, Lind I (1989) Nosocomial outbreak of group C meningococcal disease. BMJ 298:568–569
213. Cohen L, Doucet E, Bourderont D, Wackenheim P, Hubert B, Riou JY (1991) Un cas secondaire d'infection à méningocoque en milieu hospitalier. Bull Epidemiol Hebdomadaire 35:152
214. Holdsworth G, Jackson H, Kaczmarski E (1996) Meningococcal infection from saliva. Lancet 348:1443
215. Duany R, Cruz MA, Atherley S, Suarez JA, Sneller V, Vaamonde L, et al. (1998) Outbreaks of group B meningococcal disease – Florida, 1995 and 1997. MMWR Morb Mortal Wkly Rep 47:833–837
216. Gehanno JF, Kohen-Couderc L, Lemeland JF, Leroy J (1999) Nosocomial meningococcemia in a physician. Infect Control Hosp Epidemiol 20:564–565
217. Gilmore A, Stuart J, Andrews N (2000) Risk of secondary meningococcal disease in health-care workers. Lancet 356:1654–1655
218. Hunter D (1936) Saints and martyrs. Lancet ii:1131–1134
219. Anonymous (1936) Bacteriologist dies of meningitis (Medical news). JAMA 106:129
220. Feldman HA (1972) Some recollections of the meningococcal diseases: the first Harry F. Dowling lecture. JAMA 220:1107–1112
221. Pike RM (1976) Laboratory-associated infections: summary and analysis of 3921 cases. Health Lab Sci 13:105–114
222. Bhatti AR, DiNinno VL, Ashton FE, White LA (1982) A laboratory-acquired infection with *Neisseria meningitidis*. J Infect 4:247–252
223. Darchis JP, Boisivon A, Guibourdenche M, Collatz E, Riou JY (1991) Contamination de laboratoire par *Neisseria meningitidis*. Bull Epidemiol Hebdomadaire No. 35:152
224. Takata KK, Hinton BG, Werner SB, Rutherford GW, Lett SM (1991) Laboratory-acquired meningococcemia – California and Massachusetts. MMWR Morb Mortal Wkly Rep 40:46–47, 55
225. PHLS Communicable Disease Surveillance Centre (1992) Laboratory-acquired meningococcal infection. Commun Dis Rep CDR Wkly 2:39
226. Guibourdenche M, Darchis JP, Boisivon A, Collatz E, Riou JY (1994) Enzyme electrophoresis, sero- and subtyping, and outer membrane protein characterization of two *Neisseria meningitidis* strains involved in laboratory-acquired infections. J Clin Microbiol 32:701–704
227. Paradis JF, Grimard D (1994) Laboratory-acquired invasive meningococcus-Quebec. Can Commun Dis Rep 32:12–14
228. Feldman HA (1972) Meningococcal infections. Adv Intern Med 18:117–140
229. Schwartz B (1991) Chemoprophylaxis for bacterial infections: principle of and application to meningococcal infections. Rev Infect Dis 13 (Suppl 2):S170–S173
230. Jones DM (1989) Control of meningococcal disease: chemoprophylaxis for some carriers and some contact groups. BMJ 298:542–543
231. Pugsley MP, Dworzack DL, Horowitz EA, Cuevas TA, Sanders WE, Sanders CC (1987) Efficacy of ciprofloxacin in the treatment of nasopharyngeal carriers of *Neisseria meningitidis*. J Infect Dis 156:211–213
232. Schwartz B, Al-Tobaiqi A, Al-Ruwais A, Fontaine RE,

A'ashi J, Hightower AW, et al. (1988) Comparative efficacy of ceftriaxone and rifampicin in eradicating pharyngeal carriage of group A *Neisseria meningitidis*. Lancet i: 1239–1242
233. Gilja OH, Halstensen A, Didranes A, Mylvaganan H, Aksnes A, Høiby EA (1993) Use of single-dose ofloxacin to eradicate tonsillopharyngeal carriage of *Neisseria meningitidis*. Antimicrob Agents Chemother 37:2024–2026
234. Cuevas LE, Kazembe P, Mughogho GK, Tillotson GS, Hart CA (1995) Eradication of nasopharyngeal carriage of *Neisseria meningitidis* in children and adults in rural Africa: a comparison of ciprofloxacin and rifampin. J Infect Dis 171:728–731
235. Anderson MS, Glodé MP, Smith AL (2004) Meningococcal disease. In: Feigin RD, Cherry JD, Demmler GJ, Kaplan SL (eds) Textbook of pediatric infectious diseases, 5th edn. vol. 1. WB Saunders, Philadelphia, pp 1265–1280
236. Foster G, Panigrahi H, Walker M (1986) Failure of chemoprophylaxis to prevent meningococcal disease. BMJ 292:886–887
237. Cooper ER, Ellison RT III, Smith GS, Blaser MJ, Reller LB, Paisley JW (1986) Rifampicin-resistant meningococcal disease in a contact patient given prophylactic rifampin. J Pediatr 108:93–96
238. Schubiger G, Munzinger J, Dudli C, Wipfli U (1986) Meningokokken-Epidemie in einer Internatsschule: Sekundärerkrankung mit Rifampicin-Restistentem Erreger unter Chemoprophylaxe. Schweiz Med Wochenschr 116: 1172–1175
239. Yagupsky P, Ashkenazi S, Block C (1993) Rifampin-resistant meningococci causing invasive disease and failure of chemoprophylaxis. Lancet 341:1152–1153
240. Stuart JM, Cartwright KA, Robinson PM, Noah ND (1989) Does eradication of meningococcal carriage in household contacts prevent secondary cases of meningococcal disease? BMJ 298:569–570
241. Greenwood BM, Hassan-King M, Whittle HC (1978) Prevention of secondary cases of meningococcal disease in household contacts by vaccination. BMJ i:1317–1319
242. Høiby EA, Moe PJ, Lystad A, Frøholm LO, Bøvre K (1986) Phenoxymethyl-penicillin treatment of household contacts of patients with meningococcal disease. Antonie van Leeuwenhoek 52:255–257
243. Gedde-Dahl TW, Høiby EA, Brandtzaeg P, Eskerud JR, Bøvre K (1990) Some arguments on early hospital admission and treatment of suspected meningococcal disease cases. NIPH Ann 13:45–60
244. Kristiansen BE, Knapskog AB (1996) Secondary prevention of meningococcal disease: high risk contacts should be given chemoprophylaxis and preventive treatment with penicillin. BMJ 312:591–592
245. Jones DM (1996) Secondary prevention of meningococcal disease: British guidelines should have been considered. BMJ 312:1537
246. Pollard AJ, Booy R, Nadel S, Levin M (1996) Secondary prevention of meningococcal disease: penicillin is not recommended in British guidelines. BMJ 312:1536
247. Stokes T, Shukla R, Mork P (1996) Secondary prevention of meningococcal disease: no evidence exists to support use of penicillin. BMJ 312:1536–1537
248. Gotschlich EC, Goldschneider I, Artenstein MS (1969) Human immunity to the meningococcus. IV. Immunogenicity of group A and group C meningococcal polysaccharides in human volunteers. J Exp Med 129:1367–1384
249. Artenstein MS, Gold R, Zimmerly JG, Wyle FA, Schneider H, Harkins C (1970) Prevention of meningococcal disease by group C polysaccharide vaccine. N Engl J Med 282: 417–420
250. Liu TY, Gotschlich EC, Jonssen EK, Wysocki JR (1971) Studies on the meningococcal polysaccharides: I. Composition and chemical properties of the group A polysaccharide. J Biol Chem 246:2849–2858
251. Mäkelä PH, Peltola H, Käyhty H, Jousimies H, Pettay O, Rouslahti E, et al. (1977) Polysaccharide vaccines of group A *Neisseria meningitidis* and *Haemophilus influenzae* type b: a field trial in Finland. J Infect Dis 136 (Suppl):S43–S50
252. Wahdan MH, Rizk F, El-Akkad AM, El-Ghoroury AA, Hablas R, Girgis NI, et al. (1973) A controlled field trial of a serogroup A meningococcal polysaccharide vaccine. Bull World Health Organ 48:667–673
253. Wahdan MH, Sallam SA, Hassan MN, Abdel-Gawad AA, Rakha AS, Sippel JE, et al. (1977) A second controlled field trial of a serogroup A meningococcal polysaccharide vaccine in Alexandria. Bull World Health Organ 55: 645–651
254. Sanborn WR, Bencic Z, Cvjetanovic B, Gotschlich EC, Pollock TM, Sippel JE (1972) Trial of a serogroup A meningococcus polysaccharide vaccine in Nigeria. Prog Immunobiol Stand 5:497–505
255. Peltola H (1978) Group A meningococcal polysaccharide vaccine and course of the group A meningococcal epidemic in Finland. Scand J Infect Dis 10:41–44
256. Greenwood BM, Wali SS (1980) Control of meningococcal infection in the African meningitis belt by selective vaccination. Lancet i:729–732
257. Mohammed I, Zaruba K (1981) Control of epidemic meningococcal infection by mass vaccination. Lancet i: 80–83
258. Binkin N, Band J (1982) Epidemic of meningococcal meningitis in Bamako, Mali: epidemiological features and analysis of vaccine efficacy. Lancet ii:315–318
259. Cochi SL, Markowitz LE, Joshi DD, Owens RC Jr, Stenhouse DH, Regmi DN, et al. (1987) Control of epidemic group A meningococcal meningitis in Nepal. Int J Epidemiol 16:91–97
260. Masterton RG, Youngs ER, Wardle JC, Croft KF, Jones DM (1988) Control of an outbreak of group C meningococcal meningitis with a polysaccharide vaccine. J Infect 17: 177–182
261. Lennon D, Gellin B, Hood D, Voss L, Heffernan H, Thakur S (1992) Successful intervention in a group A meningococcal outbreak in Auckland, New Zealand. Pediatr Infect Dis J 11:617–623
262. Rosenstein N, Levine O, Taylor JP, Evans D, Plikaytis BD, Wenger JD, et al. (1998) Efficacy of meningococcal vaccine and barriers to vaccination. JAMA 279:435–439
263. Veeken H, Ritmeijer K, Hausman B (1998) Priority during a meningitis epidemic: vaccination or treatment? Bull World Health Organ 76:135–141
264. Hankins WA, Gwaltney JM Jr, Hendley JO, Farquhar JD, Samuelson JS (1982) Clinical and serological evaluation of a meningococcal polysaccharide vaccine groups A, C, Y, and W135 (41306). Proc Soc Exp Biol Med 169:54–57
265. Peltola H, Mäkelä HP, Käyhty H, Jousimies H, Herva E, Hallstrom K, et al. (1977) Clinical efficacy of meningococcus group A capsular polysaccharide vaccine in children three months to five years of age. N Engl J Med 297:686–691
266. Ceesay SJ, Allen SJ, Menon A, Todd JE, Cham K, Carlone GM, et al. (1993) Decline in meningococcal antibody levels in African children 5 years after vaccination and the lack of an effect of booster immunization. J Infect Dis 167:1212–1216
267. Granoff DM, Feavers IM, Borrow R (2004) Meningococ-

cal vaccines. In: Plotkin SA, Orenstein WA (eds) Vaccines, 4th edn. WB Saunders, Philadelphia, pp 959–987
268. Frasch CE (1989) Vaccines for prevention of meningococcal disease. Clin Microbiol Rev 2 (Suppl):S134–S138
269. Robbins JB, Schneerson R, Szu SC, Fattom A, Yang Y, Lagergard T, et al. (1989) Prevention of invasive bacterial diseases by immunization with polysaccharide-protein conjugates. Curr Top Microbiol Immunol 146:169–180
270. Goldblatt D (1998) Immunisation and the maturation of infant immune responses. Dev Biol Stand 95:125–132
271. Jennings HJ, Lugowski C (1981) Immunochemistry of groups A, B and C meningococcal polysaccharide-tetanus toxoid conjugates. J Immunol 127:1011–1018
272. Beuvery EC, Roy R, Kanhai V, Jennings HJ (1986) Characteristics of two types of meningococcal group C polysaccharide conjugates using tetanus toxoid as carrier protein. Dev Biol Stand 65:197–204
273. Costantino P, Viti S, Podda A, Velmonte MA, Nencioni L, Rappuoli R (1992) Development and phase 1 clinical testing of a conjugate vaccine against meningococcus A and C. Vaccine 10:691–698
274. Feavers IM (2001) Meningococcal vaccines and vaccine developments. In: Pollard AJ, Maiden MCJ (eds) Meningococcal vaccines: methods and protocols. Serie: Methods in molecular medicine 66 (JM Walker, series ed). Humana Press, Totowa, NJ, pp 1–22
275. Guo Z, Jennings H (2001) Protein-polysaccharide conjugation. In: Pollard AJ, Maiden MCJ (eds) Meningococcal vaccines: methods and protocols. Serie: Methods in molecular medicine 66 (JM Walker, series ed). Humana Press, Totowa, NJ, pp 49–54.
276. Snape MD, Pollard AJ (2005) Meningococcal polysaccharide-protein conjugate vaccines. Lancet Infect Dis 5: 21–30
277. Miller E, Salisbury D, Ramsay ME (2002) Planning, registration, and implementation of an immunisation campaign against meningococcal serogroup C disease in the UK: a success story. Vaccine 20 (Suppl 1):S58–S67
278. Bose A, Coen P, Tully J, Viner R, Booy R (2003) Effectiveness of meningococcal C conjugate vaccine in teenagers in England. Lancet 361:675–676
279. Balmer P, Borrow R, Miller E (2002) Impact of meningococcal C conjugate vaccine in the UK. J Med Microbiol 51:717–722
280. Ramsay ME, Andrews N, Kaczmarski EB, Miller E (2001) Efficacy of meningococcal serogroup C conjugate vaccine in teenagers and toddlers. Lancet 357:195–196
281. Trotter CL, Andrews NJ, Kaczmarski EB, Miller E, Ramsay ME (2004) Effectiveness of meningococcal serogroup C conjugate vaccine 4 years after introduction. Lancet 364:365–367
282. Pollard AJ, Maiden MC (2003) Epidemic meningococcal disease in sub-Saharan Africa – towards a sustainable solution? Lancet Infect Dis 3:6870
283. Stefanelli P, Fazio C, Neri A, Sofia T, Mastrantonio P (2003) First report of capsule replacement among electrophoretic type 37 *Neisseria meningitidis* strains in Italy. J Clin Microbiol 41:5783–5786
284. Hahne SJ, Gray SJ, Aguilera JF, Crowcroft NS, Nichols T, Kaczmarski EB, et al. (2002) W135 meningococcal disease in England and Wales associated with the Hajj 2000 and 2001. Lancet 359:582–583
285. Lingappa JR, Al-Rabeah AM, Hajjeh R, Mustafa T, Fatani A, Al-Bassam T, et al. (2003) Serogroup W-135 meningococcal disease during the Hajj, 2000. Emerg Infect Dis 9:665–671
286. Finne J, Leinonen M, Mäkelä PH (1983) Antigenic similarities between brain components and bacteria causing meningitis: implications for vaccine development and pathogenesis. Lancet ii:355–357
287. Finne J, Bitter-Suermann D, Goridis C, Finne U (1987) An IgG monoclonal antibody to group B meningococci cross-reacts with developmentally regulated polysialic acid units of glycoproteins in neural and extraneural tissues. J Immunol 138:4402–4407
288. Jennings HJ, Roy R, Gamian A (1986) Induction of meningococcal group B polysaccharide-specific IgG antibodies in mice by using an N-propionylated B polysaccharide-tetanus toxoid conjugate vaccine. J Immunol 137:1708–1713
289. Sierra CVG, Campa HC, Valcárcel NW (1991) Vaccine against group B *Neisseria meningitidis*: protection trial and mass vaccination results in Cuba. NIPH Ann 14: 195–207
290. Zollinger WD, Boslego J, Moran E, García J, Cruz C, Ruíz S, et al. (1991) Meningococcal serogroup B vaccine protection trial and follow-up studies in Chile. NIPH Ann 14:211–212
291. de Moraes JC, Perkins BA, Camargo MC, Hidalgo NT, Barbosa HA, Sacchi CT, et al. (1992) Protective efficacy of a serogroup B meningococcal vaccine in Sao Paulo, Brazil. Lancet 340:1074–1078
292. Milagres LG, Ramos SR, Sacchi CT, Melles CE, Vieira VS, Sato H, et al. (1994) Immune response of Brazilian children to a *Neisseria meningitidis* serogroup B outer membrane protein vaccine: comparison with efficacy. Infect Immun 62:4419–4424
293. Boslego J, García J, Cruz C, Zollinger W, Brandt B, Ruíz S, et al. (1995) Efficacy, safety, and immunogenicity of a meningococcal group B (15:P1.3) outer membrane protein vaccine in Iquique, Chile. Vaccine 13:821–829
294. Bjune G, Høiby EA, Grønnesby JK, Arnesen O, Fredriksen JH, Halstensen A, et al. (1991) Effect of outer membrane vesicle vaccine against group B meningococcal disease in Norway. Lancet 388:1093–1096
295. Herbert MA, Heath PT, Mayon-White RT (1995) Meningococcal vaccines for the United Kingdom. Commun Dis Rep CDR Rev 5:R130–R135
296. Cartwright K, Morris R, Rumke H, Fox A, Borrow R, Begg N, et al. (1999) Immunogenicity and reactogenicity in UK infants of a novel meningococcal vesicle vaccine containing multiple class 1 (PorA) outer membrane proteins. Vaccine 17:2612–2619
297. Haneberg B, Dalseg R, Oftung F, Wedege E, Høiby EA, Haugen IL, et al. (1998) Towards a nasal vaccine against meningococcal disease, and prospects for its use as a mucosal adjuvant. Dev Biol Stand 92:127–133
298. Haneberg B, Dalseg R, Wedege E, Høiby EA, Haugen IL, Oftung F, et al. (1998) Intranasal administration of a meningococcal outer membrane vesicle vaccine induces persistent local mucosal antibodies and serum antibodies with strong bactericidal activity in humans. Infect Immun 66:1334–1341
299. Oftung F, Naess LM, Wetzler LM, Korsvold GE, Aase A, Høiby EA, et al. (1999) Antigen-specific T-cell responses in humans after intranasal immunization with a meningococcal serogroup B outer membrane vesicle vaccine. Infect Immun 67:921–927
300. Rosenqvist E, Høiby EA, Wedege E, Bryn K, Kolberg J, Klem A, et al. (1995) Human antibody responses to meningococcal outer membrane antigens after three doses of the Norwegian group B meningococcal vaccine. Infect Immun 63:4642–4652
301. Hilleman MR (2000) Vaccines in historic evolution and perspective: a narrative of vaccine discoveries. Vaccine 18:1436–1447

302. Rappuoli R, del Giudice G (1999) Identification of vaccine targets. In: Paoletti LC, McInnes PM (eds) Vaccines: from concept to clinic. CRC Press, Boca Raton, pp 1 – 17
303. Adu-Bobie J, Capecchi B, Serruto D, Rappuoli R, Pizza M (2003) Two years into reverse vaccinology. Vaccine 21:605 – 610
304. Rappuoli R (2001) Reverse vaccinology, a genome-based approach to vaccine development. Vaccine 19:2688 – 2691
305. Tettelin H, Saunders NJ, Heidelberg J, Jeffries AC, Nelson KE, Eisen JA, et al. (2000) Complete genome sequence of *Neisseria meningitidis* serogroup B strain MC58. Science 287:1809 – 1815
306. Rappuoli R (2001) Conjugates and reverse vaccinology to eliminate bacterial meningitis. Vaccine 19:2319 – 2322
307. Pizza M, Scarlato V, Masignani V, Giuliani MM, Aricò B, Comanducci M, et al. (2000) Identification of vaccine candidates against serogroup B meningococcus by whole-genome sequencing. Science 287:1816 – 1820

34 Septic Shock

M. Llewelyn, J. Cohen

34.1 Sepsis Terminology

This chapter is concerned with the diagnosis and immediate treatment of patients with septic shock. Most clinicians will have a mental image of this condition and would expect to have little difficulty in recognising it from the end of the bed, but despite this there is no universally accepted definition. Indeed, when clinical investigators attempt to arrive at a consensus there are wide variations in terms. Thus, a necessary preface to this chapter is a brief discussion of the controversy surrounding the nomenclature of these syndromes.

34.1.1 Sepsis

Sepsis is the systemic response to infection, brought about by activation of the host inflammatory processes. The clinical features defining the 'systemic inflammatory response syndrome' (SIRS) seen in sepsis were identified at a consensus conference in 1991 [1]. The SIRS criteria required two or more of four features to be present: fever (or hypothermia), leucocytosis (or leucopenia), tachycardia, and tachypnoea. Although useful in that it drew attention to a common clinical pattern seen in ICU patients, SIRS has been criticised for being too sensitive and because it embraces a wide range of possible causes. Sepsis – i.e. infection – is one cause of SIRS, but many other non-infective processes (blood transfusion, trauma, pancreatitis, etc.) can cause the same clinical picture. This concern, coupled with major advances in our understanding of the pathophysiology of sepsis, led to a re-appraisal of sepsis definitions at a consensus conference in 2001 [2]. This confrence recognised the value of a wide range of clinical and laboratory parameters in the diagnosis of sepsis but saw no reason to change the fundamental definition.

34.1.2 Severe Sepsis/Sepsis Syndrome

These terms are used to describe sepsis associated with organ dysfunction, hypoperfusion or hypotension [2]. Hypoperfusion abnormalities may include, but are not limited to, lactic acidosis, oliguria, and an acute alteration in mental state. Several validated scoring systems for organ dysfunction exist for both adult and pediatric patient populations. Such systems have provided the basis for the inclusion criteria for most of the clinical trials of adjunctive agents in sepsis and as such have been the subject of much discussion. Some have argued that organ dysfunction may in fact be a protective mechanism in sepsis [3]. It may be that organ dysfunction is a marker of severity rather than an independent predictor of outcome, as has been demonstrated for sepsis related acute lung injury [4].

34.1.3 Septic Shock

Septic shock is universally recognised as the most severe end of the spectrum of systemic syndromes induced by infection. The late Roger Bone, one of the doyens of this field, wrote "Septic shock should not be viewed as a single entity...." [5]. In the same paper, Bone defined septic shock as "...simply [sic] the deranged metabolic state that arises from systemic sepsis in a hypotensive patient unresponsive to fluid management". According to the 2001 consensus conference "septic shock ... refers to a state of acute circulatory failure characterised by arterial hypotension unexplained by other causes" [2]. In adults, generally accepted cut-offs for arterial hypotension exist (systolic arterial pressure below 90 mmHg or mean arterial pressure below 60 mmHg) but in children hypotension may be a late sign in septic shock and prolonged capillary refill time (>2 s) may be an earlier marker [6].

It is not our purpose here to try to resolve dilemmas surrounding sepsis terminology, but rather to draw attention to the ongoing struggle to find a true consensus over these definitions. This has led some to suggest that it might be better to reserve 'sepsis' as a conceptual term and instead talk about specific clinical syndromes, 'severe community acquired pneumonia with organ dysfunction' for instance (J. Carlet, personal communication, 2006). At a minimum, a recent consensus conference agreed a series of definitions for specific infections in the context of sepsis and these should be used in future clinical trials [7]. Certainly there is broad agreement that septic shock first implies the presence of infection, and, secondly, describes a severe illness in which there is a multiple organ dysfunction and a mortality rate which may be as high as 75 %. This chapter will focus on the infectious diseases aspects of septic shock; other elements of the management such as cardiovascular support and monitoring are covered elsewhere (Chapters 2, 3). We will emphasise the practical approach to the diagnosis and management of patients with septic shock, in particular strategies that are currently available in routine clinical practice.

34.2 Epidemiology

Sepsis and septic shock have occurred with increasing frequency during the last 20 years, much of this being driven by an excess of hospital-acquired (nosocomial) infections [8, 9]. Accurate estimates of incidence are very difficult to generate. This is partly because of the problems with the definition that were noted above but also because of the marked variation that exists between ICUs and the inaccuracies inherent in the large scale, retrospective analyses of survival data that such estimates involve. Using data from the United States National Hospital Discharge Survey, Martin et al. gave an estimated annual sepsis incidence for the USA of 164,000 in 1979 rising nearly 9 % year on year to 660,000 in 2000 [9]. In contrast Angus et al. estimated that 751,000 cases of *severe* sepsis occurred in the USA in 1995 [10]. Although overall mortality rates have fallen (28 % to 18 % in Martin's study) the overall incidence of sepsis continues to rise and the total number of attributable deaths continues to increase.

The true incidence of septic *shock* is equally difficult to ascertain. This is principally because individual patients with sepsis will frequently have sepsis, severe sepsis and septic shock at different points in the clinical course of their illness [11]. In a prospective, multicentre study of infection on ICUs in Europe, Canada and Israel, Alberti et al. reported an infection rate of 21 % among nearly 8,400 patients staying over 24 h on the ICU. Of these patients only 18 % did not meet sepsis criteria, 24 % had severe sepsis and 30 % septic shock [12]. Annane et al. reported a rate of septic shock in French ICUs of 9.7/100 admissions in 2000, increasing from 7.0/100 admissions in 1993. This increase in septic shock incidence is consistent with Martin's study which reported an increase in the proportion of sepsis patients with multi-organ failure from 3.2 % to 9 % between the early 1980s and late 1990s. Implicit in the grading of sepsis severity is a relationship with outcome. Recent estimates of mortality associated with septic shock remain very high and very variable, broadly 40–70 % [8, 12, 13]. This wide variation may well relate to local epidemiologic factors: for instance, a study in which there were a disproportionate number of neutropenic patients would be likely to include a large number of sepsis cases caused by *Staph. epidermidis*, an organism of generally low virulence. In contrast, a unit which cared for liver transplant recipients would have relatively high rates of *Candida* infection, which is associated with a much more grave prognosis [14]. Consistent with this are the data presented in Alberti's study demonstrating differences in mortality among septic shock patients depending on whether their infection was community or hospital acquired [12]. Another factor is the complex, and at times confusing, relationship between bacteraemia, sepsis, and shock. These terms are not synonymous, but in some reports the distinction has become blurred. In the large epidemiological study of SIRS reported by Rangel-Frausto, positive blood cultures were found in 69 % of patients with shock but just 25 % of patients with sepsis [15]. However, in patients with shock the mortality was the same, irrespective of whether they were bacteraemic. In contrast, a somewhat similar study reported by Brun-Buisson et al. found that the higher mortality associated with increasing numbers of organ dysfunctions (relative risk 4.4 [95 % confidence interval 1.2–16]) *was* further increased in patients with documented infections (RR 9.4 [1.3–78]) [16].

The precise nature of the infection underlying septic shock may further influence outcome. Cohen et al. reviewed data from 510 published articles documenting >55,000 clinical infections to determine the relationship between the aetiology of sepsis in terms of microorganism and source and sepsis outcome [17]. This study confirmed the relationship between site of infection and outcome which has been documented previously [18, 19], specifically, that sepsis arising from the urinary tract, intra-vascular catheter sites and skin is less likely to be lethal than sepsis arising from pulmonary, gastrointestinal and central nervous system sources. The study also confirmed the long-held impression that certain bacteria are associated with a higher mortality across a wide range of sites of infection; *S. aureus*, *P. aeruginosa* and *S. pyogenes* were associated with higher mortality than less virulent organisms such as coagulase-negative staphylococci and *Acinetobacter* spp. [17]. Specific microbial virulence factors are not of course the only explanation for the relationship between particular pathogens and poor prognosis. The immunological state of the host is also an important factor. Bloodstream infection with *Candida* spp. has a particularly poor prognosis and this is more likely to relate to the immunocompromised state of such patients and the severity of underlying disease than to specific microbial factors.

34.3 Diagnosis

The most important reason to make a microbiologic diagnosis in septic patients is to ensure that effective antimicrobial therapy is given. There is good evidence to support the intuitive belief that patients given appropriate therapy are more likely to survive than those given inadequate or inappropriate treatment [20–23]. Obtaining microbiologic information will also contribute to the local epidemiological database, without which logical prescribing is difficult, if not impossible. There are substantial differences between intensive care units in the microbial ecology, including for example the prevalence of methicillin-resistant *Staphylococcus aureus* and vancomycin-resistant *Streptococcus faecalis*. Antimicrobial resistance patterns, too, vary widely: examples include penicillin resistance in *Streptococcus pneumoniae*, gentamicin resistance and extended spectrum beta-lactamase production in Enterobacteriaceae. Furthermore, these resistance rates are constantly changing, and an up-to-date awareness of these patterns is obviously essential when considering empiric therapy. Finally, knowledge of the microbial aetiology of sepsis may be important in the choice of adjunctive therapy. This is not yet clinical reality, but will clearly be important if, for instance, anti-endotoxin agents ever enter the clinical arena.

There are three key difficulties associated with the diagnosis of infection in patients who appear to be septic.

Establishing Infection as the Primary Cause. The controversies surrounding the definition of sepsis have been discussed above. Establishing that the patient has infection rather than a non-infective cause of SIRS can be extremely difficult. Knowledge of other pathologies that may mimic sepsis and how they may apply to the specific patient can make up for a relative paucity of clinical information. The differential diagnosis of shock due to causes other than infection includes acute myocardial infarction, massive pulmonary embolism, acute blood loss and anaphylaxis. Less common diagnoses are acute hypoadrenalism, diabetic ketoacidosis and some cases of self-poisoning. The diagnosis and management of non-infective shock is beyond the scope of this chapter.

Localising the Site of Infection. This may be confounded by the fact there are multiple pathologic processes occurring concurrently or by the frequent use of antibiotics which undermine microbiologic diagnosis. Occasionally the site of infection is occult, for instance when there is a sinusitis or deep intra-abdominal infection.

Interpreting the Microbiologic Findings. Conventional microbiology has many limitations in the ICU patient who may be septic. Principal amongst these is the fact that many organisms isolated from non-sterile sites may represent either colonisation of infection – microbiology alone cannot answer this question. Conversely, the microbiology laboratory may report negative findings in samples from sites that are in fact infected, for example because antibiotics have sterilised the specimen.

34.3.1 Clinical Approach

Fever is a common sign on the ICU and will often be the first indication of sepsis, although there are many other causes [24, 25], and practice guidelines for the evaluation of fever on the ICU have been published [26].

Focused clinical examination, guided by any risk factors relevant to the individual patient, will often reveal potential sources of sepsis and guide subsequent investigation (see Chapter 1). A number of clinical syndromes are sufficiently characteristic clinically to point to a specific diagnosis. For example, ecthyma gangrenosum, characterised by haemorrhagic, bullous lesions in the context of neutropenic sepsis is characteristic of *Pseudomonas aeruginosa* or sometimes *E. coli* sepsis. Purpura fulminans although characteristic of meningococcal sepsis may be seen in severe sepsis of other aetiologies, particularly pneumococcal sepsis. The presence of generalised erythema, conjunctival injection and mucositis may indicate staphylococcal or streptococcal toxic shock syndrome. Surgical and traumatic wounds should be exposed and examined for signs of infection. Particular attention should be paid to vascular access sites for signs of phlebitis or cellulitis and to pressure areas or injection sites for evidence of soft tissue infection. Evidence of sinusitis should be sought, and fundoscopy is invaluable in detecting candidal endophthalmitis, a pathognomonic feature of systemic fungal sepsis. Urine in the catheter may be frankly purulent, and the presence of diarrhoea may indicate *Clostridium difficile* associated colitis. The importance of repeated, complete physical examination to detect the emergence of new signs cannot be overstated.

34.3.2 Diagnostic Microbiology

Microbiological aspects of infection at specific sites are dealt with in the preceding chapters in this section. Blood cultures are considered below; a more detailed account of the microbiological investigation of sepsis is available [27].

Blood should be obtained for culture whenever there is reason to suspect a clinically significant bacteraemia. There are no good data that relate timing of blood cultures with respect to timing of fever. Nevertheless, bacteria are rapidly cleared from blood, and development of fever usually follows an episode of bacteraemia by 30–90 min, so blood cultures should be taken as soon as possible following a spike of fever.

When a decision has been made to take blood for culture, adherence to a protocol for obtaining the specimen results in lower contamination rates and will also affect yield. Skin should be sterilised prior to venepuncture by swabbing twice with either 70% isopropyl or ethyl alcohol or with an iodine containing solution [20]. Blood should be obtained by venepuncture or if necessary arterial stab. Sites associated with skin contamination (e.g. femoral site) or loss of skin integrity (e.g. dermatological disease) should be avoided. Contamination rates are not significantly higher for blood obtained through a peripheral cannula at the time of insertion and this is acceptable as a means of minimising the number of venepunctures.

An adequate volume of blood must be obtained. The concentration of bacteraemia in adult patients is frequently below one viable organism per millilitre and may be less than 0.1 organisms/ml, so it is not surprising that the volume of blood obtained for culture is an important variable determining culture yield. In adults, a minimum sample size of 10 ml will optimise yield while increasing the volume above 30 ml is not associated with significantly improved culture rates [28].

In bacteraemia associated with sources other than endocarditis, sensitivity exceeding 90% is reached with either two or three cultures. The taking of only one culture is rarely desirable. Since the rate of contamination of an individual set of blood cultures is finite, ranging from 1% to 4.6%, interpretation of a single isolate of a potentially contaminating organism may be exceedingly difficult. When clinically significant bacteraemia is suspected, two or three sets of cultures should be obtained by individual venepunctures. There is no advantage in waiting between them.

34.3.3 Non-specific Markers of Infection

Traditional markers of infection such as neutrophilia are too non-specific in the ICU setting to be of value in distinguishing sepsis, although marked neutrophilia or failure to mount a neutrophil response may be of prognostic value. Amongst the biomarkers of inflammation and infection which have been reported, C-reactive protein (CRP) and procalcitonin (PCT) have been most widely studied and are available as relatively cheap commercial assays. Both assays have been shown in numerous trials to have useful sensitivity and specificity in differentiating infection from other causes of an inflammatory response. Studies comparing CRP and PCT as markers of infection have recently been the subject of a meta-analysis [29]. This confirmed that while in most studies PCT is superior to CRP in differentiating bacterial infection from non-bacterial causes of inflammation the cut-offs applied vary markedly in different patient populations and in no setting are the sensitivities and specificities perfect. A recent comparison of the diagnostic value of PCT in medical or surgical patients with septic shock demonstrated this clearly [30]. Cut-offs of 1 ng/ml and 6 ng/ml were required to yield sensitivities/specificities of 91.7/74.2% and 76%/72.7% in medical and surgical patients respectively. There was a positive correlation of PCT level with adverse outcome as has been reported previously [31] but in this study this relationship was only apparent in medical, not surgical patients. In terms of assessing prognosis, the time course of changes in PCT may be more telling than a single point value [32]. Against the slightly better discriminatory power of PCT compared with CRP needs to be set the assay costs (PCT costs about twice as much per test) and the more robustly established biology of CRP which makes interpretation of levels in individual patients somewhat more straightforward [33]. Neither CRP nor PCT alone can differentiate sepsis from other causes of SIRS, and they should certainly never be used as the sole basis of a decision to use, or not to use, antibiotics in a patient who may be septic. Rather, they are a part of a systemic evaluation that includes clinical examination and directed diagnostic techniques. Measurement of PCT or CRP is often most valuable when done sequentially in an individual patient as an aid to following the response to treatment, or as an indicator that a focus of infection remains inadequately treated.

The possibility that direct measurement of circulating endotoxin could be used as a marker of sepsis has been the subject of long and thorough examination. Most studies have used the chromogenic limulus amebocyte lysate (LAL) assay. This has been widely used to detect endotoxin contamination of drugs and fluids; however, biological samples may contain inhibitors of the LAL reaction and fungal elements may give rise to a false positive LAL reaction [34]. However, using this assay, rates of endotoxaemia ranging from 33% to 92% have been reported in sepsis patients [35–39]. Although some studies have suggested a correlation with severity, endotoxin levels measured by LAL assay do not show good correlation with sepsis outcome. Marshall et al. recently described the measurement of endotoxaemia in ICU patients using a novel, rapid, whole-blood endotoxin assay based on neutrophil-dependent chemoluminescence [40]. Endotoxaemia was detected in the blood of 57.2% of patients on the day of ICU admission and although good correlation of endotoxin level with severity was observed, again endotoxin level did not predict outcome. Although the sensitivity

Table 34.1. Potential future biomarkers of sepsis

Marker		Ref.
sTREM (soluble triggering receptor expressed on myeloid cells)-1	Expressed by neutrophils and macrophages infected by bacteria or fungi. Plasma levels >60 mg/l indicate infection in patients with SIRS	[41]
Naturetic peptides	Brain and atrial naturetic peptide levels show correlation with severity and prognosis	[42, 43]
Monocyte HLA-DR expression	Downregulation of expression is an early marker of sepsis but data are contradictory on specificity and prognostic implications	[44]
High Mobility Group Box-1 protein (HMGB1)	Late, macrophage expressed, proinflammatory mediator. Data are conflicting as to whether levels correlate with poor prognosis	[45, 46]

(85.3%) and specificity (44.0%) of the assay for detecting gram negative sepsis were relatively poor, only 1.2% of patients with a low endotoxin level had gram negative infection and only 5.2% had infection with any organism. The authors propose that the value of the investigation of endotoxaemia on the day of admission to ICU may thus lie in its high *negative* predictive value for bacterial infection (and not exclusively gram negative infection) [40]. Nevertheless, at present there is no place for routine measurement of endotoxin levels in sepsis patients.

There has been a profusion of reports in the last 5 years of biomarkers with the potential to perform better than CRP or PCT in differentiating sepsis from non-infective SIRS, determining prognosis and stratifying patients for entry into clinical trials. Although none has yet advanced to clinical practice, some of the most promising are summarised in Table 34.1.

34.4 Management

34.4.1 General Principles

The immediate priority is to address the three potentially life-threatening issues: airway, breathing and circulation (the so-called ABC of resuscitation). There is now a clear consensus that cardiovascular resuscitation, involving fluids and in many cases vasopressors, should begin immediately septic shock is diagnosed and not be delayed until ICU admission. This has arisen out of two observations. First, that only around one-third of patients who develop sepsis do so on the ICU, while one-third develop sepsis elsewhere in the hospital and one-third outside hospital [12]. Secondly, the impressive survival benefit reported by Rivers et al. to arise from the delivery of 'goal-directed therapy' (GDT) to sepsis patients at the point of diagnosis [47]. This study used central venous oxygen saturations (>70%) as an end-point to guide cardiovascular resuscitation including administration of packed red cells and dobutamine. Detailed consideration of the physiological assessment of patients with sepsis can be found in Chapter 2. Finally, it is a sound principle of management that where there is a closed or contained focus of infection, such as an abscess, every effort is made to drain and/or remove it, as soon as it is safe and appropriate to do so. This principle is referred to as source control and is discussed in the various specific situations in which it applies in Sections IV and VI.

34.4.2 Antimicrobial Therapy

Antimicrobial therapy is self-evidently a cornerstone of the management of septic shock. For a more detailed systematic review of the literature on this subject since 1966 the reader is referred to reference [48]. The Surviving Sepsis Campaign recommends that 'intravenous antibiotic therapy should be started within the first hour...' [49]. Although randomised clinical trial data to support this practice do not exist and ethically could not be generated, there is no reason not to extrapolate from the clear survival benefit associated with early antibiotic therapy observed in animal sepsis models [50].

It is worth re-emphasising that there is now a substantial body of data supporting the, probably intuitive, view that patients who receive antibiotics which are active against the infection which is driving sepsis are less likely to die than those who receive ineffective empiric antibiotic therapy. Evidence for this comes from a series of studies dating back over 30 years and exemplified by a paper from Kreger et al. [20]. They analysed a cohort of 612 patients with gram negative bacteraemia collected over a 10-year period. Irrespective of the severity of the underlying disease, proper empirical therapy reduced by half the frequency with which shock developed, and the fatality rate was significantly less in the appropriately treated groups compared to those given inappropriate antibiotics (rapidly fatal: 29% vs. 77%, ultimately fatal 26% vs. 38%, nonfatal 11% vs. 29%). Although modern antibiotics used on the ICU generally have much wider spectra of action than 30 years ago, the spectrum of bacteria causing sepsis has also changed and antimicrobial resistance is of course a much bigger factor. Recent studies do confirm the earlier data [21–23]. In a prospective observational study of 492 bacteraemic patients on a mixed medical and surgical ICU, Ibrahim et al. observed that 29.9% received 'inadequate' antimicrobial treatment, most frequently for VRE, candida and methicillin resistant staphylococci [23]. Highly significant correlations were found between inadequate treatment of infection by each of these organisms and mortality. The overall mortality rate in patients who received 'adequate' treatment was 28.4 % compared with 61.9 %. This represents a reduction in risk of death which, at 2.18, dwarfs the impact made by the novel adjunctive treatments of sepsis discussed below. Data such as these show clearly that having a single, 'standard antibiotic regimen' for all cases of septic shock is no more logical than it would be to use a single drug for all cardiac dysrhythmias. The difficulty with sepsis however is that while an electrocardiogram will quickly identify the nature of the rhythm, microbiological diagnosis will usually be delayed 12–18 h. However, empiric therapy need not mean 'blind' therapy, as it has sometimes been called. Several factors will inform choice of empiric therapy. The focus of the infection for example will be a critical piece of information. When a patient is presumed to be septic secondary to nosocomial pneumonia, intra-abdominal sepsis or urosepsis for instance, antibiotic choice will be dictated by the local flora related to those sites. Detailed recommendations for the choice of antibiotics will be found in Section II of this book. Here we will restrict the discussion to the initial empiric antibiotic choice in patients with septic shock who are presumed to be bacteraemic and/or in whom the focus of infection is not certain.

Consideration of four simple questions will provide much valuable guidance:

1. What is the history and clinical setting? For example, what is the patient's occupation? (sewer worker, garbage disposal, etc.) Is this a post-operative infection, and if so, was it a thoracic, intra-abdominal or pelvic procedure? Was the bowel breached? Is there a history of trauma? Are there any other clues to the likely focus?
2. Is this a nosocomial or community-acquired infection? Where was this infection most likely acquired? Is there a history of travel? In certain areas of the world, primary resistance rates of common pathogens are so high that first line antibiotics cannot be trusted. The marked variation in rates of resistance of *Streptococcus pneumoniae* would be an important example of this.
3. What is the underlying disease, if any? Is the patient neutropenic, or on dialysis?
4. What is the recent microbiologic and antibiotic history? Although one cannot be certain that recent isolates are necessarily the cause of the current episode of sepsis, it is obviously important to be aware if the patient is colonised with *Pseudomonas aeruginosa* or methicillin-resistant *Staphylococcus aureus*, for instance. It is also helpful to know the recent antibiotic history, in part because one must assume that whatever is causing the current infection is presumably resistant to those drugs, but also because it may raise the possibility of fungal infection.

This basic information can be assembled quickly and will allow the choice of a suitable regimen. Rarely, the clinical picture is so unambiguous that specific therapy can be given immediately: benzyl penicillin for meningococcaemia, for instance. In general though, a broad spectrum regimen must be chosen.

Adequate cover against gram negative bacteraemia is essential, and can be achieved with a broad spectrum cephalosporin, carbapenem, quinolone or extended spectrum penicillin/beta-lactamase inhibitor combination such as piperacillin/tazobactam. A key question is whether these agents can be used alone or should be combined with an aminoglycoside. Certainly there are in vitro data which suggest synergy between beta-lactams and aminoglycosides against gram negative organisms. Furthermore aminoglycosides might broaden the antimicrobial spectrum and prevent emergence of resistance during therapy. A recent Cochrane review identified 64 trials, including 7,586 patients, which have compared beta-lactam monotherapy with beta-lactam aminoglycoside combination therapy in sepsis [51]. None addressed septic shock specifically. No survival or treatment outcome benefit was found in patients treated with aminoglycoside combination therapy but nephrotoxicity was three times more common. Of note, even in subgroup analysis of patients with urinary tract sepsis or *Pseudomonas aeruginosa* infection no benefit was found. It seems reasonable then to conclude that in patients with severe sepsis, treatment with a broad spectrum cephalosporin (such as cefotaxime or ceftazidime) or a carbapenem (e.g. imipenem, meropenem) is likely to be equally effective and less toxic than combination therapy including an aminoglycoside [48].

The empiric antibiotic regimen chosen in septic shock should always include cover for gram positive pathogens since gram positive bacteria have now surpassed gram negative bacteria as aetiological agents of sepsis [9]. Many broad spectrum agents such as carbapenems, and third generation cephalosporins have excellent gram positive activity; however if the considerations listed above suggest that the patient is at risk from sepsis caused by methicillin resistant *S. aureus* (MRSA) or *S. epidermidis*, penicillin resistant *S. pneumoniae* or the patient has a history of immediate hypersensitivity to beta-lactam agents, it may be necessary to consider additional agents such as glycopeptides or linezolid (an oxazolidinone). In localities and individual hospitals where rates of MRSA sepsis are high, inclusion of a glycopeptide in regimens for empiric management of sepsis has become routine; however the use of glycopeptides either as empiric monotherapy or in combination with drugs which lack activity against staphylococci is undesirable in view of data which suggest that glycopeptides are less effective anti-staphylococcal drugs than beta-lactams [52, 53]. Partly because of a widely held perception that treatment of *S. aureus* infection with glycopeptides is associated with poor outcome there has been considerable interest in the possible use of linezolid as an alternative in empiric regimens for sepsis. Comparative trials of regimens containing linezolid or a glycopeptide have been performed in hospital acquired pneumonia and severe soft tissue infection and have consistently shown equivalence [54–57]. In a retrospective subgroup analysis of patients with nosocomial MRSA pneumonia, Wunderlink et al. demonstrated improved survival associated with linezolid [60/75 (80%)] compared with vancomycin [54/85 (64%)] [58]. Against this report attesting to the clinical superiority of linezolid must be set concerns about the development of resistance and toxicity. The mechanism of linezolid resistance involves spontaneous mutation in the 23S rRNA. Multiple copies of this 23S rRNA gene exist in most bacterial species and resistance correlates with the proportion of the copies carrying the resistance mutation [59]. The development of resistance to linezolid during therapy is therefore both biologically plausible and has already been reported in the clinical setting [60, 61]. It is striking that after nearly half a century of widespread glycopeptide use, staphylococci with clinically relevant resistance to glycopeptides remain thankfully rare. In addition, although the toxicities associated with glycopeptide use are not trivial they are at least well known and predictable. The side-effects of linezolid are still being defined, particularly in terms of neurotoxicity and bone-marrow toxicity. For all these reasons there is no rationale for moving away from glycopeptides in the empiric management of sepsis where bacteria resistant to beta-lactams are considered likely or where the patient is allergic to beta-lactams. Linezolid should be reserved for patients who are hypersensitive to glycopeptides or where vancomycin resistant enterococci are considered to be potential aetiological agents.

Anaerobic bacteria usually occur as part of a mixed infection and rarely cause shock alone. Nevertheless, antibiotics active against anaerobes are usually included in regimens in which anaerobic bacteria might be implicated. As a general rule, metronidazole should be used for infections arising below the diaphragm and clindamycin or a penicillin/beta-lactamase inhibitor combination such as amoxicillin/clavulanate for anaerobic chest infections.

Fungi are assuming ever greater importance on the ICU, and *Candida* spp. in particular are occasionally isolated from the blood of patients with septic shock. It would be unwise to use an anti-fungal agent as the only empiric agent in a patient with septic shock, but in selected cases (for instance, neutropenic patients who had received extended courses of antibacterials and who were known to be colonised with *Candida*) the addition of an anti-fungal would be reasonable. Fluconazole is an attractive choice because of its lack of toxicity and ease of use; the potential disadvantage is that a few non-*albicans Candida* spp. have diminished sensitivity. A reasonable approach is to use a relatively high initial dose of 400–800 mg/day.

Table 34.2. First-line empiric antibiotic regimens suitable for patients with presumed septic shock in whom the primary site of infection is not apparent

Broad spectrum cephalosporin[a] (metronidazole can be added for suspected intra-abdominal infections)
Piperacillin/tazobactam (vancomycin can be added for suspected MRSA)
Vancomycin *plus* ciprofloxacin (metronidazole added for suspected intra-abdominal infections)

General comments: Several other drugs and alternative regimens exist which are equally appropriate. The lack of good RCT data means that these are only illustrative recommendations. Nevertheless, it is probably helpful to become familiar with just a small number of selected drugs and regimens rather than try to memorise many equally effective alternatives. These regimens are not intended for circumstances in which the clinical findings point clearly to a specific infection, e.g. meningococcal sepsis, necrotising fasciitis. Recommendations for these infections will be found in the relevant chapters of this book. Specialist infectious diseases/microbiological advice should be sought at an early stage, and particularly if an unusual or opportunistic infection is a possibility

Notes: [a] In patients with septic shock broad spectrum cephalosporins such as cefotaxime are preferable to commonly used second generation cephalosporins such as cefuroxime. If cover against *Pseudomonas* spp. is needed, then use ceftazidime

In summary then, there are no prospective, randomised controlled clinical trials that compare different empiric treatment strategies specifically in patients with septic shock, and recommendations must therefore be based on data drawn from other settings. Choice of the correct initial antibiotic regimen is associated with a better outcome, and under these circumstances it will rarely be possible to treat a patient with septic shock with a single drug. A summary of some suitable regimens is provided in Table 34.2.

34.4.3 Adjunctive Therapy

34.4.3.1 Steroid Therapy

Immunosuppressive doses of corticosteroids have been thoroughly evaluated as adjunctive therapy for septic shock. Used in this way steroids are of no benefit and quite possibly have harmful effects such as an increased rates of bacterial superinfection [62, 63]. Nevertheless patients with septic shock frequently have poor adrenocortical function [64]. On this basis, a series of randomised controlled trials of replacement dose corticosteroid therapy have been performed and have recently been the subject of a meta-analysis [65]. In this study Annane et al. demonstrated that while no overall mortality benefit was apparent amongst 16 randomised controlled trials of corticosteroid therapy, in five trials [66–70] of long course (5 days) low dose (< 300 mg hydrocortisone or equivalent) corticosteroid therapy a clear-cut survival benefit is present (relative risk of death 0.8 (0.67–0.9) at 28 days. Corticosteroids used in this way are also associated with increased rates of shock reversal in sepsis. There are still several areas of contention here though. Although around 50% of septic shock patients will have adrenal insufficiency as evidenced by a blunted response to adrenocorticotropic hormone challenge there is no consensus that this adequately defines adrenal insufficiency in patients with septic shock. Indeed, one view is that low dose steroids may be effective in shocked patients but that the mechanism of action is unrelated to the concept of adrenal insufficiency. The difficulty however is that in Annane's study, patients who did not have evidence of adrenal insufficiency showed no evidence of benefit. Furthermore, the need to add fludrocortisone (as in the original study [68]) has never been confirmed. Finally, although these 'low dose' steroid regimens are widely perceived to be safe, and indeed rates of adverse events in the clinical trials have been low, there are some emerging concerns relating both to herpes virus reactivation and steroid-induced myopathy resulting in difficulty in weaning [71, 72]. Although not yet fully available, preliminary data from the recently completed CORTICUS have now been presented (ref.). It appears that the CORTICUS data will not confirm a survival benefit associated with replacement-dose hydrocortisone, irrespective of adrenal function assessed by adrenocorticotropic hormone challenge, but that a decrease in time to shock reversal was observed. The role of low dose steroid regimens remains not fully defined, and this is reflected in the Surviving Sepsis Campaign (SSC) recommendation that is graded as C [49].

34.4.3.2 *Insulin Therapy*

Patients on the ICU frequently develop insulin resistance and hyperglycaemia. This has been generally regarded as a protective response to stress and historically hyperglycaemia was only treated on the ICU when levels exceeded around 12 mmol/l (~220 mg/dl). In a randomised controlled trial of tight glycaemic control in patients on a surgical intensive care unit Van den Berghe et al. demonstrated a 3.6% absolute (34% relative) reduction in mortality among patients subject to control of blood sugar between 80–110 mg/dl [73]. In view of the low control group mortality in these patients a study in medical ICU patients was performed [74]. This study failed to show a reduction in overall mortality but subgroup analysis revealed interesting differences. The study recruited patients with a predicted length of stay (LOS) on the ICU of over 3 days; however only 767 of 1,200 patients recruited *actually* stayed on the ICU 3 days. Among these patients mortality was significantly reduced by intensive glycaemic control (43% vs. 52.5%, $p = 0.009$). Patients with a LOS < 3 days had an increased mortality (27% vs. 19%). This may have been due to a failure of randomisation in the study but may also be a true effect. In an observational study of outcome on a mixed medical ICU before and after institution of a protocol for tight glycaemic control (< 140 mg/dl), Krinsley et al. demonstrated a 6.1% absolute (29% relative) reduction in mortality [75]. None of these studies has directly addressed patients with septic shock but in subgroup analysis of the Krinsley study the benefit in patients with septic shock appeared greater than in the whole study population. It seems reasonable to conclude from these data that patients with septic shock should receive insulin therapy to control blood glucose. At the current time no good data exist to determine the optimal target glucose or the optimal method for achieving and monitoring this target to avoid hypoglycaemia. Significant rates of hypoglycaemia have been associated with the 80–110 mg/dl target [74] and on the basis of the currently available data the use of a continuous insulin infusion to achieve blood glucose levels of < 150 mg/dl seems reasonable but further randomised controlled trials are underway and should report in the near future. The SSC grades the evidence in favour of tight glycaemic control as level D [49]. This grading is likely to be upgraded on the basis of the evidence outlined above.

34.4.3.3 *Activated Protein C*

Early and rapid activation of coagulation is a feature of systemic infection. Coagulopathy, manifested as disseminated intravascular coagulation, depletion of anticoagulant factors such as protein C and a bleeding diathesis, is a well recognised complication of severe sepsis. With the additional recognition that many coagulation factors also have pro-inflammatory activity, clotting pathways have become a major target for sepsis intervention. Although phase III clinical trials of antithrombin III and tissue factor pathway inhibitor failed to demonstrate survival benefit in sepsis [76, 77], the PROWESS trial of recombinant human activated Protein C (rhAPC) or drotecogin alfa activated (Xigris® Eli Lilly) demonstrated reduced 28-day all cause mortality in severe sepsis (24.7% vs. 30.8%, $p = 0.005$) [18]. Subsequent analysis of the PROWESS data has demonstrated that survival benefit was greatest in patients with more severe disease [78]. On the basis of this single trial both the US Food and Drug Administration (FDA) and the European Evaluation of Medicinal Products Agency (EMEA) approved the drug for use in severe sepsis. Extrapolating from the PROWESS data, both the FDA and the EMEA licensed rhAPC for use in severe sepsis only in patients considered to be at high risk of death. Different indicators of risk were chosen by the different agencies; the FDA approval uses an APACHE II score >25 and the EMEA the presence of two or more organ dysfunctions. The decision to licence rhAPC on the basis of a single randomised controlled trial is problematic as it makes further placebo controlled trials in a comparable patient group ethically difficult to undertake. The SSC recommendation for use of rhAPC in sepsis patients at high risk of death is, on this basis, only a grade B recommendation [49]. The ADDRESS study specifically sought to determine whether patients with severe sepsis, at low risk of death, benefit from rhAPC [79]. Patients with severe sepsis and either single organ failure or APACHE II score <25 were randomised to receive rhAPC or placebo. The trial was stopped at interim analysis when data on 2,613 patients were analysed, because of the low likelihood of a mortality benefit being detected. Investigators who have concerns about the validity of the PROWESS data point out that there was no evidence of efficacy in the subset of patients in ADDRESS who would have qualified for treatment in PROWESS, thereby failing to provide independent verification of the PROWESS data [80]. However, further supportive evidence of the efficacy of rhAPC comes from the prospective, open-label ENHANCE trial which analysed data on 2,375 patients with severe sepsis treated with rhAPC [81]. Mortality rates were similar to those found in patients who received rhAPC in the PROWESS trial. Furthermore early treatment (<24 h from sepsis onset) was associated with better outcome (odds ratio 0.782, 95% CI=0.643–0.951). The SSC recommendation that the evidence supporting rhAPC use be graded as B reflects the very considerable differences of opinion that exist among academic investigators in their assessment of the strength of the evidence in favour of its use. At the present time it seems reasonable to recommend that patients with severe sepsis at high risk of death should receive rhAPC unless relative or absolute contraindications exist which the attending clinician feels out-weigh the potential benefit of rhAPC. National and local definitions of the indications and contra-indications for rhAPC should be in place to ensure quality of care and allow valid comparisons of outcome to be made.

34.5 Future Developments

Practice guidelines for the treatment of sepsis are evolving rapidly. Further large clinical trials evaluating steroid use and insulin therapy are already in progress and will help to better define the use of these strategies. Several large phase III trials of other new adjunctive agents will report in the next few years; these include agents such as eritoran, an LPS antagonist analogue of lipid A, which produced very encouraging results in a phase II trial [82], TAK-242, a small molecule inhibitor of TLR4 [83] and TAK-242. Looking further forward, there are intriguing epidemiological data suggesting that statin use may protect patients who develop sepsis which may be extended to therapeutic trials [84]. Finally there is considerable interest in genetic profiling to identify high risk patients and in real-time immunological assessments to guide therapy [85]. It looks certain that this will remain an area of rapid change and exciting developments for the foreseeable future.

References

1. Bone RC, Balk RA, Cerra FB, et al. (1992) Definitions for sepsis and organ failure and guidelines for the use of innovative therapies in sepsis. The ACCP/SCCM Consensus Conference Committee. American College of Chest Physicians/Society of Critical Care Medicine. Chest 101:1644
2. Levy MM, Fink MP, Marshall JC, et al. (2001) SCCM/ESICM/ACCP/ATS/SIS International Sepsis Definitions Conference. Crit Care Med 31:1250
3. Singer M, De Santis V, Vitale D, Jeffcoate W (2004) Multiorgan failure is an adaptive, endocrine-mediated, metabolic response to overwhelming systemic inflammation. Lancet 364:545
4. Eggimann P, Harbarth S, Ricou B, et al. (2003) Acute respiratory distress syndrome after bacteremic sepsis does not increase mortality. Am J Respir Crit Care Med 167:1210
5. Bone RC (1994) Definitions and therapy of sepsis. In: Reinhart K, Eyrich K, Sprung C (eds) Sepsis. Current perspectives in pathophysiology and therapy. Springer-Verlag, Berlin
6. Carcillo JA, Fields AI (2002) Clinical practice parameters for hemodynamic support of pediatric and neonatal patients in septic shock. Crit Care Med 30:1365
7. Calandra T, Cohen J (2005) The international sepsis forum consensus conference on definitions of infection in the intensive care unit. Crit Care Med 33:1538
8. Annane D, Aegerter P, Jars-Guincestre MC, Guidet B (2003) Current epidemiology of septic shock: the CUB-Rea Network. Am J Respir Crit Care Med 168:165
9. Martin GS, Mannino DM, Eaton S, Moss M (2003) The epidemiology of sepsis in the United States from 1979 through 2000. N Engl J Med 348:1546
10. Angus DC, Linde-Zwirble WT, Lidicker J, Clermont G, Carcillo J, Pinsky MR (2001) Epidemiology of severe sepsis in the United States: analysis of incidence, outcome, and associated costs of care. Crit Care Med 29:1303
11. Rangel-Frausto MS, Pittet D, Hwang T, Woolson RF, Wenzel RP (1998) The dynamics of disease progression in sep-

sis: Markov modeling describing the natural history and the likely impact of effective antisepsis agents. Clin Infect Dis 27:185
12. Alberti C, Brun-Buisson C, Burchardi H, et al. (2002) Epidemiology of sepsis and infection in ICU patients from an international multicentre cohort study. Intensive Care Med 28:108
13. Vincent JL, Sakr Y, Sprung CL, et al. (2006) Sepsis in European intensive care units: results of the SOAP study. Crit Care Med 34:344
14. Crowe M, Ispahani P, Humphreys H, Kelley T, Winter R (1998) Bacteraemia in the adult intensive care unit of a teaching hospital in Nottingham, UK, 1985–1996. Eur J Clin Microbiol Infect Dis 17:377
15. Rangel-Frausto MS (1999) The epidemiology of bacterial sepsis. Infect Dis Clin North Am 13:299
16. Brun-Buisson C, Doyon F, Carlet J, et al. (1995) Incidence, risk factors, and outcome of severe sepsis and septic shock in adults. A multicenter prospective study in intensive care units. French ICU Group for Severe Sepsis. JAMA 274:968
17. Cohen J, Cristofaro P, Carlet J, Opal S (2004) New method of classifying infections in critically ill patients. Crit Care Med 32:1510
18. Bernard GR, Vincent JL, Laterre PF, et al. (2001) Efficacy and safety of recombinant human activated protein C for severe sepsis. N Engl J Med 344:699
19. Opal SM, Garber GE, LaRosa SP, et al. (2003) Systemic host responses in severe sepsis analyzed by causative microorganism and treatment effects of drotrecogin alfa (activated). Clin Infect Dis 37:50
20. Kreger BE, Craven DE, McCabe WR (1980) Gram-negative bacteremia. IV. Re-evaluation of clinical features and treatment in 612 patients. Am J Med 68:344
21. Leibovici L, Shraga I, Drucker M, Konigsberger H, Samra Z, Pitlik SD (1998) The benefit of appropriate empirical antibiotic treatment in patients with bloodstream infection. J Intern Med 244:379
22. Byl B, Clevenbergh P, Jacobs F, et al. (1999) Impact of infectious disease specialists and microbiological data on the appropriateness of antimicrobial therapy for bacteremia. Clin Infect Dis 29:60
23. Ibrahim EH, Sherman G, Ward S, Fraser VJ, Kollef MH (2000) The influence of inadequate antimicrobial treatment of bloodstream infections on patient outcomes in the ICU setting. Chest 118:146
24. Marik PE (2000) Fever in the ICU. Chest 117:855
25. Circiumaru B, Baldock G, Cohen J (1999) A prospective study of fever in the intensive care unit. Intensive Care Med 25:668
26. O'Grady NP, Barie PS, Bartlett J, et al. (1998) Practice parameters for evaluating new fever in critically ill adult patients. Task Force of the American College of Critical Care Medicine of the Society of Critical Care Medicine in collaboration with the Infectious Disease Society of America. Crit Care Med 26:392
27. Cohen J, Brun-Buisson C, Torres A, Jorgensen J (2004) Diagnosis of infection in sepsis: an evidence-based review. Crit Care Med 32:S466
28. Smith-Elekes S, Weinstein MP (1993) Blood cultures. Infect Dis Clin North Am 7:221
29. Simon L, Gauvin F, Amre DK, Saint-Louis P, Lacroix J (2004) Serum procalcitonin and C-reactive protein levels as markers of bacterial infection: a systematic review and meta-analysis. Clin Infect Dis 39:206
30. Clec'h C, Fosse JP, Karoubi P, et al. (2006) Differential diagnostic value of procalcitonin in surgical and medical patients with septic shock. Crit Care Med 34:102
31. Harbarth S, Holeckova K, Froidevaux C, et al. (2001) Diagnostic value of procalcitonin, interleukin-6, and interleukin-8 in critically ill patients admitted with suspected sepsis. Am J Respir Crit Care Med 164:396
32. Clec'h C, Ferriere F, Karoubi P, et al. (2004) Diagnostic and prognostic value of procalcitonin in patients with septic shock. Crit Care Med 32:1166
33. Pepys MB, Hirschfield GM (2003) C-reactive protein: a critical update. J Clin Invest 111:1805
34. Cohen J (2000) The detection and interpretation of endotoxaemia. Intensive Care Med 26 Suppl 1:S51
35. Danner RL, Elin RJ, Hosseini JM, Wesley RA, Reilly JM, Parillo JE (1991) Endotoxemia in human septic shock. Chest 99:169
36. Guidet B, Barakett V, Vassal T, Petit JC, Offenstadt G (1994) Endotoxemia and bacteremia in patients with sepsis syndrome in the intensive care unit. Chest 106:1194
37. Bates DW, Parsonnet J, Ketchum PA, et al. (1998) Limulus amebocyte lysate assay for detection of endotoxin in patients with sepsis syndrome. AMCC Sepsis Project Working Group. Clin Infect Dis 27:582
38. Casey LC, Balk RA, Bone RC (1993) Plasma cytokine and endotoxin levels correlate with survival in patients with the sepsis syndrome. Ann Intern Med 119:771
39. Fink PC, Grunert JH (1984) Endotoxemia in intensive care patients: a longitudinal study with the limulus amebocyte lysate test. Klin Wochenschr 62:986
40. Marshall JC, Foster D, Vincent JL, et al. (2004) Diagnostic and prognostic implications of endotoxemia in critical illness: results of the MEDIC study. J Infect Dis 190:527
41. Gibot S, Cravoisy A, Kolopp-Sarda MN, et al. (2005) Time-course of sTREM (soluble triggering receptor expressed on myeloid cells)-1, procalcitonin, and C-reactive protein plasma concentrations during sepsis. Crit Care Med 33:792
42. Brueckmann M, Huhle G, Lang S, et al. (2005) Prognostic value of plasma N-terminal pro-brain natriuretic peptide in patients with severe sepsis. Circulation 112:527
43. Morgenthaler NG, Struck J, Christ-Crain M, Bergmann A, Muller B (2005) Pro-atrial natriuretic peptide is a prognostic marker in sepsis, similar to the APACHE II score: an observational study. Crit Care 9:R37
44. Pachot A, Monneret G, Brion A, et al. (2005) Messenger RNA expression of major histocompatibility complex class II genes in whole blood from septic shock patients. Crit Care Med 33:31
45. Wang H, Bloom O, Zhang M, et al. (1999) HMG-1 as a late mediator of endotoxin lethality in mice. Science 285:248
46. Sunden-Cullberg J, Norrby-Teglund A, Rouhiainen A, et al. (2005) Persistent elevation of high mobility group box-1 protein (HMGB1) in patients with severe sepsis and septic shock. Crit Care Med 33:564
47. Rivers E, Nguyen B, Havstad S, et al. (2001) Early goal-directed therapy in the treatment of severe sepsis and septic shock. N Engl J Med 345:1368
48. Bochud PY, Bonten M, Marchetti O, Calandra T (2004) Antimicrobial therapy for patients with severe sepsis and septic shock: an evidence-based review. Crit Care Med 32:S495
49. Dellinger RP, Carlet JM, Masur H, et al. (2004) Surviving Sepsis Campaign guidelines for management of severe sepsis and septic shock. Crit Care Med 32:858
50. Kumar A, Haery C, Paladugu B, et al. (2006) The duration of hypotension before the initiation of antibiotic treatment is a critical determinant of survival in a murine model of *Escherichia coli* septic shock: association with serum lactate and inflammatory cytokine levels. J Infect Dis 193:251
51. Paul M, Silbiger I, Grozinsky S, Soares-Weiser K, Leibovici L (2006) Beta lactam antibiotic monotherapy versus beta lactam-aminoglycoside antibiotic combination therapy for sepsis. Cochrane Database Syst Rev:CD003344

52. Karchmer AW (1991) *Staphylococcus aureus* and vancomycin: the sequel. Ann Intern Med 115:739
53. Levine DP, Fromm BS, Reddy BR (1991) Slow response to vancomycin or vancomycin plus rifampin in methicillin-resistant *Staphylococcus aureus* endocarditis. Ann Intern Med 115:674
54. Rubinstein E, Cammarata S, Oliphant T, Wunderink R (2001) Linezolid (PNU-100766) versus vancomycin in the treatment of hospitalized patients with nosocomial pneumonia: a randomized, double-blind, multicenter study. Clin Infect Dis 32:402
55. Weigelt J, Itani K, Stevens D, Lau W, Dryden M, Knirsch C (2005) Linezolid versus vancomycin in treatment of complicated skin and soft tissue infections. Antimicrob Agents Chemother 49:2260
56. Wunderink RG, Cammarata SK, Oliphant TH, Kollef MH (2003) Continuation of a randomized, double-blind, multicenter study of linezolid versus vancomycin in the treatment of patients with nosocomial pneumonia. Clin Ther 25:980
57. Stevens DL, Herr D, Lampiris H, Hunt JL, Batts DH, Hafkin B (2002) Linezolid versus vancomycin for the treatment of methicillin-resistant *Staphylococcus aureus* infections. Clin Infect Dis 34:1481
58. Wunderink RG, Rello J, Cammarata SK, Croos-Dabrera RV, Kollef MH (2003) Linezolid vs vancomycin: analysis of two double-blind studies of patients with methicillin-resistant *Staphylococcus aureus* nosocomial pneumonia. Chest 124:1789
59. Marshall SH, Donskey CJ, Hutton-Thomas R, Salata RA, Rice LB (2002) Gene dosage and linezolid resistance in *Enterococcus faecium* and *Enterococcus faecalis*. Antimicrob Agents Chemother 46:3334
60. Tsiodras S, Gold HS, Sakoulas G, et al. (2001) Linezolid resistance in a clinical isolate of *Staphylococcus aureus*. Lancet 358:207
61. Wilson P, Andrews JA, Charlesworth R, et al. (2003) Linezolid resistance in clinical isolates of *Staphylococcus aureus*. J Antimicrob Chemother 51:186
62. Lefering R, Neugebauer EA (1995) Steroid controversy in sepsis and septic shock: a meta-analysis. Crit Care Med 23:1294
63. Cronin L, Cook DJ, Carlet J, et al. (1995) Corticosteroid treatment for sepsis: a critical appraisal and meta-analysis of the literature. Crit Care Med 23:1430
64. Rothwell PM, Udwadia ZF, Lawler PG (1991) Cortisol response to corticotropin and survival in septic shock. Lancet 337:582
65. Annane D, Bellissant E, Bollaert PE, Briegel J, Keh D, Kupfer Y (2004) Corticosteroids for severe sepsis and septic shock: a systematic review and meta-analysis. BMJ 329:480
66. Bollaert PE, Charpentier C, Levy B, Debouverie M, Audibert G, Larcan A (1998) Reversal of late septic shock with supraphysiologic doses of hydrocortisone. Crit Care Med 26:645
67. Briegel J, Forst H, Haller M, et al. (1999) Stress doses of hydrocortisone reverse hyperdynamic septic shock: a prospective, randomized, double-blind, single-center study. Crit Care Med 27:723
68. Annane D, Sebille V, Charpentier C, et al. (2002) Effect of treatment with low doses of hydrocortisone and fludrocortisone on mortality in patients with septic shock. JAMA 288:862
69. Yildiz O, Doganay M, Aygen B, Guven M, Keleutimur F, Tutuu A (2002) Physiological-dose steroid therapy in sepsis [ISRCTN36253388]. Crit Care 6:251
70. Chawla K, Kupfer Y, Goldman I, Tessler S (1999) Hydrocortisone reverses refractory septic shock. Crit Care Med 27:33A
71. De Jonghe B, Sharshar T, Lefaucheur JP, et al. (2002) Paresis acquired in the intensive care unit: a prospective multicenter study. JAMA 288:2859
72. Jaber S, Chanques G, Borry J, et al. (2005) Cytomegalovirus infection in critically ill patients: associated factors and consequences. Chest 127:233
73. van den Berghe G, Wouters P, Weekers F, et al. (2001) Intensive insulin therapy in the critically ill patients. N Engl J Med 345:1359
74. Van den Berghe G, Wilmer A, Hermans G, et al. (2006) Intensive insulin therapy in the medical ICU. N Engl J Med 354:449
75. Krinsley JS (2004) Effect of an intensive glucose management protocol on the mortality of critically ill adult patients. Mayo Clin Proc 79:992
76. Warren BL, Eid A, Singer P, et al. (2001) Caring for the critically ill patient. High-dose antithrombin III in severe sepsis: a randomized controlled trial. JAMA 286:1869
77. Abraham E, Reinhart K, Opal S, et al. (2003) Efficacy and safety of tifacogin (recombinant tissue factor pathway inhibitor) in severe sepsis: a randomized controlled trial. JAMA 290:238
78. Ely EW, Laterre PF, Angus DC, et al. (2003) Drotrecogin alfa (activated) administration across clinically important subgroups of patients with severe sepsis. Crit Care Med 31:12
79. Abraham E, Laterre PF, Garg R, et al. (2005) Drotrecogin alfa (activated) for adults with severe sepsis and a low risk of death. N Engl J Med 353:1332
80. Parrillo JE (2005) Severe sepsis and therapy with activated protein C. N Engl J Med 353:1398
81. Vincent JL, Bernard GR, Beale R, et al. (2005) Drotrecogin alfa (activated) treatment in severe sepsis from the global open-label trial ENHANCE: further evidence for survival and safety and implications for early treatment. Crit Care Med 33:2266
82. Rossignol DP, Wasan KM, Choo E, et al. (2004) Safety, pharmacokinetics, pharmacodynamics, and plasma lipoprotein distribution of eritoran (E5564) during continuous intravenous infusion into healthy volunteers. Antimicrob Agents Chemother 48:3233
83. Yamada M, Ichikawa T, Ii M, et al. (2005) Discovery of novel and potent small-molecule inhibitors of NO and cytokine production as antisepsis agents: synthesis and biological activity of alkyl 6-(N-substituted sulfamoyl)cyclohex-1-ene-1-carboxylate. J Med Chem 48:7457
84. Terblanche M, Almog Y, Rosenson RS, Smith TS, Hackam DG (2006) Statins: panacea for sepsis? Lancet Infect Dis 6:242
85. Prucha M, Ruryk A, Boriss H, et al. (2004) Expression profiling: toward an application in sepsis diagnostics. Shock 22:29

Respiratory Infections

Chapter 35

Tracheobronchitis in the Intensive Care Unit 35

L. Morrow, D. Schuller

35.1 Introduction

Tracheobronchitis can be broadly defined as inflammation of the airways between the larynx and the bronchioles. Clinically, this syndrome is recognized by an increase in the volume and purulence of the lower respiratory tract secretions and is frequently associated with signs of variable airflow obstruction. In the intensive care unit (ICU), tracheobronchitis is a relatively common problem with an incidence as high as 10.6% [1]. Although tracheobronchitis is associated with a significantly longer length of ICU stay and a prolonged need for mechanical ventilation, it has not been shown to increase mortality. These outcomes can be improved through the use of antimicrobial agents [1].

Tracheobronchitis results from two dominating processes: colonization of the oropharynx and its contiguous structures (dental plaque, the sinuses, the stomach) by potentially pathogenic organisms and aspiration of contaminated secretions from these anatomic sites [2]. Mechanically ventilated patients are particularly at risk for tracheobronchitis given the presence of an endotracheal tube. These devices contribute to the pathogenesis of tracheobronchitis (and pneumonia) in a variety of manners: bypassing natural host defenses, acting as a nidus for biofilm formation, allowing pooled secretions and bacteria to leak around the cuff and into the trachea, damaging the ciliated epithelium and reducing bacterial clearance directly or via frequent suctioning to maintain airway patency [3, 4].

In contrast to nosocomial pneumonia, nosocomial tracheobronchitis does not involve pulmonary parenchyma and, thus, does not cause radiographic pulmonary infiltrates. However, high quality portable chest radiographs may be difficult to obtain in the ICU, where poor patient cooperation, inconsistent technique and other obstacles lead to suboptimal studies [5]. Furthermore, common processes such as atelectasis, pulmonary edema, or pleural effusions can cause infiltrates that mimic pneumonia making the clinical distinction between pneumonia and tracheobronchitis difficult [6].

35.2 Bacterial Tracheobronchitis

Bacterial infection is the most common cause of infectious tracheobronchitis in the ICU. Infectious tracheobronchitis is clinically diagnosed when a patient develops fever, purulent respiratory secretions, and leukocytosis but the chest radiograph shows no new infiltrate [7]. Tracheobronchitis is "microbiologically confirmed" when a patient with clinically diagnosed tracheobronchitis yields culture specimens that identify a causative pathogen at appropriately high densities. When a patient lacks fever or leukocytosis (or if culture specimens reveal few organisms) the differentiation between colonization and infection is difficult and controversial. Furthermore, the significance of tracheobronchial colonization as a risk factor for subsequent lower respiratory tract infection remains unclear.

Alterations in the oropharyngeal flora of the hospitalized host have been associated with several factors including age, severity of acute illness, comorbid chronic illnesses, and duration of hospitalization [8–10]. One study of outpatients with chronic tracheostomy concluded that although these patients were routinely colonized with massive amounts of potentially pathogenic bacteria, rates of severe respiratory tract infections were low [11]. However, hospitalized patients with a tracheostomy or a translaryngeal endotracheal tube have higher rates of tracheobronchial colonization (especially with gram-negative enteric bacteria and *Pseudomonas aeruginosa*) and nosocomial pneumonia [8, 12–15].

The upper airways and proximal tracheobronchial tree provide a mechanical barrier function and a mucociliary mechanism for removing particulate matter and microbes that have been deposited within the respiratory tract. The effectiveness of mucociliary clearance depends on the composition of airway secretions, the function of the mucociliary escalator apparatus, and the presence of an effective cough reflex [16]. Artificial airways promote both colonization and the subsequent development of tracheobronchitis or pneumonia as they provide direct access for bacteria to the lower respiratory tract, reduce the effectiveness of cough reflexes, and compromise the mucociliary escalator [17, 18]. Furthermore, endotracheal tube insertion and suctioning may cause tracheal epithelial cell damage allowing bacterial adherence and increased mucus secretion and stagnation [19, 20]. Respiratory therapy devices, including medication nebulizers, ventilator spirometers, and ventilatory circuits with their attendant condensate, may play roles in harboring and transmitting bacteria [21,22].

While colonization with gram-positive organisms occurs, gram-negative bacilli are much more common colonizers in ICU patients with many studies showing *Pseudomonas* species as the most prevalent organism [1, 23–26]. While there are no useful parameters to reliably predict which colonized patients will develop infectious tracheobronchitis, it is clear that tracheobronchitis often develops in patients with tracheobronchial colonization. In one study, 7 of 15 patients with a chronic tracheostomy were colonized with various *Pseudomonas* species: all seven of them subsequently developed an episode of purulent tracheobronchitis [27]. George et al. found that tracheal colonization was a significant independent risk factor for VAP and could be documented in 93.5% of VAP cases [28]. The relationship between infectious tracheobronchitis and nosocomial pneumonia is not well defined. One relatively small study found that tracheobronchitis was not a risk factor for subsequent pneumonia [1].

Although aerobic enteric gram-negative bacilli as a group account for the majority of respiratory infections in ventilated patients, *Staphylococcus aureus* is one of the most common individual pathogens and accounts for ~20% of nosocomial respiratory infections. *S. aureus* is found in the nasopharynx in 20–40% of healthy adults and the carrier rate can be as high as 70% in hospitalized patients. Patients with structural lung diseases, such as cystic fibrosis or chronic obstructive pulmonary disease, frequently have tracheobronchial colonization with *S. aureus*. The emergence of nosocomial methicillin-resistant strains of *Staphylococcus aureus* (MRSA) and community-acquired MRSA poses a unique therapeutic problem. Infection with this pathogen is not limited to nosocomial pneumonia but also has been reported to cause fulminant tracheobronchitis [29]. MRSA tracheobronchitis may present as pseudomembranous lesions, clinically mimicking the presentation of fungal tracheobronchitis (see below) [30].

Another important nosocomial pathogen that opportunistically infects ICU patients with impaired host defenses is *Acinetobacter baumannii*. In addition to causing tracheobronchitis and pneumonia, other infectious syndromes attributable to *A. baumannii* include endocarditis, peritonitis, skin and soft tissue infection, urinary tract infection, and bloodstream infection. *A. baumannii* infections have been linked to contaminated respiratory therapy equipment, intravascular access devices, and transmission via hands of hospital personnel [31]. Seifert and coworkers observed that tracheobronchitis was the presumed portal of entry for nosocomial *A. baumannii* bacteremia in 19 of 87 (22%) episodes. This study also confirmed the results of other studies suggesting that the major determinants for developing *A. baumannii* bacteremia included treatment in an intensive care unit, major surgery, mechanical ventilation, total parenteral nutrition, broad-spectrum antimicrobial therapy, and the presence of intravascular catheters [32]. This organism's routine association with multi-drug resistance results in mortality rates as high as 46% [33, 34].

While *Mycoplasma pneumoniae* infection is best known for producing atypical pneumonia in young adults, it may result in bronchitis ~30 times more often than it causes pneumonia [35]. *M. pneumoniae* outbreaks occur sporadically but have a predilection for the late fall and early winter [36]. *M. pneumoniae* is associated with acute bronchiolitis, bronchiolitis obliterans, and bronchiolitis obliterans with organizing pneumonia (BOOP) in infants, children and adults. In children, *M. pneumoniae* is a relatively infrequent cause of bronchiolitis, accounting for 11% of cases of bronchiolitis caused by an identified agent [37]. Although acute infectious bronchiolitis requiring hospitalization is unusual in adults, *M. pneumoniae* should be considered as a cause for acute bronchitis or bronchiolitis in hospitalized patients.

Mycoplasma pneumoniae infections typically begin insidiously with fever, nonproductive cough, headache, malaise and occasional chills. Upper respiratory symptoms of rhinitis and sore throat are present in 50% of cases. Myalgias, arthralgias, skin rash or gastrointestinal symptoms are rare; bullous myringitis and ARDS occasionally develop [38]. Rare cases of profound hypoxemia with airflow obstruction and hypercapnia have been reported, presumably as a result of widespread bronchiolitis [39].

35.3 Fungal Tracheobronchitis

Fungal infections limited to the tracheobronchial tree are increasingly recognized in critically ill patients, particularly in the immunocompromised host [40–42]. Clark et al. reported that of a total of 207 patients, 15 (7%) had infection solely or predominantly within the airways [43–47]. The incidence of *Candida* infection localized to the tracheobronchial tree must be much lower as the reported cases are very rare. Furthermore, some cases are poorly documented pathologically and the diagnosis of bronchial candidiasis was made solely on the basis of repeatedly positive sputum cultures and clinical improvement after treatment with antifungal agents [48, 49]. *Candida* colonization of the respiratory tract was reported to occur in 27% of patients intubated for more than 2 days and was associated with an increased risk of *Pseudomonas* pneumonia and longer ICU and hospital stays [50]. *Aspergillus* is the predominant pathogen occurring alone or in combination with other pathogens.

Pseudomembranous and obstructive *Aspergillus* tracheobronchitis represent two different, but sometimes overlapping, clinical presentations. The first consists of intraluminal growth involving more or less the entire circumference of the airway wall with only superficial mucosal invasion. Pathologically, such infection can appear as a pseudomembrane in which a fibrinous exudate related to airway ulceration is prominent, or as tenacious mucus/fungus plugs more or less completely occluding the tracheobronchial tree. This is perhaps the most likely form of serious fungal infection to be missed clinically. Patients may complain of cough, chest pain, increasing dyspnea, fever, hemoptysis, and, possibly, signs of upper airway obstruction. Because the parenchyma is unaffected, the chest roentgenograms may be normal. Early bronchoscopy with histological examination and cultures of the bronchial casts and airway debris confirms the diagnosis [40, 43, 51].

Obstructive tracheobronchial aspergillosis may present with radiographic findings of atelectasis due to extensive obstruction of both main and subsegmental bronchi [41]. The obstruction may be severe causing acute respiratory failure [42].

Another morphological form consists of one or several discrete plaques localized to a relatively small portion of the tracheobronchial tree. Although in the early stages of infection, invasion is limited to the airway mucosa, with progression of disease fungi penetrate beyond the bronchial wall into the adjacent lung parenchyma where they may result in focal pneumonia or abscess formation. Vascular invasion is not uncommon and may lead to parenchymal or pleural hemorrhage [43].

The explanation for why fungi colonize and invade the tracheobronchial tree in certain patients is unclear. However given the underlying disorders that patients with fungal tracheobronchitis commonly have, it is clear that a deficiency in the host immune system is a common denominator among these patients. Fungal tracheobronchitis has been seen in patients with lung and bone marrow transplantation, AIDS, and hematological malignancies [52]. Prolonged neutropenia occurring either secondary to the malignancy or chemotherapy has been shown to be a risk factor for developing invasive pulmonary aspergillosis [53]. Even in the absence of neutropenia, impaired leukocyte mobilization and function may contribute to the predisposition to fungal infection in cancer patients [54]. Pseudomembranous tracheobronchitis has also been reported in patients with diabetes [40]. Corticosteroids predispose to the development of fungal invasion by inhibiting macrophage killing of spores, inhibiting phagocyte migration to the site of infection, and by suppressing antibody production, delayed hypersensitivity reaction, and wound healing [43, 55]. Broad-spectrum antibiotics change the normal flora and predispose to the development of fungal colonization. Cellular and humoral immune deficiency are additional risk factors [56].

Once the diagnosis of *Aspergillus* tracheobronchitis is established by bronchoscopy, histology, or culture, appropriate antifungal therapy should be started. In addition, multiple therapeutic bronchoscopies may be needed to debulk the intrabronchial debris.

35.4 Viral Tracheobronchitis

Many respiratory infections caused by viruses begin in the upper respiratory tract usually without producing lower respiratory symptoms. A variety of clinical syndromes including rhinitis, pharyngitis, laryngotracheitis (croup), bronchitis or tracheobronchitis, bronchiolitis and pneumonia can occur depending on the specific virus involved, the viral load, virulence, host resistance and extent of respiratory mucosal involvement [57].

The patient's age is also an important factor in the form and severity of infection; for example rhinovirus typically causes only coryza in immunocompetent adults, whereas it is a cause of croup, bronchitis, bronchiolitis and pneumonia in children. The attack rates for respiratory syncytial virus (RSV), parainfluenza virus types 1 and 3 and adenovirus are also severalfold higher in the first 2 years of life [57].

In the ICU, viral tracheobronchitis is usually seen in one of two situations: (a) primary viral infection usually acquired in the community, such as influenza, parainfluenza, adenovirus or RSV that is either severe or complicates underlying pulmonary disease or, (b) reactivation of a latent virus in the nosocomial setting, such as herpes simplex virus (HSV) or cytomegalovirus (CMV). Either situation can further be complicated by bacterial co-infection or superinfection [58].

35.4.1 Influenza Virus

The influenza viruses A, B, and C are the three most important genera of the Orthomyxoviridae, a group of single stranded RNA viruses. Hemagglutinin and neuraminidase are the major antigenic determinants of influenza A viruses and serve as the basis for their subtype classification [59]. A minor mutation in the antigenicity of hemagglutinin or neuraminidase leads to antigenic drift and explains the need for yearly changes in the influenza vaccine composition. On the other hand, genetic reassortment can result in the appearance of a novel hemagglutinin/neuraminidase combination called an antigenic shift which, due to lack of immunity in the human population, can lead to influenza pandemics.

Influenza virus infection usually involves only the upper respiratory tract, including trachea and major bronchi; however in a small percentage of patients, particularly the chronically ill or the elderly, it may be responsible for severe pneumonia. It can occur in pandemics, epidemics or sporadically. Almost all severe epidemics and all pandemics are caused by type A influenza. Typical winter outbreaks occur every year in temperate climates with a less predictable seasonal variation in tropical areas. Transmission occurs from person to person with an incubation period of 24–48 h and is highly contagious. Viral shedding and infectivity can persist for as long as 2 weeks in children, but probably less in adults [60]. Antibody formation to specific strains by either immunization or infection confers immunity for 1–2 years. Serologic studies have found a higher incidence of antibodies to influenza A and B in health care workers than controls [61]. The risk of developing a complicated course is increased in the older individuals, and those with a significant history of tobacco smoking, comorbidities and pregnancy [62–64]. Recent outbreaks of avian influenza virus infections in humans have been the source of concern for a potential influenza pandemic. Since 2004, the H5N1 influenza A virus has expanded from southern China to western China, Mongolia, Russia, and, more recently, Europe and Africa. Humans acquire avian influenza through direct contact of mucous membranes with infected secretions and excreta from infected birds or contaminated poultry. Human-to-human transmission of avian influenza has thus far only occurred sporadically and with low efficiency [65].

The clinical manifestations of human influenza are variable and depend on the virulence of the influenza virus strain, the underlying condition and response of the host. The flu-like syndrome with rapid onset of dry cough, myalgias, headache, chills and fever without major pulmonary complaints affects predominantly young adults. Another syndrome seen in influenza is bronchitis/tracheobronchitis with no radiographic abnormality but with more respiratory distress and sometimes associated with hemoptysis, exacerbation of underlying asthma or chronic obstructive pulmonary disease (COPD). In more severe cases, spread of the virus to the pulmonary parenchyma causes clinical worsening within 12–36 h with worsening dyspnea, tachypnea, cyanosis and hypoxemia [66, 67]. The radiographic abnormalities of influenza pneumonia include interstitial infiltrates, lobar consolidation with air bronchograms, and focal areas of atelectasis. Finally, it is well recognized that superinfection with *Staphylococcus aureus, Streptococcus pneumoniae, Hemophilus influenzae* or other bacteria can occur after influenza [68]. The clinical manifestations of avian influenza infection also depend on the viral subtype causing the disease. Conjunctivitis, with or without an influenza-like illness, occurs with the A/H7N7 and A/H7N3 strains. A/H5N1 strains lead to more severe presentations with frequent progression to pneumonia and a high fatality rate. Gastrointestinal complaints of abdominal pain, nausea, vomiting, and diarrhea are common. Lymphopenia and thrombocytopenia are common findings and prognostic indicators for ARDS and death [69].

The diagnosis can be confirmed by culturing the virus from respiratory secretions, a throat swab, or a nasopharyngeal aspirate. More rapid diagnostic methods available consist of direct immunofluorescence assay (DFA), polymerase chain reaction (PCR) or the rapid assays that detect activity of influenza neuraminidase or viral nucleoproteins [70]. The currently commercially available test kits do not distinguish human from avian influenza or their subtypes. The sensitivity of these kits for detecting A/H5N1 infection ranges from 33% to 86% [69, 71].

Influenza vaccination is the mainstay of protection against the disease. The older drugs available for the prevention and treatment of influenza are amantadine and rimantadine. However, their use is limited by lack of activity against influenza B, rapid emergence of resistance and, especially with amantidine, central nervous system toxicity. Agents available for the treatment of influenza A and B include the neuraminidase inhibitor zanamivir that is delivered by inhalation (10 mg bid) and oseltamivir (75 mg PO bid) [72]. Controlled clinical trials on the efficacy of neuraminidase inhibitors for the treatment and prophylaxis of human avian influenza infections have not been performed.

35.4.2 Parainfluenza Virus

In adults, parainfluenza is responsible for pharyngitis and coryza; in infants and children it is the predominant cause of severe croup. Immunocompromised individuals are at increased risk for more severe presentations. Parainfluenza type 1 and 2 occur predominantly in the autumn and early winter. Parainfluenza type 3 occurs in the spring and is an important cause of bronchiolitis or pneumonia in infants and children. Lower respiratory tract involvement in adults is uncommon.

The parainfluenza viruses cause a spectrum of respiratory illnesses similar to those caused by *Mycoplasma* infection and respiratory syncytial virus (RSV) (see below). Most are upper respiratory tract infections of which 30–50% are complicated by otitis media. In infants, about 15% of parainfluenza virus infection involves the lower respiratory tract. Croup is the signature clinical manifestation and chief cause of hospitalization in children 2–6 years of age [61].

The clinical manifestations in adults are acute pharyngitis and tonsillitis or the aggravation of an underlying cardiopulmonary problem. When complicated by pneumonia it is indistinguishable from other viral or *Mycoplasma* infection. The radiographic findings are nonspecific. The organism can be isolated by culture of sputum or nasopharyngeal secretions. Immunofluorescent antibody is useful for rapid identification.

There are currently no available antiviral agents with proven effectiveness against parainfluenza virus. Ribavirin is active against the virus in vitro, but there have been no randomized controlled trials in humans.

35.4.3 Rhinovirus

Rhinovirus causes approximately 40–50% of the common cold cases. Clinically significant lower respiratory tract infection in adults is uncommon but includes acute bronchitis, bronchiolitis and pneumonia. Perhaps more important is the indirect effect that such an infection may have in patients with asthma, COPD or other medically debilitating states. Rhinovirus infection has been associated with exacerbation of COPD and respiratory failure [73].

35.4.4 Adenovirus

Adenovirus can cause pharyngitis, pharyngoconjunctivitis, laryngotracheo-bronchitis, bronchiolitis, pneumonia or a non-specific acute respiratory syndrome; there is also some evidence that it may cause some cases of bronchiectasis, bronchiolitis obliterans and hyperlucent lung syndrome [74]. Infections can occur sporadically or in epidemics. Localized nosocomial outbreaks have also been reported.

The adenoviruses are the most common cause of the *acute respiratory disease syndrome*, a poorly defined condition consisting of fever, pharyngitis, cough, hoarseness, chest pain, and conjunctivitis. Chills and myalgias may be present. In some cases, tracheobronchitis is prominent and may be indistinguishable from the classic whooping cough caused by *Bordetella pertussis*. When pneumonia occurs it is typically mild and associated with upper respiratory symptoms. However, a few fatal cases have been seen with autopsy studies revealing extensive areas of hemorrhagic consolidation with alternating areas of atelectasis and hyperinflation. The airways frequently show marked airway congestion with mucopurulent or hemorrhagic material.

In most cases the infection is self-limited and the treatment is supportive.

35.4.5 Respiratory Syncytial Virus

Respiratory syncytial virus (RSV) is a major cause of lower respiratory tract infections (bronchiolitis and pneumonia) among young children, resulting in an estimated 51,000–82,000 hospitalizations annually in the United States. Infection occurs predominantly during the winter months and early spring. Transmission occurs by airborne droplets or hand-to-hand contact. The disease is highly contagious and there is evidence that health care workers are at increased risk for infection [61].

In adults, the disease is usually mild and limited to the upper respiratory tract. However, in the elderly, chronically ill, immunocompromised or hospitalized patient, lower tract involvement can occur [75]. Rarely, RSV can cause acute pneumonia with rapid progression to ARDS [76]. A recent prospective surveillance study of healthy elderly patients, high-risk adults, and patients hospitalized with acute cardiopulmonary conditions found RSV in 10.6% of hospitalizations for pneumonia, 11.4% for chronic obstructive pulmonary disease, 5.4% for congestive heart failure, and 7.2% for asthma [76].

The clinical manifestations reflect the extent of airway involvement. Nasal congestion and discharge usually precede the cough and wheezing by 2–3 days, but may occur simultaneously. In contrast to influenza infection, RSV is associated with relatively little risk of bacterial superinfection. The radiological findings usually reflect a disparity between the severity of respiratory symptoms and a paucity of abnormalities. However, bronchial wall thickening, peribronchial infiltrates or lobular consolidation may occur.

RSV can be cultured from nasopharyngeal or lower respiratory secretions. In adults and transplant patients, bronchoalveolar lavage is more sensitive than throat swabs [77]. The shell-vial culture has been shown to be a rapid and sensitive method. PCR and immune based assays including antigen detection by immunofluorescence or enzyme-linked immunosorbent assay (ELISA) are available for rapid diagnosis with a sensitivity and specificity of 80–90% [61].

In addition to supportive care, severe cases of RSV infection have been treated with aerosolized ribavirin (6 g reconstituted in 300 ml of sterile water to a final concentration of 20 mg/ml and administered 12–18 h/day for 3–7 days); although no clinical trials have been conducted in this patient population. There is no data regarding the use of oral ribavirin. Intravenous and inhaled human immunoglobulin RSV hyperimmune globulin and monoclonal antibody have been used to treat limited numbers of patients with RSV infection. The therapeutic effect has been marginal [61].

35.4.6 Herpes Simplex Virus

Herpes simplex virus (HSV) was first recognized as a pulmonary pathogen by Morgan and Finland almost a half century ago [78]. Stern and associates [79] first focused attention on the possibility of herpetic involvement of the trachea and its transmission via contaminated secretions from an infected patient to a health-care worker, causing herpetic whitlow. Later reports of herpetic respiratory infections have included patients with underlying diseases [80, 81], extensive burns [82], underlying malignancy, chemotherapy and radiation therapy [83], and critically ill patients with adult respiratory distress syndrome (ARDS) [84–87].

Herpetic tracheobronchitis has also been reported in immunocompetent patients without history of chronic lung disease [88–90], in patients after extracorporeal circulation for cardiac surgery [91], and following general surgery [92–94].

Despite the apparent increasing prevalence of pulmonary HSV, the relationship between respiratory HSV isolation, pulmonary function, and clinical outcome is not well documented. HSV type 1 in lower respiratory secretions has been associated with unresolved acute bronchospasm [88], prolonged requirement for mechanical ventilation [88–94], tracheal stenosis, and increased mortality [94, 95]. However, asymptomatic viral shedding of HSV also occurs in approximately 1–5% of asymptomatic normal individuals [96].

The concept of airway injury leading to viral reactivation has been reported previously in autopsy series [82, 97, 98] and in patients who have undergone surgery [88, 94]. One reason for this susceptibility of "traumatized" epithelium to viral colonization and potential subsequent inflammation may be that HSV typically infects squamous epithelium [99]. Thus, factors that promote squamous metaplasia, such as trauma, smoking, radiation therapy, or chemotherapy, may predispose the patient to lower respiratory tract infection with HSV [99].

At the present time, there are no defined criteria for the diagnosis or treatment of herpetic tracheobronchitis. Simple isolation of HSV from respiratory secretions is clearly insufficient to make this diagnosis, since HSV can be asymptomatically shed in up to 5% of asymptomatic adults, and the incidence of reactivation or shedding is increased in patients with airway injury. Thus, one usually makes the diagnosis based on a combination of the viral cultures, direct bronchoscopic examination of the endobronchial tree, cytological examination of tracheal or bronchial washings, and the clinical status of the patient.

The most frequent clinical manifestations exhibited by the patients are fever, productive cough, and dyspnea. Frequency of these symptoms does not differ between the immunocompromised and immunocompetent patients. However, immunocompetent patients have significantly more bronchospasm. These data imply that the pathogenicity of HSV in the respiratory tract may vary depending on underlying immune status and the host response [100].

In addition, the role of primary infection versus reactivation in the spectrum of clinical manifestations of tracheobronchitis is unclear. One could speculate that respiratory HSV isolation in the immunocompromised patients most often represents "asymptomatic" shedding, perhaps due to reactivation, with less airway inflammation and, consequently, less bronchial hyperactivity. For unclear reasons, the clinical manifestations of HSV infection are more severe in the immunocompetent population; this may represent a more exuberant local immune response.

Whether to treat critically ill patients with lower respiratory tract HSV isolation with acyclovir is uncertain and controversial at this time. At the present time, it seems reasonable to treat with intravenous acyclovir (8 mg/kg every 8 h for 10 days) those patients with HSV isolation from lower respiratory secretions if, in addition, they have a clinical syndrome or bronchoscopic findings consistent with tracheobronchitis. However, future prospective, randomized trials that assess the impact of treatment on the outcome of both the apparently asymptomatic HSV "carrier" and those patients with clinical HSV tracheobronchitis are needed to clarify this issue. In addition, given the risk of horizontal transmission of HSV-1 to health-care workers, full compliance with infection control measures, including use of gloves and goggles when there is any potential for contact with secretions, is recommended [101].

35.4.7 Cytomegalovirus

Cytomegalovirus (CMV) has been cultured with increasing frequency from patients on prolonged mechanical ventilatory support [102]. Similarly to the case of HSV, the clinical spectrum of CMV can range from asymptomatic viral shedding to a severe disease with profound immunosuppression, pneumonitis and multi-organ dysfunction syndrome. In contrast to HSV where the predominant involvement occurs in the airways, CMV typically involves the pulmonary parenchyma, leading to interstitial pneumonitis or diffuse alveolar damage. CMV infection has been shown to potentiate effects of bacterial infections, possibly through impairment of neutrophil migration or macrophage activation, and has been implicated in promoting bacterial translocation [94]. Cardiac surgery patients with CMV infection complicating mediastinitis have been shown to have persistence of local infection, prolonged hospitalization and increased mortality [103]. Trauma patients with HSV or CMV reactivation have also been shown to have increased ventilator dependence and increased superimposed bacterial pneumonias [104].

As with other organisms, several techniques are available to detect CMV. The virus can be isolated from various body fluids (e.g., blood, urine, respiratory secretions) and buffy coat culture may be useful. Use of shell-vial technique yields results within 24–36 h. Additional, even more sensitive techniques including immunoglobulin-labeled immunomagnetic beads, fluorescent antibody staining, in situ hybridization, and PCR have also been utilized to identify CMV antigens. However, a major limitation of these tests is that they do not differentiate infection from disease. Thus, it is sometimes necessary to obtain tissue in order to assess the cytopathic effects.

The drugs effective against CMV are ganciclovir and foscarnet. However, the decision to treat an individual patient has to balance the risk of the patient, the evidence of disease and the potential toxicity associated with treatment.

35.5 Noninfectious Etiologies

Several noninfectious processes can initiate and/or perpetuate tracheobronchitis. Potential causes include nebulized medications (*N*-acetylcysteine, colistin, tobramycin, ribavirin, and dornase alfa), microaspiration of gastric contents, prolonged exposure to high concentrations of oxygen, and repeated trauma caused by airways suctioning or procedures.

35.6 Summary

Tracheobronchitis is increasingly recognized as a distinct syndrome in the intensive care unit. The most common etiology is infection caused by bacterial, fungal, or viral pathogens. The clinical manifestations are variable and not specific for individual pathogens. The clinical distinction between incidental airway colonization and significant infection is difficult but carries important therapeutic and prognostic implications. A high index of suspicion with the appropriate diagnostic and treatment intervention can lead to an improved outcome.

Acknowledgements. We are indebted to Margie Galkowski for preparing the manuscript.

References

1. Nseir S, DiPompeo C, Pronnier P, Beague S, Onimus T, et al. (2002) Nosocomial tracheobronchitis in mechanically ventilated patients: incidence, aetiology and outcome. Eur Respir J 20:1483–1489
2. Torres A, El-Ebiary M, Rano A (1999) Respiratory infectious complications in the intensive care unit. Clin Chest Med 20:287–301
3. Craven DE, Kunches LM, Kilinsky V, Lichtenberg DA, Make BJ, McCabe WR (1986) Risk factors for pneumonia and fatality in patients receiving continuous mechanical ventilation. Am Rev Respir Dis 133:792–6
4. Adair CG, Gorman SP, Feron BM, et al. (1999) Implications of endotracheal tube biofilm for ventilator-associated pneumonia. Intensive Care Med 25:1072–6
5. Siegal MD, Tocino I (1999) Chest radiology in the intensive care unit. Clin Pulmon Med 6:347–355
6. Santos E, Talusan A, Brandestetter RD (1998) Radiographic mimics of pneumonia in the critical care unit. Crit Care Clin 14:91–104
7. Niederman MS, Craven DE, Fein AM, et al. (1984) Respiratory infection complicating long-term tracheostomy: the implication of persistent gram-negative tracheobronchial colonization. Chest 85:39–44
8. Johanson WG, Pierce AK, Sanford JP, et al. (1972) Nosocomial respiratory infections with gram-negative bacilli. Ann Intern Med 77:701–706
9. Örtqvest Å, Hammers-Berggren S, Kalin M (1990) Respiratory tract colonization and incidence of secondary infection during hospital treatment of community-acquired pneumonia. Eur J Clin Microbiol Infect Dis 9:725–731
10. Salata RA, Ellner JJ (1988) Bacterial colonization of the tracheobronchial tree. Clin Chest Med 91:623–633
11. Harlid R, Andersson G, Frostell CG, et al. (1996) Respiratory tract colonization and infection in patients with chronic tracheostomy: a one-year study in patients living at home. Am J Respir Crit Care Med 154:124–129
12. Rogers RM, Weiler C, Ruppenthal B (1972) Impact of the respiratory intensive care unit on survival of patients with acute respiratory failure. Chest 62:94–97
13. Cross AS, Roup B (1981) Role of respiratory assistance devices in endemic nosocomial pneumonia. Am J Med 70:681–685
14. Niederman MS, Ferranti RD, Zeigler A, et al. (1984) Respiratory infection complicating long-term tracheostomy. Chest 85:39–44
15. Bartlett JT, Faling, LJ, Willey S (1978) Quantitative tracheal bacteriological and cytologic studies in patients with long-term tracheostomies. Chest 74:635–639
16. Levine SA, Niederman MS (1991) The impact of tracheal intubation on host defenses and risks for nosocomial pneumonia. Clin Chest Med 12(3):523–543
17. Gal TJ (1988) How does tracheal intubation alter respiratory mechanics? Probl Anesth 2:191–200
18. Klainer AS, Turndorf H, Wu WH, et al. (1975) Surface alterations due to endotracheal intubation. Am J Med 58:674–683
19. Ramphal R, Guay P (1987) *Pseudomonas aeruginosa* adhesions for tracheobronchial mucin. Infect Immun 55:600–603
20. Ramphal R, Pyle M (1983) Adherence of mucoid and non-mucoid *Pseudomonas aeruginosa* to acid-injured tracheal epithelium. Infect Immun 41:345–31
21. Craven DE, Goularte TA, Make BJ (1984) Contaminated condensate in mechanical ventilator circuits: a risk factor for nosocomial pneumonia. Am Rev Respir Dis 129:625–628

22. Craven DE, Lichtenberg DA, Goularte TA, et al. (1984) Contaminated medication nebulizers in mechanical ventilator circuits: source of bacterial aerosols. Am J Med 77:834–838
23. Schwartz SN, Dowling JN, Benkovic C, et al. (1978) Sources of gram-negative bacilli colonizing the trachea of intubated patients. J Infect Dis 138:227–231
24. Niederman MS, Mantovani R, Schoch P, et al. (1989) Patterns and routes of tracheobronchial colonization in mechanically ventilated patients: the role of nutritional status in colonization of the lower airway by *Pseudomonas* species. Chest 95:155–161
25. Johanson WG Jr, Pierce AK, Sanford JP, et al. (1972) Nosocomial respiratory infections with gram-negative bacilli: the significance of colonization of the respiratory tract. Ann Intern Med 77:701–706
26. Nseir S, DiPompeo D, Soubrier S, Lenci H, Delour P, et al. (2005) Effect of ventilator-associated tracheobronchitis on outcome in patients without chronic respiratory failure: a case-control study. Crit Care 9:R238–245
27. Niederman MS, Ferranti RD, Ziegler A, et al. (1984) Respiratory infection complicating long-term tracheostomy: The implication of persistent gram-negative tracheobronchial colonization. Chest 85:39–44
28. George DL, Falk PS, Wunderink RG, et al. (1998) Epidemiology of ventilator-acquired pneumonia based on protected bronchoscopic sampling. Am J Respir Crit Care Med 158:1839–1847
29. Namba Y, Mihara N, Tanaka M (1997) [Fulminant tracheobronchitis caused by methicillin-resistant *Staphylococcus aureus* (MRSA)] [Japanese]. Nihon Kyobu Shikkan Gakkai Zasshi. Jpn J Thoracic Dis 35(9):969–973
30. Yamazaki Y, Hirai K, Honda T (2002) Pseudomembranous tracheobronchitis caused by methicillin-resistant *Staphylococcus aureus*. Scand J Infect Dis 34:211–213
31. Cefai C, Richards J, Gould FK, et al. (1990) An outbreak of *Acinetobacter* respiratory tract infection resulting from incomplete disinfection of ventilatory equipment. J Hosp Infect 15:177–182
32. Seifert H, Strate A, Pulverer G (1995) Nosocomial bacteremia due to *Acinetobacter baumannii*: Clinical features, epidemiology, and predictors of mortality. Medicine 74(6):340–349
33. Seifert H, Baginski R, Schulze A, et al. (1993) Antimicrobial susceptibility of *Acinetobacter* species. Antimicrob Agents Chemother 37:750–753
34. Chen YC, Chang SC, Hsieh WC, et al. (1991) *Acinetobacter calcoaceticus* bacteremia: analysis of 48 cases. J Formosan Med Assoc 90:958–963
35. Leigh MW, Clyde WA (1987) Chlamydial and mycoplasmal pneumonias. Semin Respir Infect 2:152–158
36. Rose RM, Pinkston P, O'Donnell C, et al. (1987) Viral infection of the lower respiratory tract. Clin Chest Med 8: 405–418
37. Glezen WP, Loda FA, Clyde WA, et al. (1971) Epidemiologic patterns of acute lower respiratory disease of children in a pediatric practice. J Pediatr 78:397–406
38. Fischman RA, Marschall KE, Kislak JW, et al. (1978) Adult respiratory distress syndrome caused by *Mycoplasma* pneumonia. Chest 74:471–473
39. Zack MB, Kazemi H (1973) Carbon dioxide retention in *Mycoplasma* pneumonia. Am Rev Respir Dis 107:1052–1054
40. Chang SM, Kuo HT, Lin FJ, Tzen CY, Sheu CY (2005) Pseudomembranous tracheobronchitis caused by *Aspergillus* in immunocompromised patients. Scand J Infect Dis 37:937–942
41. Routsi C, Kaltsas P, Bessis E, Rontogianni D, Kollias S, Roussos C (2004) Airway obstruction and acute respiratory failure due to *Aspergillus* tracheobronchitis. Crit Care Med 32:580–582
42. Routsi C, Platsouka E, Prekates A, Rontogianni D, Paniara O, Roussos C (2001) Aspergillus bronchitis causing atelectasis and acute respiratory failure in an immunocompromised patient. Infection 29:243–244
43. Clarke A, Skelton J, Fraser RS (1991) Fungal tracheobronchitis: report of 9 cases and review of the literature. Medicine 70(1):1–14
44. Meyer RD, Young LS, Armstrong D, et al. (1973) Aspergillosis complicating neoplastic disease. Am J Med 54:6–15
45. Orr DP, Myerowitz RL, Dubois PJ (1978) Patho-radiologic correlation of invasive pulmonary aspergillosis in the compromised host. Cancer 41:2028–2039
46. Young RC, Bennett JE, Vogel CL, et al. (1970) Aspergillosis. The spectrum of the disease of 98 patients. Medicine 49:149–173
47. Dubois PJ, Myerowitz RL, Allen CM (1977) Pathoradiologic correlation of pulmonary candidiasis in immunosuppressed patients. Cancer 40:1026–1036
48. Chakravarty SC (1967) Bronchopulmonary candidiasis: Clinical aspects. Dis Chest 51:608–613
49. Wengrower D, Or R, Segal E, Kleinman Y (1985) Bronchopulmonary candidiasis exacerbating asthma. Case report and a review of the literature. Respiration 47:209–213
50. Azoulay E, Timsit J-F, Tafflet M, et al. (2006) *Candida* colonization of the respiratory tract and subsequent *Pseudomonas* ventilator-associated pneumonia. Chest 29:110–117
51. Tasci S, Glasmacher A, Lentini S, Tschubel K, Ewig S, Molitor E, Sauerbruch T, Luderitz B, Rabe C (2006) Pseudomembranous and obstructive *Aspergillus* tracheobronchitis – optimal diagnostic strategy and outcome. Mycoses 49:37–42
52. Kramer MR, Denning DW, Marshall SE, et al. (1991) Ulcerative tracheobronchitis after lung transplantation: a new form of invasive aspergillosis. Am Rev Respir Dis 144: 552–556
53. Gerson SL, Talbot GH, Hurwitz S, et al. (1984) Prolonged granulocytopenia: the major risk factor for invasive pulmonary aspergillosis in patients with acute leukemia. Ann Intern Med 100:345–351
54. Lehrer RI, Cline MJ (1971) Leukocyte candidacidal activity and resistance to systemic candidiasis in patients with cancer. Cancer 27:1211–1217
55. Dale DC, Petersdorf RG (1973) Corticosteroids and infectious diseases. Med Clin North Am 57:1277–1287
56. Bodey GP (1984) Candidiasis in cancer patients. Am J Med 77(Suppl 4D):13–19
57. Denny FW Jr (1995) The clinical impact of human respiratory virus infections. Am J Respir Crit Care Med 152:S4
58. Ellenbogen C, Graybill JL, Silva J, et al. (1974) Bacterial pneumonia complicating viral pneumonia. Am J Med 56:169–178
59. Wong SSY, Yuen K (2006) Avian influenza virus infection in humans. Chest 129:156–168
60. Frank AL, Taber LH, Wells CR, et al. (1981) Patterns of shedding of myxoviruses and paramyxoviruses in children. J Infect Dis 144:433–441
61. Hall CB (2001) Respiratory syncytial virus and parainfluenza virus. N Engl J Med 344:1917–1928
62. Kark JD, Lebiush M, Rannon L (1982) Cigarette smoking as a risk factor for epidemic $A(H_1N_1)$ influenza in young men. N Engl J Med 307:1042–1046
63. Mullooly JP, Barker WH, Nolan TF Jr (1986) Risk of acute respiratory disease among pregnant women during influenza A epidemics. Public Health Rep 101:205–211

64. Conway SP, Simmonds EJ, Littlewood JM (1992) Acute severe deterioration in cystic fibrosis associated with influenza A virus infection. Thorax 47:112-114
65. Ungchusak K, Auewarkul P, Dowell SF, et al. (2005) Probable person-to-person transmission of Avian influenza A (H5N1). N Engl J Med 352:333-340
66. O'Brien TG, Sweeney DF (1973) Interstitial viral pneumonitis complicated by severe respiratory failure: successful management using intensive dehydration and steroids. Chest 63:314-232
67. Roberts GBS (1957) Fulminating influenza. Lancet 2:944
68. Winther B, Brofeldt S, Gronborg H, et al. (1984) Study of bacteria in the nasal cavity and nasopharynx during naturally acquired common cold. Acta Otolaryngol 98:315-320
69. Tran TH, Nguyen TL, Nguyen TD, et al. (2004) Avian influenza A (H5N1) in 10 patients in Vietnam. N Engl J Med 350:1179-1188
70. Chotpitayasunondh T, Ungchusak K, Hanshaoworatal, et al. (2005) Human disease from influenza A (H5N1). Emerg Infect Dis 11:201-209
71. Rapid diagnostic tests for influenza (1999) The Medical Letter 41:121-122
72. Calfee DP, Hayden FG (1998) New approaches to influenza chemotherapy. Neuraminidase inhibitors. Drugs 56:537-553
73. Smith CB, Kanner RE, Golden CA, et al. (1980) Effect of viral infection on pulmonary function in patients with chronic obstructive pulmonary diseases. J Infect Dis 141:271-280
74. Bateman ED, Hayashi S, Kuwano K, et al. (1995) Latent adenoviral infection in follicular bronchiectasis. Am J Respir Crit Care Med 151:170-176
75. Morales F, Calder MA, Inglis JM, et al. (1983) A study of respiratory infections in the elderly to assess the role of respiratory syncytial virus. J Infect 7:236-247
76. Falsey AR, Hennessey PA, Formica MA, et al. (2005) Respiratory syncytial virus infection in elderly and high-risk adults. N Eng J Med 352:1749-1759
77. Englund JA, Piedra PA Jewell A, Patel K, Baxter BB, Whimbey E (1996) Rapid diagnosis of respiratory syncytial virus infection in immunocompromised adults. J Clin Microbiol 34:1649-1653
87. Morgan HR, Finland M (1949) Isolation of herpes virus from a case of atypical pneumonia and erythema multiforme exudativum: with studies of four additional cases. Am J Med Sci 217:92-95
79. Stern H, Elek SD, Millar DM, Anderson HF (1959) Herpetic whitlow: a form of cross-infection in hospitals. Lancet 2:871-874
80. Lheureux P, Verhest A, Vincent JL, Liénard C, Levivier M, Kahn RJ (1985) Herpes virus infection, an unusual source of adult respiratory distress syndrome. Eur J Respir Dis 67:72-77
81. Benjamin D (1989) Herpes simplex tracheobronchitis and pneumonitis. Pediatr Pathol 9:773-777
82. Nash G, Foley FD (1970) Herpetic infection of the middle and lower respiratory tract. Am J Clin Pathol 54:857-863
83. Ramsey PG, Fife KH, Hackman RC, Mayers JD, Corey L (1982) Herpes simplex virus pneumonia: clinical, virologic, and pathologic features in 20 patients. Ann Intern Med 97:813-820
84. Frable WJ, Frable MA, Seney FD Jr (1977) Virus infections of the respiratory tract: cytopathologic and clinical analysis. Acta Cytol 21:32-36
85. Tuxen DV, Wilson JW, Cade JF (1987) Prevention of lower respiratory herpes simplex virus infection with acyclovir in patients with the adult respiratory distress syndrome. Am Rev Respir Dis 136:402-405
86. Tuxen DV, Cade JF, McDonald MI, Buchanan MR, Clark RJ, Pain MC (1982) Herpes simplex virus from the lower respiratory tract in adult respiratory distress syndrome. Am Rev Respir Dis 126:416-419
87. Prellner T, Flamholc L, Haidl S, Lindholm K, Widell A (1992) Herpes simplex virus - the most frequently isolated pathogen in the lungs of patients with severe respiratory distress. Scand J Infect Dis 24:283-292
88. Sherry MK, Klainer AS, Wolff M, Gerhard H (1988) Herpetic tracheobronchitis. Ann Intern Med 109:229-233
89. Legge RH, Thompson AB, Linder J, Woods GL, Robbins RA, Moulton AL, et al. (1988) Acyclovir-responsive herpetic tracheobronchitis. Am J Med 85:516-563
90. Chakraborty A, Forker A, Reese H, Casey J (1988) Tracheobronchitis and pneumonia due to herpes simplex virus (HSV) infection. Nebr Med J 73:347-350
91. Vaxelaire JF, Brunet F, Armaganidis A, Pochard F, Giraud T, Lanore JJ, et al. (1991) The role of herpes simplex virus in respiratory complications after cardiac surgery (abstract). Am Rev Respir Dis 143:A474
92. Porteous C, Bradley JA, Hamilton DN, Ledingham IM, Clements GB, Robinson CG (1984) Herpes simplex virus reactivation in surgical patients. Crit Care Med 12:626-628
93. Avery RK, Longworth DL (1995) Viral pulmonary infections in thoracic and cardiovascular surgery. Semin Thoracic Cardiovasc Surg 7:88-94
94. Cook CH, Yenchar JK, Kraner TO, Davis EA, Ferguson RM (1998) Occult herpes family viruses may increase mortality in critically ill surgical patients. Am J Surg 176:357-360
95. St. John RC, Pacht ER (1990) Tracheal stenosis and failure to wean from mechanical ventilation due to herpetic tracheitis. Chest 98:1520-2152
96. Corey L, Spear PG (1986) Infections with herpes simplex viruses. N Engl J Med 314:749-757
97. Nash G (1972) Necrotizing tracheobronchitis and bronchopneumonia consistent with herpetic infection. Hum Pathol 3:283-291
98. Graham BS, Snell JD Jr (1983) Herpes simplex virus infection of the adult lower respiratory tract. Medicine 62:384-393
99. Herout V, Vortel V, Vondrackova A (1966) Herpes simplex involvement of the lower respiratory tract. Am J Clin Pathol 46:411-419
100. Schuller D, Spessert C, Fraser VJ, Goodenberger DM (1993) Herpes simplex virus from respiratory tract secretions: epidemiology, clinical characteristics, and outcome in immunocompromised and nonimmunocompromised hosts. Am J Med 94:29-33
101. Perl TM, Haugen TH, Pfaller MA, Hollis R, Lakeman AD, Whitley RJ, et al. (1992) Transmission of herpes simplex virus type 1 infection in an intensive care unit. Ann Intern Med 117:584-586
102. Papazian L, Fraisse L, et al. (1996) Cytomegalovirus. An unexpected cause of ventilator-associated pneumonia. Anesthesiology 84:280-287
103. Domart Y, Trouillet JL, Fagan JY, Chastre J, Brun-Vezinet F, Gilbert C (1990) Incidence and morbidity of cytomegaloviral infection in patients with mediastinitis following cardiac surgery. Chest 97:18-22
104. Cushing D, et al. (1993) Herpes simplex virus and cytomegalovirus excretion associated with increased ventilator days in trauma patients. J Trauma 35:161

36 Severe Community-Acquired Pneumonia

M. Bodí, J. Rello

36.1 Introduction

Pneumonia is a leading cause of death in the world and the sixth most common cause of death in the United States. Indeed, in the US it is the number one cause of death from infectious diseases; each year in the US, there are from 5 to 10 million cases of community-acquired pneumonia (CAP) leading to as many as 1.1 million hospitalizations and 45,000 deaths. Management of a single in-hospital case of CAP costs around $7,500 [1].

In spite of advances in antibiotic treatments and technical improvements in the ICU, severe CAP mortality rates remain unacceptably high. In a range of studies of SCAP requiring ICU admission, crude mortality was around 20–54% [2–9].

Given the steady increase in the number of senior citizens and immunocompromised patients (those receiving steroids, organ transplant recipients, HIV patients) and the better survival rates of patients affected by chronic illness, research in this field is clearly justified. Current investigations focus on improving diagnosis, defining risk factors that influence outcome, and assessing new therapies.

In the last decade, a number of medical societies [1, 10–14] have sought to broaden our understanding of pneumonia by producing and publishing sets of guidelines. The first guidelines that avoided the traditional classification into "typical and atypical" pneumonia were published in 1993 by the American Thoracic Society (ATS) [10]. The ATS revised their guidelines in June 2001 [11], emphasizing certain modifying factors that increase the risk of infection with drug-resistant and unusual pathogens (drug-resistant *Streptococcus pneumoniae* or Gram-negative bacteria). These guidelines classify patients into four categories on the basis of the most probable etiology: (a) outpatients with no history of cardiopulmonary disease, and no modifying factors; (b) outpatients with cardiopulmonary disease (congestive heart failure or chronic obstructive pulmonary disease) and/or other modifying factors; (c) inpatients, not admitted to the ICU; and (d) patients who require intensive care admission. The IDSA (Infectious Diseases Society of America) revised their guidelines in September 2000 [1] and updated them in December 2003 [12]. In Europe similar guidelines have been produced, seeking to identify patients at risk of death or complications [13, 14]. This chapter focuses on the subgroup of CAP patients who are admitted to the ICU – approximately 10% of patients hospitalized for CAP [15] – and reviews the most important factors regarding etiology, prognosis, diagnostic tools and treatments.

36.2 Definition of Severe Community-Acquired Pneumonia

No consensus has been reached among researchers as regards the definition of severe CAP. Obviously, patients who need large volume infusions and vasopressors for shock or mechanical ventilation clearly need to be admitted to the ICU. However, patients with multilobar involvement, renal failure, confusion and other comorbidities also have lower chances of survival. Therefore, percentages of hospitalized patients requiring admission to the ICU obtained in different studies fluctuate between 5% and 35% [16], and may well reflect differences not only in clinical criteria, but in infrastructure as well. Some authors have tried to define criteria for severe pneumonia. The Pneumonia Severity Index (PSI) [17], which stratifies patients into five severity classes based on their demographic characteristics, comorbid conditions, physical findings, and diagnostic studies, is recommended as a mortality prediction rule [1, 11, 17]. The severity class is rated on a numerical scale, with lower scores associated with a lower risk of mortality. Therefore, patients in class I and II can be treated as outpatients, patients in class III can be treated either as outpatients or briefly observed in the hospital, but class IV and V (PSI ≥ 90) patients need to be hospitalized (Fig. 36.1). In 1987 the British Thoracic Association (BTS) [18] published the first guidelines based on a survey of 453 patients admitted to hospital for CAP. Using multivariate analysis the study concluded that three variables were associated with an in-

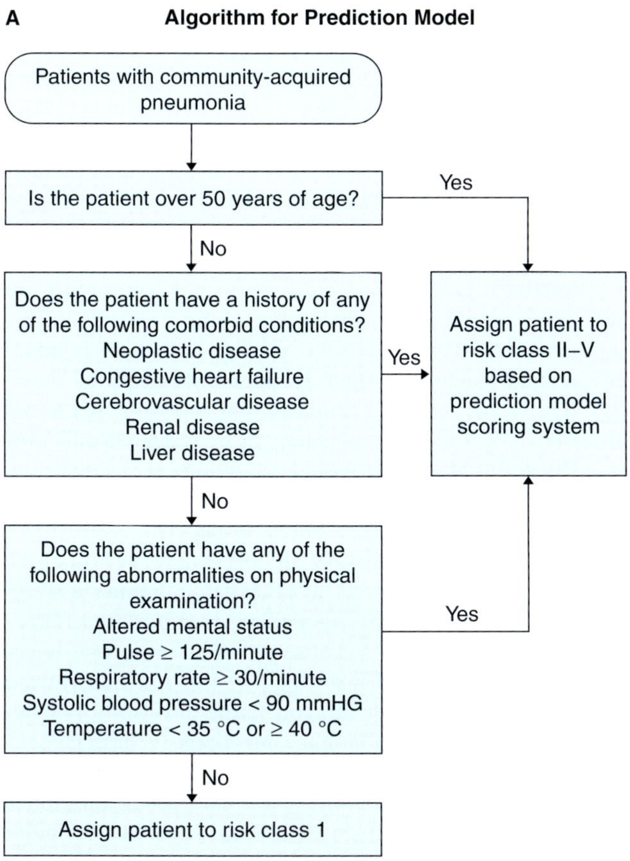

B

CHARACTERISTIC	POINTS ASSIGNED*
Demographic factor	
Age	
Men	Age (yr)
Women	Age (yr) −10
Nursing home resident	+10
Coexisting illnesses	
Neoplastic disease	+30
Liver disease	+20
Congestive heart failur	+10
Cerebrovascular disease	+10
Renal disease	+10
Physical-examination findings	
Altered mental status	+20
Respiratory rate ≥ 30/minute	+20
Systolic blood pressure < 90 mmHg	+20
Temperature < 35 °C or ≥ 40 °C	+15
Pulse ≥ 125/minute	+10
Laboratory and radiographic findings	
Arterial pH < 7.35	+30
Blood urea nitrogen ≥ 30 mg/dl (11 mmol/liter)	+20
Sodium < 130 mmol/liter	+20
Glucose ≥ 250 mg/dl (14 mmol/liter)	+10
Hematrocrit < 30 %	+10
Partial pressure of arterial oxygen < 60 mmHg	+10
Pleural effusion	+10

Fig. 36.1. A Identifying patients in Risk Class I in the Derivation of the Prediction Rule. **B** Point Scoring System for step 2 of the prediction rule for assignment to risk classes II (≤70 points), III (71–90 points), IV (91–130 points), V (>130 points)

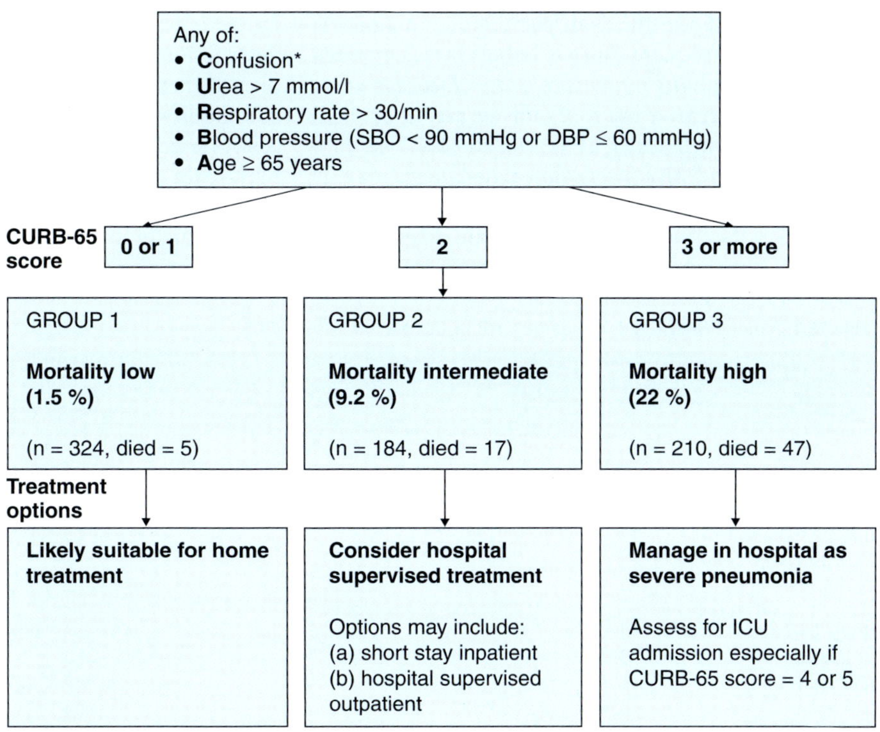

Fig. 36.2. CURB-65

creased risk of mortality: respiratory rate ≥30 breaths/min, blood urea >7 mmol/l, and diastolic blood pressure ≤60 mmHg. The association of at least two of these variables increased the mortality risk 21 times. The guidelines proposed the use of the CURB-65 severity score, comprising five "core" adverse prognostic features (Confusion, Urea, Respiratory rate, Blood pressure, Age ≥65) (Fig. 36.2) [14, 19]. The BTS approach focused on identifying high-risk patients so as not to underestimate illness severity, while the PSI approach focused on recognizing some patients as low risk, so as not to overestimate illness severity [17]. The ATS guidelines defined severe CAP as the presence of two minor criteria (systolic blood pressure <90 mmHg, PaO_2/FiO_2 <250 mmHg, involvement of >two lobes in chest radiograph), or one major criterion (need for vasopressors >4 h, or mechanical ventilation) [11].

Aside from the need to validate these rules, there is no doubt that considering pneumonia as a dynamic process (which may worsen in the first 24–48 h and require ICU admittance) can improve our approach to, and management of, this clinical entity.

36.3 Etiology and Risk Factors

The spectrum of causative agents of severe CAP is similar in hospitalized patients and in outpatients. The main difference is the relative importance of each microorganism. *S. pneumoniae* accounts for nearly 50% of cases with etiologic diagnosis [2–9, 20–24]. It accounts for about two-thirds of bacteremic pneumonia and is the most frequent cause of lethal CAP. *Legionella* species, *Haemophilus influenzae*, *Staphylococcus aureus*, and Gram-negative microorganisms are other causative pathogens in severe CAP [1–14, 20–24]. *Pneumocystis jiroveci* and *Mycobacterium tuberculosis* may be responsible for CAP in some areas [5, 20]. Table 36.1 summarizes the most prevalent etiologic diagnoses [2, 9, 20–24]. The most important risk factors for *S. pneumoniae* infection are chronic hepatic disease, alcoholism, influenza, cigarette smoking and chronic obstructive pulmonary disease (COPD) [25]. Pneumonia caused by *Legionella* spp. was the second most frequent etiology in the 1990s [2–8], though there are significant regional variations, and recent studies report a fall in its incidence, probably associated with the extended use of new fluoroquinolones and macrolides [26, 27]. It is more common in Mediterranean countries and the US than in northern Europe. The most important risk factors are smoking and corticotherapy. El-Ebiary et al. [28] reported COPD to be a more frequent risk factor in nosocomial pneumonia than in community-acquired pneumonia caused by *Legionella pneumophila* (64% vs. 41%). *H. influenzae* accounts for between 6% and 15% [2–9, 20–24] of pneumonia that require ICU admission. COPD, elderly and HIV patients are the most affected. Pneumonia caused by *S. aureus* is usually a severe infection, requiring ventilatory support in up to 90% of cases. The infection can occur after epidemic influenza or via bloodstream spread. Methicillin-resistant *Staphylococcus aureus* (MRSA) has emerged as an important infection in the community setting [29]. It has primarily been associated with skin and soft-tissue infections, but can also cause severe pulmonary infections, including pneumonia and empyema. Community-acquired MRSA is typically more susceptible to a wider class of antibiotics than healthcare-associated MRSA, but it is also more virulent. Community-acquired MRSA usually contains the gene encoding Panton-Valentine leukocidin (PVL), a toxin that creates lytic pores in the cell membranes of neutrophils and induces the release of neutrophil chemotactic factors that promote inflammation and tissue destruction (a process known as necrotizing pneumonia). The optimal antibiotic treatment for PVL-positive community-acquired MRSA is unknown; however, antibiotics with activity against MRSA and the ability to inhibit toxin production may be appropriate (linezolid or clindamycin for susceptible isolates). Enterobacteriaceae are usually involved in nosocomial pneumonia, and in some studies of CAP are the third most important

Table 36.1. Isolated pathogens of severe CAP in the period 1997–2006

Author Year Episodes	Hirani 1997 (*n*=57)	Marik 2000 (*n*=148)	El-Shol 2001 (*n*=110)	Angus 2002 (*n*=170)	Rello 2003 (*n*=204)	Mortensen 2005 (*n*=172)	Bodí 2005 (*n*=529)
Intubation	96.4	–	85	28–56	51.9	31.9	65.9
Etiological diagnosis	67	52	55	44.7	57.3	23.8	52.2
S. pneumoniae	18	13	19	14.7	35.1	36.6	48.1
Legionella spp.	16	5	9	–	19.6	–	7.7
H. influenzae	–	10	7	4.7	9.4	17.1	7.4
S. aureus	12	13	7	4.1	4.3	24.4	6.4
Enterobacteriaceae	–	13	14.5	–	1.7	7.1	6.1
P. aeruginosa	1.7	5	6	–	6.8	4.8	6.7
P. jiroveci	5.2	–	–	–	8.5	–	3.4
M. tuberculosis	1.7	–	2	–	1.7	–	2.7
Others	13.9	10	12	–	12.8	–	11.4

Table 36.2. Modifying factors that increase the risk of infection with specific pathogens

Drug-resistant *Streptococcus pneumoniae*
Age greater than 65 years
Beta-lactam therapy within the past 3 months
Immunosuppression (either as the result of an illness or induced by treatment with corticosteroids)
Multiple medical comorbidities, alcoholism
Exposure to a child in a day care center
Enteric Gram-negative organisms
Recent antibiotic therapy
Underlying cardiopulmonary disease
Residence in a nursing home
Multiple medical comorbidities
Pseudomonas aeruginosa
Structural lung disease such as bronchiectasis
Chronic obstructive pulmonary disease
Broad-spectrum antibiotic therapy that lasted for at least 7 days in the past month
Corticosteroid therapy with at least 10 mg of prednisone per day
Malignancy
Malnutrition

cause (25%) [3]. The microorganism most frequently involved is *Klebsiella pneumoniae*, which mainly affects alcoholics, COPD patients, and general patients suffering from consuming diseases. Among Gram-negative bacteria, *P. aeruginosa* stands out on account of its extreme mortality [20]. In the multicenter study by Bodí et al. [9], COPD, malignancy, previous antibiotic therapy, and rapid radiographic spread were associated with *Pseudomonas* pneumonia.

Table 36.2 shows certain modifying factors that increase the risk of infection with drug-resistant and unusual pathogens [9, 11]. Finally, in a high percentage of patients the causative agent is impossible to determine, even after extensive research. Atypical microorganisms such as *C. pneumoniae* and *M. pneumoniae* do not seem to play a role in severe pneumonia. Using PCR techniques, Menéndez et al. [30] suggested that in the subgroup of patients with unknown etiology, *S. pneumoniae* was the most probable cause.

36.4 Diagnosis

Empiricism is the usual approach in patients suffering from CAP. Indeed, some guidelines strongly recommend it [1, 11, 12]. However, a knowledge of the causative agent in severe episodes is useful, because identifying the causative agent and adjusting treatment both influence patient outcome [20]. Despite intensive etiologic research, the causative agent is not isolated in as many as 40% of cases [2–9, 20–24].

Patients hospitalized for pneumonia should have two pretreatment blood cultures and expectorated sputum Gram stain and culture [12]. The expectorated sputum specimen should be a deep-cough specimen obtained before antibiotic treatment that is rapidly transported and processed within a few hours of collection. Cytologic criteria [more than 25 neutrophils and ≤10 epithelial cells per microscopic field (×100)] should be used as a contingency for sputum culture, except with culture for *Mycobacteria* and *Legionella* species. In severe CAP a respiratory sample is available in only 40% of patients and in only 50% of these is it considered good enough for analysis [31].

Sputum induced by hypertonic saline serum has proved to be a good tool for *Pneumocystis jiroveci* and tuberculosis research, especially in AIDS patients [32]. The usefulness of this method in the detection of other pulmonary pathogens has not been established.

Blood cultures are positive in around 10–30% of patients with severe CAP [9, 33]. A prospective study of patients with CAP [34] showed that the yield of blood culture increases significantly with the severity of pneumonia, and that positive cultures only impacted on the management of critically ill patients (PSI IV and V). In spite of low sensitivity, the convincing nature of the isolation of a respiratory pathogen from blood, the opportunity to test the antimicrobial sensitivity of the isolate and the relative simplicity of drawing blood for cultures are all arguments in favor of the practice of obtaining blood cultures in patients requiring hospital admission. At least two cultures should be drawn with needlesticks at separate sites.

Other noninvasive techniques are based on antigen detection of certain microorganisms in urine, plasma or sputum. The most useful is antigen detection of *Legionella* spp. in urine: sensitivity is around 80% and specificity is near 100% [26]. Furthermore, this test is not influenced by previous use of the right antibiotic and may remain positive for several weeks after pulmonary infection. The main drawback is that only serotype 1 can be detected (though this serotype accounts for >70% of *Legionella* infection) [35]. More recently a colorimetric technique has been validated that allows antigen detection at the bedside [36]. The pneumococcal urinary antigen assay is an acceptable test to increase the standard diagnostic methods of blood culture and sputum Gram stain and culture, with the potential advantage of rapid results, similar to those for sputum. The test has a sensitivity of 80% and specificity of 94%. False positive tests can occur (nearly 10% of cases of positive results) because of colonization status without acute pneumococcal infection, more frequent among children. The main disadvantage is the need for cultures to determine susceptibility in order to guide therapy [1, 12].

Other useful diagnostic tools that can be applied in etiologic investigation are based on invasive tests. Among these, fiberoptic bronchoscopy is the most frequently used. Bronchoscopy is easy to perform when a patient is intubated, but it tends not to be widely used, because of the absence of laboratory equipment and well-trained bronchoscopic staff. Furthermore, in non-intubated patients, respiratory failure constitutes a relative contraindication, given the possibility of speeding up urgent intubation. In order to avoid this complication, a method that makes bronchoscopy safer in patients treated with CPAP has recently been described [37]. This device avoids the decline of airway pressure and maintains correct levels of PaO_2. Bronchoscopic sampling is recommended for particularly severe, selected cases with pneumonia that are unresponsive to antimicrobial therapy. The use of bronchoscopy for patients with CAP who had failed initial management has identified an infectious agent in around 30% [20]. Likewise, the correlation between bronchoalveolar lavage (BAL) and protected specimen brush (PSB) was good. In the context of immunosuppression (HIV, steroids, transplantation) or high suspicion of an atypical microorganism, performance of bronchoscopy with bronchoalveolar lavage (BAL) is the first step in the diagnostic approach. The accuracy of this test to detect *Pneumocystis jiroveci* is close to 90% [32].

Procedures based on PCR techniques can be applied to respiratory samples; sensitivity remains high, in spite of antibiotic treatment. In addition, the results are available in only a few hours. However, the high cost of these procedures and the lack of well-prepared laboratories preclude their worldwide use.

In severe CAP, a basic etiologic investigation should be performed, including at least two blood cultures, a respiratory sample (obtained by means of bronchoscope or simple BAS) and urinary antigen detection for *Legionella* and *Streptococcus pneumoniae*. Other tests can be performed depending on the equipment available at the center in question. Establishing the etiology is recommended whenever possible.

36.5 Therapy

Treatment of severe CAP involves a number of aspects that will be reviewed in this section: adequate antibiotic spectrum, shock management (discussed in Chapter 2), inflammatory response control (Chapter 16), and ventilatory support (discussed in Chapter 38). It is important to remember that mortality is due to septic shock (particularly within the first 4 days) and refractory hypoxemia (ARDS and MOF) despite adequate antibiotic treatment [5].

36.5.1 Impact of Treatment on Mortality

A range of studies using multivariate analysis have shown that inadequate antibiotic treatment is associated with a significant increase in mortality [3, 4, 7, 38–39].

In recent years, several authors have analyzed the influence of guidelines on patient prognosis [9, 40–42]. However, there are few reports of the influence of guidelines on the treatment of severely ill patients. Compliance with guidelines is lower in the most severe cases [9, 40]. Bodí et al. [9] found a low adherence (57.8%) to IDSA guidelines among 529 patients admitted to the ICU with severe CAP, and higher mortality rates when IDSA guidelines were not followed. Moreover, adherence to guidelines was the only modifiable prognosis-related factor for patients with severe CAP. Mechanical ventilation is prolonged in patients receiving non-compliant guideline therapies [43].

Timely administration of antibiotic agents to hospitalized patients with pneumonia has been associated with improved survival [44] and shorter duration of hospital stay [45]. The latest update of IDSA guidelines [12] recommends initiating antibiotic therapy within 4 h after admission for hospitalized patients with CAP.

36.5.2 Shock Management

Dyspnea, hyperventilation, oral intake intolerance, fever and sweat increase loss and limit fluid intake, causing many patients to be hypovolemic at hospital admission. Patients with hypotension should therefore receive aggressive early resuscitation. The rate of patients who meet shock septic criteria when admitted to the ICU varies [9, 23] across countries and across institutions. The specific management of patients with severe CAP and shock does not differ from that of the general population with septic shock [46, 47]. The volume repletion in patients with septic shock increases cardiac output and oxygen delivery, and is generally enough to reverse hypotension. However, the volume requirements are not easily determined in critically ill patients. Central venous pressure (CVP) is initially required to assess intravascular volume. If CVP increases or if the patient develops respiratory failure and needs mechanical ventilation, a pulmonary artery catheter is recommended before administration of vasoactive drugs. Volume repletion and norepinephrine should be the first approach to patients with septic shock. Assessment of regional and global perfusion should be evaluated by mixed venous saturation or blood lactate levels (>2 mEq/l) to guide optimum reanimation.

36.5.3 Inflammatory Response Control

Several studies have shown increased pulmonary and circulating inflammatory cytokine levels in patients with severe CAP [48]. Monton et al. reported that among patients with CAP requiring mechanical ventilation, those who received methylprednisolone had an attenuated systemic and pulmonary inflammatory response and presented a trend toward lower mortality. Recently [49], a randomized study evaluated the efficacy and safety of low-dose hydrocortisone infusion (200 mg loading bolus followed by an infusion of 240 mg for 7 days) in patients with severe CAP. Hydrocortisone treatment led to significant reductions in mechanical ventilation, length of ICU and hospital stay, and increased survival to hospital discharge and to 60 days. However, the small number of patients included ($n=46$) is the principal weakness of the study and a large randomized trial is necessary to confirm the findings.

Recombinant human activated protein C (hAPC), an anticoagulant, is an anti-inflammatory agent that has proved effective in the treatment of sepsis (the PROWESS study) [50]. In patients with sepsis, the administration of activated protein C reduced the relative risk of death by 19.4% and the absolute risk by 6.1%. However, the 90-day survival benefit of rAPH was largely attributable to an absolute reduction in mortality rate of 18.1% (from 65% to 47%) for patients who were prescribed inadequate antibiotic therapy; the reduction in mortality rate was only 4% (from 37% to 33%) for patients prescribed adequate antibiotic therapy. Laterre et al. [51] reported an additional analysis of PROWESS in patients with severe CAP. In their study, only patients with APACHE II score ≥ 25 presented a significant reduction of mortality at 90 days.

36.5.4 Treatment of Refractory Hypoxemia

Between 58% and 88% of patients admitted to the ICU for severe CAP need mechanical ventilation [9, 20–23]. In patients undergoing mechanical ventilation, the goal is to improve gas interchange and maintain plateau pressures low in order to avoid acute lung injury.

The main drawback of intubation is that it increases the possibility of superinfections. New forms of ventilation that avoid intubation have been promoted in recent years, known generically as noninvasive ventilation. Noninvasive forms of ventilation have been tested in several diseases and are very useful in COPD patients. As regards respiratory failure in severe CAP, only one controlled randomized trial has been performed to date [52], in which the authors concluded that noninvasive ventilation was associated with a significant reduction in the rate of endotracheal intubation and duration of ICU stay. In more than 50% (33/56) of the patients enrolled, COPD was the main underlying disease. Moreover, in this subgroup, a significant reduction of mortality was achieved when noninvasive ventilation was applied.

When the level of consciousness is depressed or the ability to clear secretion is impaired, intubation is indicated [53]. Delayed intubation in patients with severe CAP and noninvasive ventilation may mean worse outcome [39].

Severe CAP is associated with acute respiratory distress syndrome (ARDS) in about 10% of cases [31]. In general, when acute lung injury is present mechanical ventilation is needed, requiring high level O_2 delivery as well as higher levels of PEEP so as to ensure correct PaO_2. Two important variables in this context are FiO_2 and tidal volume. As regards FiO_2 and PEEP it is necessary to achieve a level of PEEP that maintains FiO_2 below 0.6 whenever possible. A protective ventilatory strategy for keeping plateau pressure below 30 $cmHO_2$ (using tidal volume below 6 ml/kg) improves survival in patients with ARDS and increases the number of days without ventilator use [54].

In selected cases, alveolar recruitment maneuvers and placement of the patient in prone position as rescue adjunctive therapy have been tested. These two maneuvers are used for alveolar reopening of collapsed areas of lung, but there is no conclusive evidence that they increase survival.

36.5.5 Antibiotic Treatment

Usually, antibiotic treatment is started empirically, trying to cover the most frequent microorganisms and taking into account the risk factors for specific microorganisms.

Patients who require hospitalization in the ICU with unknown etiology should be treated with combination therapy [55, 56]. This therapy should include a β-lactam and a macrolide. The goal of combination therapy in ICU patients is to provide optimal coverage for the two most commonly identified causes of lethal pneumonia – *S. pneumoniae* and *Legionella* species. For patients with hypersensitivity to β-lactams, clindamycin and fluoroquinolone antibiotics are recommended. Though based on retrospective and observational data [57–59], there is substantial evidence to support combination antibiotic therapy, at least in patients with severe bacteremic pneumococcal pneumonia. A recent study demonstrated an association for patients hospitalized with severe CAP between the empiric use of a β-lactam plus a fluoroquinolone and increased 30-day mortality [24]. A number of possible explanations for the benefit of macrolides observed by retrospective

Group	Antimicrobial agent	MIC (µg/ml) Interpretative standards		
		S	I	R
Penicillins	Penicillin	≤0.06	0.12–1	2
	Amoxicillin	≤2	4	≥8
	Amoxicillin-clavulanate	≤2/1	4/2	≥8/4
Cephalosporins (parenteral)	Cefuroxime	≤0.5	1	≥2
	Cefotaxime or ceftriaxone	≤1	2	≥4
	Cefepime	≤1	2	≥4
Cephalosporins (oral)	Cefuroxime axetil	≤1	2	≥4
	Cefaclor	≤1	2	≥4
Carbapenems	Imipenem	≤0.12	0.25–0.5	≥1
	Meropenem	≤0.25	0.5	≥1
Glycopeptides	Vancomycin	≤1	–	–
Macrolides	Erythromycin/clarithromycin	≤0.25	0.5	≥1
	Azithromycin	≤0.5	1	≥2
Fluoroquinolones	Levofloxacin	≤2	4	≥8
	Moxifloxacin/gatifloxacin	≤1	2	≥4
	Grepafloxacin/sparfloxacin	≤0.5	1	≥2
Lincosamides	Clindamycin	≤0.25	0.5	≥1

Table 36.3. MIC interpretative standards (in µg/ml) for non-meningeal pneumococcal infections according to the 2002 breakpoints [40]

studies have been put forward, including antibiotic synergy, coverage of unrecognized atypical pathogens, and immunomodulatory effects [57]. There is also some evidence that third-generation cephalosporins may be superior to penicillins as the non-macrolide component of combination therapy [60]. Cefotaxime, ceftriaxone, or amoxicillin/clavulanate are the preferred agents for pneumococcal pneumonia. Several studies found a significant association between mortality and strains with a cefotaxime MIC of 2.0 µg/ml or greater when underlying conditions were controlled for. In view of the results of this study, and following the recommendations of a panel of CDC experts, the Clinical Laboratory Standard Institute (formerly the NCCLS) raised the breakpoints for cefotaxime, ceftriaxone and amoxicillin in non-meningeal infections (Table 36.3) [61, 62].

Optimal therapy against *Legionella* infection is based on agents with high intrinsic activity and an appropriate pharmacokinetic and pharmacodynamic profile (including the ability to penetrate phagocytic cells) [26, 27]. New macroazolides and fluoroquinolones are among the first-line therapies. In severe infections, particularly those occurring in immunocompromised patients, azithromycin and later fluoroquinolones are the agents of choice.

Severe structural lung diseases, recent antibiotic therapy and recent hospitalization have been classically considered as risk factors for *Pseudomonas aeruginosa* infection [1, 10–12]. Recently, COPD, malignancy, and rapid X-ray spread were associated with severe *Pseudomonas* pneumonia [9]. Previously, in a group of patients who underwent intubation, *P. aeruginosa* was the third most frequent responsible pathogen [20]. These findings suggest that due to its high mortality rate *P. aeruginosa* should be covered in the empiric therapy of all intubated patients (especially patients with COPD, malignancy, previous antibiotic therapy or rapid X-ray spread) while awaiting bacteriology results. If *P. aeruginosa* is an issue, the recommendation is to use two antipseudomonal agents that also provide coverage for drug-resistant *Streptococcus pneumoniae* (DRSP) and *Legionella* species: an antipseudomonal agent plus ciprofloxacin, or an antipseudomonal agent plus an aminoglycoside plus a respiratory fluoroquinolone or a macrolide are recommended [1, 10–12].

Treatment options should be simplified if an etiologic diagnosis is established or highly suspected on the basis of rapid test results.

36.6 Assessment of a Nonresponding Patient

Evolution of patients with CAP within the first 2–5 days is crucial. Few data are available regarding patients who fail to respond and whose condition deteriorates after hospitalization for CAP, or regarding the impact of antibiotic resistance in respiratory pathogens on outcome.

Febrile curve, hemodynamic and respiratory failure resolution, serum concentrations of CRP (C-reactive protein), white blood cell count resolution, and chest X-ray evolution are the variables used to classify clinical response in patients with CAP [63–64]. Age and comorbid conditions have a strong influence on the course of illness [65–73]. However, when patients fail to respond or their condition deteriorates after initiation of empiric therapy, a number of possibilities should be considered. Incorrect diagnosis may be responsible for this failure: congestive heart failure, pulmonary embolus, atelectasis, sarcoidosis, neoplasms, radiation pneumonitis, pulmonary drug reactions, vasculitis, ARDS, pulmonary hemorrhage, and inflammatory lung disease. If a correct diagnosis has been made but the patient fails to respond, the physician should consider each component of the host-drug-pathogen triad. Inadequate host-pathogen responses are responsible for most treatment failures: age, multiple coexisting illnesses, severity of disease, multilobar pneumonia, bacteremia, and complications of pneumonia (metastatic infections and non-infectious extrapulmonary complications) [1, 10]. Inadequate therapy is a less frequent cause of failure, and can be prevented by rational application of the current antibiotic guidelines [1, 9–10, 63]. An additional consideration is that the patient may have CAP caused by an opportunistic organism (tuberculosis, *Nocardia* sp., *P. jiroveci*). Prevention of potential failures and early identification and treatment of their causes may improve patients' outcome [63]. When a patient fails to respond to initial empiric therapy specific tests should be considered. CT scanning and bronchoscopy may be of help, and open lung biopsy may be necessary.

Acknowledgements. Supported in part by FISS (PI04/1500) and FISS (PI05/2410).

References

1. Bartlett JG, Dowell SF, Mandell LA, File TM, Musher DM, Fine MJ (2000) Practice guidelines for the management of community-acquired pneumonia in adults. Guidelines from the Infectious Diseases Society of America. Clin Infect Dis 31:347–82
2. Hirani NA, Macfarlane JT (1997) Impact of management guidelines on the outcome of severe community acquired pneumonia. Thorax 52:17–21
3. Pachón J, Prado MD, Capote F, Cuello JA, Garnacho J, Verano A (1990) Severe community acquired pneumonia. Etiology, prognosis and treatment. Am Rev Respir Dis 142:369–373
4. Torres A, Serra-Batlles J, Ferrer A, Jiménez P, Celis R, Cobo E, et al. (1991) Severe community acquired pneumonia. Epidemiology and prognostic factors. Am Rev Respir Dis 114:312–318
5. Rello J, Quintana E, Ausina V, Net A, Prats G (1993) A three-year study of severe community acquired pneumonia with emphasis in outcome. Chest 103:232–235
6. Moine P, Vercken JB, Chevret S, Chastang C, Gajdos P, and the French Study Group for Community-Acquired Pneumonia in Intensive Care Unit (1994) Severe community-acquired pneumonia. Etiology, epidemiology and prognosis factors. Chest 105:1487–1495
7. Leroy O, Santré C, Beuscart C, Georges H, Guery B, Jacquier JM, et al. (1995) A five-year study of severe community-acquired pneumonia with emphasis on prognosis in patients admitted to an intensive care unit. Intensive Care Med 21:24–31
8. Rello J, Rodriguez R, Jubert P, Alvarez B and the Study Group of Severe Community-Acquired Pneumonia (1996) Severe community-acquired pneumonia in the elderly: epidemiology and prognosis. Clin Infect Dis 23:723–8
9. Bodí M, Rodríguez A, Solé-Violan J, Gilavert MC, Garnacho J, Blanquer J, et al., for the Community-Acquired Pneumonia Intensive Care Units (CAPUCI) Study Investigators (2005) Antibiotic prescription for community-acquired pneumonia in the intensive care unit: impact of adherence to Infectious Diseases Society of America guidelines on survival. Clin Infect Dis 41:1709–16
10. American Thoracic Society (1993) Guidelines for the initial management of adults with community-acquired pneumonia: Diagnosis, assessment of severity and initial antimicrobial therapy. Am Rev Respir Dis 148:1418–1426
11. American Thoracic Society (2001) Guidelines for the management of adults with community-acquired pneumonia. Diagnosis, assessment of severity, antimicrobial therapy, and prevention. Am J Respir Crit Care Med 163:1730–54
12. Mandell LA, Bartlett JG, Dowell SF, File TM, Musher DM, Whitney C (2003) Updated of practice guidelines for the management of community-acquired pneumonia in immunocompetent adults. Clin Infect Dis 37:1405–33
13. European Study on Community-Acquired Pneumonia (ESOCAP) Committee (1998) Guidelines for management of adult community-acquired lower respiratory tract infections. Eur Respir J 11:986
14. British Thoracic Society (2001) BTS guidelines for the management of community-acquired pneumonia in adults. Thorax 56:iv1–iv64
15. Torres A, El-Ebiary M, Zavala E, Hernández C (1996) Severe community-acquired pneumonia. Semin Resp Crit Care Med 17:265–271
16. Vallés J (1998) Severe pneumonia: sources of infection and implications for prevention. Sepsis 1:199–209
17. Fine MJ, Auble TE, Yealy DM, Hanusa BH, Weissfeld LA, Singer DE (1997) A predictive rule to identify low risk patients with community-acquired pneumonia. N Engl J Med 336:243–50
18. Research Committee of the British Thoracic Society and the Public Health Laboratory Service (1987) Community acquired pneumonia in adults in British hospitals in 1982–83: a survey of aetiology, mortality, prognostic factors and outcome. Q J Med 62:195–220
19. Lim WS, van der Eerden MM, Boersma WG, Karalus N, Town GI, Lewis SA, et al. (2003) Defining community-acquired pneumonia severity on presentation to hospital: an international derivation and validation study. Thorax 58:377–382
20. Rello J, Bodí M, Mariscal D, Navarro M, Díaz E, Gallego M, Vallés J (2003) Microbiological testing and outcome of patients with severe community-acquired pneumonia. Chest 123:174–80
21. Marik PE (2000) The clinical features of severe community-acquired pneumonia presenting as septic shock. J Crit Care 15:85–90
22. El-Sohl AA, Sikka P, Ramadan F, Davies J (2001) Etiology of severe community-acquired pneumonia in the very elderly. Am J Respir Crit Care Med 163:645–51
23. Angus DC, Marrie TJ, Obrosky DS, Clermont G, Dremsizov TT, Coley C, et al. (2002) Severe community-acquired pneumonia. Use of intensive care services and evaluation of American and British Thoracic Society diagnostic criteria. Am J Respir Crit Care Med 166:717–23
24. Mortensen EM, Restrepo MI, Anzueto A, Pugh J (2006) The impact of empiric antimicrobial therapy with a β-lactam and fluoroquinolone on mortality for patients hospitalized with severe pneumonia. Crit Care 10:R8

25. Grau I, Pallarés R (1998) Neumonía neumocócica. En Infecciones Graves. Implicaciones terapeúticas de la Neumonía Extrahospitalaria Grave. Ed Edika Med 1:17–33
26. Roig J, Rello J (2003) Legionnaires' disease: a rational approach to therapy. J Antimicrob Chemother 51:1119–29
27. Sabrià M, Pedro-Botet ML, Gómez J, Roig J, Vilaseca B, Sopena N, et al. (2005) Fluoroquinolones vs macrolides in the treatment of Legionnaire's disease. Chest 128:1401–5
28. El-Ebiary M, Sarmiento X, Torres A, Nogué S, Mesalles E, Bodí M, et al. (1997) Prognostic factors of severe *Legionella* pneumonia requiring admission to ICU. Am J Respir Crit Care Med 156:1467–1472
29. Kollef MH, Micek ST (2006) Methicillin-resistant *Staphylococcus aureus:* a new community-acquired pathogen? Curr Opin Infect Dis 19:161–8
30. Menéndez R, Córdoba J, de la Cuadra P, Cremades MJ, López-Hontagas JL, Salavert M, et al. (1999) Value of the polymerase chain reaction assay in noninvasive respiratory samples for diagnosis of community-acquired pneumonia. Am J Respir Crit Care Med 159:1868–1873
31. Leeper KV, Torres A (1995) Community-acquired pneumonia in the intensive care unit. Clin Chest Med 16: 155–171
32. Vanders Els NJ, Stover DE (1996) Approach to the patient with pulmonary disease. Clin Chest Med 17:767–785
33. Ewig S, Torres A (1999) Severe community-acquired pneumonia. Clin Chest Med 20:575–87
34. Waterer GW, Wunderink RG (2001) The influence of the severity of community-acquired pneumonia on the usefulness of blood cultures. Respir Med 95:78–82
35. Barlett JG, Breiman RF, Mandell LA, File TM (1998) Community-acquired pneumonia in adults: Guidelines for management. Clin Infect Dis 26:811–838
36. Domínguez J, Gali N, Pedroso P, Hernández A, Matas L, Manterola, et al. (1999) Evaluación del Binax now™ Legionella urinary antigen test para la detección del antígeno de *Legionella* en muestras de orina. Estudio preliminar [abstract]. Arch Bronconeumol 35(2):46
37. Antonelli M, Conti G, Riccioni L, Meduri U (1996) Noninvasive positive-pressure ventilation via face mask during bronchoscopy with BAL in high-risk hypoxemic patients. Chest 110:724–728
38. Garnacho-Montero J, García-Garmendia JL, Barrero-Almodovar Ana, Jiménez-Jiménez FJ, Perez-Paredes C, Ortiz-Leyba C (2003) Impact of adequate empirical antibiotic therapy on the outcome of patients admitted to the intensive care unit with sepsis. Crit Care Med 31:2742–51
39. Rello J, Rodríguez A, Torres A, Roig J, Solé-Violan J, Garnacho-Montero J, et al., for the CAPUCI study investigators (2006) Implications on COPD in patients admitted to the ICU by community-acquired pneumonia. A comparison with a cohort of non-COPD patients. Eur Respir J 27:1210–1216
40. Menéndez R, Ferrando D, Vallés JM, Vallterra J (2002) Influence of deviation from guidelines on the outcome of community-acquired pneumonia. Chest 122:612–17
41. Marras TK, Chan CK (1998) Use of guidelines in treating community-acquired pneumonia. Chest 113:1689–94
42. Mortensen EM, Restrepo M, Anzueto A, Pugh J (2004) Effects of guideline-concordant antimicrobial therapy on mortality among patients with community-acquired pneumonia. Am J Med 117:726–31
43. Shorr AF, Bodí M, Rodríguez A, Solé-Violan J, Garnacho-Montero J, Rello J, for CAPUCI study investigators (2006). Impact of antibiotic guideline compliance on duration of mechanical ventilation in critically ill patients with community-acquired pneumonia. Chest 130:93–100
44. Houck PM, Bratzler DW, Nsa W, Ma A, Bartlett JG (2004) Timing of antibiotic administration and outcomes for medicare patients hospitalized with community-acquired pneumonia. Arch Intern Med 164:637–44
45. Battleman DS, Callahan M, Thaler HT (2002) Rapid antibiotic delivery and appropriate antibiotic selection reduce length of hospital stay of patients with community-acquired pneumonia. Link between quality of care and resource utilization. Arch Intern Med 162:682–8
46. Vincent JL (2001) Hemodynamic support in septic shock. Intensive Care Med 27:S80–S92
47. Vidaur L, Rodríguez A, Rello J (2004) ATB therapy for sepsis, severe sepsis and septic shock. A patient based approach inspired on "The Tarragona Strategy". In: Yearbook of intensive care and emergency medicine. Springer, Berlin Heidelberg New York
48. Monton C, Torres A, El-Ebiary M, Filella X, Xaubet A, de la Bellacasa JP (1999) Cytokine expression in severe pneumonia: a bronchoalveolar lavage study. Crit Care Med 27:1745–53
49. Confalonieri M, Urbino R, Potena A, Piattella M, Parigi P, Puccio G, et al. (2005) Hydrocortisone infusion for severe community-acquired pneumonia: a preliminary randomized study. Am J Respir Crit Care Med 171:242–8
50. Dhainaut JF, Laterre PF, LaRosa SP, Levy H, Garber GE, Heiselman D, et al. (2003) The clinical evaluation committee in a large multicenter phase 3 trial of drotrecogin alfa (activated) in patients with severe sepsis (PROWESS): Role, methodology, and results. Crit Care Med 31:2291–2301
51. Laterre PF, Garber G, Levy H, Wunderink R, Kinasewitz GT, Sollet JP, et al. (2005) Severe community-acquired pneumonia as a cause of severe sepsis: Data from the PROWESS study. Crit Care Med 33:952–961
52. Confalonieri M, Potena A, Carbone G, Della Porta R, Tolley EA, Meduri GU (1999) Acute respiratory failure in patients with severe community-acquired pneumonia. A prospective randomized evaluation of noninvasive ventilation. Am J Respir Crit Care 160:1585–1591
53. Antonelli M, Conti G, Rocco M, Bufi M, De Blasi RA, Vivino G, et al. (1998) A comparison of noninvasive positive-pressure ventilation and conventional mechanical ventilation in patients with acute respiratory failure. N Engl J Med 339:429–435
54. The Acute Respiratory Distress Syndrome Network (2000) Ventilation with lower tidal volumes as compared with traditional tidal volumes for acute lung injury and the acute respiratory distress syndrome. N Engl J Med 342:1301–8
55. Waterer GW (2003) Combination antibiotic therapy with macrolides in community-acquired pneumonia. More smoke but is there any fire? Chest 123:1328–9
56. Waterer GW, Rello J (2006) Choosing the right combination therapy in severe community-acquired pneumonia. Crit Care 10:115
57. Waterer GW, Somes GW, Wunderink RG (2001) Monotherapy may be suboptimal for severe bacteremic pneumococcal pneumonia. Arch Intern Med 161:1837–42
58. Martínez JA, Horcajada JP, Almela M, Almela M, Marco F, Soriano A, et al. (2003) Addition of a macrolide to a beta-lactam based empirical antibiotic regimen is associated with lower in-hospital mortality for patients with bacteremic pneumococcal pneumonia. Clin Infect Dis 36:389–395
59. Baddour LM, Yu VL, Klugman KP, Feldman C, Ortqvist A, Rello J, et al. (2004) International Pneumococcal Study Group. Combination antibiotic therapy lowers mortality among severely ill patients with pneumococcal bacteremia. Am J Respir Crit Care Med 170:440–4
60. Brown RB, Iannini P, Gross P, Kunkel M (2003) Impact of antibiotic choice on clinical outcomes in community-acquired pneumonia. Chest 123:1503–11

61. National Committee for Clinical Laboratory Standards (2002) Performance standards for antimicrobial susceptibility testing. Twelfth informational supplement. Document M100-S12. National Committee for Clinical Laboratory Standards, Wayne, PA
62. Lujan M, Gallego M, Rello J (2006) Optimal therapy for severe pneumococcal community-acquired pneumonia. Intensive Care Med 32:971–980
63. Roson B, Carratalà J, Fernández-Sabé N, Tubau F, Manresa F, Gudiol F (2004) Causes and factors associated with early failure in hospitalized patients with community acquired pneumonia. Arch Intern Med 164:502–508
64. Almirall J, Bolíbar I, Toran P, Pera G, Boquet X, Balanzó X, et al. for The Community-Acquired Pneumonia Maresme Study Group (2004) Contribution of C-reactive protein to the diagnosis and assessment of severity of community-acquired pneumonia. Chest 125:1335–42
65. Mufson MA, Oley G, Hughey D (1982) Pneumococcal disease in a medium-sized community in the United States. JAMA 248:1486–1489
66. Marrie TJ (1990) Epidemiology of community-acquired pneumonia in the elderly. Semin Respir Infect 5:260–8
67. Riquelme R, Torres A, El-Ebiary M, Puig de la Bellacasa J, Estruch R, Mensa J, et al. (1996) Community-acquired pneumonia in the elderly. A multivariate analysis of risk and prognostic factors. Am J Respir Crit Care Med 154:1450–5
68. Almirall J, Morató I, Riera A, Verdaguer A, Priu R, Coll P, et al. (1993) Incidence of community-acquired pneumonia and *Chlamydia pneumoniae* infection: a prospective multicenter study. Eur Respir J 6:14–18
69. Lange P, Vestbo J, Nyboe J (1995) Risk factors for death and hospitalization from pneumonia. A prospective study of a general population. Eur Respir J 8:1694–1698
70. Torres A, Dorca J, Zalacaín R, Bello S, El-Ebiary M, Molinos L, et al. (1996) Community-acquired pneumonia in chronic obstructive pulmonary disease. A Spanish Multicenter Study. Am J Respir Crit Care Med 154:1456–1461
71. Seneff MG, Wagner DP, Wagner RD, Zimmerman JE, Knaus WA (1995) Hospital and 1-year survival of patients admitted to intensive care units with acute exacerbation of chronic obstructive pulmonary disease. JAMA 274:1852–1857
72. Almirall J, Mesalles E, Klamburg J, Parra O, Agudo A (1995) Prognostic factors of pneumonia requiring admission to the intensive care unit. Chest 107:511–516
73. Mundy LM, Auwaerter PG, Oldach D, Warner ML, Burton A, Vance E, et al. (1995) Community-acquired pneumonia: Impact of immune status. Am J Respir Crit Care Med 152:1309–1315

37 Legionnaires' Disease

J. Roig, M. Sabria, X. Castella

37.1 Epidemiology

37.1.1 Prevalence and Incidence in the Community and Hospital Setting

The incidence of legionnaires' disease (LD) seems to increase with age, particularly in males [36]. It was considered an infrequent cause of pneumonia in the past, but it currently ranks second to pneumococcus in the list of etiologic agents of severe community-acquired pneumonia (CAP) of bacterial origin [2, 24, 60, 89]. Considering less severe cases, in a series of 145 pneumonias in which BCYE culture, serology and the *Legionella* urinary antigen (LUA) test were systematically applied, Vergis et al. [91] reported a prevalence of LD of 13.7%. In another series of 392 adult patients with CAP treated in a university hospital, Sopena et al. found a prevalence of 12.5%, and LD was the second cause of pneumonia [83].

The incidence of LD is most likely underestimated. The number of *Legionella* spp. progressively identified as a cause of severe pneumonia is increasing and most of these species are not detected by routine laboratory tests. *Legionella waltersii* is the last *Legionella* species associated with severe pneumonia [43]. Although LD tends to occur more frequently during summertime, it seems that wet, humid weather is significantly associated with the acute appearance of this disease [27]. Although the expected rate of legionellosis in the USA ranges from 8,000 to 18,000 cases yearly [53], the mean number of cases reported to the Center for Diseases Control (CDC) from 1980 to 1998 was 360 per year [5]. According to the European Working Group for *Legionella* Infections (EWGLI), the number of cases in the European dataset provided by more than 30 countries increased from 1,255 in 1995 (annual incidence rate of 3.7 per million population) to 4,588 in 2004 (annual incidence rate of 10.1 per million population) [69]. However, in some eastern European countries, this incidence continued to be below 1 case per one million inhabitants [40]. Reporting *Legionella* infection is not mandatory in many European countries and in some geographic areas, especially those with a more depressed economy, LUA is not usually ordered in most cases of CAP.

Legionella infection has also been considered a rare cause of hospital-acquired pneumonia (HAP). However, the majority of published studies have been conducted in the ICU setting or only in mechanically ventilated patients. ICUs are usually well delimited areas with a relatively small number of patients who are not usually exposed to aerosols (showers, hot tap water). That is why LD has rarely been detected in ICUs with the only exception of those cases associated with the use of contaminated water in nasogastric tubes or mechanical ventilation equipment [11].

Legionella infection has been increasingly recognized as a cause of HAP, especially in non-ICU areas. Environmental studies have demonstrated that colonization of the potable water distribution is a common feature in many hospitals [76]. When the water supply of a hospital is known to be colonized by *Legionella*, the index of suspicion of infection by *Legionella* rises and appropriate testing is then systematically ordered. Consequently, sporadic cases of LD and nosocomial outbreaks are then more frequently reported and even historical cases, previously unrecognized, are retrospectively identified. [44, 47]. Everts et al. reported a series of HAP in which *Legionella* was the most frequent cause of nosocomial pneumonia [22]. In a multicenter study performed in 12 Spanish University hospitals, with active surveillance of HAP in non-ventilated patients and systematic use of LUA test, *L. pneumophila* was diagnosed in seven patients in five different hospitals not in an outbreak setting [78]. In one hospital, it was the first case of nosocomial legionellosis diagnosed in that center [85]. Diagnosis of *Legionella* should be considered in any case of HAP in a hospital with water distribution known to be colonized by these microorganisms [77].

37.1.2 Sources of Infection

Cooling towers and health spas continue to be the most frequently reported sources of infection in community outbreaks of LD [6, 18, 30, 31]. Potable water has been the environmental source of almost all reported hospital outbreaks [77]. However, potable water should not be neglected as a potential source of infection both in sporadic cases and small clusters detected in the community [62]. Moreover, cases of LD in newborns, most likely caused by aspiration of bath water, have also been reported [80].

37.1.3 Mode of Transmission

The most commonly accepted mechanism of transmission of *Legionella* in humans is inhalation of contaminated aerosols. However, aspiration of contaminated water could also be a major mode of transmission, especially in hospital-acquired legionellosis [77]. In a prospective study of patients with head and neck cancer undergoing tumor resection with postoperative sequelae of aspiration, 30% of postoperative pneumonias were due to *L. pneumophila* [39]. Surprisingly, several studies have failed to show a link between showering and risk of infection [23, 26, 44, 81]. Others have even reported that showering could be protective for legionnaires' disease [7]. The presumed reason for this paradoxical finding is that patients who are able to take showers are ambulatory and less likely to aspirate [77]. Nasogastric tubes [52, 90] have been linked to hospital-acquired legionellosis in several studies; the authors presumed that microaspiration of contaminated water was the cause of infection.

37.1.4 Risk Factors

In most cases of CAP caused by *Legionella,* classical risk factors such as travel or hotel accommodation are not identified. Smoking habit is, by far, the most consistently reported risk factor in most series. Underlying diseases are a major risk factor for the acquisition of *Legionella* pneumonia, especially in the hospital setting. Since aspiration is increasingly recognized as a mode of transmission, patients with swallowing disorders or those who undergo surgery requiring general anesthesia are at greater risk. The single most important factor is organ transplant. Among organ receptors heart transplants show the highest incidence and bone marrow transplants the lowest one [54, 68]. Steroid administration is an independent risk factor [44, 47]. Other forms of immunocompromise may also predispose to LD [48]. Paradoxically, AIDS patients do not appear to be at increased risk for hospital-acquired legionnaires' disease [63].

37.2 Clinical Features

The non-specific clinical data of LD cannot usually be distinguished from those found in typical bacterial pneumonia caused by other aerobic microorganisms. Initial retrospective series suggested that clinical findings such as diarrhea or central nervous system symptoms were so frequent in legionellosis that they could be considered as highly suggestive of LD [41]. Later studies have already emphasized the lack of usefulness of those allegedly distinctive clinical data [25, 70]. Prospective, randomized, comparative studies between CAP and HAP caused by *Legionella* and those caused by other bacterial etiologies have shown that there is a marked overlap between clinical, radiological and analytical signs [35, 51, 70, 92, 93]. Serum levels of inflammatory markers, such as C-reactive protein, procalcitonin and neopterin, are often high in LD [1, 28, 65]. However, the clinical or therapeutic implications of this analytical finding remain obscure. The uncertainty in clinical differential diagnosis of CAP and HAP, as well as the potential severity of LD, supports the choice of an antibiotic that is also effective against *Legionella* in the initial therapeutic approach of most instances of hospitalized CAP and at least in suspicious epidemiological situations in the case of HAP.

In some cases of Pontiac fever, usually a flu-like benign illness, shortness of breath and an abnormal oxygen saturation have been reported [13]. In the population with advanced emphysema or sevre immunocompromise that present with fever of unknown origin, a normal chest X-ray does not completely rule out pneumonia [12, 66], including that caused by *Legionella* spp. (personal observation). In this group of patients, computed tomography of the chest is recommended since an early diagnosis and therapy of radiologically unsuspected pneumonia are favorable prognostic factors.

37.3 Diagnosis

Definitive diagnosis of LD is established by recovery of the microorganism from respiratory secretions on BCYE. The selective medium recommended is BCYE-alpha supplemented with polymyxin B, anisomycin, vancomycin and dyes (PAV). To optimize the recovery of *Legionella* some authors recommend the use of two more media: BCYE media, PAV and BCYE supplemented with polymyxin, anisomycin, cefamandole and dyes (PAC) [87]. The addition of dyes facilitates the visualization of the colonies, making identification of *L. micdadei* and *L. maceachernii* easier. Pretreatment of sputum with acid is necessary to reduce the overgrowth of other bacteria. Vancomycin containing medium is preferred when *L. micdadei* is an issue since cefamandole inhibits this species [57]. The quality of sputum does not necessarily correlate with recovery of *Legionella*. This microorganism has been recovered from so-called inadequate specimens for culture (few polymorphonuclear leukocytes and numerous epithelial cells). Culture of respiratory samples continues to be the most valid diagnostic method and should be mandatory in all centers. The isolation of *Legionella* allows its microbiologic classification and subtyping by DNA studies. Molecular typing is crucial to establish an epidemiological link between environmental and clinical isolates.

Direct fluorescent antibody (DFA) is a rapid test for diagnosing LD, with results available within a few hours. DFA allows direct visualization of *Legionella*. Monoclonal antibodies against *L. pneumophila* are used in the DFA test. The sensitivity of this test is low (30–70%) due to the large respiratory inocula required. Thus, in severe pneumonia with large infiltrates, DFA is often positive. The test should always be performed by an experienced technician.

Diagnosis by serology requires a fourfold rise in antibody titers from 1 to 128 in acute and convalescent sera. A single titer of 1:256 is not, at present, considered specific enough for diagnosing LD [64]. It should not be used as criteria of definitive diagnosis of LD. Convalescent sera should be obtained at 4–6 weeks after presentation of the disease. It should be taken into account that antibody response may be delayed as long as 3 months after onset of the illness. A lack of antibody response has been observed by some authors [15]. Serology is a useful tool for epidemiological studies but it is clearly unhelpful in the acute setting.

The detection of the *Legionella* urinary antigen is a very useful technique to diagnose LD. The urinary antigen is detected very early during the course of the disease and usually disappears within 2 months, although its excretion may be longer, particularly in patients receiving immunosuppressive or steroid treatment [84].

The main limitation of the urinary antigen is that it only detects the soluble antigen of *L. pneumophila* serogroup 1. However, its usefulness is reinforced by the fact that this serogroup causes at least 80% of cases of LD [94]. Several kits are currently available for determining *Legionella* urinary antigen: Binax (*Legionella* Urinary Antigen, Binax, Portland, USA), Biotest (Biotest AG, Dreieich, Germany) and Bartels (Bartels EIA *Legionella* Urinary Antigen, Intracel, Issaquah, Washington USA). Some authors have observed an increase in the sensitivity of the test, without any decrease in specificity, if urine is concentrated [17].

A rapid immunochromatographic assay has been developed by Binax (Binax Now *Legionella* Urinary Antigen, Portland USA) to detect *L. pneumophila* serogroup 1 antigen in urine. This test has shown to be useful as a method of rapid screening in both sporadic cases and outbreaks. The sensitivity and specificity of this test are similar to those reported with ELISA. This test considerably reduces the time required for detecting *Legionella* urinary antigen with ELISA assays. It is particularly useful for small laboratories without the specialized equipment required to use ELISA or when the number of samples to be tested is small.

Some authors have suggested that, in the outbreak setting, the sensitivity of urinary antigen test is related to the degree of severity on clinical presentation [8]. However, the reported low mortality of this series (<4%) raises some concern about the actual clinical relevance of this study.

DNA amplification by polymerase chain reaction (PCR) of *Legionella* has been tested in several specimens from patients with pneumonia [58]. A rapid real-time PCR assay for *L. pneumophila* is now commercially available (BD Probe-Tec, BD Diagnostics, Sparks, Maryland, USA) [67]. However, clinical experience with the use of PCR techniques is still very limited. Although the number of cases of LD that are diagnosed exclusively on the basis of PCR testing is increasing, controlled studied are needed to establish the clinical usefulness of this technique [32, 42, 55].

37.4 Treatment

In vitro susceptibility studies do not correlate with clinical efficacy since *Legionella* is an intracellular pathogen. Treatment guidelines are supported by data obtained from in vitro studies, experimental studies with the animal model, and observational studies, some of which come from prospective clinical studies in CAP. Optimal therapy against *Legionella* infection is based on agents with high intrinsic activity, an appropriate pharmacokinetic and pharmacodynamic profile, including the ability to penetrate phagocytic cells, a low incidence of adverse reactions and an advantageous cost-efficacy relationship.

Retrospective information from the first studies of LD provided very useful clues of which antibiotics were really clinically effective [16]. It became evident that erythromycin treated patients showed the lowest mortality rate (6%) while those cases that were treated with aminoglycosides, beta-lactamic antibiotics or chloramphenicol showed a 30–40% fatality rate.

Since then, a number of clinical studies have proven that erythromycin is highly effective against *Legionella*, and until some years ago it was considered the treatment of choice. In fact, a series published in 2003 confirms that it continues to be an effective agent [37]. Route, dose and length of administration of erythromycin are critical factors in obtaining a maximum effectiveness. The recommended optimal dosing of 1 g IV

Table 37.1. Recommended therapy in legionnaires' disease[a]

Antimicrobial agents		Dosage	Route
Macro-azalides[b]	Azithromycin[d] Clarithromycin Erythromycin[c]	500 mg every 24 h 500 mg every 12 h 1 g every 6–8 h	IV, p.o. IV, p.o. IV, p.o.
Tetracyclines	Doxycycline	100 mg every 12–24 h	IV, p.o.
Fluoroquinolones	Levofloxacin[d] Moxifloxacin[d] Gemifloxacin[e] Gatifloxacin[e] Ciprofloxacin Ofloxacin	500–750 mg every 24 h 400 mg every 24 h 320 mg every 24 h 200–400 mg every 24 h 400 mg every 8–12 h 500–750 mg every 12 h 400–800 mg (total daily dose)	IV, p.o. IV, p.o. p.o. IV, p.o. IV p.o. IV, p.o.
Ketolides	Telithromycin[e]	800 mg every 24 h	p.o.

[a] Oral therapy is recommended only in those mild cases that do not require hospitalization. Some antibiotics are only commercially available in selected countries

[b] In mild cases other oral macrolides are also effective: josamycin (1 g every 12 h), roxithromycin (150 mg every 12 h), dirithromycin (500 mg every 24 h)

[c] Less active than other macrolides; risk of fluid overload, phlebitis and transitory deafness with IV administration

[d] Recommended in the more severe cases, particularly in the immunocompromised

[e] Because of short accumulated clinical experience their use is recommended only in mild to moderate cases

every 6 h is associated with some side effects [72], such as risk of fluid overload and transitory deafness.

Other more recent macrolides share with erythromycin the ability to penetrate phagocytic cells with the advantage of showing an overall better intrinsic activity against *Legionella*. Besides this superior in vitro activity against *Legionella*, they offer pharmacokinetic and pharmacodynamic advantages. Relatively minor differences in the in vitro activity among the new macrolides have also been found in different comparative studies [3]. Consequently, the treatment of choice has changed from erythromycin to the newer macrolides and fluoroquinolones (Table 37.1). Recent studies [9, 59, 79], which unfortunately show many limitations because of methodological drawbacks [46], suggest that in terms of mortality and complications both macrolides and fluoroquinolones are equivalent for most cases of LD that require hospitalization. At least in experimental studies, monotherapy with rifampicin has been associated with a rapid development of resistance.

Duration of therapy has to be decided on an individualized basis.

Combined therapy is recommended for severe episodes by some international guidelines, but there is no evidence supporting this suggestion. For most patients monotherapy with a macrolide or a selected fluoroquinolone usually leads to a more cost-effective outcome [20, 21, 73, 74].

Recent data from a Spanish multi-center severe CAP study [10] suggest that in the subset of patients with most severe legionnaires' disease [74], the majority of them under mechanical ventilation, combined therapy is most likely associated with a better outcome when compared to monotherapy. The most frequently used combined therapy in this study was clarithromycin associated with rifampicin. It is not clear which combined antibiotic approach is preferable although rifampicin is the most commonly used agent in combination therapy. Given that the risk of transient liver toxicity (hyperbilirubinemia) related to rifampicin therapy seems to increase with the length of treatment, we recommend using it for just a few days [38].

Additional toxicities of combining more than one antibiotic should be taken into account, particularly in the intensive care unit setting.

Rifampicin appears to add little to the activity of the more active drugs in cell models of infection but, at least in guinea pigs, it seems to be beneficial in combination with erythromycin, and probably clarithromycin. The combination of erythromycin and rifampicin has been reported to be more active against *L. pneumophila* than other options such as combining erythromycin and ciprofloxacin or rifampicin and ciprofloxacin [56]. In guinea pigs the addition of rifampicin causes a higher rate of bacterial killing, a decrease in the extent of pneumonia, and a lower mortality rate [19, 33].

Respiratory failure, particularly when adult respiratory distress syndrome (ARDS) is present, is a major cause of fatality [4, 29, 73]. In patients that require mechanical ventilation, the goal is to improve gas interchange and avoid causing ventilatory-induced lung injury, maintaining plateau pressures under 25. A strategy of ventilation using low tidal volumes (<7 ml/kg) is recommended to protect the lung in acute lung injury. Patients with LD and ARDS may most likely benefit from this approach. FiO_2 should be minimized to target an acceptable SaO_2 up to 90%. Recruitment maneuvers may prevent alveolar collapse and improve oxygenation. Ventilating patients in the prone position may be used as rescue therapy for the most severe episodes. Preliminary studies in the animal model have raised some concern about the risk of hyperoxia in severe legionellosis. Extra-corporeal membrane oxygenation (ECMO) has been anecdotally reported as a successful therapeutic option in treating severe *Legionella*-associated ARDS. Since many patients may recover, even without sequelae, after many days of mechanical ventilation, an aggressive approach is mandatory whenever respiratory failure appears.

Shock and acute renal failure are both associated with a high risk of death [29, 72, 73]. Hemodynamic

Table 37.2. Extrapulmonary manifestations of legionnaires' disease

Cardiovascular	Pericarditis, myocarditis,[a] endocarditis, aortic graft involvement
Neurological	Encephalitis that may mimic that caused by herpes, brain abscess, cerebellar ataxia,[a] corpus callosum involvement
Digestive	Colon involvement that may mimic ulcerative colitis, pancreatitis, digestive tract abscess, liver involvement, spleen rupture, severe diarrhea[a]
Renal	Kidney abscess, acute renal failure, interstitial nephritis[a]
Blood[a]	Thrombopenia, disseminated intravascular coagulation (DIC)
Joint and bone	Arthritis,[a] osteomyelitis
Miscellaneous	Wound infection, cellulitis, rhabdomyolysis, post-traumatic stress disorder

[a] Some of these manifestations are just reactive and they do not mean real local infection. A short course of steroid therapy may then be useful

Table 37.3. Polymicrobial infection[a] in legionellosis

Other *Legionella* spp.	Dual infections by different species of *Legionella* and different serotypes of *L. pneumophila*
Other bacteria	*Streptococcus pneumoniae, Proteus mirabilis, Staphylococcus aureus, Escherichia coli, Prevotella intermedia, Enterococcus facium, Enterobacter cloacae, Klebsiella pneumoniae, Haemophilus influenzae, Streptococcus mitis, Listeria monocytogenes, Nocardia asteroides, Neisseria meningitides*
Mycobacteria	*Mycobacterium tuberculosis*
Virus	Herpesvirus, influenza, cytomegalovirus
Fungus	*Aspergillus, Cryptococcus*
Parasites	*Pneumocystis jiroveci, Leishmania*

[a] Alleged mixed infections with *Mycoplasma pneumoniae, Chlamydia pneumoniae and Coxiella burnettii* have been reported on the basis of serology, which raises much concern about specificity

Extrapulmonary manifestations of legionellosis are uncommon and tend to occur in patients with immucontrol is the cornerstone of therapy in those patients with hemodynamic instability. If deterioration of renal function occurs, appropriate therapeutic measures including diligent administration of substitutive treatment are mandatory until complete recovery of the renal function is achieved.

It is possible that some selected, non-immunocompromised patients with severe LD may potentially benefit from a short course of steroid therapy, as has been suggested in other types of SCAP. However, there is no good evidence to recommend this approach routinely. Steroids may also be useful in the proliferative phase of diffuse alveolar damage (in patients with ARDS), in some reactive extrapulmonary manifestations (arthritis, myocarditis, renal, neurological or hematological features), and when an inflammatory pattern is identified in representative samples of lung tissue in patients with a protracted course [73, 75].
nocompromise (Table 37.2). Suppurated focus of infection should be drained by catheter insertion or performing a surgical procedure [61, 72].

Mixed infections in legionellosis should be kept in mind in the inmunocompromised population since there are many reports of death when clinicians failed to identify and treat the dual component of infection [72, 73]. A list of these mixed infections is enumerated in Table 37.3.

A proposed algorithmic approach to severe legionellosis with poor clinical resolution is suggested in Fig. 37.1. In patients with delayed resolution, superinfection by *Pseudomonas aeruginosa* should be suspected early. In patients with persisting or relapsing *Legionella* infections development of antibiotic resistance has never been reported [72, 73].

37.5 Prognostic Factors

An early, appropriate treatment usually implies a better outcome and a lower mortality rate, particularly in those cases with severe clinical presentation that require admission to the intensive care unit [29]. Severe disease itself, acute renal failure, smoking habit, and immunocompromise are the most consistently identified prognostic factors of death in LD [72, 73].

In our experience (data from the CAPUCI study presented at the 6th International Conference on Legionella, Chicago, 2005), we identify the following variables as being significantly associated with death: immunocompromise, shock, acute renal failure and APACHE II score > 15. Diabetes mellitus was another variable associated with a trend to lower survival. On univariate logistic regression analysis the following variables were

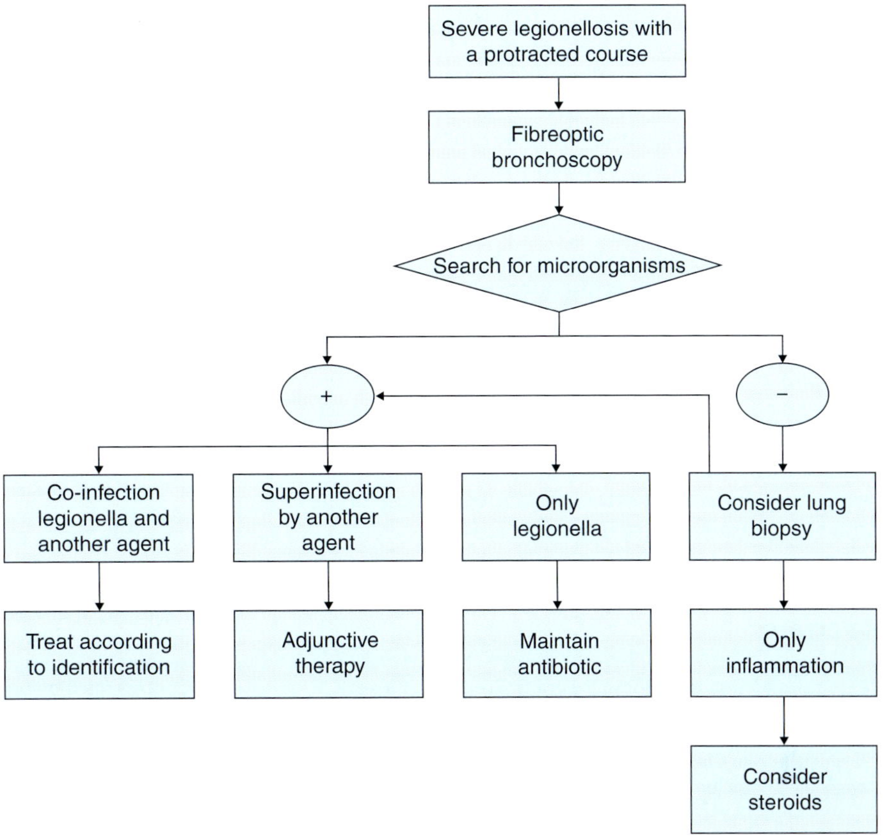

Fig. 37.1. Proposed algorithmic approach to management of intubated patients with non-resolving legionellosis. (From Roig and Rello, JAC 2003; 51:1119–1129; with permission of The British Society for Antimicrobial Therapy)

also found to be associated with death: diabetes mellitus, APACHE score and Acute Physiologic Score. The only variable that remained statistically significant on multivariate logistic regression analysis was APACHE score (OR 1.86) at UCI admission.

37.6 Prevention

The ubiquity of *Legionella* makes it very difficult to control LD, especially in the community setting, where the potential sources of infection are diverse. A correct design of the installations at risk and a strict observance of the maintenance schedules are crucial issues in preventing LD outbreaks. However, sporadic cases of LD in the community are difficult to prevent. Despite our increased knowledge about the sources, transmission and predisposing factors to acquiring *Legionella* infection, many aspects of LD prevention are still controversial. The exact role of the cooling towers in sporadic cases is insufficiently known. On the other hand, some cases of community-acquired LD may be associated with contamination of domestic water supply. Aspiration, especially in the elderly with swallowing disorders, could then play an important role in the pathogenesis of this disease.

Hot water distribution systems constitute the main reservoir for *Legionella* in hospitals. In fact, this colonization is a challenge for traditional disinfection methods. *Legionella* colonization of cold water systems is usually much lower. Disinfection with chlorine is a useful and cost effective measure in the latter setting. A strict control of the key points of water distribution supply and adequate maintenance of chlorination levels [77] is strongly recommended.

When distal sites from a hospital water distribution system are positive for *Legionella,* strategies to minimize the problem are needed, particularly if cases of HAP by *Legionella* have been eventually detected. Thus, review of hydromechanical systems, temperature control of hot water and chlorine levels, as well as maintenance procedures are mandatory. It is generally agreed that the most effective control is to keep the water temperature above 50°C. This approach does not guarantee the elimination of *Legionella* from the water supply but at least minimizes the inoculum and could be effective in preventing cases of HAP by *Legionella.* However, if cases of LD continue to appear, complementary measures of disinfection are then required. Superheat and flush methods have been used for shock disinfection in cases of heavy contamination of water or in the setting of hospital outbreaks. However, the efficacy of disinfection measures may be only transitory and recolonization of *Legionella* followed by new cases of HAP by *Legionella* has been reported [49].

The most commonly used methods for continuous hot water disinfection are copper/silver ionization [34, 50, 88]. Some experiences using chlorine dioxide have also been successful in some hospitals [86]. It has been suggested that monochloramines could be more effective than chlorine in decreasing *Legionella* colonization of potable water distribution systems of large buildings [45].

Local measures, such as filters, have been used to decrease the risk of *Legionella* infection among severely immunocompromised patients [82]. Whenever the water supply of a health care center has become colonized by *Legionella*, some relatively common hospital practices such as using tap water for oral toilet, nasogastric tubes, enteral nutrition, pureed diet, medication and respiratory devices should be prohibited because of the high risk of aspiration of inpatients [14].

References

1. Almirall J, Bolibar I, Toran P, Pera G, Boquet X, Balanzo X, et al. (2004) Contribution of C-reactive protein to the diagnosis and assessment of severity of community-acquired pneumonia. Chest 125:1335–42
2. Alvarez-Sanchez B, Alvarez-Lerma F, Jordá R, Serra J, Lopez Cambra MJ, Sandar MD (1998) Prognostic factors and etiology in patients with severe community-acquired pneumonia. Study Group on Severe Community-Acquired Pneumonia in Spain. Med Clin (Barc) 111:650–4
3. Amsden GW (2005) Anti-inflammatory effects of macrolides – an underappreciated benefit in the treatment of community-acquired respiratory tract infections and chronic inflammatory pulmonary conditions? J Antimicrob Chemother 55:10–21
4. Benhamou D, Bru JP, Chidiac C, Étienne J, Léophonte P, Marty N, et al. (2005) Legionnaires' disease: definition, diagnosis and treatment. Med Mal Infect 35:1–5
5. Benin AL, Benson RF, Besser RE (2002) Trends in legionnaires' disease, 1980–1998: declining mortality and new patterns of diagnosis. Clin Infect Dis 35:1039–46
6. Benkel DH, McClure EM, Woolard D, Rullan JV, Miller GB Jr, Jenkins SR, et al. (2000) Outbreak of Legionnaires' disease associated with a display whirlpool spa. 29:1092–8
7. Blatt SP, Parkinson MD, Pace E, Hoffman P, Dolan D, Lauderdale P, Zajac RA, Melcher GP (1993) Nosocomial Legionnaires' disease: aspirations as a primary mode of disease acquisition. Am J Med 95:16–22
8. Blázquez RM, Espinosa FJ, Alemany L, Ramos RM, Sánchez-Nieto JM, Segovia M, et al. (2005) Antimicrobial chemotherapy for Legionnaires disease: Levofloxacin versus macrolides. Clin Infect Dis 40:800–6
9. Blázquez RM, Espinosa FJ, Martinez-Toldos CM, Alemany L, García-Orenes MC, Segovia M (2005) Sensitivity of urinary antigen test in relation to clinical severity in a large outbreak of *Legionella* pneumonia in Spain. Eur J Clin Microbiol Infect Dis 24:488–91
10. Bodi M, Rodriguez A, Solé-Violan J, Gilavert MC, Garnacho J, Blanquer J, et al. (2005) Antibiotic prescription for community-acquired pneumonia in the Intensive Care Unit. Impact of adherence to IDSA guidelines and outcome. Clin Infect Dis 41:1709–16
11. Borau J, Czap RT, Strellrecht KA, Venezia RA (2000) Long-term control of *Legionella* species in potable water after a nosocomial legionellosis outbreak in an intensive care unit. Infect Control Hosp Epidemiol 21:602–3
12. Brown MJ, Miller RR, Müller NL (1994) Acute lung disease in immunocompetent patients: diagnostic accuracy of high-resolution CT. Radiology 190:247–254
13. Castor ML, Wagstrom EA, Danila RN, Smith KE, Naimi TS, Besser JM, et al. (2005) An outbreak of Pontiac fever with respiratory distress among workers performing high-pressure cleaning at a sugar-beet processing plant. J Infect Dis 191:1530–7
14. Crnich CJ, Safdar N, Maki DG (2005) The role of the Intensive Care Unit environment in the pathogenesis and prevention of ventilator-associated pneumonia. Respiratory Care 50:813–838
15. Darelid J, Lofgren S, Malmvall BE, Olinder-Nielsen MA, Briheim G, Hallander H (2003) *Legionella pneumophila* serogroup 1 antibody kinetics in patients with Legionnaires' disease: implications for serological diagnosis. Scand J Infect Dis 35:15–20
16. Davis GS, Winn WC Jr, Beaty HN (1981) Legionnaires' disease. Infections caused by *Legionella pneumophila* and *Legionella*-like organisms. Clin Chest Med 2:145–66
17. Dominguez JA, Manterola JM, Blavia R, Sopena N, Belda FJ, Padilla E, et al. (1996) Detection of *Legionella pneumophila* serogroup 1 antigen in nonconcentrated urine and urine concentrated by selective ultrafiltration. J Clin Microbiol 34:2334–2336
18. Dondero TJ, Jr, Rendtorff RC, Mallison GF, Weeks RM, Levy JS, Wong EW, et al. (1980) An outbreak of Legionnaires' disease associated with a contaminated air-conditioning cooling tower. N Engl J Med 302:365–370
19. Edelstein PH, Calarco K, Yasui VK (1984) Antimicrobial therapy of experimentally induced Legionnaires' disease in guinea pigs. Am Rev Respir Dis 130:849–56
20. Edelstein PH (1998) Antimicrobial chemotherapy for Legionnaires disease: time for a change. Ann Intern Med 129:328–330
21. Edelstein PH (2002) Chemotherapy of Legionnaires' disease with macrolide or quinolone antimicrobial agents. In: Marre R (ed) Legionella. ASM Press, Washington DC, pp 183–88
22. Everts RJ, Murdoch DR, Chambers ST, Town GI, Withington SG, Martin IR, et al. (2000) Nosocomial pneumonia in adult general medical and surgical patients at Christchurch Hospital. N Z Med J 113:221–4
23. Ezzedine H, VanOssel C, Delmee M, Wauters G (1989) *Legionella* spp. in a hospital hot water system: effect of control measures. J Hosp Infect 13:121–131
24. Falcó V, Fernández de Sevilla T, Alegre J, Ferrer A, Martínez Vázquez JM (1991) *Legionella pneumophila*. A cause of severe community-acquired pneumonia. Chest 100:1007–1011
25. Fang GD, Stout JE, Yu VL, Goetz A, Rihs JD, Vickers RM (1990) Community-acquired pneumonia caused by *Legionella dumoffii* in a patient with hairy cell leukemia. Infection 18(6):383–5
26. Farr BM, Gratz J, Tartaglino J, Getchell-White SI, Groschell DH (1988) Evaluation of ultraviolet light for disinfection of hospital water contaminated with *Legionella*. Lancet 2:669–672
27. Fisman DN, Lim S, Wellenius GA, Johnson C, Britz P, Gaskins M, et al. (2005) It's not the heat, it's the humidity: wet weather increases legionellosis risk in the greater Philadelphia metropolitan area. J Infect Dis 192:2066–73
28. Franzin L, Cabodi D (2005) *Legionella* pneumonia and serum procalcitonin. Curr Microbiol 50:43–6

29. Gacouin A, Le Tulzo Y, Lavoue S, Camus C, Hoff J, Bassen R, Arvieux C, Heurtin C, Thomas R (2002) Severe pneumonia due to *Legionella pneumophila*: prognostic factors, impact of delayed appropriate antimicrobial therapy. Intensive Care Med 28:686–691
30. Garbe PL, Davis BJ, Weisfeld JS, Markowitz L, Miner P, Garrity F, et al. (1985) Nosocomial Legionnaires' disease – epidemiologic demonstration of cooling towers as a source. JAMA 254:521–524
31. García-Fulgueiras A, Navarro C, Fenoll D, Garcia J, Gonzalez-Diego P, Jimenez-Bunuales T, et al. (2003) Legionnaires' disease outbreak in Murcia, Spain. Emerg Infect Dis 9:915–21
32. Ginevra C, Barranger C, Ros A, Mory O, Stephan JL, Freymuth F, et al. (2005) Development and evaluation of Chlamylege, a new commercial test allowing simultaneous detection and identification of *Legionella*, *Chlamydophila pneumoniae*, and *Mycoplasma pneumoniae* in clinical respiratory specimens by multiplex PCR. J Clin Microbiol 43:3247–54
33. Gibson DH, Fitzgeorge RB, Baskerville A (1983) Antibiotic therapy of experimental airborne Legionnaires' disease. J Infect 7:210–7
34. Goetz A, Yu VL (1997) Copper-silver ionization: Cautious optimism for *Legionella* disinfection and implications for environmental culturing. Am J Infect Control 25:449–51
35. Granados A, Podzamczer D, Gudiol F, Manresa F (1989) Pneumonia due to *Legionella pneumophila* and pneumococcal pneumonia: similarities and differences on presentation. Eur Respir J 2(2):130–4
36. Gutierrez F, Masia M, Mirete C, Soldan B, Rodriguez CJ, Padilla S, et al. (2006) The influence of age and gender on the population-based incidence of community-acquired pneumonia caused by different microbial pathogens in a population-based prospective cohort study. J Infect 53(3):166–74
37. Howden BP, Stuart RL, Tallis G, Bailey M, Johnson PD (2003) Treatment and outcome of 104 hospitalized patients with Legionnaires' disease. Intern Med J 33:484–8
38. Hubbard RB, Mathur RM, MacFarlaine JT (1993) Severe community acquired *Legionella* pneumonia: treatment, complications and outcome. Q J Med 86:327–32
39. Johnson JT, Yu VL, Best M, Vickers RM, Goetz A, Wagner R, et al. (1985) Nosocomial legionellosis uncovered in surgical patients with head and neck cancer: Implications for epidemiologic reservoir and mode of transmission. Lancet 2:298–300
40. Joseph C (2005) Legionnaires disease in Europe – A ten year epidemiological review 1995–2004. 6th International Conference on *Legionella*. Abstracts, p 44. Chicago, IL. October 16–20, 2005
41. Kirby BD, Snyder KM, Meyer RD, Finegold SM (1980) Legionnaires' disease: report of sixty-five nosocomially acquired cases of review of the literature. Medicine (Baltimore) 59:188–205
42. Khanna M, Fan J, Pehler-Harrington K, Waters C, Douglass P, Stallock J, et al. (2005) The Pneumoplex assays, a multiplex PCR-enzyme hybridization assay that allows simultaneous detection of five organisms, *Mycoplasma pneumoniae*, *Chlamydia* (*Chlamydophila*) *pneumoniae*, *Legionella pneumophila*, *Legionella micdadei*, and *Bordetella pertussis*, and its real-time counterpart. J Clin Microbiol 43:565–71
43. Konig C, Hebestreit H, Valenza G, Abele-Horn M, Speer CP (2005) *Legionella waltersii* – a novel cause of pneumonia? Acta Pediatr 94(10):1505–7
44. Kool JL, Fiore AE, Kioski CM, Brown EW, Benson RF, Pruckler JM, et al. (1998) More than ten years of unrecognized nosocomial transmission of Legionnaires' disease among transplant patients. Infect Contr Hosp Epidemiol 19:898–904
45. Kool JL, Carpenter JC, Fields BS (1999) Effect of monochloramine disinfection of municipal drinking water on risk of nosocomial Legionnaires' disease. Lancet 353:272–277
46. Kraus CN, Zalkikar J, Powers JH (2005) Levofloxacin and macrolides for treatment of Legionnaires' disease. Multiple comparisons give few answers. Clin Infect Dis 41:416
47. Lepine LA, Jernigan DB, Butler JC, Pruckler JM, Benson RF, Kim F, et al. (1998) A recurrent outbreak of nosocomial Legionnaire's disease detected by urinary antigen testing: evidence for long-term colonization of a hospital plumbing system. Infect Contr Hosp Epidemiol 19:905–910
48. Li Gobbi, Benucci M, Del Rosso A (2005) Pneumonitis caused by *Legionella pneumoniae* in a patient with rheumatoid arthritis treated with anti-TNF-alpha therapy (infliximab). J Clin Rheumatol 11:119–20
49. Lin YS, Stout JE, Yu VL, Vidic RD (1998) Disinfection of water distribution systems for *Legionella*. Semin Res Infect 13:147–159
50. Liu Z, Stout JE, Tedesco L, Boldin M, Hwang C, Diven WF (1994) Controlled evaluation of copper-silver ionization in eradicating *Legionella pneumophila* from a hospital water distribution system. J Infect Dis 169:919–922
51. Macfarlane JT, Miller AC, Roderick Smith WH, Morris AH, Rose DH (1984) Comparative radiographic features of community acquired Legionnaires' disease, pneumococcal pneumonia, mycoplasma pneumonia, and psittacosis. Thorax 39(1):28–33
52. Marrie TJ, Bezanson G, Haldane DJM, Burbridge S (1992) Colonization of the respiratory tract with *Legionella pneumophila* for 63 days before onset of pneumonia. J Infect 24:81–86
53. Marston BJ, Plouffe JF, File TM Jr, Hackman BA, Salstrom SJ, Lipman HB, et al. (1997) Incidence of community-acquired pneumonia requiring hospitalization. Results of a population-based active surveillance study in Ohio. The Community-Based Pneumonia Incidence Study Group. Arch Intern Med 157:1709–1718
54. Mathys W, Deng MD, Meyer J, Junge-Mathys E (1999) Fatal nosocomial Legionnaires' disease after heart transplantation: clinical course, epidemiology, and prevention strategies for the highly immunocompromised host. J Hosp Infect 43:242–246
55. McDonough EA, Barrozo CP, Russell KL, Metzgar D (2005) A multiplex PCR for detection of *Mycoplasma pneumoniae*, *Chlamydophila pneumoniae*, *Legionella pneumophila*, and *Bordetella pertussis* in clinical specimens. Mol Cell Probes 19:314–22
56. Moffie BG, Mouton RP (1988) Sensitivity and resistance of *Legionella pneumophila* to some antibiotics and combinations of antibiotics. J Antimicrob Chemother 22:457–62
57. Muder RR, Stout JE, Yu VL (2000) Nosocomial *Legionella micdadei* infection in transplant patients: fortune favors the prepared mind. Am J Med 108:346–348
58. Murdoch DR, Walford EJ, Jennings LC, Light GJ, Schousboe MI, Chereshsky AY, et al. (1996) Use of the polymerase chain reaction to detect *Legionella* DNA in urine and serum samples from patients with pneumonia. Clin Infect Dis 23:475–480
59. Mykietiuk A, Carratalà J, Fernández-Sabe N, Dorca J, Verdaguer R, Manresa F, et al. (2005) Clinical outcomes for hospitalized patients with *Legionella* pneumonia in the antigenuria era: the influence of levofloxacin therapy. Clin Infect Dis 40:794–9
60. Pachón J, Prados MD, Capote F, Cuello JA, Garnacho J, Ver-

ano A (1990) Severe community-acquired pneumonia. Etiology, prognosis, and treatment. Am Rev Respir Dis 142:369–73
61. Patel MC, Levi MH, Mahadevi P, Nana M, Merav AD, Robbins N. (2005) *L. micdadei* PVE successfully treated with levofloxacin/valve replacement: case report and review of literature. J Infect 51:265–8
62. Pedro-Botet ML, Stout JE, Yu VL (2002) Legionnaires' disease contracted from patients' homes: the coming of the third plague. Eur J Clin Microbiol Infect Dis 21:699–705
63. Pedro-Botet ML, Sabria M, Sopena N, Garcia-Nuñez M, Dominguez MJ, Reynaga E, et al. (2003) Legionnaires' disease and HIV infection. Chest 124:543–7
64. Plouffe JF, File TM, Breiman RF, Hackman BA, Salstrom SJ, Marston BJ, et al. (1995) Reevaluation of the definition of Legionnaires' disease: use of the urinary antigen assay. Community Based Pneumonia Incidence Study Group. Clin Infect Dis 20:1286–91
65. Prat C, Dominguez J, Andreo F, Blanco S, Pallares A, Cuchillo F, et al. (2006) Procalcitonin and neopterin correlation with aetiology of and severity of pneumonia. J Infect 52(3):169–77
66. Ramila E, Sureda A, Martino R, Santamaria A, Franquet T, Puzo C, et al. (2000) Bronchoscopy guided by high resolution computed tomography for the diagnosis of pulmonary infections in patients with hematologic malignancies and normal plain chest X-rays. Hematologica 85:961–966
67. Rantakokko-Jalaba K, Jalaba J (2001) Development of conventional and real-time PCR assays for detection of *Legionella* DNA in respiratory specimens. J Clin Microbiol 39:2904–2910
68. Redd SC, Schuster DM, Quan J, Pilkaytis BD, Spika JS, Cohen ML (1988) Legionellosis cardiac transplant recipients: results of a nationwide survey. J Infect Dis 158:651–653
69. Ricketts K, Joseph C (2005) Legionnaires' disease in Europe 2003–2004. Euro Surveill 10:12
70. Roig J, Aguilar X, Ruiz J, Domingo C, Mesalles E, Manterola J, et al. (1991) Comparative study of *Legionella pneumophila* and other nosocomial-acquired pneumonias. Chest 99:344–50
71. Roig J, Carreres A, Domingo C (1993) Treatment of Legionnaires' disease. Drugs 46:63–79
72. Roig J, Sabria M, Pedro-Botet ML (2003) *Legionella* spp.: community-acquired and nosocomial infections. Curr Opin Infect Dis 16:145–151
73. Roig J, Rello J (2003) Legionnaires' disease: a rational approach to therapy. JAC 51:1119–1129
74. Roig J, Rello J (2006) Treatment of Legionnaires' disease. In: Cianciotto NP (ed) Legionella. ASM Press, Washington DC (in press)
75. Roig J, Casal J, Gispert P, Gea E (2006) Antibiotic therapy of community-acquired pneumonia caused by atypical agents. Med Mal Infect (in press)
76. Sabria M, Garcia-Nuñez M, Pedro-Botet ML, Sopena N, Gimeno JM, Reynaga E, et al. (2001) Presence and chromosomal subtyping of *Legionella* species in potable water systems in 20 hospitals of Catalonia, Spain. Infect Control Hosp Epidemiol 11:673–6
77. Sabria M, Yu VL (2002) Hospital-acquired legionellosis: solutions for a preventable infection. Lancet Infect Dis 2:368–73
78. Sabria M, Modol JM, García-Núñez M, Reynaga E, Pedro-Botet ML, Sopena ML, et al. (2004) Environmental cultures and hospital-acquired Legionnaires' disease: a 5 year prospective study in 20 hospitals in Catalonia, Spain. Infect Control Hosp Epidemiol 25:1072–6
79. Sabria M, Pedro-Botet ML, Gómez J, Roig J, Vilaseca B, Sopena N, et al. (2005) Fluoroquinolones versus macrolides in the treatment of Legionnaires' disease. Chest 128: 1401–5
80. Skogberg K, Nuorti JP, Saxen H, Kusnetsov J, Mentula S, Fellman V, et al. (2002) A newborn with domestically acquired legionnaires' disease confirmed by molecular typing. Clin Infect Dis 35:82–5
81. Shands K, Ho J, Meyer R, Gorman GW, Edelstein PH, Mallison GF, et al. (1985) Potable water as a source of Legionnaires' disease. JAMA 253:1412–1416
82. Sheffer PJ, Scout JE, Wagener MM, Muder RR (2005) Efficacy of new point-of-use water filter for preventing exposure to *Legionella* and waterborne bacteria. Am J Infect Control 33(Suppl 1):S20–25
83. Sopena N, Sabria M, Pedro-Botet ML, Manterola JM, Matas L, Dominguez J, et al. (1999) Prospective study of community-acquired pneumonia of bacterial etiology in adults. Eur J Clin Microbiol Infect Dis 18:852–8
84. Sopena N, Sabria M, Pedro-Botet ML, Reynaga E, Garcia-Nuñez M, Dominguez J, et al. (2002) Factors related to persistence of *Legionella* urinary antigen excretion in patients with Legionnaires'disease. Eur J Clin Microbiol Infect Dis 21:845–8
85. Sopena N, Sabria M (2005) Multicenter study of hospital-acquired pneumonia in non-ICU patients. Chest 127:213–9
86. Srinivasan A, Bova G, Ross T, Mackie K, Paquette N, Merz W, et al. (2003) A 17-month evaluation of a chlorine dioxide water treatment system to control *Legionella* species in a hospital water supply. Infect Control Hosp Epidemiol 24:575–9
87. Stout JE, Yu VL (1997) Legionellosis. N Engl J Med 337: 682–7
88. Stout JE, Yu VL (2003) Experiences of the first 16 hospitals using copper-silver ionization for *Legionella* control: implications for the evaluation of other disinfection modalities. Infect Control Hosp Epidemiol 24:563–8
89. Torres A, Serra-Batlles J, Ferrer A, Jimenez P, Celis R, Cobo E, et al. (1991) Severe community-acquired pneumonia. Epidemiology and prognostic factors. Am Rev Respir Dis 144:312–318
90. Venezia RA, Agresta MD, Hanley E, Urquhart K, Schoonmaker D (1994) Nosocomial legionellosis associated with aspiration of nasogastric feedings diluted in tap water. Infect Control Hosp Epidemiol 15:529–533
91. Vergis E (2000) Azithromycin vs cefuroxime plus erythromycin for empirical treatment of community-acquired pneumonia in hospitalized patients: a prospective, randomized, multicenter trial. Arch Intern Med 160:1294–1300
92. Woodhead MA, Macfarlane JT (1987) Comparative clinical and laboratory features of legionella with pneumococcal and mycoplasma pneumonias. Br J Dis Chest 81(2):133–9
93. Yu VL, Kroboth FJ, Shonnard J, Brown A, McDearman S, Magnussen M (1982) Legionnaires' disease: new clinical perspective from a prospective pneumonia study. Am J Med 73(3):357–61
94. Yu VL, Plouffe JF, Pastoris MC, Stout JE, Schousboe M, Widmer A, et al. (2002) Distribution of *Legionella* species and serogroups isolated by culture in patients with sporadic community-acquired legionellosis: an international collaborative survey. J Infect Dis 186:127–8

Chapter 38

Adjunctive and Supportive Measures for Community-Acquired Pneumonia

38

G.W. Waterer, R.G. Wunderink

38.1 Introduction

The widespread introduction of penicillin in the 1940s resulted in a substantial reduction in mortality from community-acquired pneumonia (CAP). However, despite significant advances in medical science, only a small improvement has occurred since, particularly in patients with bacteremic pneumococcal pneumonia [1, 2]. Even modern intensive care has only made a small difference to the mortality in patients with severe pneumonia [3, 4]. While the aging population, increased number of patients with severe co-morbid illnesses, and the human immunodeficiency virus (HIV) epidemic have certainly contributed to the persistently high mortality rate [2, 5, 6], apparently healthy, immunocompetent patients continue to die from CAP. Disturbingly, a recent British Thoracic Society study concluded that no available therapy could substantially reduce the mortality rate from severe CAP in young adults [7].

While some causative microorganisms, such as *Pseudomonas*, and some strains of common causative microorganisms appear to be more virulent, the majority of CAP patients who die are infected with organisms sensitive to commonly prescribed antibiotics. Even the recent emergence of high level penicillin-resistant strains of *S. pneumoniae* has not significantly increased the mortality of CAP. Given that most CAP patients die despite microbiological confirmation that they received appropriate antibiotic therapy, the introduction of new antibiotic classes is unlikely to reduce mortality further. For this reason, research has been directed into non-antibiotic therapeutic measures.

Generally, supportive measures for CAP can be separated into two categories – (1) immunomodulatory therapy for the systemic inflammatory response induced by pneumonia and (2) support for the gas exchange abnormalities unique to a pulmonary source of sepsis. Chapter 16 focuses on potential immunomodulatory therapies in patients with sepsis, including pneumonia. This chapter will focus on a few pneumonia-specific immunomodulatory therapies and other advances in the intensive care management of patients with severe CAP.

38.2 Pneumonia-Specific Immune Therapies

38.2.1 Corticosteroids

Although discussed in Chapter 16, a more detailed discussion of the recent controversy over high dose corticosteroids in patients with CAP is warranted.

The best evidence of benefit for corticosteroids comes from studies in specific, narrowly defined groups of CAP patients caused by less common agents. Randomized, controlled trials have shown corticosteroids reduce mortality in AIDS patients with *Pneumocystis carinii* pneumonia and significant hypoxia, if instituted at or prior to the onset of anti-pneumocystis therapy [8, 9]. Based on a small, retrospective study of 15 subjects, corticosteroids may also improve the outcome of severe *Varicella* pneumonia [10]. Anecdotally, corticosteroids are frequently used in the setting of severe fungal pneumonia, particularly due to *Histoplasmosis* [11, 12], and a small controlled trial of 55 patients supported their use in miliary tuberculosis [13].

Following the success of pre-antibiotic corticosteroids in children with meningitis [14], Marik and colleagues [15] studied the effect of a single dose of hydrocortisone (10 mg/kg) 30 min prior to antibiotic therapy in a small randomized placebo controlled trial of 30 adult patients with severe CAP (SCAP). Hydrocortisone had no detectable effect on tumor necrosis factor alpha (TNF) production in the following 12 h, mortality (only four deaths) or length of stay in the ICU. While not encouraging, the small number of subjects studied (14 received hydrocortisone), the use of only a single dose and the measurement of only a single pro-inflammatory cytokine for only 12 h does not qualify this study to be a definitive statement on the role of corticosteroids in CAP. An important finding of this study was that beta-lactam antibiotics did not result in a significant increase in serum TNF levels, as rapid antigen release due to bacterial lysis has been postulated as a potential cause of deterioration in patients with severe CAP [16].

Also supporting a possible role for corticosteroids in severe CAP, Montón and co-workers [17] studied the effect of intravenous methylprednisolone on bronchoalveolar lavage fluid (BALF) and serum cytokines in 20 patients with severe nosocomial pneumonia or CAP. The 11 patients who received methylprednisolone had significantly lower serum and BALF TNF, interleukin (IL)-1β, IL-6 and C-reactive protein. There was also a non-significant trend to lower mortality in the steroid treated group (36% vs. 67%).

Recently, Confalonieri and colleagues compared intravenous hydrocortisone (200 mg bolus followed by 10 mg/h for 7 days) with placebo in 46 patients with severe CAP admitted to the ICU [18]. The trial was stopped early after an interim analysis showed a significant mortality benefit in the steroid group (0% vs 30%, $p=0.009$). However, the mortality difference was driven by deaths after day 8 and a high incidence of "delayed septic shock". The marked incidence of this scenario has not been seen in any other SCAP study. Significant differences in the percent of patients who received noninvasive ventilation rather than intubation and mechanical ventilation also compromise the data regarding a beneficial effect of steroids on gas exchange. Noninvasive ventilation has been shown by the same group to decrease mortality compared to invasive ventilation [19]. The statistical design of the study led to an early closure of the study, limiting the ability to exclude the possibility that other factors explain the mortality difference. The complete absence of any mortality in the corticosteroid group has also raised significant concerns about potential bias in patient selection and whether either the control or case cohort were truly representative of the general group of patients with severe CAP.

Despite the reservations, all three pilot studies suggested a trend toward benefit with steroids so further clinical studies clearly need to be conducted.

38.2.2 Prostaglandin Inhibitors

Prostaglandin antagonists are worth special comment as they have been studied in animal and human patients with pneumonia. Ibuprofen reduced the intrapulmonary shunt fraction from 29% to 21% in dogs with lobar pneumonia [20], with a corresponding decrease in the consolidated area of lung. Acetylsalicylic acid had a similar effect, reducing the shunt fraction from 38% to 23% [20]. The mechanism is unclear but may be due to reversal of prostaglandin inhibition of the hypoxia-induced pulmonary vasoconstriction.

In a small study of ten subjects with pneumonia requiring mechanical ventilation, Hanley et al. [21] studied the effect of indomethacin (1 mg/kg oral or rectal) on arterial oxygenation. Five subjects had substantial improvement in oxygenation with a small improvement in three additional patients. Improvement tended to occur in the patients with the greatest degree of hypoxemia. As ibuprofen administration appears to be relatively safe, even in the setting of sepsis [22], further studies are warranted.

In contrast, Ferrer et al. found a 2 g infusion of acetylsalicylic acid (ASA) had no effect on arterial oxygenation in seven patients with severe unilateral pneumonia [23]. Although intrapulmonary shunting did reduce by a small amount ($28\pm17\%$ vs. $23.5\pm13\%$), the lack of clinically apparent benefit was discouraging. Several possible explanations were advanced to explain the discrepancy between this study and that of Hanley et al. Clearly, a difference in efficacy between ASA and indomethacin may be the cause. However, the subjects in the study by Hanley et al. were also more severely hypoxic, with a mean $Pa0_2/Fi0_2$ of 138 compared to 168. In any event, it would seem reasonable for future studies to use indomethacin in preference to ASA.

38.2.3 Immunoglobulin Enhancement

Before the advent of antibiotic therapy, passive immunization with serum was used with some success in patients with pneumonia [24]. Mortality was reduced by approximately 10% in most age groups with a diminishing effect in patients over the age of 60. With the exception of patients with specific immunoglobulin deficiencies, this therapy has largely been abandoned due to the much greater efficacy of antibiotics in addition to the difficulty, and cost, of obtaining sufficient serum. The development of new antiviral drugs has also largely obviated the anecdotal use of hyper-immune serum in cytomegalovirus and varicella pneumonitis.

While the overall efficacy of pneumococcal immunization is unclear, especially in the elderly with some comorbid illnesses, several studies and a meta-analysis have suggested that even if pneumococcal pneumonia is not prevented, the incidence of invasive pneumococcal disease is decreased.

The use of specific anti-pseudomonal exotoxin antibodies has been tried as an adjunct to antibiotics with some success in mice [25] and guinea pigs [26], and *Pseudomonas* specific vaccines have enhanced antibiotic response in guinea pigs [27]. Anti-pseudomonal antibodies appeared safe in human subjects with evidence of increased opsonophagocytic activity in a small phase I study of 20 subjects [28], but further studies are required to determine whether they have any clinically relevant effect. In human sepsis studies, generic anti-endotoxin strategies have so far been disappointing [29, 30]. Although they have not specifically been studied in pneumonia, the primary site of sepsis in many of the patients in these studies was the lung, indicating a low likelihood of benefit.

38.2.4 Macrophage Enhancement

Legionella pneumophila is consistently identified as a leading cause of CAP, particularly in patients with severe CAP [31–34]. Unlike pneumococcal pneumonia, the immune response to *Legionella* infection is predominantly of a TH1 type [35] and bacterial killing is predominantly by macrophages [36]. Skerrett and Martin studied the effect of interferon gamma (IFNγ), a potent stimulator of macrophage function [37, 38], given as an intratracheal bolus in rats with experimental *L. pneumophila* pneumonia [39]. Intratracheal IFNγ markedly reduced the replication of *L. pneumophila* in corticosteroid treated rats, but had no detectable effect in immunocompetent rats or when given intraperitoneally.

The ability to give IFNγ by aerosol is particularly appealing since not only are systemic side effects avoided, but also a much greater effect on intrapulmonary macrophage function is seen compared to systemic administration [40]. Aerosolized IFNγ has also been shown to be safe in patients with drug resistant tuberculosis [41], and may have a role in treatment of this condition. Further studies of nebulized IFNγ, especially in patients with pulmonary legionellosis, are awaited.

38.2.5 Drotrecogin Alpha (Activated Protein C)

After many unsuccessful trials of non-antibiotic agents designed to disrupt or ameliorate the pro-inflammatory process driving septic shock and associated organ failure, activated protein C (drotrecogin alpha activated) was the first successful agent to reduce mortality in a large randomized, double blind, placebo controlled trial [42]. While 28-day mortality was clearly better in sub-groups of patients who received drotrecogin alpha activated [42], the subgroup with community-acquired pneumonia drove most of the benefit of the drug [43], with the greatest reduction in mortality seen with *Streptococcus pneumoniae* infection (RR=0.56; 95% CI 0.35–0.88). The availability of rapid urinary antigen detection for *S. pneumoniae* allows this association to enter clinical decision-making (several references for urinary antigen). Drotrecogin alpha activated appeared to have a greater effect in single organ failure than waiting for multiple (≥ two) organ failure but clearly has its greatest benefit in patients who have the highest acuity of illness. Worsening thrombocytopenia, suggestive of early disseminated intravascular coagulation, appears to be another important indicator for patients likely to respond to drotrecogin alpha activated [44]. While different criteria for the administration of drotrecogin alpha activated have been established in different institutions around the world, the presence of pneumonia and shock should prompt physicians to consider its use as early as is possible.

38.3 Other Supportive Measures

The main additional supportive therapy unique to CAP is improved oxygenation and secretion clearance. The remainder of supportive care is not different than that of other critically ill patients with infection.

38.3.1 Positioning Therapy

CAP is one of the more common causes of severe hypoxic respiratory failure. A common method to improve oxygenation, the addition of positive end expiratory pressure, may actually make oxygenation worse in patients with severe asymmetrical lung disease like CAP. The PEEP will tend to overdistend the unaffected lung, increasing pulmonary vascular resistance on the local area. This overdistension may then direct greater blood flow to the pneumonic area, especially if hypoxic vasoconstriction has been blocked by some bacterial product.

With extensive unilateral pneumonia, positioning the ventilated patient in the lateral decubitus position with the affected lung up has been demonstrated to improve oxygenation [45]. Positioning increases perfusion to the dependent, non-involved lung, increases secretion clearance from the affected lung, and may allow addition of PEEP without increasing shunt because the dependent lung is now less compliant and less likely to become overdistended. The combination of positioning and prostaglandin inhibitors is usually adequate to temporarily improve oxygenation until hypoxic vasoconstriction is restored.

38.3.2 Differential Lung Ventilation

Differentially ventilating each lung by means of a dual lumen endotracheal tube may also be beneficial [46, 47]. This allows the use of higher levels of PEEP in the affected, less compliant, lung and lower levels of PEEP in the normal lung, thus reducing the risk of barotrauma. A study by Ranieri et al. showing a correlation between the level of PEEP and pro-inflammatory cytokine production further supports this approach to protect the 'normal' lung [48]. The point at which differential ventilation is worth commencing is not clear, but Carlon and colleagues [46] suggest optimal benefit occurs when there is a 200 ml or greater difference in distribution of tidal volume between each lung.

38.3.3
Extracorporeal Membrane Oxygenation

ECMO, a modification of cardiopulmonary bypass, was designed to provide oxygenation in patients with severe respiratory failure. Although available since the 1970s, initial poor results from a National Institutes of Health sponsored prospective, multicenter randomized trial [49] limited the use of ECMO to research centers. However, a significant reduction in complications has led to resurgence in interest in ECMO as a means of providing oxygenation when all other means have failed.

The role of ECMO has most extensively been studied in neonates. In newborn infants with respiratory failure unresponsive to other therapy it has proven highly effective, having an overall survival of 80 % in over 10,000 neonates where nearly 100 % mortality would be expected [50]. Modification of the neonatal ECMO technique has also been effective in some pediatric patients with respiratory failure [51], including those with pneumonia from both bacterial [52] and viral [53] pathogens. As would be expected, as the duration of ECMO required increases, the prognosis decreases [52].

In the NIH-sponsored ECMO trial, adults with viral pneumonia did particularly poorly. In a retrospective review of 100 adults with severe acute respiratory failure supported with ECMO by Kolla and colleagues [54], a 53 % survival rate was found in the 49 patients with a primary diagnosis of pneumonia. Although this mortality seems high, patients selected for ECMO had an expected mortality in excess of 90 %. Predictors of poor response to ECMO were increasing age, days of ventilation prior to commencement of ECMO and the degree of respiratory failure as measured by the $Pa0_2/Fi0_2$ ratio. Cases of successful intervention in adults with severe *Legionella* [55, 56], pneumococcal [57] and *Varicella* pneumonia [58] have all been reported.

The clearest indication for ECMO in adults may be the Hantavirus pulmonary syndrome (HPS). With no effective antiviral therapy, care is entirely supportive. In a small series, the dramatic but time-limited cardiovascular and pulmonary hemorrhagic manifestations of HPS appeared to be well supported by ECMO [59].

ECMO would appear to have a role in some patients with severe respiratory failure secondary to pneumonia. The timing, duration and patient selection for what is an expensive, labor intensive therapy remain to be determined by prospective studies.

38.3.4
Other Therapies

Liquid ventilation with volatile hydrocarbons has been studied in the management of ARDS. Little data is currently published on its use specifically in human subjects with pneumonia. In rats given lethal doses of pneumococci, partial liquid ventilation in combination with perfluorocarbon doubled survival compared to antibiotics alone [60].

Nitric oxide (NO) inhalation has also been studied as adjunctive therapy of ARDS, as well as some other forms of severe pulmonary hypertension. While no studies specifically address human patients with pneumonia, in dogs with *Escherichia coli* pneumonia, inhaled NO had a minimal effect on oxygenation and no effect on sepsis induced pulmonary hypertension [61].

Since NO is one of the effector molecules released by macrophages to kill bacteria [62], inhaled NO has a potential antibacterial effect. Hoehn and colleagues studied the bacteriostatic effect of NO on bacterial cultures from neonates [63]. At 120 ppm (greater than the usual dose range of 40–80 ppm) NO inhibited the growth group B Streptococcus, *Staphylococcus epidermidis* and *E. coli* but not *Pseudomonas aeruginosa* or *Staphylococcus aureus*. Further studies will be required to determine whether inhaled NO has any real bacteriostatic effect in vivo, particularly as it may have deleterious effects on the function of neutrophils [64].

Aerosolized prostacyclin has also been shown by Walmrath et al. to improve oxygenation by reducing shunt and pulmonary hypertension in patients with pneumonia [65]. Twelve patients with severe pneumonia ($Pa0_2/Fi0_2 < 150$), six of whom had interstitial lung disease (ILD), received varying doses of prostacyclin. Patients with ILD required substantially larger doses of prostacyclin to produce a clinical effect. Although its efficacy has not been compared to NO in patients with pneumonia, its greater cost is a significant disadvantage.

38.3.5
Clearance of Secretions

Significant accumulation of mucopurulent secretions can occur in CAP, particularly in patients on mechanical ventilation. Mucus impaction can lead to obstruction, ranging in severity from linear atelectasis to lobar collapse.

38.3.5.1
Physical Removal

Clearly the most effective secretion clearance is a spontaneous cough. However, the respiratory compromise often attendant to severe CAP may prevent an effective cough. Support with noninvasive ventilation (NIV) may benefit the patient by both improving respiratory mechanics while allowing the patient to spontaneously expectorate [66]. However, retained secretions is also one of the causes of failure of NIV. An important strategy to avoid this complication is to avoid continuous application of NIV and actively encourage the patient to cough during periods off NIV.

In mechanically ventilated CAP patients, removal of secretions by regular suctioning is essential. The use of percussion or vibration in ventilated patients has been associated with worsening of gas exchange and the benefit in CAP patients in general is unclear.

The benefit of bronchoscopy for secretion removal is also poorly supported. Bronchoscopy for secretion removal has been associated with an increased risk of development of subsequent nosocomial pneumonia [67]. Therefore its therapeutic use should be limited. One of the few studies on this area has suggested that if lobar atelectasis is accompanied by an air bronchogram, bronchoscopy is unlikely to find a mucus plug or benefit the patient.

38.3.5.2 Mucolytics

Changing the rheologic properties of thick tenacious mucus is often attempted with little scientific support. Avoidance of dessication and inspissation of secretions does appear to be important. Adequate hydration may be the most effective therapy. Intubated CAP patients with significant secretions are poor candidates for heat and moisture exchangers and should usually have ventilation initiated with heated humidification.

The pharmacologic intervention most often ordered is *N*-acetylcysteine. Most support for this therapy is an extension of results in some cystic fibrosis patients. Whether the same benefit can be achieved in CAP patients is unclear as there is no published data of *N*-acetylcysteine use in this setting. The potential benefit is also partially offset by induction of bronchial irritation and bronchospasm in some patients. Preliminary data on agents with more physiologic support, such as UTP [68], are encouraging but need further study. Guaifenesin has limited data in non-pneumonia patients and is unlikely to have a major benefit in intubated CAP patients. Although a variety of other mucolytic agents are available, including bromhexine, rhDNase and polymyxin B, there is no data to support their use in patients with pneumonia.

38.4 Conclusion

CAP remains a significant health problem and patients continue to die despite receiving appropriate antibiotic therapy. Modification of the host immune response, both anti- and pro-inflammatory approaches, has yet to live up to the promise of improved outcome. Despite this, there is significant reason for optimism. Some immunomodulatory therapies clearly have efficacy in some patients. As our understanding of the immune response to pneumonia improves, our ability to tailor specific therapies for individual patients will also improve, hopefully avoiding the deleterious effects that have so far prevented the development of an effective immune based therapy. The possibility of delivering cytokines directly to the lung, such as with nebulized IFNγ, is a particularly promising way of achieving the desired pulmonary effect without systemic side effects.

Corticosteroids are currently unique in that they have a proven rolc in the therapy of pneumonia due to *P. carinii*. Recent research suggests there may be a much wider therapeutic indication for corticosteroids in severe CAP and further research is awaited.

Once respiratory failure has ensued, supportive measures such as patient positioning and differential lung ventilation can improve oxygenation at no additional risk in some patients, particularly those with severe unilateral pneumonia. In facilities where ECMO is available it may be beneficial in selected patients when all other means of providing respiratory support have failed. The role of inhaled NO and partial liquid ventilation is also currently unclear and awaiting further study.

References

1. Burman LA, Norrby R, Trollfors B (1985) Invasive pneumococcal infections: incidence, predisposing factors and prognosis. Rev Infect Dis 7:133–142
2. Watankunakorn C, Bailey TA (1997) Adult bacteremic pneumococcal pneumonia in a community teaching hospital, 1992–1996. Arch Intern Med 157:1965–1971
3. Hook EW, Horton CA, Schaberg DR (1983) Failure of intensive care unit support to influence mortality from pneumococcal bacteremia. JAMA 249:1055–1057
4. Franklin C, Henrickson K, Weil MH (1991) Reduced mortality of pneumococcal bacteremia after early intensive care. J Intensive Care Med 6:302–307
5. Torres JM, Cardenas O, Vasquez A, Schlossberg D (1998) *Streptococcus pneumoniae* bacteremia in a community hospital. Chest 113:387–390
6. Plouffe JF, Breiman RF, Facklam RR, Franklin County Pneumonia Study Group (1996) Bacteremia with *Streptococcus pneumoniae.* Implications for therapy and prevention. JAMA 275:194–198
7. Simpson JC, Macfarlane JT, Watson J, Woodhead MA (2000) A national confidential enquiry into community acquired pneumonia deaths in young adults in England and Wales. British Thoracic Society Research Committee and Public Health Laboratory Service. Thorax 55(12):1040–5
8. Gagnon S, Ahmad M, Boota ND, et al. (1990) Corticosteroids as adjunctive therapy for severe *Pneumocystis carinii* pneumonia in the acquired immunodeficiency syndrome. N Engl J Med 323:1444–1450
9. Bozette SA, Sattler FR, Chiu J, et al. (1990) A controlled trial of early adjunctive treatment with corticosteroids for *Pneumocystis carinii* pneumonia in the acquired immunodeficiency syndrome. N Engl J Med 323:1451–1457
10. Mer M, Richards GA (1998) Corticosteroids in life-threatening varicella pneumonia. Chest 114:426–431

11. Goldman M, Johnson PC, Sarosi GA (1999) Fungal pneumonias. The endemic mycoses. Clin Chest Med 20:507–519
12. Bradsher RW (1996) Histoplasmosis and blastomycosis. Clin Infect Dis 22:S102–S111
13. Tognian S, Jiayu Y, Liye Z, Weiwu D, Zhaoying S (1981) Chemotherapy and its combination with corticosteroids in acute miliary tuberculosis in adolescents and adults: analysis of 55 cases. Chin Med J 94:309–314
14. Lebel MH, Freij BJ (1988) Dexamethasone therapy for bacterial meningitis: results of two double-blind, placebo controlled trials. N Engl J Med 319:964–971
15. Marik P, Kraus P, Sribante J, Havlik I, Lipman J, Johnson DW (1993) Hydrocortisone and tumor necrosis factor in severe community-acquired pneumonia. Chest 104:389–392
16. Klugman K (1990) Pneumococcal resistance to antibiotics. Clin Microbiol Rev 3:171–196
17. Monton C, Ewig S, Torres A, et al. (1999) Role of glucocorticoids on inflammatory response in nonimmunosuppressed patients with pneumonia: a pilot study. Eur Respir J 14(1):218–20
18. Confalonieri M, Urbino R, Potena A, et al. (2005) Hydrocortisone infusion for severe community-acquired pneumonia: a preliminary randomized study. Am J Respir Crit Care Med 171(3):242–8
19. Confalonieri M, Potena A, Carbone G, Porta RD, Tolley EA, Umberto Meduri G (1999) Acute respiratory failure in patients with severe community-acquired pneumonia. A prospective randomized evaluation of noninvasive ventilation. Am J Respir Crit Care Med 160(5):1585–91
20. Light RB (1986) Indomethacin and acetylsalicylic acid reduce intrapulmonary shunt in experimental pneumococcal pneumonia. Am Rev Respir Dis 134:520–525
21. Hanley PJ, Roberts D, Dobson K, et al. (1987) Effect of indomethacin on arterial oxygenation in critically ill patients with severe pneumonia. Lancet 1:351–354
22. Bernard GR, Reines HD, Halushka RV, Higgins SB, Metz CA, Swindell BB, et al. (1991) Prostacyclin and thromboxane A_2 formation is increased in human sepsis syndrome. Am Rev Respir Dis 144:1095–1101
23. Ferrer M, Torres A, Baer R, Hernández C, Roca J, Rodriguez-Roisin R (1997) Effect of acetylsalicylic acid on pulmonary gas exchange in patients with severe pneumonia: a pilot study. Chest 111:1094–1100
24. Dowling HF, Lepper MH (1951) The effect of antibiotics (penicillin, aureomycin, and terramycin) on the fatality rate and incidence of complications in pneumococcic pneumonia. A comparison with other methods of therapy. Am J Med Sci 222:396–403
25. Kohzuki T, Eguchi Y, Kato M, Irie K, Ohtsuka H, Higuchi A, et al. (1993) Protective activity of anti-exotoxin A monoclonal antibody against mice infected with toxin-producing *Pseudomonas aeruginosa*. J Infect Dis 167:119–125
26. Hector RF, Collins MS, Pennington JE (1989) Treatment of experimental *Pseudomonas aeruginosa* pneumonia with a human IgM monoclonal antibody. J Infect Dis 160:483–489
27. Pennington JE, Hickey WF, Blackwood LL, et al. (1981) Active immunization with lipopolysaccharide *Pseudomonas* antigen for chronic *Pseudomonas* bronchopneumonia in guinea pigs. J Clin Invest 68:1140–1148
28. Saravolatz LD, Markowitz N, Collins MS, Bogdanoff D, Pennington JE (1991) Safety, pharmokinetics, and functional activity of human anti-*Pseudomonas aeruginosa* monoclonal antibodies in septic and nonseptic patients. J Infect Dis 167:784–785
29. Greenman RL, Schein RMH, Martin MA, et al. (1991) A controlled trial of E5 murine monoclonal IgM antibody to endotoxin in the treatment of gram-negative sepsis. JAMA 266:1097–1102
30. Ziegler EJ, Fisher CJ, Sprung CL, et al. (1991) Treatment of gram-negative bacteremia and septic shock with HA-1A human monoclonal antibody against endotoxin: a randomized, double blind, placebo-controlled trial. N Engl J Med 324:429–436
31. Klimek JJ, Ajemian E, Tontecchio S, Gracewski J, Klemas B, Jiminez L (1983) Community-acquired bacterial pneumonia requiring admission to hospital. Am J Infect Control 11:79–82
32. Aubertin J, Dabis F, Fleurett J, Bornstein N, Salamon R, Brottier E, et al. (1987) Prevalence of legionellosis among adults: a study of community-acquired pneumonia in France. Infection 15:328–331
33. Fang GD, Fine MJ, Orloff J, Arisumi D, Yu VL, Kapoor W, et al. (1990) New and emerging etiologies for community-acquired pneumonia with implications for therapy. A prospective multicenter study of 359 cases. Medicine 69: 307–316
34. Lieberman D, Schlaeffer F, Boldur I, Horowitz S, Friedman MG, Leiononen M, et al. (1996) Multiple pathogens in adult patients admitted with community-acquired pneumonia: a one year prospective study of 346 consecutive patients. Thorax 51:179–184
35. Tateda K, Matsumoto T, Ishii Y, Furuya N, Ohno A, Miyazaki S, et al. (1998) Serum cytokines in patients with *Legionella* pneumonia: relative predominance of Th1-type cytokines. Clin Diag Lab Immunol 5:401–403
36. Friedman H, Yamamoto Y, Newton C, Klein T (1998) Immunologic response and pathophysiology to *Legionella* infection. Semin Resp Infect 13:100–108
37. Murray HW (1989) Interferon-gamma, the activated macrophage, and host defense against microbial challenge. Ann Intern Med 108:608
38. Nathan CF, Prendergast TJ, Wiebe ME, Stanley ER, Platzer E, Remold HG, et al. (1984) In vivo and in vitro activation of alveolar macrophages by recombinant interferon-γ. J Exp Med 160:600–605
39. Skerrett SJ, Martin TR (1994) Intratracheal interferon-γ augments pulmonary defenses in experimental legionellosis. Crit Care Med 149:50–58
40. Jaffe R, Buhl R, Mastrangeli A, Holroyd KJ, Saltini C, Czerski D, et al. (1991) Organ specific cytokine therapy. J Clin Invest 88:297–302
41. Condos R, Rom WN, Schluger NW (1997) Treatment of multidrug-resistant pulmonary tuberculosis with interferon-gamma via aerosol. Lancet 349:1513–1515
42. Bernard GR, Vincent JL, Laterre PF, et al. (2001) Efficacy and safety of recombinant human activated protein C for severe sepsis. N Engl J Med 344(10):699–709
43. Laterre PF, Garber G, Levy H, et al. (2005) Severe community-acquired pneumonia as a cause of severe sepsis: data from the PROWESS study. Crit Care Med 33(5):952–61
44. Ely EW, Laterre PF, Angus DC, et al. (2003) Drotrecogin alfa (activated) administration across clinically important subgroups of patients with severe sepsis. Crit Care Med 31(1):12–9
45. Remolina C, Khan AU, Santiago TV, et al. (1981) Positional hypoxemia in unilateral lung disease. N Engl J Med 304:523
46. Carlon GC, Ray CR, Klein R, et al. (1978) Criteria for selective positive end-expiratory pressure and independent synchronized ventilation of each lung. Chest 74:501–507
47. Hillman KM, Barber JD (1980) Asynchronous independent lung ventilation (AILV). Crit Care Med 8:390–395
48. Ranieri VM, Suter PM, Tortorella C, De Tullio R, Dayer JM, Brienza A, et al. (1999) Effect of mechanical ventilation on

inflammatory mediators in patients with acute respiratory distress syndrome: a randomized controlled trial. JAMA 282:77–78
49. Zapol WM, Snider MT, Hill JD (1979) Extracorporeal membrane oxygenation in severe acute respiratory failure. A randomized prospective study. JAMA 242:2193
50. ECMO Registry of the Extracorporeal Life Support Organization (ELSO) (1997) ECMO Quarterly Report January 1997
51. Green TP, Timmons OD, Fackler JC, Moler FW, Thompson AE, Sweeney MF, et al. (1996) The impact of extracorporeal membrane oxygenation on survival in pediatric patients with acute respiratory failure. Crit Care Med 24:323–329
52. Masiakos PT, Islam S, Doody DP, Schnitzer JJ, Ryan DP (1999) Extracorporeal membrane oxygenation for nonneonatal acute respiratory failure. Arch Surg 134:375–379
53. Meyer TA, Warner BW (1997) Extracorporeal life support for the treatment of viral pneumonia: collective experience from the ELSO registry. J Pediatr Surg 32:232–236
54. Kolla S, Awad SS, Rich PB, Schreiner RJ, Hirschl RB, Bartlett RH (1997) Extracorporeal life support for 100 adult patients with severe respiratory failure. Ann Surg 226:544–564
55. Ichiba S, Jenkins DR, Peek GJ, Brennan KJ, Killer HM, Sosnowski A, et al. (1999) Severe acute respiratory failure due to legionella pneumonia treated with extracorporeal membrane oxygenation. Clin Infect Dis 28:686–687
56. Nakajima H, Kutsuwada T, Ohdaira T, Saito A, Satoh K, Igarashi K, et al. (1997) Extracorporeal membrane oxygenation for acute respiratory failure induced by *Legionella pneumoniae*. Nihon Kyobu Shikkan Gakkai Zasshi 35: 1363–1367
57. Codispoti M, Sanger K, Mankad PS (1995) Successful extracorporeal membrane oxygenation (ECMO) support for fulminant community-acquired pneumococcal pneumonia. Thorax 50:1317–1319
58. Lee WA, Kolla S, Schreiner RJ, Hirschl RB, Bartlett RH (1997) Prolonged extracorporeal life support for varicella pneumonia. Crit Care Med 25:997–982
59. Crowley MR, Katz RW, Kessler R, Simpson SQ, Levy H, Hallin GW, et al. (1998) Successful treatment of adults with severe Hantavirus pulmonary syndrome with extracorporeal membrane oxygenation. Crit Care Med 26:409–414
60. Dickson EW, Heard SO, Chu B, Fraire A, Brueggemann AB, Doern GV (1998) Partial liquid ventilation with perfluorocarbon in the treatment of rats with lethal pneumococcal pneumonia. Anesthesiology 88:218–223
61. Quezado ZM, Natanson C, Karzai W, Danner RL, Koev CA, Fitz Y, et al. (1998) Cardiopulmonary effects of inhaled nitric oxide in normal dogs and during *E. coli* pneumonia and sepsis. J Appl Physiol 84:107–115
62. Anggard E (1994) Nitric oxide: mediator, murderer, and medicine. Lancet 343:1199–1206
63. Hoehn T, Huebner J, Paboura E, Krause M, Leititis JU (1998) Effect of therapeutic concentrations of nitric oxide on bacterial growth *in vitro*. Crit Care Med 26:1857–1862
64. Chollet-Martin S, Gatecel C, Kermarrec N, Gougerot-Pocidalo M, Payen DM (1996) Alveolar neutrophil functions and cytokine levels in patients with the adult respiratory distress syndrome during nitric oxide inhalation. Am J Respir Crit Care Med 153:985–990
65. Walmrath D, Schneider T, Pilch J, Schermuly R, Grimminger F, Seeger W (1995) Effects of aerosolized prostacyclin in severe pneumonia. Am J Respir Crit Care Med 151: 724–730
66. Confalonieri M, Potena A, Carbone G, Della Porta R, Tolley EA, Meduri GU (1999) Acute respiratory failure in patients with severe community-acquired pneumonia. A prospective randomized evaluation of noninvasive ventilation. Am J Respir Crit Care Med 160:1585–1591
67. Joshi N, Localio AR, Hamory BH (1992) A predictive risk index for nosocomial pneumonia in the intensive care unit. Am J Med 93:135–142
68. Olivier KN, Bennett WD, Hohneker KW, Zeman KL, Edwards LJ, Boucher RC, et al. (1996) Acute safety and effects on mucociliary clearance of aerosolized uridine 5'-triphospate ± amiloride in normal human adults. Am J Respir Crit Care Med 154:217–223

39 Respiratory Infection in Immunocompromised Neutropenic Patients

S.W. Crawford

39.1 Scope of Problem

Neutropenia is increasingly common in the hospital. The rise in incidence is due to proliferation of indications for and centers performing hematopoietic stem cell transplantation, hematologic effects of AIDS, and myelosuppressive side-effects of anti-viral and cancer chemotherapies (Table 39.1). As a result, these neutropenic patients are increasingly common in the intensive care units. These patients are often lymphopenic, anemic, and thrombocytopenic. They are at risk for multiple organ failures and various infections. This chapter will focus on respiratory infections in the neutropenic patient.

Table 39.1. Some causes of neutropenia

Drug myelosuppression
Chemotherapy
Ganciclovir
Trimethaprim-sulfamethoxazole
Viral infection
Late stages of AIDS
Herpes viruses
Congenital deficiency
Inherited cyclic neutropenia
Functional defects
Corticosteroids
Chediak-Higashi syndrome
Myeloperoxidase deficiency
Chronic granulomatous diseases

39.2 Neutropenia and the Risk Factors for Infection

The neutrophil plays a key role in the host defense of extracellular bacteria (especially encapsulated organisms affected by opsonizing antibodies) and the molds and yeasts. The incidence of serious infection in neutropenic patients increases with the depth, rapidity of onset, and duration of neutropenia. The risk of infection increases with an absolute neutrophil count (ANC) $<1{,}000$ cells/mm^3, and is significantly higher with an ANC <500 cells/mm^3. A rapid decline in ANC and duration of neutropenia $>7-10$ days are associated with an increase in serious, life-threatening infection. Likewise, morbidity and mortality are increased in patients with profound neutropenia (ANC <100/mm^3) [1–3].

A study of severe, short-duration neutropenia demonstrates that fungal infections are rare when the ANC is reduced for less than 5 days. Neutropenic fever developed in 94% of patients after peripheral stem cell transplantation [4]. Profound neutropenia was short-lived (average 5 days) and most patients' fever defervesced in a median of 4 days. Although bacteremia developed in 39% (predominately Gram-positive cocci), only 5% had pulmonary infiltrates and there were no fungi identified and no infection-related deaths.

Neutrophil function before chemotherapy to treat leukemia influences infection rates [5]. Patients with a significant decrease in phagocytic activity of neutrophils developed more severe infection or died more often compared to those with no infection. Study of the neutrophil oxidative burst capacity suggested that the neutrophils may have been pre-activated and have reduced function prior to the initiation of chemotherapy.

Neutropenia associated with myelosuppression, as occurs after chemotherapy, rarely occurs in isolation from other defense defects. Lymphopenia, decreased humoral immunity, and mucosal barrier defects invariably contribute to the defense abnormalities that predispose to infection in these settings.

Both tumors and chemotherapy contribute to infection among neutropenic patients. Obstruction of the lymphatic, biliary tract, gastrointestinal or urinary systems by tumors or as a result of surgical procedures is a common cause of infections. Chemotherapy not only decreases the number of neutrophils, but also results in chemotactic and phagocytic defects. Chemotherapy, radiation, peripheral and central intravenous lines, surgery, or tumor invasion can induce breakdown of skin and mucosal barriers and can result in bacteremia. Mucositis may occur throughout the gastrointestinal system. Translocation of endogenous flora in the GI tract may explain a majority of febrile neutropenic episodes.

39.3 Trends in Infection in the Neutropenic Patient

Historically, Gram-negative bacilli, particularly *P. aeruginosa*, were the most commonly identified pathogens. Data from several sources attest to a decrease in the incidence of pseudomonal bacteremia and an increase in Gram-positive infections. The use of long-term indwelling lines accounts for some of the appearance of Gram-positive infections; the empiric antibiotic regimens that were designed to cover *P. aeruginosa* may be an additional factor. For example, the incidence of bacteremia due to Gram-negative bacilli in Japan decreased (40% to 64%) and infections due to Gram-positive bacteria increased (51% to 24%) in 1991 to 1996 compared to the prior 15 years [6]. According to the 2002 nationwide, concurrent surveillance study (Surveillance and Control of Pathogens of Epidemiological Importance [SCOPE]) Gram-positive organisms caused 65% of bloodstream infections, Gram-negative organisms caused 25%, and fungi caused 9.5%. The most-common organisms were coagulase-negative staphylococci (CoNS) (31%), *Staphylococcus aureus* (20%), enterococci (9%), and *Candida* species (9%) [7].

In the last decade there has been an increasing incidence of Gram-positive cocci infection in the neutropenic population. In these patients, infections with enterococci, viridans group streptococci and *Candida* species are significantly more common [7]. Notably, reports of *Candida* species isolates are up 20-fold since the 1980s. *Aspergillus* reports have increase 14-fold. In addition, the number of "unusual" fungal species (*Trichosporon, Fusarium, Mucor)* is also increased.

Importantly, there has been an alarming increase in the frequency of antibiotic resistant organism isolation. These pathogens include coagulase negative staphylococci, methicillin-resistant *Staphylococcus aureus* (MRSA), vancomycin-resistant enterococci (VRE), and penicillin (ceftriaxone)-resistant *S. pneumonia*.

39.4 Sites and Causes of Infections

Mortality in the febrile, neutropenic population is high, in the range of 30–50%. Early studies of empiric antibiotics in febrile neutropenia suggested that a majority of patients had occult bacterial infections. However, an infectious source is identified in only approximately 30% of febrile neutropenic episodes. Often the only evidence of infection is bacteremia, which occurs in over 20% of patients. Approximately 80% of identified infections are believed to arise from patients' own endogenous flora. The most commonly identified sources of infection in febrile neutropenic patients with leukemia are the perineal and perirectal areas, followed by the urinary tract, skin (including intravenous lines and wounds) and the lungs. However, among non-hematopoietic cancer patients pulmonary infections predominate. Many infections are detected only at autopsy, particularly disseminated fungal or combined fungal and bacterial infections.

There are numerous infections that cause pneumonia in cancer patients [8–10]. Typical bacteria are most common, accounting for over one-third of infections. Fungi, viruses, *Pneumocystis carinii* (PCP), *Nocardia asteroids*, and *Mycobacterium tuberculosis* account for a measurable number of cases each. Compounding the difficulty in establishing an etiologic agent, mixed infections may be present in up to 20% of cases.

Evidence suggests that fungal infection is a common component of neutropenic fever after chemotherapy. Pneumonia tends to develop several days after the onset of fever. Only 27% of febrile neutropenic patients *with pneumonia* respond without addition of anti-fungal agents. Over half of documented lower respiratory infections are due to fungi. Therefore, it is not surprising that the prognosis is worse for febrile neutropenic patients who develop pneumonia.

Noninfectious etiologies are common for immunocompromised patients with pulmonary infiltrates. Causes include pulmonary embolus, tumor, radiation pneumonia, atelectasis, pulmonary hemorrhage, and drug allergy or toxicity. Aspiration remains an important source of pulmonary infection in all compromised patients.

39.5 Bacterial Pathogens

Viridans streptococci (both *mitis* and *sanguis*) have become of major concern in the neutropenic host. These organisms are associated with 39% of neutropenic bacteremia after chemotherapy [11]. The complications associated with these organisms are: ARDS, shock, and endocarditis. An ANC $< 100/mm^3$ is among the strongest risk factors.

Institutional infection patterns impact the frequency and type of organisms isolated and a variety of nosocomial outbreaks in cancer patients have been reported. Some centers have reported an increased incidence of resistant pathogens such as *Candida krusei* with the routine use of prophylactic antibiotics and antifungals [12–14]. Antibiotic history, recent culture results, exposure to prophylactic antibiotics, and the susceptibility patterns for organisms in the institution should be used to help guide selection of initial antibiotic therapy.

39.6 Fungal Pathogens

Fungal infections probably represent the greatest infectious risk to neutropenic patients. Fungal infections are common among neutropenic patients, and usually arise after prolonged neutropenia and antibiotic use. Empiric antibiotics promote oral and vaginal colonization with yeast, most commonly *Candida albicans*. Hepato-splenic involvement is common in patients with disseminated candidiasis after chemotherapy. Often, symptoms are absent until the neutropenia resolves. Current diagnostic tests lack sufficient sensitivity to distinguish invasive yeast infection from colonization [15].

The incidence of nosocomial candidal infections continues to rise in the United States, and *C. albicans* is the most commonly identified species. Candidal infections are associated with the highest mortality rates of all hospital-acquired bloodstream infections, with substantial related increases in hospital costs, particularly length of stay.

The fourth most common pathogens causing nosocomial bloodstream infections in US hospitals are fungi, predominantly *Candida* species, representing 9.5% of all isolates [7, 16]. Clearly, *Candida* species are increasing in importance in the ICU as well. *Candida albicans* accounts for just over half of candidal species isolated. *C. tropicalis*, *C. glabrata*, and *C. parapsilosis* contribute 44% of isolates [17]. Speciation is importance since *C. tropicalis* and *C. krusei* are resistant to fluconazole, the agent more commonly used to treat yeast infection in the ICU. The crude mortality associated with these pathogens increases with decreasing prevalence. Mortality with the most common, coagulase-negative staphylococci is 21% and rises to 40% with the *Candida* species infections. The mortality attributable to *Candida* has been estimated at 70–88% [18, 19]. Diagnosis of candidiasis in the neutropenic host should be considered an indication for urgent therapy. The death rates among neutropenic patients with candidiasis are as high as 24% within a week of diagnosis and 63% within 3 months [20]. Although lower among patients without neutropenia, the rates are still high.

Candida is a common infection among neutropenic patients but a *rare* cause of pneumonia. Haron reported that there were only 31 cases documented at autopsy over 20 years at the MD Anderson Cancer Center [21]. The clinical and radiographic presentation of these cases was that of bronchopneumonia. There were no distinguishing features of the infection to identify the organism. Of note, most of the patients were *not* neutropenic at time of onset of pneumonia.

Candidiasis is rare in the absence of colonization of the skin, rectum or throat. Gut translocation may account for a substantial proportion of cases. The major threat to life is associated with disseminated, invasive candidiasis. Candidal invasion is associated with identified risk, and thus there are also risks for mortality. The reported risks include:

- Use of three of more antibiotics
- Neutropenia
- Immunosuppression (due to cancer/chemotherapy, steroids, other therapies)
- Concomitant infection
- Spending more than 4 days in the ICU
- Mechanical ventilation >48 h
- An elevated APACHE II score
- Abdominal surgery
- Central venous catheterization
- Total parenteral nutrition (TPN)
- Diabetes mellitus
- *Candida* colonization of more than sites
- Candiduria (>100,000 colonies/ml)
- Thrush

The therapeutic choices for treatment of systemic candida infections include fluconazole, conventional amphotericin B, liposomal amphotericin B, and lipid-complex amphotericin B. All of these are available intravenously. Only fluconazole is available orally; however, this is rarely an issue in the ICU population. There are conflicting data regarding the equivalence of fluconazole with amphotericin B in the neutropenic patient [22–24]. However, fluconazole is associated with less renal dysfunction, hypokalemia, and lower liver enzymes than amphotericin B.

Infections with molds, such as *Aspergillus* sp., vary from localized skin ulcers and invasive pneumonia, to fulminant disseminated disease. *Fusarium* sp. infections have been increasingly reported in the immunocompromised host [23–27]. Reactivation of endemic fungi (histoplasmosis, blastomycosis, and coccidioidomycosis) or tuberculosis mimics the radiographic presentation of invasive fungal pneumonia and should be considered in appropriate patients with prolonged steroids or immune suppression.

A review of the clinical presentations of invasive pulmonary aspergillosis (IPA) in a study of 35 confirmed cases demonstrated that the diagnosis of IPA was not suspected in 40% of the cases [28]. The lungs were involved in 94% and the infection was limited to lungs in 74%. Other sites of infection were the heart, CNS, liver, spleen, and skin. Only 40% were neutropenic at the time of diagnosis but 91% had used steroids in the recent past. Of importance to the management of IPA, concurrent infections were found in 83% of cases. The mortality rate was 94%.

39.7 Viral Pathogens

Viral infections, especially human herpes viruses, are common in the neutropenic population. However, neutropenia per se is not the primary risk factor for viral infection. Cell-mediated immunity (CMI) is the most important host defense against most respiratory viral pathogens. Since many patients with neutropenia also have concomitant defects in CMI, they are at risk. Herpes simplex viruses, HSV-1 and HSV-2, while common causes of skin eruptions, can also cause a wide variety of clinical syndromes, including: encephalitis, meningitis, myelitis, esophagitis, pneumonia, hepatitis, erythema multiforme, and ocular syndromes. Immunocompromised patients with disseminated varicella zoster virus (VZV) infection can have pulmonary involvement and should be placed on respiratory precautions to prevent aerosolized transmission to susceptible individuals. Cytomegalovirus remains a significant cause of diffuse pneumonia and respiratory failure among transplant recipients.

Of great concern is the emergence of respiratory viral infections including respiratory syncytial virus (RSV) as significant causes of nosocomial pneumonia. Outbreaks of infection resulting in diffuse pneumonia and respiratory failure have been reported among severely myelosuppressed patients after chemotherapy [29]. These infections should be suspected during winter and spring months, if there is associated airflow obstruction, or if upper respiratory tract symptoms preceded the onset of infiltrates. Many of the outbreaks reported appear to have been nosocomial. Visitors and hospital staff are like responsible for transmission of the virus. Prompt treatment with ribavirin (with or without immunoglobulin) has been reported as beneficial. There are few data from large series to support that these are effective treatments in severely ill neutropenic patients.

39.8 Radiographic Diagnosis

The radiographic appearance of pneumonia in the neutropenic patient carries important diagnostic information as to the possible etiology of infection. A focal or multifocal consolidation of acute onset is most commonly caused by a bacterial infection. However, similar multifocal lesions with a subacute to chronic progression may be due to fungal, tuberculous, or nocardial infections. Large nodules are usually a sign of fungal or nocardial infection in this patient population, particularly if they are subacute to chronic in onset. Viruses (especially CMV) or *P. carinii* usually cause subacute disease with diffuse abnormalities, either peri-bronchovascular or small miliary nodules. The presence of cavitation suggests a necrotizing infection that can be caused by fungi, *Nocardia*, and certain Gram-negative bacilli (most commonly *Klebsiella pneumoniae* and *Pseudomonas aeruginosa*) [9].

Table 39.2. Radiographic mimics of invasive pulmonary aspergillosis

Mucor, Fusarium, Scedosporium, etc.
Legionella
Nocardia
Rhodococcus
Gram negative enterics
Pulmonary embolism
BOOP

Chest computed tomography of the chest can help to assess the extent of the disease process and more completely define its characteristics. The morphology of the abnormalities found on CT scan can also be very useful in developing a differential diagnosis in the individual patient. Cavitary mass lesions are suggestive of infections with *Nocardia*, *Cryptococcus*, or invasive fungus, such as *Aspergillus*. The invasive fungal pneumonias classically develop cavitation and a surrounding zone of radiographic attenuation. This zone is presumably due to associated edema and hemorrhage. However, this finding is non-specific. Any process or infection resulting in lung infarction can yield similar CT findings (Table 39.2) [30]. In contrast, dense regional or lobar consolidation on CT is suggestive of bacterial pneumonia.

Chest CT scanning may identify the site for optimal sampling and assist in defining the most appropriate invasive procedure. Thus, CT can provide precise guidance for needle biopsy or for thoracoscopic or open lung excision in the case of peripheral lung nodules [31, 32]. CT can also help to predict whether bronchoscopy is likely to be useful. As an example, the demonstration of a feeding bronchus in association with a pulmonary nodule greatly increases the diagnostic yield when bronchoscopy is performed (60% versus 30% when the feeding bronchus is not visible). If CT demonstrates centrally located diffuse opacifications, a bronchoscopic approach is the procedure of choice.

39.9 Treatment

39.9.1 Antibacterial Drugs

None of the numerous antibiotic regimens studied as initial empiric therapy in febrile neutropenia has been shown to be clearly superior [33]. The majority of the tested regimens provide coverage targeted at Gram-negative bacilli, especially *P. aeruginosa*. The most common empiric treatment approaches include either "monotherapy" (with agents such as ceftazidime, imipenem, meropenem, or cefepime) or "double coverage" (with a beta-lactam and an aminoglycoside, or double beta-lactams).

Double beta-lactams are generally avoided due to the concern of overlapping toxicities. However, double coverage with the aztreonam and a beta-lactam in patients unable to tolerate an aminoglycoside may be a reasonable alternative. Two drug regimens for empiric therapy of febrile neutropenia are widely used. Clinical trials with monotherapy, either ceftazidime or imipenem cilastatin or meropenem, have demonstrated equal efficacy compared to two drug regimens [34, 35]. In one study treatment with meropenem was compared to ceftazidime in 187 patients; the number of patients on the therapy at 72 h and the completion of treatment was equivalent between the groups (50% versus 56% and 46% versus 49%, respectively) [36]. However, changes in the antibiotic regimen are more common when monotherapy is used [2, 34].

The French Febrile Aplasia Study Group report is one of the few studies to show differences in empiric antibiotic regimen [37]. The empirical use of a piperacillin/tazobactam and amikacin combination had superior response rates compared to ceftazidime and amikacin (48% versus 29%). Notably, the response rates to ceftazidime and amikacin decreased over time as the incidence of Gram-negative infections declined from 22% to 17.5%. The incidence of Gram-positive infections increased from 20% to 28%. This study provides increasing evidence of the fungal infection problem in neutropenic hosts. There was an increase in *Aspergillus*-related deaths (from 1.8% to 5.4%), while the overall infection-related mortality remained unchanged over time. It remains important to continue to monitor microbiology regardless of initial antibiotic choices.

Vancomycin is frequently considered in patients who present with hypotension, mucositis, skin or catheter site infection, a history of MRSA colonization, recent quinolone prophylaxis or persistent fever despite empiric antibiotics. However, addition of vancomycin to the initial empiric antibiotic regimen has not been shown to decrease mortality [2, 38]. The addition of empiric vancomycin did not improve outcome among febrile neutropenic patients with skin and soft tissue infections despite a higher incidence of proven Gram-positive bacteremia compared to patients with other infections (31% versus 17%) [39]. Current recommendations suggest withdrawal of vancomycin after 3 days in culture negative cases [7].

39.9.2 Antifungal Drugs

The incidence of fungal infection (especially *Candida* or *Aspergillus*) rises after patients have experienced more than 7 days of persistent fever and neutropenia [40]. Antifungal therapy is routinely added at 5–7 days of neutropenia in patients with persistent fever. While amphotericin B has been used for empiric therapy the longest, there is growing experience with fluconazole and lipid formulations of amphotericin B.

Fluconazole is well tolerated but is ineffective against *Aspergillus* and some yeast (e.g., *C. krusei* and *C. glabrata*). A retrospective study of hematogenous candidiasis from the M.D. Anderson Cancer Center found that fluconazole prophylaxis appeared to be significant in promoting a shift toward *C. krusei* and *C. glabrata* infection and away from *C. tropicalis* and *C. albicans* [14].

Fluconazole prophylaxis is frequently used in populations at risk for *Candida* infection, such as neutropenic chemotherapy or organ transplant recipients. A review of 355 autopsies after marrow transplantation detected a disturbing trend among those patients who received fluconazole prophylaxis [41]. The treatment was effective in decreasing both *Candida* infections (from 27% to 8%) and fungal liver infection (from 16% to 3%). However, *Aspergillus* infections increased from 18% to 29%. Duration of survival increased but overall mortality was unchanged. The authors surmised that the fluconazole prophylaxis increased duration of survival by decreasing early infection with *Candida* and thus increased the exposure to *Aspergillus* infections. Fluconazole is generally not recommended as empiric therapy because of this study and a meta-analysis demonstrating no benefit on mortality or systemic fungal infections [42].

Recent trials suggest that lipid formulations of amphotericin B are better tolerated and offer similar efficacy. In one large randomized, multicenter trial, 343 neutropenic patients received liposomal amphotericin B (3 mg/kg per day) and 344 amphotericin B (0.6 mg/kg per day) as empiric therapy after at least 5 days of fever and broad-spectrum antibiotics [43]. The outcomes were comparable for the two therapies for overall success (50% versus 49%), resolution of fever during neutropenia (58% versus 58%), absence of documented fungal infection (90% versus 89%), and cure of fungal infection (82% versus 73%). The liposomal preparations were better tolerated than conventional amphotericin with fewer infusion related symptoms including rigors and less nephrotoxicity. However, these new forms of amphotericin are significantly more expensive.

Recent studies suggest that itraconazole in a daily dose of 200–400 mg also may be effective treatment for aspergillosis in patients refractory or intolerant to amphotericin B. Itraconazole is available both in oral and intravenous formulations. Itraconazole was as effective as amphotericin B as empiric therapy for febrile neutropenic patients and was associated with less toxicity [44].

Two newer agents include an azole, voriconazole and an echinocandin, caspofungin. Each have been compared to liposomal amphotericin and show promise in febrile neutropenia [45, 46]. The roles of these agents remain unclear and the potential for combination therapy unexplored.

39.9.3 Colony Stimulating Factors

The role of colony stimulating factors (CSF) continues to expand. In some clinical settings, CSF have been reported to decrease the duration of neutropenia, fever, and hospitalization [47–49]. However, CSF have not been shown to decrease mortality, and are not considered routine at this time [50]. It may be appropriate to consider their use in critically ill patients such as those with pneumonia, hypotension, or organ dysfunction or in patients whose bone marrow recovery is expected to be especially prolonged.

References

1. Hathorn JW, Lyke K (1997) Empirical treatment of febrile neutropenia: evolution of current therapeutic approaches. Clin Infect Dis 24 Suppl 2:S256
2. Pizzo PA (1993) Management of fever in patients with cancer and treatment-induced neutropenia. N Engl J Med 328: 1323
3. Rubin RH, Ferraro MJ (1993) Understanding and diagnosing infectious complications in the immunocompromised host. Current issues and trends. Hematol Oncol Clin North Am 7:795
4. Kolbe K, Domkin D, Derigs HG, Bhakdi S, Huber C, Aulitzky WE (1997) Infectious complications during neutropenia subsequent to peripheral blood stem cell transplantation. Bone Marrow Transplant 19:143–147
5. Hubel K, Hegener K, Schnell R, et al. (1999) Suppressed neutrophil function as a risk factor for severe infection after cytotoxic chemotherapy in patients with acute nonlymphocytic leukemia. Ann Hematol 78:73
6. Funada H, Matsuda T (1998) Changes in the incidence and etiological patterns of bacteremia associated with acute leukemia over a 25-year period. Intern Med 37:1014
7. Wisplinghoff H, Bischoff T, Tallent SM, Seifert H, Wenzel RP, Edmond MB (2004) Nosocomial bloodstream infections in US hospitals: analysis of 24,179 cases from a prospective nationwide surveillance study. Clin Infect Dis 39:309–17
8. Ramsey PG, Rubin RH, Tolkoff-Rubin NE, et al. (1980) The renal transplant patient with fever and pulmonary infiltrates: Etiology, clinical manifestations, and management. Medicine 59:206
9. Rubin RH, Greene R (1994) Clinical approach to the compromised host with fever and pulmonary infiltrates. In: Rubin RH, Young LS (eds) Clinical approach to infection in the compromised host, 3rd edn. Plenum Press, New York, p 121
10. Chanock S (1993) Evolving risk factors for infectious complications of cancer therapy. Hematol Oncol Clin North Am 7(4):771
11. Bochud PY, Eggiman P, Calandra T, Van Melle G, Saghafi L, Francioli P (1994) Bacteremia due to viridans streptococcus in neutropenic patients with cancer: clinical spectrum and risk factors. Clin Infect Dis 18:25–31
12. Goodman JL, Winston DJ, Greenfield RA, et al. (1992) A controlled trial of fluconazole to prevent fungal infections in patients undergoing bone marrow transplantation. N Engl J Med 326:845
13. Oppenheim BA (1998) The changing pattern of infection in neutropenic patients. J Antimicrob Chemother 41:S7
14. Abi-Said D, Anaissie E, Uzun O, Raad I, Pinzcowski H, Vartivarian S (1997) The epidemiology of hematogenous candidiasis caused by different *Candida* species. Clin Infect Dis 24:1122–1128
15. Sugar AM (1990) Empiric treatment of fungal infections in the neutropenic host: review of the literature and guidelines for use. Arch Intern Med 150:2258
16. Edmond MB, Wallace SE, McClish DK, Pfaller MA, Jones RN, Wenzel RP (1999) Nosocomial bloodstream infections in United States hospitals: a three-year analysis. Clin Infect Dis 29:239–244
17. Pfaller MA, Messer SA, Hollis RJ, Jones RN, Doern GV, Brandt ME, Hajjeh RA (1999) Trends in species distribution and susceptibility to fluconazole among blood stream isolates of *Candida* species in the United States. Diagn Microbiol Infect Dis 33:217–222
18. Digiovine B, Chenoweth C, Watts C, Higgins M (1999) The attributable mortality and costs of primary nosocomial bloodstream infections in the intensive care unit. Am J Respir Crit Care Med 160:976–981
19. Fraser VJ, Jones M, Dunkel J, Storfer S, Medoff G, Dunagan WC (1992) Candidemia in a tertiary care hospital: epidemiology, risk factors, and predictors of mortality. Clin Infect Dis 15:414–421
20. Anaissie EJ, Rex JH, Uzun O, Vartivarian S (1998) Predictors of adverse outcome in cancer patients with candidemia. Am J Med 104:238–245
21. Haron E, Vartivarian S, Anaissie E, Dekmezian R, Bodey GP (1993) Primary *Candida* pneumonia. Experience at a large cancer center and review of the literature. Medicine (Baltimore) 72(3):137–42
22. Winston DJ, Hathorn JW, Schuster MG, Schiller GJ, Territo MC (2000) A multicenter, randomized trial of fluconazole versus amphotericin B for empiric antifungal therapy of febrile neutropenic patients with cancer. Am J Med 108: 282–289
23. Malik IA, Moid I, Aziz Z, Khan S, Suleman M (1998) A randomized comparison of fluconazole with amphotericin B as empiric anti-fungal agents in cancer patients with prolonged fever and neutropenia. Am J Med 105:478–483
24. Kanda Y, Yamamoto R, Chizuka A, Hamaki T, et al. (2000) Prophylactic action of oral fluconazole against fungal infection in neutropenic patients. A meta-analysis of 16 randomized, controlled trials. Cancer 89:1611–1625
23. Richardson SE, Bannatyne RM, Summerbell RC, et al. (1988) Disseminated fusarial infection in the immunocompromised host. Rev Infect Dis 10:1171
24. Boutai EI, Anaissie EJ (1997) Fusarium, a significant emerging pathogen in patients with hematologic malignancy: ten year's experience at a cancer center and implications for management. Blood 90:999
25. Krcmery V Jr, Kunova E, Jesenska Z, et al. (1996) Invasive mold infections in cancer patients: Five years' experience with *Aspergillus, Mucor, Fusarium* and *Acremonium* infections. Support Care Cancer 4:39

26. Martino P, Gastaldi R, Raccah R, et al. (1994) Clinical patterns of *Fusarium* infections in immunocompromised patients. J Infect 28:7
27. Walsh TJ, Hiemenz JW, Seibel NL, et al. (1996) Amphotericin B lipid complex for invasive fungal infections: Analysis of safety and efficacy in 556 cases. Clin Infect Dis 26:1383
28. Kaiser L, Huguenin T, Lew PD, Chapuis B, Pittet D (1998) Invasive aspergillosis. Clinical features of 35 proven cases at a single institution. Medicine 77:188
29. Whimbey E, Couch RB, Englund JA, Andreeff M, Goodrich JM, Raad II, Lewis V, Mirza N, Luna MA, Baxter B, et al. (1995) Respiratory syncytial virus pneumonia in hospitalized adult patients with leukemia. Clin Infect Dis 21:376–9
30. Won HJ, et al. (1998) Invasive pulmonary aspergillosis: Prediction at thin-section CT in patients with neutropenia – A prospective study. Radiology 208:777–782
31. Jamzen DL, Adler BD, Padley SPG, et al. (1993) Diagnostic success of bronchoscopic biopsy in immunocompromised patients with acute pulmonary disease: Predictive value of disease distribution as shown on CT. Am J Roentgenol 160:21
32. Scott WW, Kuhlman JE (1991) Focal pulmonary lesions in patients with AIDS: Percutaneous transthoracic needle biopsy. Radiology 180:419
33. Peacock JE, Herrington DA, Wade JC, Lazarus HM, Reed MD, Sinclair JW, Haverstock DC, Kowalsky SF, Hurd DD, Cushing DA, Harman CP, Donowitz GR (2002) Ciprofloxacin plus piperacillin compared with tobramycin plus piperacillin as empirical therapy in febrile neutropenic patients. A randomized, double-blind trial. Ann Intern Med 137:77–87
34. Pizzo PA, Hathorn JW, Hiemenz J, et al. (1986) A randomized trial comparing ceftazidime alone with combination antibiotic therapy in cancer patients with fever and neutropenia. N Engl J Med 315:552
35. Cometta A, Calandra T, Gaya H, et al. (1996) Monotherapy with meropenem versus combination therapy with ceftazidime plus amikacin as empiric therapy for fever in granulocytopenic patients with cancer. The International Antimicrobial Therapy Cooperative Group of the European Organization for Research and Treatment of Cancer and the Gruppo Italiano Malattie Ematologiche Maligne dell'Adulto Infection Program. Antimicrob Agents Chemother 40:1108
36. Lindblad R, Rodjeer S, Adriansson M, et al. (1998) Empiric monotherapy for febrile neutropenia – A randomized study comparing meropenem with ceftazidime. Scand J Infect Dis 30:237
37. Marie JP, et al. (1998) Neutropenic infections: Review of the French Febrile Aplasia Study Group trials in 608 febrile neutropenic patients. J Antimicrob Chemo 41 (Suppl D):57–64
38. Vardakas KZ, Samonis G, Chrysanthopoulou SA, Bliziotis IA, Falagas ME (2005) Role of glycopeptides as part of initial empirical treatment of febrile neutropenic patients: a meta-analysis of randomised controlled trials. Lancet Infect Dis 5:431–439
39. Dompeling EC, Donnelly JP, Deresinski SC, et al. Early identification of neutropenic patients at risk of grampositive bacteraemia and the impact of empirical administration of vancomycin. Eur J Cancer 32:1332
40. Kibbler CC (1997) Empirical antifungal therapy in febrile neutropenic patients: Current status. Current Topics in Medical Mycology 8:5
41. Einsele H, Hebart H, Roller G, Loffler J, Rothenhofer I, Muller CA, Bowden RA, van Burik J, Engelhard D, Kanz L, Schumacher U (1997) Detection and identification of fungal pathogens in blood by using molecular probes. J Clin Microbiol 35:1353–60
42. Kanda Y, Yamamoto R, Chizuka A, Hamaki T, Suguro M, Arai C, Matsuyama T, Takezako N, Miwa A, Kern W, Kami M, Akiyama H, Hirai H, Togawa A (2000) Prophylactic action of oral fluconazole against fungal infection in neutropenic patients. A meta-analysis of 16 randomized, controlled trials. Cancer 89:1611–1625
43. Walsh TJ, Finberg RW, Arndt C, et al. (1999) Liposomal amphotericin B for empirical therapy in patients with persistent fever and neutropenia. N Engl J Med 340:764
44. Boogaerts M, Winston DJ, Bow EJ, Garber G, Reboli AC, Schwarer AP, Novitzky N, Boehme A, Chwetzoff E, De Beule K (2001) Intravenous and oral itraconazole versus intravenous amphotericin B deoxycholate as empirical antifungal therapy for persistent fever in neutropenic patients with cancer who are receiving broad-spectrum antibacterial therapy. A randomized, controlled trial. Ann Intern Med 135:412–422
45. Walsh TJ, Pappas P, Winston DJ, Lazarus HM, Petersen F, Raffalli J, et al. (2002) Voriconazole compared with liposomal amphotericin B for empirical antifungal therapy in patients with neutropenia and persistent fever. N Engl J Med 346:225–234
46. Walsh TJ, Teppler H, Donowitz GR, Maertens JA, Baden LR, Dmoszynska A, Cornely OA, Bourque MR, Lupinacci RJ, Sable CA, dePauw BE (2004) Caspofungin versus liposomal amphotericin B for empirical antifungal therapy in patients with persistent fever and neutropenia. N Engl J Med 351:1391–1402
47. Maher DW, Lieschke GJ, Green M, et al. (1994) Filgrastim in patients with chemotherapy-induced febrile neutropenia. A double-blind, placebo-controlled trial. Ann Intern Med 121:492
48. Rowe JM (1998) Treatment of acute myeloid leukemia with cytokines: Effect on duration of neutropenia and response to infections. Clin Infect Dis 26:1290
49. Rodriguez-Adrian LJ, Grazziutti ML, Rex JH, Anaissie EJ (1998) The potential role of cytokine therapy for fungal infections in patients with cancer: Is recovery from neutropenia all that is needed? Clin Infect Dis 26:1270
50. Ozer H, Armitage JO, Bennett CL, Crawford J, Demetri GD, et al. (2000) 2000 update of recommendations for the use of hematopoietic colony-stimulating factors: evidence-based, clinical practice guidelines. American Society of Clinical Oncology Growth Factors Expert Panel. J Clin Oncol 18:3558–3585

Chapter 40

Pneumonia in Non-Neutropenic Immunocompromised Patients

J.M. Cisneros, E. Cordero, J. Pachón

40.1 Introduction

Pneumonia is a main cause of morbidity and mortality in immunocompromised patients. In general, the severity and type of immunosuppression determine both the incidence and etiology of pneumonia. In this chapter, pneumonia will be analyzed in two large groups of immunocompromised patients: patients infected by the human immunodeficiency virus (HIV) and solid organ transplant (SOT) recipients. Epidemiology, etiology, prognosis and the main clinical features of pneumonia will be reviewed in each of these two populations of patients.

40.2 Pneumonia in HIV-Infected Patients

40.2.1 Incidence, Risk Factors and Etiology

Pneumonia is one of the main causes of morbi-mortality in HIV-infected patients. The incidence of bacterial pneumonia shows a sixfold increment in HIV-infected patients when compared with the seronegative population (5.5 episodes/year vs. 0.9 episodes/year), increasing as CD4+ T-cell count decreases. In patients with a CD4 count > 500, the incidence of pneumonia is 2.3 episodes per 100 person-years; with 200–500 it is 6.8; and with < 200 the incidence reaches 10.8 episodes. Other risk factors such as intravenous drug use and cigarette smoking are associated with an increased rate of pneumonia [1].

The etiology of pneumonia in HIV-infected patients is very varied, including community, nosocomial and opportunistic pathogens, as a consequence of the large number of risk factors concurring in these patients. Table 40.1 shows the etiology of pneumonia in HIV-infected patients. In addition, the differential diagnosis of pneumonia in these patients includes other non-infectious pathologies such as lymphoma, lung cancer, bronchiolitis obliterans with organizing pneumonia, lymphocytic interstitial pneumonitis, pulmonary hypertension, and some specific entities of this chronic infection such as Kaposi's sarcoma. Etiology has changed after standardization of universal prophylaxis against *Pneumocystis jiroveci* when the T-helper cell count (CD4+) is less than 200 cells/mm^3 and the highly active antiretroviral treatment (HAART) is used.

Table 40.1. Etiology of pneumonia in HIV-infected patients

Category	Pathogen
Bacterial	*Streptococcus pneumonia* *Staphylococcus aureus* *Haemophilus influenzae* *Pseudomonas aeruginosa* *Moraxella catarrhalis* *Legionella pneumophila* *Rhodococcus equi* *Nocardia asteroides*
Mycobacterial	*Mycobacterium tuberculosis* *Mycobacterium kansasii* *Mycobacterium avium* complex
Fungal	*Pneumocystis jiroveci* *Cryptococcus neoformans* *Histoplasma capsulatum* *Coccidioides immitis* *Aspergillus* spp.
Viral	Cytomegalovirus Influenza virus Parainfluenza virus Respiratory syncytial virus
Protozoal	*Toxoplasma gondii*

For years, *P. jiroveci* pneumonia has been the first disease to indicate AIDS in HIV-infected patients, with an annual incidence of 24% in patients with CD4 counts below 200 cells/µl with no prophylaxis [2]. Currently, *P. jiroveci* pneumonia affects mainly those patients out of sanitary control who do not receive specific prophylaxis [3]. Conversely, the incidence of pneumococcal pneumonia has not decreased since the emergence of HAART and is still very high (531 cases/100,000 inhabitants per year) [4]. *Pseudomonas aeruginosa* pneumonia affects patients with low CD4 counts; it is usually community-acquired and presents a subacute course with an unfavorable evolution and frequent relapses [5]. Among the bacterial etiologies, *Staphylococcus aureus* is of relevance as a cause of community-acquired pneumonia, even methicillin-resis-

Table 40.2. Changes in the etiology of pneumonia before and after 1996–97, when HAART appeared

Etiology	Before 1996–7(%)	After 1996–7(%)
Streptococcus pneumoniae	39–40	33
Pseudomonas aeruginosa	7–18	11
Haemophilus influenzae	14	12.5
Staphylococcus aureus	6–15	12
Rhodococcus equi	6.3	2.8
Klebsiella pneumoniae	3–11	3.3
Escherichia coli	2–4	2.8
Streptococcus gr. *viridans*	4.2	0.9
Mycoplasma pneumoniae	4.2	2.8
Coxiella burnetii	1.5	1.4
Salmonella spp.	1	6.7
Nocardia asteroides	1	0.5
Legionella pneumophila	0–1	0.9
Chlamydia pneumoniae	0–7	10

tant strains, appearing in outbreaks [6]. *Haemophilus influenza* is another common bacterium [7]. Table 40.2 shows the changes in the etiology of pneumonia before and after 1996–97, when HAART appeared.

The incidence of coinfection by HIV and *Mycobacterium tuberculosis* varies according to each country's endemics. In Spain, the incidence of tuberculosis in AIDS-patients fluctuates between 3.4 and 7.6 per 100 inhabitants, being the first opportunistic infection in these patients [8]. In the USA its incidence is estimated at approximately 6,000–9,000 new cases per year [9]. Coinfection by HIV and *M. tuberculosis* is a crucial public health concern as shown by the multiresistant nosocomial tuberculosis epidemic which occurred in Florida and New York, leading to an extremely high mortality (80%) in HIV-infected patients [10]. CMV pneumonia is rare, appearing in severely immunocompromised HIV patients, and the clinical features resemble *P. jiroveci* pneumonia. The presence of extrapulmonary CMV disease should suggest the diagnosis of CMV pneumonia [11].

40.2.2 Diagnostic Approach

Integrating the information from the clinical history with that from analytical tests is the best method to guide the etiological diagnosis of this complex syndrome which comprises pneumonia in HIV-infected patients.

Among the patient's personal antecedents, the immune status, determined by the CD4+ cell count, deserves special attention. A CD4 count below 200 cells/μl is associated with a maximum risk of infection by opportunistic microorganisms such as *M. tuberculosis*, and bacteria such as *P. aeruginosa*, *H. influenzae* and *S. pneumoniae*. With CD4 counts above 200 cells/μl, the risk of infection is reduced to just bacterial etiology, including *M. tuberculosis*. The history of previous prophylaxis against *P. jiroveci* is also a relevant antecedent to consider. Finally, other factors such as intravenous drug use, sexual habits, contact with animals (cats, horses and pigeons), imprisonment and immigration from countries with a high incidence of endemic tuberculosis are of great diagnostic interest.

The distinctive clinical picture of the main entities is as follows. Bacterial pneumonias usually present acutely with fever and purulent expectoration of less than 7 days duration. On the contrary, pneumonia caused by opportunistic microorganisms usually has a more insidious presentation. Common symptoms of pneumocystis pneumonia include the subtle onset of progressive dyspnea, non-productive cough and low-grade fever. Tuberculous pneumonia has a subacute presentation in which fever, productive cough and constitutional symptoms predominate. The clinical and radiographic presentation of tuberculosis is heavily influenced by the degree of immunodeficiency. The main predictive factors are exertional dyspnea and oral thrush for *P. jiroveci* pneumonia; fever ≤ 7 days, rhonchi on examination and a 'toxic' appearance for bacterial pneumonia; and fever >7 days and weight loss for tuberculosis [12].

Typical radiographic features of pneumocystis pneumonia are bilateral perihilar interstitial infiltrates that become increasingly homogeneous and diffuse as the disease progresses. A predominantly lobar or segmentary alveolar infiltrate is the most characteristic pattern found in the bacterial etiology, and cavitation in tuberculous pneumonia. Pulmonary cavitation is also commonly found in *S. aureus*, *P. aeruginosa* and *Rhodoccocus equi* pneumonia. The chest radiograph may be normal in cases of pneumonia from *M. tuberculosis* and *P. jiroveci* in severely immunocompromised patients [12].

40.2.3 Prognosis

Pneumonia reduces survival in HIV-infected patients [13]. The average mortality of community-acquired pneumonia in the era of HAART is 9.1%, ranging from 2.3% to 40.5% depending on the severity of pneumonia at diagnosis [14]. Mortality remains high – up to 23% – in *P. jiroveci* pneumonia, even in the current era of HAART [15]. The risk of death in HIV-infected patients with tuberculosis was reported to be twice that in HIV-infected patients without tuberculosis, independently of the CD4 cell count [16].

The main factor of poor prognosis in *P. jiroveci* pneumonia is the delay in the diagnosis [17]. In community-acquired bacterial pneumonia, the factors associated with unfavorable prognosis are the occurrence of shock, CD4 counts <100, pleural effusion, cavitation and multilobar infiltrate [18]; and low CD4 counts, negativity in the tuberculin test and previous opportunistic infections in tuberculous pneumonia [16].

40.2.4 Treatment

The most relevant aspects in the treatment of pneumonia in HIV-infected patients are the following:

In patients with *P. jiroveci* pneumonia with respiratory failure (basal $pO_2 < 70$ mmHg), the administration of steroids, prednisone 40 mg/12 h, reduces mortality [19]. Similarly, in patients with severe pneumonia by *P. jiroveci*, coadministration of HAART with the specific treatment of pneumonia and early non-invasive assisted ventilation improve survival [20, 21].

Treatment of tuberculosis should follow the general principles developed for tuberculosis treatment in non-HIV-infected patients. Because of the severity of tuberculosis disease among HIV-infected patients, directly observed therapy is strongly recommended for patients with HIV-1-related tuberculosis. The optimal duration of treatment is uncertain; 6 months of therapy is probably adequate for the majority of cases, but prolonged therapy (up to 9 months) is recommended for patients with a delayed clinical or bacteriological response to therapy (symptomatic or positive culture results at or after 2 months of therapy, respectively) or perhaps with cavitary disease on chest radiograph [22]. The use of HAART is complicated by overlapping drug toxicity profiles, drug-drug interactions, and an increase in tuberculosis manifestations during immune reconstitution (paradoxical reactions). These paradoxical reactions, occurring in up to 36% of patients, usually present with fever and progression of both pulmonary lesions on the thoracic radiograph and peripheral and mediastinal lymphadenopathies, and are generally self-limited. In order to prevent these reactions, it is recommended to postpone HAART until 4–8 weeks after starting tuberculosis treatment [22, 23]. Initial guidance from the CDC stated that use of rifampin was contraindicated for persons taking nonnucleoside and protease inhibitors. Subsequent data, however, have supported the use of rifampin with certain combinations of antiretroviral agents. These include ritonavir and efavirenz with nucleoside/tide reverse transcriptase. Rifabutin could be used with most protease inhibitors, including atazanavir and fosamprenavir, provided the dose of rifabutin is reduced. Conversely, efavirenz can reduce concentrations of rifabutin, necessitating an increase in the dose of rifabutin [24].

40.2.5 Prevention

Adults and adolescents who have HIV infection should receive chemoprophylaxis against *P. jiroveci* if they have a CD4+ T-lymphocyte count of less than 200/μl or a history of oropharyngeal candidiasis. Patients with a CD4+ T-lymphocyte percentage of less than 14% or a history of an AIDS-defining illness but who do not otherwise qualify should be considered for prophylaxis. Trimethoprim-sulfamethoxazole is the recommended prophylactic agent. One double-strength tablet per day or one single-strength tablet per day is the preferred regimen. One double-strength tablet three times per week is also effective [25]. *Pneumocystis* prophylaxis should be discontinued in adult and adolescent patients who have responded to HAART with an increase in CD4+ T-lymphocyte counts to >200 cells/μl for at least 3 months [26]. All HIV-infected persons, regardless of age, who have a positive tuberculin skin test result yet have no evidence of active tuberculosis and no history of treatment for active or latent tuberculosis should be treated for latent tuberculosis infection. Isoniazid 300 mg once daily for 9 months is the option of choice [25].

Adults and adolescents who have a CD4+ T-lymphocyte count of greater than or equal to 200 cells/μl should be administered a single dose of pneumococcal conjugate vaccine if they have not received this vaccine during the previous 5 years. HIV-infected children younger than 5 years old should also be administered *H. influenzae* type b vaccine [25, 27].

40.3 Pneumonia in Solid Organ Transplant Recipients

40.3.1 Introduction

Solid organ transplant (SOT) represents a therapeutic option in patients with end-stage renal, cardiac, hepatic or pulmonary disease. In Spain, the development of transplant programs has been increasing, reaching donation rates of 34.6 per million inhabitants and with 294 heart transplants, 1,040 liver transplants and 2,125 kidney transplants performed in 2004 [28]. This continuous increase has been the consequence of the improving results. Currently, the actuarial survival at 1 year post-transplant in recipients of renal, cardiac, hepatic and pulmonary transplants is equal to or higher than 94%, 85%, 86% and 77%, respectively [29].

Pneumonia, a main cause of morbimortality in these patients, comprises a complex clinical syndrome of diverse presentations and wide etiologies, thus making early diagnosis and treatment very important and very difficult.

40.3.2 Incidence and Risk Factors

The recipient of an organ transplant is a host with a high risk of pneumonia due to multiple risk factors concurring during the post-transplant period, all of them configuring the distinctive chronology of infection in these patients.

The classification of post-SOT pneumonia – nosocomial vs. community-acquired – is harder to establish in these patients than in the general population, since the incubation period of opportunistic microorganisms is highly variable, and also because these patients, after being discharged from hospital, are still exposed to a certain degree of nosocomial infections due to the frequent explorations and follow-up visits required, so these infections should rather be considered as healthcare-associated infections [30].

The main risk factors of early post-transplant pneumonia are pulmonary colonization or infection occurring before transplant, colonization or infection of the transplanted graft, a relevant factor in lung transplant, and nosocomial infection especially when associated with mechanical ventilation. In a more specific way, reintubation and treatment with high doses of steroids have been identified as crucial risk factors of pneumonia in cardiac transplant recipients [31]. In late-onset pneumonia, after the first month post-transplant, the severity and type of immunosuppression are the main risk factors [31–33]. Up to 95% of post-transplant pneumonia episodes occur within the first 6 months [34]. The incidence of community-acquired pneumonia during the first year post-transplant is 10.7% and 5.9% in cardiac and hepatic transplant recipients respectively, while in the general population the incidence is 0.26 cases per 100 inhabitants per year [34–36].

40.3.3 Etiology

The etiology of pneumonia in SOT recipients is very varied with a high presence of opportunistic microorganisms and polymicrobial infections as shown in Table 40.3. The most frequent etiologies will be reviewed.

Cytomegalovirus (CMV) used to be the primary cause of pneumonia in SOT recipients, with a wide range of variations ranging from 2% in renal transplants to 32% in pulmonary transplants [29]. The incidence of CMV pneumonia has progressively decreased and so in cardiac transplants it has evolved from 16% in 1977–88 to 4.4–7.7% in the 1990s [33, 34, 37], and from 5% in 1984–5 to 0% in 1989–94 in liver transplant recipients [35, 38]. CMV pneumonia is frequently polymicrobial, *P. jiroveci* and *Aspergillus* spp. being the co-pathogens most commonly isolated [34]. The main risk factors are primary infection and type of immunosuppression [33, 39].

Pneumocystis jiroveci, a common cause of pneumonia in SOT recipients, has disappeared due to the generalization of prophylaxis with cotrimoxazole [40]. The risk factors for the development of *P. jiroveci* are CMV infection and previous graft rejection episodes [41].

Table 40.3. Etiology of pneumonia in solid organ transplant recipients

Early pneumonia (<30 days post-transplant)	Late pneumonia (>30 days post-transplant)
Bacterial – *Pseudomonas aeruginosa* – *Staphylococcus aureus* – *Acinetobacter baumannii* – *Burkholderia cepacia* – *Legionella pneumophila*	Bacterial – *Streptococcus pneumoniae* – *Haemophilus influenzae* – *Klebsiella pneumoniae* – *Legionella pneumophila* – *Rhodococcus equi* – *Nocardia asteroides* – *Mycobacterium tuberculosis* – Other *Mycobacterium*
Virus – Herpes simplex virus – Cytomegalovirus	Virus – Cytomegalovirus – Influenza virus A, B – Parainfluenza virus – Respiratory syncytial virus – Epstein-Barr virus
Fungi – *Aspergillus* spp. – *Mucor* spp.	Fungi – *Aspergillus* spp. – *Pneumocystis jiroveci* – *Cryptococcus neoformans* – *Histoplasma capsulatum* – *Coccidioides immitis*
Protozoal – *Toxoplasma gondii*	Protozoal – *Toxoplasma gondii*

The overall incidence of aspergillosis in SOT recipients was 1.4% in a large study [42]. The incidence of *Aspergillus* pneumonia depends on the type of transplant, severity of immunosuppression and degree of environmental exposure. Recipients of pulmonary transplant present the highest incidence (3%), followed by heart recipients (2.4%), liver recipients (2%), pancreas-kidney recipients (0.9%), and kidney recipients (0.2%) [42]. Aspergillosis during the first 3 months after transplantation is significantly associated with a more complicated postoperative period, repeated bacterial infections or cytomegalovirus disease, and renal failure. Aspergillosis after 3 months post-transplant is associated with older patients, an overimmunosuppressed state because of chronic transplant rejection or allograft dysfunction, and post-transplantation renal failure [42]. In liver transplant treatment of graft rejection with high doses of corticosteroids, OKT3 and renal impairment are the main risk factors, while neutropenia is unusual [32].

The incidence of tuberculosis in Spain in SOT recipients (0.8–1.35/100 recipients-year) is 20- to 25-fold higher than in the general population (40–45/100,000 inhabitants per year) [34, 43]. The risk factors of tuberculosis are positivity in the tuberculin skin test, pathological findings in the chest radiograph, treatment against graft rejection and the lack of prophylaxis in patients with a positive tuberculin test [44]. Pneumonia from *Nocardia* spp., mainly *Nocardia asteroides*, in SOT recipients is currently extremely unusual [45].

Community-acquired bacterial pneumonias are tenfold more frequent in cardiac transplant recipients than in the general population (2.6 cases/100 cardiac transplants vs. 258 cases/100,000 inhabitants) [34, 46]. The etiology in these patients is similar to that in the general population, and *Streptococcus pneumoniae* is the most frequent etiological agent, together with *H. influenzae* [31, 34]. *P. aeruginosa* and *Burkholderia cepacia* are a cause of recurrent pneumonia in pulmonary transplant recipients due to cystic fibrosis, a disease of difficult management and high mortality [45].

40.3.4 Diagnostic Approach

The differential diagnosis of pulmonary infiltrates in the chest radiograph in SOT recipients is very wide. Infections are by far the most common cause, but other etiologies such as atelectasis, hemorrhage, edema, pulmonary embolism and, in pulmonary transplant recipients, acute graft rejection and bronchiolitis obliterans, are possible causes as well.

The different infections have a characteristic chronology useful in making the differential diagnosis of pneumonia. CMV pneumonia presents 35 days after cardiac, 38 days after hepatic and 76 days after lung transplantation, reaching the highest incidence between the 2nd and 3rd months post-transplant. A later presentation is usually related to prolonged universal prophylaxis [47–50]. *P. jiroveci* pneumonia presents later, at 89 days post-transplant, while pneumonia from *Aspergillus* presents earlier (36 days post-transplant, range 19–139 days). The last pneumonia to occur is tuberculous pneumonia, presenting at 23 months post-transplant [34, 44].

The clinical presentation of CMV and *P. jirovecii* pneumonia is very similar, both subacutely and with common symptoms such as fever, dyspnea and non-productive cough. In lung and heart transplant recipients, however, CMV and *P. jirovecii* pneumonia may present acutely, progressing over a short period to respiratory failure [45, 51]. Hemoptoic expectoration is the most characteristic sign in *Aspergillus* spp. pneumonia [34]. Pulmonary tuberculosis presents with a subacute/chronic course with fever, cough and constitutional syndrome, similar to that in the general population, but with a higher risk of dissemination and a negative tuberculin skin test, so that frequently the diagnosis is made postmortem [43, 44]. The presentation of pneumonia by habitual pathogenic bacteria is usually acute with fever, cough and purulent expectoration [34].

Radiographic manifestations of CMV pneumonia consist of a diffuse interstitial infiltrate with bilateral extension, undistinguishable from *P. jiroveci* pneumonia [52]. Cavitation and nodules are the hallmark of pulmonary aspergillosis (Fig. 40.1) [34]. In pulmonary tuberculosis, the pulmonary infiltrate is the most common radiographic feature, followed by pleural effusion, a miliary pattern and a solitary nodule [44]. Finally, in bacterial pneumonias, the alveolar infiltrate is the predominating pattern.

The diagnostic use of these clinical and radiographic manifestations is limited; in fact only 50% of the em-

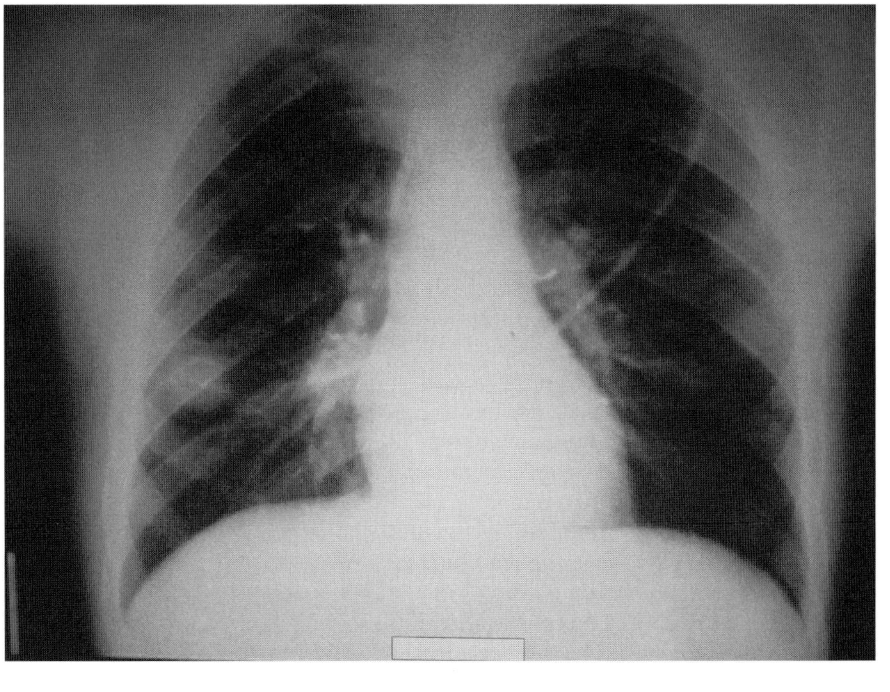

Fig. 40.1. Pulmonary aspergillosis in a liver transplant recipient

pirical treatments indicated in cardiac transplant recipients were appropriate [34]. This fact explains the need for an early and intense diagnostic approach, since the early diagnosis of pneumonia in SOT recipients improves prognosis [53]. Bronchoscopy with bronchoalveolar lavage is the diagnostic procedure of choice in SOT recipients with pulmonary infiltrates, with a diagnostic sensitivity of 63 – 70% [54].

40.3.5 Prognosis

Pneumonia reduces survival in SOT recipients. The mortality in hepatic transplant recipients with pneumonia is 53%, and 10% in those without pneumonia [31, 35]. In patients with pneumonia, poor prognosis factors are nosocomial acquisition, *Aspergillus* spp., bilateral pulmonary infiltrate and a delayed diagnosis [34, 34, 53]. According to the different etiologies, the incidence of mortality in SOT recipients with pneumonia is as follows: 12% for CMV in cardiac transplant patients [33, 34], 26% for *P. jiroveci* [51], 76% for *Aspergillus* [42] and 20% for *M. tuberculosis* [43, 44].

40.3.6 Treatment

The treatment of pneumonia in transplant recipients has two major limitations. First, there are pharmacologic interactions between antimicrobial agents and immunosuppressants, thus favoring toxicity of both groups of drugs as well as graft rejection. Second, there is a high frequency of concurring hepatic and/or renal dysfunction and/or unbalanced intestinal absorption, therefore requiring dose readjustment of antimicrobial agents. Intravenous ganciclovir is the treatment of choice in CMV pneumonia, with responses > 80% [55]. Voriconazole is the first-line treatment in pulmonary aspergillosis [56] and caspofungin is the alternative option [57]. Regarding the treatment of pulmonary tuberculosis, avoiding the use of rifampin is recommended due to the risk of severe interactions with calcineurin inhibitors [44].

40.3.7 Prevention

Valganciclovir is the agent of choice for the prophylaxis of CMV disease. The most frequent strategy used is its preemptive therapy guided by antigenemia and universal prophylaxis during the first 3 months [47, 58, 59].

Cotrimoxazole is the antimicrobial agent of choice in the prophylaxis of *P. jirovecii* pneumonia in SOT recipients. Its efficacy is nearly absolute when administered during the first 6 – 12 months post-transplant [35, 60]. In lung transplant recipients the recommended duration is 1 year in stable patients. Reinitiating or prolonging treatment is recommended whenever the dose of concomitant immunosuppressants is increased. In SOT recipients with cotrimoxazole intolerance, inhaled pentamidine, a single dose of 300 mg monthly, is a safe and effective prophylaxis [61]. Chemoprophylaxis for invasive aspergillosis is not a generalized practice in SOT recipients, with the exception of lung transplantation. In this group of patients, which is the group most frequently affected by aspergillosis, encouraging results in experimental models with aerosolized liposomal amphotericin are reported [62]. Prophylaxis against pulmonary tuberculosis is recommended in both candidates and recipients of SOT with a positive tuberculin test and/or radiographic findings compatible with previous tuberculosis. In patients with chronic hepatitis it is worth considering that the risk of severe hepatic toxicity is 11% [43, 44, 63]. Annual vaccination against influenza viruses is recommended for all candidates and recipients of SOT as well as for close relatives and sanitary staff in contact with these patients. Likewise pneumococcal vaccination is recommended for all SOT recipients [65].

Acknowledgements. We thank Ana Marín for assistance with our written English.

References

1. Hirschtick RE, Glassroth J, Jordan MC, Wilcosky TC, Wallace JM, Kvale PA, et al. (1995) Bacterial pneumonia in persons infected with the human immunodeficiency virus. Pulmonary Complications of HIV Infection Study Group. N Engl J Med 333:845 – 51
2. Phair J, Munoz A, Detels R, Kaslow R, Rinaldo C, Saah A (1990) The risk of *Pneumocystis carinii* pneumonia among men infected with human immunodeficiency virus type 1. Multicenter AIDS Cohort Study Group. N Engl J Med 322: 161 – 5
3. Stansell JD, Osmond DH, Charlebois E, LaVange L, Wallace JM, Alexander BV, et al. (1997) Predictors of *Pneumocystis carinii* pneumonia in HIV-infected persons. Pulmonary Complications of HIV Infection Study Group. Am J Respir Crit Care Med 155:60 – 6
4. Jordano Q, Falco V, Almirante B, Planes AM, del Valle O, Ribera E, et al. (2004) Invasive pneumococcal disease in patients infected with HIV: still a threat in the era of highly active antiretroviral therapy. Clin Infect Dis 38:1623 – 8
5. Schuster MG, Norris AH (1994) Community-acquired *Pseudomonas aeruginosa* pneumonia in patients with HIV infection. AIDS 8:1437 – 41
6. Mathews WC, Caperna JC, Barber RE, Torriani FJ, Miller LG, May S, McCutchan JA (2005) Incidence of and risk factors for clinically significant methicillin-resistant *Staphylococcus aureus* infection in a cohort of HIV-infected adults. J Acquir Immune Defic Syndr 40:155 – 60
7. Cordero E, Pachon J, Rivero A, Giron JA, Gomez-Mateos J, Merino MD, et al. (2000) *Haemophilus influenzae* pneumonia in human immunodeficiency virus-infected patients. The Grupo Andaluz para el Estudio de las Enfermedades Infecciosas. Clin Infect Dis 30:461 – 5

8. Vigilancia Epidemiológica del SIDA en España (2002) In: VIH y SIDA en España. Situación epidemiológica 2001. Ministerios de Sanidad y Consumo. Dirección General de Salud Pública y Consumo. Secretaría del Plan Nacional del Sida, pp 59–82
9. Markowitz N, Hansen NI, Hopewell PC, Glassroth J, Kvale PA, Mangura BT, et al. (1997) Incidence of tuberculosis in the United States among HIV-infected persons. Ann Intern Med 126:123–32
10. Nosocomial transmission of multidrug-resistant tuberculosis among HIV-infected persons – Florida and New York, 1988–1991. MMWR Morb Mortal Wkly Rep 40: 585–91
11. Salomon N, Gomez T, Perlman DC, Laya L, Eber C, Mildvan D (1997) Clinical features and outcomes of HIV-related cytomegalovirus pneumonia. AIDS 11:319–24
12. Selwyn PA, Pumerantz AS, Durante A, Alcabes PG, Gourevitch MN, Boiselle PM, Elmore JG (1998) Clinical predictors of *Pneumocystis carinii* pneumonia, bacterial pneumonia and tuberculosis in HIV-infected patients. AIDS 12:885–93
13. Osmond DH, Chin DP, Glassroth J, Kvale PA, Wallace JM, Rosen MJ, et al. (1999) Impact of bacterial pneumonia and *Pneumocystis carinii* pneumonia on human immunodeficiency virus disease progression. Pulmonary Complications of HIV Study Group. Clin Infect Dis 29:536–43
14. Arozullah AM, Parada J, Bennett CL, Deloria-Knoll M, Chmiel JS, Phan L, Yarnold PR (2003) A rapid staging system for predicting mortality from HIV-associated community-acquired pneumonia. Chest 123:1151–60
15. Benfield TL, Helweg-Larsen J, Bang D, Junge J, Lundgren JD (2001) Prognostic markers of short-term mortality in AIDS-associated *Pneumocystis carinii* pneumonia. Chest 119:844–51
16. Whalen C, Okwera A, Johnson J (1996) Predictors of survival in human immunodeficiency virus-infected patients with pulmonary tuberculosis: the Makerere University-Case Western Reserve University Research Collaboration. Am J Respir Crit Care Med 153:1977–81
17. Lundgren JD, Barton SE, Katlama C, Ledergerber B, Gonzalez-Lahoz J, Pinching AJ, et al. (1995) Changes in survival over time after a first episode of *Pneumocystis carinii* pneumonia for European patients with acquired immunodeficiency syndrome. Multicentre Study Group on AIDS in Europe. Arch Intern Med 155:822–8
18. Cordero E, Pachon J, Rivero A, Giron JA, Gomez-Mateos J, Merino MD, et al. (2000) Community-acquired bacterial pneumonia in human immunodeficiency virus-infected patients: validation of severity criteria. The Grupo Andaluz para el Estudio de las Enfermedades Infecciosas. Am J Respir Crit Care Med 162:2063–8
19. Briel M, Boscacci R, Furrer H, Bucher HC (2005) Adjunctive corticosteroids for *Pneumocystis jiroveci* pneumonia in patients with HIV infection: a meta-analysis of randomised controlled trials. BMC Infect Dis 5:101
20. Morris A, Wachter RM, Luce J, Turner J, Huang L (2003) Improved survival with highly active antiretroviral therapy in HIV-infected patients with severe *Pneumocystis carinii* pneumonia. AIDS 17:73–80
21. Confalonieri M, Calderini E, Terraciano S, Chidini G, Celeste E, Puccio G, et al. (2002) Noninvasive ventilation for treating acute respiratory failure in AIDS patients with *Pneumocystis carinii* pneumonia. Intensive Care Med 28:1233–8
22. Benson CA, Kaplan JE, Masur H, Pau A, Holmes KK (2004) Treating opportunistic infections among HIV-infected adults and adolescents: Recommendations from Centers Diseases Control, the National Institutes of Health, and the HIV Medicine Association/Infectious Diseases Society of America. MMWR Recomm Rep 53:16–21
23. Narita M, Ashkin D, Hollender ES, Pitchenik AE (1998) Paradoxical worsening of tuberculosis following antiretroviral therapy in patients with AIDS. Am J Respir Crit Care Med 158:157–61
24. Centers Diseases Control (2004) Updated guidelines for the use of rifamycins for the treatment of tuberculosis among HIV-infected patients taking protease inhibitors or nonnucleoside. MMWR 53:1–6
25. Public Health Service (USPHS), Infectious Diseases Society of America (IDSA), USPHS/IDSA Prevention of Opportunistic Infections Working Group (2001) 2001 USPHS/IDSA Guidelines for the Prevention of Opportunistic Infections in Persons Infected with Human Immunodeficiency Virus U.S. HIV Clin Trials 2(6):493–554
26. Lopez Bernaldo de Quiros JC, Miro JM, Pena JM, Podzamczer D, Alberdi JC, Martinez E, et al. A randomized trial of the discontinuation of primary and secondary prophylaxis against *Pneumocystis carinii* pneumonia after highly active antiretroviral therapy in patients with HIV infection. Grupo de Estudio del SIDA 04/98. N Engl J Med 344: 159–67
27. Madhi SA, Kuwanda L, Cutland C, Klugman KP (2005) The impact of a 9-valent pneumococcal conjugate vaccine on the public health burden of pneumonia in HIV-infected and -uninfected children. Clin Infect Dis 40:1511–8
28. Organización nacional de trasplantes. Available at: http://www.ont.es. Accessed 12 February 2006
29. Dummer JS (2005) Infections in solid organ transplant recipients. In: Mandell GL, Bennett JE, Dolin R (eds) Principles and practice of infectious diseases, 6th edn, Elsevier, Philadelphia, pp 3501–12
30. Friedman ND, Kaye KS, Stout JE, McGarry SA, Trivette SL, Briggs JP, et al. (2002) Health care-associated bloodstream infections in adults: A reason to change the accepted definition of community-acquired infections. Ann Intern Med 137:791–97
31. Gorensek MJ, Stewart RW, Keys TF, Mehta AC, McHenry MC, Goormastic MA (1988) Multivariate analysis of risk factors for pneumonia following cardiac transplantation. Transplantation 46:860–5
32. Kusne S, Torre-Cisneros J, Mañez R, Irish W, Martin M, Fung J, et al. (1992) Factors associated with invasive lung aspergillosis and the significance of positive *Aspergillus* culture after liver transplantation. Clin Infect Dis 166: 1379–83
33. Kirklin JK, Naftel DC, Levine TB, Bourge RC, Pelletier GB, O'Donnell J, et al. (1994) Cytomegalovirus after heart transplantation. Risk factors for infection and death: a multiinstitutional study. The Cardiac Transplant Research Database Group. J Heart Lung Transplant 13:394–404
34. Cisneros JM, Muñoz P, Torre-Cisneros J, Gurgui M, Rodriguez-Hernandez MJ, Aguado JM, Echaniz A, and the Spanish Transplantation Infection Study Group (1998) Pneumonia after heart transplantation: a multiinstitutional study. Clin Infect Dis 27:324–31
35. Singh N, Gayowski T, Wagener M, Marino IR, Yu VL (1996) Pulmonary infections in liver transplant recipients receiving tacrolimus. Transplantation 61:396–401
36. Marston BJ, Plouffe JF, File TM, Hackman BA, Salstrom SJ, Lipman HB, et al. (1997) Incidence of community-acquired pneumonia requiring hospitalizations: results of a population-based active surveillance study in Ohio. Arch Intern Med 157:1509–18
37. Merigan TC, Renlund DG, Keay S, Bristow MR, Starnes V, O'Connell JB, et al. (1992) A controlled trial of ganciclovir to prevent cytomegalovirus disease after heart transplantation. N Engl J Med 326:1182–6

38. Kusne S, Dummer JS, Singh N, Iwatsuki S, Makowka L, Esquivel C, et al. (1988) Infections after liver transplantation. An analysis of 101 consecutive cases. Medicine 67:132–43
39. Portela D, Patel R, Larson-Keller JJ, Ilstrup DM, Wiesner RH, Steers JL, et al. (1995) OKT3 treatment for allograft rejection is a risk factor for cytomegalovirus disease in liver transplantation. J Infect Dis 171:1014–8
40. Martinez-Marcos F, Cisneros JM, Gentil M, Algarra G, Pereira P, Aznar J, Pachón J (1994) Prospective study of renal transplant infections in 50 consecutive patients. Eur J Clin Microbiol Infect Dis 13:1023–8
41. Arend SM, Westendorp RG, Kroon FP, van't Wout JW, Vandenbroucke JP, van Es LA, van der Woude FJ (1996) Rejection treatment and cytomegalovirus infection as risk factors for *Pneumocystis jiroveci* pneumonia in renal transplant recipients. Clin Infect Dis 22:920–5
42. Gavalda J, Len O, San Juan R, Aguado JM, Fortun J, Lumbreras C, Moreno A, et al. and RESITRA (Spanish Network for Research on Infection in Transplantation) (2005) Risk factors for invasive aspergillosis in solid-organ transplant recipients: a case-control study. Clin Infect Dis 41:52–9
43. Muñoz P, Palomo J, Muñoz R, Rodriguez-Creixéms M, Pelaez T, Bouza E (1995) Tuberculosis in heart transplant recipients. Clin Infec Dis 21:398–402
44. Aguado JM, Herrero JA, Gavalda J, Torre-Cisneros J, Blanes M, Rufi G, et al. (1997) Clinical presentation and outcome of tuberculosis in kidney, liver, and heart transplant recipients in Spain. Spanish Transplantation infection Study Group, GESITRA. Transplantation 63:1278–86
45. Patel R, Paya C (1997) Infections in solid-organ transplant recipients. Clin Microbiol Rev 10:86–124
46. Bartlett JG, Breiman RF, Mandell LA, File TM (1998) Community-acquired pneumonia in adults: guidelines for management. Clin Infect Dis 26:811–38
47. Paya C, Humar A, Dominguez E, Washburn K, Blumberg E, Alexander B, et al. (2004) Efficacy and safety of valganciclovir vs. oral ganciclovir for prevention of cytomegalovirus disease in solid organ transplant recipients. Am J Transplant 4:611–20
48. Falagas ME, Snydman DR, George MJ, Werner B, Ruthazer R, Griffith J, et al. (1996) Incidence and predictors of cytomegalovirus pneumonia in orthotopic liver transplant recipients. Transplantation 61:1716–20
49. Grossi P, Minoli L, Percivalle E, Irish W, Vigano M, Gerna G (1995) Clinical and virological monitoring of human cytomegalovirus infection in 294 heart transplant recipients. Transplantation 59:847–51
50. Macdonald PS, Keogh AM, Marshman D, Richens D, Harvison A, Kaan AM, Spratt PM (1995) A double-blind placebo-controlled trial of low-dose ganciclovir to prevent cytomegalovirus disease after heart transplantation. J Heart Lung Transplant 14:32–8
51. Muñoz P, Muñoz RM, Palomo J, Rodríguez-Creixéms M, Muñoz R, Bouza E (1997) *Pneumocystis carinii* infection in heart transplant recipients. Medicine 76:415–22
52. Schulman LL, Reison DS, Austin JH, Rose EA (1991) Cytomegalovirus pneumonitis after cardiac transplantation. Arch Intern Med 151:1118–24
53. Sugimoto H, Uchida H, Nagao T, Nagao T, Tomikawa S, Mita K, et al. (1994) Improved survival of renal allograft recipients with *Pneumocystis jiroveci* pneumonia by early diagnosis and treatment. Transplant Proc 24:1556–8
54. Baselski VS, Wunderink RG (1994) Bronchoscopic diagnosis of pneumonia. Clin Microbiol Rev 7:533–58
55. Dunn DL, Mayoral J, Gillinham KJ, Loeffler CM, Brayman KL, Kramer MA, et al. (1991) Treatment of invasive cytomegalovirus disease in solid organ transplant patients with ganciclovir. Transplantation 51:98–106
56. Herbrecht R, Denning DW, Patterson TF, Bennet JE, Greene RE, Oestmann JW, et al. (2002) Voriconazole versus amphotericin B for primary therapy of invasive aspergillosis. N Engl J Med 347:408–15
57. Maertens J, Raad I, Petrikkos G, Boogaerts M, Selleslag D, Petersen FB, et al. (2004) Efficacy and safety of Caspofungin for treatment of invasive aspergillosis in patients refractory to or intolerant of conventional antifungal therapy. Clin Infect Dis 39:1563–71
58. Gane E, Saliba F, Valdecasa GJC, OǴrady J, Pescovitz MD, Lyman S, Robinson ChA (1997) Randomised trial of efficacy and safety of oral ganciclovir in the prevention of cytomegalovirus disease in liver-transplant recipients. Lancet 350:1729–33
59. Torre-Cisneros J, Fortun J, Aguado JM, de la Camara R, Cisneros JM, Gavalda J, et al. (2005) Documento de consenso. Recomendaciones GESITRA-SEIMC y RESITRA sobre prevención y tratamiento de la infección por citomegalovirus en pacientes trasplantados. Enferm Infecc Microbiol Clin 23:424–37
60. Torre-Cisneros J, de la Mata M, López-Cillero P, Sanchez-Guijo P, Miño G, Pera C (1996) Effectiveness of daily low-dose cotrimoxazole prophylaxis for *Pneumocystis jiroveci* pneumonia in liver transplantation. An open clinical trial. Transplantation 62:1519–21
61. Saukkonen K, Garland R, Koziel H (1996) Aerosolized pentamidine as alternative primary prophylaxis against *Pneumocystis jiroveci* pneumonia in adult hepatic and renal transplant recipients. Chest 109:1250–5
62. Gavalda J, Martin T, Lopez P, Gomis X, Ramirez JL, Rodriguez D, et al. (2005) Efficacy of high loading doses of liposomal amphotericin B in the treatment of experimental invasive pulmonary aspergillosis. Clin Microbiol Infect 11: 999–1004
63. Fishman JA, Rubin RH (1998) Infection in organ-transplant recipients. N Engl J Med 338:1741–51
64. Blumberg EA, Albano C, Pruett T, Isaacs R, Fitzpatrick J, Bergin J, et al. (1996) The immunogenicity of influenza virus vaccine in solid organ transplant recipients. Clin Infect Dis 22:295–302
65. Centers for Disease Control. Recommended Adult Immunization Schedule – United States, October 2005–September 2006. MMWR 54:Q1–Q4

Community-Acquired Respiratory Complications in the Intensive Care Unit: Pneumonia and Acute Exacerbations of COPD

M.I. Restrepo, A. Anzueto

This chapter will review the two most common lower respiratory tract infections in the intensive care unit (ICU), community-acquired pneumonia (CAP) and acute exacerbations of chronic obstructive pulmonary disease (AECOPD). In addition we will provide an overview of the topics including recommendations for the diagnosis and treatment.

41.1 Severe Community-Acquired Pneumonia in the ICU

Community-acquired pneumonia is the seventh leading cause of death overall and the most common cause of death from infectious diseases in the United States [1, 2]. Based on their clinical condition, patients are admitted to the medical wards, or if severely ill to the ICU. ICU patients carry the highest mortality rates among all patients with CAP [3]. Multiple sets of clinical practice guidelines have been published in the past few years addressing the treatment of CAP, and they all agree that CAP patients admitted to the hospital represent a major concern, and appropriate empiric therapy should be instituted to improve clinical outcomes [3 – 10]. We will review the current literature related to CAP patients admitted to the ICU; regarding epidemiology, risk factors, severity criteria and reasons to admit the hospitalized patient to the ICU, and the empiric and specific antibiotic therapeutic regimens employed.

41.1.1 Epidemiology

Severe CAP is defined as a clinical syndrome that develops in patients with pneumonia who require hospitalization on the ward service and/or ICU [3]. For the year 2000, over 1 million patients were hospitalized in the United States, and 65,000 deaths were attributable to CAP and influenza [11 – 13]. There is an estimated cost of approximately nine billion dollars per year [14]. Approximately 10 % of all hospitalized patients require ICU admission [15 – 17]. Hospitalized CAP patients carry significant mortality depending on the severity of illness. Several studies have reported a mortality rate of approximately 10 % in hospitalized ward patients, and 30 – 60 % mortality in patients who require ICU admission [3, 18]. CAP is burdensome to health care systems as the duration of hospitalization is 6 days at a cost of approximately $7,500 for ward patients compared to 23 days and $21,144 for ICU patients [11, 19, 20].

The most important determinants for hospitalization and assessment of severity in CAP are the patients' chronic co-morbid conditions and/or the prior antibiotic use (see Table 41.1) [3, 7, 8, 10, 21 – 27]. Prior antibiotic use has been defined in the CAP clinical practice guidelines as the use of any antibiotic regime in the past 3 months, and is also associated with increased risk of morbidity and mortality [7, 22, 28]. The most common co-morbid illnesses for CAP patients are chronic obstructive pulmonary disease (COPD), which is present in up to half of these patients, followed by alcoholism, chronic heart disease and diabetes mellitus (Table 41.1 shows the risk factors and associated microorganisms) [3, 7, 8, 10, 23 – 27]. It is important to point out that approximately one-third of patients with CAP were previously healthy [27, 29]. Elderly and nursing home patients are also at significant risk for CAP and have high mortality rates, although some experts consider pneumonia in nursing home patients as health care associated pneumonia due to the similarities in the etiologic pathogens with hospital acquired pneumonia [22, 28, 30]. Hospitalization rates for pneumonia have increased among US adults aged 64 – 74 years and aged 75 – 84 years during the past 15 years. Among those aged 85 years or older, at least 1 in 20 patients were hospitalized each year due to pneumonia [31].

The main causes of death in severe CAP patients include refractory hypoxemia, refractory shock, and other pneumonia-related complications, predominantly multi-organ failure [32 – 37].

The microbial patterns of severe CAP have been extensively studied in the past decade. Consistently, *Streptococcus pneumoniae* is recognized as the most common pathogen causing CAP. Other respiratory

Table 41.1. Risk factors associated with CAP and suggested pathogens

Risk factor	Pathogen
Alcoholism	*Streptococcus pneumoniae* and anaerobes
Cystic fibrosis and other structural lung diseases	*Pseudomonas aeruginosa, Burkholderia cepacia,* and *Staphylococcus aureus*
COPD, smoking and/or bronchiectasis	*S. pneumoniae, Haemophilus influenzae*, GNRs, *Pseudomonas aeruginosa*
Chronic aspiration	Mixed infection, anaerobes, GNRs
Chronic steroid use	*Aspergillus* spp.
Nursing home residents, recent antimicrobial therapy (considered HCAP)	*S. aureus* (MRSA), GNRs, *Pseudomonas aeruginosa*
Influenza	*Staphylococcus aureus, S. pneumoniae, Haemophilus influenzae*
Injection drug users	*S. aureus, S. pneumoniae*, anaerobes, *M. tuberculosis*
Poor dental hygiene	Anaerobes
Exposure to bats or soil with bird droppings	*Histoplasma capsulatum*
Exposure to birds	*Chlamydophila psittaci*
Exposure to cattle	*Coxiella burnetii*
Exposure to rabbits	*Francisella tularensis*
HIV infection (early with high CD4 counts)	*S. pneumoniae, Haemophilus influenza, Mycobacterium tuberculosis*
HIV infection (late with low CD4 counts)	In addition to above pathogens: *Pneumocystis jiroveci, Cryptococcus* spp., *H. capsulatum, Coccidioides* spp.
Winter	Influenza, RSV, adenovirus, parainfluenza, rhinovirus
Skin infections	Community-acquired methicillin resistant *Staphylococcus aureus* (CA-MRSA) [141, 142]
Other	Outbreaks: *Legionella* spp., viruses (avian flu, SARS coronavirus [143], metapneumovirus [144], "Sin Nombre" hantavirus [145, 146]
Additional comorbid conditions[a]	*S. pneumoniae, Haemophilus influenzae*, GNRs, atypical pathogens (*Mycoplasma pneumoniae, Chlamydophila pneumoniae*, and *Legionella* spp.)

GNRs Gram-negative rods, *HCAP* health care associated pneumonia, *MSSA* methicillin-susceptible *S. aureus, MRSA* methicillin-resistant *S. aureus, RSV* respiratory syncytial virus

[a] Include renal failure (chronic renal disease), neurological diseases (cerebrovascular diseases), malnutrition, hepatic disease (chronic liver diseases), bacteremia, smoking history and gross aspiration [23–27, 33, 68]

Table 41.2. Pneumonia severity of index score[a] (adapted from Fine et al. [39])

Criteria	Points
Age	
Male	Age (years)
Female	Age (years) –10
Nursing home resident	+10
Preexisting comorbid conditions	
Neoplastic disease	+30
Liver disease	+20
Congestive heart failure	+10
Cerebrovascular disease	+10
Renal disease	+10
Vital signs abnormalities	
Altered mental status	+20
Respiratory rate > 30 breaths per minute	+20
Systolic blood pressure < 90 mmHg	+20
Temperature < 35° or > 40 °C	+15
Heart rate > 125 per minute	+10
Laboratory or radiographic findings	
Serum blood urea nitrogen > 30 mg/dl	+20
Serum sodium < 130 meq/l	+20
Serum glucose > 250 mg/dl	+10
Hematocrit < 30 %	+10
Arterial pH < 7.35	+30
Arterial oxygen tension (PaO_2) < 60 mmHg or arterial oxygenation saturation < 90 %	+10
Pleural effusion on chest radiograph	+10

[a] For each variable present, the points indicated are added to the score, and the final score is then divided into five risk classes (see Table 41.3)

tract pathogens associated with CAP in the ICU include *Haemophilus influenza, Klebsiella pneumoniae, Legionella* species, *Staphylococcus aureus* and viral pneumonias (Table 41.2). However, there is an extensive list of pathogens associated with severe CAP in the ICU. The association of individual pathogens and certain comorbid conditions was mentioned earlier (Table 41.1), and specific treatment will be discussed at the end of this chapter.

41.1.2 Severity Assessment and Criteria for Hospital and ICU Admission

One of the most critical decisions for physicians treating patients with CAP is whether to hospitalize patients on the ward or ICU service [38]. This decision is usually made in the outpatient office or in the emergency department, and has implications for the antibiotic class selection, route, and duration of therapy.

Two tools have been developed to predict mortality and to determine the site of care for patients with CAP based on the severity of illness, the pneumonia-specific severity of illness (PSI) score and the CURB rule [39–46]. Fine and colleagues developed the PSI score as part of the pneumonia Patient Outcome Research Team Study (PORT) [39]. The PSI is based on 20 parameters including three demographic variables, five

Table 41.3. Pneumonia severity index score risk class stratification[a] (adapted from Fine et al. [39])

Risk class	Points	Mortality (%)	Recommended site of care
I	–[b]	0.1	Outpatient
II	<70	0.6	Outpatient
III	71–90	2.8	Outpatient or brief inpatient
IV	91–130	8.2	Inpatient
V	>130	29.2	Inpatient

[a] Metlay and Fine suggested a three-step process to decide the initial site of CAP treatment based on: (1) assessment of preexisting conditions that compromise safety of home care; (2) calculation of the PSI score; and (3) clinical judgment [47]

[b] Risk class I: age <50 years, no comorbidities and absence of vital-sign abnormalities

Table 41.4. CURB-65 criteria (adapted from Lim et al. [46])

Age >65 years
Altered mental status
Respiratory rate >30 breaths per minute
Diastolic blood pressure <60 mmHg
Serum blood urea nitrogen >19.6 mg/dl

Each criterion has a score of one, and the total score depends on the presence or absence of each of the five criteria. Two or more criteria suggest severe CAP and admission to the hospital is recommended.

co-morbid conditions, five physical examination findings, and seven laboratory/imaging results with the primary goal to identify low risk patients who might be managed safely at home (Tables 41.2, 41.3). In a follow-up paper, the same authors suggested a three-step process to decide the initial site of CAP treatment based on: (1) assessment of preexisting conditions that compromise safety of home care; (2) calculation of the PSI score; and (3) clinical judgment [47]. Similarly, the CURB or CURB-65 (mental status changes, increased blood urea nitrogen, increased respiratory rate, decreased blood pressure, and age above 65 years) was introduced as a much simpler rule to identify patients at low risk of dying and the possible site of care (Table 41.4) [43–46]. Both prognostic tools have been validated in several studies [48–56]. Both tools suggest that CAP patients should be hospitalized if they are included in PSI class IV and V and/or CURB or CURB-65 ≥2. It is important to recognize that these tools should not limit the clinical judgment of practicing physicians to decide site of care. In addition, these tools were not developed to identify which patients with CAP should be admitted to the ICU.

The best accepted criteria for the definition of severe CAP are those patients requiring ICU admission. However, there are recommendations based on seven clinical criteria in the 1993 American Thoracic Society (ATS) guidelines [40, 57] that were further refined by Ewig and collaborators in 1998 [42]. The ATS CAP guidelines adopted this new evidence and recommended the modified ATS criteria for severe CAP [3]. These investigators included the presence of one of the two major criteria and/or two out of three minor criteria (Table 41.5) [42]. Several studies have validated these criteria to admit patients to the ICU and applied them also in other groups of patients including elderly and HIV-infected patients [19, 42, 49, 50, 53, 58, 59].

Table 41.5. American Thoracic Society modified criteria (table adapted from Ewig et al. [3, 42])

Major criteria
Need for mechanical ventilation
Requiring vasopressors (septic shock)
Minor criteria
Respiratory rate >30 breaths per minute
PaO_2/FiO_2 ratio <250
Bilateral or multilobar infiltrates

The presence of at least one major criterion or at least two minor criteria defines a pneumonia severe enough to require ICU admission

Thus, the severity assessment criteria are useful to help physicians identify patients who may need hospitalization or ICU admission, but they are not meant to remove physicians' clinical judgment in the decision-making process.

41.1.3 Diagnosis

All patients suspected of having CAP should receive a chest radiograph to confirm the diagnosis of pneumonia. Several laboratory studies should be performed in patients with CAP admitted to the ICU in order to assess the severity of the disease and possible complications. These tests include: complete blood cell count and differential, basic blood chemistry (urea nitrogen and serum creatinine) electrolytes (sodium and potassium), glucose, and liver function tests. Evaluation of the oxygenation by pulse oxymetry or arterial blood gas analysis is extremely important and mandatory [60]. An attempt to obtain samples to identify the likely etiologic agent is indicated in severe CAP patients [61]. However, there is no supportive evidence that microbiological studies will change favorably the final outcome in these patients. Several microbiological tests are recommended in patients with CAP in the ICU (Table 41.6). In addition, other diagnostic markers including C-reactive protein (CRP) and/or procalcitonin have been used as prognostic indicators with variable results [62, 63].

41.1.4 Antimicrobial Treatment

Treatment guidelines have been developed by several professional organizations to standardize therapy for

CAP, including those patients with severe CAP [3, 6–10]. The published practice guidelines reflect the evolution of expert opinion, changes in resistance patterns and availability of new clinical data regarding the treatment and diagnosis of CAP management in immunocompetent adults. All of these guidelines support the concept that the treatment of ICU patients with CAP should be focused on the possible associated etiologic agents [3, 7, 8, 10]. Appropriate, aggressive and early therapeutic approaches including initiation of antibiotics as early as possible [36, 64] are the main interventions to decrease mortality in patients with CAP in the ICU.

Table 41.6. Laboratory studies recommended in patients with CAP admitted to the ICU

- Blood culture [147]
- Lower respiratory tract sample
  - Gram-stain and culture
    - Sputum [148]
    - Bronchoscopic or non-bronchoscopic evaluation: including either endotracheal aspirate, bronchoalveolar lavage (BAL), protected specimen brush, for quantitative cultures [149]
  - Atypical pathogens (*Mycoplasma pneumoniae*, *Chlamydophila pneumoniae* and *Legionella* spp.) culture or PCR
  - Direct immunofluorescence for influenza and RSV (winter)
  - BAL for respiratory viruses for PCR
- Urinary antigen for:
  - *Legionella* spp. [150–153]
  - *Streptococcus pneumoniae* [154–156]
- Serology testing in the initial and convalescent stages for:
  - Atypical pathogens (*M. pneumoniae*, *C. pneumoniae*, and *Legionella* spp.) if no PCR is available [157]
- Pleural fluid analysis for parapneumonic effusions
- Direct rapid viral test by nucleic acid amplification
  - Influenza, RSV, adenovirus, parainfluenza, rhinovirus

Empiric therapy should be directed against *S. pneumoniae*, *H. influenzae*, and Gram-negative bacilli with beta-lactam medications or new respiratory fluoroquinolones. *Legionella* spp. (and other atypical pathogens) should be covered with a macrolide or a fluoroquinolone [3, 6–8, 10, 65]. Mixed infections with typical and atypical pathogens occur in approximately 5–40% of cases, and should always be considered, to ensure patients are treated with appropriate empiric antimicrobial therapy [3, 6–8, 10, 56, 66, 67]. In cases in which the infecting pathogen can be identified, directed therapy should be employed [3, 6–8, 10]. In all clinical series, approximately 40–70% of patients with CAP have no pathogen identified [25, 68, 69]. The failure to identify a pathogen has not been associated with a worse outcome, but the empiric regimen should cover *S. pneumoniae* and atypical pathogens [15, 16].

The clinical practice guidelines suggest that severe CAP patients admitted to the ICU should be stratified as to whether or not the patients are at risk for *Pseudomonas* spp. infection [3, 7, 10]. If a patient has no risk factors for *Pseudomonas* infection, the treatment should always include two antibiotics, one (beta-lactam) that will cover pneumococcus (including drug resistant isolates) and another (macrolide or respiratory fluoroquinolone) that will cover atypical pathogens especially *Legionella* spp.(Table 41.7) [3, 7, 10, 70]. *Pseudomonas aeruginosa* has been reported in severe CAP patients with specific risk factors, such as chronic or

Table 41.7. Empiric antimicrobial regimen to treat severe community-acquired pneumonia in the ICU (adapted from the clinical practice guidelines [3, 6–10])

Empiric treatment	Comments
Intravenous beta-lactam – Third generation cephalosporins (ceftriaxone or cefotaxime) **or** – Beta-lactam/beta-lactamase inhibitor (ampicillin-sulbactam or piperacillin-tazobactam) **plus either**	Covers well *Streptococcus pneumoniae*, *Haemophilus influenzae*, enteric gram-negative bacilli (*Klebsiella* spp.)
Intravenous macrolide – (azithromycin or clarithromycin) **or** Intravenous fluoroquinolone[a] – (levofloxacin, or moxifloxacin)	*Legionella* spp., *Mycoplasma pneumoniae*, *Chlamydophila pneumoniae* and *C. psittaci*
Intravenous beta-lactam – Antipseudomonal beta-lactam/beta-lactamase inhibitor (aztreonam, ceftazidime, cefepime, piperacillin-tazobactam, imipenem, meropenem) **plus either** Intravenous aminoglycoside or intravenous ciprofloxacin/Levofloxacin [750] **plus** Intravenous macrolide – (azithromycin or clarithromycin) if aminoglycoside used, but not with the use of ciprofloxacin/Levofloxacin [750]	*Pseudomonas aeruginosa* (and the other pathogens above)

[a] Drug resistant *Streptococcus pneumoniae* (DRSP) is also covered by the respiratory fluoroquinolones

prolonged use of broad-spectrum antibiotic therapy, bronchiectasis, malnutrition, HIV and immunosuppression [3, 25, 59, 71, 72]. Patients with risk factors for *P. aeruginosa* admitted to the ICU require specific attention and should receive appropriate antipseudomonal agents as discussed below (Table 41.7).

Only two randomized control trials and several observational studies have evaluated the benefit of using combination therapy versus monotherapy in patients with severe CAP admitted to the ICU [73, 74]. From the limited data and significant heterogeneity between studies, we conclude that there is limited information to compare the differences in mortality for patients with CAP in the ICU. On the other hand, there is strong evidence supporting the clinical practice guidelines [3, 7, 10] by demonstrating statistically significant benefit for those patients receiving guideline concordant therapies in patients with CAP [49, 65, 75–78]. In addition, there is data to support the benefit of using a combination therapy of beta-lactamic agent plus a macrolide for initial empiric therapy to reduce mortality in patients with CAP [77].

41.1.4.1 Specific Antimicrobial Therapy

Streptococcus pneumoniae is isolated in up to one-third of all ward and ICU patients [23–26, 34, 59, 68, 69]. Several studies published by Moroney et al. [79], Kalin et al. [80], and Metlay et al. [81] evaluated clinical outcomes in patients with bacteremic pneumococcal pneumonia. Antimicrobial resistance in bacteremic *S. pneumoniae* showed no contribution to mortality or the requirement for ICU admission, but may be associated with an increased risk of adverse outcome such as suppurative complications of infection (such as empyema) [79–81]. Waterer et al. found that single effective drug therapy for severe bacteremic pneumococcal pneumonia was associated with a greater risk of death than dual effective therapy [82]. Several other studies suggested a benefit of having a macrolide added to the beta-lactam therapy in patients with bacteremic pneumococcal pneumonia [83–86]. Not adding a macrolide to a beta-lactam based initial antibiotic regimen was an independent predictor of in-hospital mortality [85]. All

Table 41.8. Specific antimicrobial therapy for patients with CAP

Pathogen specific	Recommended therapy
Streptococcus pneumoniae	
Bacteremic	Combination therapy with beta-lactam plus macrolide or fluoroquinolone
Intermediate resistance to penicillin (≤2 mg/dl)	*Third generation cephalosporin, or respiratory fluoroquinolone*
High level of resistance to penicillin (≤2 mg/dl)	*Respiratory fluoroquinolone, vancomycin, linezolid*
Staphylococcus aureus	
MSSA	Third generation cephalosporin, respiratory fluoroquinolone, or clindamycin
MRSA (CA-MRSA)[a]	Vancomycin or linezolid
Atypicals: *Chlamydophila pneumoniae*, *Mycoplasma pneumoniae* and *Legionella* spp.	Respiratory fluoroquinolone, macrolide or doxycycline (not for *Legionella* spp.)
Haemophilus influenzae	Amoxicillin
Beta-lactamase producer	Third-generation cephalosporin, beta-lactam/beta-lactamase inhibitors or a fluoroquinolone, newer macrolide (clarithromycin or azithromycin), or doxycycline
Enterobacteriaceae including *Escherichia coli*, *Klebsiella pneumoniae*, *Klebsiella oxytoca*, *Proteus mirabilis*	Third-generation cephalosporin, beta-lactam/beta-lactamase inhibitors or a fluoroquinolone
Pseudomonas aeruginosa	Intravenous antipseudomonal beta-lactam/beta-lactamase inhibitor plus either intravenous aminoglycoside or intravenous ciprofloxacin/Levofloxacin [750], plus an intravenous macrolide if aminoglycoside used, but not with the use of ciprofloxacin/Levofloxacin [750]
Coxiella burnetii or *Chlamydophila psittaci*	Macrolide or tetracycline
Influenza pneumonia [7, 158]	The newer agents oseltamivir or zanamivir cover both influenza A and B [7][b]
Aspiration pneumonia anaerobic infections	Carbapenems, clindamycin or beta-lactam/beta-lactamase inhibitors [159]

[a] CA-MRSA community-acquired methicillin-resistant *S. aureus* usually not multidrug resistant

[b] Influenza; CDC reported high levels of resistance in the 2005–2006 season [160]

other specific antimicrobial therapies for identified CAP pathogens are described in Table 41.8.

41.1.5 Duration of Therapy

Generally, the duration of therapy in patients with severe CAP is 7–10 days, but those with atypical pathogens such as *Legionella* spp. should receive longer treatment for 10–14 days [3, 87]. Several studies report the use of a critical pathway to improve the treatment for CAP patients, including those with severe disease [88–93].

Antimicrobial treatment failure or non-resolving pneumonia is usually underestimated [94]. The most common causes include microbial resistance to the initial antimicrobial regimen, suppurative complications, or the presence of nosocomial pneumonia [95].

After the initial clinical improvement, hospitalized patients should be switched from intravenous to oral antibiotic therapy, while maintaining similar antimicrobial coverage and tissue concentrations as with the parenteral form. Criteria for determining when the patient can make the transition to oral antibiotics include the ability to tolerate antibiotics by mouth, a functioning gastrointestinal tract, a stable blood pressure, a trend towards normalization of the white blood cell count, and improving symptoms such as cough, dyspnea and fevers [96–98]. A meta-analysis by Rhew et al. evaluated early intravenous to oral conversion and discharge strategies in patients with CAP, and demonstrated that these interventions are associated with a significant and safe reduction in the mean length of hospital stay [96].

Several of the quality indicators already mentioned, early administration of antibiotics, appropriate antibiotic use following the clinical practice guidelines, use of a critical pathway, switch to oral therapy and early discharge all show improved clinical outcomes in CAP [3, 7, 8, 10]. In addition, measures directed at prevention such as vaccination for pneumococcal and influenza infections, and counseling to quit smoking for patients at risk, may help to decrease the incidence of CAP [3, 7, 8, 10]. Other important processes of care include the collection of blood cultures before antibiotic administration, or in the first 24 h, a test for *Legionella* infections in ICU patients and an evaluation of oxygenation (measurement of blood gases or pulse oximetry).

41.2 Acute Exacerbations of COPD in the ICU

We will describe the diagnosis and antibiotic treatment of acute exacerbations of chronic obstructive pulmonary disease (AECOPD).

41.2.1 Epidemiology

Chronic obstructive pulmonary disease (COPD) is a condition associated with AECOPD. COPD currently accounts for approximately 110,000 deaths per year, making it, following heart disease, cancer, and stroke, the fourth leading cause of death in the United States. It has been estimated that by the year 2020, AECOPD will be the third leading cause of death [99]. The cost of treating AECOPD is very high, not only because of the economic impact, but also because of the high associated morbidity and early mortality. COPD in the United States annually accounts for 16,000,367 office visits, 500,000 hospitalizations, and 18 billion dollars in direct health care costs [100]. Despite treatment with antibiotics, bronchodilators, and corticosteroids, up to 28% of patients discharged from the Emergency Department with acute exacerbations have recurrent symptoms within 14 days [101] and 17% relapse and require hospitalization [102]. Several investigators have confirmed that relapse is more likely among patients who have lower pretreatment or post-treatment FEV_1, those who receive more bronchodilator treatments or corticosteroids during visits, and those who have higher rates of previous relapse [103].

AECOPD can be associated with significant mortality. In the Study to Understand Prognosis and Preferences for Outcomes and Rates of Treatment (SUPPORT) [104], the 180-day mortality rate was 33% and the 2-year mortality rate was 49%. Significant predictors of mortality include acute physiology and chronic health evaluation (APACHE III) score [105], body mass index, age, functional status 2 weeks prior to admission, lower ratio of PaO_2 to F_iO_2, congestive heart failure, serum albumin level, cor pulmonale, lower activities of daily living scores, lower scores on the Duke Activity Status Index, and number of hospital days before transfer to the ICU [106].

41.2.2 Etiology

Although respiratory infections are assumed to be the main risk factors for exacerbation of COPD, other factors are also involved [107]. Many patients with AECOPD are thought to have a combination of viral and bacterial infections, which contribute to their exacerbation. A variety of microorganisms have been shown to be associated with infectious bacterial AECOPD, including *Haemophilus influenzae, H. parainfluenzae, Moraxella catarrhalis,* and *Streptococcus pneumoniae* [108]. It has also been reported that these patients may be infected with atypical pathogens such as *Mycoplasma pneumoniae* and *Chlamydia pneumoniae*, but because of limitations with the diagnosis, the true prevalence of these organisms is not known [109–112]. There have been several recent studies demonstrating that patients with the most severe COPD and those that required ICU care have significantly higher prevalence of Gram-negative organisms such as Enterobacteriaceae and *Pseudomonas* species [113–115]. Several investigators have proposed that airway damage from chronic infection or colonization occurs in these patients because the bacteria cause the host to continuously release inflammatory mediators [116, 117]. Persistent infection results in lung inflammation and, as a consequence, lung function progressively decreases.

41.2.3 Diagnostic Procedures

A recent evidence base analysis has summarized the best available information related to the use of diagnostic tests in AECOPD [118, 119]. These reviews concluded that data on the utility of most diagnostic tests are limited. However, chest radiography and arterial blood gas sampling are useful while spirometry is performed at the time of the exacerbation is not [102]. Patients who require ICU care should have a chest radiograph obtained in order to rule out any other abnormalities and arterial blood gases.

41.2.4 Treatment with Antibiotics

There have been a number of clinical trials examining the use of antibiotics in the treatment of AECOPD [101, 107, 108, 120, 121]. The GOLD guideline, (GOLD website, accessed Feb. 2006) and the American Thoracic Society/European Respiratory Society (ATS/ERS) COPD consensus guidelines recommend antibiotic choices on the basis of local sensitivity patterns of the most common pathogens associated with AECOPD, and provide specific guidelines [122, 123].

There are limited number of studies that have looked at the use of antibiotics in ICU patients. Some of the recent publications, including a recent meta-analysis [124], demonstrated a benefit of antibiotics during an acute exacerbation of ambulatory patients. The study by Anthonisen et al. [125] reported that patients with all three clinical symptoms (increased shortness of breath, increased sputum production, and a change in sputum purulence) at initial presentation who received antibiotics showed a more rapid improvement in peak flow, a greater percentage of clinical successes, and a smaller percentage of clinical failures than those who received placebo. Furthermore, Allegra, et al. [126] found significant benefit with the use of amoxicillin-clavulanate acid (Augmentin) therapy compared with placebo in patients with severe disease. Patients who received this antibiotic exhibited a higher success rate (86.4% versus 50.3% in the placebo group, $p<0.01$) and a lower frequency of recurrent exacerbations.

There is only one study that has evaluated the role of antibiotics during AECOPD in ICU patients. Nouira et al. [127] published a prospective, randomized, double-blind, placebo-controlled trial, evaluating the use of ofloxacin in patients with AECOPD who required mechanical ventilation (invasive or non-invasive). This study demonstrated that a significant number of Gram-negative organisms (including *E. coli*, *P. mirabilis*, and *P. aeruginosa*) were identified in their population of patients with severe AECOPD. In addition to supporting the findings of the previously reported studies, this trial demonstrated that treating these pathogens is important for improving outcomes in this high-risk population. The antibiotic-treated group had a significantly lower in-hospital mortality rate and a significantly reduced length of stay in the hospital compared with the placebo group. In addition, the patients receiving ofloxacin were less likely to develop pneumonia than those on placebo.

There are additional potential benefits of antibiotic therapy for patients with AECOPD. Antibiotics can reduce the burden of bacteria in the airway [128]. There is a large percentage of patients with acute exacerbations (50–75% potentially pathogenic microorganisms in addition to significantly higher concentrations of frequently $\geq 10^4$ organisms) of bacteria in the large airways. Because treatment with appropriate antibiotics significantly decreases the bacterial burden at 72-h follow-up bronchoscopy, it is speculated that the proper choice of antibiotic reduces the risk of progression to more severe infections, such as pneumonia [115]. The eradication of bacteria by antibiotics is thought to break the vicious cycle of infection, i.e., lung destruction leading to progression of the lung disease.

If the use of antibiotics to treat AECOPD has all the potential benefits discussed, does it matter which agent is chosen? In the Anthonisen et al. study [125], the assumption was made that all of the antibiotics were equivalent; thus the specific agent prescribed was not considered important. Despite the problems with many of the published antibiotic trials, there are some retrospective trials that emphasize the importance of choosing the correct antibiotic for treatment of patients with AECOPD. A recent retrospective study of outpatients with documented COPD, conducted at our institution, evaluated the risk factors for therapy failure at 14 days after an acute exacerbation [129]. One group of patients received antibiotics and the second group did not. The overall relapse rate (defined as a return visit with persistent or worsening symptoms within 14 days) was 22%. After an extensive multivariate analysis, the major risk factor for relapse was lack of antibiotic therapy (32% versus 19%, $p<0.001$ compared to the antibiotic-treated group). The type of antibiotic used was also an important variable associated with the 14-day treatment failure. Patients treated with amoxicillin had a 54% relapse rate compared with only 13% for the other antibiotics ($p<0.01$). Furthermore, treatment with amoxicillin resulted in a higher incidence of failure, even when compared with those who did not receive antibiotics including amoxicillin, macrolides, and ciprofloxacin ($p=0.006$). Although there may be many explanations for these treatment failures, the most likely is that the pathogens were resistant to amoxicillin. This study showed that the use of antibiotics was associated with a significantly lower rate of therapy failure. In contrast to Anthonisen's data [125], Adams' data show that antibiotics are beneficial regardless of the severity of AECOPD. Furthermore, the patients who received antibiotics, and failed within 14 days, had a significantly higher rate of hospital admissions than those who did not receive antibiotics.

Destache et al. reported the impact of antibiotic selection, antimicrobial efficacy, and related cost in AECOPD [130]. The failure rates were significantly higher (at 14 days) for the first-line (amoxicillin, co-trimoxazole, erythromycin, and tetracycline), compared with the third-line (amoxicillin-clavulanate, azithromycin, and ciprofloxacin) agents (19% versus 7%, $p<0.05$). When compared with those who received the first-line agents, the patients treated with the third-line agents had a significantly longer time between exacerbations, overall fewer hospitalizations, and considerably lower total cost.

41.2.5 End-Point for the Treatment of AECOPD

Conventional end-points for efficacy of antibiotics treatment in AECOPD include the symptoms and bacteriological resolution measured at 2–3 weeks after the treatment was started. Most of these end-points rely solely on the subjective report of symptom improvement. It has been suggested by several investigators that other parameters such as the rate of symptom resolution, the interval between exacerbations, the improvement in quality of life, the need for hospitalization and mortality, may be more suitable end-points in this patient population [131, 132].

41.2.6 Clinical Parameters To Stratify Patients into Risk Groups

The clinical parameters that are implicated as possible risk factors for treatment failure in AECOPD and suggested therapies are summarized in Tables 41.9 and 41.10 [10, 108, 121].

41.2.7 Prevention

The two most important prevention measures in AECOPD and CAP patients are smoking cessation

Table 41.9. Patient profiles from the Canadian Chronic Bronchitis Guidelines (adapted from Balter et al. [108])

Acute tracheobronchitis (Group 0) Healthy people with cough and sputum without previous respiratory problems
"Simple" chronic bronchitis without risk factors (Group I) Increased cough and sputum, sputum purulence and increased dyspnea
"Complicated" chronic bronchitis with risk factors (Group II) As group I **plus** (at least one of the following) >4 exacerbations per year **or** Cardiac disease **or** Home oxygen **or** Chronic oral steroid use **or** Antibiotic use in the 3 months prior
Chronic "suppurative" bronchitis (Group III) As group II with constant purulent sputum, plus: Bronchiectasis (some patients) **or** FEV1<35% predicted **or** Multiple risk factors (frequent exacerbations and FEV1<50%)

Table 41.10. Recommendations for antibiotic therapy in AECOPD (adapted from Balter et al [108])

Category	Probable pathogen	Recommended therapy
Acute tracheobronchitis	Viral	Symptomatic
"Simple" AECOPD	*Haemophilus* spp. (*H. influenzae*), *M. catarrhalis*, *S. pneumoniae*	Macrolide (azithromycin or clarithromycin), amoxicillin, doxycycline, 2nd or 3rd generation cephalosporins. If treatment failure: beta-lactam/beta-lactamase inhibitor or fluoroquinolone
"Complicated" AECOPD	As above with the addition of Gram-negative organisms (*Klebsiella* spp. etc.), and multi-drug resistant (MDR) pathogens such as *Pseudomonas* spp.	3rd generation cephalosporins, beta-lactam/beta-lactamase inhibitor or fluoroquinolone (ciprofloxacin for *Pseudomonas* spp.) Parenteral inpatient therapy highly considered for MDR pathogens or treatment failures

[133–135] and active immunizations, including influenza and pneumococcal vaccinations.

Influenza is an important cause of lower respiratory tract infections. Influenza A and B often reach epidemic proportions during the winter months. The impact of influenza is critical to the development of other lower respiratory infections including AECOPD and pneumonia. Epidemiological studies have shown that the frequency of lower respiratory infections, and associated morbidity and mortality, are markedly reduced with influenza vaccination [136–138]. The polyvalent vaccine based on pneumococcal capsule serotypes has been shown to be effective in preventing pneumococcal bacteremia and pneumonia [138–140]. The vaccine is recommended in patients with COPD.

41.3 Summary

The cost, morbidity, and mortality related to CAP and AECOPD remain unacceptably high. Because these are heterogeneous groups of patients it is important to use risk-stratification based on clinical parameters and prediction tools. Appropriate antibiotic therapy is an important component in the management of both groups of patients. In particular, it is essential to administer an appropriate antimicrobial agent from the initiation of therapy, so that the risks of treatment failure and the morbidity of CAP and AECOPD may be minimized.

The views expressed in this article are those of the authors and do not necessarily represent the views of the Department of Veterans Affairs.

References

1. Anonymous (1995) Pneumonia and influenza death rates – United States, 1979–1994. [erratum appears in MMWR Morb Mortal Wkly Rep 1995 44(41):782]. MMWR 44:535–537
2. National Center for Health Statistics CfDCaP (1994) Advance report of final mortality statistics 1992. US Department of Health and Human Services, Public Health Service, Hyattsville, MD
3. Niederman MS, Mandell LA, Anzueto A, Bass JB, Broughton WA, Campbell GD, Dean N, File T, Fine MJ, Gross PA, Martinez F, Marrie TJ, Plouffe JF, Ramirez J, Sarosi GA, Torres A, Wilson R, Yu VL (2001) Guidelines for the management of adults with community-acquired pneumonia. Diagnosis, assessment of severity, antimicrobial therapy, and prevention. Am J Respir Crit Care Med 163:1730–1754
4. Anonymous (1998) ERS Task Force Report. Guidelines for management of adult community-acquired lower respiratory tract infections. European Respiratory Society. Eur Respir J 11:986–991
5. Huchon G, Woodhead M (1998) Management of adult community-acquired lower respiratory tract infections. Eur Respir Rev 8:391–426
6. Mandell LA, Marrie TJ, Grossman RF, Chow AW, Hyland RH (2000) Canadian guidelines for the initial management of community-acquired pneumonia: an evidence-based update by the Canadian Infectious Diseases Society and the Canadian Thoracic Society. The Canadian Community-Acquired Pneumonia Working Group. Clin Infect Dis 31: 383–421
7. Mandell LA, Bartlett JG, Dowell SF, File TM, Jr, Musher DM, Whitney C (2003) Update of practice guidelines for the management of community-acquired pneumonia in immunocompetent adults. Clin Infect Dis 37:1405–1433
8. Bartlett JG, Dowell SF, Mandell LA, File TM Jr, Musher DM, Fine MJ (2000) Practice guidelines for the management of community-acquired pneumonia in adults. Infectious Diseases Society of America. Clin Infect Dis 31:347–382
9. Heffelfinger JD, Dowell SF, Jorgensen JH, Klugman KP, Mabry LR, Musher DM, Plouffe JF, Rakowsky A, Schuchat A, Whitney CG (2000) Management of community-acquired pneumonia in the era of pneumococcal resistance: a report from the Drug-Resistant *Streptococcus pneumoniae* Therapeutic Working Group. Arch Intern Med 160: 1399–1408
10. Woodhead M, Blasi F, Ewig S, Huchon G, Leven M, Ortqvist A, Schaberg T, Torres A, van der Heijden G, Verheij TJM (2005) Guidelines for the management of adult lower respiratory tract infections. Eur Respir J 26:1138–1180
11. Kozak LJ, Hall MJ, Owings MF (2002) National Hospital Discharge Survey: 2000 annual summary with detailed diagnosis and procedure data. Vital & Health Statistics – Series 13: Data From the National Health Survey:1–194
12. Marston BJ, Plouffe JF, File TM, Jr, Hackman BA, Salstrom SJ, Lipman HB, Kolczak MS, Breiman RF (1997) Incidence of community-acquired pneumonia requiring hospitalization. Results of a population-based active surveillance Study in Ohio. The Community-Based Pneumonia Incidence Study Group. Arch Intern Med 157:1709–1718
13. Minino AM, Arias E, Kochanek KD, Murphy SL, Smith BL (2002) Deaths: final data for 2000. National Vital Statistics Reports 50:1–119
14. Halm EA, Teirstein AS (2002) Clinical practice. Management of community-acquired pneumonia. N Engl J Med 347:2039–2045
15. Leroy O, Santre C, Beuscart C, Georges H, Guery B, Jacquier JM, Beaucaire G (1995) A five-year study of severe community-acquired pneumonia with emphasis on prognosis in patients admitted to an intensive care unit. Intensive Care Med 21:24–31
16. Moine P, Vercken JB, Chevret S, Chastang C, Gajdos P (1994) Severe community-acquired pneumonia. Etiology, epidemiology, and prognosis factors. French Study Group for Community-Acquired Pneumonia in the Intensive Care Unit. Chest 105:1487–1495
17. Torres A, Serra-Batlles J, Ferrer A, Jimenez P, Celis R, Cobo E, Rodriguez-Roisin R (1991) Severe community-acquired pneumonia. Epidemiology and prognostic factors. Am Rev Respir Dis 144:312–318
18. Fine MJ, Smith MA, Carson CA, Mutha SS, Sankey SS, Weissfeld LA, Kapoor WN (1996) Prognosis and outcomes of patients with community-acquired pneumonia. A meta-analysis. JAMA 275:134–141
19. Angus DC, Marrie TJ, Obrosky DS, Clermont G, Dremsizov TT, Coley C, Fine MJ, Singer DE, Kapoor WN (2002) Severe community-acquired pneumonia: use of intensive care services and evaluation of American and British Thoracic Society Diagnostic criteria. Am J Respir Crit Care Med 166:717–723
20. Niederman MS, McCombs JS, Unger AN, Kumar A, Popovian R (1998) The cost of treating community-acquired pneumonia. Clin Ther 20:820–837
21. Gutierrez F, Masia M, Rodriguez JC, Mirete C, Soldan B,

Padilla S, Hernandez I, De Ory F, Royo G, Hidalgo AM (2005) Epidemiology of community-acquired pneumonia in adult patients at the dawn of the 21st century: a prospective study on the Mediterranean coast of Spain. Clin Microbiol Infection 11:788–800
22. Friedman ND, Kaye KS, Stout JE, McGarry SA, Trivette SL, Briggs JP, Lamm W, Clark C, MacFarquhar J, Walton AL, Reller LB, Sexton DJ (2002) Health care-associated bloodstream infections in adults: a reason to change the accepted definition of community-acquired infections. Ann Intern Med 137:791–797
23. Roson B, Carratala J, Dorca J, Casanova A, Manresa F, Gudiol F (2001) Etiology, reasons for hospitalization, risk classes, and outcomes of community-acquired pneumonia in patients hospitalized on the basis of conventional admission criteria. Clin Infect Dis 33:158–165
24. Garcia-Ordonez MA, Garcia-Jimenez JM, Paez F, Alvarez F, Poyato B, Franquelo M, Colmenero JD, Juarez C (2001) Clinical aspects and prognostic factors in elderly patients hospitalised for community-acquired pneumonia. Eur J Clin Microbiol Infect Dis 20:14–19
25. Luna CM, Famiglietti A, Absi R, Videla AJ, Nogueira FJ, Fuenzalida AD, Gene RJ (2000) Community-acquired pneumonia: etiology, epidemiology, and outcome at a teaching hospital in Argentina. Chest 118:1344–1354
26. Meehan TP, Chua-Reyes JM, Tate J, Prestwood KM, Scinto JD, Petrillo MK, Metersky ML (2000) Process of care performance, patient characteristics, and outcomes in elderly patients hospitalized with community-acquired or nursing home-acquired pneumonia. Chest 117:1378–1385
27. Lim WS, Macfarlane JT, Boswell TC, Harrison TG, Rose D, Leinonen M, Saikku P (2001) Study of community acquired pneumonia aetiology (SCAPA) in adults admitted to hospital: implications for management guidelines. Thorax 56:296–301
28. Kollef MH, Shorr A, Tabak YP, Gupta V, Liu LZ, Johannes RS (2005) Epidemiology and outcomes of health-care-associated pneumonia: results from a large US database of culture-positive pneumonia. Chest 128:3854–3862
29. Feldman C, Viljoen E, Morar R, Richards G, Sawyer L, Goolam Mahomed A (2001) Prognostic factors in severe community-acquired pneumonia in patients without comorbid illness. Respirology 6:323–330
30. Marrie TJ (2000) Community-acquired pneumonia in the elderly. Clin Infect Dis 31:1066–1078
31. Fry AM, Shay DK, Holman RC, Curns AT, Anderson LJ (2005) Trends in hospitalizations for pneumonia among persons aged 65 years or older in the United States, 1988–2002. JAMA 294:2712–2719
32. Tejerina E, Frutos-Vivar F, Restrepo MI, Anzueto A, Palizas F, Gonzalez M, Apezteguia C, Abroug F, Matamis D, Bugedo G, Esteban A, International Mechanical Ventilation Study G (2005) Prognosis factors and outcome of community-acquired pneumonia needing mechanical ventilation. J Crit Care 20:230–238
33. Marrie TJ, Carriere KC, Jin Y, Johnson DH (2003) Factors associated with death among adults < 55 years of age hospitalized for community-acquired pneumonia. Clin Infect Dis 36:413–421
34. Pascual FE, Matthay MA, Bacchetti P, Wachter RM (2000) Assessment of prognosis in patients with community-acquired pneumonia who require mechanical ventilation. Chest 117:503–512
35. Mehta R, Groth M (2001) Clinical application of a prognostic model for severe community-acquired pneumonia. Chest 119:312–313
36. Meehan TP, Fine MJ, Krumholz HM, Scinto JD, Galusha DH, Mockalis JT, Weber GF, Petrillo MK, Houck PM, Fine JM (1997) Quality of care, process, and outcomes in elderly patients with pneumonia. JAMA 278:2080–2084
37. Mortensen EM, Coley CM, Singer DE, Marrie TJ, Obrosky DS, Kapoor WN, Fine MJ (2002) Causes of death for patients with community-acquired pneumonia: results from the Pneumonia Patient Outcomes Research Team cohort study. Arch Intern Med 162:1059–1064
38. Dean NC, Suchyta MR, Bateman KA, Aronsky D, Hadlock CJ (2000) Implementation of admission decision support for community-acquired pneumonia. Chest 117:1368–1377
39. Fine MJ, Auble TE, Yealy DM, Hanusa BH, Weissfeld LA, Singer DE, Coley CM, Marrie TJ, Kapoor WN (1997) A prediction rule to identify low-risk patients with community-acquired pneumonia. N Engl J Med 336:243–250
40. Marrie TJ, Lau CY, Wheeler SL, Wong CJ, Vandervoort MK, Feagan BG (2000) A controlled trial of a critical pathway for treatment of community-acquired pneumonia. CAPITAL Study Investigators. Community-Acquired Pneumonia Intervention Trial Assessing Levofloxacin. JAMA 283:749–755
41. Ewig S, Schafer H, Torres A (2000) Severity assessment in community-acquired pneumonia. Eur Respir J 16:1193–1201
42. Ewig S, Ruiz M, Mensa J, Marcos MA, Martinez JA, Arancibia F, Niederman MS, Torres A (1998) Severe community-acquired pneumonia. Assessment of severity criteria. Am J Respir Crit Care Med 158:1102–1108
43. British Thoracic Society (1993) Guidelines for the management of community-acquired pneumonia in adults admitted to hospital. Br J Hosp Med 49:346–350
44. Lim WS, Lewis S, Macfarlane JT (2000) Severity prediction rules in community acquired pneumonia: a validation study. Thorax 55:219–223
45. British Thoracic Society Standards of Care Committee (2002) British Thoracic Society guidelines for the management of community acquired pneumonia in childhood. Thorax 57 Suppl 1:i1–24
46. Lim WS, van der Eerden MM, Laing R, Boersma WG, Karalus N, Town GI, Lewis SA, Macfarlane JT (2003) Defining community acquired pneumonia severity on presentation to hospital: an international derivation and validation study. Thorax 58:377–382
47. Metlay JP, Fine MJ (2003) Testing strategies in the initial management of patients with community-acquired pneumonia. Ann Intern Med 138:109–118
48. Aujesky D, Auble TE, Yealy DM, Stone RA, Obrosky DS, Meehan TP, Graff LG, Fine JM, Fine MJ (2005) Prospective comparison of three validated prediction rules for prognosis in community-acquired pneumonia. Am J Medicine 118:384–392
49. Capelastegui A, Espana PP, Quintana JM, Areitio I, Gorordo I, Egurrola M, Bilbao A (2006) Validation of a predictive rule for the management of community-acquired pneumonia. Eur Respir J 27:151–157
50. Ewig S, de Roux A, Bauer T, Garcia E, Mensa J, Niederman M, Torres A (2004) Validation of predictive rules and indices of severity for community acquired pneumonia. Thorax 59:421–427
51. Espana PP, Capelastegui A, Quintana JM, Soto A, Gorordo I, Garcia-Urbaneja M, Bilbao A (2003) A prediction rule to identify allocation of inpatient care in community-acquired pneumonia. Eur Respir J 21:695–701
52. Arnold FW, Ramirez JA, McDonald LC, Xia EL (2003) Hospitalization for community-acquired pneumonia: the pneumonia severity index vs clinical judgment. Chest 124:121–124
53. Ewig S, Kleinfeld T, Bauer T, Seifert K, Schafer H, Goke N (1999) Comparative validation of prognostic rules for

community-acquired pneumonia in an elderly population. Eur Respir J 14:370–375

54. Farr BM, Sloman AJ, Fisch MJ (1991) Predicting death in patients hospitalized for community-acquired pneumonia. Ann Intern Med 115:428–436
55. Karalus NC, Cursons RT, Leng RA, Mahood CB, Rothwell RP, Hancock B, Cepulis S, Wawatai M, Coleman L (1991) Community acquired pneumonia: aetiology and prognostic index evaluation. Thorax 46:413–418
56. Neill AM, Martin IR, Weir R, Anderson R, Chereshsky A, Epton MJ, Jackson R, Schousboe M, Frampton C, Hutton S, Chambers ST, Town GI (1996) Community acquired pneumonia: aetiology and usefulness of severity criteria on admission. Thorax 51:1010–1016
57. Niederman MS, Bass JB, Jr, Campbell GD, Fein AM, Grossman RF, Mandell LA, Marrie TJ, Sarosi GA, Torres A, Yu VL (1993) Guidelines for the initial management of adults with community-acquired pneumonia: diagnosis, assessment of severity, and initial antimicrobial therapy. American Thoracic Society. Medical Section of the American Lung Association. Am Rev Respir Dis 148:1418–1426
58. Riley PD, Aronsky D, Dean NC (2004) Validation of the 2001 American Thoracic Society criteria for severe community-acquired pneumonia. Crit Care Med 32:2398–2402
59. Cordero E, Pachon J, Rivero A, Giron JA, Gomez-Mateos J, Merino MD, Torres-Tortosa M, Gonzalez-Serrano M, Aliaga L, Collado A, Hernandez-Quero J, Barrera A, Nuno E (2000) Community-acquired bacterial pneumonia in human immunodeficiency virus-infected patients: validation of severity criteria. The Grupo Andaluz para el Estudio de las Enfermedades Infecciosas. Am J Respir Crit Care Med 162:2063–2068
60. Levin KP, Hanusa BH, Rotondi A, Singer DE, Coley CM, Marrie TJ, Kapoor WN, Fine MJ (2001) Arterial blood gas and pulse oximetry in initial management of patients with community-acquired pneumonia. J Gen Intern Med 16: 590–598
61. Rello J, Bodi M, Mariscal D, Navarro M, Diaz E, Gallego M, Valles J (2003) Microbiological testing and outcome of patients with severe community-acquired pneumonia. Chest 123:174–180
62. Boussekey N, Leroy O, Georges H, Devos P, d'Escrivan T, Guery B (2005) Diagnostic and prognostic values of admission procalcitonin levels in community-acquired pneumonia in an intensive care unit. Infection 33:257–263
63. van der Meer V, Neven AK, van den Broek PJ, Assendelft WJ (2005) Diagnostic value of C reactive protein in infections of the lower respiratory tract: systematic review. BMJ 331:26
64. Houck PM, Bratzler DW, Nsa W, Ma A, Bartlett JG (2004) Timing of antibiotic administration and outcomes for Medicare patients hospitalized with community-acquired pneumonia. Arch Intern Med 164:637–644
65. Restrepo MI, Mortensen EM, Anzueto A, Pugh JA (2003) Mortality in monotherapy versus combination therapy in severe community-acquired pneumonia: a systematic review. Chest 124:190S
66. Lieberman D, Schlaeffer F, Boldur I, Horowitz S, Friedman MG, Leiononen M, Horovitz O, Manor E, Porath A (1996) Multiple pathogens in adult patients admitted with community-acquired pneumonia: a one year prospective study of 346 consecutive patients. Thorax 51:179–184
67. Ruiz M, Ewig S, Marcos MA, Martinez JA, Arancibia F, Mensa J, Torres A (1999) Etiology of community-acquired pneumonia: impact of age, comorbidity, and severity. Am J Respir Crit Care Med 160:397–405
68. El-Solh AA, Sikka P, Ramadan F, Davies J (2001) Etiology of severe pneumonia in the very elderly. Am J Respir Crit Care Med 163:645–651
69. Afessa B, Green B (2000) Bacterial pneumonia in hospitalized patients with HIV infection: the pulmonary complications, ICU support, and prognostic factors of hospitalized patients with HIV (PIP) study. Chest 117:1017–1022
70. Shefet D, Robenshtok E, Paul M, Leibovici L (2005) Empirical atypical coverage for inpatients with community-acquired pneumonia: systematic review of randomized controlled trials. Arch Intern Med 165:1992–2000
71. Arancibia F, Bauer TT, Ewig S, Mensa J, Gonzalez J, Niederman MS, Torres A (2002) Community-acquired pneumonia due to gram-negative bacteria and *Pseudomonas aeruginosa:* incidence, risk, and prognosis. Arch Intern Med 162:1849–1858
72. Hatchette TF, Gupta R, Marrie TJ (2000) *Pseudomonas aeruginosa* community-acquired pneumonia in previously healthy adults: case report and review of the literature. Clin Infect Dis 31:1349–1356
73. Fogarty C, Siami G, Kholer R, File TM, Jr, Tennenberg AM, Olson WH, Wiesinger BA, Scott Marshall JA, Oross M, Khan JB (2004) Multicenter, open label, randomized study to compare the safety and efficacy of levofloxacin versus ceftriaxone sodium and erythromycin followed by clarithromycin and amoxicillin-clavulanate in the treatment of serious community-acquired pneumonia in adults. Clin Infect Dis 38:S16–23
74. Leroy O, Saux P, Bedos JP, Caulin E (2005) Comparison of levofloxacin and cefotaxime combined with ofloxacin for ICU patients with community-acquired pneumonia who do not require vasopressors. Chest 128:172–183
75. Bodi M, Rodriguez A, Sole-Violan J, Gilavert MC, Garnacho J, Blanquer J, Jimenez J, de la Torre MV, Sirvent JM, Almirall J, Doblas A, Badia JR, Garcia F, Mendia A, Jorda R, Bobillo F, Valles J, Broch MJ, Carrasco N, Herranz MA, Rello J, Community-Acquired Pneumonia Intensive Care Units Study I (2005) Antibiotic prescription for community-acquired pneumonia in the intensive care unit: impact of adherence to Infectious Diseases Society of America guidelines on survival. Clin Infect Dis 41:1709–1716
76. Dean NC, Silver MP, Bateman KA, James B, Hadlock CJ, Hale D (2001) Decreased mortality after implementation of a treatment guideline for community-acquired pneumonia. Am J Med 110:451–457
77. Garcia Vazquez E, Mensa J, Martinez JA, Marcos MA, Puig J, Ortega M, Torres A (2005) Lower mortality among patients with community-acquired pneumonia treated with a macrolide plus a beta-lactam agent versus a beta-lactam agent alone. Eur J Clin Microbiol Infect Dis 24:190–195
78. Mortensen EM, Restrepo M, Anzueto A, Pugh J (2004) Effects of guideline-concordant antimicrobial therapy on mortality among patients with community-acquired pneumonia. Am J Med 117:726–731
79. Moroney JF, Fiore AE, Harrison LH, Patterson JE, Farley MM, Jorgensen JH, Phelan M, Facklam RR, Cetron MS, Breiman RF, Kolczak M, Schuchat A (2001) Clinical outcomes of bacteremic pneumococcal pneumonia in the era of antibiotic resistance. Clin Infect Dis 33:797–805
80. Kalin M, Ortqvist A, Almela M, Aufwerber E, Dwyer R, Henriques B, Jorup C, Julander I, Marrie TJ, Mufson MA, Riquelme R, Thalme A, Torres A, Woodhead MA (2000) Prospective study of prognostic factors in community-acquired bacteremic pneumococcal disease in 5 countries. J Infect Dis 182:840–847
81. Metlay JP, Hofmann J, Cetron MS, Fine MJ, Farley MM, Whitney C, Breiman RF (2000) Impact of penicillin susceptibility on medical outcomes for adult patients with bacteremic pneumococcal pneumonia. Clin Infect Dis 30:520–528
82. Waterer GW, Somes GW, Wunderink RG (2001) Monother-

apy may be suboptimal for severe bacteremic pneumococcal pneumonia. Arch Intern Med 161:1837–1842

83. Baddour LM, Yu VL, Klugman KP, Feldman C, Ortqvist A, Rello J, Morris AJ, Luna CM, Snydman DR, Ko WC, Chedid MB, Hui DS, Andremont A, Chiou CC, International Pneumococcal Study G (2004) Combination antibiotic therapy lowers mortality among severely ill patients with pneumococcal bacteremia. Am J Respir Crit Care Med 170:440–444
84. Lujan M, Gallego M, Fontanals D, Mariscal D, Rello J (2004) Prospective observational study of bacteremic pneumococcal pneumonia: Effect of discordant therapy on mortality. Crit Care Med 32:625–631
85. Martinez JA, Horcajada JP, Almela M, Marco F, Soriano A, Garcia E, Marco MA, Torres A, Mensa J (2003) Addition of a macrolide to a beta-lactam-based empirical antibiotic regimen is associated with lower in-hospital mortality for patients with bacteremic pneumococcal pneumonia. Clin Infect Dis 36:389–395
86. Mufson MA, Stanek RJ (1999) Bacteremic pneumococcal pneumonia in one American City: a 20-year longitudinal study, 1978–1997. Am J Med 107:34S–43S
87. Sabria M, Pedro-Botet ML, Gomez J, Roig J, Vilaseca B, Sopena N, Banos V, Legionnaires Disease Therapy G (2005) Fluoroquinolones vs macrolides in the treatment of Legionnaires disease. Chest 128:1401–1405
88. Dresser LD, Niederman MS, Paladino JA (2001) Cost-effectiveness of gatifloxacin vs ceftriaxone with a macrolide for the treatment of community-acquired pneumonia. Chest 119:1439–1448
89. Halley HJ (2000) Approaches to drug therapy, formulary, and pathway management in a large community hospital. Am J Health Syst Pharm 57 Suppl 3:S17–21
90. Yost NP, Bloom SL, Richey SD, Ramin SM, Cunningham FG (2000) An appraisal of treatment guidelines for antepartum community-acquired pneumonia. Am J Obstet Gynecol 183:131–135
91. Palmer CS, Zhan C, Elixhauser A, Halpern MT, Rance L, Feagan BG, Marrie TJ (2000) Economic assessment of the community-acquired pneumonia intervention trial employing levofloxacin. Clin Ther 22:250–264
92. Fogarty CM, Greenberg RN, Dunbar L, Player R, Marrie TJ, Kojak CM, Morgan N, Williams RR (2001) Effectiveness of levofloxacin for adult community-acquired pneumonia caused by macrolide-resistant *Streptococcus pneumoniae:* integrated results from four open-label, multicenter, phase III clinical trials. Clin Ther 23:425–439
93. Clark LC, Davis CW (2000) Experiences at a large teaching hospital with levofloxacin for the treatment of community-acquired pneumonia. Am J Health Syst Pharm 57 Suppl 3:S10–13
94. Menendez R, Perpina M, Torres A (2003) Evaluation of nonresolving and progressive pneumonia. Semin Respir Infect 18:103–111
95. Arancibia F, Ewig S, Martinez JA, Ruiz M, Bauer T, Marcos MA, Mensa J, Torres A (2000) Antimicrobial treatment failures in patients with community-acquired pneumonia: causes and prognostic implications. Am J Respir Crit Care Med 162:154–160
96. Rhew DC, Tu GS, Ofman J, Henning JM, Richards MS, Weingarten SR (2001) Early switch and early discharge strategies in patients with community-acquired pneumonia: a meta-analysis. Arch Intern Med 161:722–727
97. Ramirez JA, Bordon J (2001) Early switch from intravenous to oral antibiotics in hospitalized patients with bacteremic community-acquired *Streptococcus pneumoniae* pneumonia. Arch Intern Med 161:848–850
98. Eron LJ, Passos S (2001) Early discharge of infected patients through appropriate antibiotic use. Arch Intern Med 161:61–65
99. Murray CJ, Lopez AD (1997) Alternative projections of mortality and disability by cause 1990–2020: Global Burden of Disease Study. Lancet 349:1498–1504
100. Feinleib M, Rosenberg HM, Collins JG, Delozier JE, Pokras R, Chevarley FM (1989) Trends in COPD morbidity and mortality in the United States. Am Rev Respir Dis 140:S9–18
101. Ball P, Tillotson G, Wilson R (1995) Chemotherapy for chronic bronchitis. Controversies. Presse Medicale 24: 189–194
102. Emerman CL, Effron D, Lukens TW (1991) Spirometric criteria for hospital admission of patients with acute exacerbation of COPD. Chest 99:595–599
103. Murata GH, Gorby MS, Kapsner CO, Chick TW, Halperin AK (1992) A multivariate model for the prediction of relapse after outpatient treatment of decompensated chronic obstructive pulmonary disease. Arch Intern Med 152:73–77
104. Connors AF, Jr, Dawson NV, Thomas C, Harrell FE, Jr, Desbiens N, Fulkerson WJ, Kussin P, Bellamy P, Goldman L, Knaus WA (1996) Outcomes following acute exacerbation of severe chronic obstructive lung disease. The SUPPORT investigators (Study to Understand Prognoses and Preferences for Outcomes and Risks of Treatments). Am J Respir Crit Care Med 154:959–967
105. Knaus WA, Wagner DP, Draper EA, Zimmerman JE, Bergner M, Bastos PG, Sirio CA, Murphy DJ, Lotring T, Damiano A, et al. (1991) The APACHE III prognostic system. Risk prediction of hospital mortality for critically ill hospitalized adults. Chest 100:1619–1636
106. Seneff MG, Wagner DP, Wagner RP, Zimmerman JE, Knaus WA (1995) Hospital and 1-year survival of patients admitted to intensive care units with acute exacerbation of chronic obstructive pulmonary disease. JAMA 274: 1852–1857
107. Ball P (1995) Epidemiology and treatment of chronic bronchitis and its exacerbations. Chest 108:43S–52S
108. Balter MS, La Forge J, Low DE, Mandell L, Grossman RF, Canadian Thoracic S, Canadian Infectious Disease S (2003) Canadian guidelines for the management of acute exacerbations of chronic bronchitis. Can Respir J 10 Suppl B:3B–32B
109. Blasi F, Damato S, Cosentini R, Tarsia P, Raccanelli R, Centanni S, Allegra L (2002) *Chlamydia pneumoniae* and chronic bronchitis: association with severity and bacterial clearance following treatment. Thorax 57:672–676
110. Seemungal TA, Wedzicha JA, MacCallum PK, Johnston SL, Lambert PA (2002) *Chlamydia pneumoniae* and COPD exacerbation. Thorax 57:1087–1088; author reply 1088–1089
111. Smieja M, Leigh R, Petrich A, Chong S, Kamada D, Hargreave FE, Goldsmith CH, Chernesky M, Mahony JB (2002) Smoking, season, and detection of *Chlamydia pneumoniae* DNA in clinically stable COPD patients. BMC Infect Dis 2:12
112. Smieja M, Mahony J, Petrich A, Boman J, Chernesky M (2002) Association of circulating *Chlamydia pneumoniae* DNA with cardiovascular disease: a systematic review. BMC Infect Dis 2:21
113. Eller J, Ede A, Schaberg T, Niederman MS, Mauch H, Lode H (1998) Infective exacerbations of chronic bronchitis: relation between bacteriologic etiology and lung function. Chest 113:1542–1548
114. Miravitlles M, Espinosa C, Fernandez-Laso E, Martos JA, Maldonado JA, Gallego M (1999) Relationship between bacterial flora in sputum and functional impairment in

patients with acute exacerbations of COPD. Study Group of Bacterial Infection in COPD. Chest 116:40–46
115. Soler N, Torres A, Ewig S, Gonzalez J, Celis R, El-Ebiary M, Hernandez C, Rodriguez-Roisin R (1998) Bronchial microbial patterns in severe exacerbations of chronic obstructive pulmonary disease (COPD) requiring mechanical ventilation. Am J Respir Crit Care Med 157:1498–1505
116. Murphy TF, Sethi S (1992) Bacterial infection in chronic obstructive pulmonary disease. Am Rev Respir Dis 146: 1067–1083
117. Sethi S, Muscarella K, Evans N, Klingman KL, Grant BJ, Murphy TF (2000) Airway inflammation and etiology of acute exacerbations of chronic bronchitis. Chest 118: 1557–1565
118. Bach PB, Brown C, Gelfand SE, McCrory DC, American College of Physicians-American Society of Internal M, American College of Chest P (2001) Management of acute exacerbations of chronic obstructive pulmonary disease: a summary and appraisal of published evidence. Ann Intern Med 134:600–620
119. Snow V, Lascher S, Mottur-Pilson C, Joint Expert Panel on Chronic Obstructive Pulmonary Disease of the American College of Chest Physicians and the American College of Physicians-American Society of Internal M (2001) Evidence base for management of acute exacerbations of chronic obstructive pulmonary disease. Ann Intern Med 134:595–599
120. Ball P, Harris JM, Lowson D, Tillotson G, Wilson R (1995) Acute infective exacerbations of chronic bronchitis. QJM 88:61–68
121. Balter MS, La Forge J, Low DE, Mandell L, Grossman RF, Chronic Bronchitis Working G, Canadian Thoracic S, Canadian Infectious Disease S (2003) Canadian guidelines for the management of acute exacerbations of chronic bronchitis: executive summary. Can Respir J 10:248–258
122. Celli BR, MacNee W, Force AET (2004) Standards for the diagnosis and treatment of patients with COPD: a summary of the ATS/ERS position paper. Eur Respir J 23: 932–946
123. Pauwels RA, Buist AS, Calverley PM, Jenkins CR, Hurd SS, Committee GS (2001) Global strategy for the diagnosis, management, and prevention of chronic obstructive pulmonary disease. NHLBI/WHO Global Initiative for Chronic Obstructive Lung Disease (GOLD) Workshop summary. Am J Respir Crit Care Med 163:1256–1276
124. Saint S, Bent S, Vittinghoff E, Grady D (1995) Antibiotics in chronic obstructive pulmonary disease exacerbations. A meta-analysis. JAMA 273:957–960
125. Anthonisen NR, Manfreda J, Warren CP, Hershfield ES, Harding GK, Nelson NA (1987) Antibiotic therapy in exacerbations of chronic obstructive pulmonary disease. Ann Intern Med 106:196–204
126. Allegra L, Blasi F, de Bernardi B, Cosentini R, Tarsia P (2001) Antibiotic treatment and baseline severity of disease in acute exacerbations of chronic bronchitis: a re-evaluation of previously published data of a placebo-controlled randomized study. Pulm Pharmacol Ther 14:149–155
127. Nouira S, Marghli S, Belghith M, Besbes L, Elatrous S, Abroug F (2001) Once daily oral ofloxacin in chronic obstructive pulmonary disease exacerbation requiring mechanical ventilation: a randomised placebo-controlled trial. Lancet 358:2020–2025
128. Cabello H, Torres A, Celis R, El-Ebiary M, Puig de la Bellacasa J, Xaubet A, Gonzalez J, Agusti C, Soler N (1997) Bacterial colonization of distal airways in healthy subjects and chronic lung disease: a bronchoscopic study. Eur Respir J 10:1137–1144
129. Adams SG, Melo J, Luther M, Anzueto A (2000) Antibiotics are associated with lower relapse rates in outpatients with acute exacerbations of COPD. Chest 117:1345–1352
130. Destache CJ, Dewan N, O'Donohue WJ, Campbell JC, Angelillo VA (1999) Clinical and economic considerations in the treatment of acute exacerbations of chronic bronchitis. J Antimicrob Chemother 43 Suppl A:107–113
131. Wilson R, Allegra L, Huchon G, Izquierdo JL, Jones P, Schaberg T, Sagnier PP, Group MS (2004) Short-term and long-term outcomes of moxifloxacin compared to standard antibiotic treatment in acute exacerbations of chronic bronchitis [see comment]. Chest 125:953–964
132. Wilson R, Schentag JJ, Ball P, Mandell L, Study G (2002) A comparison of gemifloxacin and clarithromycin in acute exacerbations of chronic bronchitis and long-term clinical outcomes. Clin Ther 24:639–652
133. Anthonisen NR, Connett JE, Kiley JP, Altose MD, Bailey WC, Buist AS, Conway WA, Jr, Enright PL, Kanner RE, O'Hara P, et al. (1994) Effects of smoking intervention and the use of an inhaled anticholinergic bronchodilator on the rate of decline of FEV1. The Lung Health Study. JAMA 272:1497–1505
134. Fiore MC, Jorenby DE, Baker TB (1997) Smoking cessation: principles and practice based upon the AHCPR Guideline, 1996. Agency for Health Care Policy and Research. Ann Behav Med 19:213–219
135. Fiore MC, Jorenby DE, Baker TB, Kenford SL (1992) Tobacco dependence and the nicotine patch. Clinical guidelines for effective use. JAMA 268:2687–2694
136. Centers for Disease Control and P (2004) Influenza and pneumococcal vaccination coverage among persons aged > or =65 years and persons aged 18–64 years with diabetes or asthma – United States, 2003. MMWR 53:1007–1012
137. Centers for Disease Control and P (2005) Influenza vaccination levels among persons aged > or =65 years and among persons aged 18–64 years with high-risk conditions – United States, 2003. MMWR 54:1045–1049
138. Nichol KL, Mallon KP, Mendelman PM (2003) Cost benefit of influenza vaccination in healthy, working adults: an economic analysis based on the results of a clinical trial of trivalent live attenuated influenza virus vaccine. Vaccine 21:2207–2217
139. Butler JC, Breiman RF, Campbell JF, Lipman HB, Broome CV, Facklam RR (1993) Pneumococcal polysaccharide vaccine efficacy. An evaluation of current recommendations. JAMA 270:1826–1831
140. Centers for Disease Control and P (2004) Updated recommendations on the use of pneumococcal conjugate vaccine: suspension of recommendation for third and fourth dose. MMWR 53:177–178
141. Francis JS, Doherty MC, Lopatin U, Johnston CP, Sinha G, Ross T, Cai M, Hansel NN, Perl T, Ticehurst JR, Carroll K, Thomas DL, Nuermberger E, Bartlett JG (2005) Severe community-onset pneumonia in healthy adults caused by methicillin-resistant *Staphylococcus aureus* carrying the Panton-Valentine leukocidin genes. Clin Infect Dis 40:100–107
142. Micek ST, Dunne M, Kollef MH (2005) Pleuropulmonary complications of Panton-Valentine leukocidin-positive community-acquired methicillin-resistant *Staphylococcus aureus:* importance of treatment with antimicrobials inhibiting exotoxin production. Chest 128:2732–2738
143. Kahn JS (2003) Human metapneumovirus: a newly emerging respiratory pathogen. Curr Opin Infect Dis 16: 255–258
144. Peiris JS, Yuen KY, Osterhaus AD, Stohr K (2003) The severe acute respiratory syndrome. N Engl J Med 349: 2431–2441

145. Hawes S, Seabolt JP (2003) Hantavirus. Clin Lab Sci 16:39–42
146. Ramos MM, Overturf GD, Crowley MR, Rosenberg RB, Hjelle B (2001) Infection with Sin Nombre hantavirus: clinical presentation and outcome in children and adolescents. Pediatrics 108:E27
147. Metersky ML, Ma A, Bratzler DW, Houck PM (2004) Predicting bacteremia in patients with community-acquired pneumonia. Am J Respir Crit Care Med 169:342–347
148. Garcia-Vazquez E, Marcos MA, Mensa J, de Roux A, Puig J, Font C, Francisco G, Torres A (2004) Assessment of the usefulness of sputum culture for diagnosis of community-acquired pneumonia using the PORT predictive scoring system. Arch Intern Med 164:1807–1811
149. Rodriguez RM, Fancher ML, Phelps M, Hawkins K, Johnson J, Stacks K, Rossini T, Way M, Holland D (2001) An emergency department-based randomized trial of nonbronchoscopic bronchoalveolar lavage for early pathogen identification in severe community-acquired pneumonia. Ann Emerg Med 38:357–363
150. Dominguez J, Gali N, Matas L, Pedroso P, Hernandez A, Padilla E, Ausina V (1999) Evaluation of a rapid immunochromatographic assay for the detection of *Legionella* antigen in urine samples. Eur J Clin Microbiol Infect Dis 18:896–898
151. Harrison BD, Farr BM, Connolly CK, Macfarlane JT, Selkon JB, Bartlett CL (1987) The hospital management of community-acquired pneumonia. Recommendations of the British Thoracic Society. J R Coll Physicians Lond 21:267–269
152. Helbig JH, Uldum SA, Bernander S, Luck PC, Wewalka G, Abraham B, Gaia V, Harrison TG (2003) Clinical utility of urinary antigen detection for diagnosis of community-acquired, travel-associated, and nosocomial legionnaires' disease. J Clin Microbiol 41:838–840
153. Yzerman EP, den Boer JW, Lettinga KD, Schellekens J, Dankert J, Peeters M (2002) Sensitivity of three urinary antigen tests associated with clinical severity in a large outbreak of Legionnaires' disease in The Netherlands. J Clin Microbiol 40:3232–3236
154. Dominguez J, Blanco S, Rodrigo C, Azuara M, Gali N, Mainou A, Esteve A, Castellvi A, Prat C, Matas L, Ausina V (2003) Usefulness of urinary antigen detection by an immunochromatographic test for diagnosis of pneumococcal pneumonia in children. J Clin Microbiol 41: 2161–2163
155. Dominguez J, Gali N, Blanco S, Pedroso P, Prat C, Matas L, Ausina V (2001) Detection of *Streptococcus pneumoniae* antigen by a rapid immunochromatographic assay in urine samples. Chest 119:243–249
156. Smith MD, Derrington P, Evans R, Creek M, Morris R, Dance DA, Cartwright K (2003) Rapid diagnosis of bacteremic pneumococcal infections in adults by using the Binax NOW *Streptococcus pneumoniae* urinary antigen test: a prospective, controlled clinical evaluation. J Clin Microbiol 41:2810–2813
157. Templeton KE, Scheltinga SA, van den Eeden WCJFM, Graffelman AW, van den Broek PJ, Claas ECJ (2005) Improved diagnosis of the etiology of community-acquired pneumonia with real-time polymerase chain reaction. Clin Infect Dis 41:345–351
158. Khater F, Moorman JP (2003) Complications of influenza. South Medic J 96:740–743
159. Marik PE (2001) Aspiration pneumonitis and aspiration pneumonia. N Engl J Med 344:665–671
160. Centers for Disease Control and P (2006) High levels of adamantane resistance among influenza A (H3N2) viruses and interim guidelines for use of antiviral agents – United States, 2005–06 influenza season. MMWR 55: 44–46

Chapter 42

Management of Hospital-Associated Pneumonia in the Intensive Care Unit

42

J. Rello, L. Vidaur, E. Díaz, A. Rodríguez

42.1 Introduction

Ventilator-associated pneumonia (VAP) is the leading nosocomial infection in the intensive care unit (ICU) [1] and represents up to 80 % of episodes of hospital-acquired pneumonia (HAP). The true attributable mortality of VAP episodes in critically ill patients has been debated [2]. However, well designed matched cohort studies have demonstrated the association between late onset VAP and higher mortality, particularly when caused by virulent bacteria such as *Pseudomonas aeruginosa* producing type III secretory proteins [3]. Virulence rather than resistance is a key feature.

However, associated mortality and morbidity in VAP is increased in those patients with wrong or delayed initial antibiotic treatment, which is frequently associated with the presence of resistant strains [4, 5]. Nonfermenting Gram-negative bacteria (GNB) other than *P. aeruginosa* are usually resistant to multiple antibiotics, but they have a tendency to colonize rather than cause invasive disease.

The universal colonization of *P. aeruginosa* in patients intubated longer than 5 days [6] and the evidence that methicillin-resistant *Staphylococcus aureus* (MRSA) is currently the most common identified antibiotic-resistant pathogen focus the problem mainly on these two pathogens. Mortalities as high as 50 % have been consistently reported for MRSA pneumonia and *P. aeruginosa* pneumonia. The highest mortality rates are reported if the patient is immunocompromised or has renal failure.

When a VAP episode is suspected in the ICU, the attending physician needs to solve three questions. First, does this patient actually have a VAP? Second, are microbiologic studies indicated? And which antibiotic regimen is the best option for this patient? Once those questions have been answered, the attending physician should follow the evolution of these patients with the aims of evaluating the response to therapy and optimizing antibiotic treatment in order to limit the emergence of multi-resistant bacteria.

We have previously published four reviews on the management of VAP [7–10], and here we expand upon and update our recommendations.

42.2 Confirming the Suspicion of HAP

The suspicion of a new episode of HAP has to be established in hospitalized patients who develop pulmonary infiltrates plus fever and in all intubated patients with clinical signs of sepsis. The physicians must promptly identify the source of infection in order to: (1) start adequate antibiotic therapy for sepsis and (2) control the source of infection if needed [11].

The pathophysiology of VAP includes the spread of infecting organisms to the lower respiratory tract, overwhelming the local respiratory defenses. A local inflammatory response is developed in the respiratory tract, manifested as respiratory purulent secretions. In fact, the absence of purulent secretions in the respiratory tract makes the diagnosis of VAP unlikely [12], except in neutropenic patients or in aspergillosis, but the presence of purulent respiratory secretions may be due to other conditions, frequently with tracheobronchitis.

The differential diagnosis between tracheobronchitis and HAP should be based on radiographic tools, usually chest X-ray. To establish a definite diagnosis of HAP, a radiological opacity with alveolar condensation has to be present. The pre-test probability of the development of ventilator-associated pneumonia has been measured by the Clinical Pulmonary Infection Score (CPIS) [13]. CPIS measures the degree of fever, volume and appearance/characteristics of tracheal secretions, chest radiograph, white blood cell count, oxygenation and tracheal aspirate culture. This score establishes the likelihood of having VAP. Serial measurements of this score have been used to establish clinical resolution of VAP [14]. Singh et al. used a modification of the CPIS and reported that low-risk patients (CPIS <6) with suspected VAP could be treated with 3 days of antibiotic and had better clinical outcomes and fewer antibiotic-resistant superinfections when compared with 10–21 days of therapy [15]. Unfortunately, some variables are subjective, and the value given to each element of the score is arbitrary.

42.3 Confirming the Causative Pathogens

The decision to start antibiotic therapy depends on the microorganisms presumed to be involved. The choice of empirical antibiotic treatment can be improved if the decision is based on direct staining of respiratory samples. Gram stains are available for protected specimen brush samples [16], bronchoalveolar lavage [17] or tracheal aspirates [18]. The quality of the lower respiratory tract samples is also crucial in the interpretation of the microorganisms involved in the etiology of HAP. The presence of >1% of epithelial cells in bronchoscopic samples suggests heavy oropharyngeal contamination [19], so does >10% of epithelial cells if a tracheal aspirate has been obtained [20]. The microbiologic information is of vital importance in order to assure the appropriateness of antibiotic therapy and to optimize therapy from broad to narrow spectrum if the patient is responding to therapy. Direct staining of respiratory secretions is a simple procedure and can give valuable information (in less than an hour) to guide initial therapy. Moreover, Gram staining is useful for determining the quality of the respiratory sample. Regarding this issue some important problems have been detected, for example the use of previous antibiotic therapy, steroids, or the presence of *Pseudomonas aeruginosa* have been associated with negative direct staining [21]. In an international consensus conference [22] on the diagnosis and treatment of VAP, some experts agreed that microbiological findings are useful mainly based on two rules: first, the presence of intracellular bacteria and a positive Gram stain (or other direct tests) may be of great help in selecting the initial antibiotic regimen but not in making the diagnosis of pneumonia. The diagnostic technique used, bronchoscopic or tracheal aspirate with quantitative cultures, did not influence either the rate of de-escalation or of mortality in a recent report [23].

Performing an e-test sensitivity analysis on respiratory or blood samples before microorganism identification anticipates the delivery of sensitivity information the following day of pneumonia onset, with an important shortening of the period of inadequate therapy [24]. Indeed, starting antibiotic therapy quickly, avoiding the delay of microbiologic sampling, has more impact on outcome than the type of semiquantitative or quantitative technique used [23, 25–27].

42.4 Management of VAP

Cardiovascular support and supportive measures to improve hemodynamics and oxygenation are critical to overcome a severe infection. The most important concept that we have learned in the last decade is probably that delay in administration of effective therapy for intubated patients with VAP is associated with increases in mortality rate [28], length of stay and cost [29]. Early implementation of adequate antibiotics correctly and expeditiously, as soon as there is clinical suspicion of HAP, should increase the likelihood of early reduction of bacterial burden of the pathogens responsible, thus minimizing the risks and the potential consequences of delayed therapy [27]. In addition, information regarding risk factors/comorbidities, previous antibiotic exposure and length of hospitalization can provide useful assistance in selecting the initial antibiotic agent. The use of broad spectrum antibiotics should be quickly narrowed based on microbiologic information whenever possible. Initial narrow-spectrum antibiotics are at risk of increasing the probability of death due to inadequate therapy if resistant pathogens are implicated.

Second, quantitative microbiological findings can make it possible to change, adjust, or reduce the administration of antibiotics in some patients. The majority of experts have agreed that the use of broad-spectrum antibiotics for less than 48 h would not induce a significant risk of multiresistance [22, 30]. Classifying patients according to prior duration of mechanical ventilation or prior exposure to antibiotics provided a basis for anticipating the pathogens [31]. Considerable information is available on the influence of certain comorbidities or risk factors such as steroids, head trauma, structural lung disease, and immunocompromise on the spectrum of the pathogens responsible for an infectious event [32]. However, we must take into account that the causes of VAP vary across different hospitals and between different ICUs in the same hospital [33, 34], as indicated in Figs. 42.1 and 42.2. These differences can be explained by differences in patient demographics, strategies for prophylaxis, methods of diagnosis and local patterns of resistant organisms [34]. Table 42.1 summarizes the points that determine the

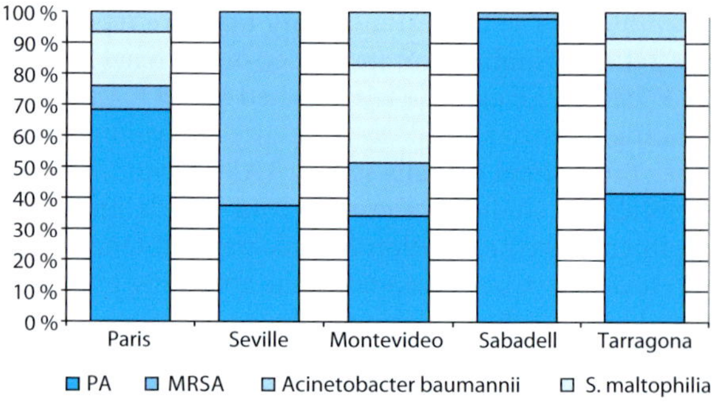

Fig. 42.1. Distribution of pathogens for late onset VAP and antibiotic exposure subset across five different institutions (modified from ref [34]). PA: *Pseudomonas aeruginosa*; MRSA: methicillin-sensitive *Staphylococcus aureus*; S. maltophilia: *Stenotrophomonas maltophilia*

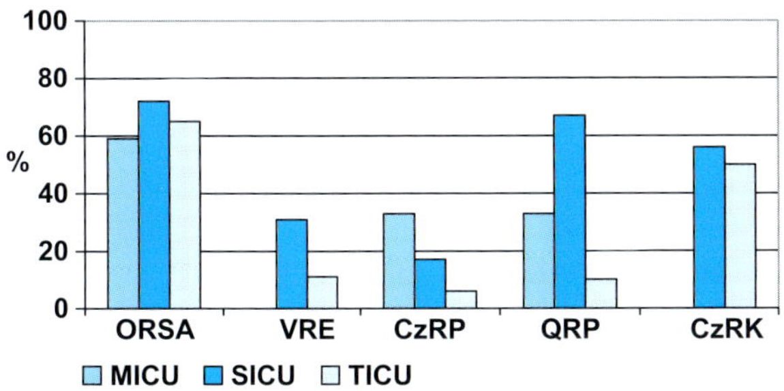

Fig. 42.2. Distribution of different resistant microorganisms causing VAP between three ICUs in a single teaching hospital [modified from ref. [33]). MICU: medical intensive care unit; SICU: surgical intensive care unit; TICU: trauma intensive care unit; ORSA: oxacillin-resistant *Staphylococcus aureus*; VRE: vancomycin-resistant *Enterococcus* species; CzRP: ceftazidime resistant *Pseudomonas* species; QRP: quinolone resistant *Pseudomonas* species; CzRK: ceftazidime resistant *Klebsiella* species

Table 42.1. The "Tarragona strategy" for the therapy of VAP (modified from ref. [64])

1. Antibiotic therapy should be started immediately
2. Antibiotic choice can be targeted, in some cases, based on direct staining
3. The prescription should be modified in the light of microbiologic findings
4. Prolonging antibiotic treatment does not prevent recurrences
5. Patients with chronic obstructive pulmonary disease or 1 week of intubation should receive combination therapy, due to the risk of ventilator-associated pneumonia caused by *Pseudomonas aeruginosa*
6. Methicillin-resistant *Staphylococcus aureus* is not expected in the absence of antibiotic exposure, whereas methicillin-sensitive *S. aureus* should be strongly suspected in comatose patients
7. Therapy against yeast is not required, even in the presence of *Candida* species colonization
8. Vancomycin administration for Gram-positive pneumonia is associated with a very poor outcome
9. The specific choice of agent should avoid any regimen to which a patient has been exposed previously
10. Guidelines should be regularly updated and customized to local patterns

management of VAP in our institution. Knowledge of the local microbial epidemiology and susceptibility patterns is crucial for the initial choice of antibiotics [35].

Overall, some patients (who develop their infection within 5 days of hospitalization, who are free of recent antibiotic exposure and who have not had hospitalization in the previous 3 months) are at low risk from resistant organisms. In this subset, adequate initial selection would be a non-pseudomonal third generation cephalosporin because antibiotics should target common community-acquired organisms in addition to some Enterobacteriaceae and methicillin-sensitive *Staphylococcus aureus* (MSSA). The presence of MSSA should be strongly suspected in comatose patients. Several reports have demonstrated a higher incidence of MSSA in patients with altered levels of consciousness [36]. Drugs effective against *S. aureus* should be included in the empirical regimen for treating nosocomial pneumonia in patients in coma.

Methicillin-resistant *Staphylococcus aureus* (MRSA) pneumonias are common in patients with prolonged intubation periods and prior use of antibiotics. This pathogen is the second most frequently isolated from patients who die of pneumonia. The treatment options for this pathogen are still limited. A high mortality rate among patients treated with vancomycin for pneumonia caused both by MRSA and MSSA has been consistently reported [37]. It might probably be due to the poor lung penetration of vancomycin which results from prescribing label doses (1 g/12 h) [38]. In addition, underdosification of antibiotics is frequent in ventilated hyperdynamic patients who have an increase in the volume of distribution (see Chapter 12 by Lipman). Achieving adequate steady state levels usually takes 4 days for teicoplanin [39]. This evidence suggested that current glycopeptides are suboptimal for MRSA pneumonia [37, 40]. Daptomycin is ineffective in the treatment of pneumonia. It has not only limited penetration into pulmonary epithelial fluid, but its activity is inhibited by pulmonary surfactant. In a randomized trial, patients with nosocomial MRSA pneumonia [41] who received quinupristin/dalfopristin had a clinical response rate of 19.4% compared with 40% in vancomycin recipients. Post hoc analysis of randomized clinical trials has suggested the potential superiority of linezolid therapy over vancomycin therapy using label doses in treating nosocomial pneumonia (and VAP) [42, 43]. Continuous administration of vancomycin has been associated with improved survival of MRSA pneumonia compared with standard dosification [44].

Pseudomonas aeruginosa is frequent in patients with structural pulmonary disease, 1 week of prior hospitalization, prolonged periods of intubation (>5 days), and prior exposure to antibiotics [45]. Empirical treatment in patients meeting these criteria should include combination therapy with drugs with antipseudomonal activity until a microbiological diagnosis is established to reduce the risk of initial therapy with a resistant agent. Carbapenems are the drugs of choice for patients suspected of being infected by *P. aeruginosa* who are receiving beta-lactam agents. If the patient is receiving a carbapenem, an antipseudomonal fluoroquinolone is a reasonable option. Finally, if a patient with VAP is receiving a fluoroquinolone, combination therapy based on piperacillin-tazobactam should be considered [46].

Acinetobacter baumannii has specific risk factors that differ from *P. aeruginosa* or other nonfermenters. Baraibar et al. [47] identified risk factors for *A. baumannii* VAP that included neurosurgery, ARDS, head trauma and large-volume pulmonary aspiration. Resistance is increasing, carbapenems, sulbactam, tigecycline and colistin being the most sensitive agents. Sulbactam is bacteriostatic and is suitable for mild infections using an 8-g/day dosification. Colistin can be used aerosolized. Tygecycline would be a reliable alternative in the future and clinical trials are ongoing. *A. baumannii* tends to cause polymicrobial infections colonizing the respiratory tract of patients with artificial airways rather than causing invasive disease. If the risk of *Acinetobacter baumannii* exists, experimental models have suggested that antimicrobial therapy should include a carbapenem, alone or associated with rifampin or tobramycin [48].

42.5 Optimization of Antimicrobial Therapy for VAP

Once a patient has been diagnosed of having HAP and an empirical broad spectrum antibiotic has been started, the evaluation of resolution of different clinical parameters of HAP is a useful tool to tailor the response to treatment. The most widely used variables to evaluate the response to treatment in VAP are clinical, microbiological or biochemical [8, 47–56]. Assessment of clinical resolution and the recommended approach to patients with poor resolution is described in detail in the next chapter.

The main goal of treatment of HAP in critically ill patients is the start of appropriate initial antibiotic therapy as early as possible in order to diminish mortality related to this nosocomial infection [57–59]. The initial antibiotic therapy has to cover all the responsible pathogens involved. However, the overuse of antibiotics is associated with the emergence of resistant bacteria [60]. An approach to the treatment of HAP based on de-escalation of antimicrobial therapy, once the microorganism responsible for VAP is isolated, diminishes the overuse of antibiotics and the emergence of resistant bacteria.

De-escalation requires the implementation of initial broad-spectrum empirical antibiotic therapy and aims to avoid the overuse of antibiotics [23]. The first stage involves administering broad spectrum antibiotics. The second stage focuses on simplifying the antibiotic therapy. This approach to the management of HAP involves: (a) changing the focus from multiple agents to single agent if *Pseudomonas aeruginosa* is not present; (b) shortening the therapy to <5 days if the culture is negative and there is >48 h of defervescence; and (c) changing from a broad to a narrow agent based on culture data. In the absence of *P. aeruginosa*, patients with combination therapy must be switched to monotherapy after withholding ciprofloxacin or amikacin. Interestingly, the mortality of patients with de-escalation has been reported to be lower than that observed in the group of patients with initial antibiotic therapy unchanged [23].

42.6 Duration of Antibiotic Courses for HAP

A course of 14–21 days of antibiotic treatment has been advocated to treat HAP [61], but the length of antibiotic treatment has not been clearly defined. Long courses of antibiotics can increase costs, side effects, and resistant phenotypes but do not prevent recurrences [62]. Shorter antibiotic regimens have been used to reduce antimicrobial costs, adverse events and the emergence of antibiotic-resistant pathogens [15]. Chastre et al. [63] have demonstrated that an 8-day course of antibiotics is comparable to 15 days in terms of mortality, superinfections and relapses of pneumonia.

42.7 Conclusion

Management of HAP needs to balance the avoidance of unnecessary antibiotic overuse with adequate initial empiric therapy. A clinical diagnosis based on new pulmonary opacity and purulent respiratory secretions plus other signs of inflammation is valuable in screening for patients with suspected HAP. A rational strategy starts with immediate initiation of adequate antibiotics and collection of respiratory secretions to evaluate for a causative organism. A respiratory specimen with direct staining and quantitative cultures in intubated patients should be obtained as a minimum. Overall, the need to choose adequate antibiotics correctly and expeditiously is fundamental in the use of broad spectrum antibiotics, but needs to be quickly narrowed based on microbiologic information. However, some patients (who develop their infection within 5 days of hospitalization, who are free of recent antibiotic exposure and who have not had hospitalizations in the previous 3 months) are at low risk for resistant organisms. In this subset, adequate initial selection could be a non-pseudomonal third generation cephalosporin, since antibiotics should target usual community-acquired organisms in addition to some Enterobacteriaceae and *Staphylococcus aureus*. Coverage of MRSA should be limited only to wards with concomitant index cases and to patients under antibiotic exposure. Patients at risk of *Pseudomonas aeruginosa* (e.g., 1 week of prior hospitalization, COPD, etc.) require the initial use of a combination of piperacillin/tazobactam and ciprofloxacin, or amikacin plus imipenem, meropenem or an antipseudomonal cephalosporin. If the risk of *Acinetobacter baumannii* exists, one of these agents should be a carbapenem. Af-

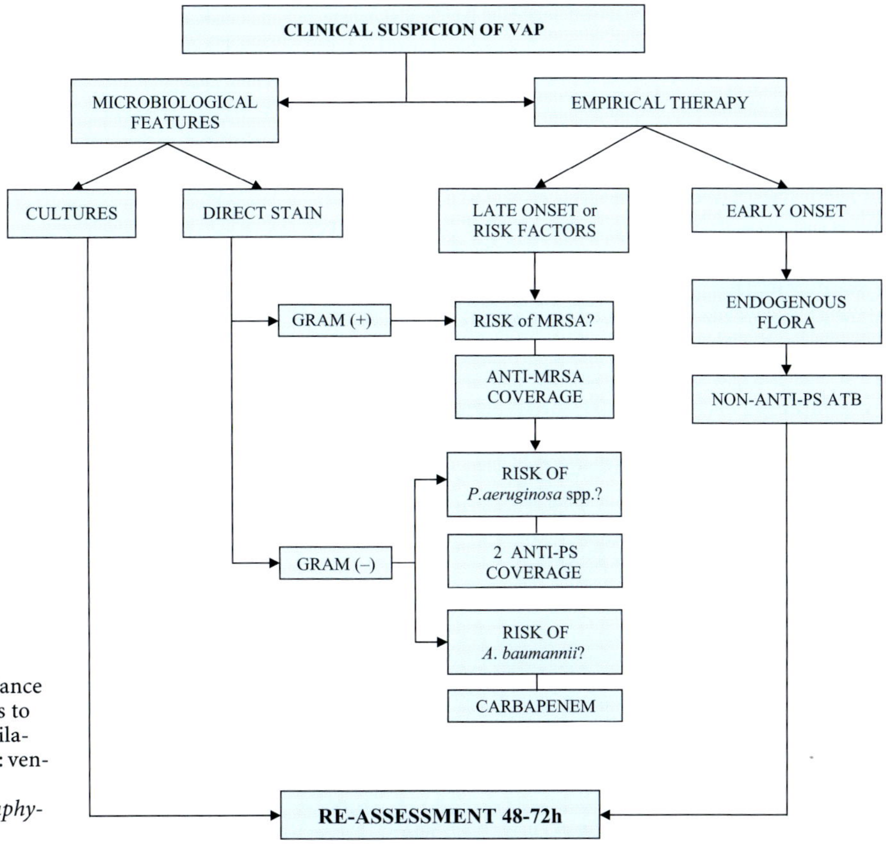

Fig. 42.3. Flow diagram for guidance in initial management decisions to the patient with suspected ventilator-associated pneumonia. VAP: ventilator-associated pneumonia; MRSA: methicillin-resistant *Staphylococcus aureus*

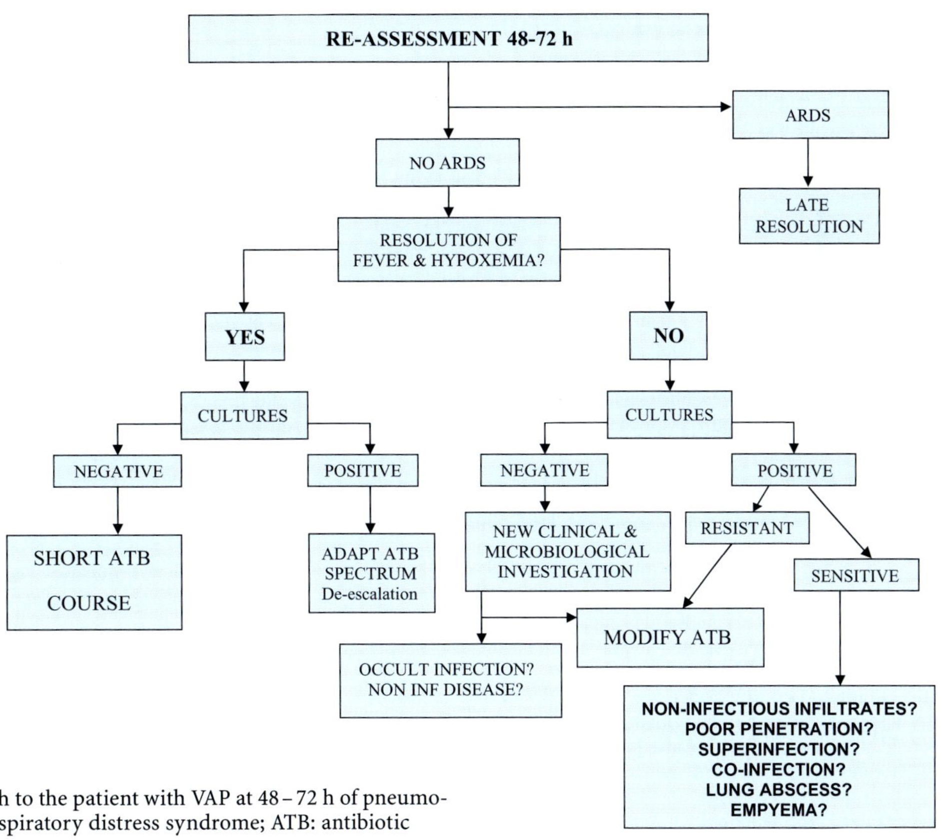

Fig. 42.4. Clinical approach to the patient with VAP at 48–72 h of pneumonia onset. ARDS: acute respiratory distress syndrome; ATB: antibiotic

ter 48 h of therapy, each patient should be re-evaluated based mainly on resolution of hypoxemia and fever plus initial microbiologic information. Whereas broad-spectrum therapy is warranted in many patients initially, that treatment may be narrowed considerably as culture results identify the causative organism and its sensitivity. Recent data suggest that reducing overall treatment duration to a maximum of 1 week is safe, effective and is less likely to promote the growth of resistant organisms in patients who are clinically improving. An algorithm summarizing the management approach to a patient with suspected VAP is given in Figs. 42.3 and 42.4. Optimal management should be based on a strategy combining early high doses of an effective agent for a short period of time, which is further simplified based on microbiologic information.

Acknowledgements. Supported in part by grants from CIRIT SGR 2005/920, Distincio Recerca Universitaria (JR), RED RESPIRA (ISCiii-RTIC 03/11), and FISS PI 05/2410.

References

1. Vincent JL, Bihari DJ, Suter PM, et al. (1995) The prevalence of nosocomial infection in intensive care units in Europe: Results of the European Prevalence of Infection in Intensive Care (EPIC study). JAMA 274:639–644
2. Rello J (1999) Impact of nosocomial infections on outcome: Myths and evidence. Infect Control Hosp Epidemiol 20:392–394
3. Hauser AR, Cobb E, Bodi M, et al. (2002) Type III protein secretion is associated with poor clinical outcomes in patients with ventilator-associated pneumonia caused by *Pseudomonas aeruginosa*. Crit Care Med 30:521–8
4. Rello J, Gallego M, Mariscal D, et al. (1997) The value of routine microbiological investigation in ventilator-associated pneumonia. Am J Respir Crit Care Med 156:196–200
5. Luna CM, Vujacich P, Niederman MS, et al. (1997) Impact of BAL data on the therapy and outcome of ventilator-associated pneumonia. Chest 111:676–685
6. Valles J, Mariscal D, Cortes P, et al. (2004) Patterns of colonization by *Pseudomonas aeruginosa* in intubated patients: a 3-year prospective study of 1,607 isolates using pulsed-field gel electrophoresis with implications for prevention of ventilator-associated pneumonia. Intensive Care Med 30:1768–75
7. Sandiumenge A, Diaz E, Bodi M, Rello J (2003) Therapy of ventilator-associated pneumonia. A patient based approach based on the ten rules of "The Tarragona strategy". Intensive Care Med 29:876–883
8. Rello J, Diaz E (2003) Pneumonia in the intensive care unit. Crit Care Med 31:2544–2551
9. Díaz E, Rodriguez AH, Rello J (2005) Ventilator-associated pneumonia: Issues related to the artificial airway. Respir Care 50:900–906
10. Vidaur L, Sirgo G, Rodriguez AH, Rello J (2005) Clinical approach to the patient with suspected ventilator-associated pneumonia. Respir Care 50:965–974
11. Vidaur L, Rodriguez A, Rello J (2004) Antibiotic therapy for sepsis, severe sepsis and septic shock: The "Tarragona" strategy. In: Yearbook of intensive care and emergency medicine. Springer, Berlin Heidelberg New York, pp 229–241
12. Gallego M, Rello J (1999) Diagnostic testing for ventilator-associated pneumonia. Clin Chest Med 20:671–79
13. Pugin J, Auckentaler R, Mili N (1991) Diagnosis of ventilator-associated pneumonia by bacteriologic analysis of bronchoscopic and nonbronchoscopic "blind" bronchoalveolar lavage fluid. Am Rev Respir Dis 143:1121–1129
14. Luna C, Blanzaco D, Niederman M, et al. (2003) Resolution of ventilator-associated pneumonia: Prospective evaluation of the clinical pulmonary infection score as an early clinical predictor of outcome. Crit Care Med 31:676–82
15. Singh N, Rogers P, Atwood CW, et al. (2000) Short course empiric antibiotic therapy for patients with pulmonary infiltrates in the intensive care unit. Am J Respir Crit Care Med 162:505–511
16. Rello J, Mariscal D, Gallego M, et al. (2002) Effect of thioglycolate as transport medium in the direct examination of respiratory samples and guiding initial antibiotic treatment in intubated patients with pneumonia. Crit Care Med 30:311–314
17. Chastre J, Fagon JY, Soler P (1998) Diagnosis of nosocomial bacterial pneumonia in intubated patients undergoing ventilation: Comparison of the usefulness of bronchoalveolar lavage and the protected specimen brush. Am J Med 84:499–506
18. Morris AJ, David CT, Reller LB (1993) Rejection criteria for endotracheal aspirates from adults. J Clin Microbiol 31:1027–1029
19. Mertens AH, Nagler JM, Galdermans DI, et al. (1998) Quality assessment of protected specimen brush samples by microscopic cell count. Am J Respir Crit Care Med 157: 1240–1243
20. Salata RA, Lederman MM, Shlaes DM, et al. (1987) Diagnosis of nosocomial pneumonia in intubated, intensive care unit patients. Am Rev Respir Dis 135:426–32
21. Valles J, Rello J, Fernández R, et al. (1994) Role of bronchoalveolar lavage in mechanically ventilated patients with suspected pneumonia. Eur J Microbiol Infect Dis 13:549–558
22. Rello J, Paiva A, Baraibar J, et al. (2001) International conference for the development of Consensus on the Diagnosis and Treatment of Ventilator-associated pneumonia. Chest 120:955–70
23. Rello J, Vidaur L, Sandiumenge A, et al. (2004) De-escalation therapy in ventilator-associated pneumonia. Crit Care Med 32:2183–90
24. Bouza E, Torres MV, Burillo A (2005) Aportación del laboratorio de microbiología al diagnóstico de la neumonía asociada a la ventilación mecánica. Enferm Infecc Microbiol Clin 23 (Suppl 3):2–9
25. Rello J, Gallego M, Mariscal D, et al. (1997) The value of routine microbial investigation in ventilator-associated pneumonia. Am J Respir Crit Care Med 156:196–200
26. Gallego M, Valles J, Rello J (1997) New perspectives in the diagnosis of ventilator-associated pneumonia. Curr Opin Pulm Med 23:116–119
27. Iregui M, Ward S, Sherman G, et al. (2002) Clinical importance of delays in initiation of appropriate antibiotic treatment for ventilator-associated pneumonia. Chest 122:262–268
28. Kollef MH, Ward S (1998) The influence of mini-BAL cultures on patient outcomes: implications for the antibiotic management of ventilator-associated pneumonia. Chest 113:412–20
29. Dupont H, Mentec H, Sollet JP, Bleichner G (2001) Impact of appropriateness of initial antibiotic therapy on the outcome of ventilator-associated pneumonia. Intensive Care Med 27:355–62

30. Soo Hoo GW, Wen E, Nguyen TV, et al. (2005) Impact of clinical guidelines in the management of severe hospital-acquired pneumonia. Chest 128:2778–87
31. Trouillet JL, Chastre J, Vuagnat A, et al. (1998) Ventilator-associated pneumonia caused by potentially drug-resistant bacteria. Am J Respir Crit Care Med 157:531–39
32. Rello J, Ausina V, Ricart M, et al. (1994) Risk factors for infection by *Pseudomonas aeruginosa* in patients with ventilator-associated pneumonia. Intensive Care Med 20:193–8
33. Namias N, Samiian L, Nino D, et al. (2000) Incidence and susceptibility of pathogenic bacteria vary between intensive care unit within a single hospital: implications for empiric antibiotic strategies. J Trauma 49:638–45
34. Rello J, Sa-Borges M, Correa H, et al. (1999) Variations in etiology of ventilator-associated pneumonia across four treatment sites: implications for antimicrobial prescribing practices. Am J Respir Crit Care Med 160:608–13
35. Sandiumenge A, Diaz E, Bodi M, Rello J (2003) Therapy of ventilator-associated pneumonia. A patient-based approach based on the ten rules of "The Tarragona Strategy". Intensive Care Med 29:876–83
36. Rello J, Ausina V, Castella J, et al. (1992) Nosocomial respiratory tract infections in multiple trauma patients. Influence of level of consciousness with implications for therapy. Chest 102:525–9
37. Gonzalez C, Rubio M, Romero-Vivas J, et al. (1999) Bacteremic pneumonia due to *Staphylococcus aureus:* A comparison of disease caused by methicillin-resistant and methicillin-susceptible organisms. Clin Infect Dis 29:1171–7
38. Lamer C, de Beco V, Soler P, et al. (1993) Analysis of vancomycin entry into pulmonary lining fluid by bronchoalveolar lavage in critically ill patients. Antimicrob Agents Chemother 37:281–6
39. Pea F, Brollo L, Viale P, et al. (2003) Teicoplanin therapeutic drug monitoring in critically ill patients: a retrospective study emphasizing the importance of a loading dose. J Antimicrob Chemother 51:971–975
40. Rello J, Torres A, Ricart M, et al. (1994) Ventilator-associated pneumonia by *Staphylococcus aureus.* Comparison of methicillin-resistant and methicillin-sensitive episodes. Am J Respir Crit Care Med 150:1545–49
41. Fagon J, Patrick H, Haas DW, et al. (2000) Treatment of gram-positive nosocomial pneumonia. Prospective randomized comparison of quinupristin/dalfopristin versus vancomycin. Nosocomial Pneumonia Group. Am J Respir Crit Care Med 161:753–62
42. Kollef MH, Rello J, Cammarata SK, et al. (2004) Retrospective analysis of two double-blind studies comparing linezolid with vancomycin. Intensive Care Med 30:388–94
43. Wunderink R, Rello J, Cammarata SK, et al. (2003) Linezolid vs Vancomycin. Analysis of two double-blind studies of patients with methicillin-resistant *Staphylococcus aureus* nosocomial pneumonia. Chest 124:1789–97
44. Rello J, Sole-Violan J, Sa-Borges M, et al. (2005) Pneumonia caused by oxacillin-resistant *Staphylococcus aureus* treated with glycopeptides. Crit Care Med 33:1983–7
45. Rello J, Jubert P, Valles J, et al. (1996) Evaluation of outcome for intubated patients with pneumonia due to *Pseudomonas aeruginosa.* Clin Infect Dis 23:973–8
46. Rello J, Diaz E (2001) Optimal use of antibiotics for intubation-associated pneumonia. Intensive Care Med 27:337–9
47. Baraibar J, Correa H, Mariscal D, et al. (1997) Risk factors for infection by *Acinetobacter baumannii* in intubated patients with nosocomial pneumonia. Chest 112:1050–4
48. Montero A, Ariza J, Corbella X, et al. (2004) Antibiotic combinations for serious infections caused by carbapenem-resistant *Acinetobacter baumannii* in a mouse pneumonia model. J Antimicrob Chemother 54:1085–91
49. Denessen PJW, van der Ven AIAM, Kessels AGH, et al. (2001) Resolution of infectious parameters after antimicrobial therapy in patients with ventilator-associated pneumonia. Am J Respir Crit Care Med 163:1371–75
50. Ioanas M, Ferrer M, Calvacanti M, et al. (2004) Causes and predictors of nonresponse to treatment of intensive care unit-acquired pneumonia. Crit Care Med 32:938–45
51. Ioanas M, Ewig S, Torres A (2003) Treatment failure in patients with ventilator-associated pneumonia. Infect Dis Clin North Am 17:753–71
52. Garrard CS, A'Court CD (1995) The diagnosis of pneumonia in the critically ill. Chest 108:17S–25S
53. Vidaur L, Gualis B, Rodríguez A, et al. (2005) Clinical resolution in patients with suspicion of ventilator-associated pneumonia: A cohort study comparing patients with and without acute respiratory distress syndrome. Crit Care Med 33:1248–1253
54. Wunderink RG (1995) Ventilator-associated pneumonia. Failure to respond to antibiotic therapy. Clinics Chest Med 16:173–193
55. American Thoracic Society (2005) Guidelines for the management of adults with hospital-acquired, ventilator-associated, and healthcare-associated pneumonia. Am J Respir Crit Care Med 171:388–416
56. Luyt CE, Guerin V, Combes A, et al. (2005) Procalcitonin kinetics as a prognostic marker of ventilator-associated pneumonia. Am J Respir Crit Care Med 171:48–53
57. Luna CM, Vujacich P, Niederman MS, et al. (1997) Impact of BAL data on the therapy and outcome of ventilator-associated pneumonia. Chest 111:676–85
58. Kollef MH (2000) Inadequate antimicrobial treatment an important determinant of outcome for hospitalized patients. Clin Infect Dis 31:S131–S138
59. Wunderink RG (2003) Tis a gift to be simple. Chest 124: 777–78
60. Hoffken G, Niederman MS (2002) Nosocomial pneumonia: The importance of a de-escalation strategy for antibiotic treatment of pneumonia in the ICU. Chest 122: 2183–2196
61. American Thoracic Society (1995) Hospital-acquired pneumonia in adults: Diagnosis, assessment of severity, initial antimicrobial therapy, and preventive strategies. A consensus statement. Am J Respir Crit Care Med 153: 1711–25
62. Rello J, Mariscal D, March F, et al. (1998) Recurrent *Pseudomonas aeruginosa* pneumonia in ventilated patients. Relapse or reinfection. Am J Respir Crit Care Med 157: 912–916
63. Chastre J, Wolff M, Fagon JY, et al. (2003) Comparison of 8 to 15 days of antibiotic therapy for ventilator-associated pneumonia in adults: a randomized trial. JAMA 290:2588–2598
64. Sandiumenge A, Díaz E, Bodi M, Rello J (2003) Therapy of ventilator-associated pneumonia. A patient-based approach based on the ten rules of "The Tarragona Strategy". Intensive Care Med 29:876–83

43 Assessment of Resolution of Ventilator Associated Pneumonia

M.L. Groth, M.S. Niederman

Ventilator associated pneumonia (VAP) is the most frequent infectious complication in critically ill patients, associated with a prolonged length of stay in the intensive care unit (ICU) and a significantly increased risk of death [1, 2]. The attributable mortality of VAP varies with the infecting organism and with the patient population [3]; for example, mortality is higher in patients with acute respiratory distress syndrome (ARDS) [4], as well as in medical compared to surgical patients with VAP. The natural history of resolution of VAP is not well defined, but mortality of VAP has been well studied, and the clinical predictors of mortality have also been characterized [5–7]. It is reasonable to assume that patients at a high risk of death from VAP are more likely to have delayed resolution, or prolonged recovery, if they survive an episode of VAP [7].

In this chapter, we review the available data about the time course of resolution of VAP, including the definition of resolution and the clinical features that correlate with outcomes in this illness. Once the natural history of VAP is better defined, we may be able to identify patients with a good clinical response early in the course of illness, and then possibly shorten the duration of antibiotic in this group. On the other hand, if we can also identify patients with a poor response to initial antibiotic therapy, at an early time point, based on a knowledge of the natural history of illness, it may be possible to intervene with aggressive diagnostic and therapeutic maneuvers that could improve outcome.

Once a patient is suspected of having VAP, it is essential to collect a lower respiratory tract culture, preferably before any change or initiation of antibiotic therapy. The culture can be collected invasively [bronchoscopic protected specimen brush (PSB) or bronchoalveolar lavage (BAL)] or non-invasively (endotracheal aspirate or blind brush or lavage samples). In addition, the respiratory sample can be cultured quantitatively or semi-quantitatively (light, moderate or heavy growth being reported) [2]. Initial empiric therapy may need to be changed once results of respiratory tract secretions or blood cultures are available, with the goal of using as focused and specific a regimen as possible. Repeat cultures of respiratory tract secretions are subsequently needed to evaluate for microbiologic resolution on the infection.

43.1 How To Define the Resolution of VAP

Resolution of VAP can be based on either clinical or microbiological end points [8]. The risk of death in patients with VAP is similar whether VAP is diagnosed clinically or bronchoscopically [3, 6, 9, 10]. Clinical end points, such as improvement, resolution, delayed resolution, relapse, failure and death, can be defined, but it is important to specify how the pneumonia was diagnosed.

If we use a clinical definition of disease, some patients with non-infectious causes of lung infiltrates and clinical abnormalities will be included. The absence of response to antibiotics may indicate that the infiltrates were not caused by infection, but were due to acute lung injury, atelectasis, pulmonary edema, pulmonary contusion, hemorrhage, chemical pneumonitis, drug toxicity or other inflammatory conditions [8]. Clinical response to therapy can be defined in terms of temperature, purulence of secretions, leukocytosis, indices of oxygenation, such as PaO_2/FiO_2 ratio, and radiographic abnormalities. Many of these parameters have been combined into the Clinical Pulmonary Infection Score, which when measured serially, has been used to clinically define the presence of VAP resolution [5].

If we use a microbiologic definition of VAP, cultures of respiratory tract secretions must be obtained to establish the etiologic pathogen. Microbiologic end points are primarily the eradication or persistence of the organisms, and can also include the emergence of resistance or superinfection with a new organism that was not present initially.

If the correct diagnosis is VAP, then resolution can be defined using clinical or bacteriologic measurements, or sometimes both types of information can be combined to define the course of illness. Clinical improvement in VAP is usually apparent after 48–72 h of therapy, as discussed below, and therefore the selected antibiotic regimen should not be changed during this time, unless there are signs of progressive deterioration or it is dictated by the initial culture results. The exact time course of normal resolution is not well defined, but the available data are summarized below. Delayed resolution is present if the time response to therapy is longer than expected. Relapse and recurrence are similar and imply an initial clinical improvement followed by a subsequent clinical deterioration. If the event involves the same organism (the inclusion of microbiologic information), then a relapse or recurrence is present, while a superinfection is present, if the etiologic organism is a newly acquired pathogen [8]. The ultimate non-resolution is death, but not all mortalities are the direct result of VAP, and approximately one-third to one-half of all mortalities are attributable to the pneumonia itself [3, 7, 11].

43.2 Clinical Predictors of Mortality in VAP

A number of clinical findings have been identified that increase the risk for mortality from VAP and these same risk factors are associated with poor response to antibiotic therapy, and presumably a slower response rate in patients who do recover. They include underlying severe systemic illness and complex pre-existing comorbid conditions. Multivariate analysis of several studies suggests that these risk factors could be categorized as patient factors, bacteriologic factors, or therapy-related features (Table 43.1). The patient factors include: age >60 years, prolonged duration of mechanical ventilation, coma on admission, shock, creatinine >1.5, transfer from another ward to the ICU, bilateral infiltrates, an ultimately fatal underlying condition, multiple system organ failure, and a non-surgical primary diagnosis [7, 12–16]. The bacteriologic factors that predict mortality include the presence of "high risk" or resistant pathogens [*P. aeruginosa* or *S. aureus* including methicillin-resistant organisms (MRSA)], the emergence of resistance during therapy, or the presence of superinfection. The therapy related predictors of mortality include: inappropriate initial therapy and prior antibiotic therapy (particularly for a previous pneumonia so that therapy is being given for superinfection) [6, 7, 17, 18].

Table 43.1. Risk factors for an adverse outcome (mortality) from VAP

Patient risk factors
Prolonged mechanical ventilation before pneumonia
Underlying fatal or serious illness
APACHE score of 11–30
Severe pneumonia (with sepsis, or ARDS)
Bilateral lung infiltrates
Medical (vs. surgical) diagnosis
Age >60
Bacteriologic risk factors
High risk pathogen
Pseudomonas aeruginosa
Acinetobacter sp.
S. maltophilia
Methicillin-resistant *S. aureus*
Antibiotic resistant pathogen
Especially if acquired during therapy
Superinfection after a first course of therapy
Therapy-related risk factors
Prior antibiotic therapy
Inadequate initial therapy (organism not sensitive to therapeutic agent)
Inadequate dose or dosing regimen

While most studies have looked only at mortality, there are some limited data about the predictors of non-response to VAP therapy, that include both those who died and those who were slow to improve. Ionas and colleagues [19] evaluated 71 patients with VAP, and found that 44 had a non-response, defined by a lack of clinical improvement, or worsening, after 72 h of therapy, and 22 of these patients subsequently died. In a univariate analysis, the predictors of non-response were: male sex, initial hypotension, use of corticosteroids, prior pneumonia in the preceding year, and signs of systemic inflammation (elevated IL-6 and IL-8 levels) on the day of VAP onset. Only an initial elevation of IL-6 was associated with non-response in a multivariate analysis. In the non-survivors in this study, the only predictor of mortality in a multivariate analysis was persistent elevation of IL-6 on day 3 of therapy. Other factors predicting mortality in the univariate analysis included: inappropriate antimicrobial therapy, MRSA as a cause of pneumonia, persistent hypoxemia on day 3, and reintubation. In another study, Combes et al. found that 28 of 124 patients had a VAP recurrence [20]. Recurrence was defined when there were clinical signs of pneumonia, with a new or progressive infiltrate and in the study, recurrence was defined as either "persistence" if the original pathogen was present on a repeat quantitative culture of a protected brush or BAL sample (persistence), or as "relapse" if the finding of pathogens occurred after the completion of therapy. The presence of recurrence was unrelated to the etiology of the first episode of VAP but was correlated in a multivariate analysis with: severity of the initial radiographic abnormality, persistent fever at day 8, and the presence of ARDS on day 8. Recurrence prolonged the duration of ventilation, the hospital stay and the ICU stay, and was also correlated with an increased mortality rate, emphasizing the close relation between mortality and non-response to therapy.

A summary of the available data about risk factors for mortality from VAP is included below.

43.2.1 Patient Risk Factors

43.2.1.1 *Duration of Mechanical Ventilation*

Late onset VAP (after 4 days of mechanical ventilation) has a much higher mortality than early onset VAP (within the first 4 days of mechanical ventilation) [2, 18]. This probably reflects the fact that *P. aeruginosa*, *Acinetobacter* sp. and methicillin-resistant *S. aureus* (MRSA) and other resistant organisms are more common in late onset VAP and are more difficult to treat [2, 21, 22]. In addition, these organisms are commonly multi-resistant and they may persistently colonize intubated patients (especially *P. aeruginosa*), and thus microbiologic eradication may be impossible [23]. In contrast, early onset VAP is caused by *S. pneumoniae*, *H. influenzae*, and methicillin-sensitive *S. aureus* [2], organisms that can be eradicated rapidly by readily available antimicrobial therapy, and a short course of antibiotics may be effective [24]. Another confounding factor is that the patients who develop late-onset infections have more severe underlying illness, as reflected by the need for prolonged ventilation. It is, therefore, unclear whether it is the types of bacteria present in late onset VAP or the disease-related factors that predispose to late onset infection, that lead to a relatively worse outcome. These effects are difficult to separate, and the problem is further confounded by the fact that not all investigators have been able to demonstrate that patients with late-onset VAP have a higher mortality than those with early-onset pneumonia [3]. More recently, some insight into this issue has emerged with the recognition that some patients with "healthcare related pneumonia" (HCAP) are at risk for infection with multi-drug resistant (MDR) pathogens, regardless of the time of pneumonia onset. This is because, by definition, these patients are in contact with the healthcare environment prior to hospitalization (such as those who reside in nursing homes, those recently hospitalized in the past 90 days, and those undergoing hemodialysis) [2], and thus when they develop VAP, the pathogens can be the same early in the hospital stay as are present later in the hospital stay.

43.2.1.2 *Severity of Illness on Admission*

Scoring systems, such as the APACHE (Acute Physiology And Chronic Health Evaluation) score, have been used to define severity of illness on admission to the ICU. In one study of 279 ICU patients, of whom 93 had infection, the development of infection was associated with an increased risk of death. However, the greatest mortality attributable to nosocomial infection occurred in patients with moderate degrees of illness, and not in those with very mild or very severe disease [25]. The odds ratio of attributable death was 4.5 in patients with an APACHE score of 11 – 20, and 2.2 in those with a score of 21 – 30. These findings suggest that patients who have very mild illness on admission will recover regardless of the presence of infection, while those with very severe illness have their outcome defined by factors other than infection. In spite of these findings, Rello et al. did observe that the development of nosocomial pneumonia has a direct impact on severity of illness as measured by the APACHE score [26]. They followed 26 patients with antibiotic sensitive VAP due to *P. aeruginosa*, and defined a population of 18 patients who responded to therapy and a group of 6 who did not. Although both groups had similar APACHE scores on admission, the responders had a serial drop in the APACHE score, even when pneumonia was diagnosed, and as it was treated. However, the non-responders had a serial increase in APACHE score, which was measured at the time of VAP diagnosis, and the score rose even higher 72 h after treatment. If the score at this time was ≥ 20, the mortality rate was nearly 100 % [26].

43.2.1.3 *Severity of Pneumonia*

Pneumonia-related risk factors associated with an increased risk of death include worsening hypoxemia, shock or severe sepsis, bilateral radiographic involvement and persistent respiratory failure [7]. The impact of bacteremia on outcome is unclear since different studies have had conflicting results [27, 28]. As mentioned above, initial radiographic abnormality, as well as persistence on day 8, were predictors of recurrence in one study, and recurrence in turn was a mortality predictor [20].

43.2.1.4 *Age*

In some studies, age has been identified as a mortality risk in both univariate and multivariate analysis. However, the impact of age itself has been variable, with studies implying that the association of age with other disease processes may be the most important explanation for the observed risk. The relevant age for mortality has varied from > 45 years to > 60 or > 70 years [14, 15, and 16].

43.2.1.5 *Type of Patient*

Chastre et al. found that in patients with acute respiratory distress syndrome (ARDS) the presence of VAP significantly increased the duration of mechanical ventilation but not mortality, while mortality was increased by VAP in patients without ARDS [29]. The effect of VAP on mortality is different for medical compared to surgical patients: surgical and trauma patients have a lower attributable mortality rate from VAP than other populations [3, 30]. This could be explained because trauma patients are often young, without underlying comorbidities, and often have early-onset VAP, caused by sensitive organisms that are relatively easy to treat.

43.2.2 Bacteriologic Risk Factors

43.2.2.1 High Risk and Antibiotic Resistant Pathogens

Pseudomonas aeruginosa, Acinetobacter sp., *Stenotrophomonas maltophilia* and methicillin-resistant *Staphylococcus aureus* are considered "high risk" pathogens and are associated with higher mortality [17, 22, 31, 32, 33], although one study did not find them to be a risk factor for relapse or persistence [20]. These organisms tend to be antibiotic-resistant, and are difficult to treat, and the patients who are affected are often seriously ill. Fagon and colleagues observed that the overall attributable mortality of VAP was 27%, but rose to 43% when VAP was due to *P. aeruginosa* or *Acinetobacter* sp. [22]. Similarly, Kollef et al. found 65% mortality among the patients with late-onset VAP when the pathogens were *P. aeruginosa, Acinetobacter* sp. or *S. maltophilia* [17]. Mortality from VAP is also increased if initial antibiotic therapy is inadequate, and the frequency of inadequate therapy is highest for antibiotic-resistant organisms. A review by Kollef indicated that nearly 40% of empiric antibiotic choices were inadequate when VAP was due to *P. aeruginosa*, 25% with *S. aureus* and 20% with *Acinetobacter* spp. [34]. There are studies showing no excess mortality for respiratory infections with resistant bacteria, but it is likely that these patients did so well because of the use of adequate antibiotic therapy [35]. A recent report from Zahar and colleagues found no increased mortality in VAP due to MRSA [36]. However, Rello and colleagues performed a case-control study of 75 patients with MRSA VAP, and found an odds ratio of mortality of 3.8 with MRSA, and the absolute mortality for MRSA VAP was 48%, compared to 25% for the ventilated controls [37]. Therapy may have had some impact on the findings, since those who received continuous infusion of vancomycin had a lower mortality than those treated with non-continuous vancomycin or teicoplanin.

Other microbiologic features, such as the number of organisms isolated from bronchoscopically retrieved specimens and the influence of prior antibiotic use on the number of organisms recovered, may be important but have not been adequately studied. Some studies have suggested worse outcomes when bronchoscopic samples had high bacterial counts [38]. In addition, one study suggested that if BAL samples showed no growth, then the prognosis was excellent and that antibiotics could be safely stopped after 3 days, even if there was a clinical suspicion of VAP, although for most patients in this study, there was a low clinical suspicion of infection [39].

Although *P. aeruginosa* VAP is associated with a high attributable mortality, a study by Carmeli et al. showed a dramatic mortality impact for the acquisition of resistance during therapy for patients with *P. aeruginosa* infection [40]. Although resistance at baseline was associated with a delay in effective therapy for some patients, those with resistant organisms had the same mortality rate as those with sensitive organisms (7.6%). However, if emergence of resistance occurred during therapy, mortality rose threefold, and the incidence of secondary bacteremia increased ninefold.

43.2.3 Therapy Related Risk Factors

Because VAP is a severe infection, the prompt institution of antibiotics is expected to favorably influence survival. However, antimicrobial therapy can have two other effects. In patients with very severe illness, there may be limited efficacy, as these patients cannot benefit from effective therapy. In addition, the development of pneumonia, especially with resistant organisms, can occur due to extensive use of antibiotics [6, 14].

43.2.4 Inadequate and Inappropriate Initial Antibiotic Therapy

Mortality in VAP has been associated with inadequate empiric antibiotic therapy. In the new ATS/IDSA guidelines for nosocomial pneumonia, the terms "inadequate" and "inappropriate" were defined, with the term "inappropriate" being used to refer to the failure to select an antibiotic to which the etiologic organism is sensitive [2]. In general, most studies of VAP therapy have evaluated whether therapy is appropriate or not, by this definition. "Inadequate" refers to not only using the correct antibiotic, but doing so in the correct dose and timing, and doing all the other things necessary to achieve successful therapy. In general, studies have not examined inadequate vs. adequate therapy.

Several authors have observed significantly lower mortality rate in patients receiving appropriate antibiotic therapy, compared to inappropriate therapy [3, 6, 41, 42, 43]. However, not all studies found a difference in mortality rate for patients receiving appropriate antibiotic therapy [44, 45]. Whether it is possible to modify therapy based on microbiologic data and have a favorable result remains an open question [6, 42].

Kollef and colleagues evaluated the relationship between inappropriate antimicrobial treatment and hospital mortality in 2,000 patients admitted to the intensive care unit of an urban teaching hospital [18]. Inappropriate antimicrobial therapy, defined as the microbiologic documentation of an infection that was not being effectively treated at the time of identification, was being used in a total of 169 (8.5 %) patients and the hospital mortality rate for these patients was 52.1 % compared to 12.2 % mortality for those receiving appropriate therapy. Luna and colleagues conducted a prospective observational study in 132 patients with VAP [6]. All patients underwent a bronchoscopy with BAL within 24 h of establishing a clinical diagnosis of VAP, and most received antibiotic therapy prior to bronchoscopy. When therapy was appropriate (16/50 patients), the mortality rate was 38 %. In patients receiving inappropriate therapy, the mortality rate was significantly greater (91 %) and did not improve when they were switched to appropriate therapy based on BAL data. This emphasizes the need to choose initial empiric therapy accurately.

In a more recent study, Micek and colleagues used a protocol of initial broad-spectrum empiric therapy, after a clinical diagnosis of VAP, which included cefepime, ciprofloxacin or gentamicin, and vancomycin or linezolid [46]. Using this therapy protocol, 93.5 % of patients received initially effective therapy. The authors recommended discontinuation of antibiotics when patients with suspected VAP were found to have a non-infectious cause of lung infiltrates or to have resolution of clinical signs of pneumonia and they were able to reduce duration of therapy to as low as 5.8 days following this protocol, even though resistant gram-negative bacteria were commonly present. Interestingly, they found that the total duration of therapy (a measurement of how rapidly patients had resolution of VAP) was correlated with the initial CPIS, with those patients having a high initial score requiring a longer duration of therapy than those with a lower initial score.

Several studies have shown [47, 48] that it is not enough to administer the correct therapy, but that this therapy must be administered in a timely fashion, and that mortality increases if the correct therapy is not given in the first 24 h of illness. In another study, the impact of delays in therapy was progressive, with mortality being 7.4 % if the correct therapy was given at the onset of VAP, but rising to 25.8 % if the correct therapy was first given on day 1, and 50 % if given on day 2 or later [49]. In that same study, the impact of appropriate therapy also interacted with severity of illness, being able to reduce mortality only in those VAP patients with less severe illness. Patients with very severe illness, as measured by an organ dysfunction score, had the same high mortality regardless of the appropriateness of therapy, implying that they were too ill to recover.

43.2.4.1 *Prior Antibiotic Therapy*

Use of antibiotics prior to the development of pneumonia has been associated with a higher mortality rate in patients who later develop pneumonia [6, 14, 17]. The use of antibiotics may lead to emergence of antibiotic resistant pathogens. It has been shown that when bronchoscopy was positive while patients were receiving antibiotics for VAP, the organisms were generally antibiotic resistant [50]. Conversely, the lack of use of prior antibiotics has been associated with lower mortality and more sensitive organisms such as gram-positives and *Haemophilus influenzae* [51].

43.2.4.2 *Adequate Antibiotic Dosing*

When antimicrobial therapy is administered, it must be dosed in a manner that takes into account mechanism of action, activity relative to the MIC of the target organism, and penetration to the site of infection. Some antibiotics, like aminoglycosides, linezolid, and quinolones, are bactericidal in a concentration dependent fashion, while others (beta-lactam antibiotics and vancomycin) kill in relation to how long the serum concentration exceeds the minimum inhibitory concentration (MIC) of the target organism [52]. Antibiotics that kill in a concentration-dependent fashion may be best administered as once daily doses. This approach achieves high peak concentrations in the serum, thus maximizing efficacy, but with low trough concentrations, which may minimize the toxicity of agents such as the aminoglycosides. When an antibiotic kills in a time-dependent fashion, the optimal antibacterial effect with the minimal total dose of antibiotic could be achieved by continuous infusion administration, but this approach has not been proven to have any benefit [53].

In addition to the timing of administration, an antibiotic must be used at a high enough dose to treat the likely pathogens present in a severely ill patient with VAP. In the ATS/IDSA nosocomial pneumonia guidelines, recommendations are given for the dosing of antibiotics for VAP in patients with normal renal function [2]. These doses were chosen based on studies of pneumonia in severely ill patients and include: cefepime 1 – 2 g every 8 – 12 h; imipenem 500 mg every 6 h or 1 g every 8 h; meropenem 1 g every 8 h, piperacillin-tazobactam 4.5 g every 6 h; levofloxacin 750 mg daily or ciprofloxacin 400 mg every 8 h; vancomycin 15 mg/kg every 12 h leading to a trough level of 15 – 20 mg/l; linezolid 600 mg every 12 h; and aminoglycosides of 7 mg/kg per day of gentamicin or tobramycin and 20 mg/kg of amikacin.

43.3 Time Course of Resolution of Ventilator Associated Pneumonia

43.3.1 Resolution of Clinical Parameters

While the resolution of pneumonia can be defined both clinically and microbiologically, most patients are observed in a serial fashion using readily available bedside information. Many of the features of VAP have been combined into a scoring system, the clinical pulmonary infection score (CPIS) of Pugin et al., and the resolution of illness can be defined by serial measurements of the CPIS [54]. Using a modification of this system, Garrard et al. measured a daily CPIS in 83 patients with nosocomial pneumonia [55]. Pneumonia was diagnosed when the score was ≥6 out of a possible score of 10, based on assessing five variables, each of which received a score from 0 to 2. These variables were: temperature, white blood cell count, purulence of secretions, oxygenation, and extent of radiographic infiltrates. The CPIS increased progressively from a baseline value <6, to a value >6 over the 2 days preceding the day that the diagnosis was made and antibiotics were started [55]. Once therapy was initiated, the CPIS fell gradually over the next 9 days, generally falling below 6 by the 5th day of therapy. When the CPIS did not fall, the clinical deterioration was usually due to infection with *P. aeruginosa*.

Singh and colleagues have used serial measurements of the CPIS to describe the time course of illness in patients with VAP. In that study, patients were clinically evaluated with a CPIS that included five variables, scored on a scale of 0–2: fever, leukocytosis, appearance of tracheal secretions, radiographic patterns and oxygenation to assess the likelihood of pneumonia [56]. If the score was >6, patients were diagnosed as having VAP and were treated for 10–21 days. However, those with a clinical diagnosis of VAP but a score of <6 were randomized to either "standard care" or 3 days of ciprofloxacin at 400 mg every 8 h. After 3 days, for the patients treated with ciprofloxacin, the CPIS was measured again, adding two other criteria: radiographic progression and the results of respiratory cultures, and if the score remained< 6, antibiotics were stopped. Using this approach, 42 patients received standard therapy, and 39 received 3 days of ciprofloxacin therapy. Only 11 of the 39 patients needed continued antibiotics after 3 days (because the CPIS had increased to >6), and the rest of the group had the antibiotic stopped after 3 days. Their outcomes were similar to the patients who received standard duration of therapy. These data showed that many patients have a rapid clinical response associated with a good outcome with a short course of antibiotic therapy, which can reduce antibiotic resistance. However, it is still unclear if the findings mean that some patients with early pneumonia can respond rapidly to timely and appropriate therapy, or if some of these patients appeared to respond so well because they never actually had pneumonia to begin with.

A study by Luna and colleagues followed ventilated patients prospectively with serial calculations of the CPIS before the onset of VAP, and then at the time of diagnosis and during therapy. In this study, microbiologic confirmation required the growth of 10^4 colony forming unit/ml (cfu/ml) of a pathogen from a bronchoscopically obtained BAL or from blood cultures [57]. Sixty-three patients developed clinical evidence and had microbiologic confirmation of VAP. An increase in CPIS score was seen prior to the onset of VAP, which fell progressively with treatment. The decrease was significant on all 31 patients who survived, but not significant in the non-survivors. The only clinical parameter that distinguished survivors from non-survivors was the PaO_2/FiO_2 ratio. Patients receiving adequate antibiotics had a decrease in CPIS and a significant improvement in oxygenation by day 3 of treatment, whereas those receiving inadequate therapy did not.

An observational study by Vidaur and colleagues [4] compared the resolution of VAP in patients with and without ARDS. Seventy-five episodes of VAP without ARDS were identified and compared with 20 episodes with ARDS at the time of diagnosis of VAP. They found that resolution of fever, increase in the PaO_2/FiO_2 >250 mmHg, and white blood cell count in episodes of VAP occurred by the 3rd day of therapy in 73.3%, 74.7%, and 53.3% of patients. In the absence of ARDS, resolution of fever and PaO_2/FiO_2 >250 occurred within the 1st day of therapy in 50% of the patients. Radiographic resolution and clearance of secretions were late events (median of 14 and 6 days of resolution). In patients with ARDS, resolution of fever remained the earliest response variable and radiologic resolution was an extremely poor indicator, being present in only 10% of ARDS patients after 15 days of follow-up. Sixty-five percent of ARDS patients failed to improve after 48 h of therapy as compared to 14.7% of controls. Again, this study suggests that improvement in oxygenation and core temperature occurs early and can help clinicians shorten the duration of therapy in non-ARDS VAP. In patients with ARDS, resolution of VAP takes twice as long and is associated early on, only with improvement in temperature, and not oxygenation.

43.3.2 Resolution of Bacteriologic Abnormalities

Serial quantitative microbiologic studies of lower respiratory tract secretions can also define resolution end [24]. Garrard et al. have correlated their clinical assessment using the CPIS, with serial quantitative cultures of nondirected, non-bronchoscopic lung lavage samples in 89 episodes of VAP in 83 patients [55]. A rise in culture counts was seen during the 2 days preceding the clinical onset of pneumonia, and the counts decreased with the initiation of therapy. Clinical and microbiologic parameters were well correlated, and patients who showed a good clinical response to therapy had a rapid fall in colony counts, usually by 48–72 h. Treatment failures were often due to the presence of *P. aeruginosa* VAP, with a higher mortality rate and a persistence of colony counts $>10^3$ cfu/ml. A microbiologic non-response to therapy could be defined at 24–72 h, while recognition of a clinical non-response generally took longer. This may not be clinically relevant in practice because of the delay in obtaining the results of bacterial cultures.

Serial bronchoscopy has also been used to evaluate the resolution of nosocomial pneumonia. Dreyfuss et al. performed serial protected specimen brush (PSB) sampling in 34 patients with a clinical suspicion of pneumonia, all of whom had initial quantitative cultures that showed "borderline" results, with organisms present at a concentration of between 10^2 and 10^3 cfu/ml [58]. None of these patients was treated with antibiotics, but repeat bronchoscopy was performed within 72 h if there was persistent suspicion of pneumonia and if patients were maintained off antibiotics. In 12 patients, the same organism was isolated on the repeat bronchoscopy, but now at a $>10^3$ concentration and antibiotics were administered, while in 22 patients, the diagnosis of pneumonia was excluded. The mortality rate in the population having a positive repeat bronchoscopy (75%) was significantly higher than the mortality rate of those with a negative repeat bronchoscopy, suggesting that some patients may have had early pneumonia, even with relatively low colony counts, at a time when clinical features of pneumonia were present, and that when left untreated, counts rise rapidly in those with VAP.

Montravers et al. obtained repeat PSB samples 72 h after starting therapy to define the bacteriologic response to therapy. The results of these microbiologic evaluations were compared with the clinical outcome [59]. When the follow-up PSB sample showed no growth or $<10^3$ cfu/ml, a clinical therapeutic failure occurred only 7% of the time, whereas a microbiologic failure to eradicate, indicated by $>10^3$ cfu/ml, was associated with clinical failure in 55.8% of the patients. Sixty-seven percent of patients had sterilization of pulmonary secretions by day 3; 21% had persistent low-grade infection; and 12% had persistent high-level infection. Clinical improvement was present in 96% of those with microbiologic eradication, and in 81% of those with persistent low-level infection, but in only 44% of those with persistent high-level infection. These data suggest that most patients with VAP have a rapid clinical and microbiologic response to therapy, and that the two parallel one another, but it remains uncertain whether the identification of a non-response can lead to modification of therapy that could improve outcome. Baughman and colleagues confirmed this general idea, by doing serial non-quantitative BAL samples in 32 patients with VAP, with samples collected at the time of diagnosis and between days 2 and 5 of therapy [60]. They found that 18 of 32 patients with VAP had persistent high bacterial counts and they had a significantly increased mortality that was twice as high as those with sterile cultures on the repeat sample.

43.3.3 Resolution of Specific Abnormal Findings

Several recent studies have looked at the resolution of VAP. Dennesen et al. examined the resolution of symptoms and signs in 27 patients with VAP diagnosed clinically and microbiologically, all of whom were receiving adequate and appropriate antibiotic therapy [24]. Resolution was defined as the first day that four endpoints were achieved: absence of fever, decrease in leukocyte count to $\leq 10{,}000/mm^3$, improvement in PaO_2/FiO_2 ratio ≥ 250, and no growth or 1+ growth of bacteria in cultures of respiratory tract secretions The mean time to resolution was 5 days for fever, 6 days for oxygenation, 8 days for leukocyte count, and 10 days for bacterial cultures. The mean time for resolution of all parameters for the group as a whole was 9 days, but only 6 days if clinical and not microbiologic criteria were used to define response (Fig. 43.1). Again, the best predictor of resolution was improvement in oxygenation as measured by PaO_2/FiO_2 ratio ≥ 250 and duration of antibiotic therapy was generally longer than required to achieve resolution. An interesting finding in this study was that clinical resolution preceded microbiologic response; this may have reflected the fact that organisms such as *P. aeruginosa* persist in culture even with an adequate clinical response. Thus, microbiologic endpoints may be unrealistic for certain organisms. A recent comparison of 8 days vs. 15 days of treatment for VAP [61] demonstrated that resolution, mortality and recurrence were similar when patients received a shorter duration of antibiotics, except in those with non-fermenting gram negative bacilli, who tended to have a slightly higher recurrence rate. In this study, all patients received appropriate antibiotic therapy, and the investigators followed resolution of individual VAP parameters (Fig. 43.1). They found that at day 7, the mean temperature was 37.9 °C, the leukocyte count remained above $10{,}000/mm^3$, the PaO_2/FiO_2 ratio was above 225, and the radiograph continued to be abnormal. The findings in this study are very similar to the findings by Dennesen et al. [24].

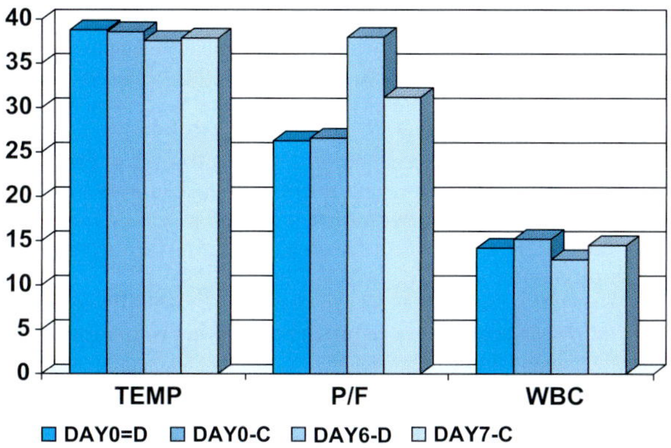

Fig. 43.1. Shown is the time course of resolution of clinical features in patients with VAP, showing the mean white blood cell count (WBC) in units of thousands per cubic millimeter; the PaO_2/FiO_2 (P/F) ratio in units of kPa; and the temperature (TEMP) in degrees centigrade. The data are shown on day 0 (day of diagnosis) and day 6 of therapy for the 27 patients in the study by Dennesen et al. (Day 0-D, Day 6-D) and on day 0 and day 7 for the 401 patients in the study by Chastre et al. (Day 0-C, Day 7-C). In both studies, the findings are similar

43.3.4 Changes in Biologic Markers During Resolution of VAP

An interesting study by Luyt and colleagues [62] evaluated the evolution of serum procalcitonin levels in patients with VAP during therapy. Procalcitonin, the precursor molecule of calcitonin, has no hormonal activity. Procalcitonin levels increase during bacterial infections and are associated with prognosis in patients with sepsis and septic shock [63, 64]. They obtained serial serum procalcitonin levels (day 1, 3 and 7) in 63 patients with microbiologically proven VAP. During treatment serum procalcitonin levels decreased in all patients, but were significantly higher in the 38 patients with an unfavorable outcome, which included death, VAP recurrence or extrapulmonary infection. Using receiver operating characteristic curves, a procalcitonin cut-off value of 1 ng/ml on day 1 had a sensitivity of 83% and a specificity of 64% to predict an unfavorable outcome. On day 3, a procalcitonin level >1.5 ng/ml and a PaO_2/FiO_2 <210 were similarly predictive of poor outcome with odds ratios of 24.6 and 25.9 respectively. On day 7, a procalcitonin level >0.5 ng/ml was the strongest predictor of adverse outcome with an odds ratio of 64.2 [62]. They concluded that serum procalcitonin levels may be helpful in early risk stratification in patients with VAP. However, a clinical parameter, the $Pa0_2/Fi0_2$ ratio on day 3 was also a good predictor of adverse outcomes.

Plasma and BAL levels of soluble triggering receptor expressed on myeloid cell (sTREM-1) have been recently measured in ventilated patients in the search for an early indicator of the development of VAP [65]. Twenty-eight ventilated patients were prospectively followed with serial plasma and non-directed BAL fluid levels of sTREM-1. Nine patients were subsequently diagnosed and treated for VAP and 19 patients did not develop VAP. Plasma levels did not change significantly in either group, but BAL fluid sTREM-1 levels rose sharply in the nine VAP patients before the diagnosis and declined quickly after initiation of antibiotic treatment. In this study, however, all patients with VAP responded well to treatment. Thus, further investigation is clearly necessary to determine whether local sTREM-1 levels may be useful in monitoring response to therapy in VAP.

43.4 Non-Response to VAP Therapy: Definitions and Differential Diagnosis

There is no uniformly accepted definition of non-response or non-resolution of VAP, but recent investigations have given us a good understanding of the natural history of VAP, a good overview of the expected response to therapy, and an appreciation of the variety of factors associated with a delayed response or mortality. As we have seen, patient factors, clinical findings and microbiologic data can be used to identify those who are likely to do well and those who are unlikely to respond. Using a combination of clinical finding and microbiologic criteria for resolution, such as serial measurements of the CPIS, we may be able to identify those patients who are responding well to therapy and shorten the duration of antibiotic treatment, or we could identify at an early time point those who need further evaluation because of a poor response to therapy. Studies evaluating changes in the concentration of biologic markers during resolution of VAP have shown promising results and may become useful in early risk stratification. Future studies are needed to determine whether proactive management and evaluation, based on any of these parameters, will be able to impact the outcome of patients with VAP.

In the studies that have been done, the definition of non-response has been made by 72 h [5, 19], while relapse or recurrence generally starts at day 9 or later [20]. Causes of non-response in the study by Ionas et al. were sometimes multiple and included: use of inappropriate therapy (10/44), superinfection (6/44), concomitant infection (13/44), non-infectious cause (7/44) or no known cause (16/44) [19]. Those without a known cause commonly had serious underlying illnesses such as ARDS, sepsis or multiple organ dysfunction.

If the patient is not improving by day 3 then a broad differential diagnosis is needed, focusing on several broad areas: treatment of the wrong organism, treatment of the wrong diagnosis, or the presence of a complication of VAP [2]. Organism considerations include the presence of a resistant or unsuspected pathogen, including fungi and mycobacteria. The diagnosis may not be pneumonia, but could be atelectasis, congestive heart failure, inflammatory lung disease, pulmonary embolus, pulmonary hemorrhage, a non-pulmonary infection or malignancy. Complications of VAP that can lead to a non-resolution of clinical findings include pulmonary embolus, antibiotic-induced diarrhea, drug fever or empyema. The first step in evaluating these patients is to check respiratory tract cultures, just to be sure that the therapy is active against the pathogen(s) isolated. In addition, more cultures and diagnostic testing are needed to evaluate the patient properly, depending on the likely explanation, after performing a careful differential diagnosis. When a patient is not responding to initial therapy, based on our understanding of the natural history of disease resolution, a change in antibiotics, combined with an aggressive diagnostic re-evaluation, should be done no later than day 3.

References

1. Vincent JL, Bihari DJ, Suter PM, et al. (1995) The prevalence of nosocomial infection in intensive care units in Europe. Results of the European Prevalence of Infection in Intensive Care (EPIC) Study. JAMA 274:639 - 644
2. Niederman MS, Craven DE, Bonten MJ, et al. (2005) Guidelines for the management of adults with hospital-acquired, ventilator-associated, and healthcare-associated pneumonia. Am J Respir Crit Care Med 171:388 - 416
3. Heyland DK, Cook DJ, Griffith L, et al. (1999) The attributable morbidity and mortality of ventilator associated pneumonia in the critically ill patient. Am J Respir Crit Care Med 159:1249 - 56
4. Vidaur L, Gualis B, Rodriguez L, et al. (2005) Clinical resolution in patients with suspicion of ventilator-associated pneumonia: a cohort study comparing patients with and without acute respiratory distress syndrome. Crit Care Med 33:1248 - 53
5. Luna CM, Niederman MS (2002) What is the natural history of resolution of ventilator associated pneumonia. Semin Respir Crit Care Med 23:471 - 470
6. Luna CM, Vujacich P, Niederman MS, et al. (1997) Impact of BAL data on the therapy and outcome of ventilator associated pneumonia. Chest 111:676 - 85
7. Niederman MS (2000) Bronchoscopy in non-resolving nosocomial pneumonia. Chest 117:121S–218S
8. Lowenkron S, Niederman MS (1992) Definition and evaluation of the resolution of nosocomial pneumonia. Semin Respir Infect 7:271 - 281
9. Timsit JF, Chevret S, Valcke J, et al. (1996) Mortality of nosocomial pneumonia in ventilated patients: influence of diagnostic tools. Am J Resp Crit Care Med 154:116 - 23
10. Bregeon F, Papazian L, Visconti A, et al. (1997) Relationship of microbiologic diagnostic criteria to morbidity and mortality in patients with ventilator associated pneumonia. JAMA 277:655 - 662
11. Kollef MH, Shorr A, Tabak YP, et al. (2005) Epidemiology and outcomes of health-care-associated pneumonia. Chest 128:3854 - 3862
12. Torres A, Aznar R, Gatell JM, et al. (1990) Incidence, risk, and prognosis factors of nosocomial pneumonia in mechanically ventilated patients. Am Rev Respir Dis 142: 523 - 528
13. Malangoni M, Crafton R, Mocek FC (1994) Pneumonia in the surgical intensive care unit: Factors determining successful outcome. Am J Surg 167:250 - 255
14. Rello J, Ausina V, Ricart M, et al. (1993) Impact of previous antimicrobial therapy on the etiology and outcome of ventilator-associated pneumonia. Chest 104:1230 - 1235
15. Kollef MH (1993) Ventilator associated pneumonia – a multivariate analysis. JAMA 270:1965 - 70
16. Almirall J, Mesalles E, Klamburg J, et al. (1995) Prognostic factors of pneumonia requiring admission to the intensive care unit. Chest 107:511 - 6
17. Kollef MH, Silver P, Murphy DM, Trovillion E (1995) The effect of late-onset ventilator-associated pneumonia in determining patient mortality. Chest 108:1655 - 62
18. Kollef MH, Sherman G, Ward S, Fraser V (1999) Inadequate antimicrobial treatment of infections: a risk factor for hospital mortality among critically ill patients. Chest 115:462 - 474
19. Ionas M, Ferrer M, Cavalcanti M, et al. (2004) Causes and predictors of nonresponse of intensive care unit-acquired pneumonia. Crit Care Med 32:938 - 945
20. Combes A, Figliolini C, Trouillet JL, et al. (2003) Factors predicting ventilator-associated pneumonia recurrence. Crit Care Med 31:1102 - 1107
21. Rello J, Torres A, Ricart M, et al. (1994) Ventilator-associated pneumonia by *Staphylococcus aureus*: comparison of methicillin-resistant and methicillin-sensitive episodes. Am J Resp Crit Care Med 150:1545 - 49
22. Fagon JY, Chastre J, Hance AJ, et al. (1993) Nosocomial pneumonia in ventilated patients: a cohort study evaluating attributable mortality and hospital stay. Am J Med 94:281 - 88
23. Rello J, Mariscal D, March F, et al. (1998) Recurrent *Pseudomonas aeruginosa* pneumonia in ventilated patients: relapse or reinfection? Am J Resp Crit Care Med 157:912 - 16
24. Dennesen PJW, van der Van A, Kessels AGH, et al. (2001) Resolution of infectious parameters after antimicrobial therapy in patients with ventilator-associated pneumonia. Am J Respir Crit Care Med 163:1371 - 1375
25. Bueno-Cavanillas A, Delgado-Rodriguez M, Lopez-Luque A, et al. (1994) Influence of nosocomial infection on mortality rate in an intensive care unit. Crit Care Med 22: 55 - 60
26. Rello J, Jubert P, Valles J, et al. (1996) Evaluation of outcome for intubated patients with pneumonia due to *Pseudomonas aeruginosa*. Clin Infect Dis 23:973 - 978
27. Pittet D, Woolson RF, Wenzel RP (1997) Microbiological factors influencing the outcome of nosocomial bloodstream infection: a 6-year, validated, population-based model. Clin Infect Dis 24:1068 - 1078
28. Luna C, Videla A, Matera J, et al. (1999) Blood cultures have limited value in predicting severity of illness and as a diagnostic tool in ventilator-associated pneumonia (VAP). Chest 116:1075 - 84
29. Chastre J, Vaugnat A, Joly-Guillou ML, et al. (1998) Nosocomial pneumonia in patients with acute respiratory distress syndrome. Am J Resp Crit Care Med 157:1165 - 72
30. Baker AM, Meredith JW, Haponik EF (1996) Pneumonia in intubated trauma patients. Microbiology and outcomes. Am J Respir Crit Care Med 153:343 - 9
31. Crouch Brewer S, Wunderink RG, Jones CB, Leeper KV Jr (1996) Ventilator-associated pneumonia due to *Pseudomonas aeruginosa*. Chest 109:1019 - 29
32. Prod'hom G, Leuenberger P, Koerfer J, et al. (1994) Nosocomial pneumonia in mechanically ventilated patients receiving antiacid, ranitidine, or sucralfate as prophylaxis

for stress ulcer: A randomized controlled trial. Ann Intern Med 120:653 - 662

33. Trouillet JL, Chastre J, Vuagnat A, et al. (1998) Ventilator-associated pneumonia caused by potentially drug-resistant bacteria. Am J Respir Crit Care Med 157:531 - 539
34. Kollef MH (2000) Inadequate antimicrobial treatment: An important determinant of outcome for hospitalized patients. Clin Infect Dis 31 (Suppl 4):S131–S138
35. Vanhems P, Lepape A, Savey A, et al. (2000) Nosocomial pulmonary infection by antimicrobial-resistant bacteria of patients hospitalized in intensive care units: Risk factors and survival. J Hosp Infect 45:98 - 106
36. Zahar JR, Clec'h C, Tafflet M, et al. (2005) Is methicillin resistance associated with a worse prognosis in *Staphylococcus aureus* ventilator-associated pneumonia? Clin Infect Dis 41:1224 - 31
37. Rello J, Sole-Violan J, Sa-Borges M, et al. (2005) Pneumonia caused by oxacillin resistant *Staphylococcus aureus* treated with glycopeptides. Crit Care Med 33:2127 - 2128
38. Brunson M, Meduri GU, Leeper KV (1993) Pneumonia in ARDS: diagnostic and prognostic value of bilateral bronchoscopic sampling. Am Rev Respir Dis 147:A355
39. Kollef MH, Kollef KE (2005) Antibiotic utilization and outcomes for patients with clinically suspected ventilator-associated pneumonia and negative quantitative BAl culture results. Chest 128:2706 - 2713
40. Carmeli Y, Troillet N, Karchmer AW, Samore MH (1999) Health and economic outcomes of antibiotic resistance in *Pseudomonas aeruginosa*. Arch Intern Med 159:1127 - 1132
41. Alvarez-Lerma F (1996) Modification of empiric antibiotic treatment inpatients with pneumonia acquired in the intensive care unit: ICU-Acquired Pneumonia Study Group. Intensive Care Med 22:387 - 94
42. Rello J, Gallego M, Mariscal D, et al. (1997) The role of routine microbial investigation in ventilator-associated pneumonia. Am J Respir Crit Care Med 156:196 - 200
43. Kollef MH, Ward S (1998) The influence of mini-BAL cultures on patients outcomes: Implications for the antibiotic management of ventilator-associated pneumonia. Chest 113:412 - 420
44. Sanchez-Nieto JM, Torres A, Garcia-Cordoba F (1998) Impact of non invasive versus invasive quantitative culture sampling on outcome of ventilator-associated pneumonia: a pilot study. Am J Respir Crit Care Med 157:371 - 6
45. Ruiz M, Torres A, Ewig S, et al. (2000) Non-invasive versus invasive microbial investigation in ventilator associated pneumonia: evaluation of outcome. Am J Respir Crit Care Med 162:119 - 25
46. Micek ST, Ward S, Fraser V, Kollef MH (2004) A randomized controlled trial of an antibiotic discontinuation policy for clinically suspected ventilator-associated pneumonia. Chest 125:1791 - 1799
47. Luna CM, Aruj P, Niederman MS, et al. (2006) Appropriateness and delay to initiate therapy in ventilator-associated pneumonia. Eur Resp J 27:158 - 164
48. Iregui M, Ward S, Sherman G, et al. (2002) Clinical importance of delays in the initiation of appropriate antibiotic treatment for ventilator-associated pneumonia. Chest 122:262 - 268
49. Clec'h C, Timsit JF, De Lassense A, et al. (2004) Efficacy of adequate early antibiotic therapy in ventilator-associated pneumonia: Influence of disease severity. Intensive Care Med 30:1327 - 1333
50. Souweine B, Veber B, Bedos JP, et al. (1998) Diagnostic accuracy of protected specimen brush and bronchoalveolar lavage in nosocomial pneumonia: impact of previous antimicrobial treatments. Crit Care Med 26:236 - 44
51. Rello J, Ricart M, Ausina V, et al. (1992) Pneumonia due to *Haemophilus influenzae* among mechanically ventilated patients: Incidence, outcome, and risk factors. Chest 102:1562 - 65
52. Niederman MS (1997) The principles of antibiotic use and the selection of empiric therapy for pneumonia. In: Fishman A (ed) Pulmonary diseases and disorders, 3rd edn. McGraw-Hill, New York, pp 1939 - 1949
53. Hanes SD, Wood GC, Herring V, et al. (2000) Intermittent and continuous ceftazidime infusion for critically ill trauma patients. Am J Surg 179:436 - 440
54. Pugin J, Auckenthaler R, Mili N, et al. (1991) Diagnosis of ventilator-associated pneumonia by bacteriologic analysis of bronchoscopic and non-bronchoscopic "blind" bronchoalveolar lavage fluid. Am Rev Respir Dis 143:1121 - 29
55. Garrard CS, A'Court CD (1995) The diagnosis of pneumonia in the critically ill. Chest 108:17S–25S
56. Singh N, Rogers P, Atwood CW, et al. (2000) Short-course empiric antibiotic therapy for patients with pulmonary infiltrates in the intensive care unit: A proposed solution for indiscriminate antibiotic prescription. Am J Respir Crit Care Med 162:505 - 511
57. Luna CM, Blanzaco D, Niederman MS, et al. (2003) Resolution of ventilator-associated pneumonia: prospective evaluation of the clinical pulmonary infection score as an early clinical predictor of outcome. Crit Care Med 31:676 - 682
58. Dreyfuss D, Mier L, Le Bordelles G, et al. (1993) Clinical significance of borderline quantitative protected specimen culture results. Am Rev Respir Dis 147:946 - 951
59. Montravers P, Fagon JY, Chastre J, et al. (1993) Follow-up protected specimen brushes to assess treatment in nosocomial pneumonia. Am Rev Respir Dis 147:38 - 44
60. Baughman RP, Kerr MA (2003) Ventilator-associated pneumonia patients who do not reduce bacteria from the lungs have a worse prognosis. J Intensive Care Med 18: 269 - 274
61. Chastre J, Wolff M, Fagon JY, et al. (2003) Comparison of 8 vs 15 days of antibiotic therapy for ventilator-associated pneumonia in adults: a randomized trial. JAMA 290: 2588 - 2598
62. Luyt CE, Guerin V, Combes A, et al. (2005) Procalcitonin kinetics as a prognostic marker of ventilator-associated pneumonia. Am J Respir Crit Care Med 171:48 - 53
63. Assicot M, Grendel D, Carsin H, et al. (1993) High serum procalcitonin concentrations in patients with sepsis and infection. Lancet 341:515 - 518
64. Wanner GA, Keel M, Steckholzer U, et al. (2002) Relationship between procalcitonin plasma levels and severity of injury, sepsis, organ failure, and mortality in injured patients. Crit Care Med 28:950 - 957
65. Determan RM, Millo JL, Gibot S, et al. (2005) Serial changes in soluble triggering receptor expressed in myeloid cells in the lung during development of ventilator-associated pneumonia. Intensive Care Med 31:1495 - 1500

44 Invasive Devices in the Pathogenesis of Nosocomial Pneumonia

M. Valencia, T.T. Bauer, A. Torres

44.1 Introduction

Nosocomial pneumonia remains a common complication in patients who require mechanical ventilation. On various occasions endotracheal intubation has been identified as a risk factor for nosocomial pneumonia. Levine and Niederman [1] described four different device/host interactions that may be responsible. First, an endotracheal tube can have direct effects on the airway, resulting in an impairment of local host defense mechanisms. Mucosal injury can reduce mucociliary function, while upper airway defenses are bypassed and the effectiveness of cough is reduced. Second, intubation can result in an enhanced capacity of tracheobronchial cells to bind Gram-negative bacteria, an effect that favors airway colonization and, thus, pneumonia. Third, the airway injury can create binding sites for bacteria in the basement membrane of the bronchial tree. Fourth and most important in relation to bacterial biofilm, endotracheal tubes may serve as a reservoir for bacteria [1].

Recent studies have suggested that microorganisms can adhere to the surface of endotracheal tubes. Some species produce an exopolysaccharide that acts as a slime-like adhesive and the surface lining has been referred to as bacterial biofilm [2].

Other invasive devices such as bronchoscopes and tracheal suction systems can also introduce microorganisms into the patient's lower respiratory tract. Although transmission of infections by bronchoscopy depends on many factors, the cleaning and disinfection process is the single element that the clinician can most influence. In spite of disinfection measures several cases of nosocomial transmission of infections and pneumonia have been detected [3].

This manuscript will review the basic research related to bacterial biofilm formation on abiotic surfaces and the possible role of bacterial biofilm on the inner lumen of endotracheal tubes and the possible role of other invasive devices for the pathogenesis of ventilator-associated pneumonia.

44.2 Bacterial Biofilm: Definition and Formation

Bacterial biofilms are defined as matrix-enclosed bacterial populations adherent to each other and/or to surfaces or interfaces. This definition includes microbial aggregates and also adherent populations within the pore spaces in porous media [4].

The biofilm can be regarded as a complex matrix with channels that allow nutrients to circulate analogous to tissues of higher organisms [5]. The sessile forms of the bacteria coated in biofilm can give rise to *planktonic* bacteria that may eventually leave the biofilm and disperse into the environment. Some of the bacterial species that may generate biofilms are currently regarded to have only low pathogenic potential in the context of nosocomial pneumonia such as *Staphylococcus epidermidis*. However, *P. aeruginosa* and *Streptococcus pneumoniae* are common nosocomial pulmonary pathogens and their potential to aggregate in biofilms has been well described [6]. Four fundamental steps have been identified during the process of biofilm formation and are best described for *P. aeruginosa* [6]. Flagella play an important role for the *initial attachment* to abiotic surfaces of *P. aeruginosa* during the first step of biofilm formation. Type IV pilli and twitching motility further leads to the *formation of microcolonies* of these bacteria. Recent research has shown that strains of *P. aeruginosa* unable to form these initial microcolonies were also unable to form a mature biofilm on a polyvinylchloride (PVC) plastic surface [7]. Once microcolonies are formed, the attached bacteria have to *mature into a differentiated biofilm* [5]. Bacteria secrete small molecule pheromones at this stage to determine whether there are enough bacteria to initiate the expression of a particular phenotype ("*quorum sensing*") [8]. If this step is successful, the microcolonies differentiate into a structured, thick, biocide-resistant biofilm.

44.3 Bacterial Biofilm: Antibiotic Drug Resistance

Biofilm-covered bacteria in the inner lumen of endotracheal tubes have a decreased susceptibility to antibiotic drugs for three reasons [9]. First, the biofilm reaches into an air-filled lumen that provides almost no host defense mechanisms. Ultrastructural analysis of biofilm in endotracheal tubes has been shown to harbor polymorphonuclear leukocytes as well; however, until now it has been unclear whether this reflects directed migration or simply a contaminating mechanism during coughing or endotracheal suctioning [10]. Second, the biofilm protects the sessile forms of the bacteria physically from antibiotic action. Antibiotics may be either unable to penetrate the biofilm [11, 12] or the decreased diffusing capacity increases the likelihood of deactivation prior to target contact [13]. The third reason for antibiotic resistance is the slow-growing or starved state of the sessile bacteria and some researchers hypothesize that the bacteria may even adopt a distinct phenotype as a biological response to growth on a surface [14–16].

44.4 Bacterial Biofilm in Endotracheal Tubes

To date only few studies have addressed bacterial biofilm formation in endotracheal tubes of mechanically ventilated patients. Most studies have attempted to prove three important points about biofilm in this medical device: presence and quantity, the ultrastructure, and the viability of the observed microorganisms. In 1986 Sottile and associates studied 25 ventilation tubes (PVC, endotracheal or tracheostomy) that had been removed from patients in one multidisciplinary ICU after an average of 9.2 days (range 1–46 days) of respiratory support [17]. By means of scanning electron microscopy (SEM), they could identify amorphous material on the inner surface that was confluent in 21/25 tubes (84%) and intermittent in 4/25 endotracheal tubes (16%). Rod shaped or coccoid bacteria were seen on the surface of 17/25 devices (68%). Qualitative bacterial cultures were obtained from 23 endotracheal tubes and showed bacterial growth on 19/23 occasions (83%). A total of 92% of the patients had received antibiotic drugs and the following microorganisms were cultured: *S. aureus, P. aeruginosa, Proteus mirabilis, and S. epidermidis*. Diaz-Blanco and colleagues observed coccoid structures through SEM on all 29 endotracheal tubes from neonates after mechanical ventilation for 0.5–14 days (100%) [18]. *S. epidermidis* was cultured from 12/29 tubes (41%) and group B hemolytic *S. epidermidis, P. aeruginosa*, and *Klebsiella pneumoniae* from 1/29 tubes (3%), respectively. All patients had received antibiotics (100%).

An attempt was made to quantify the amount of material deposited on endotracheal tubes by Inglis and associates [19]. Cotton swabs of all tubes were subjected to quantitative bacterial cultures and the scraped-off material was also weighed. The researchers found more than 50 mg of biofilm dry weight in 30/40 tubes (75%), but the absolute weight did not seem to be associated with the duration of use. In 33/45 tubes (73%), bacteria were cultured (*P. aeruginosa, K. pneumoniae, Proteus mirabilis, E. coli, and Enterobacter cloacae*) and the bacterial counts were as high as 10^6 colony forming units (cfu) per centimeter of tube length.

In 1993, Inglis and coworkers radiographically detected biofilm in 45 of 50 endotracheal tubes (90%) removed from patients in a general ICU [20]. The integrity of the tube was maintained in this study and the amount of deposited material was analyzed according to tube shape. Biofilm thickness was measured with a dial gauge caliper and the distribution assigned to a Magill curve template. They could clearly demonstrate that the presence of biofilm was more likely at the tip of the endotracheal tube (proximal segment, 45/50 tubes, 90%) and decreased towards the proximal end of the tube (distal segment, 14/50 tubes, 28%). No correlation was found with the duration of use for this distribution pattern. The biofilm in vivo is probably a combination of microbial biofilm generation and ventilatory secretion deposition during expiration, coughing or endotracheal suctioning. This hypothesis is further supported by the fact that endoluminal biofilm from endotracheal tubes of mechanically ventilated patients is composed not only of bacteria and exopolysaccharides but also contains neutrophils in varying stages of disintegration with an amorphous matrix most likely corresponding to respiratory mucus [10].

44.5 Sequence of Colonization of Endotracheal Tubes

It has been shown that oropharyngeal colonization precedes pulmonary infection and is an independent risk factor of nosocomial pneumonia [21–23]. Microaspiration is probably the most important pathogenic mechanism [1, 24], but oropharyngeal colonization may also facilitate biofilm development in the endotracheal tube [19]. Feldman and coworkers investigated biofilm formation in 21 ICU patients undergoing 24 extubations (mean length of intubation 0.5–12 days) [25]. They identified biofilm on the inner surface of all endotracheal tubes by SEM (24/24, 100%) and viable – mostly Gram-negative – bacteria were identified from secretions of all but three tubes (21/24, 88%). In a second part of this study they attempted to identify the sequence of colonization by sampling of the oropharynx, the nasogastric tube, the interior of the airway tube and endotracheal secretions in ten uninfected patients on at least five consecutive days [25]. It was interesting that the appearance of microorganisms in lower respiratory tract secretions almost invariably preceded their appearance in the interior of the endotracheal tube. This finding strongly suggests that the sequence of colonization is oropharynx – tracheobronchial tree – endotracheal tube and that the biofilm formation only plays a minor role, at least for the etiology of the first pulmonary infection. This assumption is also supported by the more prominent biofilm formation near the tip of the endotracheal tube in this [25] and previous studies [10]. Another interesting finding of this study was that various microorganisms showed a definitive pattern of the colonization process. There appeared to be a tendency for Gram-positive isolates to colonize the oropharynx early (12–36 h), and to appear rapidly thereafter in the stomach and then in the lower respiratory tract secretions. The colonization pattern of Gram-negative isolates occurred somewhat later. Colonization of the oropharynx begins between 36 and 48 h and then progressively colonizes the stomach, thereafter appearing in the endotracheal secretions and all these isolates are subsequently noted within the endotracheal tube by 69 h [25].

44.6 Bacterial Biofilm on Endotracheal Tubes and Nosocomial Pneumonia

It has been proposed that bacteria from the biofilm lining of the endotracheal tube might be scattered into the lungs during ventilation gas flow, since dissemination of bacteria from the tube has been demonstrated in vitro [19]. Dynamic studies simulating the scattering of tracheal tube biofilm have shown that bacteria can be disseminated many centimeters from the orifice of the endotracheal tube, far into the lung [20].

Sottile and associates were among the first to suggest that there may be a relationship between nosocomial pneumonia and bacterial adherence to the interior of the endotracheal tube [17]. A study in neonates undergoing prolonged mechanical ventilation failed to demonstrate a clinical relationship between endotracheal tube colonization and nosocomial pneumonia [18]. However, this study may have lacked sufficient power, because the children were screened for nosocomial infections after extubation. In a recently published case control study, endotracheal tubes from patients with ventilator-associated pneumonia were more often covered with biofilm (20/20, 100%) than those of uninfected control patients (6/20, 30%) [26]. Of those patients with ventilator-associated pneumonia, 14/20 (70%) had pathogens that were indistinguishable by genotyping in both endotracheal tubes and tracheal secretions. In contrast, no matching pairs of pathogens were isolated from control patients. However, this study leaves the question unanswered whether the bacteria at the inner lumen of the endotracheal tube contribute to the development of ventilator-associated pneumonia or whether they are spread from the tracheobronchial tree to the tube during coughing or endotracheal suctioning.

The contribution of endotracheal tube biofilm in the pathogenesis of ventilator-associated pneumonia is controversial [27, 28], especially if the magnitude of the problem is related to that of other risk factors of ventilator-associated pneumonia [29–32]. Nevertheless, it may be of crucial importance to the pathogenesis of recurrent ventilator-associated pneumonia [6, 25]. Rello and coworkers investigated recurrent episodes of pneumonia caused by *P. aeruginosa* in 37 mechanically ventilated patients [33]. They analyzed 16 isolates of five patients and all but one were considered relapses because of the concordance in chromosomal fingerprinting. As pointed out above, *P. aeruginosa* is known to produce bacterial biofilm with reduced antibiotic susceptibility and even withstands topical antibiotic therapy in a clinical setting [34]. In the study performed by Feldman and coworkers, these authors found that colonization of the endotracheal tube with microorganisms potentially causing pneumonia appears to persist in many cases despite apparently successful treatment of the previous pneumonia. These microorganisms may represent a persistent source of organisms causing recurrent infections [25].

44.7 Control of Endotracheal Tube Colonization

Since the colonization of ETT biofilm may serve as a reservoir from which bacteria are continuously seeded into the lower respiratory tree, an effective method of decreasing the ETT colonization is first required to thereby support the hypothesis that biofilm is a potential contributing factor to the pathogenesis of VAP. Methods implemented to control ETT colonization are the use of tubes impregnated with antiseptics, anti-adherent coatings and nebulized antibiotics, among others. As has been described previously, the effectiveness of systemic antibiotics to decrease colonization may be limited by their inability to penetrate the biofilm. The small amount of antibiotic that actually does penetrate the biofilm may increase the risk of the emergence of resistant bacteria that may subsequently colonize the respiratory tract of the patient [25].

In a laboratory airway model, Pacheco-Fowler and coworkers assessed the effect of ETT impregnated with chlorhexidine (CHX) and silver carbonate (antiseptic ETT) against several microorganisms [35]. Antiseptic and control ETT were inserted in culture tubes half-filled with agar media previously contaminated at the surface with 10^8 cfu/ml of the selected test organism. Swabs of proximal and distal ends of the agar tract in the models were subcultured. Initial and residual CHX levels (5 days post-implantation) were determined. Cultures of antiseptic ETT revealed colonization by the tested pathogens ranging from 1 to 100 cfu/ml compared with approximately 10^6 cfu/ml for the control ETT ($p<0.001$). The amount of CHX retained in the antiseptic ETT after 5 days of implantation was an average of 45% of the initial level. There were important differences between the several organisms colonizing the impregnated and control ETTs. It remains to be determined how these coated tubes interact with the live tissues around them and the effect that such interaction may ultimately have on the release, concentration and/or effectiveness of the ETT. In another study, Berra et al. investigated bacterial colonization of the ventilator circuit, the ETT, and the lungs when the ETT was coated with silver-sulfadiazine and chlorhexidine in polyurethane, using no bacterial/viral filter [36]. Sixteen sheep were randomized to receive either a standard ETT or a coated ETT and were ventilated for 24 h. At autopsy, the authors sampled the trachea, bronchi, lobar parenchyma, and ETT for quantitative bacterial cultures. Qualitative bacterial cultures were obtained from the filter, humidifier, inspiratory and expiratory lines, and water trap. ETTs were analyzed with light microscopy, SEM and laser scanning confocal microscopy. In the control group, all eight ETTs were heavily colonized (10^5–10^8 cfu/g), forming a thick biofilm. The ventilator circuit was always colonized. Pathogenic bacteria colonized the trachea and the lungs in five out of eight sheep (up to 10^9 cfu/g). In the study group, seven out of eight ETTs and their ventilator circuits showed no growth, with absence of biofilm with the last ETT and the respective ventilator circuit showing low bacterial growth (10^3–10^4 cfu/g). The trachea was colonized in three sheep, although no bacterial growth was observed in the lungs and bronchi, except for one bronchus in one sheep. The authors concluded that coated ETT induced a nonsignificant reduction in trachea colonization, eliminated or reduced bacterial colonization of the ETT and ventilator circuits and prevented lung bacterial colonization. The use of silver-sulfadiazine and chlorhexidine has the advantage that bacteria are not known to develop resistance to these antiseptics [37]. Changing the surfactant coating of the ETT may prevent the colonization to the ETT surface. Jones and coworkers [38] performed a study to describe the physicochemical and microbial anti-adherent properties of surfactant blends as candidate coatings for ETTs. Organic solutions of surfactants containing a range of ratios of cholesterol and lecithin (0:100, 25:75, 50:50, 75:25, dissolved in dichloromethane) were prepared and coated onto ETT PVC using a multiple dip-coating process. Adherence of *S. aureus* and *P. aeruginosa* to surfactant-coated PVC at each successive time period (0.5, 1, 2, 4, 8 h) was significantly lower than to uncoated PVC, with the extent of the reduction frequently exceeding 90%. Interestingly, the microbial anti-adherent properties of the coatings were dependent on lecithin content. Based on the impressive microbial anti-adherence properties and durability of the surfactant coating on PVC following dip coatings, it has been proposed that these systems may usefully reduce the incidence of ventilator-associated pneumonia when employed as luminal coatings of the ETT. Finally, although systemic antibiotics do not reach high concentrations on the ETT biofilm, the use of nebulized antibiotics may be effective in preventing the formation of microbial biofilm. Gentamicin, nebulized via the ETT, was compared with parenteral cefuroxime as a prevention measure. The authors concluded that nebulized gentamicin attained high concentrations in the ETT lumen and was more effective in preventing the formation of biofilm than two parenterally administered cephalosporins. This therapy may be useful in preventing VAP [39].

44.8 Bronchoscopy

Bronchoscopy can occasionally transmit infectious lung diseases. The bronchoscope traverses the nasopharynx or oropharynx and may thus inoculate the tracheobronchial tree and possibly the pulmonary parenchyma. Another potential complication is the bronchoscopic spread of infection from an infected to an uninfected patient.

Although transmission of infections by bronchoscopy depends on many factors, the cleaning and disinfection process is the single key measure to avoid transmission of infections. Some organisms such as mycobacteria are inherently more resistant to disinfectants. In addition, the effectiveness of the germicide depends on its type, concentration, and duration of exposure. If residual patient material, such as blood or sputum, remains in the bronchoscope after cleaning, the effectiveness of any subsequent disinfection procedure will dramatically diminish. Moreover, the complexity of the instrument, with crevices, joints or pores, creates problems for both cleaning and disinfecting.

Several studies have estimated this risk of developing lung infection after bronchoscopy. In a large retrospective study of 24,521 patients who underwent bronchoscopy, Credel and associates found only two cases of pneumonia [40]. In a prospective study, Pereira and coworkers reported the development of fever in 16% of the patients, parenchymal infiltrates in 6%, and one patient developed rapidly progressive pneumonia and died after bronchoscopy. No organisms were isolated from cultures of blood drawn at the time of the procedure or during complications. Among the patients who developed pneumonia, the isolates from sputum generally consisted of aerobic and anaerobic microorganisms normally found in the mouth [41]. In a third study, using two types of disinfection solutions to clean the bronchoscope, Suratt and associates surveyed 249 bronchoscopic procedures and no patient developed pneumonia in either period [42].

Although these few studies imply that bronchoscopy may be free of the risk of transmitting microorganisms, several studies have reported the transmission of infectious agents by bronchoscopy. In 1978, Hussain reported transmission of *Pseudomonas* species in seven patients who had undergone bronchoscopy. Infection was related to the biopsy-suction attachment and resulted in one patient developing lower right pulmonary lobe pneumonia [43]. In 1982 Sammartino described the development of infection in 11 patients after a bronchoscopic procedure due to the presence of *P. aeruginosa* in the inner channel of the bronchoscope, despite appropriate cleaning [44]. The contamination was eliminated after sterilizing the bronchoscope with ethylene oxide. Boisjoly and associates reported a case in which bronchoscopy for the evaluation of hemoptysis was followed by uveitis 2 weeks later and by endophthalmitis after 4 weeks [45]. Both sputum and vitreous cultures yielded *P. aeruginosa*. Despite aggressive medical treatment, enucleation was eventually performed.

Bronchoscopic transmission of bacteria other than *Pseudomonas* spp. has also been described. In one report, investigators isolated a *Proteus* spp. from an index patient and eight subsequent patients, although no patient developed pneumonia [46]. In an outbreak that had serious consequences, Webb and Vall-Spinoza reported three patients who developed infection by *S. marcescens* after undergoing bronchoscopy: Two of these patients died of necrotizing pneumonia caused by this organism, and an index patient infected by *S. marcescens* was identified [47].

Beyt and coworkers [48] published a case of fatal streptococcal pneumonia and septicemia following flexible bronchoscopic examination and endobronchial biopsy in a patient with severe chronic congestive heart failure although a causal relationship was unclear.

Anecdotal reports of the development of pneumonia and lung abscess after transbronchial biopsy of a peripheral mass lesion are noteworthy [49, 50]. Watts and Green reported that transbronchial fine-needle aspiration of a subcarinal lymph node was followed by bacteriemia secondary to *Streptococcus viridans* infection [51]. The increasing incidence of tuberculous and nontuberculous mycobacterial infection has increased the likelihood that bronchoscopy may spread these organisms. In addition, mycobacteria are inherently more resistant to disinfectants. In 1980 Leers [52] and Nelson and colleagues in 1983 [53] reported one case each of cross-contamination with *Mycobacteriun* tuberculosis although the patients did not show evidence of tuberculosis. In a subsequent report, Wheeler and coworkers described three cases of bronchoscopic transmission of *M. tuberculosis* that resulted in clinically significant infection [54]. Recently, Agerton and coworkers reported that fatal multidrug resistant tuberculosis was transmitted by bronchoscopy [55]. In the four mentioned reports problems were detected in the disinfection procedure. Mycobacteria other than *M. tuberculosis* such as *M. chelonae* have been implicated in bronchoscopic transmission of infections [56, 57]. In both cases, problems were detected with the disinfection procedure.

Spread of preexisting pulmonary infections is more common than the propagation of patient to patient infection by bronchoscopy. Fortunately, in most cases, patients have not shown clinical evidence of infection. Although transmission of infections to an uninfected patient by bronchoscopy depends on many factors such as the immunological status of the patient or the duration of the procedure, the cleaning and disinfection process is the single key measure to control. Routine procedures to prevent contamination include compliance with recommended cleaning and disinfecting regimens and regular maintenance of bronchoscopes [58].

According to our experience, the high incidence of airway colonization in intubated patients makes bronchoscopy a clear potential transmitter of nosocomial infections. Bronchoscopes in the ICU should follow a very strict policy of cleaning, aeration and disinfection. A specific ICU nursing team should be responsible for these practices and monthly microbiological surveillance of the inner channel and outer parts of the bronchoscope is strongly recommended.

44.9 Tracheal Suction Catheter

Endotracheal suctioning is an essential and common supportive procedure for patients requiring mechanical ventilation. This procedure removes respiratory secretions and maintains the permeability of the upper airways. Currently, there are two types of suction-catheter systems, the open single-use catheter system and the closed multiuse in-line catheter system (Fig. 44.1).

Open suctioning uses a single use catheter that can be rapidly inserted and withdrawn from the ETT. Sterile gloved technique is mandatory when using the open system because of the risk of environmental cross-contamination. Closed multiuse systems have less risk of cross-contamination. However, the multiuse catheter can be contaminated after the initial pass through the

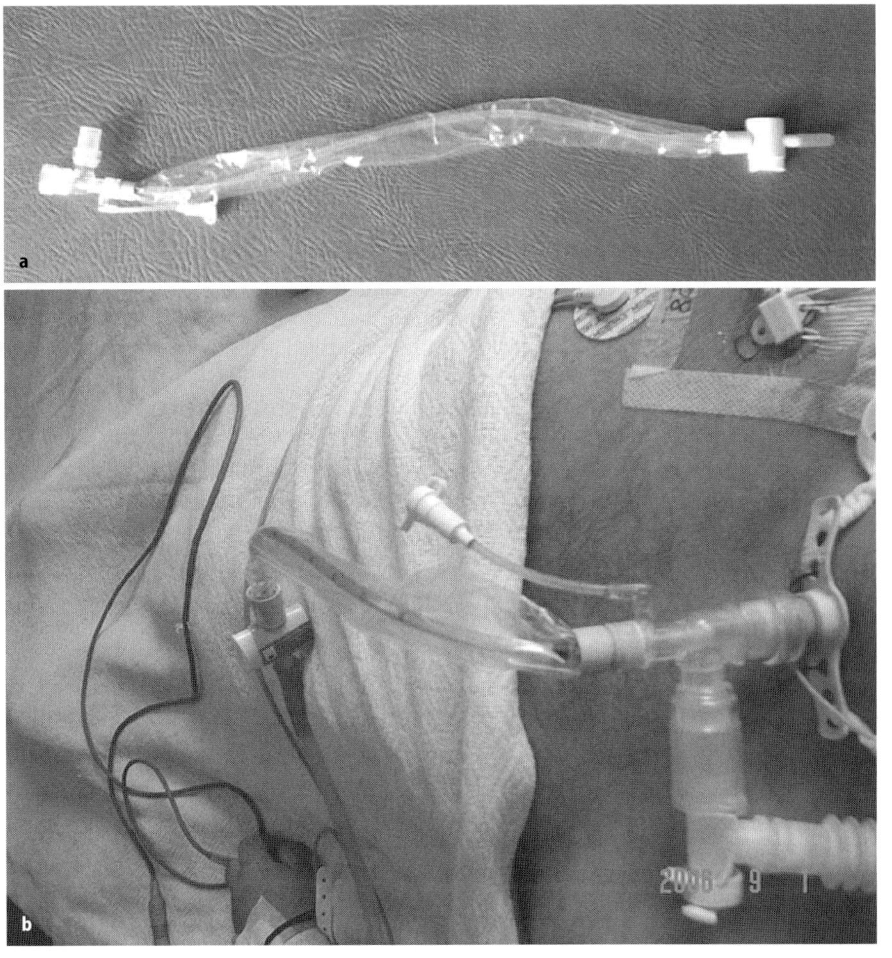

Fig. 44.1. The closed multiuse in-line catheter system

ETT and repeated insertions may increase the chance of lower airway colonization from the suction-catheter tip and ETT. Suction catheters may introduce microorganisms into the lower respiratory tract increasing the risk of colonization of the lower airways, and thus the risk of ventilator-associated pneumonia. Moreover, in patients with respiratory instability, the complications associated with this technique include arterial oxygen desaturation, cardiac arrhythmias, inability to maintain PEEP, and sudden death [59].

Closed suction catheter devices are now used in many hospitals, decreasing the risk of environmental cross-contamination, saving time and eliminating the need to disconnect the patient from the ventilator [60–63]. However, on comparing the two systems it has been suggested that the risk of catheter contamination or pneumonia is not different comparing the standard procedure with the multiuse system [64, 65] and few studies have shown favorable results for the closed systems.

The endpoints of the study by Topeli et al. were to determine the rate of VAP and colonization of the ventilator tubing [66]. They prospectively compared the effect of closed versus open suction systems and found that the type of suction system used had no effect on development of VAP. Moreover, the closed system increased the rate of colonization of the ventilator tubing, especially by multidrug resistant microorganisms. Another prospective, randomized study with negative results including 443 patients has recently been published by a Spanish group [67]. The closed-tracheal suction system did not decrease the incidence of VAP incidence or even exogenous pneumonia, which may be easier to reduce with this system.

Combes and coworkers [68] performed a prospective randomized study in 104 patients to compare the VAP incidence rates in patients according to the type of endotracheal suctioning (closed versus open) and used the Stericath closed suctioning system. The non-adjusted incidence rate of VAP was lower (although not significant) for the closed than for the open system (7.32 vs. 15.89/1,000 patient-days, $p=0.07$): Multivariate analysis showed an adjusted risk of VAP 3.5 times higher in the closed system (95% CI: 11.0–12.33). The suctioning procedure was performed once every 2 h and the Stericath was changed every 24 h.

There is currently no rigorous scientific evidence to recommend one practice over another, similar to the recommendation reported in the most recent guidelines for the prevention of nosocomial pneumonia published by the Centers for Disease Control and prevention [69].

The optimal procedure of the closed multiuse catheter system is still not clear. On one hand, it is recommended to change the in-line suction catheter every 24 h. This recommendation is based on the ability of bacteria to aggregate on the surface of suction catheters and ETTs to form a biofilm that protects the bacteria from the action of microbial agents or host defenses [10, 17]. Dislodgement of these bacterial aggregates into the lung has been proposed as a possible mechanism for the development of VAP [19]. Others investigators have suggested that increased manipulation of the ventilator circuit can predispose the development of VAP [31, 70]. Recently, Kollef and coworkers reported the same incidence of VAP in two groups of patients with or without daily changes of in-line suction catheters during mechanical ventilation [71].

In our opinion, the closed multiuse system is useful in unstable patients requiring mechanical ventilation with high oxygen concentrations or high levels of PEEP and in immunosuppressed patients because of the extremely high risk of infections that these patients have. The in-line suction catheter must be changed when a mechanical failure of the devices is detected (e.g., malfunction of the valve resulting in the leakage of air into the protected covering sheath of the catheter) or when visible soil is clotting the inner catheter (such as resulting from aspiration of blood or aspired emesis). Except in the above mentioned situations we use the open system with single use catheters in routine suctioning procedures.

44.10 Conclusions

Bacterial biofilm has been demonstrated on the inner surface of ETTs in a high percentage of these tubes removed from mechanically ventilated patients. Biofilm formation seems to be independent of the duration of mechanical ventilation. However, whether this is due to the rapid formation of biofilm or whether there or other factors involved has not been systematically investigated. Endoluminal biofilm seems to form either more rapidly or more frequently at the distal end of the ETT. However, in vivo pure biofilm does not develop and factors such as mucus deposition should also be taken into account. Recent research indicates that bacterial biofilm may form more frequently in the ETTs of patients with VAP. Nevertheless, this may represent contamination, and the magnitude of the contribution of endoluminal bacterial biofilm to the pathogenesis of VAP may be minimal when other risk factors are taken into account. In contrast, bacterial biofilm of ETTs may play an important role as a persistent source of infectious material for recurrent episodes of VAP. However, changing the ETT after *P. aeruginosa* pneumonia cannot be recommended at this stage, since re-intubation itself represents an independent risk factor for nosocomial pneumonia [72]. Coated ETTs or the use of exchangeable inner linings may be a more suitable way to prevent re-infection.

Other invasive devices such as bronchoscopes and tracheal suction catheters may also play a role in the pathogenesis of nosocomial pneumonia. The use of adequate methods of clearing and disinfection of the bronchoscope is mandatory to prevent infections.

References

1. Levine SA, Niederman MS (1991) The impact of tracheal intubation on host defenses and risks for nosocomial pneumonia. Clin Chest Med 12:523–543
2. Costerton JW (1999) Introduction to biofilm. Int J Antimicrob Agents 11:217–221
3. Prakash UB (1993) Does the bronchoscope propagate infection? Chest 104:552–559
4. Costerton JW, Lewandonski Z, Caldwell DE, Korber DR, Lapin-Scott HM (1995) Microbial biofilms. Annu Rev Microbiol 44:711–745
5. Costerton JW, Cheng KJ, Geesey GG, Ladd TI, Nickel JC, Dasgupta M, Marrie TJ (1987) Bacterial biofilms in nature and disease. Annu Rev Microbiol 41:435–464
6. Costerton JW, Stewart PS, Greenberg EP (1999) Bacterial biofilms: a common cause of persistent infections. Science 21:1318–1322
7. O'Toole GA, Kolter R (1998) Flagellar and twitching motility are necessary for *Pseudomonas aeruginosa* biofilm development. Mol Microbiol 30:295–304
8. Parsek MR, Greenberg EP (1999) Quorum sensing signals in development of *Pseudomonas aeruginosa* biofilms. Methods Enzymol 310:43–55
9. Gorman SP, McGovern JG, Woolfson AD, Adair CG, Jones DS (2001) The concomitant development of poly(vinyl chloride)-related biofilm and antimicrobial resistance in relation to ventilator-associated pneumonia. Biomaterials 22:2741–2747
10. Inglis TJ, Lim TM, Ng ML, Tang EK, Hui KP (1995) Structural features of tracheal tube biofilm formed during prolonged mechanical ventilation. Chest 108:1049–1052
11. Vorachit M, Lam K, Jayanetra P, Costerton JW (1993) Resistance of *Pseudomonas pseudomallei* growing as a biofilm on silastic discs to ceftazidime and co-trimoxazole. Antimicrob Agents Chemother 37:2000–2002
12. Shigeta M, Tanaka G, Komatsuzawa H, Sugai M, Suginaka H, Usui T (1997) Permeation of antimicrobial agents through *Pseudomonas aeruginosa* biofilms: a simple method. Chemotherapy 43:340–345
13. Dibdin GH, Assinder SJ, Nichols WW, Lambert PA (1996) Mathematical model of beta-lactam penetration into a biofilm of *Pseudomonas aeruginosa* while undergoing simultaneous inactivation by released beta-lactamases. J Antimicrob Chemother 38:757–769

14. Ishida H, Ishida Y, Kurosaka Y, Otani T, Sato K, Kobayashi H (1998) In vitro and in vivo activities of levofloxacin against biofilm-producing *Pseudomonas aeruginosa*. Antimicrob Agents Chemother 42:1641–1645
15. Fletcher M (1991) The physiological activity of bacteria attached to solid surfaces. Adv Microb Physiol 32:53–85
16. Bagge N, Ciofu O, Skovgaard LT, Hoiby N (2000) Rapid development in vitro and in vivo of resistance to ceftazidime in biofilm-growing *Pseudomonas aeruginosa* due to chromosomal beta-lactamase. APMIS 108:589–600
17. Sottile FD, Marrie TJ, Prough DS, Hobgood CD, Gower DJ, Webb LX, Costerton JW, Gristina AG (1986) Nosocomial pulmonary infection: possible etiologic significance of bacterial adhesion to endotracheal tubes. Crit Care Med 14:265–270
18. Diaz-Blanco J, Clawson RC, Roberson SM, Sanders CB, Pramanik AK, Herbst JJ (1989) Electron microscopic evaluation of bacterial adherence to polyvinyl chloride endotracheal tubes used in neonates. Crit Care Med 17: 1335–1340
19. Inglis TJ, Millar MR, Jones JG, Robinson DA (1989) Tracheal tube biofilm as a source of bacterial colonization of the lung. J Clin Microbiol 27:2014–2018
20. Inglis TJ (1993) Evidence for dynamic phenomena in residual tracheal tube biofilm. Br J Anaesth 70:22–24
21. Coalson JJ, Gerstmann DR, Winter VT, Delemos RA (1991) Bacterial colonization and infection studies in the premature baboon with bronchopulmonary dysplasia. Am Rev Respir Dis 144:1140–1146
22. Rubenstein JS, Kabat K, Shulman ST, Yogev R (1992) Bacterial and fungal colonization of endotracheal tubes in children: a prospective study. Crit Care Med 20:1544–1549
23. Garrouste-Orgeas M, Chevret S, Arlet G, Marie O, Rouveau M, Popoff N, Schlemmer B (1997) Oropharyngeal or gastric colonization and nosocomial pneumonia in adult intensive care unit patients. A prospective study based on genomic DNA analysis. Am J Respir Crit Care Med 156:1647–1655
24. Estes RJ, Meduri GU (1995) The pathogenesis of ventilator-associated pneumonia: I. Mechanisms of bacterial transcolonization and airway inoculation. Intensive Care Med 21:365–383
25. Feldman C, Kassel M, Cantrell J, Kaka S, Morar R, Goolam Mahomed A, Philips JI (1999) The presence and sequence of endotracheal tube colonization in patients undergoing mechanical ventilation. Eur Respir J 13:546–551
26. Adair CG, Gorman SP, Feron BM, Byers LM., Jones DS, Goldsmith CE, Moore JE, Kerr JR, Curran MD, Hogg G, Webb CH, McCarthy GJ, Milligan KR (1999) Implications of endotracheal tube biofilm for ventilator-associated pneumonia. Intensive Care Med 25:1072–1076
27. Koerner RJ (1997) Contribution of endotracheal tubes to the pathogenesis of ventilator-associated pneumonia. J Hosp Infect 35:83–89
28. Van Saene HKF, Damjanovic V, Williets T, Mostafa SM, Fox MA, Petros AJ (1998) Pathogenesis of ventilator-associated pneumonia: is the contribution of biofilm clinically significant? [letter]. J Hosp Infect 38:231–240
29. Torres A, Aznar R, Gatell JM, Jiménez P, González J, Ferrer M, Celis R, Rodriguez-Roisin R (1990) Incidence, risk, and prognosis factors of nosocomial pneumonia in mechanically ventilated patients. Am Rev Respir Dis 142:523–528
30. Bonten MJ, Bergmans DC, Ambergen AW, de Leeuw PW, van der Geest S, Stobberingh EE, Gaillard CA (1996) Risk factors for pneumonia, and colonization of respiratory tract and stomach in mechanically ventilated ICU patients. Am J Respir Crit Care Med 154:1339–1346
31. Craven DE, Kunches LM, Kilinsky V, Lichtenberg DA, Make BJ, McCabe WR (1986) Risk factors for pneumonia and fatality in patients receiving mechanical ventilation. Am Rev Respir Dis 133:792–796
32. Fernández-Crehuet R, Diáz-Molina C, De Irala J, Martínez-Concha D, Salcedo-Leal I, Masa-Calles J (1997) Nosocomial infection in an intensive-care unit: Identification of risk factors. Infect Control Hosp Epidemiol 18:825–830
33. Rello J, Mariscal D, Marco F, Jubert P, Sanchez F, Valles J, Coll P (1998) Recurrent *Pseudomonas aeruginosa* pneumonia in ventilated patients: relapse or reinfection? Am J Respir Crit Care Med 157:912–916
34. Gorman S, Adair C, O'Neill F, Goldsmith C, Webb H (1993) Influence of selective decontamination of the digestive tract on microbial biofilm formation on endotracheal tubes from artificially ventilated patients. Eur J Clin Microbiol Infect Dis 12:9–17
35. Pacheco-Fowler V, Gaonkar T, Wyer PC, Modak S (2004) Antiseptic impregnated endotracheal tubes for the prevention of bacterial colonization. J Hosp Infect 57:170–174
36. Berra L, De Marchi L, Yu Z, Laquerriere P, Baccarelli A, Kolobow T (2004) Endotracheal tubes coated with antiseptics decrease bacterial colonization of the ventilator circuits, lungs, and endotracheal tube. Anesthesiology 100:1446–56
37. Fox CL, Modak SM, Sampath LA (1991) Infection-resistant compositions, medical devices and surfaces and methods for preparing and using same. United States of America, May 28, 1991, patent no. 5019096
38. Jones DS, McMeel S, Adair CG, Gorman SP (2003) Characterisation and evaluation of novel surfactant bacterial anti-adherent coatings for endotracheal tubes designed for the prevention of ventilator-associated pneumonia. J Pharmacy Pharmacol 55:43–52
39. Adair CG, Gorman SP, Byers LM, Jones DS, Feron B, Crowe M, Webb HC, McCarthy GJ, Milligan KR (2002) Eradication of endotracheal tube biofilm by nebulized gentamicin. Intensive Care Med 28:426–431
40. Credle WF Jr, Smiddy JF, Elliot RC (1974) Complications of fiberoptic bronchoscopy. Am Rev Respir Dis 109:67–72
41. Pereira W, Kovnat DM, Khan MA, Iacovino JR, Spivack ML, Sneider GL (1975) Fever and pneumonia after flexible bronchoscopy. Am Rev Respir Dis 112:59–64
42. Surta PM, Gruber B, Wellons HA, Wenzel RP (1977) Absence of clinical pneumonia following bronchoscopy with contaminated and clean bronchofiberscopes. Chest 71: 52–54
43. Hussain SA (1978) Fiberoptic bronchoscope-related outbreak of infection with *Pseudomonas*. Chest 74:483
44. Sanmartino MT, Israel RH, Magnussen CR (1982) *Pseudomonas aeruginosa* contamination of fiberoptic bronchoscopes. J Hosp Infect 3:65–71
45. Boisjoly HM, Jotterand VH, Brazin R, Bergeron MG (1987) Metastatic *Pseudomonas* endophthalmitis following bronchoscopy. Can J Ophthalmol 22:378–380
46. Weinstein HJ, Bone RC, Ruth WE (1977) Contamination of a fiberoptic bronchoscope with a *Proteus* species. Am Rev Respir Dis 116:541–543
47. Webb SF, Vall-Spinosa A (1975) Outbreak of *Serratia marcescens* associated with flexible fiberoptic bronchoscope. Chest 68:703–705
48. Beyt BE Jr, King DK, Glew RH (1977) Fatal pneumonitis and septicemia after bronchoscopy. Chest 72:105–107
49. Hsu JT, Barret CR Jr (1981) Lung abscess complicating transbronchial biopsy of a mass lesion. Chest 80:230–232
50. Muers M, Lane D (1980) Acute pneumonia and pneumothorax as a complication of transbronchial biopsy. Endoscopy 12:183–187
51. Watts WJ, Green RA (1984) Bacteremia following transbronchial fine needle aspiration. Chest 85:295

52. Leers WD (1980) Disinfecting endoscopes: how to not transmit *Mycobacterium* tuberculosis by bronchoscopy. Can Med Assoc J 123:275–283
53. Nelson KE, Larson PA, Schraufnagel DE, Jackson J (1983) Transmission of tuberculosis by flexible fiberbronchoscopes. Am Rev Respir Dis 127:97–100
54. Wheeler PW, Lancaster D, Kaiser AB (1989) Bronchopulmonary cross-colonization and infection related to mycobacterial contamination of suction valves of bronchoscopes. J Infect Dis 159:954–958
55. Agerton T, Walway S, Gore B, Pozsik C, Plikaytis B, Woodley C, Honorato I (1999) Transmission of a highly drug resistant strain (strain W1) of *Mycobacterium* tuberculosis. Community outbreak and nosocomial transmission via a contaminated bronchoscope. JAMA 278:1073–1077
56. Pappas SA, Schaaff DM, DiCostanzo MB, King FW, Sharp JT (1983) Contamination of flexible fiberoptic bronchoscopes. Am Rev Respir Dis 127:391–392
57. Uttley AHC, Honeywell KM, Fitch LE, Yates MD, Collins CH, Simpson RA (1990) Cross contamination of bronchial washings. Br Med J 301:1274
58. Mehta AC, Minai OA (1990) Infection control in the bronchoscopy suite. Clinics Chest Med 20:19–32
59. Brown SE, Stansbury DW, Merril EJ, Linden GS, Light RW (1983) Prevention of suctioning-related arterial oxygen desaturation. Comparison of off-ventilator and on-ventilator suctioning. Chest 83:621–627
60. Mayhall CG (1988) The Trach Care closed tracheal suction system: a new medical device to permit tracheal suctioning without interruption of ventilatory assistance. Infect Control Hosp Epidemiol 9:125–126
61. Baker T, Taylor M, Wilson M, Rish J, Brazeal S (1989) Evaluation of a closed system endotracheal suction catheter. Am J Infect Control 17:97
62. Johnson KL, Kearney PA, Johnson SB, Niblett JB, McMillan NL, McClain RE (1994) Closed versus open endotracheal suctioning: costs and physiologic consequences. Crit Care Med 22:658–666
63. Cobley M, Atkins M, Jones FL (1991) Environmental contamination during tracheal suction. A comparison of disposable conventional catheters with a multiple-use closed system device. Anaesthesia 46:957–961
64. Deppe SA, Kelly JW, Thoi LL, Chudy JH, Longfield RN, Ducey JP, Truwit CL, Antopol MR (1990) Incidence of colonization, nosocomial pneumonia, and mortality in critically patients using a Trach Care closed-suction system versus an open-suction system: prospective, randomized study. Crit Care Med 18:1393
65. Ritz R, Scott LR, Coyle MB, Pierson DJ (1986) Contamination of a multiple-use suction catheter in a closed-circuit system compared to contamination of a disposable, single-use suction catheter. Respir Care 31:1087–1091
66. Topeli A, Harmanci A, Cetinkaya Y, Akdeniz S, Unal S (2002) Comparison of the effect of closed versus open endotracheal suction systems on the development of ventilator-associated pneumonia. J Hosp Infect 58:14–19
67. Lorente L, Leucona M, Martín MM, García C, Mora ML, Sierra A (2005) Ventilator-associated pneumonia using a closed versus an open tracheal suction system. Crit Care Med 33:115–119
68. Combes P, Fauvage B, Oleyer C (2001) Nosocomial pneumonia in mechanically ventilated patients, a prospective randomised evaluation of the Stericath closed suctioning system. Intensive Care Med 26:878–882
69. Tablan OC, Andreson LJ, Arden NH, Breiman RF, Butler JC, McNeil MM (1994) Guideline for prevention of nosocomial pneumonia. The Hospital Infection Control Practices Advisory Committee, Centers for Disease Control and Prevention. Infect Control Hosp Epidemiol 15:588–625
70. Kollef MH, Shapiro SD, Fraser VJ, Silver P, Murphy M, Trovillon E, Hearns ML, Richards RD, Cracchilo L, Hossin L (1995) Mechanical ventilation with or without 7-day circuit changes: a randomized controlled trial. Ann Intern Ved 123:168–174
71. Kollef MH, Prentice D, Shapiro SD, Fraser VJ, Silver P, Trovillion E, Weilitz P, von Harz B, St John R (1997) Mechanical ventilation with or without daily changes of in-line suction catheters. Am J Respir Crit Care Med 156:466–472
72. Torres A, Gatell JM, Aznar R, El-Ebiary M, Puig de la Bellacasa J, González J, Ferrer M, Rodriguez-Roisin R (1995) Re-intubation increases the risk of nosocomial pneumonia in patients needing mechanical ventilation. Am J Respir Crit Care Med 152:137–141

Infections with Surgical Implications

VI

Chapter 45

Multiple Organ Dysfunction Syndrome

45

F.M. Pieracci, S.R. Eachempati, P.S. Barie

The multiple organ dysfunction syndrome (MODS) is defined as the progressive, potentially reversible dysfunction of two or more organ systems following acute, life-threatening disruption of systemic homeostasis. Now nearly 40 years since its initial description [1], MODS remains the leading cause of mortality among patients requiring ICU care. Furthermore, the financial burden to both individual hospitals and the health care system as a result of caring for patients with MODS is astronomical. Currently, MODS is believed to represent the most severe manifestation of dysregulated or uncontrolled systemic inflammation. Despite a sophisticated understanding of the pathogenesis of MODS, effective therapies have remained elusive; prevention is crucial if lives are to be spared. This is likely due to the underlying heterogeneity of the syndrome itself; organ dysfunction may arise following a vast array of physiologic insults, and MODS may affect variable numbers of organ systems to varying degrees at different times. Further frustrating the development of targeted therapeutics are the redundancy and interrelationships of the dysregulated immune response characteristic of MODS. However, an increased appreciation of these interrelationships has resulted in advancements in the treatment of MODS. This chapter will review current conceptualizations of MODS as well as present and future therapeutic strategies.

45.1 Historical Perspectives

Multiple organ failure following severe physiologic insult arose during the late 1960s as the unwanted consequence of advancements in the recognition and treatment of shock. Patients resuscitated successfully following shock were often noted to succumb to a novel disease process characterized by the progressive, irreversible failure of several organ systems. In 1975 Baue synthesized early case reports of organ failure following severe injury [1–3] into the concept of multiple organ failure as a distinct entity, which he described as "the progressive failure of many or all systems after an overwhelming injury or operation" [4]. In his initial description, Baue gleaned two concepts fundamental to mortality during critical illness. First, he recognized that mortality in the ICU was the consequence of the interaction of multiple failing organs. Furthermore, he appreciated the interrelationships of individual organ systems; injury to one organ system could cause dysfunction of another. These observations were eventually validated in numerous clinical series. For example, pulmonary failure was found more often than not to occur along with dysfunction of at least one other organ system [5]. Moreover, mortality of acute respiratory failure is usually determined by the magnitude of non-pulmonary organ dysfunction; the combination of respiratory and hepatic dysfunction is especially deleterious [5]. Furthermore, improvements in the treatment of the acute respiratory distress syndrome (ARDS), such as ventilation at low tidal volumes, also decreased the likelihood of additional, subsequent organ failure [6]. Soon after Baue's initial description of multiple organ failure, Fry et al. reported a linear relationship between the number of failed organs and mortality during critical illness; whereas mortality following failure of a single organ was 30%, mortality following failure of four or more organs was 100% [7].

The etiology of multiple organ failure was initially believed to be always infectious in nature [8]. However, clinical, pathologic, and experimental findings soon called this theory into question. Autopsies of patients with multiple organ failure did not always demonstrate an obvious source of infection; sometimes infection was never present, or organ dysfunction progressed despite successful anti-infective therapy [9, 10]. Furthermore, more often than not, trauma patients with organ failure were not infected [11]. When infection did occur during critical illness, it sometimes followed organ failure, rather than preceding it [12]. Under experimental conditions, the characteristic hemodynamic and inflammatory derangements could be replicated in the absence of infection [13, 14].

Some investigators attempted to reconcile this discrepancy by suggesting that an occult reservoir of pathogens, such as the proximal gastrointestinal tract, could serve to perpetuate sepsis and organ failure in the absence of another, identifiable source of infection [15,

16]. According to the "gut-motor" hypothesis, bacterial overgrowth during critical illness (secondary to antacid therapy, impaired intestinal immunity, or both) provided the fuel to sustain organ dysfunction. However, subsequent investigations revealed that selective gut decontamination neither attenuated the severity of organ dysfunction nor improved mortality, calling this theory into question [14, 17].

The realization that infection was a sufficient, but unnecessary cause of organ damage resulted in a reevaluation of the pathophysiology of multiple organ failure. In a seminal article, Goris et al. suggested "massive activation of inflammatory mediators by severe tissue trauma or intra-abdominal sepsis" as the etiology of multiple organ failure [11]. Marshall et al. reinforced this theory by observing that the degree of the inflammatory response to infection predicted ICU mortality, rather than the type or degree of infection itself [18]. Eventually, the hypothesis developed that a hypodynamic, excessive, or otherwise dysfunctional immune response was the principal cause of organ damage, rather than the cytotoxic effects of invading microorganisms per se. This theory synthesized the myriad, seemingly unrelated, causes of organ failure into a unifying hypothesis, and was consistent with both clinical and experimental observations. In recognition of this advancement, and in an attempt to standardize it, an American College of Chest Physicians/Society of Critical Care Medicine consensus statement put forth diagnostic criteria for what was termed the systemic inflammatory response syndrome (SIRS) in 1992 [19]. The diagnosis of SIRS involved fulfillment of two or more of the following criteria: (1) core body temperature >38 °C or <36 °C, (2) heart rate >90 beats per minute, (3) respiratory rate >20 breaths per minute (not ventilated) or $PaCO_2$ <32 mmHg (ventilated), (4) WBC >12,000, <4,000, or >10% immature forms (bands). When the cause of SIRS was infection, it was termed sepsis.

Organ dysfunction was also recognized as a common complication of SIRS, and the term MODS signified the presence of altered organ function in critically ill patients such that homeostasis could not be achieved without intervention. Specifically, SIRS correlates with both incidence and magnitude of MODS, and ultimately mortality [20]. Currently, MODS remains the acronym used most commonly to describe organ dysfunction during critical illness. However, several other terms have been used, and may remain in use (Table 45.1).

Table 45.1. Historic synonyms for what is referred to currently as the multiple organ dysfunction syndrome

Sequential organ failure
Progressive systems failure
Remote organ failure
Multiple organ failure
Multiple organ failure syndrome
Multiple organ systems failure

45.2 Epidemiology

The MODS is widely believed to be the leading cause of death among ICU patients [21–24]. As many as 19% of ICU patients will develop MODS [21–25], and MODS is responsible for 50% [26, 27] to 80% [23] of ICU mortality. Patients who develop MODS suffer over a 20-fold increase in mortality and a doubled length of stay (LOS) compared to critically ill patients who do not develop MODS [28]. A recent report noted MODS to be the most common diagnosis in ICU patients who required a prolonged LOS (>21 days) [29], but even modest degrees of organ dysfunction prolong hospitalization.

Any biological stress that activates systemic inflammation may precipitate SIRS, thus placing the patient at risk for MODS. Known causes of MODS are listed in Table 45.2. Our group found hypoperfusion/ischemia without shock to be the most common etiologic insult responsible for MODS, followed by sepsis without shock, and shock regardless of etiology [28]. Moreover, Sauaia et al. found that an injury severity score (ISS) of ≥25 points along with a transfusion requirement of ≥6 units of red blood cell concentrates was associated with a 46% likelihood of developing MODS [30]. More recently, Cryer et al. broadened these risk factors, reporting a 66% incidence of MODS in patients with an ISS ≥25, regardless of transfusion requirement [31].

For any given etiologic mechanism, both increased age [24] and number of comorbidities [24, 32] increase the likelihood of developing MODS. Furthermore, recent work has shown that certain individuals may harbor a genetic predisposition to MODS in the form of an exaggerated inflammatory response to illness [33, 34].

Table 45.2. Causes of the multiple organ dysfunction syndrome

Sepsis
Multiple trauma
Burns
Pancreatitis
Pulmonary aspiration of gastric contents
Massive hemorrhage
Massive transfusion
Ischemia-reperfusion
Ischemic necrosis
Microvascular thrombosis
Interleukin-2 therapy
Salicylate intoxication
Multiple sequential physiologic insults

45.3 Pathophysiology

Three unique mechanisms for the precipitation of MODS have been proposed [35]. According to the one-hit model, organ failure develops as the direct result of a massive initial insult (e.g., burn or multi-trauma), which is of itself sufficient to cause MODS. By contrast, the two-hit model describes sequential insults, usually isolated temporally. According to the two-hit model, a priming insult (e.g., burn) is followed by a subsequent insult (e.g., catheter-related blood stream infection) that, in the setting of inflammation, induces further immune dysfunction and eventual organ failure. Finally, according to the "sustained-hit" model, a continuous, smoldering insult, such as multi-drug resistant, ventilator-associated pneumonia, both causes and sustains organ failure. In reality, any combination of these three mechanisms may result in MODS.

Organ failure may or may not follow a particular temporal sequence. Cardiovascular instability is often the first manifestation of dysfunctional homeostasis, resulting in ischemia-reperfusion (I-R) injury after resuscitation. The splanchnic and renal circulations are particularly susceptible to I-R injury. Pulmonary failure is equally common and is usually an early manifestation, whereas hepatic, hematologic, gastrointestinal and renal failure are usually later manifestations that may or may not become apparent [4, 7, 36]. In particular, hepatic dysfunction may not be recognized promptly because the liver has redundant metabolic capacity and substantial dysfunction may precede elevation of the serum bilirubin concentration. Furthermore, certain combinations of organ failure have been shown to be especially deleterious (e.g., hepatic and pulmonary, or renal and pulmonary) [5].

Organ damage following severe injury is believed to occur secondary to uncontrolled activation of the inflammatory response caused by tissue hypoxia. Following tissue injury, the early stage of the inflammatory response is characterized by macrophage activation as well as secretion of inflammatory cytotoxins and cytokines. Cytotoxins are released primarily by CD8+ T-lymphocytes and act locally by causing damage to cell walls and tight junctions [37]. By contrast, cytokines mediate primarily the CD4+ T-cell response and may be secreted by a variety of cell types in addition to those of the immune system. Cytokines act both locally (including on the cells that secrete them) and systemically. Although cytokines may be classified broadly into groups by function (Table 45.3), the cytokine-mediated inflammatory response is redundant; each cytokine has multiple activities on different cell types, some of which are salutary. The balance of pro and anti-inflammatory responses is not always self-regulatory and balanced; predominance of either influence may be deleterious. As such, the inflammatory response has been challenging to manipulate for therapeutic effect.

Recruitment of polymorphonuclear (PMN) leukocytes into tissue represents a second prominent feature of MODS. Postmortem examinations of patients with ARDS have demonstrated massive PMN leukocyte infiltration into lung parenchyma [38]. Furthermore, depletion [39] or inhibition [40] of PMN leukocytes decreases the severity of lung injury in animal models of ARDS. Infiltration of PMN leukocytes is accompanied by upregulation of both hepatic inflammatory proteins (e.g., C-reactive protein) and the complement system [41], increased capillary permeability, and the formation of reactive oxygen and nitrogen species. The clinical manifestations of increased capillary permeability

Table 45.3. Major classes of inflammatory cytokines, representative members, their receptors, and their main action(s). (Adapted from [102])

Cytokine	Producer cell	Main actions
Hematopoietins		
IL-1	Macrophages, epithelial cells	Fever, T-cell activation, macrophage activation
IL-2	T cells	T-cell proliferation
IL-6	T cells, macrophages	T- and B-cell growth and differentiation, acute phase protein production
IL-7	Bone marrow stroma	Growth of immature T cells and B cells
Chemokines		
IL-8	Macrophages, others	Chemotactic for neutrophils, T cells
MCP-1	Macrophages, others	Chemotactic for monocytes
Modulators of immune response		
TNF-α	Macrophage, NK cells	Local inflammation, endothelial activation
TNF-β	T cells, B cells	Killing, endothelial activation
IL-12	B cells, macrophages	NK-cell activation, T-cell differentiation
IFN-γ	T cells, natural killer cells	Macrophage activation, increased MHC production
Anti-inflammatory		
IL-10	T cells, macrophages	Inhibition of macrophage function
IL-13	T cells	Inhibition of macrophage cytokine production
TGF-β	Monocytes, T cells	Inhibition of cell growth, anti-inflammatory

IL interleukin, *MCP* macrophage chemoattractant protein, *TNF* tumor necrosis factor, *NK* natural killer, *INF* interferon, *MHC* major histocompatibility complex, *TGF* transforming growth factor are peripheral edema, pulmonary edema (characteristic of ARDS), and cerebral edema.

Apoptosis, or programmed cell death, is deranged in MODS. Increased markers of apoptosis such as Fas [42] and nuclear matrix proteins [43] have been found in patients with MODS. Interestingly, whereas some cell types such as splenic lymphocytes and hepatocytes demonstrate accelerated apoptosis, other cell types, such as circulating PMN leukocytes, exhibit inhibited apoptosis. Still other tissues, such as the kidney and lung, show only minimal changes in rates of cellular death [44–46].

The uncontrolled inflammation characteristic of MODS is accompanied by microvascular thrombosis [47]. Indeed, the inflammatory and coagulation systems are intimately related, and often impossible to distinguish. Several pro-inflammatory cytokines [e.g., tumor necrosis factor-alpha (TNF-α)] may activate tissue factor and initiate the coagulation cascade [46]. In turn, the thrombin receptor is known to activate nuclear factor kappa beta (NF-κB), which causes increased transcription of pro-inflammatory gene products [48]. Microvessel coagulation results in further hypoxia, thus perpetuating the inflammatory response. Early coagulopathy increases the risk of developing MODS [49].

Whereas the initial phase of MODS is characterized by a disruption of homeostatic mechanisms to favor inflammation, a second, distinct later period is characterized by *impaired* inflammation and increased susceptibility to infection. During this period, there is an increase in serum concentrations of anti-inflammatory cytokines such as interleukin (IL)-10, IL-13, and transforming growth factor (TGF)-β, impaired antibody synthesis, and anergy of T-lymphocytes [50–52]. This response has been termed the compensatory anti-inflammatory response system (CARS), and the result referred to as immunoparalysis [52]. This acquired immunodeficiency state is believed to lead to the high incidence of late nosocomial infections that is characteristic of critical illness and the development of organ dysfunction.

In summary, two distinct periods of altered immune function characterize MODS. The first is dominated by uncontrolled inflammation, increased endothelial permeability, microvessel coagulopathy, altered apoptosis, and disruption of parenchymal cellular integrity. The second involves a predominance of anti-inflammatory cytokines, immunosuppression, and an increased risk of infection. This general disruption of the normal regulation of the immune system during MODS has been termed immunologic dissonance [53].

An alternative theory describes the pathogenesis of MODS as a disruption of inter-organ or intercellular communication [54]. Accordingly, each organ system is viewed as a stochastic (random) biologic oscillator, whose activity varies periodically with time. The dynamic behavior of any one organ necessarily reflects the state of the organism as a whole. During normal homeostasis, variability within each oscillator is preserved through mechanical, neural, hormonal, and immune (e.g., cytokine and prostaglandin) inputs. As a result of massive physiologic insult, inter-oscillator communication becomes uncoupled, resulting in a regularization of normally variable organ outputs.

The majority of research in the area of biologic oscillators has been conducted using loss of normal heart rate variability as a marker of uncoupling. Recent investigations have reported increased cardiac regularity after administration of endotoxin to healthy volunteers [55], as well as in emergency department patients with sepsis [56]. Furthermore, low heart rate variability correlates with both ICU mortality [57, 58] and mortality from MODS [59, 60]. As a result, measurement of heart rate variability has emerged recently as a non-invasive, accurate, and validated tool to predict outcomes during critical illness [61].

The uncoupling of stochastic biologic oscillators offers an intriguing alternative theory for the pathogenesis of MODS, and has been used to explain the failure of anti-mediator trials aimed at attenuating the inflammatory response in these patients (discussed below) [62]. However, substantial additional research, as well as a fundamental shift in the current conceptualization of MODS, will be required to provide tangible options for the treatment of patients with MODS. One such example suggested by Buchman involves a shift from traditional random or scheduled sampling of physiologic parameters to continuous sampling strategies in order to better capture loss of organ variability [59].

45.4 Organ System Manifestations

Although uncontrolled inflammation exerts distinct, predictable effects on each organ system, organ dysfunction rarely occurs in isolation. Moreover, it is important to note that organ dysfunction in critical illness is usually multifactorial. For example, renal dysfunction is often iatrogenic, resulting from the use of either nephrotoxic medications or radiocontrast media. Listed below are the known consequences of systemic inflammation on individual organ systems.

Although cardiovascular failure manifested as shock is often the cause of SIRS and ultimately MODS, inflammation also results in impaired cardiac function. Tumor necrosis factor and reactive oxygen and nitrogen species inhibit cardiac contractility [63]. Inflammation also causes increased endothelial permeability and vasodilation, decreasing blood volume and systemic vascular resistance, respectively. Thus, each component of blood pressure is affected (preload, contractility, and afterload), resulting in hypotension that may be refractory to aggressive volume replacement, thus necessitating the use of vasopressor therapy.

Lung inflammation results in impaired gas diffusion that is manifested primarily as hypoxia rather than hypercarbia. The most severe pulmonary manifestation of MODS is ARDS, characterized by a PaO_2:F_iO_2 of less than 200, and diffuse bilateral pulmonary infiltrates on chest radiography in the presence of a pulmonary capillary wedge pressure of less than 18 mmHg. The ARDS is a relatively common complication of SIRS, and has been described in detail elsewhere [64].

In addition to alterations in leukocyte production and function, both thrombopoiesis and erythropoiesis are inhibited during MODS. Thrombocytopenia is a well-recognized sequela of both SIRS and sepsis and results not only from bone marrow suppression, but also from increased consumption and sequestration within the reticuloendothelial system. Furthermore, IL-1, TNF-α, and TGF-β inhibit erythropoietin synthesis and action [65–68]. Recombinant TNF-α induces anemia and hypoferremia associated with decreased iron release from the reticuloendothelial system and incorporation into red blood cells [69, 70]. Interleukin-1 and TNF-α also induce ferritin production as part of the "acute-phase reaction," sequestering iron that might otherwise be available for erythropoiesis [71]. Both generalized inflammation and microvascular thrombosis lead to the widespread consumption of clotting factors, which, in its most severe form, may cause disseminated intravascular coagulation.

Manifestations of gastrointestinal I-R injury range from stress-related gastric mucosal hemorrhage ("stress gastritis") to acute acalculous cholecystitis. Furthermore, ileus, malabsorption, and diarrhea are common sequelae of mucosal inflammation. Disruption of intestinal mucosal integrity as a result of splanchnic I-R injury or due to the actions of inflammatory cytokines may facilitate the translocation of invading microorganisms and cause both bacteremia and infection (i.e., "gut-motor" hypothesis, discussed previously) [15, 72]. Increased intestinal permeability has been associated with the subsequent development of both SIRS and MODS [73].

Hepatic dysfunction in patients with MODS is characterized by cholestatic jaundice [74]. Leakage of bilirubin from the hepatic canalicula into the intracellular and eventually intravascular space may be due to the disruption of tight junctions by cytotoxic inflammation [37]. Hepatic synthetic function during inflammation is characterized by early upregulation of positive acute-phase reactants (e.g., C-reactive protein and ferritin), and downregulation of negative acute-phase reactants (e.g., albumin and transferrin). This initial period is followed by generalized impairment, including decreased synthesis of coagulation factors manifest as an elevation of the prothrombin time that is not corrected by the administration of vitamin K.

Hypoperfusion, microvascular thrombosis, and cerebral edema combine to cause encephalopathy in MODS. Furthermore, the recently described critical illness polyneuropathy syndrome, characterized by debility, muscle weakness, and eventual atrophy, has been associated with the development of MODS [75]. As mentioned previously, alternations of autonomic tone manifested as loss of normal heart rate variability, baroreflex sensitivity, and chemoreflex sensitivity are common in patients with MODS, and the degree of autonomic dysfunction correlates with mortality. Critical illness polyneuropathy may be a better indicator of neurologic dysfunction than encephalopathy in that it may be quantified by electromyography and is not affected by sedatives.

Hypoxic/ischemic insults to the kidney are the most common cause of acute renal failure, characterized by oliguria, azotemia, fluid overload, and accumulation of metabolites normally excreted via the urine. Other common causes of acute renal failure include rhabdomyolysis and drug toxicity (e.g., iodinated contrast media, antibiotics). Electrolyte abnormalities are not a prominent feature of renal injury unless caused by rhabdomyolysis (where potassium and phosphate accumulate rapidly), likely because they are monitored and corrected readily by the clinician. Although renal dysfunction usually becomes apparent (i.e., elevated serum creatinine concentration) later in the course of MODS, sub-clinical hypoxic damage likely occurs at the time of the initial insult. Even mild degrees of renal impairment (well short of the need for renal replacement therapy) translate into substantial morbidity and mortality. Pro-inflammatory cytokines such as TNF-α may also activat the renin-angiotensin-aldosterone axis [28]. Finally, as mentioned previously, IL-1, TNF-α and TGF-β inhibit erythropoietin synthesis and function, which essentially ceases below a glomerular filtration rate <25 ml/min.

45.5 Diagnosis

Early attempts at diagnosis depicted organ failure as an "all-or-nothing response." Organ failure was recorded as a dichotomous, categorical variable for each organ. Moreover, failure of each organ was given the same weight, regardless of severity. Organ failure was considered present if an iatrogenic intervention to support organ function was necessary (e.g., hemodialysis in the setting of acute renal failure). Prognosis was related solely to the number of failed organs, rather than the severity and the timing of failure. The former observation remains true, but more subtle gradations of organ dysfunction are now recognized.

Organ system	Score 0	1	2	3	4
Respiratory (PaO_2/FiO_2)[a]	>300	226–300	151–225	76–150	≤75
Renal (serum creatinine)[b]	≤100	101–200	201–350	351–500	>500
Hepatic (serum bilirubin)[c]	≤20	21–60	61–120	121–240	>240
Cardiovascular (PAR)[d]	≤10	10.1–15.0	15.1–20.0	20.1–30.0	>30.0
Hematologic (platelet count)[d]	>120	81–120	51–80	21–50	≤20
Neurologic (GCS)	15	13–14	10–12	7–9	≤6

[a] PaO_2:FiO_2 is calculated without reference to the use or mode of mechanical ventilation, and without reference to the use or level of positive end-expiratory pressure
[b] The serum creatinine concentration is measured in μmol/l, without reference to the use of dialysis
[c] The serum bilirubin concentration is measured in μmol/l
[d] The platelet count is measured in platelets/ml × 10^{-3}
PAR pressure adjusted heart rate, *GCS* Glasgow Coma Scale Score

Table 45.4. The Multiple Organ Dysfunction Score. To convert the serum creatinine concentration from μmol/l to mg/dl, divide by 88.4. To convert the serum bilibrubin concentration from μmol/l to mg/dl, divide by 17.1. (Reproduced from [78])

The current conceptualization of MODS is more mature: MODS is not an "all-or-nothing" phenomenon, not every organ "fails" even when dysfunction develops, and not every organ becomes dysfunctional to the same extent [76]. Rather, organ dysfunction is recognized to occur in a continuum of altered physiology. In response to this conceptualization, several scoring systems have been developed to quantify the extent of organ dysfunction associated with MODS.

Organ systems typically considered in the scoring of MODS are: (1) respiratory, (2) cardiovascular, (3) renal, (4) hepatic, (5) hematologic, and (6) central nervous system (CNS). Notably absent from this list are both the gastrointestinal and endocrine systems, which currently suffer from a lack of objective measurements of organ failure. Four scoring systems are currently employed with frequency [77–80]. Central to each is a gradation of organ dysfunction based on mostly objective measurements of altered physiologic function.

One such scoring system, the multiple organ dysfunction (MOD) score, is shown in Table 45.4 [77]. The MOD score was developed from a Medline review of clinical studies involving patients with MODS between 1969 and 1993. Five organ systems were evaluated using available physiologic markers: (1) respiratory (PaO_2:FiO_2), (2) renal (serum creatinine concentration), (3) hepatic (serum bilirubin concentration), (4) hematologic (platelet count), and (5) CNS (Glasgow Coma Scale score – the most subjective of the measurements). Cardiovascular dysfunction is quantified by the pressure-adjusted heart rate, which is defined as the product of the heart rate and the ratio of central venous pressure to mean arterial pressure. Each organ system is graded on a scale from 0 to 4 points for a maximum total score of 24. A MOD score of 0 for any organ system corresponds to a mortality of less than 5%, whereas a score of 4 correlates with a mortality of greater than 50%. The aggregate MOD score for survivors is calculated using the worst value for each organ system for each day, or can be scored on a cumulative basis for the episode of care.

Other scoring systems follow similar patterns and include the Brussels score [78], the sepsis-related organ failure assessment (SOFA) [79], and the logistic organ dysfunction system (LODS) [80]. These scoring systems have been validated similarly using cohorts of critically ill patients.

Data obtained using scoring systems may be used in a variety of ways for prognostication. Initial, aggregate, and mean scores have all been correlated with mortality. For example, the total MOD score correlates in a linear fashion with ICU mortality both when calculated on ICU day 1 and when the maximum score is compared to the score on day 1 [77]. Similarly, calculations of the initial, highest, and mean SOFA score all correlate with ICU mortality [81]. Due to variability of daily scores, the cumulative or aggregate scores are generally believed to possess the greatest prognostic ability. For example, daily MOD scores have been shown to decrease from peak values in patients who eventually die of MODS [31].

Because patients may demonstrate altered physiology in the immediate postoperative period related to anesthesia and recovery or transient, stereotypical surgical "stress," some authors have criticized both SIRS and MODS scoring systems as being oversensitive during this time period. Furthermore, some scoring systems have traditionally omitted data obtained during the first 48 h. However, more recent evidence suggests that both SIRS and MODS scores calculated as early as 48 h [20], and even 24 h after injury [24, 31], can predict mortality from MODS. These results have called into question the traditional pathophysiologic framework that depicts MODS as an occurrence relatively late in the ICU course (i.e., the two-hit model), and suggest that substantial organ dysfunction actually occurs much earlier. For these reasons, early and aggressive resuscitation to avoid or minimize the consequences of I-R injury are of paramount importance [82]. Indeed, markers of organ dysfunction observed as early as post-injury day 1 are perhaps better viewed as outcome measures rather than risk factors.

Although scoring systems are useful prognostic tools, they are limited by both a lack of standardization and omission of certain organ systems due to a lack of objective criteria of dysfunction. Furthermore, certain markers used in scoring systems (e.g., serum bilirubin concentration) may serve as poor proxies for organ function [28]. However, the development and refinement of current scoring systems highlights a fundamental improvement in the understanding of the pathophysiology of MODS.

45.6 Management

Management of MODS may be classified broadly as either prophylaxis or treatment, which in turn is either supportive care or attenuation of the pro-inflammatory response. Supportive care involves early recognition, resuscitation, and artificial maintenance of organ function. Evidence-based strategies include ventilation with lower tidal volumes for ARDS [6], aggressive renal replacement therapy for acute renal failure [83, 84], and stringent glycemic control (serum glucose concentration of 80–110 mg/dl) through the use of intensive insulin therapy [85]. In a population of critically ill surgical patients, this last intervention resulted in a striking reduction in infection, acute renal failure, critical illness polyneuropathy, blood transfusions, organ failure, and mortality.

Of note, although tissue hypoxia plays an important role in the initial pathophysiology of MODS, resuscitation to supranormal levels of tissue oxygenation to prevent or attenuate MODS using high FiO_2, inotropes (e.g., dobutamine), or blood transfusion has not improved outcomes, and may in fact worsen the severity of organ dysfunction during MODS [86–89]. Exacerbation of tissue damage following the introduction of supranormal concentrations of oxygen may be explained by increased substrate for the generation of cytotoxic oxygen free radicals.

Efforts to manipulate the dysregulated immune response characteristic of MODS have constituted a substantial portion of experimental research in the field of critical care over the last 2 decades. Early attempts sought to achieve generalized immunosuppression. However, treatment with non-specific inhibitors of inflammation such as non-steroidal anti-inflammatory drugs [90], corticosteroids [91], or dietary fish oil [92, 93] did not improve outcomes. Indeed, non-steroidal anti-inflammatory agents may worsen organ dysfunction, particularly renal function and gastric mucosal integrity.

As an understanding grew of the role of individual cytokines in the inflammatory response, attention turned towards targeted, mediator-directed therapy for MODS. Nearly 100 such clinical trials have been conducted to date. These interventions fall broadly into two categories: (1) monoclonal antibodies (e.g., anti-TNF-α, anti-endotoxin) or (2) receptor antagonists [e.g., IL-1 (IL-1ra)]. However, targeted interventions aimed at cytokine neutralization have been largely disappointing [94]. A recent, combined analysis of clinical trials of mediator-directed therapy in patients with SIRS reported only a modest (3%) overall reduction in 28-day mortality [91], and no mediator-directed treatment has been licensed specifically for use in patients with established MODS in the U.S.

The failure of mediator-directed therapy is likely multifactorial. Measurement of elevated serum concentrations of inflammatory cytokines during MODS does not confirm causality. Expression of mediators may vary over time, and is regulated by a variety of complementary mediators, each of which has several targets. Furthermore, measurement of serum concentrations may not reflect tissue activity. Finally, regional variations in ICU practice may explain partially the discrepancy between efficacy and effectiveness observed when comparing clinical trials.

Recently, drotrecogin alfa (activated) [recombinant activated protein C (APC)], an endogenous coagulation factor with anti-inflammatory, anticoagulant, and fibrinolytic properties, gained approval worldwide for the treatment of severe sepsis associated with a high risk of death [95]. The development of APC for this purpose galvanized appreciation of the interrelationship between the inflammatory and coagulation systems in the pathophysiology of both SIRS and MODS. Although the primary outcome variable reported following therapy with APC was a reduction in 28-day mortality [19.4% relative risk reduction in death compared with placebo ($p=0.005$)] [95], a subsequent analysis also revealed a significant improvement in mean SOFA scores at 28 days in patients treated with drotrecogin alfa (activated) vs. placebo [96].

The success of APC represents a major advance in the treatment of severe sepsis, SIRS, and MODS. Furthermore, despite initially discouraging results with mediator-directed therapy, novel diagnostics have since emerged in recognition of the importance of temporal variation in expression of inflammatory cytokines. Bedside tests to measure IL-6, TNF-α, and IL-1 concentrations have refined the window for intervention in patients with MODS. For example, Panacek et al. recently used the rapid IL-6 test to identify patients during periods of high TNF-α expression [97]. Treatment with monoclonal antibody to TNF-α in this patient population resulted in a significant reduction in both 28-day mortality and severity of organ failure in patients with severe sepsis. Finally, the characterization of novel cytokines, such as IL-18, may provide additional targets for mediator-directed therapy [98].

Additional therapies for the management of sepsis, distinct from mediator-based efforts, continue to emerge. Corticosteroids, once believed to worsen outcomes during sepsis, appear to decrease mortality when administered in lower doses to patients with relative adrenal insufficiency [99]. Furthermore, experimental trials investigating GR270773, a novel phospholipid emulsion that binds and neutralizes circulating endotoxin, have produced encouraging results [100, 101], and phase III clinical trials are currently in progress.

In summary, supportive care remains the mainstay of therapy for MODS. However, reduced severity of organ failure following treatment with APC, as well as encouraging results combining rapid cytokine tests, mediator-directed therapy, and novel strategies to combat sepsis, ensure that effective pharmacologic treatment of patients with MODS is both a realistic and imminent prospect. Finally, alternative conceptualizations of the pathogenesis of MODS, such as the theory of uncoupling of biologic oscillators (discussed above), provide exciting areas for future research.

Both the heterogeneous patient population and lack of standardized scoring systems limit the tracking of progress in the management of MODS. Furthermore, both temporal and spatial comparisons are hindered by variations in severity of illness and thus the likelihood of developing MODS. An earlier report of mortality following MODS reported no difference in either the incidence of (14%) or mortality from (60%) MODS when comparing patients admitted from 1979–1982 to those admitted from 1988–1990 [24]. However, a significant decrease in mortality was noted in those patients with what was considered severe organ failure (≥ three organs failed on day 4 or later). A more recent study (March 1997 – December 1997) found that mortality from MODS, defined as a MOD score of ≥2 for two organ systems and the necessity of an active ICU intervention, was 53% [29]. A still more recent (January 2005) prospective study reported a 17% incidence of MODS and 45% mortality in over 7,000 patients from 79 ICUs [21]. Thus, mortality from MODS may be decreasing over time. However, future studies using both standardized, incremental scoring systems and similar subject populations to compare outcomes in patients with organ failure are warranted.

45.7 Conclusion

The multiple organ dysfunction syndrome arose as the unwanted byproduct of advancements in the field of intensive care medicine. The common result of survival following severe physiologic insult, MODS continues to be the leading cause of mortality and resource expenditure in the ICU. Current conceptualization of the etiology of MODS has evolved from uncontrolled systemic infection to uncontrolled systemic inflammation. The MODS is best conceptualized as occurring on a continuum; rather than dichotomizing organ failure into "MODS-present" or "MODS-absent," use of scoring systems that include standardized, incremental values for each organ system is preferred. Tissue hypoxia, deranged cellular apoptosis, impaired cellular integrity, microvascular thrombosis, increased vascular permeability, and disrupted cell-cell communication are all prominent pathophysiologic features of MODS. These features exert predictable effects on each organ system. Although current treatment of MODS remains primarily supportive, exciting developments based on an appreciation of the interrelationships between the inflammatory and coagulation systems, as well as the temporal importance of products of the inflammatory cascade, provide hope for eventual victory in the battle against this frequent, elusive, costly, and deadly syndrome.

References

1. Ashbaugh DG, Bigelow DB, Petty TL, Levine BE (1967) Acute respiratory distress in adults. Lancet 319–323
2. Skillman JJ, Goldman H, Silen W (1969) Respiratory failure, hypotension, sepsis and jaundice. Am J Surg 117:523–530
3. Tilney NL, Morgan AP (1969) Sequential system failure after rupture of abdominal aortic aneurysms: An unsolved problem in postoperative care. Ann Surg 178:117–122
4. Baue AE (1975) Multiple, progressive, or sequential systems failure: A syndrome of the 1970s. Arch Surg 110:779–781
5. Schwartz DB, Bone RC, Balk RA, et al. (1989) Hepatic dysfunction in the adult respiratory distress syndrome. Chest 95:871–875
6. Brower RG, Matthay MA, Morris A, et al. (2000) Ventilation with lower tidal volumes as compared with traditional tidal volumes for acute lung injury and the acute respiratory distress syndrome. N Engl J Med 342:1301–1308
7. Fry DE, Fulton RL, Polk HC Jr (1980) Multiple system organ failure: The role of uncontrolled infection. Arch Surg 115:136–140
8. Fry DE (2000) Multiple organ dysfunction syndrome: Past, present and future. Surg Infect 1:155–161
9. Rowlands BJ, Soong CV, Gardiner KR (1999) The gastrointestinal tract as a barrier in sepsis. Br Med Bull 55:196–211
10. Sinanan M, Maier RV, Carrico CJ (1984) Laparotomy for intra-abdominal sepsis in patients in an intensive care unit. Arch Surg 1:652–658
11. Goris RJA, te Boekhorsh TPA, Nuytinic JKS, Gimbrere JSF (1985) Multiple organ failure: Generalized autodestructive inflammation? Arch Surg 120:1109–1115
12. Marshall JC, Christou NV, Horn R, et al. (1988) The microbiology of multiple organ failure: The proximal gastrointestinal tract as an occult reservoir of pathogens. Arch Surg 123:309–313
13. Goris RJA, Boekholtz WKF, van Bebber IPT, et al. (1986) Multiple organ failure and sepsis without bacteria: An experimental model. Arch Surg 121:897–901

14. Goris RJ, van Bebber IP, Mollen RM, Koopman JP (1991) Does selective decontamination of the gastrointestinal tract prevent multiple organ failure? An experimental study. Arch Surg 126:561–565
15. Carrico CJ, Meakins JL, Marshall JC, et al. (1986) Multiple-organ failure syndrome: The gastrointestinal tract: The motor of MOF? Arch Surg 121:197–201
16. Marshall JC, Christou NV, Horn R, Meakins JL (1988) The microbiology of multiple organ failure. Arch Surg 123:309–315
17. Cerra FB, Maddaus MA, Dunn DL, et al. (1992) Selective gut decontamination reduces nosocomial infections and length of stay but not mortality or organ failure in surgical intensive care unit patients. Arch Surg 127:163–169
18. Marshall JC, Sweeney D (1990) Microbial infection and the septic response in critical surgical illness: Sepsis, not infection, determines outcome. Arch Surg 125:17–23
19. American College of Chest Physicians/Society of Critical Care Medicine Consensus Conference (1992) Definitions for sepsis and organ failure, and guidelines for the use of innovative therapies in sepsis. Crit Care Med 20:864–874
20. Talmor M, Hydo L, Barie PS (1999) Relationship of systemic inflammatory response syndrome to organ dysfunction, length of stay, and mortality in critical surgical illness: Effect of intensive care unit resuscitation. Arch Surg 134: 81–87
21. Cabre L, Mancebo J, Solsona JF, et al. (2005) Multicenter study of the multiple organ dysfunction syndrome in intensive care units: The usefulness of Sequential Organ Failure Assessment scores in decision making. Intensive Care Med 31:927–933
22. Heard SO, Fink MP (1991) Multiple organ system failure syndrome – Part I: Epidemiology, prognosis, and pathophysiology. J Intensive Care Med 6:279–294
23. Deitch EA (1992) Multiple organ failure: Pathophysiology and potential future therapy. Ann Surg 216:117–134
24. Zimmerman JE, Knaus WA, Wagner DP, et al. (1996) A comparison of risks and outcomes for patients with organ system failure. Crit Care Med 24:1633–1641
25. Wheeler AP, Bernard G (1999) Treating patients with severe sepsis. N Engl J Med 340:207–214
26. Tran DD, Groeneveld ABJ, van der Meulen J, et al. (1990) Age, chronic disease, sepsis, organ system failure, and mortality in a medical intensive care unit. Crit Care Med 18:474–479
27. Tran DD, Cuesta MA, van Leeuwen PA, et al. (1993) Risk factors for multiple organ system failure and death in critically injured patients. Surgery 114:21–30
28. Barie PS, Hydo LJ (2000) Epidemiology of multiple organ dysfunction syndrome in critical surgical illness. Surg Infect 1:173–183
29. Martin CM, Hill AD, Burns K, Chen LM (2005) Characteristics and outcomes for critically ill patients with prolonged intensive care unit stays. Crit Care Med 33: 1922–1927
30. Sauaia A, Moore FA, Moore EE, et al. (1994) Early predictors of postinjury multiple organ failure. Arch Surg 129: 39–45
31. Cryer HG, Leong K, McArthur DL, et al. (1999) Multiple organ failure: By the time you predict it, it's already there. J Trauma 46:597–604
32. Perl TM, Dvorak L, Hwang T, Wenzel RP (1995) Long-term survival and function after suspected gram-negative sepsis. JAMA 274:338–45
33. Knight JC, Kwiatkowski D (1999) Inherited variability of tumor necrosis factor production and susceptibility to infectious disease. Proc Assoc Am Physicians 111:290–298
34. Humphries SE, Luong LA, Montgomery HE, et al. (1999) Gene-environment interaction in the determination of levels of plasma fibrinogen. Thromb Haemost 82:818–825
35. Moore FA, Moore EE (1995) Evolving concepts in the pathogenesis of postinjury multiple organ failure. Surg Clin North Am 75:257–77
36. Cryer HG (2000) Advances in the understanding of multiple organ failure. Surg Infect 1:165–170
37. Fink MP, Delude RL (2005) Epithelial barrier dysfunction: a unifying theme to explain the pathogenesis of multiple organ dysfunction at the cellular level. Crit Care Clin 21: 177–196
38. Sessler CN, Bloomfield GL, Fowler AA (1996) Current concepts of sepsis and acute lung injury. Clin Chest Med 17:213–235
39. Stephens KE, Ishizaka A, Wu ZH, et al. (1988) Granulocyte depletion prevents TNF-mediated acute lung injury in guinea pigs. Am Rev Respir Dis 138:1300–1307
40. Nathans AB, Marshall JC, Watson RWG, et al. (1996) Diethylmaleate ameliorates endotoxin-induced acute lung injury. Surgery 120:360–366
41. Roumen RM, Redl H, Schlag G, et al. (1995) Inflammatory mediators in relation to the development of multiple organ failure in patients after severe blunt trauma. Crit Care Med 23:474–480
42. Papathanassoglou ED, Moynihan JA, Vermillion DL, et al. (2000) Soluble Fas levels correlate with multiple organ dysfunction severity, survival, and nitrate levels, but not with cellular apoptotic markers in critically ill patients. Shock 14:107–112
43. Yamada Y, Endo S, Nakae H, et al. (1999) Nuclear matrix protein levels in burn patients with multiple organ dysfunction syndrome. Burns 25:705–708
44. Hotchkiss RS, Schmieg RE Jr, Swanson PE, et al. (2000) Rapid onset of intestinal epithelial and lymphocyte apoptotic cell death in patients with trauma and shock. Crit Care Med 28:3207–3217
45. Jimenez MF, Watson RWG, Parodo J, et al. (1997) Dysregulated expression of neutrophil apoptosis in the systemic inflammatory response syndrome (SIRS). Arch Surg 132: 1263–1270
46. Hotchkiss RS, Swanson PE, Freeman BD, et al. (1999) Apoptotic cell death in patients with sepsis, shock, and multiple organ dysfunction. Crit Care Med 27:1230–1251
47. Dorinsky PM, Gadek JE (1989) Mechanisms of multiple nonpulmonary organ failure in ARDS. Chest 96:885–92
48. Ryu J, Pyo H, Jou I, et al. (2000) Thrombin induces NO release from cultured rat microglia via protein kinase C, mitogen-activated protein kinase, and NF-KB. J Biol Chem 275:29955–2999
49. Gando S, Nanzaki S, Kemmotsu O (1999) Disseminated intravascular coagulation and sustained systemic inflammatory response syndrome predict organ dysfunctions after trauma: Application of clinical decision analysis. Ann Surg 229:121–127
50. Marchant A, Alegre ML, Hakim A, et al. (1995) Clinical and biological significance of interleukin-10 plasma levels in patients with septic shock. J Clin Immunol 15:266–273
51. Miller-Graziano CL, Szabo G, Griffey K, et al. (1991) Role of elevated monocyte transforming growth factor β (TGF-β) production in posttrauma immunosuppression. J Clin Immunol 11:95–102
52. Volk, Reinke P, Döcke WD (1999) Immunostimulation with cytokines in patients with 'immunoparalysis.' In: Marshall JC, Cohen J (eds) Immune response in the critically ill. Springer-Verlag, Berlin, pp 393–404
53. Bone RC (1996) Immunologic dissonance: a continuing evolution in our understanding of the systemic inflammatory response syndrome (SIRS) and multiple organ dys-

function syndrome (MODS). Ann Intern Med 125:680–687
54. Godin PJ, Buchman TG (1996) Uncoupling of biologic oscillators: A complementary hypothesis concerning the pathogenesis of multiple organ dysfunction syndrome. Crit Care Med 24:1107–1116
55. Godin PJ, Fleisher LA, Eidsath A, et al. (1996) Experimental human endotoxemia increases cardiac regularity: Results from a prospective, randomized, crossover trial. Crit Care Med 24:1117–1124
56. Barnaby D, Ferrick K, Kaplan D, et al. (2002) Heart rate variability in emergency department patient with sepsis. Acad Emerg Med 9:661–670
57. Winchell RJ, Hoyt DB (1996) Spectral analysis of heart rate variability in the ICU: A measure of autonomic function. J Surg Res 63:11–16
58. Winchell RJ, Hoyt DB (1997) Analysis of heart-rate variability: A noninvasive predictor of death and poor outcome in patients with severe head injury. J Trauma 43: 927–933
59. Buchman TG (2004) Nonlinear dynamics, complex systems, and the pathobiology of critical illness. Curr Opin Crit Care 10:378–382
60. Schmidt H, Muller-Werdan US, Hoffman T, et al. (2004) Autonomic dysfunction predicts mortality in patients with multiple organ dysfunction syndrome of different age groups. Crit Care Med 33:1994–2004
61. Buchman TG, Stein PK, Goldstein B (2002) Heart rate variability in critical illness and critical care. Curr Opin Crit Care 8:311–315
62. Seely AJ, Christou NV (2000) Multiple organ dysfunction syndrome: Exploring the paradigm of complex nonlinear systems. Crit Care Med 28:2193–2200
63. Ungureanu-Longrois D, Balligand J, Kelly RA, et al. (1995) Myocardial contractile dysfunction in the systemic inflammatory response syndrome: a cytokine-inducible nitric oxide synthase in cardiac myocytes. J Mol Cell Cardiol 27:155–167
64. Garber BG, Herbert PC, Yelle J-D, et al. (1996) Adult respiratory distress syndrome: A systematic overview of incidence and risk factors. Crit Care Med 24:687–695
65. Jelkmann W, Pagel H, Wolff M, Frandrey J (1992) Monokines inhibiting erythropoietin production in human hepatoma cultures and in isolated perfused rat kidneys. Life Sci 50:301–308
66. Jelkmann W (1998) Proinflammatory cytokines lowering erythropoietin production. J Interferon Cytokine Res 18: 555–559
67. Faquin WC, Schneider TJ, Goldberg MA (1992) Effect of inflammatory cytokines on hypoxia-induced erythropoietin production. Blood 79:1987–1994
68. Frede S, Fandrey J, Pagel H, et al. (1997) Erythropoietin gene expression is suppressed after lipopolysaccharide or interleukin-1 beta injections in rats. Am J Physiol 273: R1067–R1071
69. Moldawer LL, Marano MA, Wei H, et al. (1989) Cachectin/tumor necrosis factor alters red blood cell kinetics and induces anemia in vivo. FASEB J 3:1637–1643
70. Alvarez-Hernandez X, Liceaga J, McKay IC, Brock JH (1989) Induction of hypoferremia and modulation of macrophage iron metabolism by tumor necrosis factor. Lab Invest 61:319–322
71. Rogers JT, Bridges KR, Durmowicz GP, et al. (1990) Translational control during the acute phase response. Ferritin synthesis in response to interleukin-1. J Biol Chem 265:14572–14578
72. Davis MG, Hagen PO (1997) Systemic inflammatory response syndrome. Br J Surg 84:920–935
73. Faries PL, Simon RJ, Martella AT, et al. (1998) Intestinal permeability correlates with severity of injury in trauma patients. J Trauma 44:1031–1036
74. Franson TR, LaBrecque DR, Buggy BP, et al. (1989) Serial bilirubin determinations as a prognostic marker in clinical infections. Am J Med Sci 297:149–152
75. Leijten FS, Harineck-de Werd JE, Poortvliet DC, de Weerd AW (1991) The role of polyneuropathy in motor convalescence after prolonged mechanical ventilation. JAMA 274:1221–1225
76. Bone RC, Balk RA, Cerra FB, et al. (1992) Definitions for sepsis and organ failure and guidelines for the use of innovative therapies in sepsis. Chest 101:320–326
77. Marshall JC, Cook DJ, Christou NV, et al. (1995) Multiple Organ Dysfunction Score: A reliable descriptor of a complex clinical outcome. Crit Care Med 23:1638–1652
78. Bernard G (1997) The Brussels score. Sepsis 1:43–44
79. Vincent JL, Moreno R, Takala J, et al. (1996) The SOFA (Sepsis-related Organ Failure Assessment) score to describe organ dysfunction/failure. On behalf of the Working Group of Sepsis-Related Problems of the European Society of Intensive Care Medicine. Intensive Care Med 22:707–710
80. Le Gall JR, Klar J, Lemeshow S, et al. (1996) The logistic organ dysfunction system. A new way to assess organ dysfunction in the intensive care unit. JAMA 276: 802–810
81. Ferreira FL, Peres Bota D, Bross A, et al. (2001) Serial evaluation of the SOFA score to predict outcome in critically ill patients. JAMA 86:1754–1758
82. Rivers E, Nguyen B, Navstad S, et al. (2001) Early goal-directed therapy in the treatment of severe sepsis and septic shock. N Engl J Med 345:1368–1377
83. Ronco C, Bellomo R, Homel P, et al. (2000) Effects of different doses in continuous veno-venous haemofiltration on outcomes of acute renal failure: A prospective randomized trial. Lancet 356:26–30
84. Schiffl H, Lanf SM, Fischer R (2002) Daily hemodialysis and the outcome of acute renal failure. N Engl J Med 346:305–310
85. Van den Berghe G, Wouters P, Weekers F, et al. (2001) Intensive insulin therapy in critically ill patients. N Engl J Med 345:1359–1367
86. Hayes MA, Timmins AC, Yau EF, et al. (1994) Elevation of systemic oxygen delivery in the treatment of critically ill patients. N Engl J Med 330:1717–1722
87. Gattinoni L, Brazzi L, Pelosi P, et al. (1995) A trial of goal-oriented hemodynamic therapy in critically ill patients. N Engl J Med 333:1025–1032
88. Herbert PC, Wells G, Blajchman MA, et al. (1999) A multicenter, randomized, controlled clinical trial of transfusion requirements in critical care: Transfusion Requirements in Critical Care Trials Group. N Engl J Med 340:409–417
89. Alia I, Esteban A, Gordo F, et al. (1999) A randomized and controlled trial of the effect of treatment aimed at maximizing oxygen delivery in patients with severe sepsis or septic shock. Chest 115:453–461
90. Bernard GR, Wheeler AP, Russell JA, et al. (1997) The effects of ibuprofen on the physiology and survival of patients with sepsis. The Ibuprofen in Sepsis Study Group. N Engl J Med 336:912–918
91. Zeni F, Freeman B, Natanson C (1997) Anti-inflammatory therapies to treat sepsis and septic shock: A reassessment. Crit Care Med 25:1095–1100
92. Rosman C, Grond J, Buurman WA, de Smet BJ, de Jonge R, Sietsma M, van Schilfgaarde R, Bleichrodt RP (1993) Fish oil increases the release of tumour necrosis factor and interleukin-6, and has no effect on the incidence of multiple organ failure in rats with peritonitis. Eur J Surg 159:563–570

93. Gielen CJ, van As AB, Goris RJ (1993) Do diets enriched with oil prevent multiple organ failure in mice? Eur J Surg 159:609–612
94. Marshall JC (2000) Clinical trials of mediator-directed therapy in sepsis: What have we learned? Intensive Care Med 26:S75–S83
95. Bernard GR, Vincent J, Laterre P, et al. (2001) Efficacy and safety of recombinant human activated protein C for severe sepsis. N Engl J Med 344:699–709
96. Vincent JL, Angus DC, Artigas A, et al. (2003) Effects of drotrecogin alfa (activated) on organ dysfunction in the PROWESS trial. Crit Care Med 31:834–40
97. Panacek EA, Marshall JC, Albertson TE, et al. (2004) Efficacy and safety of the monoclonal anti-tumor necrosis factor antibody F(ab')2 fragment afelimomab in patients with severe sepsis and elevated interleukin-6 levels. Crit Care Med 32:2173–2182
98. Tschoeke SK, Oberholzer A, Moldawer LL (2006) Interleukin-18: A novel prognostic cytokine in bacteria-induced sepsis. Crit Care Med 34:1225–1233
99. Annane D, Sebille V, Charpentier C, et al. (2002) Effect of treatment with low doses of hydrocortisone and fludrocortisone on mortality in patients with septic shock. JAMA 288:862–871
100. Gordon BR, Parker TS, Levine DM, et al. (2003) Safety and pharmacokinetics of an endotoxin-binding phospholipid emulsion. Ann Pharmacother 37:943–950
101. Goldfarb RD, Parker TS, Levine DM, et al. (2003) Protein-free phospholipid emulsion treatment improved cardiopulmonary function and survival in porcine sepsis. Am J Physiol Reg Int Comp Physiol 284:R550–R557
102. Janeway CA, Travers P (1997) Immunobiology: The immune system in health and disease, 3rd edn. Garland Publishing, New York

46 Sepsis in Obstetrics

D. Koulenti, H. Correa

46.1 Introduction

The management of critically ill obstetric patients presents a challenge for the critical care physician because they have significant physiological differences compared to the average patient admitted to the intensive care unit (ICU) [1, 2]. The fact that two lives are endangered simultaneously makes this challenge even greater. Besides, obstetric infections are more commonly related to emotional, moral, legal, social and sanitary factors compared to other severe infections and are significantly dependent on the economic and technical development, community patterns and traditions of each country.

In this chapter we will not discuss all the infections that may occur in pregnancy and the postpartum period, but only obstetric sepsis and septic shock. Obstetric sepsis (OS) refers to the severe infectious conditions that place a mother's life at risk. The OS may be caused by: (a) endometritis/myometritis/panmetritis and myometrial abscess following the evacuation of pregnancy at term, spontaneously through the vagina or by caesarean section, complicated or not by peritonitis; (b) infections secondary to the evacuation of an early pregnancy: provoked abortion or, less often, miscarriage; (c) infections of the amniotic fluid during pregnancy (chorioamnionitis, e.g. following amniocentesis or related to the cervical cerclage's complications); (d) septic pelvic thrombophlebitis; (e) episiotomy infections; or (f) necrotizing fasciitis.

It should be highlighted that the critically ill patient is at high risk from sources of infection not commonly encountered by the obstetrician-gynaecologist. A careful physical examination and selected imaging studies are important in excluding uncommon sources. In addition, non-infectious illnesses can mimic septic shock.

The principles of management of obstetric sepsis and septic shock do not differ from those of septic shock from other causes, with the addition of the possible need of evacuation of the uterus. The prompt initiation of appropriate antibiotics, eradication of the focus of infection and supportive care are the mainstay of management.

46.2 Epidemiology

Maternal mortality (MM) due to delivery varies greatly between countries, especially between developed and developing countries. The trend of OS mortality is descending, but the rate varies depending on the level and the rhythm of development in each country. In the USA during the 1990s the MM was 9.8/100,000 live births, having decreased 90 % since the 1950s, while in Sweden it was 6.6 per 100,000 live births [3, 4]. On the other hand, overall postpartum infection has decreased from 15 % in the 1950s to 1 – 8 % of all deliveries, while the incidence of bacteraemia is approximately 8 – 10 % in obstetric patients with clinical evidence of local infection [4 – 6]. These patients rarely progress to more significant complications, such as septic shock [7]. However, when care is delayed or inadequate, infection can progress quickly to generalized sepsis, which can result in infertility, chronic disability and even death. In developed countries maternal death rates associated with infection range from 4 % to 8 %, or approximately 0.6 maternal deaths per 100,000 live births [8 – 10]. Despite the fact that pregnancy is traditionally considered an immunocompromised state, the dramatic increase in pelvic vascularity during pregnancy promotes maternal survival after infection by improving the perfusion of the infected organs. Additional reasons for the more favourable outcomes in the parturient include: younger age group, transient nature of bacteraemia, type of organism involved, and primary site of infection (the pelvis is more amenable to both surgical and medical intervention).

46.3 Physical Examination, Laboratory and Imaging Studies

Clinical symptoms and signs of OS vary depending on the source of infection and may include the following: fever and chills, lower abdominal tenderness on one or both sides of the abdomen, guarding or rebound (in the presence of pelvic or generalized peritonitis), adnexal and/or parametrial tenderness elicited with bimanual examination, enlarged uterus, foul-smelling lochia or pus in the cervical os, vaginal or cervical lacerations (induced abortion), erythema, oedema, tenderness, and discharge from the surgical incision or episiotomy site, in cases of post-surgical wound infections. Patients with septic thrombophlebitis, although rare, may have palpable pelvic veins and tachycardia that is out of proportion to the fever. Respiratory symptoms, such as cough, pleuritic chest pain, or dyspnoea, may be present in cases of septic ARDS or septic pulmonary embolus. Maternal and fetal tachycardia, hypotension, cold and pale skin, and sweating are present in severe sepsis and septic shock.

Diagnostic work-up for finding the focus of infections includes blood, urine, cervical, and wound (if appropriate) specimens for culture. A Gram's stain of potentially infected material could guide the initial treatment. Tissue obtained during an endometrial biopsy or uterine aspiration or surgery provides a better specimen for culture than does cervical discharge. Abnormal findings on pelvic ultrasound may overlap with those of retained products from conception (RPOC) and intrauterine haematoma. Pather et al. [11] reported that the sensitivity and specificity of ultrasound in detecting retained product of conception were 94% and 16%, respectively; the presence of an echogenic focus together with a thickened endometrium of more than 10 mm was the most accurate ultrasound feature of RPOC (positive predictive value 80%) [11]. Contrast computed tomography (CT) examination of the abdomen and pelvis may be helpful in detecting a pelvic abscess or an infected haematoma.

46.4 Obstetric Infections

46.4.1 Peripartum Endometritis/Myometritis/Panmetritis Myometrial Abscess

Endometritis is infection of the endometrium or decidua (retained products of conception), with extension into the myometrium and parametrial tissues that usually results from an ascending infection from the lower genital tract. Postpartum endometritis is mostly polymicrobial (70% of cases) [1], primarily caused by the vaginal bacterial flora (anaerobic bacteria, Gram-negative facultative bacteria, and streptococci), but can also result from sexually transmitted organisms (e.g. *Chlamydia trachomatis* and *Neisseria gonorrhoeae*) [12, 13]. In the developed countries, most postpartum infections are related to caesarean section, while in the developing countries, postpartum endometritis more often follows vaginal delivery. Incidence varies depending on the route of delivery and the patient population. Major risk factors of peripartum endometritis include caesarean delivery, especially preterm, previous caesarean sections, prolonged rupture of membranes, long labour with multiple vaginal examinations, extremes of patient age, and low socioeconomic status [9, 14].

Early postpartum endometritis is defined as occurring within the first 48 h, and late endometritis as occurring between 3 days and 6 weeks following delivery. In acute endometritis neutrophils are present within the endometrial glands, while in chronic endometritis plasma cells and lymphocytes are present within the endometrial stroma. Chronic endometritis in the obstetric population is usually associated with retained products of conception after delivery or elective abortion.

The diagnosis of endometritis is usually based upon clinical findings [1]: fever (usually occurring within 36 h of delivery), lower abdominal pain, foul-smelling lochia, abnormal vaginal bleeding, abnormal vaginal discharge, malaise, and tachycardia. Abdominal distention and absent bowel sounds may occur. A temperature greater than 38 °C (104 °F) in the absence of other causes of fever is the most common sign. Regarding the laboratory data, leucocytosis may be present, but it is difficult to interpret. Due to physiologic changes associated with pregnancy, the leucocyte count and segmented neutrophil percentage do not predict infection. Therefore clinical findings are most important in diagnosing postpartum infections [15]. Blood culture may be positive in 10–30% of cases. Endocervical cultures (or DNA probe) should be obtained for gonorrhoea and *Chlamydia* infections. Ultrasound may help the diagnostic approach [11]. CT and MRI of the abdomen and pelvis may be helpful for excluding broad ligament masses, septic pelvic thrombophlebitis, ovarian vein thrombosis, and phlegmon.

Immediately after making the diagnosis of endometritis and excluding other sources of infection, empirical broad-spectrum antibiotic treatment should be initiated. Improvement is anticipated within 48–72 h in nearly 90% of women treated with an appropriate regimen. Surgical management is not usually necessary in acute endometritis in the obstetric population. Dilatation and curettage may be advised for retained products of conception, however. A classic regimen for severe pelvic sepsis is penicillin (5 million units/6 h/i.v.) or ampicillin (2–3 g/6 h/i.v.) combined with clindamycin (900 mg/8 h/i.v.) and an aminoglycoside, either gentamicin or tobramycin (a loading dose of 2 mg/kg, followed by 1.5 mg/kg/8 h, depending on the blood level and renal status) [19]. A meta-analysis demonstrated a trend towards a decrease in the incidence of postpartum endometritis in women who received treatment with ampicillin, gentamicin and clindamycin compared to those who received ampicillin and gentamicin alone, but this did not reach statistical significance [16]. Intravenous antibiotic therapy should be continued until the patient is afebrile for 24–48 h, the white blood cell count returns to normal, and the patient is tolerating oral liquids and solids, and ambulating without difficulty, without the need for additional days of oral antibiotic therapy [17, 18]. Patients failing to respond to the initial antibiotic treatment should be thoroughly evaluated for the possible emergence of a resistant bacterium or the development of an abscess or septic pelvic thrombophlebitis.

Patients with microabscesses in the myometrium typically do not respond to medical therapy. On examination the uterus is large, tender, and boggy with a dilated cervix. Radiographic imaging may demonstrate gas or fluid in the myometrium (gas in the uterine cavity is normal after a caesarean delivery).

46.4.2 Septic Abortion

Septic abortion is defined as sepsis in association with recent pregnancy termination, spontaneous or induced. Morbidity and mortality from septic abortion are infrequent in the developed countries but very common in the developing countries, remaining a primary cause of maternal death. Overall mortality from legal abortion in Europe is less than 1 death per 100,000 procedures [19]. The World Health Organization (WHO) estimates that 25–50% of the 500,000 maternal deaths occurring every year are the result of illegal abortion, the vast majority occur in the developing countries, and are primarily due to sepsis [19]. In the USA the rate of hospitalization for septic abortion (0.21 per 1,000 abortions) is remarkably low. The risk of death from postabortion sepsis is highest for young unmarried women, and those who undergo procedures who do not directly evacuate the contents of the uterus [19, 20]. With more advanced gestation, there is a higher risk of uterine perforation and retained products of conception [19].

The diagnosis of septic abortion must be considered for any woman of reproductive age with vaginal bleeding or serosanguineous to purulent discharge, lower abdominal pain or pelvic pain, and fever. Some women have a milder illness with low-grade fever, mild lower abdominal pain, and moderate vaginal bleeding, and they usually have either incomplete or failed abortion (continuing pregnancy) or haematometra (retained clotted and liquid blood) [21]. A common feature in reported cases of death from septic abortion is delayed treatment; a delay in treatment allows the infection to progress to bacteraemia, pelvic abscess, septic pelvic thrombophlebitis, disseminated intravascular coagulopathy, septic shock, renal failure, and death [19]. Illegal abortion performed by insertion of rigid foreign objects increases the risk of perforation, and intrauterine instillation of soap solutions containing cresol and phenol poses the risk of uterine necrosis, renal failure, toxicity to the central nervous system, cardiac depression, and respiratory arrest [19]. In case of perforation, radiographic studies of the abdomen may help identify free air or foreign bodies. Disseminated sepsis is suggested by high fever and prostration, tachycardia, tachypnoea, respiratory difficulty, and low blood pressure [18].

Septic abortion is usually polymicrobial, derived from the normal flora of the vagina and endocervix, with the important addition of sexually transmitted pathogens. Gram-positive and gram-negative aerobes and facultative or obligate anaerobes, *Neisseria gonorrhoeae* and *Chlamydia trachomatis* are all possible pathogens, while in the USA *Clostridium perfringens* is mostly associated with illegal abortion [19]. It is noteworthy that in developing countries, tetanus remains a cause of mortality from septic abortion [19].

Patients with septic abortion should be hospitalized. Any tissue remaining from the pregnancy must be evacuated without delay as soon as broad-spectrum empirical antibiotic therapy and fluid resuscitation have been started. Delay in the evacuation of the uterus because of the poor patient's condition is a common mistake in the management of septic abortion with fatal consequences [19]. The evacuation of the uterus can be done successfully with curettage guided by ultrasonography or with medical means [19]. The 15-methyl analogue of prostaglandin F_{2a}, or high doses of oxytocin, can also be used, while prostaglandin E_2 or dinoprostone is contraindicated in patients with sepsis because of the elevation of body temperature that they produce [19]. If there is no response to uterine evacuation and to adequate medical therapy (see antibiotic treatment of endometritis), in the presence of clostridial myometritis, in the presence of pelvic abscess, and in the cases of uterine perforation with suspected bowel perforation, a laparotomy should be performed. Indications for total hysterectomy with removal of both adnexa include a discoloured, woody appearance of the uterus and adnexa, suspicion of clostridial sepsis, crepitation of the pelvic tissue, and radiographic evidence of air within the uterine wall [19].

Mifepristone is a progesterone antagonist that is increasingly used as an abortifacient. The original FDA approval of mifepristone included a "black-box" warning that the use of this drug could result in incomplete abortion requiring surgical intervention and potentially fatal complications (ruptured ectopic pregnancy and septic shock) [22]. Recent reports have highlighted the occurrence of infrequent but serious complications. Deaths due to endometritis and toxic shock syndrome associated with *Clostridium sordellii*, a rarely encountered microorganism in clinical specimens (1% of *Clostridium* species), that occurred within 1 week after mifepristone-induced abortions, have been described.

Two toxins of *C. sordellii* toxins, a lethal one and a haemorrhagic one (that antigenically and pathophysiologically appear similar to *Clostridium difficile* toxins B and A, respectively), are responsible for this potential [23]. The physician should be aware of the unusual and rather distinctive signs and symptoms: an absence of fever, but presence of tachycardia, refractory hypotension, haemoconcentration, oedema, effusions in multiple serum cavities, and dramatic leucocytosis. In all the reported cases the patients were young and healthy, they had apparently successful procedures (no evidence on autopsy of retained products of conception), their clinical presentations were somewhat cryptic because they had cramping, which is very common after the procedure, and no fever, and they all died remarkably rapidly after presentation. These cases indicate the need for physician awareness and the early recognition of this syndrome and the need for further study of its association with mifepristone-induced abortion. A possible pathophysiologic explanation of *C. sordellii* induced septic shock is that mifepristone, by blocking both progesterone and glucocorticoid receptors, interferes with the controlled release and functioning of cortisol and cytokines [24]. Failure of physiologically controlled cortisol and cytokine responses results in an impaired innate immune system that causes the disintegration of the body's defence system necessary to prevent the endometrial spread of *C. sordellii* infection. The abnormal cortisol and cytokine responses due to mifepristone coupled to the release of potent exotoxins and an endotoxin from *C. sordellii* seem to be the major contributors to the rapid development of lethal septic shock [24].

46.4.3 Chorioamnionitis

Intra-amniotic infections can complicate up to 10% of deliveries [25] and they are associated with maternal morbidity and neonatal sepsis, pneumonia and death. Studies from the United Kingdom, Australia, and the United States reported a 6–14% incidence of villitis. Villitis does not indicate placental infection but only inflammation. Classical teaching holds that chorioamnionitis occurs in 1% of all deliveries. This probably is a very conservative incidence. Lower socioeconomic groups are expected to have a higher incidence of maternal chorioamnionitis. Malnourished pregnant women in the developing countries have a higher risk of ascending urogenital infection with subsequent amniotic fluid infection, possibly because of a decrease in host defence factors regularly present in the amniotic fluid [26]. Maternal chorioamnionitis is more commonly observed in prolonged labours and/or prolonged rupture of the fetal membranes. The latter is considered the highest risk factor related to the pathogenesis of maternal chorioamnionitis. Sepsis complicates 0.5–1.3% of the cases of chorioamnionitis [1].

Diagnosis of chorioamnionitis can be confirmed by culture, amniotic fluid Gram stain, white cell count, glucose and cytokine levels [1]. However, needle aspiration of amniotic fluid is an invasive procedure that can be risky with intact fetal membranes because rupture of the fetal membranes can occur during or after the procedure. Bleeding or placental abruption can also be a consequence of the procedure. Fetal injury must be avoided by performing the procedure using ultrasonographic guidance.

Antibiotics reduce maternal and fetal mortality [1]. Regarding intrapartum administration of antibiotics, the current consensus is in favour when the diagnosis of intra-amniotic infection has been made; however, the results of a recent meta-analysis neither support nor deny it, although a trend has been reported towards improved neonatal outcomes when antibiotics are administered intrapartum [16]. No recommendations can be made on the most appropriate antimicrobial regimen to treat intra-amniotic infection [16] (see antibiotic treatment of endometritis).

46.4.4 Septic Pelvic Thrombophlebitis

Septic pelvic thrombophlebitis (SPT) is a rare condition associated with the postpartum period and is thought to be preceded by a pelvic infection. It was first reported by Collins et al. in 1951, when he reported data from 70 cases [27]. The overall incidence of SPT has been reported as 1:3,000 deliveries; 1:9,000 after vaginal delivery and 1:800 after caesarean section [28]. Postpartum endometritis may spread throughout the pelvic venous system, including the inferior vena cava. The embolic disease process is more common in the right ovarian vein, whereas left ovarian vein thrombosis with renal vein involvement is less common [29, 30]. Patients often present with pain and fever in the postpartum period. There may be initial clinical improvement with antibiotic therapy, but patients with SPT will continue to "spike" fevers daily, usually in the evening, despite the resolution of pain, with or without toxic appearance, except for persistent fever. Septic pulmonary emboli may occur and cause chest pain. Diagnosis is made clinically and can be confirmed by CT scanning or MRI, which demonstrate the affected vessels, usually hypogastric or ovarian [31]. Antibiotic therapy and anticoagulation with heparin (e.g. 10,000 units intravenously followed by 1,000 units/h) should result in defeverscence within 48 h; rarely surgical ligation and removal of the infected veins is required with the insertion of a vena cava filter [32]. As patients respond quickly to heparin anticoagulant therapy, long-term anticoagulation is seldom needed. Most clinicians continue antibiotic therapy along with anticoagulation, although research has failed to show a quicker resolution of the febrile course. It is interesting that a randomized control trial demonstrated that women given heparin in addition to antimicrobial therapy for septic thrombophlebitis did not have better outcomes compared to those who continued with antimicrobial therapy alone. Furthermore, the findings of a retrospective study conducted by Witlin et al. [33] did not support the time-honoured rule that septic pelvic thrombophlebitis responds within 24–48 h to therapeutic anticoagulation with heparin, and suggested that criteria other than imaging studies or immediate defervescence following heparin therapy should be implemented for diagnosis of septic pelvic thrombophlebitis [33].

46.4.5 Episiotomy Infections

Episiotomy, the site of perineal surgical incision at the time of parturition, can be infected [1]. Complicated infection may lead to dehiscence and fistula formation or even cellulitis, myonecrosis and septic shock. Uncomplicated infection may manifest with fever, swelling, purulent discharge and local pain and tenderness. The treatment consists of intravenous antibiotics, drainage and debridement [1].

46.4.6 Necrotizing Fasciitis

Necrotizing fasciitis is a severe suppurative infection of the superficial and deep fascia, mostly due to group A beta-haemolytic streptococci and clostridia, and it is often polymicrobial [1]. It should be suspected in cases with high spiking fevers and prostration. The affected area is usually tender to palpation but may otherwise appear normal. Skin discolouration and crepitus occur as later findings. Antibiotic therapy usually includes a penicillin and clindamycin. However, the cornerstone of treatment is the entire surgical excision of the necrotic area until healthy bleeding tissue [1]. Hyperbaric oxygenation in combination with effective surgical and antibiotic therapy may improve the outcome [34].

46.5 Conclusion

Sepsis is an infrequent yet important cause of death in the gravida. A high index of suspicion and early recognition of sepsis may decrease maternal and fetal morbidity and mortality. Prompt initiation of empirical broad-spectrum antibiotic therapy and control of the focus of infection is the mainstay of treatment. In the case of severe sepsis or septic shock the patient should be admitted to the ICU. In pregnant women priorities of treatment should be directed first towards maternal well-being, especially early in the course of resuscitation, because fetal compromise results mainly from maternal decompensation during sepsis. If the source of infection is the fetus or residua, delivery and (re)evacuation of uterus are indicated, respectively.

References

1. Soubra S, Guntupali K (2005) Critical illness in pregnancy. Crit Care Med 33(10):248–255
2. Fernandez-Perez E, Salman S, Pendem S, Farmer JC (2005) Sepsis during pregnancy. Crit Care Med 33(10):286–293
3. Hogberg U (1986) Maternal death in Sweden, 1971–1980. Acta Obstet Gynecol Scand 65:161–167
4. Fein AM, Duvivier R (1992) Sepsis in pregnancy. Clin Chest Dis 13:709–22
5. Blanco JD, Gibbs RS, Castaneda YS (1981) Bacteremia in obstetrics: clinical course. Obstet Gynecol 58:621
6. Bryan CS, Reynolds KL, Moore EE (1984) Bacteremia in obstetrics and gynecology. Obstet Gynecol 64:155–158
7. Duff P (1986) Pathophysiology and management of post-cesarean endomyometritis. Obstet Gynecol 67:269–76
8. Atrash HK, Koonin LM, Lawson HW, et al. (1990) Maternal mortality in the United States, 1979–1986. Obstet Gynecol 76(6):1055–60
9. Chaim W, Bashiri A, Bar-David J, et al. (2000) Prevalence and clinical significance of postpartum endometritis and wound infection. Infect Dis Obstet Gynecol 8(2):77–82
10. Rochat RW, Koonin LM, Atrash HK, Jewett JF (1998) Maternal mortality in the United States: report from the Maternal Mortality Collaborative. Obstet Gynecol 72(1):91–7
11. Pather S, Ford M, Reid R, Sykes P (2005) Postpartum curettage: an audit of 200 cases. Aust N Z J Obstet Gynaecol 45(5):368–71
12. Rosene K, Eschenbach DA, et al. (1986) Polymicrobial early postpartum endometritis with facultative and anaerobic bacteria, genital mycoplasms, and *Chlamydia trachomatis:* Treatment with piperacillin or cefoxitin. J Infect Dis 153:1028–37
13. Sherman D, Lurie S, Betzer M, et al. (1999) Uterine Flora at cesarean and its relationship to postpartum endometritis. Obstet Gynecol 94:787–91
14. Dare FO, Bako AU, Ezechi OC (1988) Puerperal sepsis: a preventable post-partum complication. Tropical Doctor 28(2):92–5
15. Partlow DB, Chauhan SP, Justice L, et al. (2004) Diagnosis of postpartum infections: clinical criteria are better than laboratory parameters. J Miss State Med Assoc 45(3):67–70
16. Hopkins L, Smaill F (2002) Antibiotic regimens for management of intra-amniotic infection. Cochrane Database Syst Rev (3):CD003254
17. French LM, Smaill FM (2000) Antibiotic regimens for endometritis after delivery. Cochrane Database Syst Rev (2):CD001067
18. Faro S (2005) Postpartum endometritis. Clin Perinatol 32(3):803–14
19. Stubblefield PG, Grimes DA (1994) Septic abortion. N Engl J Med 331(5):310–4
20. Amy JJ (1994) Management of septic abortion. N Engl J Med 331(25):1716–7
21. Hakim-Elahi E, Tovell HMM, Burnhill MS (1990) Complications of first-trimester abortion: a report of 170,000 cases. Obstet Gynecol 76:129–135

22. Greene MF (2005) Fatal infections associated with mifepristone-induced abortion. N Engl J Med 353(22):2317–8
23. Rorbye C, Petersen IS, Nilas L (2000) Postpartum *Clostridium sorellii* infections associated with fatal toxic shock syndrome. Acta Obstet Gynecol Scand 79(12):1134–5
24. Miech RP (2005) Pathophysiology of mifepristone-induced septic shock due to *Clostridium sordellii*. Ann Pharmacother 39(9):1483–8
25. Soper DE, Mayhall CG, Dalton HP (1989) Risk factors for intraamniotic infection. A prospective epidemiologic study. Am J Obstet Gynecol 161:562–6
26. Naeye RL, Blanc WA (1970) Relation of poverty and race to antenatal infection. N Engl J Med 283:555–60
27. Collins CG, MacCallum EA, Nelson EW, et al. (1951) Suppurative pelvic thrombophlebitis. I. Incidence, pathology and etiology. Surgery 30: 298–310
28. Brown CE, Stettler RW, Twickler D, Cunningham FG (1999) Puerperal septic pelvic thrombophlebitis: incidence and response to heparin therapy. Am J Obstet Gynecol 181(1):143–8
29. Munsick RA, Gillanders LA (1981) A review of the syndrome of puerperal ovarian vein thrombophlebitis. Obstet Gynecol Surv 36:57–61
30. Bahnson RR, Wendel EF, Vogeizang RL (1985) Renal vein thrombosis following puerperal ovarian vein thrombophlebitis. Am J Obstet Gynecol 152:290–293
31. Brown CEL, Lowe TW, Cunningham FG, et al. (1986) Puerperal pelvic thrombophlebitis: impact on diagnosis and treatment using x-ray computed tomography and magnetic resonance imaging. Obstet Gynecol 68:789–795
32. Livengood CH Septic pelvic thrombophlebitis and ovarian vein thrombosis. Uptodate on line 13.2.
33. Whitlin AG, Mercer BM, Sibai BM (1996) Septic pelvic thrombophlebitis or refractory postpartum fever of undetermined etiology. J Matern Fetal Med 5(6):355–8
34. Grim PS, Gottlieb LJ, Boddie A, Batson E (1990) Hyperbaric oxygen therapy. JAMA 263:2216–2220

47 Diagnosis and Management of Intra-abdominal Sepsis

T.L. Husted, E.W. Mueller, T.M. Lasky, M.A. Jafri, J.S. Solomkin

47.1 Introduction

Intra-abdominal infections are commonly encountered in the general medical/surgical intensive care unit (ICU). Perhaps the largest group of these patients has recently undergone or will shortly undergo some form of interventional procedure. There have been important advances in supportive care, diagnostic tools, anti-infective therapy, and interventional techniques; resulting in both improved care and new controversies in the management of these critically ill patients. Most notable is the role of routine non-invasive imaging for suspected intra-abdominal infections, its use in monitoring success of therapy, and the role of percutaneous or laparoscopic intervention to replace formal laparotomy. The continuing development of antibiotics has provided a novel opportunity for tailoring therapy to the requirements of the individual.

The primary effect of these innovations has been a more accurate diagnosis and lessened morbidity – measured as length of stay. It is likely that percutaneous abscess drainage for various diseases has decreased mortality. However, even with application of state of the art care, intra-abdominal infections can result in considerable morbidity and mortality.

Additional complexity surrounds the care of hospitalized patients for whom intra-abdominal infection occurs following elective or emergent abdominal operation. These patients are typically infected with a difficult to treat flora and represent the current frontier in therapeutic research.

47.1.1 Pathophysiology of the Local and Systemic Response to Intra-abdominal Infections

Patients with intra-abdominal infections are a subset of sepsis syndrome patients.

Diffuse peritonitis may, however, present with a more fulminant physiologic disturbance because the anatomy of the peritoneum may allow a very rapid and very large absorption of toxins (both foreign and host-generated). Well-defined diaphragmatic stomata provide mechanical clearance of particulates and solutes from the intraperitoneal space. Diaphragmatic lymphatic channels provide a means for entry of peritoneal fluid (including any bacteria or proinflammatory mediators) via the thoracic duct into the venous circulation (Fig. 47.1). Lymphatic capillaries are distributed in the subperitoneal connective tissue of the diaphragm. The average area of a stoma is approximately 10 μm^2, although peritonitis will increase the diameter of these stomata. Inspiration decreases intrathoracic pressure thereby creating a pressure gradient for fluid movement across the diaphragm, out of the abdomen and into the systemic circulation [1–4].

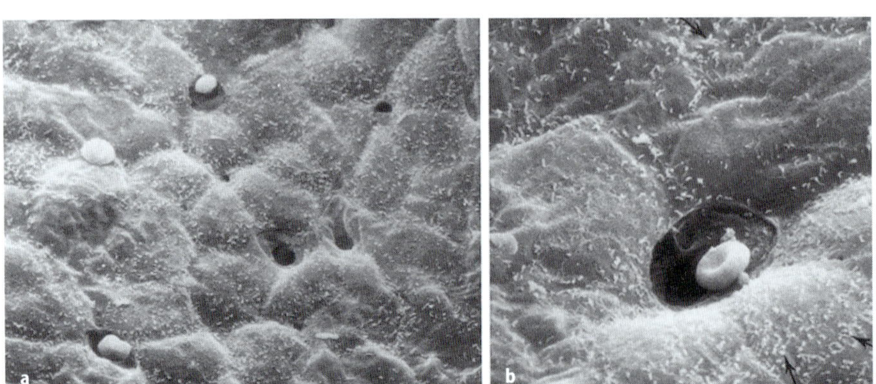

Fig. 47.1. Scanning electron microscopy of a bat diaphragm demonstrating the peritoneal surface with stomata and free orifice, occupied by erythrocyte (**a**, ×1,250; **b**, ×2,500). (Reprinted with permission from: The lymphatic vessels and the so-called "lymphatic stomata" of the diaphragm: A morphologic ultrastructural and three-dimensional study. Giacomo Azzali, *Microvascular Research* 57:30, 1999)

An additional issue is encountered during creation of the pneumoperitoneum required for laparoscopy; increased intra-abdominal pressure during a laparoscopic procedure for established intra-abdominal infection would be expected to increase such transdiaphragmatic flow. However, the local intraperitoneal immune system is impaired during carbon dioxide pneumoperitoneum, evidenced by suppression of intraperitoneal cell-mediated immunity. This feature may be clinically important and should be acknowledged when considering laparoscopic surgery in patients with sepsis [5–8].

Other peritoneal defense mechanisms include resident peritoneal macrophages and large recruitable pools of circulating neutrophils and monocytes, which participate in bacterial killing and abscess formation. Ingestion of microorganisms by these cells results in secretion of a variety of proinflammatory mediators, including chemokines, cytokines, lipid derivatives, reactive oxygen species, and lysosomal enzymes. Manipulation of the number and function of these resident and recruited cells is now possible through the use of colony-stimulating factors but has not been found beneficial in clinical trials. Similarly, manipulation of the expression of proinflammatory mediators from these inflammatory cells has been postulated to modulate the sepsis response, but clinical trials have been disappointing [9].

The release of proinflammatory products of peritoneal origin into lymphatic and vascular channels may also be responsible for significant hepatic dysfunction. Liver dysfunction is common during the course of intra-abdominal infection and occasionally progresses to fatal hepatic failure [10]. Acute-phase proteins generated by the liver during sepsis contribute to the procoagulant, antifibrinolytic state believed important in the development of multiple organ dysfunction syndrome and host survival [11]. Primary hepatic dysfunction results from hepatocellular injury, ostensibly due to poor perfusion during shock. This clinical entity, labeled ischemic hepatitis, occurs in the period immediately after shock and resuscitation, and is manifested by transaminase elevation, decreased lactate clearance, and often hypoglycemia.

Considerable evidence supports the notion that various macrophage products, including interleukins-1 and -6 and tumor necrosis factor-alpha, substantially alter hepatocyte function [10]. Aside from conversion of hepatic synthetic function to acute-phase reactants, serum chemistries reveal evidence of ductal epithelial cytotoxicity, including elevated alkaline phosphatase levels and elevated bilirubin levels. The large number of fixed tissue phagocytes in the liver (Kupffer cells) that are capable of responding to endotoxin absorbed from systemic or mesenteric blood vessels represents a potentially important source of chemokines, cytokines, and other hepatocyte regulatory substances, although portal endotoxemia has not been detected in humans [12].

Virulence determinants present on the organisms participating in these mixed flora infections, encompassing aerobic, anaerobic, and facultative Gram-negative organisms, explain the physiologic response seen in sepsis. Facultative and aerobic Gram-negative organisms express and release endotoxin and endotoxin-associated proteins spontaneously, although shedding is not likely intensified by administration of antibiotics. Aside from the potential for inducing the release of cytokines and other inflammatory mediators, these substances induce local thrombosis through a variety of endothelial and macrophage-mediated processes.

Synergistic interactions between certain anaerobes, most notably *Bacteroides fragilis* and endotoxin-bearing Gram-negative organisms, suppress local host defense mechanisms and facilitate the establishment of infection. *B. fragilis* produces a capsular polysaccharide that interferes with complement activation and inhibits leukocyte function. These phenomena are thought to restrict the delivery of phagocytes to the site of infection, permitting a more rapid rate of bacterial growth than would otherwise be seen.

47.2 Clinical Aspects of Care for Patients with Intra-abdominal Infections

47.2.1 Initial Therapeutic Goals

Acute perforations of the gastrointestinal tract with subsequent peritonitis often present with sepsis or septic shock and may mandate initial treatment in an intensive care environment. Physical findings and the patient's history routinely provide sufficient diagnostic support to obviate further diagnostic testing. Plain radiographs of the abdomen may reveal free air, a uniform indicator of visceral perforation in the absence of prior intervention. Other findings from plain radiographs that support the diagnosis of intra-abdominal infection include pneumatosis intestinalis, bowel obstruction, and a mass effect. Pneumatosis has rare benign causes. More dramatic but less common findings are air in the portal vein or extra-luminal gas collections indicative of an abscess; these radiographic signs are sufficiently specific to justify immediate intervention (Fig. 47.2). The only reason to obtain plain films rather than a computed tomographic study is to lessen the time the patient is away from the intensive care environment. Patients with diffuse peritonitis require laparotomy to deal with the enteric perforation and to perform peritoneal lavage. Radiographic studies are then intended only to support the need for emergent

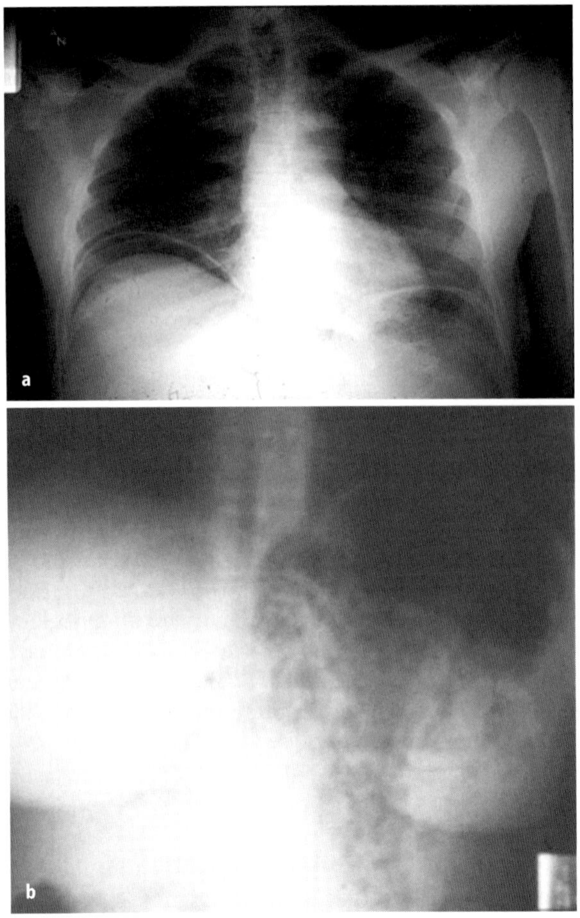

Fig. 47.2. a Plain radiographs demonstrating free air on an upright film of the abdomen; and **b**: taken with the patient's right side down showing blebs of gas in the wall of the colon at the splenic flexure (pneumatosis caused by vascular compromise). The center of radius of the gas bubbles does not lie in the lumen of the bowel, indicating that the colon is most likely perforated

operation, not define the process or provide anatomic information.

Perforations of the upper gastrointestinal tract cause impressive physical findings of peritonitis but rarely manifest evidence of septic shock. Conversely, perforations of the colon result in such substantial bacterial contamination that it is often accompanied by a hypotensive reaction. In either setting, progressive clinical deterioration cannot be reversed until soiling of the peritoneal cavity is terminated. Therefore, resuscitation cannot be completely achieved until operative intervention is performed. Patients with acute perforation of the gastrointestinal tract should be sufficiently resuscitated to be able to undergo induction of anesthesia and resuscitation should continue during the operation. The primary point is rapid volume loading to counter the vasodilatory effects of anesthetics coupled with the pre-existing vasodilation of peritoneal soilage. More refined parameters of completed resuscitation, such as optimization of cardiac output or oxygen delivery, should not be used until the patient has undergone intervention.

47.2.2 Surgical Management of Diffuse Peritonitis

Procedures used for management of intra-abdominal infections have at least five possible components: (a) drainage of any fluid collections, (b) closure of perforations of the GI tract by resection or diversion, (c) debridement of devitalized tissue, (d) drain placement, and (e) surgical wound management. Each of these elements is the subject of some debate [13–15].

Under certain circumstances, the procedure performed may not be optimal for control of infection. This may occur because anatomic conditions do not allow the procedure of choice to be performed (e.g., extensive adhesions or tumor infiltration preventing mobilization of the bowel for resection or ostomy creation), unrecognized disease elements (e.g., multiple abscesses), misdiagnosis, or technical error such as inadvertent and unrecognized bowel perforation. Inadequate procedures may therefore be significant determinants of outcome that may make clinical cure less likely even with aggressive supportive and appropriate anti-infective therapy. These patients are a critical subgroup because they may in fact disproportionately benefit from highly effective antibiotic and anti-sepsis therapy.

A complex mix of factors affect a decision to perform a specific procedure, including variables such as the underlying condition of the patient, the acute physiologic response to infection, the duration of infection prior to diagnosis and treatment, the anatomic extent of disease, patient anatomy, and the availability of both post-operative intensive care support and radiographic reassessment. The complexity of this decision-making process makes the development of an algorithm quite difficult.

Operative management of peritonitis involves immediate evacuation of all purulent collections, with particular attention to subphrenic, subhepatic, interloop, and pelvic collections. It is well established that the perforated bowel should be resected. This notion has evolved from studies over several decades of mortality following surgical treatment of perforated diverticulitis. Resection with end-colostomy was shown to decrease mortality significantly as compared to transverse loop colostomy and drainage. Despite recent reports of low rates of anastomotic dehiscence with primary anastomosis, surgeons have not universally accepted this concept because previously reported complication rates from primary anastomosis are staggering. Controversies in the operative management of peritonitis primarily surround wound closure techniques and scheduled re-laparotomy. Abdominal wall edema typically develops in patients with diffuse peritonitis secondary to colonic perforation or anastomotic dehiscence as part of a generalized syndrome of increased capillary permeability. This syndrome is worsened by the accepted need to provide aggressive restoration and in many cases supranormal expansion of intravascular volume. Primary closure of the abdominal incision in such patients may be difficult or even unwise. Increased intra-abdominal pressure can result in compression of mesenteric and renal veins, leading in some instances to acute renal failure or bowel necrosis. This clinical entity is commonly referred to as *abdominal compartment syndrome*. To avoid this early postoperative complication, insertion of fascial prostheses can be performed. A variety of materials have been used, including Marlex, Silastic, polytetrafluoroethylene, or more recently an opened 3-L sterile intravenous bag. Each approach has its own virtues and problems [16].

Impermeable materials can exacerbate peritonitis and should be used only if planned re-laparotomy is to be undertaken. However, multiple laparotomies for abdominal sepsis have been correlated wih increased mortality and poor outcomes, especially because of increased incidence of fistula formation [17]. Reoperation to control intra-abdominal pathology has also been shown to cause substantial hypotension in the perioperative period due to increased cytokine release; demonstrating an inverse correlation between serum interleukin-6 levels and postoperative mean arterial pressure.

The mesh materials, particularly in patients with diffuse peritonitis, effectively create an open abdominal wound that allows continual abdominal drainage. However, these patients require extensive wound care. An alternative to definitive closure of the abdominal wall incision includes temporary abdominal closure using the clear Bogota bag. This clear 3-L saline intravenous solution bag is drained and opened to offer a one-ply impermeable dressing. This bag is sutured at the seam to the fascial edges to prevent contraction and provide a non-adherent surface to prevent development of adhesion. Additionally, with a clear bag on each side of the fascia, the edges can be closed together to provide a semi-sterile environment for the abdominal wound.

The advantages of such a temporary closure are twofold. One, the fascia edges remain fresh, avoiding the injury encountered with re-laparotomy. Two, the bag can be cinched periodically to preclude fascial retraction, which may lead to difficult hernia closure in the future. This method has been used with success at our institution, often allowing for beside washout of intra-abdominal fluid collection and frequent re-assessment of the peritoneal cavity, while preserving and extending the viability of the abdominal fascia.

These techniques are often used when the patient is so hemodynamically unstable that bowel anastamoses are not performed (if resections have been done). Because of concerns for absence of sufficient mesenteric blood flow to allow for anastomotic healing, bowel ends may be left stapled. Anastamoses are then performed when shock has been reversed.

47.2.3 Diagnostic Imaging for Suspected Intra-abdominal Infections Other than Peritonitis

In the absence of physical findings of diffuse peritonitis, diagnostic imaging with either computed tomography (CT) or ultrasound should be routinely performed in seriously ill patients with intra-abdominal infection. The urgency of investigation is dictated by the degree of hemodynamic instability present. Most patients should be evaluated within hours of clinical diagnosis. This initial imaging study has become central to therapeutic decision-making since interventional radiology has replaced operative treatment for many localized processes, including diverticular abscesses. Double contrast CT is the single best modality for fully evaluating the extent of disease in most situations. Ultrasound is also quite versatile and has the added advantage of being portable, thus allowing certain procedures to be performed in the ICU. However, ultrasonography is limited by bowel gas, body habitus, and a lower sensitivity for retroperitoneal processes or parenchymal infection. Usually the choice of modality is based on the experience and preference of the interventional radiologist.

47.3 Percutaneous Abscess Drainage

Percutaneous abscess drainage (PAD) and operative intervention are best viewed as complementary rather than competitive techniques. When feasible, non-operative (i.e., percutaneous) drainage of abscesses is preferable to open surgical intervention due to the initial patient condition decline that nearly universally accompanies operative manipulation of intra-abdominal infection. The exact basis for this is unclear, but a substantial proportion of patients undergoing emergency operation for intra-abdominal infection experience acute hemodynamic compromise in the early post-operative period. When used for appropriate indications PAD is at least as effective as operation and is associated with less morbidity.

Inflammation may manifest as a phlegmon (viable inflamed tissue), a liquefied abscess, infected necrotic (nonviable) tissue, or a combination of all. Liquefied abscesses are drainable, whereas phlegma and necrotic tissue are not. Decisions regarding which modality to use are largely based on CT findings and require experience, clinical judgment, and careful consideration of underlying and coexistent disease processes. Close cooperation between the surgeon, interventional radiologist and other physicians involved in the patient's care is mandatory. Specific indications for PAD have expanded significantly and now include many conditions that were previously thought undrainable, such as multiple or multiloculated abscesses, abscesses with enteric communication and infected hematomas [18, 19].

It is important to define the goals of the procedure in evaluating indications and success. Potential outcomes include cure, temporization, palliation and failure. A cure is achieved when the abscess is resolved by the drainage procedure. Temporization allows resolution of an abscess and clinical improvement, with operative intervention needed to treat the underlying cause or resect necrotic tissue. The benefits of temporizing relate to the improved physiologic condition of the patient and the reduction in the extent of infection as initial healing occurs. Palliation is achieved with improvement in the patient's condition due to abscess drainage, despite the presence of a fatal underlying condition. We consider temporizing and palliative results to represent success.

The basic requirements for PAD include a safe route of percutaneous access and the presence of a fluid collection of drainable consistency. Bleeding dyscrasias are a relative contraindication, similar for any interventional procedure. Safe percutaneous access is attainable in most cases. It is generally possible to distinguish drainable fluid from phlegmon or necrotic tissue using a combination of imaging and fine-needle aspiration. Not all fluid collections require drainage, although it is generally required for those that are infected and for sterile collections that cause symptoms due to mass effect. This determination must be made on an individual basis.

47.3.1 Technical Aspects

It is important that the drainage route not cross a sterile fluid collection or other infected space because of the risk of cross-contamination. Crossing the pleural space for thoracic and upper abdominal drainage carries the risk of empyema formation. It is acceptable to cross the peritoneal space to drain an extraperitoneal abscess. Placement of a catheter through the small bowel or colon should always be avoided. Transgastric drainage of lesser sac pseudocysts has been advocated by some authors and appears to be safe, although this approach remains controversial. Lesser sac collections also can be approached transhepatically through the left lobe of the liver, although traversing solid organs should be avoided whenever possible. Obviously, it is important to be aware of, and avoid, major vascular structures.

After catheter placement, the cavity should be evacuated as completely as possible and irrigated with saline until the fluid is clear. Initial manipulation of the catheter(s) and irrigation should be done as gently as possible to minimize the induction of transient bacteremia and subsequent potential hemodynamic instability. Immediate imaging determines the need for repositioning of the catheter, placing a larger-bore catheter or placing additional drains. For cavities that are completely evacuated at the initial drainage and for which there are no abnormal communications to viscera, simple gravity drainage generally suffices. For larger or more viscous collections and those with ongoing output due to fistulous connections, suction drainage with sump catheters is more effective. Thoracic drains always should be placed to water-seal suction to avoid the complication of simple or tension pneumothorax.

Proper catheter management following the initial placement is a critical determinant of success and requires the interventional radiologist to become an active member of the management team. Drains should be checked regularly (at least daily) to monitor the volume and nature of the output, ensure adequate function and clinical response, and quickly recognize and correct any catheter-related problems. Most authorities recommend periodic irrigation of the drains, once or several times per day, with sterile saline. This can be performed by either physicians or trained nurses. In general, irrigation with proteolytic agents or antibiotics is of no value, although fibrinolytic agents may be useful for evacuation of fibrinous or hemorrhagic collections. No standard protocol has been established for follow-up imaging. Repeat imaging studies and catheter injections are frequently used to document progress and identify problems. It is occasionally necessary to replace or reposition drains or add additional catheters. The need for follow-up imaging studies should be determined on a case-by-case basis by monitoring clinical progress and drainage output.

Catheters should be removed when criteria for abscess resolution are met. Clinical criteria of success include resolution of symptoms and indicators of infection (fever and leukocytosis). Catheter-related criteria include a decrease in daily drainage to less than 10 ml and a change in the character of the drainage from purulent to serous. Radiographic criteria include documentation of abscess resolution and closure of any fistulous communications. If catheters are maintained until these criteria are satisfied, the likelihood of recurrence of the abscess is minimized. Although some authorities recommend gradual catheter removal over several days, we usually remove the drain in one step and have had no significant problem with recurrence.

For sterile fluid collections, the drain should be removed as soon as possible, generally within 24–48 h, to minimize the risk of superinfection.

47.3.2 Causes of Failure

In evaluating the causes of PAD failure, a number of factors are consistently identified. Among these factors is fluid that is too viscous for drainage or the presence of phlegmon or necrotic debris. Technical modifications such as increasing the drain size and irrigation can salvage some of these drainage procedures. Recognition of phlegmon or necrotic tissue on follow-up imaging studies may lead to cessation of attempts at PAD or a modification of the expected goal. Multi-loculated collections and multiple abscesses are another cause of failure that can be minimized by using an adequate number of catheters along with mechanical disruption of adhesions with a guidewire. Fistulous communications, either unrecognized or persistent, are yet another potential cause of failure, as is drainage of a necrotic tumor mistaken by imaging to represent an abscess. Recognition of a significant soft tissue component, maintenance of a high index of suspicion and the use of percutaneous biopsies can minimize the risk of failing to appreciate the presence of tumor. Suspicious fluid also can be sent for cytologic assessment. The success rate for PAD tends to be lower in immunocompromised patients.

The results of PAD for abscesses complicating Crohn's disease are less encouraging. Patients without fistulous communications to the bowel are usually cured by PAD, whereas those with fistulas generally require bowel resection. Among patients requiring operation, initial PAD usually leads to significant clinical improvement and permits performance of a one-stage operation. No iatrogenic entero-cutaneous fistulas have been reported. CT scan or MRI imaging is necessary in the clinical setting where an abscess is suspected.

Low pelvic abscesses in contact with the rectum or vagina can be treated surgically by incision and drainage through these organs. The same approach can be taken using sonographic guidance, and advances in endoluminal ultrasound techniques have facilitated such procedures. Experience with ultrasound-guided transrectal and transvaginal drainage is growing, and these procedures appear to be effective and well tolerated. Good success also has been achieved in the management of tubo-ovarian abscesses complicating pelvic inflammatory disease that are refractory to medical management. In most cases, the need for hysterectomy and oophorectomy due to pelvic abscess has been outdated.

47.4 Management of Specific Intra-abdominal Infections

47.4.1 Infected Necrotizing Pancreatitis

Perhaps the most challenging problem in intra-abdominal infections has been the management of infected pancreatic necrosis. Since the last update of this chapter, considerable information has become available regarding new interventional strategies, and the requirements for empiric therapy for documented infected pancreatic necrosis have been clarified [20–22].

47.4.2 Origin of Infection in Pancreatic Necrosis

Microbial translocation may represent an important cause of septic morbidity in patients with acute pancreatitis. Alterations in intestinal permeability may also predispose to translocation. The extent of gastric colonization and intestinal permeability has been examined in patients with acute pancreatitis [18]. There was a significantly higher incidence of colonization with potentially pathogenic enteric bacteria in patients with severe disease compared to those with mild disease.

47.4.2.1 Role of Antibacterial Prophylaxis in Pancreatic Necrosis

There has been some further progress in understanding antibiotic therapy for pancreatitis and its complications. This area has received increasing intention because of the trend to provide prophylactic broad spectrum antibiotic agents therapy for non-infected acute necrotizing peritonitis. Death from acute severe pancreatitis results from infection and multiple organ system failure occurring late in the course of illness. Patients with necrotizing pancreatitis involving at least one-third of the organ are at highest risk of secondary infection and death. A recent review has summarized the findings of available trials [24]. Antibiotics have demonstrated benefit in four recently completed studies despite a recent consensus panel convened by the Society of Critical Care Medicine having reviewed the available data and recommended against routine prophylaxis [20, 24–28].

47.4.2.2 Indications for Intervention in Pancreatitis with Necrosis

The at-risk population for infection is those with necrosis of approximately 30% or more of the pancreas as determined by contrast enhanced CT scanning. While advances in supportive and adjunctive care have resulted in decreased mortality rates, death still occurs in

10–20% of patients. Recent data suggest that patients with pancreatic necrosis without infection can be managed with a conservative strategy, reserving surgery or other forms of intervention for documented infection. Conservative management produces a subset of patients with persistent pain, malaise, and an inability to tolerate a diet or return to activities of daily life. These patients with organized necrosis do well with delayed debridement. Further, infection may develop late after weeks of sterility, and is diagnosed by fine needle aspiration of pancreatic necrosis [29].

Computed tomography is the procedure of choice for localizing and characterizing complications of acute pancreatitis, and fine-needle aspiration is invaluable in documenting infection. Percutaneous drainage is a therapeutic option for evacuation of infected fluid but is not capable of removing infected necrotic tissue. Factors that would mitigate against this approach include the presence of multiple small lesser sac abscesses or concerns about erosion of the inflammatory mass into the colon or major blood vessels. Drainage of central (pancreatic bed and lesser sac) collections is less often successful than is drainage of peripheral collections due to the frequent presence of a phlegmon and/or necrosis in the central regions.

The surgical management of infected necrosis has evolved from a strategy of planned re-explorations until no further evidence of necrosis was identified to a more recent approach of a single procedure with CT scan follow-up if clinical signs suggest recurrent infection [30, 31]. In the recent past, an expanding experience with laparoscopic procedures in the management of pancreatic necrosis has been reported. These reports have detailed different approaches, including transmesocolic, transgastric transgastrocolic and retroperitoneoscopic approaches [32–35]. These approaches likely offer management of these conditions without the added problems of a large abdominal incision. Given the relative infrequency of this condition (infected necrosis) it is unlikely that a comparative trial will be performed.

For localized (acute or chronic) fluid collections, percutaneous drainage is successful in a high percentage of cases. Fistulous communications to the pancreatic duct are commonly present but may be difficult to document radiographically. To minimize the risk of recurrence with pancreatic fluid collections, it is especially important to document complete cessation of drainage before removing drains. Endoscopic retrograde cholangiopancreatography (ERCP) is valuable to document patency of the pancreatic duct, since fistulas associated with downstream obstruction are unlikely to heal and generally require operation.

47.4.3 Biliary Tract Infections

47.4.3.1 Acute Cholecystitis (Calculous and Acalculous)

Acute cholecystitis in the intensive care setting is unique compared with disease seen in ambulatory populations or hospitalized patients. Most cases are acalculous and likely represent complications of microvascular and mucosal dysfunction with more significant epithelial degeneration and muscle necrosis than calculous cholecystitis. Incidence has been seen to increase with length of ICU stay and mortality is related to degree of organ failure. Associations with prolonged shock, use of vasopressors, narcotic use, and mechanical ventilation have all been proposed. An impairment of smooth muscle contractility marked by decreases in calcium influx and release has been found in animal models, with corresponding gallbladder atony characterized by earlier and more frequent development of sludge in gallbladders of ICU patients [36].

This condition often presents as occult sepsis, with or without physical findings of right upper quadrant tenderness. Liver transaminase levels are abnormal in about half of the patients and therefore are not reliable as screening tests [37, 38]. Imaging modalities to diagnose acute cholecystitis include ultrasound, CT, and cholescintigraphy. Ultrasound is used most commonly to identify this condition and has the advantage of bedside application by a variety of users in the critically ill. Sonographic findings include increases in wall thickness, striated intramural gallbladder lucencies, pericholecystic fluid or sonolucency. Increased gallbladder wall thickness can be due to a variety of benign conditions, including hypoalbuminemia and right heart failure, and is a poor indicator of acute cholecystitis alone. Intramural lucencies reflect subserosal inflammation and are therefore believed to be relatively specific for acute cholecystitis [37–39]. Similarly, pericholecystic fluid is specific but uncommon. CT, often used as an early diagnostic test for patients with unidentified postoperative sepsis, is sensitive and specific for acute cholecystitis. As with ultrasound, increased gallbladder wall thickness, intramural low-attenuation areas, and pericholecystic fluid collections in the absence of ascites are important findings. Cholescintigraphy can be employed in cases where ultrasound and CT are not conclusive and with the use of morphine enhancement can be up to 100% sensitive and 88% specific. Treatment focuses on relief of biliary obstruction by means of cholecystectomy, cholecystostomy or rarely nasobiliary drainage with lavage. The use of cholecystostomy in the critically ill provides a safe alternative for patients who cannot tolerate operative intervention and can often be preformed at the bedside with ultrasound guidance. An interval cholecystectomy can be done when the patient's condition allows [40–43].

47.4.3.2
Ascending Cholangitis

Ascending cholangitis, which results from biliary obstruction and secondary bacterial infection, classically presents with the clinical triad of fever, chills and jaundice; although rarely seen in clinical practice. Relief of obstruction should be performed on an emergent basis. Common causes of biliary obstruction include ductal calculi, benign strictures, adenopathy and neoplastic diseases (e.g., pancreatic carcinoma, cholangiocarcinoma). The diagnosis of biliary obstruction is based on demonstration of abnormal dilation of the common bile duct or its tributaries, or both. Ultrasound is the best modality for demonstrating biliary dilation. It may also demonstrate supportive findings such as ductal wall thickening, intraluminal gas or pericholecystic fluid collections. Sonography is extremely sensitive in detecting stones in the gallbladder but is less sensitive in detecting common duct calculi. CT is less sensitive than ultrasound in identifying stones, as stones often have the same radiographic density as the surrounding bile, but is superior in imaging underlying pancreatic diseases, be they inflammatory or neoplastic.

The diagnostic imaging of cholangitis has several pitfalls. Early obstruction may present without demonstrable biliary dilation. Conversely, a dilated bile duct may not be functionally obstructed, but rather the dilation may be due to prior biliary obstruction with resultant ectasia. Clinical and laboratory signs of biliary obstruction (e.g., jaundice, hyperbilirubinemia or elevated serum alkaline) phosphatase are generally adequate to distinguish between obstructive and nonobstructive biliary dilation. Gas in the biliary tree is often a sensitive sign of infection, though this may be nonpathologic in patients who have undergone prior biliary bypass or endoscopic instrumentation.

Direct visualization of the biliary tree, via percutaneous transhepatic cholangiography (PTC) or ERCP, is often used for diagnostic and therapeutic purposes. A thorough discussion of the relative merits of these two techniques is beyond the scope of this chapter. In most cases, cross-sectional imaging is sufficient for diagnostic purposes, and intervention is used for therapy. If biliary obstruction is strongly suspected on clinical grounds and imaging does not demonstrate dilation, direct visualization of the duct may be warranted to identify early nondilated obstruction. ERCP is less invasive and generally is the initial procedure of choice for distal obstruction, whereas PTC may be more useful for proximal obstructions. To a large extent, the choice of modalities rests with the expertise of available personnel.

47.4.4
Intestinal Ischemia

Ischemic disease of the bowel may result from arterial or venous occlusion or from a nonocclusive low-flow state in the mesenteric vessels. Enteric ischemia is a frequent diagnostic consideration in the acutely ill patient. Plain radiography and CT scanning should be performed to seek evidence of advanced ischemia such as pneumatosis or portal vein gas. When acute embolic enteric ischemia is strongly suspected, angiography is the procedure of choice for confirmation and identification of the site and cause of ischemia [44].

In patients whose symptoms are less specific, CT is a very useful modality for evaluating suspected enteric ischemia as well as for identifying other abdominal pathology contributing to the patient's critical illness. The

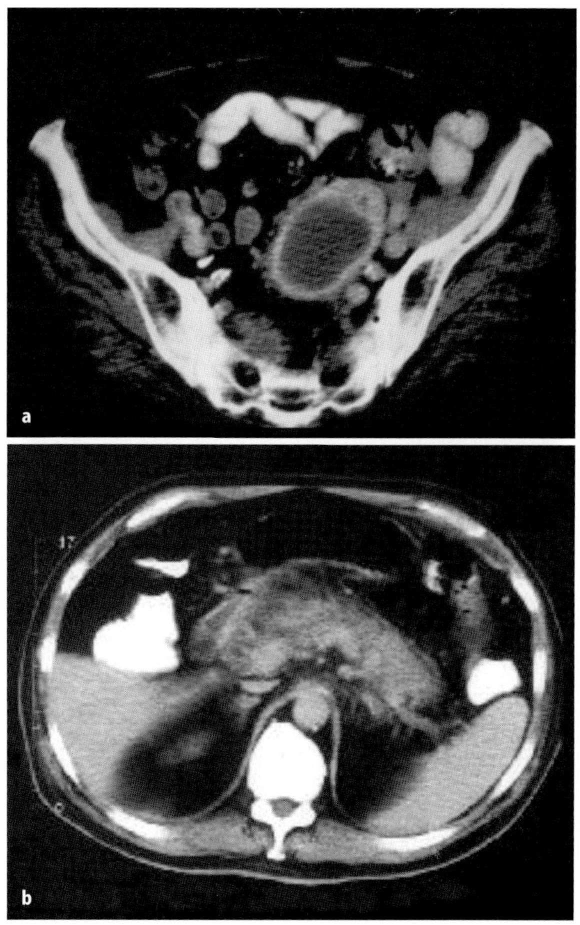

Fig. 47.3. a Abscess from perforated colonic diverticulum identified by CT scan with double contrast. (Note enhancement of abscess rim, caused by hypervascularity and the interface of bacterial growth and the host.) **b** CT scan with double contrast demonstrating necrotizing pancreatitis with evidence of abscess formation by virtue of air bubbles in edematous peripancreatic tissue (*arrow*)

earliest changes of ischemia are nonspecific and include bowel dilation and mural thickening. With transmural ischemia, inflammatory changes are seen in the mesenteric fat. However, these findings are nonspecific and CT has limited sensitivity for detecting early and potentially reversible cases of mesenteric ischemia. The findings are more specific when transmural necrosis has developed and include air within the bowel wall and portal venous system (Fig. 47.3).

If ischemic disease is suspected on the basis of the clinical evaluation or imaging studies, but the findings remain nonspecific, angiography should be performed. The oral and intravenous contrast used for CT may compromise the subsequent performance of angiography; however, CT can detect other forms of pathology in the abdomen and is less invasive. Accordingly, the choice between CT and angiography depends on the degree of clinical suspicion of ischemia.

47.4.5 Intra-abdominal Infections in Postoperative Patients

Postoperative peritonitis generally is a consequence of anastomotic leakage. This is a highly lethal condition, in part because it often is diagnosed late due to the reluctance to entertain the possibility of a suture line dehiscence. This diagnosis should be considered in any patient with signs of sepsis who has undergone a gastrointestinal anastomosis. Typical findings of diffuse abdominal tenderness may be masked by incisional pain. Because laparotomy itself introduces free air into the abdominal cavity, pneumoperitoneum is a nonspecific finding in patients during the first few days after celiotomy. The most common error is to ascribe clinical deterioration to pulmonary processes that often are a consequence of peritonitis.

Ultrasound or CT reveals peritoneal fluid, which, if present, should lead to ultrasound-guided aspiration for diagnostic purposes. Surgical treatment should include either re-anastomosis or end-colostomy. Postoperative abscesses are managed as detailed above. The postoperative patient deserves the highest degree of suspicion for anastomotic leak upon any suggestion that an intra-abdominal process has begun.

47.4.6 Enteric Fistulas

Intestinal fistulas are among the most challenging and morbid complications following intra-abdominal operations. The most common source is the small intestine, followed by the colon, stomach, duodenum, biliary tract and pancreas. Occult sepsis is often the initial clinical finding resulting from a systemic response due to inflammation surrounding the nascent fistula. The foundation of diagnosis and treatment involve early control of sepsis by identifying the source of fistula and draining any associated abscess, aggressive fluid resuscitation with special attention to electrolyte imbalances, nutritional support and appropriate fistula control with wound and skin care.

Mortality from fistulas is most closely associated with concomitant sepsis. It is this area in which aggressive ICU intervention is paramount. The initial stabilization maneuvers of fluid resuscitation and electrolyte correction, early nutritional support, and judicious and targeted antibiotics remain mainstays. Recognizing the presence of a fistula is the first step in management. Presumably, the abnormal communication is initially occluded with debris or adequate maneuvers to demonstrate the leak and its tract are not performed. A sudden change in the character of drainage or persistent output greater than 50 ml/day should alert the clinician to the presence of a fistula. Injection of contrast into the drainage catheter or other imaging studies (upper gastrointestinal contrast study, barium enema, ERCP or radionuclide biliary scan) is useful for demonstrating a fistula, assessing the adequacy of catheter placement and later documenting closure of the fistula.

Abscesses with fistulous communication to the alimentary canal, biliary tree, or pancreatic duct represent a special problem for percutaneous drainage. Fistulas are loosely characterized as high (greater than 100 ml/day) or low (less than 100 ml/day) output. Low-output fistulas can be managed easily with PAD in most cases, while most high-output fistulas can be quickly converted to low-output fistulas through the same maneuver.

The importance of aggressive nutritional support cannot be overemphasized. If possible, enteric nutrition should be provided through catheters placed distal to the fistula. For proximal high-output fistulas, parenteral nutrition is often required unless a surgically or endoscopically placed catheter can be placed distal to the perforation. Somatostatin appears useful in the management of patients with fistulas.

A critical aspect to fistula management is wound care, especially challenging with high-output fistulas. Use of synthetic, nonabrasive bandages with frequent dressing changes is often helpful. Recent debate has centered on the use of porous sponges with vacuum assisted closure devices. Though the application of direct suction on a fistula may seem counterintuitive, several case reports have demonstrated decreased cost, increased patient satisfaction, shorter hospital stays, decreased skin breakdown and earlier re-initiation of enteral feedings [45–47].

The presence of active underlying inflammatory disease (e.g., Crohn's disease, diverticulitis, etc.) ischemia or neoplasia is associated with a higher rate of failure, and temporization in these cases is often a more reasonable goal. It is important to exclude downstream obstruction, as this invariably prevents closure of the fistula. Proximal diversion of bowel contents to diminish flow (by means of gastric or intestinal tube suction) and maintenance of nutrition (enteral feeding distal to fistula or parenteral nutrition) are critical determinants of success. Proximal diversion is recommended for all gastroduodenal and small bowel fistulas and for all high-volume leaks. The perils of treatment often come when repeated operative interventions are performed prior to control of infection, appropriate drainage and nutritional stabilization. In the largest and longest series tracking enteric fistulas, patients with the greatest success rates were in good nutritional state, had no signs of sepsis, were out of an ICU setting and usually underwent definitive repair months after diagnosis of the fistula [48–51].

47.5 Antimicrobial Therapy for Intra-abdominal Infections

The goals of antibiotic therapy for intra-abdominal infections that are to be treated by either percutaneous or operative intervention are: (1) to hasten the elimination of infecting microorganisms, (2) minimize the risk of recurrent intra-abdominal infection, (3) (perhaps) shorten the clinical manifestations of infection, and (4) limit the extension of abdominal wound infection (e.g., necrotizing fasciitis). In patients with localized abscesses, antibiotics reduce fever and other manifestations of systemic response, but only after a 24- to 36-h interval. Antibiotics should be administered after fluid resuscitation has been initiated to restore adequate visceral perfusion and provide better drug distribution. Moreover, antimicrobial side effects may be exacerbated with impaired organ perfusion.

Antimicrobial agents are often begun empirically when the diagnosis of intra-abdominal infection is suspected, before the establishment of an exact diagnosis and before results of appropriate cultures are available. Accordingly, the clinician often must make a presumptive diagnosis and anticipate the pathogens that are most likely to be encountered at the site of infection. Empiric antibiotics used for intra-abdominal infections should be active against enteric Gram-negative facultative and obligate anaerobic bacilli (Table 47.1). The microbiology of intra-abdominal infection has been well defined. The identity and density of microorganisms depend on the site of the gastrointestinal tract perforation. In general, gastric, duodenal, and proximal jejunal perforations release small numbers of Gram-positive aerobic and Gram-negative anaerobic organisms into the peritoneal cavity. These organisms are generally susceptible to first-line agents such as cephalosporins and are rapidly eradicated by defense mechanisms in intact hosts. *Candida albicans* or other fungi are cultured from approximately 20% of patients with acute perforations of the gastrointestinal tract. Even when fungi are recovered, antifungal agents are unnecessary unless the patient has recently received immunosuppressive therapy for neoplasm, transplantation or inflammatory disease or has recurrent intra-abdominal infection.

Table 47.1. Organisms identified in three recently completed clinical trials in intra-abdominal infections

Study	Cipro/ Imi [59]	Clina/ Imi [57]	Erta/Pip-tazo [67]
Number of patients	330	312	396
Facultative/aerobic Gram-negatives	81%	84%	83%
Any anaerobes	50%	67%	–
Any Gram-positive cocci	61%	67%	50%
Escherichia coli	59%	68%	70%
Klebsiella species	19%	16%	13%
Pseudomonas aeruginosa	12%	15%	13%
Proteus species	7%	6%	4%
Enterobacter species	5%	5%	5%
Citrobacter species	5%	4%	–
Other Gram-negatives	12%	8%	12%
Bacteroides fragilis	31%	32%	36%
Bacteroides thetaiotaomicron	–	19%	20%
Bacteroides uniformis	–	14%	11%
Bacteroides vulgatus	–	9%	7%
Bacteroides distasonis	–	8%	11%
Bacteroides ovatus	–	–	11%
Other *Bacteroides*	11%	13%	17%
Clostridium species	12%	20%	33%
Prevotella		14%	10%
Peptostreptococci	9%	18%	16%
Fusobacterium	2%	11%	7%
Eubacterium spp.		15%	18%
Other anaerobes	12%	24%	19%
Streptococci	16%	58%	22%
Streptococcus viridans	17%	–	8%
Hemolytic streptococci	5%	–	–
Staphylococcus aureus	5%	5%	2%
Other *Staphylococcus*	4%	–	6%
Coagulase-negative staphylococci	6%	–	–
Enterococcus, not speciated	17%	2%	12%
Enterococcus faecalis	4%	13%	11%
Enterococcus faecium	2%	4%	3%
Enterococcus avium		6%	–
Group D *Streptococcus*	5%	–	–

Cultures from patients with distal small bowel perforations grow Gram-negative facultative organisms with variable density. Perforations of the distal small bowel often evolve to localized abscess formation and present with peritonitis only after rupture of the abscess. Colonic anaerobes such as *B. fragilis* are variably present. Patients with colon-derived intra-abdominal infections show contamination of the peritoneal cavity with large numbers of facultative and obligate anaerobic Gram-negative organisms.

Decisions regarding definitive antimicrobial therapy should be guided by the results of cultures obtained by operative or percutaneous drainage. For critically ill patients with intra-abdominal infections, fluid collections, particularly if purulent, should be sampled for Gram's stain followed by culture and sensitivity. If the Gram's stain reveals a predominance of Gram-positive cocci, which may indicate that enterococci or other fecal streptococci are significant co-pathogens at the site of infection, the clinician should consider alterations in the antibiotic regimen to include agents that are specifically active against enterococci (see below). This selection should be guided by local susceptibility patterns and may require addition of vancomycin [52].

47.5.1 Rationale for Selection of Antibacterial Agents

47.5.1.1 Pharmacokinetic and Pharmacodynamic Considerations

Two broad categories describe microbial pharmacodynamics: concentration-dependent or time-dependent killing. Both of these classifications relate specific host pharmacokinetic parameters to the minimum-inhibitory concentration (MIC) of the antimicrobial for the respective pathogen. Briefly, concentration-dependent agents exhibit maximal antimicrobial activity when the ratio of the magnitude of antimicrobial exposure-to-MIC is higher (e.g., peak serum concentration-to-MIC or area under the curve [AUC]-to-MIC ratios). Agents included in this category for most relevant microorganisms include aminoglycosides, fluoroquinolones, metronidazole, amphotericin B, and echinocandin antifungals. Conversely, the antimicrobial activity of time-dependent agents is more closely related to the duration of microbial exposure to concentrations above the MIC, rather than the magnitude of microbial exposure. This principle describes the activity of β-lactams, carbapenems, monobactams, vancomycin, linezolid, and azole antifungals.

Dosing of antimicrobial agents should be optimized based on their pharmacokinetic and pharmacodynamic properties. Concentration-dependent agents should be given as increased doses at more extended intervals (as permitted by host toxicity), whereas time-dependent agents should be given with increased frequency (based on host pharmacokinetics) to limit or eliminate the duration of time that antimicrobial concentrations are below the microorganism MIC. The logical extension of this notion is continuous infusion of cell wall active agents. This becomes particularly attractive for organisms with high MICs and where mutation rates to resistance may be increased.

Critically ill patients often exhibit pharmacokinetic alterations which include expanded volumes of distribution of most antimicrobial agents. Some may exhibit more rapid clearance while impaired renal function is a well-recognized complication of sepsis. Additionally, effects of renal replacement therapies should be anticipated to optimize adequate tissue exposure. Thus, it is important to anticipate these changes when selecting antimicrobial dose, interval, and infusion time.

47.5.2 Specific Antibiotic Recommendations

Outcomes are heavily influenced by the rapidity of diagnosis and appropriate intervention, and the timeliness and efficacy of anti-infective therapy. There are a wide range of individual antimicrobial agents and combinations of agents available for use in complicated intra-abdominal infections. There are convincing data that absent or inadequate empiric and definitive antibiotic therapy results in both increased failure rates and increased mortality [53]. Conversely, unnecessary or needlessly broad therapy carries its own problems. Various patient and agent-specific toxicities of therapy may occur, including superinfection, microbial resistance and organ toxicity. Acquisition of intrinsically resistant organisms and selective pressure for resistance within the unit, hospital or community is of increasing concern [54, 55].

Antimicrobial susceptibility patterns within each hospital and the local ICU should be noted when selecting initial empiric antibiotic therapy. In vitro data, especially antimicrobial susceptibility tests, are predictive of the in vivo response of infecting bacteria to particular antibacterial agents. Although a variety of susceptibility testing techniques are available, disk or automated testing is appropriate for bacteria isolated from intra-abdominal infections except in extraordinary circumstances.

Evidence from in vitro data, animal studies and clinical trials has led to widespread acceptance of the need to provide empiric antimicrobial therapy directed against *Escherichia coli* and other common members of the Enterobacteriaceae family. In addition, *B. fragilis*. *B. fragilis* and *E. coli* are the most common isolates from intra-abdominal infections and are the organisms that are most likely to cause bacteremia in abdominal sepsis, further attesting to their pathogenicity.

The evidence in support of broadening therapy to cover organisms other than common facultative and obligate anaerobes such as *E. coli* and *B. fragilis* is more controversial. Initial empiric coverage of *Pseudomonas aeruginosa* has been associated with a decreased likelihood of persistent or recurrent abdominal infection when these organisms were isolated from the site of infection. Other trials, however, using antimicrobial agents not effective against *P. aeruginosa*, have not found a high incidence of treatment failure when this organism was isolated. The severity of infection, comorbid illnesses (e.g., immunosuppressed states, diabetes, etc.) and previous geographic location of the presenting patient (i.e., community vs. healthcare-associated) should guide the breadth of empiric antimicrobial therapy.

A large number of agents are broadly active against the bacteria found in intra-abdominal infection. These are best discussed as classes of drugs and include aminoglycosides, carbapenems, cephalosporins, penicillins plus β-lactamase inhibitors, and quinolones. Aztreonam, a monobactam, can be considered as a cephalosporin-class agent.

47.5.2.1 *Identification of High Risk Patients*

Several attempts have been made to identify clinical features in patients with peritonitis that increase the risk of adverse outcomes. These analyses have identified parameters prognostic of mortality rather than the risk of recurrent infection, including higher APACHE II scores, poor nutritional status, significant cardiovascular disease, and inability to obtain adequate source control [56]. Similarly, patients immunosuppressed by medical therapy for transplantation, cancer, or inflammatory disease should receive a broader spectrum of therapy. Patients with other acute and chronic diseases may also be immunosuppressed although this is difficult to define. For such patients, antimicrobial regimens with expanded spectra may be warranted, including meropenem, imipenem/cilastatin, piperacillin/tazobactam, a quinolone plus metronidazole, or a third/fourth generation cephalosporin plus metronidazole.

Prolonged pre-hospital length of stay and prolonged (> 2 days) pre-operative antimicrobial therapy are significant predictors of failure from recurrent infection, and suggest that organisms resistant to the empiric antimicrobial regimen may be responsible [42, 43]. Such patients should be treated for healthcare-associated infection. Appropriate regimens for such patients will mirror therapy provided for other ICU-acquired infections such as ventilator-associated pneumonia, and typically include a carbapenem and vancomycin. Individual units may harbor multi-resistant organisms and require even more focused therapy.

47.5.2.2 *Duration of Therapy*

Antimicrobial therapy for established infections should be continued until resolution of clinical signs of infection occurs, including normalization of temperature and white blood cell count, and return of gastrointestinal function. The risk of subsequent treatment failure appears to be quite low in patients who have no clinical evidence of infection at the time of cessation of antimicrobial therapy [57].

In patients who have persistent or recurrent clinical evidence of intra-abdominal infection after 5 – 7 days of therapy, appropriate diagnostic investigation should be undertaken. This should include CT or ultrasound imaging, and antimicrobial therapy effective against the organisms initially identified should be continued. Patients with persistent or recurrent intra-abdominal infections will likely require additional intervention to achieve source control. If a patient has persistent clinical symptoms and signs, but no evidence of a new or persistent infection is uncovered after a careful investigation, termination of antimicrobial therapy is warranted.

47.5.2.3 *Indications for Anti-Enterococcal Therapy*

Although the appropriate role of anti-enterococcal therapy is controversial, most authorities believe that specific therapy directed towards this organism should be given only when enterococci are the only organisms isolated from abdominal samples or are isolated from blood. Numerous prospective, blinded and randomized trials have compared regimens active against routine isolates of *Enterococcus* for community-acquired infections. In at least six of these studies, the comparator regimen did not have similar coverage [58, 59]. Nonetheless, none of these trials demonstrated an advantage to treatment for enterococci. Routine coverage of *Enterococcus* is therefore not necessary for patients with community acquired intra-abdominal infections.

Antimicrobial therapy for enterococci should be given when enterococci are recovered from patients with healthcare-associated infections. The selection of appropriate antimicrobials should be guided by susceptibility testing. Local ICU antibiograms and antimicrobial resistance patterns should be known due to the emergence of ampicillin and vancomycin resistant enterococci. If the sample reveals Gram-negative bacilli, failure to isolate either facultative or obligate anaerobes on culture does not obviate the need to continue providing antimicrobial agents against both.

47.5.2.4 *Indications for Antifungal Therapy*

Candida albicans or other fungi are cultured from about 20 % of patients with acute perforations of the gastrointestinal tract. Even when fungi are recovered, antifungal agents are unnecessary unless the patient has recently received immunosuppressive therapy for neoplasm, transplantation, or inflammatory disease, or has post-operative or recurrent intra-abdominal infection.

Anti-infective therapy for *Candida* should be withheld until the infecting species is identified. If *Candida albicans* is found, fluconazole is an appropriate choice. For fluconazole-resistant *Candida* species, therapy with amphotericin B, caspofungin or voriconazole is appropriate. The latter two agents cause substantially less toxicity than amphotericin B, and are specifically indicated for patients with renal dysfunction or transplantation.

47.5.2.5
Aminoglycosides

Aminoglycosides have been the mainstay of therapy for serious Gram-negative infections for the past 40 years. Due to their potential for nephrotoxicity and ototoxicity and their narrow therapeutic range, however, there has been considerable movement away from aminoglycosides as first-choice agents for community-acquired intra-abdominal infections. Several classes of agents, all highly active and effective against the anticipated infected flora of intra-abdominal infections, are available. The use of β-lactams or quinolones in combination with metronidazole, β-lactams combined with β-lactamase inhibitors, or carbapenems in mixed flora infections has given clinical results equivalent to or better than those seen with aminoglycoside-based combinations [60]. Aminoglycosides no longer represent the gold standard for therapy of intra-abdominal infections and need not be used for community-acquired intra-abdominal infections. The use of aminoglycosides as first-choice agents for empiric treatment of healthcare-associated intra-abdominal infections should depend on local susceptibility patterns of healthcare-associated isolates.

Considerable movement has been seen toward high-dose intermittent therapy with aminoglycosides. Patients with major infections have expanded volumes of distribution for aminoglycosides and commonly require at least 2.5 mg/kg gentamicin or tobramycin to achieve therapeutic levels. Regimens involving high doses (5 – 10 mg/kg) of gentamicin or tobramycin given once every 24 h have been evaluated. The rationale for this form of treatment is based on the concentration-dependent bactericidal activity and post-antibiotic effect phenomenon observed with aminoglycosides.

47.5.2.6
Lactams

An alternative strategy to the use of penicillinase-resistant cephalosporins is to use currently available penicillins (e.g., ampicillin and piperacillin) in combination with a β-lactamase inhibitor, such as sulbactam, clavulanic acid or tazobactam. These agents are potent inhibitors of penicillinases and other non-extended spectrum β-lactamases from Gram-positive and anaerobic Gram-negative organisms. They have less activity against the chromosomal β-lactamases (e.g., extended-spectrum β-lactamases or ESBL) seen in many strains of Enterobacteriaceae and do not completely compensate for the marginal Gram-negative activity of the penicillin derivative. The primary concern has to do with organisms that constitutively express β-lactamases. Organisms that typically express this activity include *Enterobacter* species, *P. aeruginosa, Citrobacter, Serratia* and *Acinetobacter* species. These particular organisms are most commonly encountered in healthcare-associated infections but are also present in approximately 15% of community-acquired infections. Clinical trials with these agents for intra-abdominal infections have been generally confined to patients with acutely perforated gastroduodenal ulcers and acute appendicitis. These β-lactamase inhibitors add considerable anti-staphylococcal and anti-*Bacteroides* activity to the base penicillin.

47.5.2.7
Carbapenems

Imipenem and meropenem, carbapenem derivatives, have broad activity against facultative and obligate Gram-negative anaerobes and excellent Gram-positive activity (excluding methicillin-resistant staphylococci) [61 – 66]. In particular, these agents are more active against ESBL-producing Enterobacteriaceae. Imipenem is formulated with cilastatin, a renal dehydropeptidase inhibitor that prevents renal tubular epithelial metabolism of the drug. In situations in which plasma accumulation of imipenem occurs (high dose levels or renal failure), the drug has been associated with seizures. With lower dose levels and appropriate adjustments for renal failure, however, seizures are rare. Meropenem has not been associated with such neurotoxicity. Moreover, the in vitro activity of meropenem is slightly broader than imipenem, whereby the MICs of many organisms (e.g., *P. aeruginosa*) are one dilution lower. Another carbapenem derivative recently introduced is ertapenem. Unlike imipenem and meropenem, this agent is more appropriately utilized for the empiric management of community-acquired or mild-to-moderate intra-abdominal infections. Ertapenem has similar activity against Gram-negative anaerobes as imipenem and meropenem; however, this agent is less broad for healthcare-associated obligate Gram-negative and certain Gram-positive organisms (i.e., enterococci) [67].

47.5.2.8
Fluoroquinolones

As clinical experience has accumulated, quinolone antibiotics appear to be useful for intra-abdominal infections. These agents act by inhibiting deoxyribonucleic acid (DNA) replication and have shown similar activity to imipenem in clinical trials for pneumonia and intra-abdominal infection. Available quinolones have little anti-*B. fragilis* activity and should be combined with metronidazole to include obligate Gram-negative anaerobic coverage. There has been a concerning rise in the incidence of quinolone resistance, often paired with extended spectrum-lactamase production, in healthcare associated infections. While fluoroquinolones remain suitable for management of mild to moderate community-acquired infections, local susceptibility patterns should be reviewed prior to their use in high severity intra-abdominal infections, especially following prior antimicrobial therapy or operation.

47.5.2.9 Imidazoles

As outlined previously, metronidazole has remained highly effective against *Bacteroides* species, in contradistinction to clindamycin, and is now the preferred agent for combination therapy with later-generation cephalosporin or aztreonam-based therapy.

References

1. Oya M, Shimada T, Nakamura M, et al. (1993) Functional morphology of the lymphatic system in the monkey diaphragm. Arch Histol Cytol 56:37
2. Li JC, Yu SM (1991) Study on the ultrastructure of the peritoneal stomata in humans. Acta Anat 141:26
3. Levine S, Saltzman A (1988) Postinflammatory increase of lymphatic absorption from the peritoneal cavity: role of diaphragmatic stomata. Microcirc Endothelium Lymphatics 4:399
4. Elk JR, Adair T, Drake RE, et al. (1990) The effect of anesthesia and surgery on diaphragmatic lymph vessel flow after endotoxin in sheep. Lymphology 23:145
5. Clary EM, Bruch SM, Lau CL, et al. (2002) Effects of pneumoperitoneum on hemodynamic and systemic immunologic responses to peritonitis in pigs. J Surg Res 108:32
6. Holub Z (2002) Impact of laparoscopic surgery on immune function. Clin Exp Obstet Gynecol 29:77
7. Novitsky YW, Callery MP (2002) Laparoscopic surgery and the nuances of systemic immunity. J Clin Gastroenterol 34:109
8. Ure BM, Niewold TA, Bax NM, et al. (2002) Peritoneal, systemic, and distant organ inflammatory responses are reduced by a laparoscopic approach and carbon dioxide versus air. Surg Endosc 16:836
9. van Deventer SJ, Knepper A, Landsman J, et al. (1988) Endotoxins in portal blood. Hepatogastroenterology 35:223
10. Gimson AE (1987) Hepatic dysfunction during bacterial sepsis. Intensive Care Med 13:162
11. Cerra FB (1992) Multiple organ failure syndrome. Dis Mon 26:816
12. Moore FA, Moore EE, Poggetti R (1991) Gut bacterial translocation via the portal vein: a clinical perspective with major torso trauma. J Trauma 31:629
13. Wachs ME, Wolfgang HS (1991) Primary intestinal anastomosis is unsafe in the presence of generalized peritonitis. In: Simmons RL, Udekwu AO (eds) Debates in clinical surgery. Mosby-Year Book, St. Louis, p 228
14. Liebert C, Deweese BM (1981) Primary resection without anastomosis for perforation of acute diverticulitis. Surg Gynecol Obstet 152:30
15. Debas H, Thomson FB (1972) A critical review of colectomy with anastomosis. Surg Gynecol Obstet 135:747
16. Buck JR, Fath JJ, Chung SK, et al. (1995) Use of absorbable mesh as an aid in abdominal closure in the emergent setting. Am Surg 61:655
17. Sautner T, Gotzinger P, Red-Wenzel EM, et al. (1997) Does reoperation for abdominal sepsis enhance the inflammatory host response? Arch Surg 132:250
18. vanSonnenberg E, D'Agostino HB, Casola G, et al. (1991) Percutaneous abscess drainage: current concepts. Radiology 181:617
19. Solem CA, Loftus EV (2004) Management of refractory inflammatory bowel disease. Gastroenterol Clin North Am 33:319
20. Nathens AB, Curtis JR, Beale RJ, et al. (2004) Management of the critically ill patient with severe acute pancreatitis. Crit Care Med 32:2524
21. Whitcomb DC (2006) Acute pancreatitis. N Engl J Med 354:2142
22. Shankar S, vanSonnenberg E, Silverman SG, et al. (2004) Imaging and percutaneous management of acute complicated pancreatitis. Cardiovasc Intervent Radiol 27:567
23. McNaught CE, Woodcock NP, Mitchell CJ, et al. (2002) Gastric colonization, intestinal permeability and septic morbidity in acute pancreatitis. Pancreatology 2:463
24. Kramer KM, Levy H (1999) Prophylactic antibiotics for severe acute pancreatitis: the beginning of an era. Pharmacotherapy 19:592
25. Pederzoli P, Bassi C, Vesentini S, et al. (1993) A randomized multicenter clinical trial of antibiotic prophylaxis of septic complications in acute necrotizing pancreatitis with imipenem. Surg Gynecol Obstet 176:480
26. Sainio V, Kemppainen E, Puolakkainen P, et al. (1995) Early antibiotic treatment in acute necrotising pancreatitis. Lancet 346:663
27. Delcenserie R, Yzet T, Ducroix JP (1996) Prophylactic antibiotics in treatment of severe acute alcoholic pancreatitis. Pancreas 13:198
28. Lankisch PG, Lerch MM (2006) The role of antibiotic prophylaxis in the treatment of acute pancreatitis. J Clin Gastroenterol 40:149
29. Clancy TE, Ashley SW (2002) Current management of necrotizing pancreatitis. Adv Surg 36:103
30. Bradley E III, Olson RA (1991) Current management of pancreatic abscess. Adv Surg 24:361
31. Mithofer K, Mueller PR, Warshaw AL (1997) Interventional and surgical treatment of pancreatic abscess. World J Surg 21:162
32. Ammori BJ (2002) Laparoscopic transgastric pancreatic necrosectomy for infected pancreatic necrosis. Surg Endosc 16:1362
33. Cuschieri A (2002) Pancreatic necrosis: pathogenesis and endoscopic management. Semin Laparosc Surg 9:54
34. Horvath KD, Kao LS, Wherry KL, et al. (2001) A technique for laparoscopic-assisted percutaneous drainage of infected pancreatic necrosis and pancreatic abscess. Surg Endosc 15:1221
35. Park JJ, Kim SS, Koo YS, et al. (2002) Definitive treatment of pancreatic abscess by endoscopic transmural drainage. Gastrointest Endosc 55:256
36. Gomez-Pinilla PJ, Morales S, Camello-Almaraz C, et al. (2006) Changes in guinea pig gallbladder smooth muscle Ca^{2+} homeostasis by acute acalculous cholecystitis. Am J Physiol Gastrointest Liver Physiol 290:G14
37. Laurila JJ, Syrjala H, Laurila PA, et al. (2004) Acute acalcu-

lous cholecystitis in critically ill patients. Acta Anaesthesiol Scand 48:986
38. Laurila JJ, Ala-Kokko TI, Laurila PA, et al. (2005) Histopathology of acute acalculous cholecystitis in critically ill patients. Histopathology 47:485
39. Owen CC, Jain R (2005) Acute acalculous cholecystitis. Curr Treat Options Gastroenterol 8:99
40. Basaran O, Yavuzer N, Selcuk H, et al. (2005) Ultrasound-guided percutaneous cholecystostomy for acute cholecystitis in critically ill patients: One center's experience. Turk J Gastroenterol 16:164
41. Akyurek N, Salman B, Yuksel O, et al. (2005) Management of acute calculous cholecystitis in high-risk patients: percutaneous cholecystotomy followed by early laparoscopic cholecystectomy. Surg Laparosc Endosc Percutan Tech 15:315
42. Welschbillig-Meunier K, Pessaux P, Lebigot J, et al. (2005) Percutaneous cholecystostomy for high-risk patients with acute cholecystitis. Surg Endosc 19:1256
43. Macri A, Scuderi G, Saladino E, et al. (2006) Acute gallstone cholecystitis in the elderly: treatment with emergency ultrasonographic percutaneous cholecystostomy and interval laparoscopic cholecystectomy. Surg Endosc 20:88
44. Park WM, Gloviczki P, Cherry KJ, et al. (2002) Contemporary management of acute mesenteric ischemia: Factors associated with survival. J Vasc Surg 35:445
45. Medeiros AC, Aires-Neto T, Marchini JS, et al. (2004) Treatment of postoperative enterocutaneous fistulas by high-pressure vacuum with a normal oral diet. Dig Surg 21:401
46. Hyon SH, Martinez-Garbino JA, Benati ML, et al. (2000) Management of a high-output postoperative enterocutaneous fistula with a vacuum sealing method and continuous enteral nutrition. ASAIO J 46:511
47. Cro C, George KJ, Donnelly J, et al. (2002) Vacuum assisted closure system in the management of enterocutaneous fistulae. Postgrad Med J 78:364
48. Haffejee AA (2004) Surgical management of high output enterocutaneous fistulae: a 24-year experience. Curr Opin Clin Nutr Metab Care 7:309
49. Lynch AC, Delaney CP, Senagore AJ, et al. (2004) Clinical outcome and factors predictive of recurrence after enterocutaneous fistula surgery. Ann Surg 240:825
50. Hollington P, Mawdsley J, Lim W, et al. (2004) An 11-year experience of enterocutaneous fistula. Br J Surg 91:1646
51. Kaur N, Minocha VR, Mundu M (2004) Improving outcome in patients of high output small bowel fistula. Trop Gastroenterol 25:92
52. Solomkin JS, Mazuski JE, Baron EJ, et al. (2003) Guidelines for the selection of anti-infective agents for complicated intra-abdominal infections. Clin Infect Dis 37:997
53. Falagas ME, Barefoot L, Griffith J, et al. (1996) Risk factors leading to clinical failure in the treatment of intra-abdominal or skin/soft tissue infections. Eur J Clin Microbiol Infect Dis 15:913
54. Wilton P, Smith R, Coast J, et al. (2002) Strategies to contain the emergence of antimicrobial resistance: a systematic review of effectiveness and cost-effectiveness. J Health Serv Res Policy 7:111
55. Shlaes DM, Gerding DN, John JF Jr, et al. (1997) Society for Healthcare Epidemiology of America and Infectious Diseases Society of America Joint Committee on the Prevention of Antimicrobial Resistance: guidelines for the prevention of antimicrobial resistance in hospitals. Clin Infect Dis 25:584
56. Wacha H, Hau T, Dittmer R, et al. (1999) Risk factors associated with intraabdominal infections: a prospective multicenter study. Peritonitis Study Group. Langenbecks Arch Surg 384:24
57. Solomkin JS, Wilson SE, Christou NV, et al. (2001) Results of a clinical trial of clinafloxacin versus imipenem/cilastatin for intraabdominal infections. Ann Surg 233:79
58. Ohlin B, Cederberg A, Forssell H, Solhaug JH, Tveit E (1999) Piperacillin/tazobactam compared with cefuroxime/metronidazole in the treatment of intra-abdominal infections. Eur J Surg 165:875
59. Solomkin JS, Reinhart HH, Dellinger EP, et al. (1996) Results of a randomized trial comparing sequential intravenous/oral treatment with ciprofloxacin plus metronidazole to imipenem/cilastatin for intra-abdominal infections. The Intra-Abdominal Infection Study Group. Ann Surg 223(3):303–15
60. Solomkin JS, Dellinger EP, Christou NV, et al. (1990) Results of a multicenter trial comparing imipenem/cilastatin to tobramycin/clindamycin for intra-abdominal infections. Ann Surg 212:581
61. Brismar B, Malmborg AS, Tunevall G, et al. (1995) Meropenem versus imipenem/cilastatin in the treatment of intra-abdominal infections. J Antimicrob Chemother 35:139
62. Basoli A, Meli EZ, Mazzocchi P, et al. (1997) Imipenem/cilastatin (1.5 g daily) versus meropenem (3.0 g daily) in patients with intra-abdominal infections: results of a prospective, randomized, multicentre trial. Scand J Infect Dis 29:503
63. Berne TV, Yellin AE, Appleman MD, et al. (1996) Meropenem versus tobramycin with clindamycin in the antibiotic management of patients with advanced appendicitis. J Am Coll Surg 182:403
64. Condon RE, Walker AP, Sirinek KR, et al. (1995) Meropenem versus tobramycin plus clindamycin for treatment of intraabdominal infections: results of a prospective, randomized, double-blind clinical trial. Clin Infect Dis 21:544
65. Geroulanos SJ (1995) Meropenem versus imipenem/cilastatin in intraabdominal infections requiring surgery. Meropenem Study Group. J Antimicrob Chemother 36(Suppl A):191
66. Huizinga WK, Warren BL, Baker LW, et al. (1995) Antibiotic monotherapy treatment guidelines for intra-abdominal infections with meropenem in the surgical management of intra-abdominal infections. J Antimicrob Chemother 36(Suppl A):179
67. Solomkin JS, Yellin AE, Rotstein OD, et al. (2003) Ertapenem versus piperacillin/tazobactam in the treatment of complicated intraabdominal infections: results of a double-blind, randomized comparative phase III trial. Ann Surg 237:235

Chapter 48

Surgical Site Infection Control in the Critical Care Environment

C.E. Edmiston, Jr, P.J. Wilson, B.F. Grahn

48.1 Introduction

Over the past 20 years there has been a significant change in the demographics of hospitalized patients, reflected in patients being admitted with more severe disease processes resulting in a higher risk for infection. This is especially true for surgical patients, many of whom require admission to the ICU and are the recipient of various lines, catheters and other intravascular devices. The number of surgical procedures performed annually in the United States approaches 30 million and based upon data derived from the CDC's National Nosocomial Infection Surveillance (NNIS) program, surgical site infections (SSIs) are the third most frequently reported healthcare-associated infection (HAI) [1, 2]. Several studies suggest that surgical site infections are associated with both an increased length of stay (up to 7.3 days) and increased total hospital charges, which in the case of selected surgical pathogens such as methicillin-resistant *Staphylococcus aureus* (MRSA) can result in excess charges amounting to several thousands of dollars [3, 4]. In addition, the acquisition of an SSI has been suggested to be associated with increased mortality when compared to closely matched hospitalized patients without an SSI.

The National Nosocomial Infection Surveillance (NNIS) program developed through cooperation with the Centers for Disease Control and Prevention is an operation specific index with a fairly high discriminatory power compared to previous risk stratified index systems. Currently, within most institutions in the United States the infection control team monitors those surgical procedures which, by virtue of historical experience, possess the greatest risk for postoperative infection. At Froedtert Memorial Lutheran Hospital, the major teaching affiliate institution associated with the Medical College of Wisconsin, decisions as to which procedures are to be monitored are made by an interdisciplinary committee, the Surgical Wound Taskforce. The efforts of this group to reduce/prevent postoperative surgical site infections may, however, be impacted by external risk factors such as antimicrobial resistance. In addition, ignorance or disregard for appropriate infection control practces is often equally to blame for failure to prevent HAI in both the medical and surgical ICU.

Strategies for preventing postoperative surgical site infections require attention to infection control practices and appropriate patient care management. Three factors have been identified as influencing the development of a postoperative surgical site infection: (a) the patient's intrinsic risk factor, (b) extrinsic factors associated with the operation itself, and finally (c) microbial virulence. The following discussion will focus upon these three factors and also emphasize the recent Guidelines for the Prevention of Surgical Site Infections that have been developed by the Hospital Infection Program of the Centers for Disease Control and Prevention.

48.2 Microbiology and Pathogenesis of Surgical Site Infections

Surgical site infections may be caused by endogenous or exogenous microbial contamination. Table 48.1 demonstrates the distribution of pathogens associated with surgical site infections in the United States. This data from the NNIS program encompasses two study intervals, 1986 – 1989 and 1990 – 1996 [5]. In addition to

Table 48.1. Predominant microbial pathogens associated with surgical site infections (NNIS 1986 – 1996)

Organism	Percentage of isolates 1986 – 1989	1990 – 1996
Staphylococcus aureus	17	20
Coagulase negative staphylococci	12	14
Enterococcus spp.	13	12
Escherichia coli	10	8
Pseudomonas aeruginosa	8	8
Enterobacter spp.	8	7
Proteus mirabilis	4	3
Klebsiella pneumoniae	3	3
Streptococcus spp.	3	3
Candida albicans	2	3
Miscellaneous gram-positives	–	4
Bacteroides fragilis	–	2

understanding the etiology and pathogenesis of the predominant pathogens associated with SSIs, it is also important to recognize that the emergence of antimicrobial resistance among both gram-positive and gram-negative microorganisms has a profound impact on the care of the surgical patient in the ICU, limiting therapeutic options and emphasizing reinforcement of stringent infection control practices [6, 7].

48.2.1 Gram-Positive Microorganisms

Staphylococcus aureus is the most common surgical site pathogen at 20%, followed by *Staphylococcus epidermidis* (14%) and *Enterococcus* species at 12%. Overall, gram-positive pathogens are responsible for 53% of surgical site infections. *Staphylococcus aureus* has been recognized to be a significant HAI pathogen since the late 19th century. According to data derived from the National Nosocomial Infection Surveillance (NNIS) program, the incidence of methicillin-resistant *Staphylococcus aureus* (MRSA) has increased from less than 2.5% in the mid-1970s to greater than 50% in 2005 [6, 8]. While early reports placed the greatest incidence of MRSA in tertiary medical centers, it is now obvious that this organism is ubiquitous within the healthcare environment, with even small hospitals (less than 200 beds) reporting rates greater than 25%. It is important to note that quite often these organisms will express resistance to antibiotics other than the beta-lactam group such as the fluoroquinolones. For example, it has been pointed out in one study that resistance to methicillin is often accompanied by resistance to both the 2nd and 3rd generation quinolone, such as ciprofloxacin and levofloxacin [9]. In addition, the emergence of community-acquired MRSA as colonizing flora in patients undergoing elective surgical procedures threatens the potential efficacy of our current surgical prophylaxis regimen for clean/clean-contaminated procedures [10]. At present, vancomycin remains the drug of choice for the treatment of MRSA. However, a growing number of institutions are reporting intermediate level resistance to vancomycin, due to the presence of a thick exopolysaccharide capsular material surrounding the bacterial cell [11]. This nontraditional mechanism of resistance is rather problematic, especially since routine susceptibility testing often suggests that these organisms are fully sensitive to vancomycin. Fortunately, newer gram-positive active agents such as linezolid and daptomycin have emerged as viable therapeutic options for selective MRSA infections in high-risk patient populations [12, 13].

It is important to note that the development of antimicrobial resistance among the staphylococci may involve a myriad of genetic mechanisms including transposon, plasmid or chromosomal mediated resistance. While *Staphylococcus aureus* is recognized as the most virulent member of this genus, *Staphylococcus epidermidis* is presently the most common pathogen recovered from biomedical device-related infections [14]. In addition, 73% of the *Staphylococcus epidermidis* strains at our institution express resistance to the 1st generation cephalosporins. This has significant implications for the selection of a surgical prophylactic agent for high-risk patients undergoing clean surgical procedure and has prompted the substitution of a 2nd generation agent for patients undergoing surgery. The presence of MRSA in the surgical ICU and other units of the hospital has necessitated the adoption of strict isolation guidelines that while controversial, these policies have been successful in limiting or preventing microbial dissemination to other patients or units of the healthcare environment.

The enterococci have been traditionally viewed as a second class pathogen in surgery, often found as a component of normal flora and recovered in mixed infections. However, many enterococci express multidrug resistance and drug susceptibility is highly variable, dependent upon the microbial species. In most institutions, *Enterococcus faecalis* is still highly sensitive to ampicillin (>90%), while greater than 80% of *Enterococcus faecium* strains will express resistance to ampicillin. Prior to 1994, the vast majority of hospital microbiology laboratories in the United States did not speciate the enterococci, but rather reported their results to genus level. It is obvious that with the emergence of these multi-resistance strains greater efforts are needed to document the epidemiology of these organisms within the hospital environment. Susceptibility to other beta-lactam agents may also demonstrate significant variation. While in some surveys sensitivities to piperacillin may exceed 90%, high rates or resistance (>95%) are demonstrated against many of the 3rd generation cephalosporins [9]. In the last 10 years, the appearance of high level aminoglycoside resistance has reduced the therapeutic efficacy of the synergistic combination of penicillin and gentamicin for the treatment of enterococcal bacteremias. In the face of high level beta-lactam and aminoglycoside resistance, vancomycin has emerged as the therapy of choice for many enterococcal infections.

However, in 1989 reports suggested that selected strains of enterococci were developing resistance to the glycopeptides, in particular among strains of *Enterococcus faecium*. Over the past 10 years there have been numerous studies demonstrating nosocomial outbreaks associated with vancomycin-resistant enterococcal (VRE) strains expressing high level (Van A) vancomycin resistance [15, 16]. This high level type of resistance is carried on a single transposable element that is incorporated into a bacterial plasmid. A moderate and low level resistance to vancomycin has also been identified but the precise genetic mechanisms are presently unclear. In an effort to reduce the risk of vancomycin resistance among the enterococci and to prevent the spread of this resistance to the more virulent staphylococci, the CDC has developed criteria for the appropriate use of vancomycin through the Hospital Infection Control Practice Advisory Committee [17]. This important document encompasses four separate areas: (a) development of microbiologic criteria for the identification, susceptibility testing to detect vancomycin resistance and screening for VRE in hospitalized patients, (b) development of educational programs that enhance healthcare workers' understanding of the epidemiology and pathogenesis of VRE, (c) development of prevention and control strategies to reduce the incidence of VRE in the healthcare environment, and finally (d) criteria for the prudent use of vancomycin.

48.2.2 Gram-Negative Microorganisms

Data from the NNIS hospitals suggest that gram-negative microorganisms continue to be a significant source of morbidity and mortality for surgical patients. *Pseudomonas aeruginosa* is currently responsible for approximately 9% of surgical site infections, while *Enterobacter, Escherichia coli* and *Klebsiella pneumoniae* occur as nosocomial SSI pathogens approximately 8.8%, 7.1%, and 3.5% of the time, respectively. Anaerobic bacteria on the other hand such as the gram-negative *Bacteroides fragilis* occur as surgical site pathogens less than 3% of the time [5]. Members of the Enterobacteriaceae and *Pseudomonas aeruginosa* have all been associated with selected mechanisms of resistance, some of which have occurred quite rapidly over the past 10 years [6]. Strains of *Klebsiella pneumoniae* that express resistance to the 3rd generation cephalosporins including ceftriaxone, cefotaxime or ceftazidime are increasing at a rate of 1–2% a year [9]. This resistance is due to an extended spectrum beta-lactamase (ESBL) enzyme that is capable of hydrolyzing not only the 3rd generation cephalosporin antibiotics but also aztreonam. Unfortunately, under laboratory conditions these organisms will often appear to be sensitive to these agents, therefore rendering false-positive antibiogram data [18, 19]. This type of resistance is occurring at a much faster pace among ICU patients than the general hospital population. It has been proposed that increased duration of stay in the ICU is associated with acquisition of this type of resistance in strains of *Klebsiella pneumoniae* [9, 19]. Quinolone resistance in *Pseudomonas aeruginosa* has increased more dramatically over the past 10 years, with resistance rates ranging from 20% to 35%. However, it is important to note that it does not appear that the increase in quinolone resistance among strains of *Pseudomonas aeruginosa* is solely an ICU phenomenon, but rather occurs throughout the hospital [6]. At present, in our institution we are seeing a 20% rate of resistance among *Pseudomonas aeruginosa* to the carbapenems which is due to an altered bacterial membrane porin, preventing the entry of the antimicrobial into the bacterial cell. It is obvious that the increase in resistance that is currently being seen in the SICU is related to several important variables. First the high-risk status of the patient population coupled with their severity of illness contributes to the overall problem of host susceptibility to HAI. Second, the failure to ascribe to basic infection control practices exacerbates the problem of acquisition and dissemination. Finally, a less than prudent pattern of antimicrobial use has intensified the pressure placed upon patients in the critical care environment.

48.3 Endogenous Versus Exogenous Sources of Contamination

Historically most SSIs have been viewed as derived from the patient's own endogenous flora, whether from the skin, or pharyngeal or gastrointestinal tract. For instance, vascular, orthopedic or plastic surgical procedures often involve the skin or skin structures and therefore tend to involve a gram-positive flora if infection occurs, while general surgical procedures involving the gastrointestinal tract have a more gram-negative focus [20, 21]. Alternatively, exogenous contamination may occur within the intraoperative environment as a result of contaminated instruments, breaks in aseptic technique or from members of the surgical team. Studies conducted in our institution have shown that potential HAI pathogens, both gram-positive and gram-negative, are present in the air of the operating room environment [14, 22]. As a result of these findings a special effort is undertaken to ensure that implantable biomedical devices are immediately covered upon removal from sterile packaging so as to reduce the potential for intraoperative contamination.

The infecting dose required to produce a postoperative surgical site infection has been determined to be in the order of magnitude of 5.0 $\log_{10}$ colony forming units or greater per gram of tissue [23]. This value was from studies conducted in experimental animal models of infection. The inoculum size, however, required to produce an infection is diminished when an inert foreign body is present in the wound. It has been suggested that 100 microorganisms or less per gram of tissue may be sufficient to produce a biomedical-associated infection [24]. Unfortunately, patients presenting for surgery in the year 2006 are often high-risk, exhibiting multi-organ disease states and demonstrating varying levels of anergy. Therefore, it is likely that patients with diminished phagocytic cell function and poor wound healing characteristics, such as in the diabetic patient, are at higher risk for infection and that the microbial threshold dose for producing a postoperative infection is less well defined in this patient population.

48.4 Problematic Risk Factors Associated with Surgical Site Infections

Multivariant analysis has been used to analyze the association of two or more risk factors upon development of surgical site infection. Table 48.2 identifies several intrinsic (patient) and extrinsic (operation) factors that may influence the risk of developing a surgical site infection. While it is reasonable to assume that diminished nutritional status (severe-protein calorie malnutrition) may predispose one to development of a surgical site infection, it has been very difficult to assess the benefit of nutritional supplementation on decreasing the risk of SSI [5, 25–27]. The diabetic patient offers another case in point. Previous scientific studies have demonstrated that diminished leukocytic cell function and poor wound healing occurs in patients with hyperglycemia [28–30]. Recent studies have documented the relationship of hyperglycemia to infection in the critically ill patient population [31–33]. The risk factors associated with surgical site infection can be categorized as either intrinsic or extrinsic.

Another area of continued controversy is the role that *Staphylococcus aureus* nares colonization plays in the development of a postoperative surgical site infection. Studies have documented the impact of preoperative nares colonization of *S. aureus* on the subsequent development of surgical site infections [34]. Mupirocin, a topical antibiotic, has been shown to be effective for eliminating *S. aureus* from the anterior nares of both patients and healthcare professionals. The response to this phenomenon has been the implementation of decolonization protocol for selected patients. A study utilizing cardiothoracic patients has suggested that mupirocin when applied preoperatively to the nares resulted in reduced risk of SSIs [35]. However, a recent report from a Veterans Administration Hospital quite clearly demonstrated that the use of mupirocin to control endemic MRSA resulted in the recovery of MRSA *S. aureus* isolates exhibiting high level resistance to mupirocin [36]. In addition, recent reports have documented that mupirocin is only marginally effective in reducing MRSA nasal colonization and infections within an endemic environment. The precise role for this compound in the surgical patient population is yet to be determined. Clearly, *S. aureus* carriage appears to be a significant independent risk factor for surgical site infection following selected surgical procedures; however, further studies are needed to assess the most effective and judicious use of mupirocin in surgical patients. While it may be difficult to assess the relative importance of these intrinsic factors in the development of a postoperative surgical site infection, it is prudent to view each of these characteristics such as obesity, smoking and even age as factors that may potentially engender the risk of infection for our patients.

Table 48.2. Intrinsic (patient) and extrinsic (operation) risk factors that may influence the development of a surgical site infection

Intrinsic factors	Extrinsic factors
Patient gender	Site of surgery
Patient age	Surgical scrub
Nutritional status	Surgical skin prep
Diabetes – hyperglycemia	Hair removal
Smoking	Duration of surgery
Severity of disease – ASA score	Perioperative prophylaxis
Immunocompetence	OR ventilation
Weight	Drains and packs
Presence of other infections	Surgical attire and drapes
Microbial colonization	Surgical technique
Duration of preoperative stay	Poor hemostasis
Perioperative hypothermia	Dead space
	Tissue trauma

Several extrinsic factors have also been suggested as contributing to the risk of surgical site infections. The surgical site is an obvious factor since procedures involving the gastrointestinal tract will expose the wound to potential contamination involving a myriad of microbial population, while a breast biopsy will have a much lower risk for contamination. Skin asepsis and perioperative prophylaxis will be discussed in a separate section since both of these issues merit careful consideration when determining sentinel events that result in an increase in surgical site infection rates. Ongoing efforts to reduce the microbial burden in the operating room are viewed as a priority among healthcare professions. Current standards that direct a minimum of 15 air changes per hour in the operating room indicate the relative importance placed upon operating room ventilation as a potential risk factor for infection [37]. The standards that address room ventilation as well as policies and procedures for the disinfection and sterilization of surgical equipment and devices have reduced the iatrogenic sources of intraoperative contamination [38]. The importance of surgical attire as a risk factor for infection is a topic of some debate. The use of gowns, gloves and masks actually plays a twofold role in the operation room: (a) it protects the healthcare worker from contamination by blood and body fluids, and (b) it reduces the potential for microbial shedding, which may contaminate the operative field or devices inserted at the time of surgery [5]. Unlike the intrinsic or patient risk factors, many of the extrinsic risk factors influence the intraoperative level of microbial contamination. Efforts to reduce the level of microbial contamination in the OR have been universally viewed as appropriate and beneficial to reducing the overall risk of postoperative infection. Finally, the cornerstone for good surgical care resides with exquisite surgical technique and when coupled with judicious infection control practices results in reduced wound morbidity and favorable patient outcomes.

48.5 Strategies for the Prevention of Surgical Site Infections

48.5.1 Preoperative Skin Preparations

For over 100 years, surgeons, infectious disease experts and other health professionals have recognized that infections may be transmitted to patients within the operating room environment. Because of the luxurious nature of the microbial flora colonizing the surface of the skin, great attention has been paid to the surgical site and several antiseptic agents are available for preoperative disinfection of the incisional site. In general, preoperative skin preps should provide a broad spectrum of activity against both gram-positive and gram-negative bacteria. This is also true for agents that are used as hand and forearm scrubs. Table 48.3 lists the three agents currently used as surgical site preparations. Alcohol, chlorhexidine and iodine/iodophors all demonstrate excellent activity against gram-positive bacteria such as the staphylococci or enterococci. Alcohol demonstrates the best antiseptic activity against gram-negative bacteria compared to chlorhexidine and iodine/iodophor. At our institution we require our patients to bath the night before surgery with an antiseptic agent, which in most cases involves using a chlorhexidine gluconate soap. This is done to reduce the microbial burden on the surface of the body. While this may appear prudent, there are however no scientific studies validating this practice as efficacious in reducing the incidence of surgical site infections. Of all the various compounds that are used as antiseptic agents in the OR, chlorhexidine gluconate has the greatest residual activity and is not inactivated by blood or other body fluids [5].

Studies conducted in our laboratory using an FDA endorsed protocol demonstrate that a 3-min surgical prep with chlorhexidine results in at least 8 h of suppressed growth on the surface of unexposed skin (unpublished data). While chlorhexidine gluconate has been viewed as most effective as a surgical skin-preparation at a concentration of 4%, a recent clinical study has suggested that a chlorhexidine gluconate impregnated cloth at a concentration of 2% may be highly effective at reducing the microbial skin burden of selected HAI pathogens within a critical care patient population [39]. Further studies are warranted to determine the efficacy of this unique device in reducing the risk of surgical site infections. Likewise, aqueous alcohol at a concentration of 70–90% is germicidal against bacteria, fungi and viruses [40]. However, a distinct problem associated with using alcohol solutions in the operating room is the issue of flammability. Alcohol fires are dramatic when they occur and can be catastrophic within the operating room [41]. Alcohol, chlorhexidine and iodine/iodophors have also been formulated into surgical hand scrub solutions, and chlorhexidine in isopropyl alcohol has been found to exhibit excellent residual activity as a surgical hand scrub [42–45].

48.5.2 Antimicrobial Prophylaxis in Surgery

The perioperative use of antibiotic has become an essential standard of care for all operations or classes in which it has been shown to reduce the rate of SSI [46, 47]. The rules or principles governing the appropriate use of antimicrobial prophylaxis include the following [48, 49]:

1. There is a probable risk of infection in the absence of a prophylactic agent.
2. There is knowledge of the probable contaminating flora associated with operative wound or organ/space site.
3. The activity of the chosen prophylactic agent should encompass the majority of pathogens likely to contaminate the wound or organ/space site.
4. The prophylactic agent must be administered as a dose which provides an effective tissue concentration prior to intraoperative bacterial contamina-

Table 48.3. Antiseptic agents currently available for preoperative surgical skin prep (SSP) and surgical scrub (SS)

Agent	Spectrum of activity				Rapidity	Residual	Uses
	GP	GN	FN	VR			
Alcohol	E	E	G	G	Fast	None	SSP/SS
Chlorhexidine	E	G	F	G	Moderate	E	SSP/SS
Iodine/iodophors	E	G	G	G	Moderate	Minimal	SSP/SS
PCMX	G	F	F	F	Moderate	G	SS
Triclosan	G	G	P	U	Moderate	E	SS

GP gram-positive bacteria, *GN* gram-negative bacteria, *FN* fungi, *VR* virus, *E* excellent, *G* good, *F* fair, *P* poor, *U* unknown, *PCMX* parachlorometaxylenol

tion. Administration must occur 30–60 min prior to incision (usually with the induction of anesthesia).
5. The effective dose must be governed by the weight of the patient. For example with the cephalosporins, and patients weighing >70 kg, dosage should be doubled.
6. If the surgical procedure lasts ≤3 h, a single prophylactic dose is usually sufficient. However, procedures lasting >3 h require an additional effective dose. Procedures in which there is rapid blood loss and/or fluid administration will dictate more frequent dosing. Postoperative prophylaxis is strongly discouraged; there is no evidence to suggest that multiple doses are more efficacious at preventing postoperative surgical site infections than a single effective dose.

The first generation cephalosporin, cefazolin or the 2nd generation agent cefuroxime are frequently used as prophylactic agents for many clean-contaminated operations. In general, antimicrobial prophylaxis is discouraged for elective clean surgical cases. However, patients with comorbid risk factors such as diabetes, obesity or who are receiving concomitant immunosuppressive therapy may receive a single prophylactic dose when undergoing an elective surgical procedure. Patients undergoing an elective operation involving the distal gastrointestinal tract will usually receive one to two doses of either cefoxitin or cefotetan (2nd generation agents) which provides broad-spectrum coverage for any anticipated contaminants. The use of antibiotic prophylaxis for the insertion of a biomedical device is in general an exception to the clean surgery rule. Biomedical device-associated infections are often seen as catastrophic and recalcitrant to traditional antibiotic therapy; therefore administration of one to two perioperative antimicrobial doses is viewed as prudent in light of the perceived risk. Patients unable to receive a cephalosporin because of previous hypersensitivity reactions can be given either clindamycin or vancomycin for gram-positive coverage or aztreonam as an alternative for effective gram-negative coverage. Finally, vancomycin should never be used as a routine agent for prophylaxis unless there is evidence of MRSA clustering on the selected surgical service.

48.5.3 Administration of Blood, Oxygen and Normothermia in the Surgical Patient

It has been widely reported that the administration of blood perioperatively is associated with a twofold increase in the surgical wound infection rate in patients undergoing elective colon resection for cancer [50]. However, a closer examination of the data suggests that the rationale for withholding whole blood or blood products is fundamentally flawed since multivariate analysis was not performed on a myriad of confounding variables that may have influenced the study's outcome. Therefore, it is generally viewed as safe and appropriate to administer whole blood or blood products to patients during the intraoperative period.

Two recent multicentered studies have suggested that the intraoperative use of 80% supplemental oxygen followed by hyperoxia 2–6 h postoperatively results in a 50% reduction in the surgical site infection rate in selected clean/clean-contaminated surgical procedures [51, 52]. Elevating the percentage of inspired oxygen was viewed as beneficial for tissue perfusion and neutrophil function. This is a provocative hypothesis and while this technique may be viewed as somewhat avant-garde, the scientific foundation upon which it is based is fundamentally sound and merits further serious consideration by surgical practitioners.

Hypothermia in a surgical patient is defined as a body core temperature <36.0°C (96.8°F). Conditions and practices that contribute to surgical patient cooling include:

Skin prep solution	Thin gowns	Body surface exposure
Cool operating room table	Anesthesia	Cold irrigation (IV) fluids
Open wounds		

Hypothermia alters the body's ability to resist infection and therefore preserving core body temperature has been shown to reduce the risk of postoperative morbidity due to infection. The earliest study to document the relationship between hypothermia and SSIs was published in 1996, documenting that patients undergoing colorectal surgery with a mean intraoperative core temperature of 34.7°C had a 12% infection rate compared to 6% in the normothermia group [53]. Two recent studies in clean and clean-contaminated surgical cases clearly demonstrate that even mild hypothermia was associated with an increased risk for surgical site infections [54, 55]. These studies have suggested that, regardless of the type of surgery, maintaining normothermic temperatures (36.0–38.0°C) throughout the peri-, intra- and immediate postoperative period improves patient outcome by reducing morbidity due to infection.

48.6 Classification of Surgical Site Infections

Surgical wounds are classified into four groups based upon selected criteria developed by the National Academy of Science/National Research Council (NAS/NRC) [56]. *Class I* or "Clean" wounds represent an uninfected operative wound in which there is no inflammation and the hollow viscus sites such as the GI, urinary, respiratory or genital tract have not been breached. Clean wounds are primarily closed with closed drainage. *Class II* or "Clean-Contaminated" wounds may involve controlled entry into the GI, urinary, respiratory or genital tract in a manner where there is little or no contamination. Elective procedures involving the oropharynx, appendix or biliary tract are typical of Class II procedures providing no break in aseptic technique is encountered. *Class III* or "Contaminated" wounds involve procedures in which there has been a major break in sterile technique or there has been gross spillage of gastrointestinal contents. This classification includes: open, fresh, accidental wounds in which there may be evidence of acute inflammation. Finally, *Class IV* or "Dirty-Infected" wounds involve perforated viscera, tissues in which there is an existing infection, or traumatized devitalized tissues. In most cases, patients with Class IV wounds are already receiving antimicrobial therapy.

While the NAS/NRC classification has been helpful in defining which patients would benefit from antimicrobial prophylaxis, it does not provide us with standardized criteria for defining the site of infection. The Centers for Disease Control and Prevention have developed the National Nosocomial Infection Surveillance program, which utilizes standardized surveillance criteria for defining surgical site infections. Surgical site infections are now classified as either superficial incisional, deep incisional or organ space infection. Designation to one of three sites is defined as follows:

48.6.1 Superficial Incisional Surgical Infections

Any infection that occurs within 30 days postsurgical procedure and involves only the skin or subcutaneous tissue of the incision. In addition, at least one of the following must occur:

1. Purulent drainage from the superficial incisional site with or without laboratory confirmation.
2. Microorganisms are recovered from culture of tissue or fluid from the incisional site.
3. The wound is deliberately opened by the surgeon because of one of the following signs or symptoms of infection: pain or tenderness, swelling, redness or heat.
4. Surgeon or attending physician renders a diagnosis of infection.

Simple stitch abscesses, episiotomy wounds, infection burn wounds or SSI that involve the fascia and muscle layers are not defined as superficial SSIs.

48.6.2 Deep Incisional Surgical Site Infection

Any infection involving the deep soft tissues (fascia and muscle layers) that occurs within: (a) 30 days postsurgical procedure provided no biomedical device has been inserted, or (b) up to 1 year if a biomedical device has been inserted and the infection appears related to that device. In addition, at least one of the following must occur:

1. Purulent drainage originating from the deep incision.
2. Wound dehisces or is deliberately opened in response to fever, localized pain or tenderness.
3. There is an abscess or other clinical evidence of an infection of the deep incisional site.
4. A diagnosis of infection is made by the attending physician.

When the infection involves both the superficial and deep incision sites, the infection is reported as a deep incisional. Any organ/space surgical site infection that drains through the incision is reported as deep incisional.

48.6.3 Organ Space Surgical Site Infection

Any infection involving any part of the anatomy (organ or cavity space) other than the incision that occurs within: (a) 30 days postsurgical procedure provided no biomedical device has been inserted, or (b) up to 1 year if a biomedical device has been inserted and the infection appears related to that device. In addition, at least one of the following must occur:

1. Evidence of purulent drainage from a drain position through a stab wound into the organ space.
2. Recovery of bacterial from organ/space culture.
3. Evidence of abscess of infection of organ/space
4. A diagnosis of organ/space infection is made by the attending physician.

Examples of the classification of site-specific organ/spaces are presented in Table 48.4.

Table 48.4. Classification of site-specific organ/spaces for surveillance of surgical site infections

Arterial/venous infection	Eye (orbit)	Meningitis
Breast abscess	GI tract	Myocarditis
Ear, mastoid	Intracranial	Oral cavity
Endocarditis	Osteomyelitis	Sinusitis
Endometritis	Joint/bursa	Spinal abscess
Upper respiratory tract	Vaginal cuff	

48.7 Surveillance of Surgical Site Infections

Surveillance of surgical site infections is a sentinel component of an overall infection control strategy that involves collection, management, analysis and reporting of wound infection data in an effort to determine baseline HAI rates, which are reported to surgeons in an effort to reduce the surgical site infection risk. In the development of a surgical site surveillance program the overall goals must be clearly focused, addressing the priorities and objectives of the healthcare institution's infection control program. The National Nosocomial Infection Surveillance program has been an important resource for: (a) identifying the role of sentinel patient risk factors through stratification strategies, (b) establishing benchmark rates for specific surgical procedures, and (c) providing a primary reference for precise definitions of selected surgical site infections.

48.7.1 Predictors of Surgical Site Infections

Three categories have been established which are recognized as accurate predictors of surgical site infections. First, the level of potential microbial contamination of the surgical site during the intraoperative period is an important variable when assessing the relative risk of an SSI. This was briefly discussed in an earlier section and essentially involves classifying the surgical procedures based upon the NAS/NRC definitions of clean, clean-contaminated, contaminated and dirty. The second predictor is the duration of the operative procedure and the final predictor is the physiologic status of the host as measured by the ASA (American Society of Anesthesiology) score [57].

These three predictors in essence provide a risk index that is operation specific. The index ranges from 0 to 3 and is derived through assigning points based upon the following:

1. One point is assigned when the ASA score is ≥3; the ASA score ranges from 1 to 5 with a score of 1 defining a normally healthy patient, while a score of 5 is reflective of a patient who is not expected to survive for 24 h
2. One point is assigned whenever the operation is classified as either a "contaminated" or a "dirty" one based upon the NAS/NRC classification scheme.
3. One point is assigned if the surgical procedure lasts greater than a defined time interval, reflective of the 75th percentile durational period of the specific operation being performed.

Therefore, a patient with a risk index score of 0 would by definition have the lowest risk of infection for the specific surgical procedure. On the other hand, a score of 3 would place the patient within the highest risk category for that specific operation.

48.7.2 Surveillance Strategies

One of the weaknesses of the current surveillance program in US hospitals is that our data collection strategies are based upon reviewing inpatient surgical procedures. In our own institution, over 40% of surgical procedures are performed in the outpatient or ambulatory environment. This percentage is growing daily and presently in many communities there are free-standing facilities both pubic and private that exclusively perform outpatient surgeries. This has created a dilemma in the infection control communities; how do we best target our surveillance efforts in the current healthcare environment? In addition, most of the operations upon which the NNIS benchmark data is based involve data derived from traditional surgical (open) procedures. Rapid advances in the field of laparoscopic surgery within all of the surgical professions are not reflected within the NNIS data pool. Therefore, few if any benchmark rates are currently available for minimally invasive surgical procedures. This deficiency is currently under study; however, it will be several years before our surveillance teams have stratification rates reflective of these new minimally invasive technologies.

48.7.3 Inpatient Surveillance

Few if any healthcare facilities have the luxury of time, personnel and monetary resources to indulge in global surgical site surveillance. Many institutions practice a "targeted" type of surveillance of selected surgical procedures which may in part be based upon: (a) knowledge of surgical procedures performed upon high-risk patient populations, (b) concerns associated with selected surgical techniques (biomedical implantation), and (c) recognition of increased incidence of infection in selected patient or procedure specific populations [58]. Table 48.5 reports the surgical procedures currently selected for surveillance with our institution in 2000 and 2005. Selected surgical procedures are added or deleted from surveillance based upon volume, intrinsic risk of patient population, and prior history of surgical site infections. While "targeted" surveillance may address the historical or current infection trends, care must be taken so that no clusters or outbreaks are overlooked within those non-selected surgical procedures. It is also prudent to design your surveillance strategies so that a broad band of surgical disciplines are included in the census. Finally, flexibility is an inherent characteristic of a successful program since re-

Table 48.5. Surgical procedures selected for surveillance at Froedtert Memorial Lutheran Hospital, 2000 and 2005

Procedures	Operation cutpoint (h)	2000	2005
Abdominal hysterectomy	2	Yes	Yes
Hernia repair with mesh	2	Yes	No
Gastric bypass	4	Yes	Yes
Coronary bypass (chest)	5	Yes	Yes
Coronary bypass/valves	5	No	Yes
Valve replacement	5	No	No
Cesarean section	1	Yes	Yes
Colon surgery	3	Yes	Yes
Craniotomy/craniectomy	4	Yes	Yes
Vascular surgery	3	Yes	Yes
Fusion – cervical with implant	4	No	Yes
Fusion – lumbar with implant	4	Yes	Yes
Fusion – thoracic with implant	4	No	No
Hip replacement	2	Yes	Yes
Knee replacement	2	No	Yes
Kidney/pancreas transplant	7	Yes	No
Liver transplant	7	Yes	No

sources may have to be rapidly shifted in response to a dynamic change in surgical site infection rates, albeit service or procedure selected.

The preferred method as documented in the surgical literature for identifying a surgical site infection is direct observation of the surgical site by a trained practitioner. Infection control personnel (ICP) should be regular visitors to the clinical wards or units since visibility is essential for promoting trust and collegiality. It is also possible at this time for the ICP to interact with the attending physician and nursing staff or answer questions relative to specific policy or procedures. Also a visible presence in the patient care areas allows the infection control staff to observe sentinel infection control practices such as hand washing or adherence to isolation policies. Often the ICP is viewed as the harbinger of bad news rather than a colleague who is available as a clinical resource. Surgical site infections represent an adverse outcome that may upon reflection have been prevented. Direct observation is also beneficial since it allows the ICP to observe whether appropriate wound care practices are being used.

While direct observation represents the "best" of infection control practices, much of the data reported within the infection control literature is actually derived from indirect case-finding studies. Indirect measurements are represented by chart reviews, daily review of laboratory reports, pharmacy reports and "curbside" discussions with healthcare professions. Essentially any clinical resource is available for indirect audit; however, many of these strategies are stagnant in time since infections detected retrospectively after the patient has been discharged often leave a "cold trail" especially if the infection falls outside of a traditional cluster. Sorting out all of the potential intrinsic and extrinsic variables that may contribute to a surgical site infection after the patient has been discharged often leads to more questions than answers, if not inconclusive findings. Regardless of the surveillance strategy, institutions that utilize NNIS benchmarks tend to collect similar data such as date of operation, NNIS operative procedure category, surgeon and patient identifier, the usual patent demographics, duration of operation, wound class, ASA score, discharge date, etc.

48.7.4 Postdischarge and Outpatient Surveillance

Several studies have suggested that between 12% and 84% of SSIs can be detected after the patient has been discharged from the hospital [59, 60]. This creates a problem for most hospital-based infection control programs, especially if postdischarge follow-up occurs at a site remote to where the original operation was performed [61]. It would not be heretical to suggest that even the most diligent of infection control programs likely fails to capture anywhere from 25% to 40% of their surgical site infections, the majority of which are probably superficial incisional site infections. It is interesting to note that institutions which emphasize the use of clinical pathways to manage the routine "clinical continuum" are experiencing shorter hospital stays for selected procedures than hospitals relying upon traditional order and patient care directives. It is ironic that in an effort to improve the efficiency and quality of patient care, we are omitting significant outcome data for surgical patients. Several strategies have been proposed for capturing postdischarge data that include remote reviewing of clinic charts, and physician and/or patient surveys utilizing the mail or direct telephone contact. It is unsettling to contemplate that the credibility of an institution's surgical site surveillance program could possibly rest squarely upon the shoulders of a patient population that is required to assess their own wounds for infection [62].

One investigator has proposed that "electronic surveillance" of pharmacy records within an integrated health information system may offer the best possibilities for tracking surgical site infections after the patient has left the hospital [63]. At present, even under the best of scenarios, surveillance strategies that rely upon questionnaires or telephone surveys are probably failing to capture anywhere from 15% to 60% of infections postdischarge [64, 65]. It is evident that leadership is needed in this arena since at this time the CDC and other professional bodies can offer no clear guidance regarding which detection method should be used for postdischarge or outpatient surveillance. It is possible that future efforts may be focused on selecting a few "targeted" surgical procedures which are then intensely monitored with the result of this surveillance used to interpolate (indicator) the overall quality of the combined surgical services within the institution. While this approach may have several potential minefields, it may come to pass that selecting a few key surgical procedures with sufficient statistical power coupled to electronic surveillance may, in fact, be a plausible way to assess surgical site infection rates in the postdischarge and outpatient environments.

48.8 Some Final Thoughts on Wound Management and Infection Control Practices

The basic principles of effective surgical wound management are also grounded in appropriate infection control practices. It has long been recognized that the presence of necrotic debris in the wound can facilitate the growth of microorganisms [66]. Abscesses should be drained and any sinus tract excised. The principle that wounds that are kept moist, heal better than wounds left open has been a source of constant debate. When caring for the wound the clinical practitioner must avoid at all cost any contamination between themselves, other patients or multiple wounds on the same patient. All disposable or contaminated material must be placed in an appropriate labeled (biohazard) container [67].

Infection control practices vary widely between institutions. The use of sterile gloves and aseptic technique is well documented for the prevention of wound sepsis during the postoperative period. The Centers for Disease Control and Prevention has suggested that sterile gloves be used for the first 24 h of incisional care. However, no specific glove recommendations are offered for the management of postoperative wounds beyond this period. A recent survey found that nurses in acute care facilities were more likely to wear sterile gloves when managing postoperative surgical wounds beyond the 24-h postoperative window [68]. The use of chemically clean versus sterile gloves for managing wounds has emerged as a major discussion point primarily because of the issue of cost. The use of chemically clean but nonsterile gloves has been shown within our institution to be a major cost saving over sterile, individually wrapped surgical gloves. The impact of this strategy on infection control practices within an institution is debatable and subject to individual interpretation. Whether or not sterile or chemically clean gloves are used when caring for an open wound is likely dependent upon the type of wound or clinical setting. Sterile technique is indicated when managing wounds in immunosuppressed patients or open surgical wounds involving exposed organ/space sites.

There are at present several emerging technologies, which may impact upon infection control practices by reducing the potential for wound colonization/contamination in acute wounds. This includes the use of dressings that attempt to manipulate the biology of the wound and thereby accelerate normal wounds, which will have measurable infection control benefits. Another strategy has been the incorporation of antimicrobial or antiseptic substances into the matrix of the wound dressing. The incorporation of selected metals with antiseptic activity such as silver has potential intrinsic value in reducing wound contamination postoperative wounds such as sternal incisions. The ideal strategy might involve application of an active dressing that exhibits antiseptic properties while stimulating the activation of various cell types such as neutrophils or macrophages within the wound itself, thereby augmenting both the native inflammatory and maturation processes that occur as part of normal wound healing. Finally, over the past 15 years numerous antiseptic technologies have been applied to selected biomedical devices (central lines, Foley catheters, shunts, etc.), documenting a reduced risk for selected HAI in high-risk patient populations. This strategy has recently been applied to a surgical suture in an effort to reduce the risk of surgical wound infection [69]. Triclosan, a broad-spectrum antiseptic agent, has been applied to the surface of a selected braided suture, inhibiting the adherence of staphylococci to the surface of that device. The presence of a safe, antiseptic device within the wound bed has great appeal, especially in those surgical procedures where the risk of wound contamination is high [70, 71]. While innovative technology can play an important role in risk reduction, it should in all likelihood be an adjunctive component of a comprehensive strategy based upon the following surgical cornerstones, timely and appropriate antimicrobial prophylaxis, effective skin antisepsis and exquisite surgical technique.

It is obvious that the morbidity and mortality associated with surgical site infections has had an impact not only on patient care but also on those infection control practices that attempt to limit or reduce the acquisition/dissemination of HAI pathogens within the hospital environment.

References

1. Centers for Disease Control and Prevention, National Center for Health Statistics (1997) Vital and health statistics, detailed diagnoses and procedures, National Hospital Discharge Survey, 1994, vol 127. DHHS Publication, Hyattsville, MD
2. Emori TG, Gaynes RP (1993) An overview of nosocomial infections, including the role of the microbiology laboratory. Clin Microbiol Rev 6:428–432
3. Boyce JM, Potter-Bynoe G, Dziobek L (1990) Hospital reimbursement patterns among patients with surgical wound infections following open heart surgery. Infect Control Hosp Epidemiol 11:89–94
4. Engemann JJ, Carmeil Y, Cosgrove SE, Fowler VG, Bronstein MZ, Trivette SL, Briggs JP, Sexton DJ, Kaye KS (2003) Adverse and economic outcomes attributable to methicillin-

resistance among patients with *Staphylococcus aureus* surgical site infections. Clin Infect Dis 36:592 – 598
5. Mangram AJ, Horan TC, Pearson ML, Silver LC, Jarvis WR (1999) Hospital Infection Program, National Center for Infectious Diseases, Center for Disease Control and Prevention. Guidelines for prevention of surgical site infection. Am J Infect Control 27:97 – 132
6. National Nosocomial Infection Surveillance System (2004) National Nosocomial Infections Surveillance (NNIS) System report, data summary from January 1992 through June 2004, issues October 2004. Am J Infect Control 32:470 – 485
7. Troche G, Joly LM, Guibert M, Zazzo JF (2005) Detection and treatment of antibiotic-resistant bacterial carriage in a surgical intensive care unit: a 6-year prospective survey. Infect Control Hosp Epidemiol 26:161 – 165
8. Gaynes RP (1997) Surveillance of nosocomial infections: a fundamental ingredient for quality. Infect Control Hosp Epidemiol 18:475 – 478
9. Fridkins SK, Gaynes RP (1999) Antimicrobial resistance in intensive care units. Clin Chest Med 20:303 – 316
10. Kourbatova EV, Halvosa JS, King MD, Ray SM, White N, Blumberg HM (2005) Emergence of community-associated methicillin resistant *Staphylococcus aureus* USA 300 clone as a cause of healthcare-associated infections among patients with prosthetic joint infections. Am J Infect Control 33:385 – 391
11. Turco TF, Meldo GP, Williams R (1998) Vancomycin intermediate-resistant *Staphylococcus aureus*, Ann Pharmacother 32:758 – 760
12. Kollef MH, Rello J, Cammarata SK, et al. (2004) Clinical cure and survival of Gram-positive ventilator-associated pneumonia: retrospective analysis of two double-blind studies comparing linezolid with vancomycin. Intensive Care Med 30:388 – 394
13. Steenbergen JN, Alder J, Thorne GM, Tally FP (2005) Daptomycin: a lipopeptide antibiotic for the treatment of serious Gram-positive infections. J Antimicrob Agents Chemother 55:283 – 288
14. Edmiston CE, Seabrook GR, Cambria RA, Brown KR, Lewis BD, Sommers JR, Krepel CJ, Wilson PJ, Sinski SA, Towne JB (2005) Molecular epidemiology of microbial contamination in the operating room environment: is there a risk for infection? Surgery 138:572 – 588
15. Centers for Disease Control and Prevention (1993) Nosocomial enterococci resistant to vancomycin – United States, 1989 – 1993. MMWR 42:597 – 599
16. Gin AS, Zhanel GG (1996) Vancomycin-resistant enterococci. Ann Pharmacother 30:615 – 624
17. Hospital Infection Program, Hospital Infection Control Advisory Committee (1995) Recommendations for preventing the spread of vancomycin-resistance. Infect Control Hosp Epidemiol16:105 – 113
18. Tenover FC, McGowan JE (1996) Reasons for the emergence of antibiotic resistance. Am J Med Sci 311:9 – 16
19. Fridkin SK, Hill HA, Volkova NV, Edwards JR, Lawton RM, Gaynes RP, McGowan JE (2002) Temporal changes in prevalence of antimicrobial resistance in 23 US hospitals. Emerg Infect Dis 8:697 – 701
20. Altemeier WA, Culbertson WR, Hummel RP (1968) Surgical consideration of endogenous infections – sources, types, and methods of control. Surg Clin North Am 48:227 – 240
21. Wiley AM, Haleri GB (1979) Routes of infection: a study of using "tracer particles" in the operating room. Clin Orthop 139:150 – 155
22. Edmiston CE, Sinski S, Seabrook G, Simons D, Goheen M (1999) Airborne particulates in the OR environment. AORNJ 69:1169 – 1183
23. Krizek TJ, Robson MC (1975) Evolution of quantitative bacteriology in wound management. Am J Surg 130: 579 – 584
24. James RC, MacLeod CJ (1961) Induction of staphylococcal infections in mice with small inoculum introduced on sutures. Br J Exp Pathol 42:266 – 277
25. Mullens JL, Gertner MH, Buzby GP, Goodhart GL, Rosato EF (1979) Implications of malnutrition in the surgical patient. Arch Surg 114:121 – 125
26. Campos AC, Mequid MM (1992) A critical appraisal of the usefulness of perioperative nutrition support. Am J Clin Nutr 55:117 – 130
27. Winsor JA, Hill GL (1988) Protein depletion and surgical risk. Aust NZ J Surg 58:711 – 715
28. Lilienfeld DE, Vlahov D, Tenney JH, McLaughlin JS (1988) Obesity and diabetes as risk factors for postoperative wound infections after cardiac surgery. Am J Infect Control 16:3 – 6
29. Terranova A (1991) The effect of diabetes mellitus on wound healing. Plast Surg Nurs 11:20 – 25
30. Talbot TR (2005) Diabetes mellitus and cardiothoracic surgical site infections. Am J Infect Control 33:353 – 359
31. Zerr KJ, Furnay AP, Grunkemeier GL, Bookin S, Kanhere V, Starr A (1997) Glucose control lowers the risk of wound infection in diabetics after open heart operations. Ann Thorac Surg 63:356 – 361
32. Krinsley JS (2004) Effect of an intensive glucose management protocol on mortality of critically ill adult patients. Mayo Clin Proc 79:992 – 1000
33. Sung J, Bochicchio GV, Joshi M, Bochicchio K, Tracy K, Scalea M (2005) Admission hyperglycemia is predictive of outcome in critically ill trauma patients. J Trauma 59: 80 – 83
34. Kluytmans JA, Mouton JW, Ijzerman EP, Vandenbroucke-Grauls CM, Maat AW, Wagenvoot JH, et al. (1995) Nasal carriage of *Staphylococcus aureus* as a major risk factor for wound infections after cardiac surgery. J Infect Dis 171: 216 – 219
35. Kluytmans JA, Mouton JW, VandeBergh MF, Manders MJ, Maat AP, et al. (1996) Reduction of surgical site infections in cardiothoracic surgery by elimination of nasal carriage of *Staphylococcus aureus*. Infect Control Hosp Epidemiol 17:780 – 785
36. Vasquez JE, Walker ES, Franzus BW, Overbay BK, Reagan DR, Sarubbi FA (2000) The epidemiology of mupirocin resistance among methicillin-resistant *Staphylococcus aureus* at a Veterans' Affairs Hospital. Infect Control Hosp Epidemiol 21:459 – 464
37. American Institute of Architects (1999) Guidelines for design and construction of hospitals and health care facilities. American Institute of Architects Press, Washington, DC
38. Centers for Disease Control and Prevention (1992) Postsurgical infections associated with nonsterile implantable devices. MMWR 41:263
39. Vernon MO, Hayden MK, Trick WE, Hayes RA, Blom DW, Weinstein RA (2006) Chlorhexidine gluconate to cleanse patients in a medical intensive care unit. Arch Intern Med 166:306 – 312
40. Larson E (1988) Guidelines for use of topical antimicrobial agents. Am J Infect Control 16:253 – 266
41. Hardin WD, Nichol RL (1997) Handwashing and patient skin preparation. In: Malangoni MA (ed) Critical issues in operating room management. Lippincott-Raven, Philadelphia, pp 133 – 149
42. Larson EL (1995) APIC guidelines for handwashing and hand antisepsis in health care settings. Am J Infect Control 23:251 – 269

43. Wade JJ, Casewell MW (1991) The evaluation of residual antimicrobial activity on hands and its clinical relevance. J Hosp Infect 18 (Suppl B):23 – 28
44. Grabsch EA, Mitchell DJ, Hooper J, Turnidge JD (2004) In-use efficacy of a chlorhexidine in alcohol surgical rub: a comparative study. ANZ J Surg 74:769 – 772
45. Adams D, Quayum M, Worthington T, Lambert P, Elliot T (2005) Evaluation of a 2 % chlorhexidine gluconate in 70 % isopropyl alcohol skin disinfectant. J Hosp Infect 61: 287 – 290
46. Wittman DH, Condon RE (1991) Prophylaxis of postoperative infections. Infection 19:S337–S344
47. Nichols RL (1982) Postoperative wound infections. N Engl J Med 307:1701 – 1710
48. FMLH Suggested Recommendations and Guidelines for Surgical Prophylaxis (2005) Froedtert Memorial Lutheran Hospital Antibiotic Utilization Guidelines. Froedtert Memorial Lutheran Hospital, Milwaukee, WI
49. Bratzler DW, Houck PM, Richard C, Steele L, Dellinger EP, Fry DE, Wright C, Ma A, Carr K, Red L (2005) Use of antimicrobial prophylaxis for major surgery. Arch Surg 140: 174 – 182
50. Vamvakas EC, Carven JH, Hibberd PL (1996) Blood transfusion and infection after colorectal surgery. Transfusion 36:1000 – 1008
51. Grief R, Akca O, Horn EP, Kurz A, Sessler DL (2000) Supplemental perioperative oxygen to reduce the incidence of surgical-wound infections. Outcomes Research Group. N Engl J Med 342:161 – 167
52. Belda EJ, Aguilera L, de la Asuncion JG, Alberti J, Vicente R, Ferrandiz L, Rodriguez R, Company R, Sessler DI, Aguilar G, Botello SG, Orti R (2005) Supplemental perioperative oxygen and the risk of surgical wound infection. JAMA 294:2035 – 2042
53. Kurz A, Sessler DI, Lenhardt R (1996) Perioperative normothermia to reduce the incidence of surgical wound infection and shorten hospitalization. N Engl J Med 334: 1209 – 1215
54. Melling AC, Ali B, Scott EM, Leaper DJ (2001) Effects of preoperative warming on the incidence of wound infection after clean surgery: a randomized controlled trial. Lancet 358:876 – 880
55. Flores-Maldonado A, Medina-Escobedo C, Rios-Rodriguez HMG, Fernandez-Dominguez R (2001) Mild perioperative hypothermia and the risk of wound infection. Arch Med Res 32:227 – 231
56. Berard F, Gandon J (1964) Postoperative wound infections: the influence of ultraviolet irradiation of the operating room and various other factors. Ann Surg 160 (Suppl 1): 1 – 192
57. SHEA, APIC, CDC, SIS (1992) Consensus paper on the surveillance of surgical wound infections. Infect Control Hosp Epidemiol 13:599 – 605
58. Pottinger JM, Herwaldt LA, Perl TM (1997) Basics of surveillance – an overview. Infect Control Hosp Epidemiol 18:513 – 527
59. Law DJ, Mishriki SF, Jeffery PJ (1990) The importance of surveillance after discharge from the hospital in the diagnosis of postoperative wound infection. Ann R Coll Surg Engl 72:207 – 209
60. Weigelt JA, Dryer D, Haley RW (1992) The necessity and efficiency of wound surveillance after discharge. Arch Surg 127:77 – 82
61. McKibben L, Horan T, Tokars JI, Fowler G, Cardo DM, Pearson ML, Brennan PJ (2005) Guidance on public reporting of healthcare-associated infections: recommendations of the healthcare infection control practices advisory committee. Am J Infect Control 33:217 – 226
62. Seaman M, Lammers R (1991) Inability of patients to self-diagnose wound infections. J Emerg Med 9:215 – 219
63. Sands K, Vineyard G, Platt R (1996) Surgical site infections occurring after hospital discharge. J Infect Dis 173: 963 – 970
64. Fanning C, Johnston BL, MacDonald S, LeFort-Jost S, Dokkerty E (1999) Postdischarge surgical site surveillance. Can J Infect Control 10:75 – 79
65. Zoutman D, Pearce P, McKenzie M, Taylor G (1990) Surgical wound infections occurring in day surgery patients. Am J Infect Control 18:277 – 282
66. Robson MC (1997) A failure of wound healing caused by an imbalance of bacteria. Surg Clin N Am 77:637 – 650
67. Witte MB, Barbul A (1997) General principles of wound healing. Surg Clin N Am 77:509 – 529
68. Wise LC, Hoffman J, Grant L, Bostrum J (1997) Nursing wound care survey: sterile and nonsterile glove choice. J Wound Ost Cont Nurs 24:144 – 150
69. Storch ML, Rothenburger SJ, Jacinto SJ (2004) Experimental efficacy study of coated Vicryl Plus® antibacterial sutures in guinea pigs challenged with *Staphylococcus aureus*. Surg Infect 5:281 – 288
70. Ford HR, Jones P, Gaines B, Reblock K, Simpkins DL (2005) Intraoperative handling and wound healing: controlled clinical trial comparing coated Vicryl Plus® suture. Surg Infect 6:313 – 321
71. Edmiston CE, Seabrook GR, Goheen MP, Krepel C, Lewis BD, Brown KR, Towne JB (2006) Bacterial adherence to surgical sutures: can antibacterial-coated sutures reduce the risk of microbial contamination? J Am Coll Surgeons 203:481 – 489

Chapter 49

Severe Soft Tissue Infections: A Syndrome-Based Approach

49

A. Sitges-Serra

49.1 Introduction

Severe soft tissue infections (SSTI) rank among the most common and potentially dangerous infections that can be acquired either in the community or in the hospital. Community-acquired SSTI may occur in previously healthy people but most often are diagnosed in immunocompromised patients, in patients with advanced cancer, with diabetes, receiving steroids or with AIDS. Diabetic patients are particularly susceptible to SSTI acquired at home probably as a result of tissue ischemia secondary to micro- or macroangiopathy. Healthy individuals may develop SSTI either spontaneously, after trauma or after insect or animal bites. SSTI developing in hospitalized patients often represent a postoperative complication, particularly of emergency operations, in patients with severe trauma, intra-abdominal infections or vascular disease. Patients undergoing solid organ transplantation may also develop insidious and severe infections of the soft tissues, for example, mucormycosis. Finally, bed-ridden patients may develop SSTI complicating decubitus ulcers.

49.2 Depth of Infection and Time Evolution

There are several well-characterized clinical syndromes revealing the presence of an SSTI. These should be familiar to all practitioners dealing with ill patients since appropriate recognition and early treatment may be live saving or, at least, may prevent the development of severe systemic complications. For this reason, SSTI will be presented in this chapter as separate clinical syndromes characterized by four fundamental parameters: the presence of systemic symptoms, the macroscopic appearance, the depth of microbial invasion (assessed by physical examination and/or surgical exploration) and the time from onset to overt disease. These are the most useful clinical guides helping the clinician in making a good differential diagnosis and appropriately treating SSTI. In particular, clinicians should be able to recognize the layer or layers of soft tissue involved: the skin, the fatty subcutaneous tissue, the muscular fascia and the muscle itself. In addition, an appropriate assessment of the *tempo* (a musical term used to designate the speed and *brio* that should be employed to interpret a score) of the infection is also of paramount importance. Many SSTI progress quite rapidly and may cause serious systemic complications if therapy is not instituted early enough.

49.3 When Should a Severe Soft Tissue Infection Be Suspected?

Mild dermal and subdermal infections are rather common in primary care and are usually the result of minor trauma (superficial wound infections, puerperal mastitis, paronychia) or may develop into abnormal anatomical structures (pilonidal sinus, omphalitis, perianal abscess). These are well-circumscribed suppurative lesions that respond to standard therapy with oral antibiotics and/or surgical drainage. These minor common infections are to be distinguished from the most severe forms that may either complicate an apparently superficial infection in an immunocompromised host or start de novo with an aggressive clinical picture. When examining a patient with a soft tissue infection, there are several hints that should lead the clinician to suspect that he or she is dealing with an SSTI rather than a mild one. These can be summarized as follows:

49.3.1 Systemic Symptoms

High fever, tachycardia and prostration are often found in patients with SSTI such as streptococcal gangrene, necrotizing fasciitis or gas gangrene. In addition, these patients may progress rapidly to septic/toxic shock and die within a few hours no matter what treatment they receive.

49.3.2
Skin Lesions: Necrosis or Bullae

The presence of skin lesions, particularly of bullae or necrosis, is typical of some syndromes of SSTI such as necrotizing cellulitis or severe *Streptococcus pyogenes* infections. Necrotic tissues are often gray to black colored, do not bleed and are not painful when incised with a scalpel. Bullae are also found in some SSTI and in these cases the skin lesion usually reveals a deeper involvement.

49.3.3
Crepitation

Crepitus is a typical sign of SSTI due to gas-producing microorganisms. Once mechanical causes of crepitation are ruled out (lung lesion, magnesium salts, accidental subdermal air injection), infection is the most probable cause of this ominous sign. Crepitation is not a pathognomonic sign of *Clostridium* spp. infections since it can also be observed in infections due to gas-forming Enterobacteriaceae such as *E. coli* (i.e., crepitant cellulitis). A mixed flora producing necrotizing fasciitis causes subcutaneous crepitation in roughly 25% of cases.

49.3.4
Progressing Disease

Skin lesions that do not heal after an "appropriate" initial treatment characterize some SSTI. A non-healing perineal incision after debridement of a seemingly banal perianal abscess may signal the presence of a necrotizing fasciitis due to a mixed enteric flora, particularly in diabetic or immunocompromised patients. In other circumstances, as happens in cases of Meleney's synergistic gangrene, necrosis progresses and the lesion tends to expand centrifugally despite a seemingly appropriate antibiotic therapy.

49.3.5
Absence of Pus

From the Hippocratic empiric days to the days of Ambroise Paré in the sixteenth century, suppuration of a wound was considered an essential phase of the normal healing process and regarded as a good prognostic sign (*pus bonum et ludabile)*. Time has proved that surgeons of the classical period were essentially right since most SSTI are not associated with the production of pus. Instead, they are characterized by the presence of a gray or brown fluid discharge that in the case of *Clostridium* spp. infections or mixed infections with anaerobic gram negative bacilli is typically foul smelling.

49.4
Physical Exploration

Adequate assessment of the extension and depth of an SSTI cannot be achieved if the lesions are not thoroughly explored. If there is not a preexistent surgical wound and surgical drainage is not indicated, soft tissue infections are explored superficially. Tenderness, edema and dermal necrosis should be looked for. If present, crepitation is a revealing sign of the severity of a soft tissue infection. If SSTI arise in a preexistent surgical wound or if surgical drainage is indicated, a thorough exploration is mandatory. Inspecting a wound should be carried out with sterile gloves. Stitches must be removed. The wound margins should be opened wide and the color and consistency of the fatty tissue noted. Necrotizing cellulitis is characterized by a grayish to black discoloration of the subcutaneous fat. The index finger should be used to look for separation of the subcutaneous fat from the muscular fascia, an ominous sign typical of necrotizing fasciitis. Gentle lateral pressure with the fingertip is exerted deep in the wound. If the tissues do not offer resistance, the gloved finger easily dissects the plane existing between the subcutaneous fat and the muscle. Muscle state should be assessed by opening the fascia. There may be massive muscular edema with a compartmental syndrome and then the muscle herniates through the fascial incision. This happens preferentially in whole-thickness Group A streptococcal infections (often called streptococcal "gangrene"). In cases of muscle necrosis (clostridial myonecrosis), the muscle appears gray instead of pink red and does not bleed when cut.

In all circumstances, physical exploration of an SSTI should reach the limits of the lesion until healthy tissues are found. This is an essential part of the surgical treatment of SSTI. Failure to identify the limits of the infection also means failure to actually debride and excise all the infected or necrotic tissue, a common cause of treatment failure.

49.5
Microbiology and Pathogenesis

Many microorganisms may cause SSTI. The gram-positive cocci *S. aureus* and *Str. pyogenes* rank among the most commonly involved bacteria. *S. aureus* is usually implicated in less severe forms of tissue infections above the diaphragm such as puerperal mastitis, anthrax or paronychia, but it is also commonly involved in more severe lower limb infections in old people and in diabetics, often as the MRSA variant. In immunocompromised hosts, it may cause pyomyositis or extensive soft tissue infections as a result of surgical wound or catheter site infections ("tunnelitis"). *Str. pyogenes* is responsible for relatively minor superficial infections (impetigo, erysipelas) but is also responsible for whole-thickness extremely SSTI in previously healthy individuals, in surgical wounds, in limbs with lymphedema and in neutropenic patients. Other gram-positive cocci involved, mostly in infections developing after animal or human bites, are the anaerobic streptococci (peptostreptococci) and *Str. viridans*. The particularly virulent association of anaerobic or microaerophilic streptococci with *S. aureus* was originally reported by Frank Meleney [1] as the cause of one of the most representative SSTI: progressive synergistic gangrene.

A mixed flora involving enteric bacteria (*B. fragilis*, Enterobacteriaceae, *E. faecalis*) is often found in necrotizing infections arising in the perineal area due to anal or urogenital disease. Other gram negative non-fermenting bacilli may be recovered from SSTI. Dog bites may be occasionally complicated by *Capnocytophaga canimorsus* infection. *P. aeruginosa* may be recovered from mixed necrotizing infections.

Anaerobic gram-positive bacilli of the genus *Clostridium* (*C. perfringens*, *C. septicum*, *C. novyi*) are both involved in severe suppurative infections or as part of a mixed enteric flora causing necrotizing fascitis and in gas gangrene, a fulminant, predominantly muscular, highly lethal necrotizing infection.

Finally, fungus of the order Mucorales are involved in whole thickness infections in severely immunocompromised hosts, usually receptors of solid organ transplantation.

The pathogenesis of SSTI is multifactorial. The three most important determinant factors influencing the clinical manifestations and the time evolution are the following:

49.5.1 Intrinsic Virulence of the Microorganism: Toxic Shock

Some of the bacteria involved in SSTI are extremely virulent due to their having exotoxins that can trigger both a systemic inflammatory reaction and a local devastating disease due to extensive and rapidly spreading inflammation and superimposed ischemia due to vascular compression or thrombosis. Apparently superficial or even occult skin infections (up to 20% of cases) due to *Str. pyogenes* or *S. aureus* may cause a severe systemic response characterized as the toxic shock syndrome. Patients are profoundly ill and may develop sudden shock and rash associated with multiorgan failure, particularly acute renal failure. Other clinical findings include fever, diffuse macular erythroderma and desquamation.

Some Group A *Str. pyogenes* secrete potent pyrogenic exotoxins that play a major role in the pathogenesis of toxic shock. The production of these exotoxins is enhanced by the M protein, also an inhibitor of phagocytosis. The *spe* exotoxins exert their effects in two ways: they stimulate mononuclear cells and they interact with T lymphocytes as "superantigens," namely, antigens that do not require pre-processing by monocytes and bind directly to the major histocompatibility complex class II molecules on the surface of T cells. This occurs in a much higher proportion of T cells (5–20%) than would happen in a regular pre-processed antigen presentation. Clonal proliferation of this large T-cell subset results in the massive release of lymphokines. As a consequence of mononuclear and T-cell activation, production of TNF-α and β, IL-1, IL-2 and IL-6 is triggered, resulting in multiple organ dysfunction and shock [2, 3].

49.5.2 Tissular or Environmental Factors

Good tissue perfusion is an essential component of the local defense mechanisms preventing bacterial proliferation and invasion by providing the necessary elements to support the in situ antibacterial response: leukocytes, macrophages, complement, nutrients and oxygen. Tissue ischemia is an essential determinant factor for invasive *Clostridium* spp. infections and infections complicating ischemic limbs, particularly in the diabetic patient. Gas gangrene almost always develops on necrotic and devitalized tissues resulting from severe trauma, vascular disease, inappropriate surgery or unresected gangrenous bowel. More rarely, clostridial myonecrosis may develop spontaneously due to *C. septicum* bacteremia arising from an unsuspected colonic cancer [4] or minor injuries such as intramuscular injections. Once *Clostridium* spp. proliferate in the ischemic tissues, they release many potent exotoxins such as lecithinase, which destroys cell membranes and causes hemolysis and diffuse tissue damage, or θ-toxin, which seems to be the main factor responsible for muscle tissue necrosis.

Foreign bodies facilitate the proliferation of bacteria within the biofilm formed on their surfaces that, in addition, protects the microorganisms from local host defenses. Prosthetic materials or foreign bodies in close contact with the bowel may induce bacterial translocation through local inflammation of the intestinal wall [5] Thus, in some circumstances foreign materials may be the main trigger of an SSTI initiated in deep tissues or cavities.

Defective lymphatic drainage is a well-known tissue factor increasing the susceptibility to infections. *Str. pyogenes*, in particular, shows a marked preference for edematous limbs (arm edema after mastectomy, lower limb edema and ulcer due to venous insufficiency).

Obesity may also play a major role in favoring bacterial proliferation in the relatively hypovascularized fatty tissue. In addition, SSTI may be more difficult to

Table 49.1. Associated conditions which may impair the inflammatory response and facilitate the origin and spreading of soft tissue infections

Treatment with steroids
Treatment with immunosuppressors
Disseminated cancer
AIDS
Organ transplantation
Neutropenia
Chemotherapy
Polytrauma
Multiorgan failure
Diabetes mellitus
Old age

eradicate in obese individuals for obvious anatomical reasons.

49.5.3 The Host Factor

Patients with a blunted inflammatory/immune response (Table 49.1) are at high risk of developing an SSTI even after a minor injury or as a complication of a superficial infection (i.e., perirectal abscess, phlebitis, appendectomy wound). Absence of a cellular and humoral immune and inflammatory response at the site of a primary infection results in failure of the host to circumscribe the septic focus, rapid spreading of bacteria and impressive skin lesions. Patients with neutropenia or on high-dose steroids may harbor a spontaneous or postoperative SSTI with few, if any, local inflammatory changes.

49.6 Initiating Factors

49.6.1 Spontaneous Infections

Absence of a definite, clinically obvious, portal of entry is not uncommon for necrotizing fasciitis, pyomyositis or severe streptococcal infections. In some of these cases minor breaches allowing bacteria to penetrate the tissues can be identified such as perianal fistula, prostatitis or minimal dermal abrasions on the upper or lower extremities. In necrotizing perineal infections, anal, urological or genital disease is the usual responsible cause of the infection. A perirectal abscess, as the initial septic focus, is involved in about 50% of cases [6]. Necrotizing fasciitis of the neck region, potentially extending to the mediastinum, is usually secondary to a protracted dental infection involving the second or third mandibular molars or to a progression of a retropharyngeal abscess secondary to trauma [7]. Exceptionally, even gas gangrene may occur without an apparent focus in patients with colonic malignancies (see below).

49.6.2 Postoperative Infections

Almost all syndromes of SSTI can develop in surgical wounds. Severe streptococcal infections may complicate minor surgical interventions such as meniscectomy or herniorrhaphy. Gas gangrene may occur after surgery of the appendix, small bowel or colon. Necrotic bowel left in situ and conservative limb amputation for ischemic vascular disease are two of the procedures that carry a higher risk of postoperative gas gangrene. Necrotizing fasciitis can follow abdominal surgery, often of the septic type, mostly in debilitated and diabetic patients.

49.6.3 Post-traumatic Infections

SSTI often follow complex trauma of the extremities or trauma involving the abdominal viscera. Clostridial myonecrosis was once the paradigm of this syndrome and was responsible for many deaths, particularly following war injuries. Modern trauma management, including broad spectrum antibiotic therapy and early excision of all devitalized tissues, has almost eliminated this dreaded infection. In the late 1970s, however, it was still the first cause of gas gangrene in a referral unit [6]. Insect or dog bites may cause Meleney's gangrene in healthy individuals. Dog and human bites are also a well known antecessor of SSTI due to the very high bacterial colonization of the oral cavity in which anaerobes outnumber aerobes by $1/10^3$–10^6.

49.6.4 Drug Abuse

An increasing number of cases of SSTI, usually of the upper extremities, are observed in parenteral drug abusers with or without AIDS. These may present initially as a local subcutaneous abscess that may lead the clinician to ignore a deeper infection involving the fascia and muscle. Mortality in this type of patients can be as high as 20% [8].

49.6.5 Fistula Arising from the Gastrointestinal Tract

Colonic cancer, acute appendicitis and sigmoid diverticulitis may give rise to a necrotizing infection as a first clinical manifestation. This is preceded by inflammatory adhesion to the abdominal wall and fistulization of the bowel lumen to the muscles and subcutaneous fat of the lower abdomen, the groin or even the upper third of the thigh if the infection follows the plane of the psoas muscle [9].

49.7 Classification, Etiology and Management of the Main Clinical Syndromes

There have been numerous attempts to classify SSTI to help clinicians better diagnose and treat these disorders. Some authors have used a microorganism-based approach but this is not entirely satisfactory since some SSTI syndromes are due to a specific bacterium (i.e., streptococcal severe infections or clostridial myonecrosis) while others are not (Meleney's gangrene, necrotizing fasciitis). In Table 49.2 we put forward a classification that combines depth of infection (layer or layers predominantly affected) with the time course. Some bacteria-specific syndromes such as pyoderma gangrenosum due to *P. aeruginosa*, carbuncle due to *B. anthracis* or erysipeloid will not be discussed.

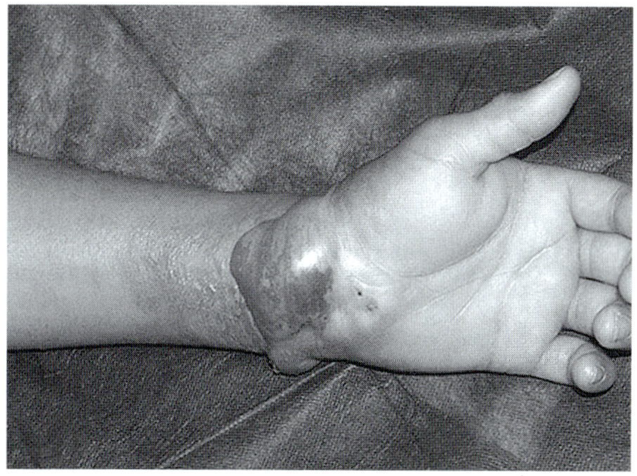

Fig. 49.1. Whole thickness *Streptococcus pyogenes* infection after local trauma. The patient was treated with debridement, penicillin and clindamycin

49.7.1 Cellulitis (Dermal and Subdermal Infections)

Group A *Streptococcus pyogenes* is a relatively common cause of less severe cellulitis (erysipelas) which is easily diagnosed on the basis of a typical clinical picture (high fever, erythema and pain) and responds to penicillin therapy (4 million units/4 h). Streptococcal cellulitis should be differentiated from *S. aureus* purulent infection. Presence of regional enlarged nodes and systemic symptoms (high fever and malaise) with a short incubation period are most often found in streptococcal infections. Blisters or bullae can also be found although, in our experience, these are more characteristic of whole-thickness streptococcal infections (Fig. 49.1).

Suprafascial SSTI are represented mainly by three major syndromes: necrotizing cellulitis, crepitant cellulitis and Meleney's gangrene.

Necrotizing cellulitis is a rare rapidly progressing skin and subcutaneous fat necrosis usually due to a mixed flora involving Enterobacteriaceae, gram positive cocci, *Bacteroides* spp. and even *Clostridium* spp. It is characterized by necrosis of the deep fatty subcutaneous tissue layer progressing centrifugally and to the skin. Dermal involvement is seen with patchy areas of necrosis and erythema. There is no necrosis of the underlying fascia or muscle. Severe toxicity is the rule and the disease usually runs a rapid and fatal course. It has been reported as a postoperative complication of different surgical procedures often involving the abdominal wall (cholecystectomy, colectomy, hysterectomy). It can also involve the extremities as a result of trauma. Wide spectrum antibiotic therapy (i.e., piperacillin-tazobactam 12 g/day plus vancomycin 500 mg/8 h) needs to be instituted immediately and appropriate samples for culture obtained as soon as possible. Extensive excision of the skin and subcutaneous tissue needs to be carried out leaving exposed wide fascial surfaces requiring a local treatment similar to that of infected burn wounds after scar excision.

Table 49.2. A classification of severe soft tissue infections based on the depth of infection and the time course

	Rapid (<72 h)	Subacute (<7 days)
Skin and dermis	Erysipelas Necrotizing cellulitis Crepitant cellulitis	Meleney's gangrene (progressive synergistic gangrene)
Fascia	Necrotizing fasciitis	Necrotizing fasciitis
Muscle	Gas gangrene Post-traumatic Postoperative Spontaneous	Pyomyositis
All layers	Gas gangrene Streptococcal gangrene	Diabetic foot/leg Mucormycosis

Crepitant cellulitis is usually due to gas-forming *E. coli*, *Streptococcus* spp., *Bacteroides fragilis* or *Clostridium* spp. The hallmark of this syndrome is absence of skin lesions in a febrile patient with local tenderness and crepitation. These are most commonly found in: (1) surgical wounds of the abdomen, and (2) in lower limbs of diabetic patients [10]. Deeper microbial invasion should be ruled out and a gram stain of the exudate may help to establish the diagnosis between clostridial and non-clostridial crepitant cellulitis. Treatment consists of antibiotics, debridement and, eventually, limb revascularization or amputation.

Meleney's synergistic gangrene is a form of progressive subacute necrotizing cellulitis characterized by an enlarging wound which demarcates into three zones (Fig. 49.2): a wide peripheral zone of erythema surrounding a tender purple zone, the center of which becomes black and necrotic with subsequent ulceration (Meleney's "ulcer"). There may be no or little systemic

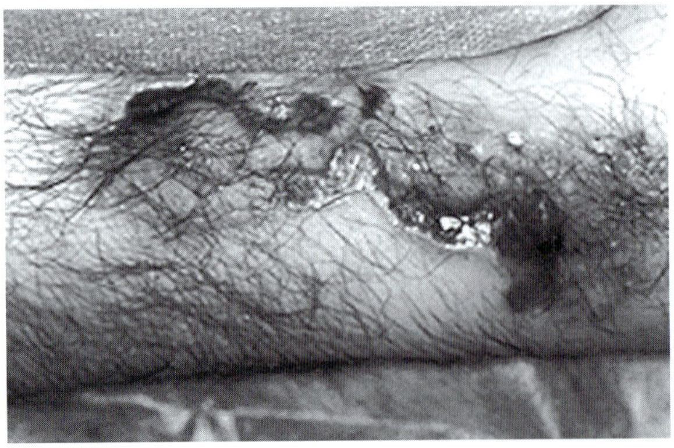

Fig. 49.2. Meleney's gangrene around a radial arterial catheter skin entry site in a patient with head trauma treated with high-dose steroids. Culture grew *Enterococcus faecalis*

toxicity. In healthy people, SSTI may be caused by insect or dog bites. Meleney's gangrene may also complicate a surgical or a venipuncture wound. From the bacteriological point of view, Meleney's ulcer usually results from the synergistic action of an anaerobic or microaerophilic microorganism with an aerobic one. A characteristic combination is that of *Peptostreptococcus* with *S. aureus*, but Enterobacteriaceae and other anaerobes may also be involved. Meleney's ulcer enlarges in a period of days and may not respond to antibiotic therapy if the central necrosis is not excised. The muscle fascia is usually preserved. Decubitus ulcers typically evolve to Meleney's gangrene when they get infected. They enlarge progressively uncovering large surfaces of the affected body areas. Debridement of the necrotic and "purple" zones is essential to stop the progression of the skin and subcutaneous fat necrosis.

49.7.2 Necrotizing Fasciitis

In some studies, severe streptococcal infections are often included under this heading. For example, Bisno and Stevens [3] term as necrotizing fasciitis type 2, the whole-thickness infections due to Group A streptococcus, whereas they classify as necrotizing fasciitis type 1 those mixed infections with predominance of anaerobes and enteric bacteria characterized almost exclusively by fascial necrosis. In a historical paper, Rea and Wyrick [11] described as necrotizing fasciitis those infections caused mostly by hemolytic streptococci and *S. aureus*. In more recent studies, however, the term necrotizing fasciitis has been reserved preferentially for mixed infections associated almost exclusively with fascial necrosis and subcutaneous undermining in connection with trauma, surgery or originating spontaneously around the oral or perineal areas [6, 7, 12, 13]. This seems appropriate since the clinical presentation, evolution, bacteriology, treatment and prognosis of these mixed infections are very different than those of SSTI caused by *Str. pyogenes*. Necrotizing fasciitis is often seen in patients with associated conditions such as diabetes, cancer or receiving steroids. In necrotizing fasciitis involving the male genitalia (Fournier's gangrene), two-thirds of the patients are diabetic, alcoholic or both [14].

In about 25% of the cases skin lesions (ecchymosis, bullae) and/or crepitation may be present. In general, however, superficial lesions are not prominent and this may erroneously lead to an underestimation of the severity of the disease. The hallmark of necrotizing fasciitis is extensive skin undermining of the deep subcutaneous tissue. This is easily diagnosed by physical exploration with a gloved finger or with a surgical instrument. Underlying muscle is usually spared. The lesion content is usually dark-brown, liquid and devoid of frank pus.

The incubation period of necrotizing fasciitis is usually less than a week and by the time the diagnosis is made, fasciitis usually extends more than 10 cm around the initiating focus and severe systemic symptoms are present. Renal failure, jaundice, metabolic acidosis and hypoalbuminemia are very often found. About 20% of patients are in septic shock and almost all of them will die of the disease despite aggressive treatment.

The most common origins of necrotizing fasciitis are surgical wounds (usually after abdominal surgery for a septic condition), spontaneous perineal wounds due to anorectal or genitourinary disease, spontaneous cervical wounds (secondary to an odontogenic infection) and post-traumatic wounds, after accidental trauma or illicit drug injection.

Treatment of necrotizing fasciitis includes three major phases: wide surgical debridement and drainage, antibiotic therapy and metabolic support. Surgical debridement usually implies extensive fascia resection through wide skin "windows." Aggressive skin resection is seldom required. Drains should be placed in all the skin incisions and these should follow as far from the initiating focus as indicated by the presence of undermining. Frozen-section biopsies have been proposed to better identify the margins of the infection [15] but they are probably unnecessary if debridement is appropriately guided by the presence of skin undermining and gross appearance of the muscular fascia.

Cultures should be taken from the deepest infected areas and empiric wide spectrum antibiotic therapy initiated as soon as possible. The microorganisms most often involved are the *E. coli*, *K. pneumoniae*, *Proteus* spp., *P. melaninogenica*, *Fusobacterium* spp., *B. fragilis*, *Streptococcus* spp., *P. aeruginosa* and *E. faecalis*. About 30% of necrotizing fasciitis are monomicrobial and a case due to *S. enteritidis* was reported by our group [16]. Because these patients are often in renal failure, piperacillin-tazobactam (12 g/day) is administered as the antibiotic of choice. It has the additional advantage of being active against *Enterococcus* spp. and *P. aeruginosa*, two bacterial species commonly found in patients with necrotizing fasciitis of the perineal region. Depending on the local resistance patterns, amikacin or aztreonam should be added to ensure appropriate coverage of gram-negative rods. If the presence of *S. aureus* is highly likely (institutionalized patients, repeated admissions to hospital), vancomycin or linezolid should also be added.

Metabolic and nutrition support is essential in these debilitated often-malnourished patients [17]. Hydroelectrolytic balance should be reestablished, diabetes should be controlled with insulin and artificial nutrition considered in all cases, if possible, by the enteral route.

Mortality ranges from 10 % to 30 % and is negatively influenced by any delay in performing a prompt and radical surgical debridement [18].

49.7.3 Muscle Infections: Pyomyositis and Clostridial Myonecrosis

Pyomyositis is the presence of an abscess within the skeletal muscle. It may be a secondary metastatic infection due to *S. aureus* bacteremia of any origin, or present as a primary muscular abscess developing spontaneously or after trauma. Pyomyositis has been extensively reported in tropical countries but is rare in Europe and the USA [19].

Clinically, pyomyositis presents with pain and swelling over a muscle group, typically in the proximal regions of the upper or lower extremities (thighs, buttocks and shoulder). Fever is usually present. Pain, limitation of motion and local inflammatory signs may precede the development of systemic symptoms. Differential diagnosis should be made with thrombophlebitis, bone trauma, septic arthritis, fibrillar rupture and soft tissue sarcoma. Nuclear magnetic resonance or computed tomography have proved extremely useful for the diagnosis of all musculoskeletal mass lesions and usually give the correct diagnosis. Although most commonly pyomyositis is due to *S. aureus*, other bacteria have been associated with this syndrome such as the Enterobacteriaceae. Thus, initial empiric antibiotic therapy should cover both gram-positive cocci and gram-negative rods. A Gram stain and appropriate cultures of a pus sample should be taken as soon as possible either by puncture or at the time of surgical intervention.

In addition, surgical debridement is often required when an abscess cavity can be delineated. The skin and the muscle fascia should be treated conservatively. Drainage of the purulent cavity and excision of necrotic muscle is usually limited to the muscle compartment. Cloxacillin (2 g/6 h) is the drug of choice against methicillin-sensitive *S. aureus*. If MRSA is suspected then linezolid or vancomycin should be administered.

Clostridial myonecrosis or "gas gangrene" is the most dramatic form of SSTI. Strictly speaking, gas gangrene should be described under the heading of "whole-thickness infections" since it usually involves also the skin and subcutaneous tissue, causing extensive necrosis and bullae of the superficial layers of the soft tissues. However, because the hallmark of gas gangrene is myonecrosis, it is better included in the group of infections affecting primarily the skeletal muscle.

Gas gangrene is due to *Clostridium* spp., a strictly anaerobic gram-positive sporulated rod easily identifiable on a Gram stain. Most of the post-traumatic and postoperative clostridial myonecroses are due to *C. perfringens*, while the spontaneous or bacteremic form is caused by *C. septicum*. As mentioned earlier, clostridial myonecrosis is fundamentally an "exotoxin" disease caused by the proliferation of *Clostridium* spp. under anaerobic conditions favored by the presence of ischemic and necrotic tissues either as a result of trauma or surgery. The organism is characterized by its ability to produce numerous extracellular toxins including alpha-toxin or phospholipase C, theta-toxin or perfringolysin O, kappa-toxin or collagenase, as well as a sporulation-associated enterotoxin. Alpha-toxin is the key virulent determinant exotoxin. It is a 370-residue, zinc metalloenzyme that has phospholipase C activity, and can bind to membranes in the presence of calcium [20, 21].

Clostridial myonecrosis presents under three major syndromes: post-traumatic, postoperative and spontaneous. Post-traumatic gas gangrene has become an uncommon complication of trauma and has the lowest mortality (15–20%). In the recent Bosnian war (1991–1992), no amputation for gas gangrene was carried out on over 1,200 lower extremity war wounds [22]. Clostridial myonecrosis may also follow apparently minor trauma such as in inappropriately given intramuscular injections or parenteral drug abuse. Postoperative gas gangrene is usually secondary to abdominal septic operations – often involving the small bowel or the colon – or to contaminated vascular or orthopedic procedures that leave behind devascularized muscle (Fig. 49.3). It has a mortality of 50 %. Spontaneous gas gangrene is due to a *C. septicum* bacteremia arising from a malignancy in the gastrointestinal tract, usually a colonic carcinoma, or observed in patients with leukemia or severe enteritis due to chemotherapy induced mucosal damage, and is a fatal disease [23, 24]. It has a mortality close to 100 %, and patients usually die within 24–36 h of onset.

Gas gangrene is a fulminant disease. It has a very short time of incubation and may cause death within the first 48 h. Thus, the only chance for survival is early recognition and appropriate treatment. Clinical signs

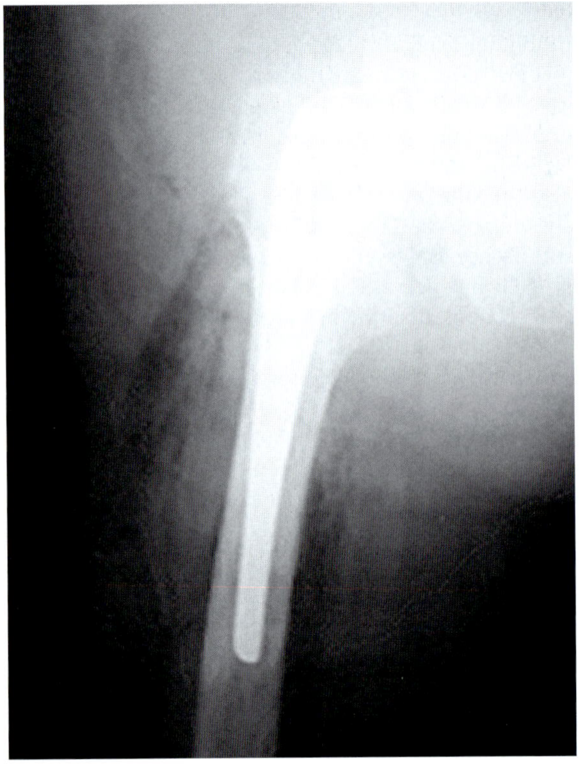

Fig. 49.3. Postoperative gas gangrene after emergency hip replacement with massive gas production within the thigh muscular compartment

that may help in the diagnosis of gas gangrene are severe general deterioration (hypotension, oliguria, disorientation, jaundice and local pain) beginning early after trauma or surgery, extensive crepitation and an ominous purple discoloration of the skin with bullae containing blackish exudates. The necrotic skin is not painful. Hemoglobinuria secondary to massive intravascular hemolysis can also be found. Multisystem organ failure may develop rapidly and the patient dies of uncontrollable hypotension, anuria and hemolysis.

Treatment is based in wide tissue excision and debridement, high dose penicillin and intensive care support. The addition of hyperbaric oxygen has been shown to have a synergistic effect in reducing morbidity and mortality in both canine and murine models. Although no prospective human data are available, retrospective data indicate that concomitant hyperbaric oxygen therapy has resulted in a twofold reduction in mortality. It has also been shown that production of alpha-toxin stops at high pO_2 (240 mmHg). Where feasible, hyperbaric oxygen therapy should be incorporated into the treatment plan for gas gangrene.

49.7.4 Whole-Thickness Infections: Streptococcal "Gangrene" and Mucormycosis

Streptococcus pyogenes may be the cause of severe, invasive and rapidly evolving whole-thickness soft tissue infections. In a recent epidemiological study in Ontario, Canada, about 1.5 cases of severe streptococcal infections were observed per 100,000 inhabitants/year, 50% of them being of invasive Group A streptococcal soft tissue infections [26]. Most of these affect the children and the elderly. The most extreme clinical manifestation of SSTI due to *Str. pyogenes* is the toxic shock syndrome. In a recent report, Wood et al. [27] have reviewed the main clinical manifestations in 59 patients (Table 49.3).

Initially described by McLennan [28], deep streptococcal infections cause diffuse swelling of the involved muscle (usually in the extremities), often associated with a compartmental syndrome and inflammatory changes in the overlying fascia, subcutaneous fat and skin. Superficial signs suggestive of streptococcal infection (erythema, edema and bullae) are the rule but deeper invasion should be suspected if there is limited motion, limb swelling and systemic symptoms suggestive of toxic shock. Immediate recognition and differential diagnosis with streptococcal cellulitis is important since delay in surgical debridement carries a poor prognosis. In situations where superficial signs are scarce, measurement of muscle compartment pressure may be helpful, and, if pressures are above 40 mmHg, fasciotomy is indicated [3]. Surgical intervention is indicated if patients do not respond to penicillin, present with already established acute renal failure or there is vascular compromise due to massive muscle swelling. It also helps in making a definitive diagnosis by obtaining deep samples for bacteriological culture and Gram's

Table 49.3. Streptococcal toxic shock syndrome: summary of clinical manifestations of 59 patients (from ref. [27])

	No. of patients (%)
Major criteria	
Shock	52 (88%)
Fever	50 (85%)
Rash	48 (81%)
Desquamation	24 (41%)
Associated systemic dysfunction criteria	
Renal	51 (86%)
Gastrointestinal	35 (59%)
CNS	31 (52%)
Myalgia or elevated CPK	27 (46%)
Mucous membrane	27 (46%)
Hepatic	26 (44%)
Hematologic	25 (42%)
Operation required	41 (69%)
Death	14 (24%)

staining. Debridement may be conservative (sparing the overlying skin) with excision of necrotic tissues and wide fasciotomy to relieve compartmental hypertension [27].

Streptococcus pyogenes is exquisitely sensitive to penicillin, which is the agent of choice for most streptococcal infections. For patients with allergy to beta-lactam antibiotics, linezolid is probably the drug of choice. In deep-seated infections, however, doubts have been expressed about the efficacy of single drug therapy [3]. This may be related to the presence of massive bacterial inoculum or the lack of expression of penicillin-binding proteins. A potent effect against *Str. pyogenes* has been ascribed to clindamycin because it appears to facilitate *Str. pyogenes* phagocytosis and to inhibit the synthesis of bacterial toxins. Thus, in view of the severity of the disease it is advisable to add clindamycin (600 mg/6–8h) to penicillin when treating whole-thickness streptococcal infections [3].

Mucormycosis (zygomycosis) is an uncommon, subacute, frequently fatal, fungal infection which rarely arises in otherwise healthy people. Different species of the order Mucorales are responsible for this disease such as *Mucor* spp., *Rhizopus* spp., *Apophysomyces* spp., and *Saksenaea* spp. [29–31]. An underlying disease, frequently diabetes mellitus or immunosuppression after solid organ transplantation, is almost always present. It appears in different anatomic sites: paranasal, cerebral, pulmonary, and gastrointestinal areas; and in the soft tissue of the extremities. It can also progress to disseminated disease by vascular invasion. Tissue infiltration by the hyphae of mucormycosis must be seen microscopically to establish the diagnosis, but culture is required to identify the fungal species involved. A study of 33 cases seen in one hospital over 5 decades [32] suggests that the incidence of this infection is increasing. There has been an improvement in outcome, which has been paralleled by a major shift from postmortem to premortem diagnosis. Premortem diagnosis gives the opportunity for metabolic stabilization, surgical excision, and liposomal amphotericin-B therapy appropriate to this disease. Successful use of hyperbaric oxygen has been reported in rhinocerebral mucormycosis, and it may be of benefit in high-risk patients with soft tissue infections by preventing local and systemic spreading of the fungus.

49.8 Prognostic Factors

Some studies have recently addressed the major determinants of death or limb loss in patients with SSTI. Wilson et al. [33] developed a scoring system using data from a randomized prospective trial on antibiotic treatment of hospitalized patients with SSTI. Elevated BUN, hyponatremia, anemia, lesion size and surgical wound infections were independent predictors of treatment failure. The presence of at least one associated comorbid condition also influenced outcome.

In another study on SSTI of the limbs, Anaya et al. [34] analyzed risk factors for limb loss and death. The overall mortality rate in their study was 16.9%, and 26% of the patients lost their affected limb. The independent predictors of death were leukocytosis $>30{,}000/mm^3$, *S*-creatinine >2 mg/dl and heart disease. Hypotension (systolic TA <90 mmHg) and heart disease at admission predicted limb loss. In addition, these authors found that the presence of *Clostridium* spp. was an independent predictive factor for both limb loss (OR 3.9) and mortality (OR 4.1) and that it was commonly associated with intravenous drug use and leukocytosis $>30{,}000/mm^3$.

References

1. Sandusky WR (1983) Frank L. Meleney: pioneer surgeon-bacteriologist. Arch Surg 118:151–155
2. Baker MD, Acharya KR (2004) Superantigens: structure-function relationships. Int J Med Microbiol 293:529–37
3. Bisno AL, Stevens DL (1996) Streptococcal infections of skin and soft tissues. N Engl J Med 334:240–5
4. Case 49 (1979) Fulminant illness with subcutaneous crepitance. N Engl J Med 301:1276–81
5. Mora EM, Cardona MA, Simmons RL (1991) Enteric bacteria and ingested inert particles translocate to intraperitoneal prosthetic materials. Arch Surg 126:157–63
6. Bubrick MP, Hitchcock CR (1979) Necrotizing anorectal and perineal infections. Surgery 86:655–62
7. Estrera AS, Landay MJ, Grisham JM, Sinn DP, Platt MR (1983) Descending necrotizing mediastinitis. Surg Gynecol Obstet 157:545–52
8. Callahan TE, Schecter WP, Horn JK (1998) Necrotizing soft tissue infection masquerading as cutaneous abscess following illicit drug injection. Arch Surg 133:812–7
9. Nicell P, Tabrisky J, Lindstrom R, Peter M (1975) Thigh emphysema and hip pain secondary to gastrointestinal perforation. Surgery 78:555–59
10. Bessman AN, Wagner W (1975) Nonclostridial gas gangrene. Report of 48 cases and review of the literature. JAMA 233:958–63
11. Rea WJ, Wyrick WJ (1970) Necrotizing fasciitis. Ann Surg 172:957–64
12. Changyul OH, Chongwook L, Jacobson JH (1982) Necrotizing fasciitis of perineum. Surgery 91:49–51
13. Rouse ThM, Malangoni MA, Schulte WJ (1982) Necrotizing fasciitis: A preventable disaster. Surgery 92:765–70
14. Clayton MD, Fowler JE, Sharifi R (1990) Causes, presentation and survival of fifty seven patients with necrotizing fasciitis of the male genitalia. Surg Gynecol Obstet 170: 49–55
15. Stamenkovic I, Lew PD (1984) Early recognition of potentially fatal necrotizing fasciitis. The use of frozen section biopsy. N Engl J Med 310:1689–1693
16. Sánchez C, Capell S, Casanovas A, Admetlla M, Sitges-Serra A (1984) Necrotizing fasciitis caused by *Salmonella enteritidis*. Scand J Infect Dis 16:321–2
17. Majeski JA, Wesley Alexander J (1983) Early diagnosis, nutritional support and immediate extensive debridement

improve survival in necrotizing fasciitis. Am J Surg 145:784–7
18. McHenry CR, Piotrowski JJ, Petrinic D, Malangoni MA (1995) Determinants of mortality for necrotizing soft-tissue infections. Ann Surg 221:558–65
19. Schlech WF, Moulton P, Kaiser AB (1981) Pyomyositis: Tropical disease in a temperate climate. Am J Med 71: 900–2
20. Rood JI (1998) Virulence genes of *Clostridium perfringens*. Annu Rev Microbiol 52:333–60
21. Naylor CE, Eaton JT, Howells A, Justin N, Moss DS, Titball RW, Basak AK (1998) Structure of the key toxin in gas gangrene. Nat Struct Biol 5:738–46
22. Jovanovic S, Wertheimer B, Zelic Z, Getos Z (1999) Wartime amputations. Mil Med 164:44–7
23. Kudsk KA (1992) Occult gastrointestinal malignancies producing metastatic *Clostridium septicum* infections in diabetic patients. Surgery 112:765–72
24. Bodey GP, Rodríguez S, Fainstein V, Elting LS (1991) Clostridial bacteremia in cancer patients. A 12-year experience. Cancer 67:1928–42
25. Stephens MB (1996) Gas gangrene: potential for hyperbaric oxygen therapy. Postgrad Med 99:217–20
26. Davies HD, McGeer A, Schwartz B, Green K, Cann D, Simor AE, Low DE (1996) Invasive Group A streptococcal infections in Ontario, Canada. N Engl J Med 335:547–54
27. Wood ThF, Potter MA, Jonasson O (1993) Streptococcal toxic shock-like syndrome. The importance of surgical intervention. Ann Surg 217:109–14
28. MacLennan JD (1943) Streptococcal infections of muscle. Lancet 1:582–4
29. Bearer EA, Nelson PR, Chowers MY, Davis CE (1994) Cutaneous zygomycosis caused by *Saksenaea vasiformis* in a diabetic patient. J Clin Microbiol 32:1823–4
30. Chakrabarti A, Kumar P, Padhye AA, Chatha L, Singh SK, Das A, Wig JD, Kataria RN (1997) Primary cutaneous zygomycosis due to *Saksenaea vasiformis* and *Apophysomyces elegans*. Clin Infect Dis 24:580–3
31. Holland J (1997) Emerging zygomycoses of humans: *Saksenaea vasiformis* and *Apophysomyces elegans*. Curr Top Med Mycol 8:27–34
32. Parfrey NA (1986) Improved diagnosis and prognosis of mucormycosis. A clinicopathologic study of 33 cases. Medicine (Baltimore) 65:113–23
33. Wilson SE, Solomkin JS, Le V, Cammarata SK, Bruss JB (2003) A severity score for complicated skin and soft tissue infections derived from phase III studies of linezolid. Am J Surg 185:369–75
34. Anaya DA, McMahon K, Nathens AB, Sullivan SR, Foy H, Bulge E (2005) Predictors of mortality and limb loss in necrotizing soft tissue infections. Arch Surg 140:151–7

Chapter 50

Vascular Graft Infections

50

R. Hasanadka, G.R. Seabrook, C.E. Edmiston

Infection of a vascular reconstruction is an infrequent, but ominous, complication. The patient is at risk not only from the infection but also from the potential for ischemia if the conduit must be interrupted, replaced or removed. Because vascular grafts function as substitute conduits in the arterial circulation, vascular graft infections are approached with a greater sense of gravity than other surgical wound or prosthetic implant infections. A vascular graft infection may be associated with sepsis, erosion of the graft into the gastrointestinal tract, dehiscence of the graft-artery suture line, and result in hemorrhage or false aneurysm formation or rupture of the graft itself. The incidence of infection is less when autologous tissue is used for artery replacement or bypass compared with prosthetic bypass grafting, and this observation remains a compelling reason to use autologous conduits in the management of arterial trauma where contamination is frequent. However, routine replacement of aortic segments for aneurysmal or occlusive disease cannot use autologous tissue, as there is no large enough segment of conduit that can be sacrificed. The inflammatory response associated with implantation of a foreign body appears to potentate the risk of infection, even when minimal bacterial contamination of a vascular bioprosthesis occurs.

The biology and epidemiology of vascular graft infections correlate with their clinical presentation, and provide direction for diagnostic and treatment strategies. It is important to understand how vascular grafts become contaminated, how bacteria resist host defense mechanisms, and the spectrum of symptoms and signs associated with a vascular prosthesis infection. A classification of vascular graft infections based on pathogenesis and timing after operation also helps guide the management of this complication.

50.1 Pathogenesis

Bacterial contamination of prosthetic vascular grafts is a frequent, if not routine, occurrence. Contamination may occur when the graft is placed or at a time remote from surgical implantation. Contamination before implantation, due to improper sterilization or packaging of the graft, is a rare cause of graft infection. Prostheses may become infected after implantation by inoculation of the external graft surface or by hematogenous seeding. Moore et al. showed that bacteremia could induce a graft infection up to 6 months after implantation if the lumen of the graft did not become lined with a well-developed pseudointima [1]. The evidence in humans for vascular graft infection caused by bacteremia is anecdotal. Szilagyi and colleagues at Henry Ford Hospital pioneered work in aortic replacement, and in 1972 observed an infection of an aortic graft in a patient with an abscess of the hand, and postulated that it was hematogenous seeding of the prosthesis [2]. Goldstone and Moore postulated that prosthetic graft infections could be linked to a prior gram-negative urinary tract infection [3]. It has been well documented that bacteremia follows diagnostic instrumentation of the oral, gastrointestinal, and genitourinary tracts, but there have been few clinical reports of vascular graft infections as a consequence of dental or endoscopic procedures.

The greatest risk of vascular graft contamination occurs at the time of graft implantation. There are several routes by which microorganisms may come into contact with a vascular graft. A gross break in operative technique, permitting the graft to touch unprepared skin, would result in obvious contamination. Bacteria are also present within the dermal layer of skin, and are thereby protected from the bactericidal effects of the surgical scrub. Incisional margins, therefore, are theoretically contaminated sites, although the number of organisms is low. Colonization of prosthetic vascular grafts by bacteria residing in diseased arterial walls, to which the graft is anastomosed, has been implicated as an etiology of late graft infections. Ernst et al. reported that the incidence of graft infection in patients undergoing aortic surgery increased from 2% to 10% when aortic wall cultures were positive [4]. Macbeth et al. studied the arterial wall microbiology in patients undergoing elective aortic and extremity vascular reconstructions [5]. Cultures of the native artery, arterial thrombus, atheroma, and peri-arterial tissues were positive in 43% of the specimens studied. In a group of patients with clinical graft infections, there was a 57% incidence of anastomotic dehiscence in 14 of 20 patients with positive arterial wall cultures, compared with no occurrence of graft-artery disruption in patients with negative cultures. These data suggest that occult infection of diseased native arteries contributes to infection of vascular prostheses and may complicate the excision of infected grafts. Performance of a concomitant surgical procedure (e.g., incidental appendectomy, cholecystectomy, or colon resection) at the time a vascular graft is implanted may dramatically increase the risk of infecting the bioprosthesis with the patient's enteric flora. Newer evidence indicates that microbial aerosols can routinely be recovered from the operating room environment, and that the spectrum of organisms recovered closely matches the profile commonly responsible for vascular graft infections [6]. However, no direct link has been established with airborne bacteria and wound or prosthetic device infections.

The lymphatic system may also provide a route of contamination leading to the infection of a vascular graft. In the immediate postoperative period, prosthetic grafts implanted in the groin are bathed by lymphatic drainage from the distal extremity. These lymphatics may be draining the tissue of chronically infected ulcers or ischemic tissue where the normal protective barriers have been compromised. The potential for graft contamination by lymphatics is compounded by the transection of multiple lymphatic channels during routine arterial dissection, particularly in the femoral region where lymphatic drainage follows the course of venous tributaries. The graft thus may be contaminated by bacteria traveling through lymphatic and venous channels to the systemic circulation or by directly bathing the graft in contaminated fluid from disrupted lymphatic channels. Rubin et al. showed experimentally in a canine model that lymphatics could collect *Escherichia coli* and *Staphylococcus aureus*, and transport them to the site of a vascular graft [7].

Biomaterial implantation, bacterial contamination, and operative dissection will each incite an inflammatory response by the host. Inflammation is characterized by a local reaction of injured tissue and more importantly the blood vessel endothelium. The inflammatory response has two missions: neutralization of the offending agent, and repair of the injury. The inflammatory response usually eradicates any bacterial inocula and provides the framework for wound healing, which eventually results in vascular graft incorporation by surrounding structures. That the process is effective is evidenced by the low rate (<2%) of vascular graft infections in "clean" cases. In response to a bacterial challenge, an inflammatory reaction develops and stimulates the recruitment of leukocytes (primarily neutrophils and monocytes), plasma cells, and macrophages. Vasodilatation occurs at the site of the infection, with the opening of new arteriolar and venular beds, followed by an increase in vascular permeability. The activated neutrophils enclose the bacteria in a phagocytic vacuole, into which cytoplasmic granules containing collagenase, elates, and plasminogen activator are discharged. Derived from blood monocytes, tissue macrophages act against foreign matter, including bacteria, by phagocytosis and degradation with hydrolytic enzymes released from lysosomes. Mobile phagocytes are attracted to bacteria and to all sites of inflammation even in the absence of microbes.

Through the excretion of chemotaxins, bacteria and injured tissue stimulate the migration of leukocytes by means of a process that is chemically modulated through intracellular cyclic nucleotides. Phagocytosis is facilitated by coating the microorganisms or foreign material with serum factors called opsonins. These immunoglobulins exhibit a specificity for the surface receptors on macrophages and neutrophils. Antigenic binding also causes the foreign particle or bacterium to become situated in close proximity to the phagocyte, permitting it to be engulfed. Antibodies that attach to the surfaces of bacteria may alter ionic charges on the cell surfaces, so they are more easily ingested by the phagocyte. Biologically active components of the complement system participate in the inflammatory response by increasing vascular permeability and acting as chemotactic agents.

A bacterial infection occurring in the environment of a prosthetic vascular graft results in a pathological condition, in which the host is attempting to eradicate the infection as well as direct an inflammatory response against the foreign body. Both the bacteria and foreign body stimulate similar responses of the immune system. However, the presence of a foreign body also serves as a "decoy" by creating a reactive environment, and expending cellular energy of the inflammatory response while diminishing available reserves of phagocytic activity against bacterial invasion. The cellular and enzymatic activity at the site of the vascular prosthesis results in increased oxidative metabolism with the generation of oxygen free radicals that may be injurious to adjacent cells. The cytotoxic enzymes are more likely to damage or destroy host tissue than the vascular prosthesis.

50.2 Bacteriology

Initial reports of prosthetic graft infections identified *S. aureus* as the predominant pathogen [8, 9]. Szilagyi, in an early comprehensive study of vascular graft infections, identified coagulase-positive staphylococci as the infecting organism in 13 of 40 graft infections [2]. Gram-negative organisms, including *E. coli*, *Proteus*,

Bacteroides, and *Pseudomonas*, accounted for another 14 graft infections. Liekweg and Greenfield also identified *S. aureus* as the most common organism cultured, but observed an increased recovery of enteric pathogens through the course of the series [10]. The mean time interval to presentation was 27 weeks. All investigators have emphasized that the majority (two-thirds) of graft infections involve the femoral component of the vascular prosthesis.

The organisms involved in early graft infections tend to exhibit virulent characteristics. Coagulase produced by staphylococcal species, such as *S. aureus*, coats the microorganisms with a film of fibrin that allows them to clump together, organize within a wound or abscess cavity, and thus inhibit phagocytosis. Coagulase-positive staphylococci also produce lysins, which are hemolytic and responsible for cell necrosis and the killing of mobilized leukocytes. Coagulase production may contribute to antibiotic resistance.

Pseudomonas species have been notoriously associated with virulent infections involving vascular grafts. Geary et al. reported a significant increased incidence of anastomotic disruption and vein graft wall necrosis in a canine model when *Pseudomonas aeruginosa* was used to infect prosthetic and autologous vascular grafts [11]. The virulence of *Pseudomonas* species is associated with their ability to produce destructive endotoxins [12]. Elastase and alkaline protease, produced by the bacteria, act against the elastin and collagen in artery or vein graft walls, compromising structural integrity.

The presence of the prosthetic implant potentiates the infection when bacterial contamination is present. The vascular graft is not an innocent bystander to the infection; it amplifies the inflammatory response and enhances the pathological process. The environment created by the inflammatory reaction in response to a foreign body is conducive to bacterial survival and proliferation. Cellular debris surrounding the vascular prosthesis provides an acidic, relatively ischemic environment that provides appropriate nutritional sources for the bacteria, and protects them from the action of other phagocytes and from lysosomal enzymes that would normally be bactericidal.

Bacteria may also become sequestered in the interstices of a vascular graft and be further protected from polymorphonuclear leukocytes and macrophages by being incorporated in a mesh of fibroblasts, collagen, platelets, and fibrin. Proteolytic enzymes released during this inflammatory process may have little effect on sequestered microcolonies, and rather may injure normal surrounding tissue, including the artery wall to which the graft material is anastomosed.

Surface characteristics of a vascular prosthesis, including porosity, hydrophobicity, and texture, influence the magnitude of the inflammatory response that occurs following implantation. More porous structures allow contiguous tissue ingrowth over the surface of the prosthetic, rather than the formation of a fibrous capsular plane at the interface of the graft and host tissue. A prosthetic with a high degree of porosity permits tissue invasion with a decreased inflammatory response. Expanded polytetrafluoroethylene (PTFE) vascular grafts are formed by an extrusion process and have a structure that permits tissue incorporation but a porosity low enough to obviate the need for preclotting before insertion in the arterial stream. These characteristics also result in the formation of a pseudointima that is less thrombogenic than the lining of the more porous woven or knitted Dacron vascular grafts.

Colonization of a vascular graft with bacteria ensures that an ongoing inflammatory interaction within the host will occur. The resultant cellular and tissue response is manifest by clinical signs of inflammation including pain, fever, swelling, leukocytosis, and autolysis of surrounding tissue. The inflammatory response is successful if the foreign body and bacteria are digested and eliminated, as might occur after placement of an absorbable surgical suture, but such a benign outcome would not be expected following infection of a vascular prosthesis. For the latter, the inflammatory response results in the progressive involvement of surrounding tissue with graft erosion, sinus tract formation, or suture line dehiscence due to loss of tensile strength of the adjacent artery wall.

Over the past 3 decades, the opportunity to study a large population of patients with prosthetic grafts has become available. The incidence of early graft infection has decreased, and with long-term follow-up, a significant incidence of late graft infection has been chronicled. Late-appearing infections are more subtle in their presentation, and progress in a more indolent fashion than classic surgical wound infections. A decade after Szilagyi's review of graft infections, Bandyk et al. reported a series of aortofemoral graft infections that identified a mean time interval from operation to treatment of 41 months (range 14–80 months) [13]. The contrasting feature of this series, compared with prior reports, was that *Staphylococcus epidermidis* prevailed as the organism responsible for the infection in 60% of the cases. The clinical presentation of these infections differed from the familiar combination of pain, swelling, erythema, and incision breakdown characteristic of a surgical wound infection and observed in most graft infections caused by *S. aureus* or gram-negative organisms. Clinical features associated with *S. epidermidis* graft infections included anastomotic false aneurysm, a sinus tract communicating between the graft and the skin, and failure of the graft to become incorporated in the adjacent tissue with formation of a perigraft cavity containing an exudate. Typically, the perigraft fluid was composed of many polymorphonuclear leukocytes, but no bacteria. A more recent review of 45 anastomotic femoral pseudoaneurysms, which presented with no clinical signs of graft infection, also documented that many of the patients have characteristics associated with *S. epidermidis* graft infections, as described previously [14]. The recovery of *S. epidermidis* organisms from abnormal arterial tissue is not unusual. Macbeth et al., in their survey of arterial wall microbiology, reported *S. epidermidis* was the most common (71 % of isolates) organism cultured from arteries, arterial thrombus, and atheroma of patients undergoing elective aortic and extremity arterial reconstruction [5].

The involvement of coagulase-negative staphylococci (CNS) with vascular graft infections involving the inguinal site is not unexpected. The highest staphylococcal concentrations on body skin surfaces are found in the axilla and the groin where the temperature and humidity provide an optimum environment for growth. Although CNS had previously been dismissed as nonpathogenic skin contaminants when recovered from prosthetic material, their role in infections involving implanted devices in humans has been confirmed. In addition to infecting vascular grafts, CNS have been implicated as the pathogenic organisms in infections of cardiac valves, cerebrospinal fluid shunts and intravascular catheters [15–17].

We have shown that many vascular patients entering the hospital are colonized with multiple strains of slime-producing CNS. Twenty-one patients admitted to our institution for lower extremity arterial revascularization had body surface cultures of planned incision sites performed on admission, immediately preoperatively and 5 days postoperatively. A large number ($n=327$) of CNS isolates were recovered, and *S. epidermidis* was the predominant species isolated at all three sample times [18]. On admission to the hospital, the incidence of methicillin resistance was 15 % for *S. epidermidis* and 10. 1 % for the other CNS isolates. However, 5 days after operation, the incidence of *S. epidermidis* methicillin resistance increased to 50 % and the overall and methicillin resistance of CNS strains increased to 57 %. The hospital environment, including perioperative antibiotic administration, results in an increased frequency of antibiotic-resistant CNS strains. This selection process can contribute to the pathogenicity of these organisms, especially in patients with prolonged hospitalization before surgery or those requiring reoperation, since routine antibiotic prophylaxis may not be as effective.

As vascular surgeons have become suspicious of occult infection, more sophisticated culture techniques have been used. Enhanced recovery of CNS is achieved when graft material is submitted for culture in trypticase soy broth and further improved by disrupting adherent bacteria from the graft fabric by using ultrasonic oscillations. Glucose supplementation of the cryptic soy broth used for staphylococcal incubation may be required to recover colonies when only a few organisms are present in the initial sample of graft material submitted for culture. A prolonged (up to 14 days) incubation period for slow growing, fastidious organisms may be required.

There is no evidence that vegetative lesions occur within arterial conduits infected by CNS similar to those that may be located on infected cardiac valves. Fever is seldom a presenting symptom with late graft infections, nor are other stigmata of cardiac valve infections typically present, such as Osler's lesions, Janeway's lesions, Roth's spots, petechiae, or splinter hemorrhages. The lack of these signs in graft infection caused by CNS points against a seeding and showering process as an etiologic factor in most late graft infections.

50.3 Natural History of Graft Infections

Szilagyi et al. classified graft infections in a three-tiered system based on the anatomic level of invasion. Grade I infections involved only the dermis; Grade II infections extended into the subcutaneous region but did not involve the prosthetic material; Grade III infections involved the arterial implant [2]. Because the Grade I and II infections are not involved with significant sequelae, they have not been studied in detail. Most Grade III infections result as a consequence of a surgical wound infection and probably evolve through the two previous phases during their clinical presentation. Szilagyi's classification scheme centered on the concept that contamination of the vascular graft occurs primarily through the surgical wound or via an enteric erosion. Indeed, these are the important mechanisms of early graft infections. More recent reports on graft infection have focused on pathogenesis and treatment of late-appearing infections, particularly graft-enteric erosions or fistulas. Investigators have emphasized the concept of bacterial adherence to the vascular graft material as a critical initial step in the infectious process. The time of onset following the primary operation for a graft infection to appear frequently predicts which pathogens are involved. The classification of graft infections as early (less than 6 months following implantation) or late is useful clinically, since different diagnostic and treatment strategies are required.

Early graft infections follow a clinical course of a surgical wound infection which, in fact, is the likely etiology. During the perioperative period, the surgical wound is inoculated with bacteria and the graft becomes colonized. A local inflammatory response occurs, and an abscess involving the vascular conduit forms. The surgical wound, itself, is the focus of the infection, and any portion of the graft may be involved. The infection may extend along the external surface of the graft, to involve the suture line between the graft and the native arterial tissue, with a significant risk of anastomotic dehiscence.

Infections of autologous grafts occurring in the early perioperative period are frequently related to technical error, adjacent ischemic tissue, or a concomitant infectious process. Infected autologous tissue (e.g., vein grafts or patches, endarterectomized arterial segments) may necrose and rupture either at, or away from, suture lines. Most infections involving autologous conduits occur early and present as wound infections. They are treated with classic surgical techniques for wound management: drainage of abscess cavities; debridement of devitalized tissue; coverage of an uninfected conduit with viable tissue; or excision of an infected conduit. Late graft infections involving autologous vascular grafts are rare, and the incidence is not great enough to define etiologies and to formulate management within a classification scheme.

Early prosthetic vascular graft infections are usually the result of local wound contamination. These infections may be associated with a wound-healing complication such as dehiscence, hematoma, seroma, lymphatic leak, or skin edge necrosis. The graft becomes inoculated through the disrupted surgical incision or via an adjacent abscess cavity. The anastomotic suture lines of prosthetic grafts are dependent on the integrity of the native artery, because a union between the prosthetic and the implanted material via a proliferative process does not occur. In the early postoperative period, dehiscence of the suture line is associated with hemorrhage because the prosthetic material will not have become incorporated by surrounding tissue to contain the force of arterial pressure.

As surgical technique and perioperative antibiotic therapy have become increasingly rigorous, the relative incidence of early graft infection has decreased. Infections involving prosthetic grafts are more likely to occur late in the postoperative course. One group of these infections involves a previously incorporated, uninfected graft becoming contaminated by direct exposure (graft enteric erosion) or hematogenous seeding from another systemic septic focus (e.g., pneumonia, urinary tract infection, dental abscess). These infections are likely to present with the patient exhibiting clinical signs of sepsis (e.g., fever, chills, lethargy, leukocytosis, vasodilatation, hyperdynamic cardiac activity, septic shock). Signs of wound infection may be absent and timely diagnosis delayed, because the infection is focused at the site of the graft that is located deep to the overlying healed surgical incision. The contaminated graft is targeted by host defenses as a septic focus, and an acute inflammatory response ensues. An exudative process will encircle the vascular prosthesis. As the infection extends along the external surface of the prosthetic material, the vascular anastomosis may become involved in the infection. The infecting organisms are virulent gram-positive cocci or gram-negative enteric pathogens. Successful treatment involves aggressive intervention with resection of the prosthetic material, extra-anatomic bypass, systemic antimicrobial therapy, and multisystem support of a critically ill patient.

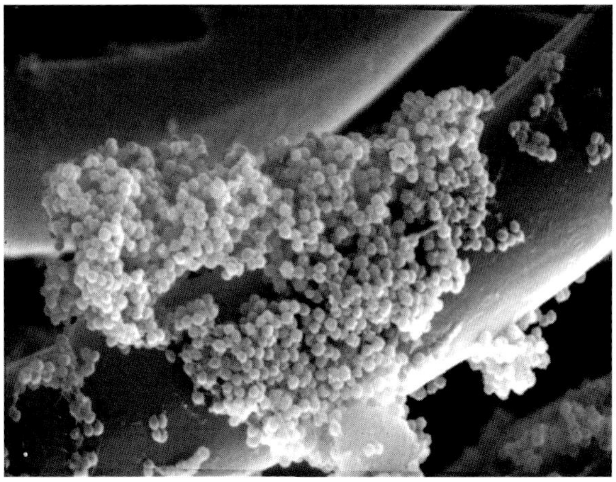

Fig. 50.1. Scanning electron micrograph of *Staphylococci epidermidis* on Dacron graft fabric. Numerous adherent bacterial microcolonies are enclosed within an extracellular surface biofilm. These mucin-producing organisms become sequestered within the interstices of the prosthetic graft fabric leading to occult infection

The second group of late vascular graft infections follows a more cryptic process. Bacterial microcolonies contaminate the graft, are sequestered within the interstices of the prosthetic fabric, and become adherent to the graft surface at the time of implantation. These infections are most frequently caused by CNS. As the body incorporates the prosthetic graft, the contaminating bacteria are entrapped, and may be surrounded by an exopolysaccharide biofilm (mucin or slime), which protects the organisms from the host's immune defense system and systemic antibiotics (Fig. 50.1).

There may be a latent period extending from months to years following prosthetic implantation when no clinical signs of infection are exhibited, and the integrity of the prosthetic anastomosis remains unaltered. Eventually, the microbial population grows beyond the surface of the graft, is recognized by host defenses, and a chronic inflammatory process develops. Cytolysins released from macrophages break down the matrix of collagen and fibroblasts that has coalesced around the prosthetic material, resulting in the graft becoming unincorporated from the host tissue. In this environment, the artery wall may become inflamed with a decreased anastomotic tensile strength at the graft-artery interface [20]. Persistence of the chronic inflammatory state may lead to the development of a pseudoaneurysm at the anastomotic site. This low-grade inflammatory process does not present as systemic sepsis, but is more commonly manifest by subtle changes at graft implantation. The incorporated graft becomes surrounded with a perigraft exudate or fluid collection and, with a continuous stimulus for inflammation, a sinus tract may form between the perigraft cavity and the skin surface, or a pseudoaneurysm may form at the graft-artery interface due to disruption of the anastomosis. If a pseudoaneurysm is explored during the evolution of this inflammatory reaction, signs of infection (perigraft fluid, leukocytes, or bacteria on gram stain) may be evident. Treatment strategy depends on the recognition that these anatomic changes are due to an infectious process, rather than host vessel degeneration or an immune-mediated reaction directed at the vascular prosthesis. Identification of the pathogen in these circumstances requires the culture of the biomaterial itself, rather than culture of perigraft tissue or fluid. Failure to recognize a graft infection invariably leads to a future graft-healing complication, typically manifesting at an anastomotic site as either rupture or thrombosis of a false aneurysm.

Fabric-covered stent graft infection is a less studied complication following endovascular exclusion of aneurysmal disease. Anecdotically, the infection rate of bare metal stents is extremely rare. Stent grafts, however, are constructed with synthetic fabric which, similar to surgically placed prosthetic grafts, could be inoculated either through the surgical site – for femoral artery cutdown – or during episodes of subsequent bacteremia. It is unknown if the bacterial colonization of residual mural thrombus between the graft and the native aneurysm wall would affect stent graft infection rates.

The Dutch Randomized Endovascular Aneurysm Management (DREAM) trial reported a graft infection rate of 0.6% (1 of 171 patients), which was not statistically different than the treatment arm for open repair [19]. The limitation of the DREAM trial in regards to infection rate, which is true with most stent graft series, is that the operative complication follow-up was short term and not geared towards analyzing infection risk factors. Ducasse et al. contacted 40 centers worldwide to gather data on a cohort of 65 cases of stent graft infection during exclusion of aortic or iliac aneurysms [20]. Placement for aortoenteric fistula or infection-related pseudoaneurysm was excluded, leading to a reported overall graft infection rate of 0.43%. The majority of patients presented with symptoms of high grade infection (retroperitoneal fluid collection, cutaneous fistula, septic embolization, or hemorrhagic shock) as opposed to the more indolent course of *S. epidermidis*. In the 44 cases that a positive culture could be identified, 54.5% were *S. aureus*.

50.4 Diagnostic Imaging

Computerized tomography is the most useful and accurate modality to diagnose a vascular graft infection. Findings that will lead to the diagnosis of graft infection are perigraft air, perigraft fluid collections, and inflammatory changes in the retroperitoneal structures (Fig. 50.2). Although residual intra-abdominal air may be present in the early post-operative period, particularly following aneurysm repair, after 2 months any air in the region of the graft should be considered pathologic. When perigraft air is found late (greater than 6 months) following implantation, the diagnosis of graft infection is almost certain. When vascular contrast is administered in association with axial imaging, the CT provides information to define the arterial anatomy that should obviate the need for angiography. Although CT scanning will seldom demonstrate an aorto-enteric fistula, it may provide information to argue against that diagnosis if it can be demonstrated that the duodenum is separated from the vascular structures by normal tissue planes with no inflammatory tissue changes.

Arteriography has more potential in formulating operative strategy than in establishing a diagnosis of prosthetic graft infection. An arteriogram may locate a graft infection by demonstrating a nonpalpable proximal pseudoaneurysm, but this modality never identified a fistulous tract independently diagnosed as primary graft infection. Arteriographic imaging of the native vascular anatomy allows the surgeon to plan the extra-anatomic arterial reconstruction.

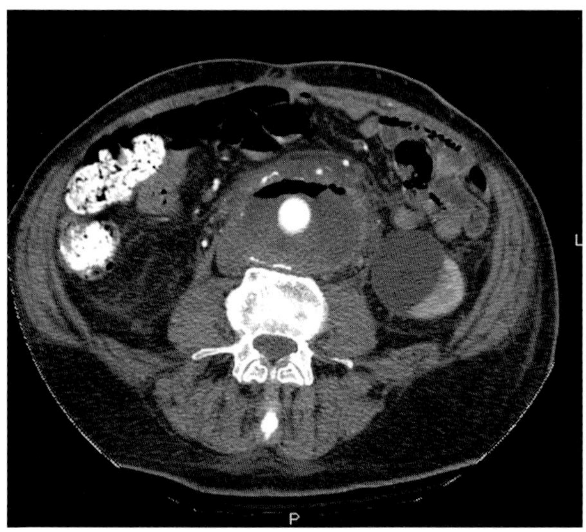

Fig. 50.2. CT scan of a patient 33 months following emergent aortic graft placement for a ruptured abdominal aortic aneurysm. The graft is surrounded in fluid with a gas pocket located anteriorly. A large left renal cyst is also seen. At operation an aorto-enteric fistula was identified. Operative cultures grew *Enterococcus* species, *K. pneumoniae*, and *C. albicans*

Attempts to firmly establish the diagnosis of aorto-enteric fistula can be an arduous task. Patients with aorto-enteric fistula usually present with some form of gastrointestinal bleeding. It may be acute and severe making the diagnosis obvious; however, patients may initially present with only anemia or guaiac positive stools. Upper GI endoscopy is the most frequently performed diagnostic intervention, but it actually establishes the diagnosis in only a few patients. Endoscopy is more commonly employed to identify other pathology responsible for a source of significant blood loss in the esophagus, stomach, or duodenum. Most patients with vascular grafts and GI bleeding have GI sources of bleeding and not aorto-enteric fistulae. However, the clinician must be wary not to implicate "esophagitis, gastritis, gastric erosions or duodenitis" when there is actually major blood loss. In such a setting avoiding the diagnosis of aorto-enteric fistula will only lead to a delay in establishing the correct diagnosis. Only an actively bleeding lesion or other demonstrable GI pathology that can account for the patient's symptoms should be considered a true source of hemorrhage as an alternative to an aorto-enteric fistula during this evaluation.

50.5 Treatment Aortic Graft Sepsis

Principles of operative management consist of total excision of the infected aortic graft, debridement of the aorta to reach normal artery wall, debridement of retroperitoneal structures associated with the infectious process, longitudinal closure of the duodenum, oversewing the aorta followed by an onlay omental patch, placement of retroperitoneal drains if there had been an abscess cavity, and revascularization through an extra-anatomic route. Such an operation is one of the most taxing surgical procedures performed for both the patient and surgeon. If the patient is stable, it is preferable to perform the extra-anatomic revascularization as a staged procedure, followed in 24 h with excision of the infected graft. This allows for two shorter operations with better ability to manage the patient's fluid status and the associated risk to the cardiac and pulmonary systems. In our reported series of 20 patients, 14 underwent aortic graft excision followed by extra-anatomic revascularization, while 5 patients had extra-anatomic revascularization performed prior to excision of the aortic prosthesis. Whether revascularization was performed before or after aortic graft excision did not alter the eventual outcome of the patients in our series. Although performing the revascularization prior to graft excision avoids the obligatory ischemic time to the lower extremities, there is the theoretical risk of bacteremic seeding of the new graft material if it is placed prior to removal of the infected prosthesis. However, the one patient in our series who developed an infection of his axillofemoral graft had it placed after excision of the aortic graft [21].

The most common technique for lower extremity revascularization is axillofemoral, femoral-femoral bypass constructed with PTFE graft material, which has the lowest incidence of bacterial adherence [22]. If the aortic procedure has been confined to the abdomen, then the common femoral arteries can be used for the extra-anatomic reconstruction with little risk of contamination. However, when the aortic graft has been extended to the femoral segments, the revascularization must be taken more distally through uninfected tissue. If the patient's superficial femoral artery is open, the lower extremities are usually not at risk for ischemia; however, when there is arterial occlusion of the superficial femoral segment, the reconstruction must target the profunda femoris or even the popliteal artery for runoff.

In our series, cultures from two patients who presented with clinical signs of sepsis recovered a polymicrobial mixture of aerobic and anaerobic organisms. Five of the nine patients with late-onset primary graft infection had only *Staphylococcus epidermidis* recovered. Despite having clinical evidence of graft infection (draining wound sinus, perigraft exudate, poor graft incorporation, anastomotic pseudoaneurysm), the four remaining patients had no isolates recovered [21].

Despite broad advances in medical technology, operative mortality (14–50%) and morbidity (25–70%, primarily from lower limb amputations) have remained considerable, when the standard treatment of excision of the infected graft and revascularization via an extra-anatomic approach is followed [23, 24]. This has led some authors to suggest alternative approaches such as simple repair of the fistula without regrafting, or in situ replacement of the prosthesis in the infected field [25, 26]. Although it may be necessary for vascular surgeons to have these options available in their treatment armamentarium, prosthetic material should not be permanently placed in an infected field.

Aortic stump dehiscence remains a significant late cause of death in patients surviving surgical treatment of aortic vascular graft infections. In situ replacement of grafts from patients with aorto-enteric fistulae resulted in a 16% incidence of recurrent fistula or dehiscence, and exsanguination at the proximal anastomosis [21]. Reilly et al. reported a 25% dehiscence and mortality in 25 patients following perioperative treatment for aorto-enteric fistulas, but no cases of aortic stump problems in patients treated for primary graft infection [24].

There are two factors that play a role in the pathogenesis of late aortic stump problems: persistent periaortic infection and bacterial virulence. The aorta must be debrided back to normal arterial wall to enable a secure closure. Attempts to close friable, edematous aorta predispose the patient to future complications. In addition, an attempt must be made to debride the surrounding retroperitoneal structures involved in the infectious process to remove sources of contamination. The second factor related to subsequent infectious problems with the aortic stump is related to the virulence of the organisms involved in the infectious process. Late stump dehiscence is more common following aorto-enteric fistulas than primary graft infections. Isolates from aorta-enteric fistulae are polymicrobial and involve more virulent organisms such as *Escherichia coli, S. aureus, and Pseudomonas.* In contrast, *Staphylococcus epidermidis* is the most common isolate recovered from late onset primary graft infections. The inherent low virulence of *S. epidermidis*, when combined with complete excision of the prosthesis, has resulted in the failure of this organism to be implicated in aortic stump dehiscence.

Following excision of an aortic graft the patient should be maintained on a course of antibiotic therapy to protect the patient from infection from residual microscopic contamination and to irradiate organisms still in the lymphatic system. If pre-operative blood cultures were positive, the susceptibility data from these cultures will guide therapy. However, the nature of biofilm infections may result in negative cultures from specimens collected at the procedure. Empiric therapy must then be instituted. We use a semi-synthetic penicillin with a beta-lactam inhibitor or a quinolone, with additional coverage to both of these regimens if there is an indication that an anaerobic process is involved. Vancomycin is not routinely used. Intravenous therapy is routinely continued for 2 weeks and then the patient is converted to an oral agent, which is continued until there is evidence on follow-up CT scan that all of the intra-abdominal inflammatory process has resolved (Fig. 50.3).

When long-term antibiotic therapy is prescribed, the consequences of this therapy must be considered, including the development of drug allergies, specific organ dysfunction such as nephrotoxicity, the development of supra-infections including pseudomembranous colitis, and the emergence of bacterial resistant organisms.

The most common risk factor that predisposes to infectious complications is multiple previous vascular procedures. Repetitive exposure of the graft increases the risk of contamination and a subsequent infection. Archer and Tenenbaum have demonstrated the emergence of antibiotic resistance in staphylococcal strains recovered from cardiac surgery patients in the postoperative period [27]. The necessity for graft revision in the early postoperative period may greatly increase the risk of graft colonization by more virulent or resistant strains of the commensal skin flora.

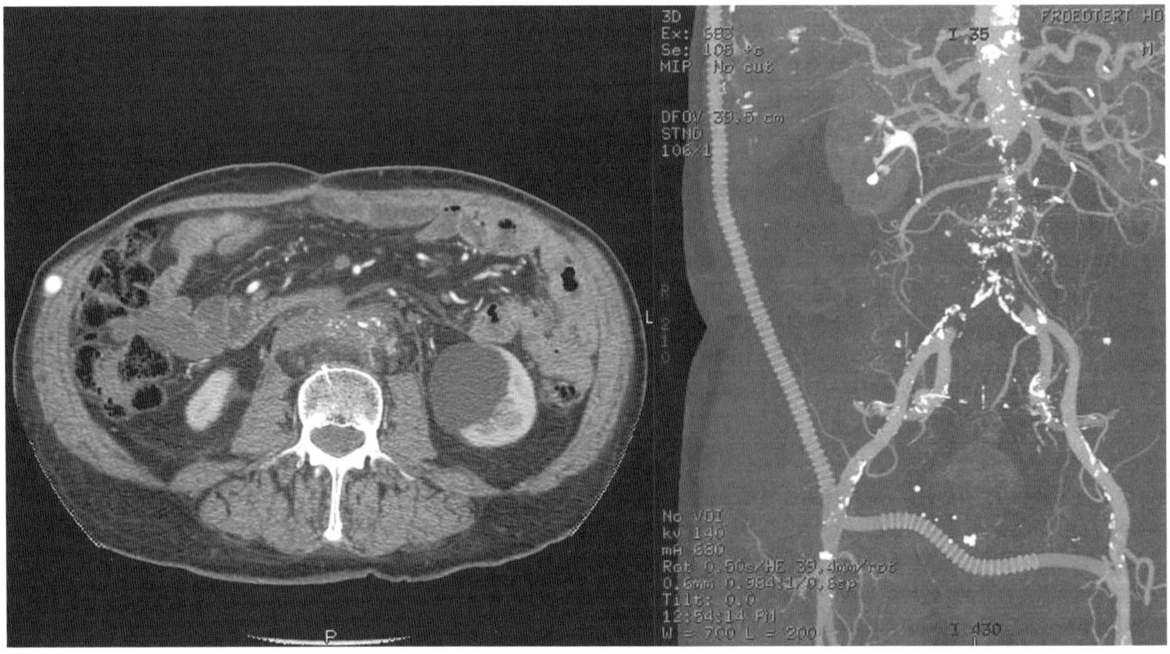

Fig. 50.3. CT scan of the patient (Fig. 50.2) 11 weeks following excision of the infected aortic graft and oversewing of the infrarenal aorta. Resolution of the inflammatory changes is seen on the axial image (*left*). An axillofemoral bypass was constructed to perfuse the lower extremities, seen on a maximum intensity projection image (*right*)

50.6 In Situ Replacement of Infected Grafts

The low virulence of coagulase-negative staphylococci and their unique characteristics of colonization via a surface biofilm permit treatment of some infected grafts by excision of the grossly involved graft segments, debridement of perigraft tissue and adjacent artery, and in situ replacement of another prosthesis. Several caveats must be emphasized in selecting this treatment option. First, it is essential that the patient has the correct microbiologic diagnosis. This technique is not appropriate or recommended for patients who have gram-negative bacteria infections. The role of coagulase-positive staphylococci in these infections is not yet defined. In latent, indolent infections where coagulase-positive staphylococci are cultured, in situ replacement may be successful. Why some patients with coagulase-positive staphylococcal infections fail to mount the systemic reaction that is more classically associated with this infection is not understood. There may be a spectrum of virulence in these species in which some isolates act like the more benign coagulase-negative staphylococci.

Graft biofilm infections involving the femoral anastomosis are the cases where an in situ replacement technique will be most appropriately used. When an in situ technique is employed, the operative treatment must include total excision of the biofilm cavity and the involved graft. Because this often results in an extensive groin dissection, there is an increased incidence of lymphatic wound complications, particularly the occurrence of lymphoceles in the post-operative period. The use of muscle coverage is important because it provides vascularized tissue to surround the graft and be interposed between the skin and the conduit if wound complications occur. The treatment of a lymphocele should be aggressive, with operative ligation and drainage if they do not promptly resolve or begin to leak through the wound creating a potential tract for secondary infections.

Expanded PTFE is usually selected as a replacement interposition graft because our laboratory data has demonstrated that the bacterial adherence of slime-producing bacteria is significantly less to ePTFE than to knitted or woven Dacron [28]. Slime-producing coagulase-negative staphylococci adhered to the knitted Dacron 100 times greater than to PTFE. Because bacterial adhesion is the important first step in biofilm graft infection, the relative resistance to bacterial adhesion possessed by PTFE has significant potential advantages as an in situ replacement conduit.

A special note of caution needs to be raised for patients who have femoral limbs of their aorto-bifemoral grafts resected. Even after the replacement grafts have healed well and have demonstrated no evidence of recurrent infection, the residual aortic graft segment in the patient may subsequently develop changes suggestive of coagulase-negative staphylococcus infection manifested by the development of a perigraft cavity and fluid. Should this clinical presentation occur, it probably represents a latent infection that existed even at the time of the initial resection. Since replacement of the intra-abdominal portion of an aortobifemoral graft is fraught with the greatest potential for complications, it is reasonable to be cautious in making a decision to remove the aortic segment.

Because biofilm infections occur months and years after an initial vascular reconstructive procedure, the mortality rate from associated cardiovascular disease is high in this cohort of patients. The mortality rate for most series of patients with graft infections is at or above 50 %, most of it caused by cardiovascular causes. Because of this high mortality rate, clinicians are curtailed in studying extended durability of this repair technique.

In our series of infected aortic grafts, patients were treated with complete graft excision and extra-anatomic bypass, which were compared to patients treated with partial graft excision, in situ reconstruction, or other methods of graft salvage [29]. Overall perioperative mortality was 27 % and the recurrent infection rate was 20 %, which is comparable to other values reported in the literature. Neither mortality or recurrent infection was statistically different between the two groups. However, this series was not randomized and the options for treatment were at the surgeon's discretion. Until the surgical outcomes of infected aortic grafts can be better studied, our recommendation is still to hold true to the principle of complete excision and extra-anatomic bypass with consideration for in situ reconstruction only in the presence of the more indolent infections.

50.7 Treatment of Endovascular Graft Sepsis

Because the incidence of stent graft infection is very low, the clinical outcomes are not well studied. Ducasse et al. found in their multicenter cohort of infected stent grafts that surgical excision with reconstruction had less mortality than treatment with antibiotics and drainage (14% vs. 36.4%, $p=0.086$) [20]. They also found that the mortality was significantly lower with in situ reconstructions than extra-anatomical bypass (5.8% vs. 16%, $p=0.32$). Because the aneurysm sac is not violated, complete excision may be more feasible allowing the more durable reconstruction to be created. However, caution should be taken in that the surgical subgroups were small and were treated in multiple centers with varying conduit for the in situ reconstruction.

Similar to surgical grafts, the principle of complete excision, debridement, and operative reconstruction holds true for stent graft infections. The option to perform an in situ reconstruction versus an extra-anatomical bypass needs to be further studied.

50.8 Conclusions

The most important factor in selecting treatment regimens for vascular graft infections is the proper analysis of the patient. The role of the infecting organism is primary in selecting less radical treatment of in situ repair as opposed to the traditional treatment of graft excision and extra-anatomic bypass to restore distal flow.

The pathobiology of graft infections is affected by the microorganisms colonizing the graft, the site of implantation, and the character of the prosthetic material used in the reconstruction. Sensitive culture techniques are necessary to recover bacteria from graft infections when overt signs of sepsis are absent.

It is critical for the surgeon to identify patients with biofilm infections during follow-up surveillance. Because of the indolent nature of the infection and the low virulence of the organisms, the diagnosis can rarely be made definitely before graft removal and culture. The clinical presentation is typical enough so that a tentative diagnosis can be reliably made. The principal components of this diagnosis include an infection occurring at a time remote from the previous vascular procedure (at least 6 months) and the absence of systemic evidence of toxicity. The use of CT scanning and duplex scanning is valuable to detect perigraft fluid and the presence of intra-abdominal false aneurysms.

Late prosthetic graft infections differ from classical surgical wound infections, and management of these complications requires the vascular surgeon to understand the etiology and natural history of the process. We do not recommend in situ replacement for gram-negative infection and for coagulase-positive staphylococcus infections where the patient has systemic effects of infection and bacteria can be seen on gram stains of the perigraft fluid. In these situations traditional techniques of graft removal and autogenous or extra-anatomic revascularization are still the treatments of choice.

References

1. Moore WS, Rosson CT, Hall AD, et al. (1969) Transient bacteremia: a cause of infection in prosthetic vascular grafts. Am J Surg 7:342–343
2. Szilagyi DE, Smith RF, Elliott JP, et al. (1972) Infection in arterial reconstruction with synthetic grafts. Ann Surg 176:321–333
3. Goldstone J, Moore WS (1968) Infection in vascular prostheses. Arch Surg 97:872–888
4. Ernst CB, Campbell HC, Daugherty ME, et al. (1977) Incidence and significance of intraoperative bacterial cultures during abdominal aortic aneurysmectomy. Ann Surg 185: 626–633
5. Macbeth GA, Rubin JR, McIntyre KE, et al. (1984) The relevance of arterial wall microbiology to the treatment of prosthetic graft infections: graft infection vs. arterial infection. J Vasc Surg 1:750–756
6. Edmiston CE, Sinski S, Seabrook GR, Simons D, Goheen M (1999) Airborne particulates in the OR environment. AORN 69:1169–1183
7. Rubin JR, Malone JM, Goldstone J (1985) The role of the lymphatic system in acute arterial prosthetic graft infections. J Vasc Surg 2:92–98
8. Javid H, Julian OC, Dye WS, et al. (1962) Complications of abdominal aortic grafts. Arch Surg 85:142–153
9. Fry WJ, Lindenauer SM (1967) Infection complicating the use of plastic arterial implants. Arch Surg 94:600–609
10. Liekweg WG, Greenfield LJ (1977) Vascular prosthetic infections: collected experience and results of treatment. Surgery 81:335–342
11. Geary KJ, Tomkiewicz ZM, Harrison HH, et al. (1990) Differential effects of a gram-negative and a gram-positive infection on autogenous and prosthetic grafts. J Vasc Surg 11:339–347
12. Rotschafer JC, Shikuma LR (1986) *Pseudomonas aeruginosa* susceptibility in a university hospital: recognition and treatment. Drug Intell Clin Pharm 20:575–581
13. Bandyk DF, Berni GA, Thiele BL, et al. (1984) Aortofemoral graft infection due to *Staphylococcus epidermidis*. Arch Surg 119:102–108
14. Seabrook GR, Schmitt DD, Bandyk DF, Edmiston CE, Towne JB (1990) Anastomotic femoral pseudoaneurysm: A prospective investigation of occult infection as an etiologic factor. J Vasc Surg 11:629–634
15. Slaughter L, Morris JE, Starr A (1973) Prosthetic valvular endocarditis: a 12 year review. Circulation 47:1319–1325
16. Bayston R, Pennym SR (1972) Excessive production of mucoid substance in staphylococcus SIIA: a possible factor in colonization of Holter shunts. Dev Med Child Neurol 14:25–28
17. Peters G, Locci R, Pulverer G (1982) Adherence and growth of coagulase-negative staphylococci on surfaces of intravenous catheters. J Infect Dis 146:479–482
18. Levy MF, Schmitt DD, Edmiston CE, Bandyk DD, Krepel CJ, Seabrook GR, Towne JB (1989) Sequential analysis of staphylococcal colonization by body surface cultures on patients undergoing vascular surgery. J Clin Microbiol 28:664–669
19. Prinssen M, Verhoeven ELG, Buth J, Cuypers PWM, van Sambeek MRHM, Balm R, Buskens E, Grobbee DE, Blankensteign JD (2004) A randomized trial comparing conventional and endovascular repair of abdominal aortic aneurysms. N Engl J Med 351:1607–18
20. Ducasse E, Calisti A, Speziale F, Rizzo L, Misuraca M, Fiorani P (2004) Aortoiliac stent graft infection: current problems and management. Ann Vasc Surg 18:521–6
21. Schmitt DD, Seabrook GR, Bandyk DF, Towne JB (1990) Graft excision and extra-anatomic revascularization: the treatment of choice for the septic aortic prosthesis. J Cardiovasc Surg 31:327–332
22. Schmitt DD, Bandyk DF, Pequet AJ, Malangoni MA, Towne JB (1986) Mucin production by *Staphylococcus epidermidis*. Arch Surg 121:89–95
23. O'Hara PJ, Hertzer NR, Beven EG, Krajewski LP (1986) Surgical management of infected abdominal aortic grafts: review of a 25 years experience. J Vasc Surg 3:725–31

24. Reilly LM, Altman H, Lusby RJ, Kersh RA, Eherenfeld WK, Stoney RJ (1984) Late results following surgical management of vascular graft infection. J Vasc Surg 1:36–44
25. Walker WE, Cooley DA, Duncan JM, Hallman GL, Ott DA, Reul GJ (1987) The management of aortoduodenal fistula by *in situ* replacement of the infected abdominal aortic graft. Ann Surg 205:727–32
26. Thomas WEG, Baird RN (1986) Secondary aortoenteric fistulae: towards a more conservative approach. Br J Surg 73:875–8
27. Archer GL, Tenenbaum MJ (1980) Antibiotic-resistant *Staphylococcus epidermidis* in patients undergoing cardiac surgery. Antimicrob Agents Chemother 17:269–72
28. Schmitt DD, Bandyk DF, Pequet AJ, Towne JB (1986) Bacterial adherence to vascular prostheses. J Vasc Surg 3:732–740
29. Hart JP, Eginton MT, Brown KR, Seabrook GR, Lewis BD, Edmiston CE, Towne JB, Cambria RA (2005) Operative strategies in aortic graft infections: is complete graft excision always necessary? Ann Vasc Surg 19:154–60

51 Acute Mediastinitis

K.P. Bhavan, D.K. Warren

51.1 Introduction

Mediastinitis is an infection of the structures in the thorax excluding the lungs and pleural space. Most cases of mediastinitis are secondary to spread of infection from a distant site or direct inoculation of organisms secondary to trauma or esophageal perforation due to malignancy. The last 30 years have seen a dramatic increase in the annual number of cardiac surgical procedures performed. Consequently, post-sternotomy surgical site infections have accounted for an increasing number of cases of mediastinitis. Despite significant advances in antibiotic therapy, surgical technique, and intensive care management, mediastinitis continues to have a high morbidity and mortality. This chapter will focus on three major categories of mediastinitis, including descending necrotizing infections, mediastinitis secondary to esophageal perforations, and post-sternotomy surgical site infections, and will discuss the pathogenesis, presentation, diagnosis, and management associated with each. The anatomy of the neck and mediastinum, which is crucial to understanding the pathogenesis and complications of mediastinitis, as well as unusual causes of mediastinitis will also be reviewed.

51.1.1 Historical Overview

The first major review of suppurative mediastinitis was by Pearse [1] in 1938 involving 110 cases. In this series, 58% of cases were due to esophageal perforation and the remainder were secondary to descending infections of the head and neck, along with post-surgical complications. Mortality in the pre-antibiotic era without surgical drainage was 85%; with surgery mortality decreased to 35%.

With the increasing use of the median sternotomy incision, a new cause of mediastinitis rapidly became apparent. Overall, the infection rate for median sternotomy is low, but given the volume of patients who undergo this procedure for cardiac surgery each year, even a low rate translates into a potentially large number of patients with post-operative mediastinal infections. In a 1976 review by Culliford [2], mortality ranged from 7% in the group that was recognized early to 20% among patients diagnosed late post-operatively. The surgical management of these infections has evolved from initial debridement with closure by secondary intention, to primary closure with closed irrigation, to the use of omental and muscle flaps.

The advent of antibiotics did little alone to change the outcome of mediastinitis. In 1983, Estera et al. [3] reviewed 21 cases of descending necrotizing mediastinitis from 1960 to 1980 and reported a mortality of 42.8%, with the majority of these cases being diagnosed at autopsy. This high mortality rate was attributed to the frequent lack of physical and radiographic findings early in the course of the disease. The development of computerized tomography (CT) has increased the capacity for earlier diagnosis and improved pre-operative planning of surgical management. An analysis of 48 cases of mediastinitis from 1990 to 1998 revealed that the mortality for descending infections had improved to 23% [4], which the authors attributed to the availability of CT.

51.1.2 Anatomy of the Neck and Mediastinum

Understanding the pathogenesis, complications, and successful management of mediastinal infections requires knowledge of the anatomical relationships between the organs and vascular structures of the neck and mediastinum. The mediastinum contains the heart, great vessels, trachea, esophagus, paratracheal lymph nodes, and the thymus. This is bordered anatomically by the thoracic inlet superiorly, the diaphragm inferiorly, the sternum anteriorly, the vertebral bodies posteriorly, and the pleural cavities laterally. The fascial planes of the head and neck are of great importance in understanding the spread of infection in the chest. The most important of these fascial planes are the retropharyngeal, visceral, prevertebral, lateral pharyngeal, and previsceral spaces which communicate directly with the mediastinum, and determine the mechanism by which perforations in the cervical esophagus and infections of the oropharynx can spread to the thorax.

The clinically important areas in the neck are divided into three sections determined by their relationship to the hyoid bone (Fig. 51.1). The retropharyngeal and the visceral spaces extend both above and below the hyoid bone. The retropharyngeal space, or retrovisceral space, is limited anteriorly by the middle layer of the

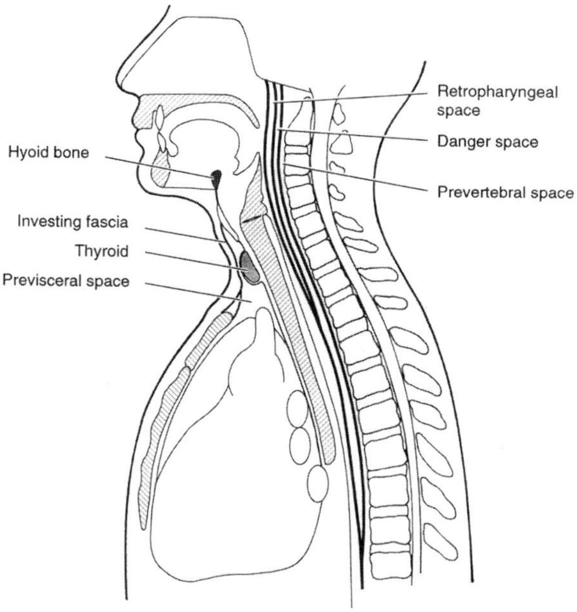

Fig. 51.1. The deep fascial layers of the neck and their relationship to the mediastinum

deep cervical fascia and the deepest layer of the deep cervical fascia, or the alar fascia posteriorly. This space exists behind the hypopharynx and esophagus from the base of the skull to the superior mediastinum. Retropharyngeal infections in this space can descend easily into the superior mediastinum. This was recognized early to be the space most likely involved in cervical esophageal perforations [1, 5]. This space is often involved in extension of infections of the cervical vertebra. Just posterior to the retropharyngeal space, between the alar fascia and the prevertebral fascia, is an area called by some authors the "danger space" [5], which extends from the base of the skull to the crus of the diaphragm and is a source of potential dissemination of retropharyngeal or lateropharyngeal infection to the base of the posterior mediastinum and the retroperitoneal space [3, 5].

The visceral space is located within the carotid sheath and includes all three layers of the deep cervical fascia. Infections in this space less commonly extend down to the mediastinum, but given their location in relationship to the great vessels, can cause internal jugular vein septic thrombophlebitis and carotid artery rupture. Classically, suppurative lymphadenitis, peritonsillar abscess, and Ludwig's angina were causes of infections in this space; however, any of the structures of the pharynx and neck can serve as a source.

Above the hyoid bone are the submandibular space, the lateral pharyngeal space, the masticator space, and the parotid space. The submandibular and masticator spaces are most involved with dental infections, with Ludwig's angina being a result of submandibular space infection. The lateral pharyngeal space communicates with many of the spaces in the neck and is associated with infections of the pharynx, teeth, tonsils, or parotids. The parotid space communicates directly with the "danger space" and the lateral pharyngeal space. Therefore, infections in the parotids can rapidly extend throughout the mediastinum.

Below the hyoid bone is the anterior visceral or previsceral space. This extends from the hyoid bone superiorly to the anterior mediastinum inferiorly. It is bordered by the strap muscles anteriorly, and surrounds the trachea, with the esophagus forming its posterior border. The pretracheal investing fascia is attached to the pericardium and the parietal pleura, which can result in pericarditis and empyema from infection in this space. The most common causes of infection in this space include tracheal or esophageal disruption. Finally, the course of the esophagus is important to review, as esophageal perforation is a significant cause of mediastinitis and the complications of this can be predicted partially from the site of the perforation. The upper two-thirds of the thoracic esophagus lies in close proximity to the right pleural space, while the distal third deviates to the left to enter the diaphragmatic hiatus. Perforations of the lower thoracic esophagus are more likely to cause left-sided empyemas and possible retroperitoneal extension.

51.1.3 Pathogenesis

The causes of mediastinitis are multiple (Table 51.1). However, cases can be divided by source, which explains the microbiology of the infection and also in part determines treatment strategies. Head and neck infections, esophageal perforations, and post-sternotomy infections are the primary causes of mediastinitis. Other more unusual causes of mediastinal infection will also be addressed.

51.2 Descending Necrotizing Mediastinitis

Descending necrotizing mediastinitis is an unusual infection arising from the structures of the mouth, neck, and pharynx. This begins as a localized infection, which then descends inferiorly via the fascial planes of the neck into the thorax. Several factors facilitate the spread of these infections to the mediastinal structures, including gravitational drainage, negative intrathoracic pressure with inspiration, and the lack of significant barriers in the retropharyngeal space. The fascial planes of the neck can be penetrated by these infections, and subsequently involve all compartments of the neck and mediastinum. Often, patients can rapidly

Table 51.1. Selected causes of mediastinitis

Descending necrotizing mediastinitis	**Esophageal perforation**
Odontogenic [5, 7–9]	Emesis [39, 55]
Ludwig's angina [13]	Carcinoma [40, 41, 46]
Peritonsillar abscesses [5, 13–15]	Foreign body [49, 50]
Parotitis [17]	Penetrating trauma [45, 52, 53]
Facial cellulitis [20]	Blunt trauma [48, 49, 52]
Epiglottitis [19]	Traumatic hyperextension [44]
Pharyngitis [13–16]	*Iatrogenic*
Infectious mononucleosis [16]	Esophagogastroduodenoscopy [46]
Cervical lymphadenitis [1]	Esophageal dilation [44]
Iatrogenic	Nasogastric tube [46]
Tooth extraction [11, 12]	Esophageal sclerotherapy [46]
Air-turbine dental equipment [11, 12]	Esophageal surgery [43, 46]
Oral [7] or nasal intubation	Dislodged cervical fixation device [47]
Post-tracheotomy [19]	**Cardiothoracic surgery**
Thyroidectomy [1]	Coronary artery bypass grafting [57]
Central venous catheterization [126]	Cardiac valve replacement [61–63, 66, 87–90]
	Cardiac transplantation [72–74, 84, 85]
	Disseminated spread
	Bacteremia [116–119]
	Pneumonia or empyema [1, 113–118, 121]

progress to septic shock, multi-system organ failure, and death unless adequate surgical therapy is initiated. Descending necrotizing mediastinitis has been classified as diffuse or localized type based on the level of infection seen on diagnostic CT imaging. Surgical treatment of descending mediastinitis varies accordingly with this classification system. In Type I descending mediastinitis, the infection is localized to the upper mediastinal space in the area above the tracheal bifurcation and treatment involves transcervical drainage to evacuate pus. Type II infection is diffuse in nature and subclassified as IIA involving the anterior lower mediastinum and IIB, involving infection in the lower posterior mediastinum. Treatment of Type IIA infection includes irrigation through the subxiphoidal and cervical incisions in addition to percutaneous thoracic drainage as needed. Finally, Type IIB infection is treated with complete irrigation and debridement of the mediastinum through a right standard thoracotomy followed by left minimal thoracotomy [6].

Odontogenic infections account for 30–70% of all cases of descending mediastinitis [3, 5, 7, 8]. Infections involving the 2nd and 3rd mandibular molars are particularly dangerous, since the roots of these teeth extend below the hyoid ridge. Thus, apical abscesses in the 2nd and 3rd molar roots can often rupture through the mandibular bone into the submandibular space, causing Ludwig's angina or gaining access to the deeper spaces of the neck. Occasionally, these infections will be occult or minor [10, 11]. Dental procedures such as tooth extraction, root canal therapy, high speed air-turbine dental equipment, and laceration of oral soft tissue have been also associated with mediastinitis [11, 12].

Peritonsillar and retropharyngeal infections account for most of the remaining cases of descending necrotizing mediastinitis. Peritonsillar abscesses complicating bacterial tonsillitis [3, 5, 13–15] or infectious mononucleosis [16] are frequently reported. Retropharyngeal abscesses may develop from extension of a peritonsillar disease, penetrating trauma to the pharynx [3], parotitis [17], epiglottitis [18], oral or nasotracheal intubation [7], and post-tracheotomy [19]. In one study 50% of patients with parapharyngeal neck infections had some evidence of mediastinal involvement by CT [20].

Other rare causes of descending necrotizing mediastinitis include facial cellulitis [21] and transnasal sinus drainage [8]. Though common in the pre-antibiotic era, suppurative cervical lymphadenitis, cervical discitis, and post-thyroidectomy surgical site infections rarely cause mediastinitis currently.

51.2.1 Microbiology

Descending necrotizing mediastinitis is generally a polymicrobial infection, caused by aerobic and anaerobic oropharyngeal flora. Mediastinal tissue, pericardial fluid, and pleural fluid have multiple organisms seen on Gram stain. Typical anaerobic bacteria include *Bacteroides* spp., *Fusobacterium* spp., anaerobic *Streptococcus* spp. *Peptostreptococcus* sp., and *Prevotella denticola* [12]. Aerobic organisms most frequently recovered include aerobic streptococci, *Staphylococcus aureus*, and the family Enterobacteriaceae. Several authors [3, 22, 23] have theorized that the altered redox potential and the closed spaces of the fascial planes of the neck lead to an environment in which organisms can thrive, resulting in a high organism count and rapid tissue destruction.

51.2.2
Signs and Symptoms

Many patients with mediastinitis present with fever, neck and chest pain or non-specific symptoms. Often, individuals are on antibiotics for dental infections or presumed bacterial pharyngitis [3]. Mediastinitis can be missed initially unless clinical suspicion is high. Development of chest pain in individuals with infections of the head and neck should arouse suspicion of mediastinal spread [5]. As mediastinal infection progresses, brawny induration of the upper chest and neck can occur, along with pitting edema and subcutaneous crepitus. This process can then extend to the upper extremities in some cases [8]. Loss of the sternal notch and the clavicular landmarks can also be seen. These signs, while highly suggestive of mediastinitis, are insensitive [8]. Though dysphagia is more commonly associated with esophageal perforation, it can be seen in cases of posterior mediastinitis in which the esophagus is compressed by abscess formation [24]. Airway compromise due to compression of the central airway and pharynx from inflammation is common and can lead to dyspnea and ultimately respiratory collapse. Epigastric and abdominal pain mimicking an acute abdomen has been reported with descent of the necrotizing process into the retroperitoneum [3].

Because descending necrotizing mediastinitis can progress rapidly and diagnosis is frequently delayed, patients often present with complications. As discussed earlier, complications are dependent on the anatomy of the mediastinum. The most frequent complication is empyema due to rupture of a mediastinal abscess through the parietal pleura. Transudative pleural effusions have been reported; however, purulent fluid from direct extension of the infection is more common. Bacterial pericarditis with friction rub or tamponade has been described, which is also believed to be secondary to direct extension. This is especially true of infections in the pretracheal space. Involvement of the cranial nerves in the neck can lead to focal neurological deficits. As the disease progresses, tracheal and esophageal fistulas can develop [25]. Vascular structures in both the neck and thorax are also susceptible to involvement, including thrombosis of the internal jugular vein or the carotid artery rupture [9]. The great vessels in the thorax, particularly the innominate vein and artery, can erode from direct infection [3, 8], resulting in rapid exsanguination. Anterior mediastinitis can rarely result in superior vena cava obstruction with head and neck cyanosis, edema, and neck vein distention [24].

51.2.3
Diagnosis

Rapid diagnosis of descending necrotizing mediastinitis is crucial. While 60% of patients with necrotizing mediastinitis due to an odontogenic infection present for medical attention within 48 h of onset of symptoms, the delay may be as long as 15 days [5]. Several reviews have noted a delay from admission to diagnosis on average of 2.5 days [3, 5, 8]. As clinical signs are often non-specific or do not become apparent until widespread tissue destruction has already occurred, radiological diagnosis is paramount [3, 5, 8, 27]. Radiographic findings in descending necrotizing mediastinitis can be identified in both lateral simple neck and standard chest X-rays. Lateral neck radiographs may reveal subcutaneous air in the soft tissue of the neck, swelling of the prevertebral soft tissue (suggestive of retropharyngeal abscess), loss of cervical spine lordosis, or air in the retropharyngeal space. Chest radiographs can show mediastinal widening, pneumomediastinum, anterior displacement of the thoracic trachea due to abscess formation, mediastinal air-fluid levels, enlarged cardiac silhouette, and pleural effusion. Plain radiography, however, is usually negative early in the disease, with findings only becoming present after sepsis has developed [27].

Most authors agree that the most rapid and effective way to diagnose descending mediastinitis is by CT [3, 5, 8, 27]. Magnetic nuclear resonance (MRI) can similarly show fascial planes and chest involvement; however, patients often are too unstable to undergo MRI. CT is particularly helpful in assessing extent of disease and guiding surgical therapy. The benefit of CT became apparent in the review by Estrera et al. in 1983 [3] when mediastinal involvement was noted in these patients by CT when plain films had been unrevealing. Fluid collections, loss of distinct tissue planes, mediastinal inflammation, and air in the mediastinum are easily seen by CT. Pericarditis and empyemas can also be assessed by this method. Serial CT imaging with contrast has been shown to be useful in identifying progression of descending necrotizing mediastinitis into the neck and chest. As a surveillance tool, CT allows for earlier diagnosis and directed operative drainage [28].

51.2.4
Treatment

The effective management of descending necrotizing mediastinitis requires rapid recognition of the extent of disease. Aggressive fluid resuscitation, stabilization of the compromised airway, early empiric antibiotic therapy, and surgical drainage are the mainstays of therapy.

The dramatic inflammatory reaction often seen in mediastinal infections results in a significant amount of third space sequestration. This requires volume resuscitation with intravenous fluids. The extensive amount of pharyngeal edema and inflammation seen in descending necrotizing mediastinitis can rapidly compromise the airway. Many authors recommend tracheotomy for all patients with descending necrotizing mediastinitis to assure airway patency, and to avoid the risk of accidental dislodgement of an endotracheal tube, which may be impossible to replace in the face of tissue edema [3, 8, 27, 29, 30]. Endotracheal intubation causing the traumatic rupture of a parapharyngeal abscess into the pharynx, with subsequent aspiration pneumonia, has been reported [8]. More recent authors, however, have taken the approach of performing a tracheotomy only when there is evidence of impending airway compromise by clinical criteria or CT [7]. This is in part due to the risk of introducing infection into the lower airway perioperatively during the procedure [7, 31–33]. Regardless, a low threshold for performing tracheotomy is a prudent approach in these patients.

Descending necrotizing mediastinitis is a surgical emergency. As noted previously, despite the onset of improved imaging, the mortality of this disease has not changed dramatically in the last 20 years. This is felt in part by many to be a result of inadequate initial surgical drainage and debridement. Though there are some reports of successful antibiotic management alone [20] and CT-guided drainage of focal mediastinal abscesses [34], most agree that aggressive surgical drainage is the cornerstone of therapy [3, 5, 8, 25–27, 35]. Transcervical drainage was the traditional approach to descending necrotizing mediastinitis; however, this was felt by many to be inadequate, particularly when there was extension of necrosis below the level of the fourth thoracic vertebrae [3]. In cases that involve the anterior mediastinum a subxiphoid incision combined with submandibular incisions has been used [26, 27]. However, most surgeons advocate drainage by thoracotomy when mediastinitis involves either the pleural space, pericardial cavity, or the inferior mediastinum [8, 35]. Several risks are associated with standard thoracotomy including osteomyelitis, phrenic nerve palsy, and sternal dehiscence [36]. Some authors have reported successful treatment of descending necrotizing mediastinitis, involving the posterior and lower mediastinum, using video-assisted thoracoscopic surgery [6, 36]. In patients suspected to have posterior mediastinitis, particularly in the case of post-esophagectomy, transesophageal echocardiography and guided fine-needle aspiration has also been reported to be useful in both diagnostic and therapeutic management of the disease [37]. More recently, some authors have reported favorable results in the treatment of descending necrotizing mediastinitis using percutaneous catheter drainage versus the conventional surgical approach. Percutaneous catheter drainage is a less invasive procedure associated with a decreased propensity to develop secondary infections [38]. Post-operative fever that persists, or lack of clinical improvement, should prompt a repeat CT to search for undrained sources of infection [8].

Empiric antibiotic therapy coverage should be initiated as soon as possible. Antibiotic coverage should be broad and directed toward those organisms most likely to be implicated in this infection. Regimens with activity against Gram-positive organisms, including *Streptococcus* and *Staphylococcus* spp., parapharyngeal facultative anaerobes, and Gram-negative aerobic organisms, are most appropriate. Penicillin G has activity against the oral flora both aerobic and the facultative anaerobic bacteria and can be used as part of an initial regimen. However, many of the *Prevotella* spp. have acquired β-lactam resistance, so clindamycin or metronidazole would be necessary, along with another antibiotic with Gram-negative activity. Alternatively, single-agent empiric therapy with a broad spectrum β-lactamase resistant penicillin, such as imipenem, piperacillin/tazobactam, ticarcillin/tazobactam, or ampicillin/sulbactam, can be used. Antibiotic therapy can be further refined once surgical culture results become available. Anaerobic coverage should be continued regardless of culture results, however, given that anaerobic bacteria are frequently difficult to recover. The duration of antibiotic therapy must be tailored to the clinical response of the patient but frequently is on the order of weeks.

51.3 Mediastinitis Resulting from Esophageal Perforation

Disruption of the esophagus results in the spillage of salivary secretions and food particles directly into the mediastinum. Prior to the onset of modern cardiothoracic surgery, esophageal perforation was the most common cause of mediastinitis in the first half of the twentieth century [1]. While oropharyngeal flora plays a role in the pathogenesis of mediastinitis due to esophageal perforation, there remain significant differences in presentation, diagnosis, and surgical management between this entity and mediastinitis arising from head and neck infections.

The most common causes of esophageal perforation are iatrogenic [39–41] and secondary to endoscopy, esophageal dilation procedures, complications of variceal banding or electrocautery, breakdown of surgical anastomoses after esophageal resection, or inadvertent perforation during head and neck surgery [42–44]. Patients who develop perforation after instrumentation generally have some underlying esophageal disease [46]. Case reports of migration of dislodged cervical fixation devices or cervical bone fragments eroding into the esophagus have been noted [47]. Hyperextension injuries of the cervical spine and other trauma to the neck and chest are also causes of esophageal rupture. Deceleration injury resulting in thoracic esophageal perforation has also been reported [48]. Glatterer et al. [45] reviewed 26 cases of esophageal perforation and found that 21 of these cases were due to cervical injury, of which four were due to blunt trauma. Another cause of esophageal injury is erosion due to foreign bodies lodged within the esophagus, particularly in patients with underlying esophageal pathology [49]. Finally, malignancy, ingestion of caustic substances, and emesis are well-recognized sources of perforation. Perforation due to malignancy has a worse outcome and may be related to a tendency towards a more conservative approach [40, 46].

Because esophageal injury results in the spillage of oropharyngeal secretions into the mediastinum, the microbiology is very similar to that found in mediastinitis secondary to odontogenic disease. These infections are generally polymicrobial in nature. Gram-positive organisms such as *Streptococcus* and *Staphylococcus* spp. along with facultative and obligate anaerobes from the oropharyngeal flora are frequent causative pathogens. Gram-negative enteric bacteria have also been identified from culture. *Candida* spp. frequently colonizes the human esophagus and has also been identified in infections [42].

51.3.1 Signs and Symptoms

Mediastinitis arises as a complication of esophageal perforation often because the perforation is missed. Immediately after an injury occurs, the classic symptoms of chest pain and subcutaneous emphysema are often absent. In individuals with head and neck trauma, the diagnosis may be obscured by more apparent injuries. Patients may present with chest pain, shortness of breath, nausea, and malaise. Dysphagia and odynophagia have been reported, especially in cases involving foreign bodies. Pediatric cases of foreign body ingestion can have excessive salivation or what appears to be new onset asthma [50]. Cervical esophageal injury can present with pain and tenderness in the neck, resistance in the neck to passive motion, cough, stridor, hoarseness, or bleeding in the mouth. Lower thoracic injuries can present as a rigid or tender abdomen, along with a mediastinal crunch on auscultation due to pneumomediastinum. In individuals with blunt or penetrating trauma to the neck or chest, subcutaneous emphysema, hematoma of the neck, and blood return from nasogastric tube have also been associated with perforation [45]. As the process advances, neck erythema, swelling, and fever become apparent, finally progressing to septic shock and multisystem organ failure.

As with infections arising from the head and neck, mediastinitis from esophageal perforation will often present with complications of infection. Extension into the pleural space can lead to pneumothorax, hemothorax, and empyema. Purulent pericarditis can be seen. Esophageal fistula formation is a late complication of infection, which can result in communication with the skin, respiratory tract, or vascular structures in the mediastinum and neck [45, 51]. Exsanguination from aortoesophageal fistulas has been reported [50].

51.3.2 Diagnosis

There is no single best test to diagnose esophageal perforation. Oral contrast studies performed with a water-soluble material, such as Gastrografin, will often reveal a disruption. This is generally the safest method for rapid diagnosis and should be the first step in evaluation of a suspected esophageal perforation. However, in several reviews water-soluble contrast studies have been associated with a false-negative rate of between 20 % and 50 % [45, 52, 53]. This has led some authors to recommend performing barium swallow studies or endoscopy if the initial water-soluble study is negative [45, 50]. Other imaging modalities, such as CT and MRI, are useful in defining the extent of mediastinal involvement, but lack detailed visualization of esophageal anatomy. Plain radiography can give some clues to the underlying diagnosis of an esophageal perforation and mediastinitis, but lacks adequate sensitivity [45]. Cervical or mediastinal air, mediastinal widening, pleural effusion, pneumothorax, or mediastinal air-fluid levels all can be seen. Occasionally, a foreign body can be identified on plain film.

51.3.3 Treatment

Success in treating mediastinitis secondary to esophageal perforation rests partially on the rapid diagnosis of the underlying perforation. A detailed history is important to identify risk factors for disruption such as violent emesis, recent endoscopic procedures, and ingestions. Often in trauma cases a history is unavailable and instead a high index of suspicion must be present, particularly in injuries to the neck and penetrating chest wounds. Contamination of the paraesophageal space with saliva and bacteria occurs early in the course of injury, and delay in diagnosis leads to extension of infection. Several authors have shown increased mortality if the delay in diagnosis is greater than 12–24 h [42, 51]. However, more recent studies have shown less of an association with outcome and time to diagnosis [40, 46]. When esophageal perforation is suspected, the patient should be made NPO to minimize further contamination and empiric antimicrobial therapy should be instituted.

As with descending head and neck infections rapid institution of broad-spectrum antimicrobials is essential. *Candida* spp., as noted above, is frequently isolated from culture and empiric antifungal therapy, particularly in patients at high risk for invasive fungal disease (e.g., prolonged ICU stay, prior broad-spectrum antibiotic use, and neutropenia), should be considered [39].

Surgical management of esophageal perforation remains somewhat controversial. Some have advocated conservative management with antibiotic therapy, nothing by mouth, and interventional radiology-placed drainage, nasogastric drainage, and supplemental enteral or parenteral nutrition for contained perforations without sepsis [46]. The use of esophageal stents [55] to contain perforations and thorascopic drainage of the mediastinum [56] have also been reported. Most do agree, however, that in patients with circumferential or multiple disruptions of the esophagus, intra-abdominal perforations, uncontained perforations, and evidence of mediastinitis or sepsis, surgical intervention is warranted [40]. Surgical techniques of repair perforations vary by surgeon and center. The techniques are influenced by the underlying co-morbidities and overall operative risk in a particular patient. These procedures include primary repair with or without pleural or muscular buttress, esophagectomy, T-tube drainage, and cervical esophagostomy.

Recent studies have shown some improvement in mortality from infections due to esophageal leaks, with current rates of 4–25% [40, 46], versus 15–44% [42, 45] in the late 1980s. There has not been a significant change in the time to diagnosis [46], however. Whether advances in intensive care management or refinement in selection of surgical approach account for the decreased death rate is unclear. Despite this, infections due to esophageal perforation remain a significant source of morbidity and mortality.

51.4 Mediastinitis as a Complication of Cardiac Surgery

With the advent of cardiopulmonary bypass, the modern era of cardiothoracic surgery became a reality. It was recognized early that infections of the sternum could easily extend into the mediastinum and carry serious consequences. Though the incidence of post-operative deep wound infection has been between 0.23% and 2.7% in most large studies [59–65], the mortality has been between 14% and 41% [59, 61–63, 67]. These infections are associated with significant morbidity; median hospital length-of-stay for an infected patient is double that of non-infected patients [67]. Additionally, many infected patients need to undergo repeated surgical procedures. Often, patients who survive the infection are left with chronic pain and significant chest wall deformity. Despite the relatively low incidence of mediastinitis from cardiac surgery, the sheer number of procedures performed each year have made it the most common cause of acute mediastinitis today.

Host risk factors for mediastinitis after cardiac surgery include diabetes mellitus [63, 64], obesity [63, 65], and extended preoperative hospital length of stay [66]. Perioperative risk factors include use of intra-aortic balloon pump or other inotropic support [65], excessive aortic cross-clamp and by-pass time [69], re-exploration or emergent surgery [63, 65, 69], prolonged post-operative mechanical ventilation [70, 71], and concurrent saphenous vein graft harvest site infection [63]. Several other procedures such as pre-operative chest hair removal by razor shaving [64], reliance on electrocautery for dissection [69], and use of bilateral internal mammary arterial grafting in diabetics [65] have all been associated with increased risk of deep sternal wound infections.

Cardiac transplantation procedures warrant special discussion. Several studies have documented sternal wound infection rates following cardiac transplant of approximately 2.5% [72, 73]. Risk factors specifically associated with mediastinitis after cardiac transplant include prior mediastinotomy, ischemic cardiomyopathy, and early acute rejection requiring the use of steroids and murine-monoclonal CD-3 antibody (OKT3) [72, 73]. Donor-to-recipient transmission of bacteria has also been reported as a cause of mediastinitis [74].

51.4.1 Microbiology

The microbiology of mediastinitis following cardiac surgical procedures differs from infections which arise from head and neck or esophageal sources. This is due to the skin being the supposed primary site of entry. Several studies have noted an approximately 60% positive culture rate when sternal wounds were explored. Gram-positive organisms are the predominate organism isolated in sternal wound cultures [59, 61, 63, 65, 67, 75], with *Staphylococcus aureus* as the most common organism isolated, followed by coagulase-negative *Staphylococcus* and *Enterococcus* spp. Some more unusual organisms, such as *S. pneumoniae* and *Aspergillus flavus,* have been reported as causative agents [76, 77]. Gram negative bacteria are present in approximately 20–40% of infections and commonly include *E. coli*, *Enterobacter* spp., *Serratia* spp., *Klebsiella* spp., and *Pseudomonas* species [62, 63, 67, 75]. Post-operative infections with *Candida* spp. [78] have been associated with prolonged pre-operative antibiotic use. The rate of candidemia in these patients was 75% in one study [78]. Anaerobes, such as *Proprionobacterium acne*, *Bacteroides* spp. [80, 81], have been identified as causative agents in a number of cases. Other more unusual pathogens, such as *Corynebacterium xerosis* [82] and *Mycoplasma hominis* [83], have been rarely reported. *M. hominis* can be missed due to slow growth in anaerobic media. Compared to mediastinitis due to head and neck or esophageal sources, post-operative mediastinitis is polymicrobial in nature only 10% of the time [66, 75]. Bacteremia occurs in 23–57% of patients with mediastinitis and has been associated with increased mortality [58]. Conversely, in individuals who are bacteremic after coronary artery by-pass, deep sternal wound infections were the cause in 67% of the cases in one study [79]. There have been cases of hematogenous seeding of the wound site from catheter-associated bacteremia [86]. Mediastinitis after cardiac transplantation also is most frequently due to *Staphylococcus* spp., followed by Gram-negative bacilli; however, some opportunistic organisms, such as *Nocardia* spp. [73, 74, 84] and *Aspergillus* spp. [85], have been reported.

Rapid-growing mycobacterium are an unusual group of pathogens associated with post-sternotomy mediastinitis. *M. fortuitum*, *M. chelonei*, and *M. smegmatis* have all caused deep sternal wound infections. Porcine heterograft valves contaminated with *M. chelonei* [87–89], and ice for cooling cardioplegic solution contaminated with *M. fortuitum* [90], have been responsible for epidemic outbreaks of mediastinitis in cardiothoracic units. Clinically, infections with the rapid-growing mycobacterium tend to be more indolent, with the formation of cold abscesses and fistulas [91] or minimal inflammatory signs [92]. However, infections with these organisms can result in breakdown of vein graft anastomotic sites and aortic pseudoaneurysms due to vasculitis [90]. Rapid-growing mycobacterium should be considered in those patients with evidence of deep sternal wound infection post-sternotomy, but negative routine cultures [93].

51.4.2 Signs and Symptoms

Mediastinitis after cardiac surgery can present as late as 3–6 months after surgery; however, the average time to presentation is 7–15 days post-procedure [61, 67]. Wound drainage, which occurs in 70–100% of cases, erythema, increased pain at the operative site, and fever have been observed in case reviews of post-surgical mediastinitis [61, 94]. Though wound drainage is frequently present, it is non-specific. Sternal instability and sternal dehiscence, either partial or complete, are indicators of underlying deep infection; however, they are reportedly present in only 25–60% of mediastinitis patients [57]. In one study dehiscence was observed to occur 24–48 h after onset of wound drainage [64]. Drainage through the sternotomy wound that bubbles with respiratory chest wall motion is indicative of deep infection in the mediastinum; in one pediatric series all patients with this finding had anterior mediastinal involvement [80]. Laboratory data is generally limited in usefulness. Leukocytosis [62, 64, 95] is the most common laboratory finding in mediastinitis. In a small percentage of patients, leukocytosis and persistent fever may be the only presenting signs of mediastinal infection.

Post-sternotomy mediastinitis can be associated with serious complications. Empyema and pericarditis from direct extension of infection can be seen, along with sepsis, and multisystem organ failure. Endocarditis has been seen in valve replacement surgery and cardiac transplantation. Coronary artery graft anastomotic breakdown and aortic graft dehiscence with fatal exsanguination have also been reported [68].

51.4.3 Diagnosis

The diagnosis of post-operative mediastinitis is based on a high clinical index of suspicion. No single test is definitive. Several studies have looked at the utility of wound and epicardial lead cultures in the diagnosis of mediastinitis. Surface wound cultures in one review were not sensitive, yielding the causative pathogen in only 6 of 15 cases [68]. Cultures of epicardial pacemaker leads, given their position in the anterior mediastinum and ease at which they can be removed under sterile conditions for culture, have been looked at as a diagnostic tool. However, one large study showed that the overall positive predictive value of epicardial cultures was only 11.6%, and only slightly better with *S. aureus*-positive cultures [60]. The role of chest radiography is limited in the diagnosis of deep sternal wound infections. Indium scanning has been evaluated in a small study, which showed an 83% sensitivity rate [96]. Computerized tomography can be used for diagnostic purposes [73, 96], but again there are conflicting reports of the sensitivity and specificity of the technique. Yamaguchi et al. studied the diagnostic validity of CT for mediastinitis following cardiac surgery and found a sensitivity of 67% and specificity of 83% in a small case series of patients. By post-operative day 14, the authors found both the sensitivity and specificity of CT as a diagnostic modality to reach 100% [96]. CT can identify fluid collections to sample for evidence of infection (Fig. 51.2). It is also useful in following patients after debridement and drainage. Benlolo reports the use of sternal puncture as a diagnostic procedure to be helpful in achieving an earlier diagnosis of post-sternotomy mediastinitis, thereby leading to decreased morbidity/mortality and shorter length of ICU stay [97]. Bedside sternal aspiration can therefore be useful in making a diagnosis and obtaining early culture results to guide antibiotic therapy [98].

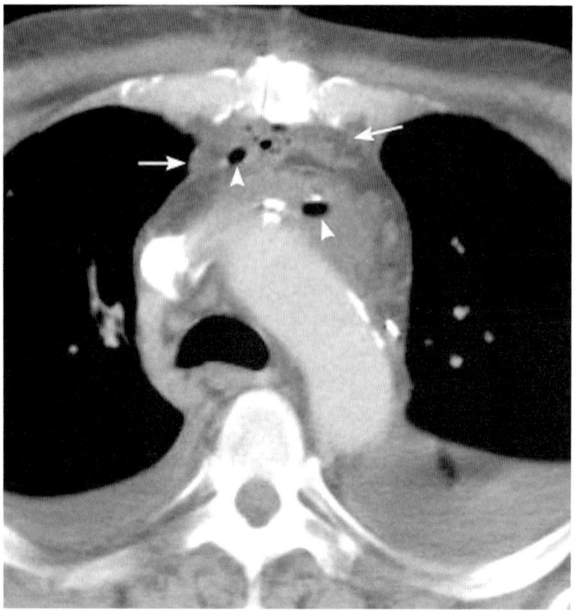

Fig. 51.2. Mediastinal abscess following median sternotomy. Computed tomography scan 3 weeks following coronary artery bypass grafting shows soft tissue stranding of the retrosternal fat (*arrows*). A prevascular fluid collection is also present as well as abundant gas bubbles (*arrowheads*). (From Lee KT, Sagel SS, Stanley RJ, Heiken JP. In: Computed body tomography with MRI correlation, vols 1, 2. 4th edn. 2006, Lippincott Williams and Wilkins, with permission)

51.4.4 Treatment

Antibiotic therapy alone for mediastinitis is generally inadequate, and should be viewed as an adjuvant to surgical treatment. Antimicrobial therapy should be empirically started when post-operative infection is suspected. Coverage should include anti-staphylococcal coverage and, given the significant proportion of cases in which Gram-negative organisms are isolated, a broad-spectrum antibiotic with activity against cephalosporinase-producing organisms, such as *Enterobacter* spp., should be given. Therapy should then be tailored to cover organisms found in intra-operative specimens and is generally on the order of 4–6 weeks of intravenous therapy, or longer in cases with significant sternal osteomyelitis. Initial surgical management of mediastinitis in the past consisted of debridement of necrotic or infected tissue, especially sternal bone, with the mediastinum left packed open to close by secondary intention. This approach resulted in a high morbidity, often complicated by pneumonia [94], prolonged hospital stay, abnormal thoracic wall mechanics, and cosmetic deformity.

Surgical treatment at present varies, and is partially dependent on the viability of the sternum at the time of surgery. Approaches in which the sternum is relatively intact include debridement with rewiring of the sternum, and percutaneous drainage, either as a single staged procedure, or after several days of open irrigation. Some have also advocated the use of continuous sternal irrigation with antibiotic or povidone-iodine solutions either in a closed procedure [99], or as follow-up of open debridement and re-wiring. Closed continuous sternal irrigation is able to maintain normal chest wall mechanics compared to open procedures, however, has been reported to have a high failure rate and an association with iodine toxicity when povidone-iodine was used as an irrigant [100, 101]. Several studies have looked at rigid fixed closure or modified re-wiring of the sternum after open debridement [102]. When there has been significant evidence of sternal destruction or recurrence of infection, frequently a large dead space is present after debridement. This often requires the use of muscle or omental flaps to both obliterate the dead space and achieve closure of the wound. Generally, this has been done as a staged procedure, particularly if a significant amount of infected, devitalized tissue is present, but in some series patients with relatively clean wound margins have had closure with myocutaneous flaps at the time of initial debridement and irrigation [103]. More recently, vacuum assisted closure therapy post-medial sternotomy has been advocated by some as first line therapy. This method has been shown to decrease wound edema, decrease the time to definitive closure and decrease bacteria colony counts in the wound, leading to lower rates of infection [104]. Others have examined the use of omental flaps as an adjunct to pectoralis muscle flaps. The advantages of using omentum include both availability and a characteristic highly vascular nature. In the small group of patients who underwent this procedure, the authors report no major post-operative complications and report the laparoscopic technique used in the study to be less invasive and useful in harvesting omentum [105]. While major plastic surgery allows for chest wall closures, long-term it can result in chronic pain, paresthesia, sternal instability, or shoulder weakness [106]. There are also rare reports of myocardial hemorrhage post-debridement, with puncture of the myocardium by the sternal edge [107, 108]. The ideal surgical management for patients with post-sternotomy mediastinitis remains to be defined.

51.5 Chronic Fibrosing Mediastinitis and Other Uncommon Causes of Mediastinitis

There are several infectious causes of mediastinitis, which can present with a more insidious course consisting of adenopathy and progressive fibrosis of mediastinal structures. This can result in pulmonary artery fibrosis with pulmonary hypertension, tracheobronchial stenosis, esophageal obstruction or esophago-respiratory fistulas, and superior vena caval obstruction. *Histoplasmosis capsulatum* is the organism most frequently associated with mediastinal fibrosis [109], though *Mycobacterium tuberculosis* [110], *Blastomyces dermatitidis* [112], and *Wuchereria bancrofti* [113] have been reported to result in similar syndromes. *H. capsulatum* is thought to cause mediastinal fibrosis from ongoing seepage of fungal antigens from granulomas in the mediastinal tissue resulting in a host hypersensitivity response [114]. Patients with chronic fibrosing mediastinitis can present with symptoms of cough, dyspnea, pleuritic chest pain, hemoptysis, dysphagia and superior vena cava syndrome, but the time between presentation of initial symptoms and late sequelae may last several years. In areas associated with endemic TB and histoplasmosis, a high level of clinical suspicion is warranted due to the nonspecific nature of symptoms and findings on exam. The definitive diagnosis is made through mediastinoscopy or thoracotomy [115]. There are various case reports on treating idiopathic fibrosing mediastinitis with corticosteroid therapy, but management of this disease overall remains unclear [115]. Inhalational exposure to the spores of *B. anthracis* may result in a mediastinitis. This has received attention in recent years due to concerns of the use of anthrax in biological warfare [120–122]. The infection results in a primary focal hemorrhagic, necrotizing pneumonia and can cause bloody pleural effusions [123]. Another striking finding in the clinical course of inhalational anthrax is the development of rapidly progressive hemorrhagic thoracic lymphadenitis and mediastinitis [121]. The significant amount of third-space fluid shift into the mediastinum can result in stridor, chest pain, and cyanosis from compression of the tracheobronchial tree [124]. Inhalational anthrax generally follows a biphasic clinical course. In the initial stage, patients can present with a nonspecific prodrome of malaise, myalgia, nonproductive cough, and fever followed by a short period of improvement. The second stage lasts up to 24 h and is marked by significant clinical deterioration, with the development of acute respiratory distress, hypoxemia, large pleural effusions septic shock and multiple organ dysfunction [123, 125]. Patients can rapidly progress to intravascular collapse and death. A widened mediastinum and significant pleural effusions may be seen on chest radiographs.

Hematogenous seeding of the mediastinum is unusual but has been reported. *Salmonella* spp. has been associated with mediastinitis from hematogenous dissemination [117]. *S. pyogenes* [118] and *S. aureus* [119] have also resulted in mediastinitis after bacteremia.

Finally, mediastinitis has been observed as a complication of central venous catheterization. Migration of the catheter out of the vessel into the mediastinum results in an infiltration of the infusate and chemical mediastinitis [126].

Mediastinitis continues to be a challenge for the clinician. For descending necrotizing mediastinitis an understanding of the anatomy of the head and neck is important in recognizing mediastinal infections which originate in these structures. Likewise, in patients with either esophageal disease or procedures performed on the esophagus, signs or symptoms of infection should warn the clinician of possible perforation. Understanding risk factors for mediastinitis after cardiac surgery and that deep sternal wound infections can often lack clear clinical indicators is important. Computerized tomography still remains the diagnostic test of choice for mediastinitis secondary to descending infection. For cases in which esophageal perforation is suspected, an oral contrast radiographic study can aid in diagnosis. While no single diagnostic test has proven superior for post-cardiac surgery mediastinitis, CT is helpful in guiding the surgical approach. The treatment of mediastinitis requires a high index of suspicion and prompt initiation of both broad antimicrobial therapy and surgical evaluation. This currently offers the best chance of survival in these critically ill patients.

References

1. Pearse HE, Jr (1938) Mediastinitis following cervical suppuration. Surg Gynecol Obstet 157:588–607
2. Culliford AT, Cunningham JN, Jr, Zeff RH, Isom OW, Teiko P, Spencer FC (1976) Sternal and costochondral infections following open-heart surgery. A review of 2,594 cases. J Thorac Cardiovasc Surg 72:714–726
3. Estrera AS, Landay MJ, Grisham JM, Sinn DP, Platt MR (1983) Descending necrotizing mediastinitis. Surg Gynecol Obstet 157:545–552
4. Kiernan PD, Hernandez A, Byrne WD, Bloom R, Dicicco B, Hetrick V, Graling P, Vaughan B (1998) Descending cervical mediastinitis. Ann Thorac Surg 65:1483–1488
5. Marty-Ane CH, Alauzen M, Alric P, Serres-Cousine O, Mary H (1994) Descending necrotizing mediastinitis. Advantage of mediastinal drainage with thoracotomy. J Thoracic Cardiovasc Surg 107:55–61
6. Min HK, Choi YS, Shim YM, Sohn YI, Kim J (2004) Descending necrotizing mediastinitis: A minimally invasive approach using video-assisted thorascopic surgery. Ann Thoracic Surg 77:306–310
7. Temes RT, Crowell RE, Mapel DW, Ketai L, Pett SB, Jr, Wernly JA (1998) Mediastinitis without antecedent surgery. Thorac Cardiovasc Surg 46:84–88
8. Colmenero RC, Labajo AD, Yanez VI, Paniagua J (1993) Thoracic complications of deeply situated serous neck infections. J Craniomaxillofac Surg 21:76–81
9. Zachariades N, Mezitis M, Stavrinidis P, Konsolaki-Agouridaki E (1988) Mediastinitis, thoracic empyema, and pericarditis as complications of a dental abscess: report of a case. J Oral Maxillofacial Surg 46:493–495
10. Haraden BM, Zwemer FL, Jr (1997) Descending necrotizing mediastinitis: complication of a simple dental infection. Ann Emerg Med 29:683–686
11. Phelps R, Jacobs RA (1985) Purulent pericarditis and mediastinitis due to *Peptococcus magnus*. JAMA 254:947–948
12. Rubin MM, Cozzi GM (1987) Fatal necrotizing mediastini-

tis as a complication of an odontogenic infection. J Oral Maxillofacial Surg 45:529 - 533
13. Gilchrist BF, Valerie EP, Nguyen M, Coren C, Klotz D, Ramenofsky ML (1997) Pearls and perils in the management of prolonged, peculiar, penetrating esophageal foreign bodies in children. J Pediatr Surg 32:1429 - 1431
14. Wills PI, Vernon RP, Jr (1981) Complications of space infections of the head and neck. Laryngoscope 91:1129 - 1136
15. Albertsen J, Thomsen EM (1970) Nonclostridial deep gas-producing infection in the neck. Arch Otolaryngol 92: 383 - 385
16. Kopec SE, Irwin RS, Mello CJ, Umali CB (1997) Bilateral anaerobic empyemas complicating infectious mononucleosis. Chest 112:833 - 835
17. Guardia SN, Cameron R, Phillips A (1991) Fatal necrotizing mediastinitis secondary to acute suppurative parotitis. J Otolaryngol 20:54 - 56
18. Chong WH, Woodhead MA, Millard FJ (1990) Mediastinitis and bilateral thoracic empyemas complicating adult epiglottitis. Thorax 45:491 - 492
19. Bishop MJ (1981) Epiglottitis in the adult. Anesthesiology 55:701 - 702
20. de Marie S, Tjon ATR, van der Mey AG, Meerdink G, van Furth R, van der Meer JW (1989) Clinical infections and nonsurgical treatment of parapharyngeal space infections complicating throat infection. Rev Infect Dis 11:975 - 982
21. Perfect JR (1980) Mediastinitis complicating cellulitis of the head and neck. South Med J 73:1378 - 1380
22. Economopoulos GC, Scherzer HH, Gryboski WA (1983) Successful management of mediastinitis, pleural empyema, and aortopulmonary fistula from odontogenic infection. Ann Thorac Surg 35:184 - 187
23. Stone HH, Martin JD, Jr (1972) Synergistic necrotizing cellulitis. Ann Surg 175:702 - 711
24. Pane GA, Hamilton GC, Call E (1983) Nontraumatic suppurative mediastinitis presenting as acute mediastinal widening. Ann Emerg Med 12:777 - 779
25. Kruyt PM, Boonstra A, Fockens P, Reeders JW, van Lanschot JJ (1996) Descending necrotizing mediastinitis causing pleuroesophageal fistula. Successful treatment by combined transcervical and pleural drainage. Chest 109:1404 - 1407
26. al Ebrahim KE (1995) Descending necrotising mediastinitis: a case report and review of the literature. Eur J Cardiothoracic Surg 9:161 - 162
27. Wheatley MJ, Stirling MC, Kirsh MM, Gago O, Orringer MB (1990) Descending necrotizing mediastinitis: transcervical drainage is not enough. Ann Thoracic Surg 49: 780 - 784
28. Freeman RK, Vallieres E, Verrier ED, Karmy-Jones R, Wood DE (2000) Descending necrotizing mediastinitis: An analysis of the effects of serial surgical debridement on patient mortality. J Thoracic Cardiovasc Surg 119(2):260 - 267
29. Lalwani AK, Kaplan MJ (1991) Mediastinal and thoracic complications of necrotizing fasciitis of the head and neck. Head Neck 13:531 - 539
30. Maisel RH, Karlen R (1994) Cervical necrotizing fasciitis. Laryngoscope 104:795 - 798
31. Zeitoun IM, Dhanarajani PJ (1995) Cervical cellulitis and mediastinitis caused by odontogenic infections: report of two cases and review of literature. J Oral Maxillofacial Surg 53:203 - 208
32. Ogiso A, Tamura M, Minemura T, Kurashina K, Kotani A (1992) Mediastinitis caused by odontogenic infection associated with adult respiratory distress syndrome. Oral Surg Oral Med Oral Pathol 74:15 - 18
33. Harrison GA, Schultz TA, Schaberg SJ (1983) Deep neck infection complicated by diabetes mellitus. Report of a case. Oral Surg Oral Med Oral Pathol 55:133 - 137
34. Marsh MD, Amorosa JK, Abassi M, Nosher JL, Gross SC, Alcid DV (1984) Salmonella mediastinitis - a rare disease. Comput Radiol 8:375 - 377
35. Bonapart IE, Stevens HP, Kerver AJ, Rietveld AP (1995) Rare complications of an odontogenic abscess: mediastinitis, thoracic empyema and cardiac tamponade. J Oral Maxillofac Surg 53:610 - 613
36. Ho MW, Dhariwal DK, Chandrasekhar J, Patton DW, Silvester KC, Sadiq S, Evans RM (2005) Use of interventional radiology in the management of oral and maxillofacial surgery. October 15.
37. Fritscher-Ravens A, Schirrow L, Pothmann W, Knofel WT, Swain P, Soehendra N (2003) Critical care TEE and guided FNA for diagnosis and management of posterior mediastinitis. Crit Care Med 31(1):126 - 132
38. Nakamori Y, Fujimi S, Ogura H, Kuwagata Y, Tanaka H, Shimazu T, Ueda T, Sugimoto H (2004) Conventional open surgery versus percutaneous catheter drainage in the treatment of cervical necrotizing fasciitis and descending necrotizing mediastinitis. Am J Roentgenol 182:1443 - 1449
39. Bauer TM, Dupont V, Zimmerli W (1996) Invasive candidiasis complicating spontaneous esophageal perforation. Am J Gastroenterol 91:1248 - 1250
40. Bufkin BL, Miller JI, Jr, Mansour KA (1996) Esophageal perforation: emphasis on management. Ann Thorac Surg 61:1447 - 1451
41. Reeder LB, DeFilippi VJ, Ferguson MK (1995) Current results of therapy for esophageal perforation. Am J Surg 169:615 - 617
42. Burnett CM, Rosemurgy AS, Pfeiffer EA (1990) Life-threatening acute posterior mediastinitis due to esophageal perforation. Ann Thoracic Surg 49:979 - 983
43. Holinger PH, Schild JA (1969) The Zenker's (hypopharyngeal) diverticulum. Ann Otol Rhinol Laryngol 78:679 - 688
44. Gertler JP, Brophy C, Elefteriades J (1986) Esophageal rupture after routine Maloney dilatation. A proposed mechanism. J Clin Gastroenterol 8:175 - 176
45. Glatterer MS, Jr, Toon RS, Ellestad C, McFee AS, Rogers W, Mack JW, Trinkle JK, Grover FL (1985) Management of blunt and penetrating external esophageal trauma. J Trauma 25:784 - 792
46. Lawrence DR, Moxon RE, Fountain SW, Ohri SK, Townsend ER (1998) Iatrogenic oesophageal perforations: a clinical review. Ann R Coll Surg Engl 80:115 - 118
47. Lew TW, Darby J, Marion DW (1995) Candida mediastinitis and septic shock following occult esophageal perforation in a patient with posttraumatic quadriplegia. J Trauma 39:805 - 808
48. Micon L, Geis L, Siderys H, Stevens L, Rodman GH, Jr (1990) Rupture of the distal thoracic esophagus following blunt trauma: case report. J Trauma 30:214 - 217
49. Kamath MP, Shanmugam, Shetty AB, Prasad KC (1998) A rare complication of an impacted foreign body in the cricopharynx. Am J Otolaryngol 19:61 - 65
50. Komatsu ES, Costa F, Marchese LT, Villari FS (1989) Abscess of the mediastinum: a case report. J Pediatr Surg 24:1125
51. Salo JA, Isolauri JO, Heikkila LJ, Markkula HT, Heikkinen LO, Kivilaakso EO, Mattila SP (1993) Management of delayed esophageal perforation with mediastinal sepsis. Esophagectomy or primary repair? J Thorac Cardiovasc Surg 106:1088 - 1091
52. Splener CW, Benfield JR (1976) Esophageal disruption from blunt and penetrating external trauma. Arch Surg 111:663 - 667

53. Weaver AW, Sankaran S, Fromm SH, Lucas CE, Walt AJ (1971) The management of penetrating wounds of the neck. Surg Gynecol Obstet 133:49 - 52
54. Buecker A, Wein BB, Neuerburg JM, Guenther RW (1997) Esophageal perforation: comparison of use of aqueous and barium-containing contrast media. Radiology 202:683 - 686
55. Eubanks PJ, Hu E, Nguyen D, Procaccino F, Eysselein VE, Klein SR (1999) Case of Boerhaave's syndrome successfully treated with a self-expandable metallic stent. Gastrointest Endosc 49:780 - 783
56. Roberts JR, Smythe WR, Weber RW, Lanutti M, Rosengard BR, Kaiser LR (1997) Thoracoscopic management of descending necrotizing mediastinitis. Chest112:850 - 854
57. Bitkover CY, Gardlund B (1998) Mediastinitis after cardiovascular operations: a case-control study of risk factors. Ann Thoracic Surg 65:36 - 40
58. Munoz P, Menasalvas A, Bernaldo de Quiros JC, Desco M, Vallejo JL, Bouza E (1997) Postsurgical mediastinitis: a case-control study. Clin Infect Dis 25:1060 - 1064
59. Maroto LC, Aguado JM, Carrascal Y, Perez A, Perez-de-la-Sota E, Cortina JM, Delgado R, Rodriguez E, Molina L, Rufilanchas JJ (1997) Role of epicardial pacing wire cultures in the diagnosis of poststernotomy mediastinitis. Clin Infect Dis 24:419 - 421
60. El Oakley RM, Wright JE (1996) Postoperative mediastinitis: classification and management. Ann Thoracic Surg 61:1030 - 1036
61. Kutsal A, Ibrisim E, Catav Z, Tasdemir O, Bayazit K (1991) Mediastinitis after open heart surgery. Analysis of risk factors and management. J Cardiovasc Surg (Torino) 32: 38 - 41
62. Engelman RM, Williams CD, Gouge TH, Chase RM, Jr, Falk EA, Boyd AD, Reed GE (1973) Mediastinitis following open-heart surgery. Review of two years' experience. Arch Surg 107:772 - 778
63. El Oakley R (1997) Mediastinitis in patients undergoing cardiopulmonary bypass: risk analysis and midterm results. J Cardiovasc Surg (Torino) 38:595 - 600
64. Ko W, Lazenby WD, Zelano JA, Isom OW, Krieger KH (1992) Effects of shaving methods and intraoperative irrigation on suppurative mediastinitis after bypass operations. Ann Thorac Surg 53:301 - 305
65. Hazelrigg SR, Wellons HA, Jr, Schneider JA, Kolm P (1989) Wound complications after median sternotomy. Relationship to internal mammary grafting. J Thorac Cardiovasc Surg 98:1096 - 1099
66. The Parisian Mediastinitis Study Group (1996) Risk factors for deep sternal wound infection after sternotomy: a prospective, multicenter study. J Thorac Cardiovasc Surg 111:1200 - 1207
67. Bor DH, Rose RM, Modlin JF, Weintraub R, Friedland GH (1983) Mediastinitis after cardiovascular surgery. Rev Infect Dis 5:885 - 897
68. Sethi GK, Copeland JG, Moritz T, Henderson W, Zadina K, Goldman S (1991) Comparison of postoperative complications between saphenous vein and IMA grafts to left anterior descending coronary artery. Ann Thorac Surg 51: 733 - 738
69. Nishida H, Grooters RK, Merkley DF, Thieman KC, Soltanzadeh H (1990) Postoperative mediastinitis: a comparison of two electrocautery techniques on presternal soft tissues. J Thorac Cardiovasc Surg 99:969 - 976
70. Kouchoukos NT, Wareing TH, Murphy SF, Pelate C, Marshall WG, Jr (1990) Risks of bilateral internal mammary artery bypass grafting. Ann Thorac Surg 49:210 - 217
71. Farinas MC, Gald PF, Bernal JM, Rabasa JM, Revuelta JM, Gonzalez-Macias J (1995) Suppurative mediastinitis after open-heart surgery: a case-control study covering a seven-year period in Santander, Spain. Clin Infect Dis 20:272 - 279
72. Karwande SV, Renlund DG, Olsen SL, Gay WA, Jr, Richenbacher WE, Hawkins JA, Millar RC, Marks JD (1992) Mediastinitis in heart transplantation. Ann Thoracic Surg 54:1039 - 1045
73. Baldwin RT, Radovancevic B, Sweeney MS, Duncan JM, Frazier OH (1992) Bacterial mediastinitis after heart transplantation. J Heart Lung Transplant 11:545 - 549
74. Burket JS, Chenoweth CE, Meyer TL, Barg NL (1999) Donor-to-recipient transmission of bacteria as an unusual cause of mediastinitis in a heart transplant recipient. Infect Control Hosp Epidemiol 20:132 - 133
75. Gottlieb LJ, Beahm EK, Krizek TJ, Karp RB (1996) Approaches to sternal wound infections. Adv Card Surg 7: 147 - 162
76. Maroto LC, Aguado JM, Carrascal Y, Rodriguez JE, Cortina JM, Rufilanchas JJ (1996) Fulminant mediastinitis due to *Streptococcus pneumoniae* following cardiac surgery: report of a case. Clin Infect Dis 22:594 - 595
77. Vandecasteele SJ, Boelaert JR, Verrelst P, Graulus E, Gordts BZ (2002) Diagnosis and treatment of *Aspergillus flavus* sternal wound infections post-cardiac surgery. Clin Infect Dis 35:887 - 890
78. Clancy CJ, Nguyen MH, Morris AJ (1997) Candidal mediastinitis: an emerging clinical entity [review]. Clin Infect Dis 25:608 - 613
79. Kohman LJ, Coleman MJ, Parker FB, Jr (1990) Bacteremia and sternal infection after coronary artery bypass grafting. Ann Thorac Surg 49:454 - 457
80. Czachor JS, Hawley HB (1988) Anaerobic wound infection: *Bacteroides* mediastinitis after cardiovascular surgery. Heart Lung 17:335 - 338
81. Cerat GA, McHenry MC, Loop FD (1976) Median sternotomy wound infection and anterior mediastinitis caused by *Bacteroides fragilis*. Chest 69:231 - 232
82. King CT (1994) Sternal wound infection due to *Corynebacterium xerosis*. Clin Infect Dis 19:1171 - 1172
83. Sielaff TD, Everett JE, Shumway SJ, Wahoff DC, Bolman RM, III, Dunn DL (1996) *Mycoplasma hominis* infections occurring in cardiovascular surgical patients. Ann Thoracic Surg 61:99 - 103
84. Thaler F, Gotainer B, Teodori G, Dubois C, Loirat P (1992) Mediastinitis due to *Nocardia asteroides* after cardiac transplantation. Intensive Care Med 18:127 - 128
85. Byl B, Jacobs F, Antoine M, Depierreux M, Serruys E, Primo G, Thys JP (1993) Mediastinitis caused by *Aspergillus fumigatus* with ruptured aortic pseudoaneurysm in a heart transplant recipient: case study. Heart Lung 22: 145 - 147
86. Weinstein RA, Jones EL, Schwarzmann SW, Hatcher CR, Jr (1976) Sternal osteomyelitis and mediastinitis after open-heart operation: pathogenesis and prevention. Ann Thorac Surg 21:442 - 444
87. Tyras DH, Kaiser GC, Barner HB, Laskowski LF, Marr JJ (1978) Atypical mycobacteria and the xenograft valve. J Thorac Cardiovasc Surg 75:331 - 337
88. Levy C, Curtin JA, Watkins A, Marsh B, Garcia J, Mispireta L (1977) *Mycobacterium chelonei* infection of porcine heart valves. N Engl J Med 297:667 - 668
89. Laskowski LF, Marr JJ, Spernoga JF, Frank NJ, Barner HB, Kaiser G, Tyras DH (1977) Fastidious mycobacteria grown from porcine prosthetic-heart-valve cultures. N Engl J Med 297:101 - 102
90. Kuritsky JN, Bullen MG, Broome CV, Silcox VA, Good RC, Wallace RJ, Jr (1983) Sternal wound infections and endocarditis due to organisms of the *Mycobacterium fortuitum* complex. Ann Intern Med 98:938 - 939
91. Sethi GK, Simons WJ, Scott SM (1985) *Mycobacterium*

fortuitum infections of the mediastinum. J Cardiovasc Surg (Torino) 26:307–309

92. Robicsek F, Hoffman PC, Masters TN, Daugherty HK, Cook JW, Selle JG, Mauney CU, Hinson P (1988) Rapidly growing nontuberculous mycobacteria: a new enemy of the cardiac surgeon. Ann Thorac Surg 46:703–710
93. Hoffman PC, Fraser DW, Robicsek F, O'Bar PR, Mauney CU (1981) Two outbreaks of sternal wound infection due to organisms of the *Mycobacterium fortuitum* complex. J Infect Dis 143:533–542
94. Jimenez-Martinez M, Arguero-Sanchez R, Perez-Alvarez JJ, Mina-Castaneda P (1970) Anterior mediastinitis as a complication of median sternotomy incisions: diagnostic and surgical considerations. Surgery 67:929–934
95. Browdie DA, Bernstein RV, Agnew R, Damle A, Fischer M, Balz J, Bernstein RV (1991) Diagnosis of poststernotomy infection: comparison of three means of assessment [published erratum appears in Ann Thorac Surg 1991 52(4):900]. Ann Thoracic Surg 51:290–292
96. Yamaguchi H, Yamauchi H, Yamada T, Ariyoshi T, Aikawa H, Kato Y (2001) Diagnostic validity of computed tomography for mediastinitis after cardiac surgery. Ann Thorac Cardiovasc Surg 7(2):94–98
97. Benlolo S, Mateo J, Raskine L, Tibourtine O, Bel A, Payen D, Mebazaa A (2003) Sternal puncture allows an early diagnosis of poststernotomy mediastinitis. J Thoracic Cardiovasc Surg 125(3):611–617
98. Rosenbaum GS, Klein NC, Cunha BA (1990) Poststernotomy mediastinitis. Heart Lung 19:371–372
99. Albat B, Trinh-Duc P, Boulfroy D, Picard E, Wintrebert P, Thevenet A (1993) Mediastinitis in heart transplant recipients: successful treatment by closed local irrigation. Cardiovasc Surg 1:657–659
100. Campistol JM, Abad C, Nogue S, Bertran A (1988) Acute renal failure in a patient treated by continuous povidone-iodine mediastinal irrigation. J Cardiovasc Surg (Torino) 29:410–412
101. Glick PL, Guglielmo BJ, Tranbaugh RF, Turley K (1985) Iodine toxicity in a patient treated by continuous povidone-iodine mediastinal irrigation. Ann Thorac Surg 39:478–480
102. Gottlieb LJ, Pielet RW, Karp RB, Krieger LM, Smith DJ, Jr, Deeb GM (1994) Rigid internal fixation of the sternum in postoperative mediastinitis. Arch Surg 129:489–493
103. Nahai F, Rand RP, Hester TR, Bostwick J III, Jurkiewicz MJ (1989) Primary treatment of the infected sternotomy wound with muscle flaps: a review of 211 consecutive cases. Plast Reconstr Surg 84:434–441
104. Agarwal JP, Ogilvie M, Wu LC, Lohman RF, Gottlieb LJ, Franczyk M, Song DH (2005) Vacuum-assisted closure for sternal wounds: A first-line therapeutic management approach. Plastic Reconstr Surg 116(4):1035–1040
105. Acarturk TO, Swartz WM, Luketich J, Quinlin RF, Edington H (2004) Laparoscopically harvested omental flap for chest wall and intrathoracic reconstruction. Ann Plastic Surg 53(3):210–216
106. Ringelman PR, Vander Kolk CA, Cameron D, Baumgartner WA, Manson PN (1994) Long-term results of flap reconstruction in median sternotomy wound infections. Plast Reconstr Surg 93:1208–1214
107. Piwnica A, Abdelmeguid I, Mesnildrey P, Laborde F, Menasche P, Romano M, Guedon C (1988) Rupture of the right ventricular free wall. An unusual complication of mediastinitis after cardiac surgery. Eur J Cardiothoracic Surg 2:172–175
108. Georgiade G, Levan TA, Anthony J, Oldham N, Julio H, Milano C, Ritter E (1998) Management and prevention of cardiovascular hemorrhage associated with mediastinitis. Ann Surg 227:145–150
109. Camacho MT, Edelman M, Rozenblit A, McKitrick JC, Pinsker K, Fell SC (1996) Mediastinal histoplasmosis causing massive hematemesis. J Thorac Cardiovasc Surg 111:1283–1286
110. Suzuki T, Suzuki S, Kamio Y, Hori G, Endo S, Suzuki H (1997) Mediastinal tuberculous lymphadenitis diagnosed and treated by thoracoscopy. Thorac Cardiovasc Surg 45:140–142
111. Ramakantan R, Shah P (1990) Dysphagia due to mediastinal fibrosis in advanced pulmonary tuberculosis. AJR Am J Roentgenol 154:61–63
112. Lagerstrom CF, Mitchell HG, Graham BS, Hammon JW, Jr (1992) Chronic fibrosing mediastinitis and superior vena caval obstruction from blastomycosis. Ann Thorac Surg 54:764–765
113. Gilbert HM, Hartman BJ (1996) Short report: a case of fibrosing mediastinitis caused by *Wuchereria bancrofti*. Am J Trop Med Hyg 54:596–599
114. Goodwin RA Jr, Nickell JA, Des Perez RM (1972) Mediastinal fibrosis complicating healed primary histoplasmosis and tuberculosis. Medicine 51:227–246
115. Manali ED, Saad CP, Krizmanich G, Mehta AC (2003) Endobronchial findings of fibrosing mediastinitis. Respir Care 48(11):1038–1042
116. Nordmann P, Commare MC, Ronco E, Barois A, Nauciel C (1994) Mediastinitis due to non-typhi *Salmonella* [letter]. Clin Infect Dis 18:255–256
117. Snider JM, Hannah H, McNabney WK, Pemberton LB (1993) Salmonella mediastinal abscess. Ann Thorac Surg 56:556–558
118. Henkel JS, Armstrong D, Blevins A, Moody MD (1970) Group A beta-hemolytic *Streptococcus* bacteremia in a cancer hospital. JAMA 211:983–986
119. Dreyfuss D, Djedaini K, Bidault-Lapomme C, Coste F (1992) Nontraumatic acute anterior mediastinitis in two HIV-positive heroin addicts. Chest 101:583–585
120. Centers for Disease Control and Prevention (1999) Bioterrorism alleging use of anthrax and interim guidelines for management – United States, 1998. MMWR Morb Mortal Wkly Rep 48:69–74
121. Abramova FA, Grinberg LM, Yampolskaya OV, Walker DH (1993) Pathology of inhalational anthrax in 42 cases from the Sverdlovsk outbreak of 1979. Proc Natl Acad Sci U S A 90:2291–2294
122. Atlas RM (1998) The medical threat of biological weapons. Crit Rev Microbiol 24:157–168
123. Mina B, Dym JP, Kuepper F, Tso R, Arrastia C, Kaplounova I, Faraj H, Kwapniewski A, Krol CM, Grosser M, Glick J, Fochios S, Remolina A, Vasovic L, Moses J, Robin T, DeVita M, Tapper ML (2002) Fatal inhalational anthrax with unknown source of exposure in a 61 year old woman in New York City. JAMA 287(7):858–862
124. Sekhar PC, Singh RS, Sridhar MS, Bhaskar CJ, Rao YS (1990) Outbreak of human anthrax in Ramabhadrapuram village of Chittoor district in Andhra Pradesh. Indian J Med Res 91:448–452
125. Shafazand S, Doyle R, Ruoss S, Weinacker A, Raffin TA (1999) Inhalational anthrax: epidemiology, diagnosis, and management. Chest 116(5):1369–1376
126. Anderson CM, Walters RS, Hortobagyi GN (1996) Mediastinitis related to probable central vinblastine extravasation in a woman undergoing adjuvant chemotherapy for early breast cancer. Am J Clin Oncol 19:566–568

Chapter 52

Pancreatic Infection

52

R. Hasanadka, C.P. Johnson, C.E. Edmiston, Jr

Pancreatic infection occurs most often as a complication of acute pancreatitis. The unique aspects of pancreatic inflammation predispose to secondary bacterial infection, which occurs in approximately 5% of all cases of acute pancreatitis. This review focuses on the pathogenesis, microbiology and surgical management of pancreatic infections, which occur as a complication of acute pancreatitis.

52.1 Pathophysiology of Acute Pancreatitis

Acute pancreatic inflammation leads to a spectrum of pathologic conditions ranging from mild edematous pancreatitis which is usually self limited, to severe necrotizing pancreatitis, a fulminant illness associated with mortality rates approaching 50–70%. Clinical and pathological severity of acute pancreatitis correlate with the development of pancreatic and peripancreatic necrosis. The unique predilection of the pancreas to undergo autodigestive necrosis during acute inflammation is due to the high content of lipolytic and proteolytic enzymes that are contained within this exocrine gland. Although these enzymes are normally stored in an inactivated precursor form, they may become activated following various physiologic stressors such as toxin exposure, direct trauma, viral infection and ischemia.

The two most common causes of acute pancreatitis are alcohol ingestion and biliary tract disease (gallstones). These two etiologies comprise over 90% of cases. The relative frequencies of alcohol and biliary disease vary depending on the population studied. In rural areas of the United States and in Europe, gallstone-pancreatitis predominates, while in large urban areas alcohol is the primary cause of acute pancreatitis [1].

Additional etiologies for acute pancreatitis include the postoperative state (following abdominal or thoracic operations, especially coronary bypass procedures), hypercalcemia, hypertriglyceridemia and drug-associated pancreatitis. Of the latter, asparaginase, azathioprine, valproic acid, sulfonamides, pentamidine, mercaptopurine, mesalamine, and various nucleoside analogues used to treat the human immunodeficiency virus are the most commonly implicated agents. Other commonly prescribed drugs that have been implicated in drug-induced pancreatitis include oral opiate preparations, furosemide, hydrochlorothiazide, estrogen preparations, steroids, and metformin [2]. Endoscopic retrograde cholangiopancreatography (ERCP) is the cause of acute pancreatitis in up to 5% of cases. Finally, in 10% of cases, no obvious inciting agent can be identified. However, about two-thirds of idiopathic pancreatitis has been shown to be due to microlithiasis of the biliary tract [3].

Pancreatitis also occurs as a result of ischemia reperfusion injury in association with pancreas transplantation. The outcome in this situation may be loss of the allograft, as the management of peripancreatic infection in conjunction with immunosuppressive therapy is especially difficult.

The exact mechanisms by which various insults trigger pancreatic inflammation are not known. Regardless, the clinical and pathologic severity appear related to the extent of pancreatic enzyme activation and autodigestion which results in pancreatic and peripancreatic necrosis. In addition to local release of pancreatic enzymes and consequent tissue damage, significant systemic release (and toxicity) occurs as reflected by elevated serum levels of amylase, lipase, and protease [4]. The clinical course in acute pancreatitis is typically not related to the magnitude of serum enzyme elevation, but rather other factors or criteria that may be present on admission to the hospital or develop within the first 48 h of illness.

The most widely used classification system, initially presented by Ranson [5], identified 11 factors that were predictive of poor outcomes for acute pancreatitis. Using the classification as presented in Table 52.1, patients with 0–2 criteria experienced almost no mortality. Patients with three or four had an expected mortality of 15% and approximately 40% require intensive care support. Patients with five or six criteria had mortality rates of approximately 50% and essentially all require intensive care support. Patients with seven or more criteria experienced mortality rates approaching 100%. It

Table 52.1. Ranson's early prognostic signs for acute pancreatitis. (Data from [5])

At admission
Age older than 55 years
WBC > 16,000 cells/mm^3
Blood glucose > 200 mg/dl
Serum LDH > 350 U/l
AST > 250 U/dl
During initial 48 h
Hematocrit fall > 10 points
BUN elevation > 5 mg/dl
Serum Ca^{2+} fall to < 8 mg/dl
Arterial pO_2 < 60 mmHg
Base deficit > 4 mEq/l
Estimated fluid sequestration > 6 l

WBC white blood cell, *BUN* blood urea nitrogen, *LDH* lactate dehydrogenase, *AST* aspartate amino transferase

is important to recognize that these criteria were published in 1974. Modern day outcomes are expected to be better. Nonetheless, Ranson's criteria are useful because patients can be identified early on for more aggressive management which may include hemodynamic monitoring, frequent computed tomography (CT) scans and prophylactic antibiotics.

Other classification systems have been used in acute pancreatitis. These include the Glasgow (or Imrie) criteria [6], Acute Physiology and Chronic Health Enquiry (APACHE) [7] and the Atlanta Symposium criteria [8]. These criteria and classification systems all have similar predictive value for assessment of acute pancreatitis.

The complications of acute pancreatitis can be divided into two phases: early and late. In both phases the severity of complications is related to the intensity of inflammation and the associated development of pancreatic and peripancreatic necrosis.

Early complications are related to extravascular fluid shifts that are associated with edema in the peripancreatic region and intestinal ileus. Additional fluid shifts may occur in the form of pulmonary edema as the lung serves as a target organ for released cytokines and other mediators of pancreatic inflammation. Elevated levels of interleukin-6 and C-reactive protein (> 150 mg/l) have been shown to be associated with more severe forms of pancreatitis [9]. Pulmonary capillary dysfunction has been linked to abnormalities of circulating phospholipase A [10] to increased levels of free fatty acids generated from the action of pancreatic lipase [11] and to alteration of pulmonary surfactant [12]. Up to 50% of patients with acute pancreatitis show demonstrable impairment of pulmonary function, usually in the form of hypoxemia. This may be subtle and manifest only as tachypnea or may be dramatic as occurs in adult respiratory distress syndrome (ARDS). Despite advances in critical care medicine, patients with respiratory failure associated with acute pancreatitis experience a high mortality rate [13, 14].

Bacterial translocation and/or alteration of the gut mucosal barrier may be important in the pathophysiology of early organ dysfunction in acute pancreatitis. Endotoxin, a lipopolysaccharide derived from the outer membrane of gram negative bacteria and a potent activator of inflammation, can be detected in the serum of patients with severe pancreatitis [15]. Elevated endotoxin levels correlate with the syndrome of multiple organ failure. However, it is not known whether this relationship represents cause or effect.

Patients with severe acute pancreatitis may also experience renal insufficiency. In many cases this is due in part to hypovolemia. In animal models, renal tubular cells have been shown to undergo apoptosis within several hours of acute pancreatitis suggesting the role of humoral mediators [16]. Acute renal failure, which does not respond to fluid replacement, is a grave complication generally associated with overwhelming illness and multiple organ failure. Mortality rates approach 100%.

Late complications of acute pancreatitis occurring after 7 days are generally due to the development of secondary infection or pseudocyst formation. Of these, pancreatic infection is associated with much greater morbidity and will be the focus for the remainder of this review.

52.2 Pancreatic Infection – Definitions

Secondary pancreatic infections occur in 2–5% of all cases of acute pancreatitis and are responsible for more than 80% of the late deaths associated with this disease. The risk of infection is proportional to the severity of illness as determined by Ranson's criteria. Three kinds of pancreatic infection occur: pancreatic abscess, infected pancreatic necrosis and infected pancreatic pseudocyst. *Pancreatic abscess* is a discrete, often circumscribed collection of purulent material within or around the pancreas that contains little or no necrotic tissue. *Infected pancreatic necrosis*, on the other hand, is an infection within or around the pancreas that contains nonviable tissue of pancreatic or peripancreatic origin. Most commonly, it is the peripancreatic fat that undergoes necrosis in response to acute pancreatic inflammation. Infected necrosis is by far the most common form of infection accompanying acute pancreatitis, constituting approximately 90% of infections [17]. Pure pancreatic abscess is relatively rare.

Both pancreatic abscess and infected pancreatic necrosis occur as a progression or continuation of pancreatic inflammation and, therefore, develop within 2–4 weeks of the onset of initial illness. *Pancreatic pseudocyst* develops after resolution of the acute illness, usually after 4 weeks. By definition, pancreatic pseudocyst is a localized collection of pancreatic tissue, fluid, debris, enzymes, and blood enclosed by a wall of fibrous granulation tissue and, thus, requires time to develop. Most pancreatic pseudocysts are sterile, but they may become secondarily infected either spontaneously or as a consequence of instrumentation.

52.3 Pathogenesis of Infection

The pathogenesis of pancreatic infection in acute pancreatitis may be multifaceted, as there are several potential pathways by which microorganisms can reach the pancreas or peripancreatic tissue during acute inflammation. The most direct pathway is through the biliary ducts, which contain bacteria in up to 90% of cases of choledocholithiasis [4]. This would seem to be the most likely pathway in gallstone pancreatitis. Another pathway appears to be by way of translocation through the adjacent transverse colon, either through direct spread or via lymphatic channels [18]. Other possible routes include hematogenous [19, 20], via lymphatic channels to the circulation [21, 22], and via ascites to the pancreas [19, 21]. Experimental studies support both direct extension from the colon and transperitoneal migration. Widdison et al. demonstrated in a feline model of acute pancreatitis that radioactively labeled intestinal *E. coli* were not recovered from the site of acute necrotizing pancreatitis when the colon was enclosed in an impermeable plastic bag which prohibited direct bacterial translocation [18]. Using a model of caerulein-induced pancreatitis in rats, Medich et al. [23] concluded that bacterial translocation leads to transperitoneal infection of the pancreas. These authors suggested that selective decontamination of the gut and peritoneal lavage may prevent secondary pancreatic infection in acute pancreatitis. In contrast, Arendt et al., using the same model of acute pancreatitis, found that bacteria did not spread through the peritoneal route [24].

In humans the mechanism for pancreatic and peripancreatic infection in acute pancreatitis is not known. However, the results of a prospective randomized trial by Luiten et al. suggest a prominent role for enteric organisms [25]. These investigators examined the use of selective gut decontamination in severe acute pancreatitis. Patients were entered into this trial according to clinical or radiographic criteria that placed them at high risk for development of secondary pancreatic infection. The treatment group received oral colistin sulfate 200 mg, amphotericin 500 mg and norfloxacin 50 mg every 6 h until the episode of pancreatitis resolved clinically. The control group did not receive any prophylactic antibiotics. The groups were equally matched with respect to severity of pancreatitis as judged by clinical and CT criteria. Secondary pancreatic infection occurred in 20/52 (38%) of the control group vs. 9/50 (18%) of the selective decontamination group ($p=0.03$). Gram negative infection predominated in the control group (33%) whereas only 8% of patients in the selective decontamination group developed gram negative pancreatic infection. Patients in the control group developed more frequent complications such as requirement for bowel resections and fistula formation and trended toward a higher mortality rate (35% vs. 22%) although the latter difference did not reach statistical significance ($p=0.19$). However, when early mortality (due to the initial phase of acute pancreatitis) was excluded, the difference in late mortality was impressive: 10/44 (23%) for control and 3/42 (7%) for selective decontamination. The authors of this study also demonstrated convincingly that gram negative pancreatic infection in the control group was preceded by intestinal colonization with the same gram negative organisms. The results from this multicenter trial reported by Luiten et al. provide strong evidence for the role of gut-derived organisms in the pathogenesis of secondary infection in acute pancreatitis.

The risk of pancreatic infection rises steadily during the course of illness from acute pancreatitis [26–28]. Beger et al. reported that 24% of patients undergoing surgery within the first week for severe acute pancreatitis were infected and this figure rose to 46% after the second week and 71% after the third week [26]. Similar rates of infection were reported by Gerzof et al., who performed CT-guided percutaneous aspirates [27], and by Bassi et al., who examined smears taken intra-operatively [28]. One should note that these figures are derived from a selected subset of acute pancreatitis patients who are more ill and therefore undergoing diagnostic and surgical procedures.

The risk of secondary pancreatic infection in acute pancreatitis is clearly related to the extent of pancreatic and peripancreatic necrosis [29–31]. Using contrast-enhanced CT scanning, Berger et al. demonstrated that an increasing percentage of pancreatic necrosis was associated with an increasing risk of infection. Patients with more than 50% necrosis had a 66% incidence of infection, whereas patients with less than 30% necrosis had a 38% incidence of infection (Table 52.2).

Because of the association between pancreatitis and peripancreatic necrosis, one of the therapeutic goals in

Table 52.2. Correlation of the extent of pancreatic necrosis (as determined from contrast enhanced CT scanning) and risk of infection in 226 patients with severe acute pancreatitis. (From [34])

Extent of necrosis	Sterile ($n=155$)	Infected ($n=71$)
<30%	57	35
30–50%	22	23
>50%	21	42

the management of acute pancreatitis should be to decrease tissue necrosis. A variety of strategies have been tried, including the use of high molecular weight dextran [32], somatostatin [33, 34] and protease inhibitors such as gabexate mesilate. The latter inhibits phospholipase A2 [35, 36]. Unfortunately, none of these agents has been found to be effective when administered in the clinical setting.

Another strategy to decrease pancreatic and peripancreatic necrosis may be early jejunal feeding. Targarona et al. have shown that 44 patients, who received total enteral nutrition, had less morbidity and mortality than 43 patients, who received TPN, in cases of severe pancreatitis based on CT criteria [37]. The rate of infected pancreatic necrosis was 20% when receiving enteral nutrition compared to 74% with TPN ($p<0.001$). This was associated with lower rates of surgical intervention (25% vs. 88%, $p<0.001$) and lower mortality rates (5% vs. 35%, $p<0.001$). The mechanism for this may be related to release of inhibitory GI hormones such as PYY during jejunal feeding [38] and decreased bacterial translocation [39].

52.4 Microbiology of Pancreatic Infection

Pancreatic or peripancreatic infection in the setting of acute pancreatitis is most often caused by gram negative enteric bacteria [40–42]. As many as 50% of infections are polymicrobial [43]. Table 52.3 illustrates the spectrum of bacteria involved. The most common organism isolated is *E. coli*, which occurs in 25–40% of cases. The next most common organisms tend to be *Pseudomonas* spp. [25, 40], although in some studies *Enterobacter* spp. are more common [41]. *Klebsiella* spp., *Proteus* spp., *Acinetobacter* spp. and *Citrobacter* spp. have also been noted [25]. *Staphylococcus epidermidis* and *Staphylococcus aureus* are the most common gram positive organisms isolated. Enterococci are increasingly isolated as are *Candida* (usually *Candida albicans*) in more recent reports [25, 41]. Infections with gram negative organisms seem to carry a higher mortality rate than infections with gram positive organisms [44]. It should be noted that the preponderance of *Pseudomonas* and *Staph.* infections in some series may be related to the use of percutaneous drainage catheters.

Table 52.3. Bacteriology in severe acute pancreatitis ($n=87$ patients). (Adapted from [34])

Escherichia coli	25%
Staphylococcus aureus	17%
Pseudomonas spp.	15%
Klebsiella spp.	9%
Proteus spp.	9%
Candida	4%
Streptococcus faecalis	3%
Enterobacter spp.	3%
Anaerobes	16%
Monomicrobial	76%
Polymicrobial	24%

The use of selective gut decontamination may modify the bacterial flora found in secondary pancreatic infections. When a regimen of colistin, amphotericin and norfloxacin was used, the percentage of gram isolates decreased from 61% to 21% [25]. However, of four gram negative infections from 50 patients treated with this combination of antibiotics, three of these involved resistant strains of *Pseudomonas aeruginosa* or *Klebsiella*.

Anaerobic species have not been cultured frequently from infections complicating acute pancreatitis. This is perhaps surprising considering the close proximity of the colon and a postulated role for direct extension of organisms. The paucity of anaerobes could be in part related to technical difficulties in culturing anaerobes from intra-abdominal infections [45].

52.5 The Role of Prophylactic Antibiotics

The potential role of prophylactic antibiotics in preventing secondary pancreatic infections in acute pancreatitis has been demonstrated in experimental studies [15]. In a rat model of caerulein-induced pancreatitis, Foitzik et al. compared several prophylactic regimens: intravenous cefotaxime, intravenous imipenem, selective gut decontamination (with polymyxin E, tobramycin and amphotericin) and full gut decontamination (the same oral antibiotics plus intravenous cefotaxime). None of these regimens affected early mortality, but animals receiving imipenem or full gut decontamination demonstrated decreased bacterial counts in the pancreas relative to controls [46].

Additional studies with the rat caerulein-induced pancreatitis model have examined the prophylactic use of intravenous ciprofloxacin and imipenem [47]. At 7 days, 75% of control rats (not receiving antibiotics) had developed pancreatic infection with organisms similar to those found in humans. Both ciprofloxacin and imipenem significantly reduced the incidence of secondary infection in these animals by roughly 50%. However, due to the low numbers of animals surviving, the authors were not able to show a difference in mortality.

In a feline model of pancreatic infection, Widdison et al. demonstrated that cefotaxime was effective in reducing bacterial counts in the pancreas when administered 12 h after induction of pancreatitis [48]. However, this model is clearly different from other experimental models as pancreatitis is induced by ductal infusion of glycodeoxycholic acid and live *E. coli*. Animals in this study did not develop necrotizing pancreatitis and mortality did not occur in any of the groups. Therefore, the relevance to human pancreatitis is uncertain.

The efficacy of antibiotic prophylaxis in acute pancreatitis is related to the properties of tissue penetration for specific agents. Trudel et al. demonstrated that ampicillin does not achieve adequate concentrations in pancreatic tissue in a model of canine pancreatitis [49]. Roberts and Williams also investigated penetration of ampicillin into pancreatic tissue by measuring ampicillin levels in pancreatic ductal fluid at the time of ERCP [50]. In six of seven subjects, ampicillin was undetectable in the fluid.

In contrast, ciprofloxacin and imipenem consistently achieve good penetration into pancreatic tissue. Buchler et al. examined pancreatic tissue levels for ten different antibiotics in patients undergoing elective pancreatic surgery [51]. They found that aminoglycosides consistently failed to achieve significant tissue levels in the pancreas. Extended-spectrum penicillins including mezlocillin, piperacillin and third generation cephalosporins such as ceftizoxime and cefotaxime achieved minimum inhibitory concentrations that inhibited most, but not all, of the common infecting organisms. Ciprofloxacin and imipenem achieved bactericidal levels against most organisms.

Acute inflammation may alter the penetration characteristics of antibiotics. Foitzik et al. demonstrated in a rat model of acute pancreatitis that cefotaxime tissue levels may vary according to changes in capillary blood flow and pancreatic edema [52]. Interestingly, tissue imipenem levels do not seem to be altered by changes in blood flow or inflammation. It has been shown, in addition, that ofloxacin (from the fluoroquinolone class) achieves bactericidal tissue levels in normal and inflamed pancreas, but, more importantly, in pancreatic necrosis.

In human studies, Drewelow et al. have shown that ceftazidime achieved adequate antimicrobial concentrations in both viable and necrotic pancreatic tissue in three human subjects with acute necrotizing pancreatitis [53]. Bassi et al. examined penetration of several antibiotics including aminoglycosides, perfloxacin, imipenem, mezlocillin and metronidazole into infected pancreatic necrosis [54]. These samples were collected by CT-guided needle aspiration or at the time of surgical intervention. The authors found that perfloxacin and metronidazole consistently attained levels greater than the MICs for the organisms found in necrotic tissue. Aminoglycoside levels were consistently inadequate. Mezlocillin and imipenem were intermediate, although imipenem tissue levels increased with time.

In summary, the third generation cephalosporins, piperacillin, mezlocillin, fluoroquinolones, imipenem and metronidazole achieve adequate pancreatic tissue concentrations when given as prophylactic agents for acute pancreatitis. The aminopenicillins (ampicillin), first generation cephalosporins and aminoglycosides do not achieve effective concentrations in pancreatic tissue. It should be noted, however, that the relevance of pancreatic tissue penetration to clinical efficacy in acute pancreatitis is debatable since, in most cases, secondary infection occurs in peripancreatic necrosis.

52.6 Clinical Trials of Antibiotic Prophylaxis

The rationale for prophylactic antibiotic therapy in acute pancreatitis is based on the widely accepted premise that severe acute pancreatitis is commonly associated with pancreatic and peripancreatic necrosis, which is, in turn, susceptible to secondary infection. Thus, prevention of infection should have a measurable impact on clinical outcomes. Unfortunately, it has not been possible to demonstrate unequivocal benefit for the use of prophylactic antibiotics in acute pancreatitis. There are many reasons for this. Many cases of pancreatitis are mild and these patients are not at high risk for secondary infection. Studies which fail to include sufficient numbers of patients with severe pancreatitis as determined by clinical (Ranson, Imrie) or CT criteria may not show a difference in outcome with antibiotic prophylaxis. Furthermore, if enrollment criteria for antibiotic studies are based on CT criteria that require establishment of pancreatic or peripancreatic necrosis, it may be too late for antibiotics to alter the outcome. Nonetheless, Norback et al. have been able to show a benefit with imipenem prophylaxis using CT criteria for enrollment (see below). The failure of early trials may have been related to use of ampicillin and similar drugs that do not achieve good tissue penetration. Recent studies provide stronger evidence for a beneficial role of prophylactic antibiotics.

In 1993, Pederzoli et al. from Italy reported the results of a multicenter randomized controlled trial [55]. Seventy-four patients with severe pancreatitis, as judged by Ranson's criteria and with pancreatic necrosis proven by CT scan, were randomized to receive imipenem 0.5 g intravenously every 8 h for 14 days or to a control group receiving no antibiotics. Pancreatic infection was confirmed by fine needle aspiration or at operation. Imipenem reduced the incidence of secondary pancreatic infection from 30% in control to 12% in treated patients ($p<0.001$). However, multiple organ failure, need for operative intervention and mortality were not reduced to an equal extent and none of the differences in these outcome measures achieved statistical significance. Of note, there was a trend toward decreased mortality in the imipenem group (7.3% vs. 12.1%). Also, the rates of non-pancreatic infection were significantly reduced in the antibiotic treated group (14.6% vs. 48.5%). A weakness of this study is the small number of patients overall and a selection bias whereby only two of 16 patients with extensive (>50%) pancreatic necrosis were randomized to the control group. Thus, infection and mortality in the control group were lower than expected making it difficult to detect a difference between control and treatment arms.

In 1995, Sainio from Finland reported a randomized controlled trial evaluating the use of cefuroxime, a second generation cephalosporin, for prophylaxis of pancreatic infection in patients with alcohol-induced severe pancreatitis [56]. Sixty patients were randomized to receive either intravenous cefuroxime 1.5 g three times daily or no antibiotics. Cefuroxime did not reduce the incidence of pancreatic sepsis, but significantly decreased both the number of surgical interventions (8 vs. 36, $p=0.012$) and mortality from 23% in the control group to 3% in the antibiotic group ($p=0.028$). The reason for this dramatic effect on mortality is not clear, especially in view of the fact that cefuroxime did not alter the incidence of secondary pancreatic infection.

In another small study, Schwarz et al. in 1997 reported 26 patients with necrotizing pancreatitis proven by CT scan, randomized to a regimen of ofloxacin plus metronidazole versus no antibiotics [57]. The antibiotic regimen did reduce the number of gram negative pancreatic infections (1/13 vs. 6/16), but the overall infection rate and mortality were not significantly different.

Several uncontrolled studies support the use of prophylactic antibiotics in severe acute pancreatitis. In the previously cited study by Bassi [54], a series of 60 patients receiving either prophylactic perfloxacin or imipenem for severe pancreatitis were compared. Although perfloxacin more consistently penetrated pancreatic tissue and exceeded the MICs for commonly isolated organisms, imipenem was more effective at preventing pancreatic infections (10% vs. 34%; $p<0.05$) and lowering mortality (10% vs. 24%) although the latter did not reach statistical significance.

In a retrospective review, Ho and Frey [17] also supported the use of prophylactic antibiotics for severe acute pancreatitis. These authors reviewed 180 patients treated over 14 years and grouped them into three periods. During 1982–1989 (50 patients) no prophylactic antibiotics were used; during 1990–1992 ($n=55$) patients were given antibiotics in a non-uniform manner. From 1993 to 1996, 75 patients with severe pancreatitis and APACHE II scores greater than 6 associated with abnormal CT findings were given a 4-week course of intravenous imipenem. A progressive decrease in the incidence of secondary pancreatic infection was noted over the three time periods. During the most recent period, 20 of 75 (27%) patients developed pancreatic infection. Moreover, mortality was progressively lowered from 16% during 1983–1989, to 7% during 1990–1992, to 5% during 1993–1996. Due to the increasing numbers of patients observed during these three time periods and use of the APACHE scoring system, which may have included patients with slightly milder forms of pancreatitis, it is difficult to compare the results of this retrospective study to the prospective studies which have been based on Ranson or Imrie criteria. Also, these authors included significant numbers of patients with peripancreatic fluid collections only (without necrosis) whereas most of the randomized trials have included primarily patients with necrosis. Nonetheless, the overall results suggest a beneficial role for prophylactic antibiotics in severe acute pancreatitis.

In 1998, Golub et al. performed a meta-analysis of eight published trials of prophylactic antibiotics in acute pancreatitis [58]. Using an endpoint of death, their analysis revealed a positive benefit for prophylactic antibiotics when limited to cases of severe pancreatitis and using antibiotics that achieve therapeutic pancreatic tissue levels such as imipenem and the fluoroquinolones. However, the validity of meta-analysis as used to define the role of prophylactic antibiotics in acute pancreatitis has been questioned [15] as varying antibiotic regimens have been used and the majority of studies have not been sufficiently powered to detect important clinical differences.

More recently, several prospective, randomized trials have been published using various regimens of imipenem and the fluoroquinolones. In 2001, Nordback et al. showed a decrease in morbidity and mortality using a prophylactic course of imipenem when compared to waiting for signs and symptoms of infected necrosis [59]. Ninety patients identified to have necrotizing pancreatitis based on serum C-reactive protein (>150 mg/l) and CT scan findings were randomized to receive imipenem (1.0 g with cilastatin intravenously three times a day) started within 48 h of admission versus waiting until the diagnosis of infected necrosis was made either noninvasively (recurrent fever, >30% rise in WBC, and >30% rise in C-reactive protein, ruling out other infectious etiologies) or invasively with CT guided needle aspiration. It was found that prophylactic administration of imipenem decreased the need for surgery from 36% ($n=14$) to 8% ($n=25$) when compared to the control subgroup that received delayed treatment ($p=0.04$). The rate of major organ complications (pseudocyst, diabetes, acute respiratory distress syndrome, pulmonary embolus, oliguria >1 day, and need for hemodialysis) also reduced from 64% to 20% ($p=0.008$), and mortality was reduced from 36% to 8% ($p=0.04$).

Nordback's group terminated antibiotic therapy when patients were afebrile with a normal WBC count and a C-reactive protein below 50 mg/l. The average duration of prophylactic imipenem was not measured but was believed to be greater than 2 weeks [59]. Maravi-Poma et al. attempted to address whether prophylactic imipenem needed to be given until resolution of symptoms or if a 14-day course was sufficient [60]. There was no significant difference between the number of infectious complications or mortality in patients randomized to a 14-day course of imipenem vs. patients treated until resolution of all infectious complications.

In 2003, Manes et al. questioned whether imipenem was the best carbapenem for prophylactic therapy of acute pancreatic necrosis [61]. In their study, 176 patients were prospectively randomized between receiving meropenem (500 mg intravenously every 8 h) and imipenem (500 mg intravenously every 6 h). There was no difference between the two groups. The incidence of infected pancreatic necrosis was 11.4% ($n=88$) in the meropenem group and 13.6% ($n=88$) in the imipenem group. The incidence of extrapancreatic infections was 21.6% in the meropenem group compared to 23.9% for the patients treated with imipenem. The rate of multi-organ failure (7.9%) and mortality (12.5%) for the two groups were similar. Manes et al. then concluded that meropenem could be used as an alternative to imipenem for prophylactic therapy.

Despite the large body of literature supporting the use of prophylactic antibiotics in severe acute pancreatitis, there remains some disagreement. Isenmann et al. argue that the prior randomized trials are not appropriately blinded [62]. In 2004, their group published results of a multicenter, placebo-controlled, double-blinded trial randomizing 119 patients between receiving prophylactic antibiotics (ciprofloxacin 400 mg intravenously twice daily and metronidazole 500 mg intravenously twice daily) and placebo in patients with severe acute pancreatitis, defined as necrosis seen on CT imaging and a C-reactive protein > 150 mg/l. Patients were allowed to receive open antibiotic therapy if they developed a systemic inflammatory response, two or more organ failure, extrapancreatic infection, or an increase in serum C-reactive protein. They found no benefit with prophylactic ciprofloxacin/metronidazole under these conditions. The incidence of infected pancreatic necrosis in patients with necrotizing pancreatitis was 17% ($n=41$) in the treatment group and 14% ($n=35$) in the placebo group. Mortality was 7% and 11% respectively. With equivocal morbidity and mortality, the authors argue an economic basis for reserving antibiotic therapy to treating signs of sepsis rather than as prophylaxis.

It is commonly thought that prophylactic broad-spectrum antibiotics will lead to increased numbers of fungal infections. In an evidenced based review in 2006, Heinrich et al. found no increased risk for fungal infection [63]. Their analysis also resulted in odds ratios favoring the prophylactic use of antibiotics for infected necrosis with imipenem ($p=0.002$) but not with a quinolone and metronidazole ($p=0.57$). The odds ratios for sepsis ($p=0.01$) and mortality ($p=0.04$) also favored prophylactic antibiotics.

Finally, the question of fostering antibiotic resistance is raised when advocating prophylactic antibiotics. Howard and Temple evaluated their single center experience by comparing operative cultures from treating 34 consecutive patients with infected pancreatic necrosis before routine antibiotic use (1977–1992) and 61 patients during the era of routine antibiotic use (1993–2001) [64]. While they did notice a shift from predominant gram-negative species prior to routine prophylactic use to mostly gram-positives when using imipenem for prophylaxis, they did not notice a significant difference in beta-lactam resistance or fungal infections.

In summary, there remains substantial evidence, experimental and clinical, to provide a rationale for prophylactic antibiotics in severe acute pancreatitis. The majority of published reports indicate a benefit and, to date, there are no reports to suggest a worse outcome due to infection with resistant strains or other adverse outcomes. By using various clinical and radiographic criteria, it is relatively easy to identify patients who are at greatest risk for secondary pancreatic infection. It would seem prudent to identify these patients as early as possible and to administer prophylactic antibiotics such as imipenem or meropenem.

52.7 Clinical Management of Pancreatic Infections

52.7.1 Presentation

Abdominal pain, tenderness and fever are the most common symptoms and signs of pancreatic infection. Unfortunately, these findings are neither sensitive nor specific. Fever may be absent in up to 35% of patients [65, 66]. Additional findings may include prolonged nausea or vomiting and a palpable mass. In general, patients who do not resolve their symptoms of acute pancreatitis within 1 week should be suspected of developing pancreatic infection.

52.7.2 Diagnosis

There are no sensitive or specific laboratory markers for pancreatic infection. Leukocytosis to a variable degree is almost uniformly seen, but is certainly not pathognomonic for infection. Amylase and lipase values may return to normal despite the presence of pancreatic infection. Elevated serum levels of C-reactive protein, phospholipase A_2 and trypsinogen activation peptides have been shown to correlate with the development of pancreatic and peripancreatic necrosis [67–72]. However, none of these assays is specific for infection nor are they readily available in most hospitals, with the exception of C-reactive protein. Currently, the diagnosis of pancreatic infection requires radiologic imaging.

Contrast-enhanced computed tomography (CT scanning) has become the gold standard for evaluating the pancreas in acute pancreatitis. The value of CT

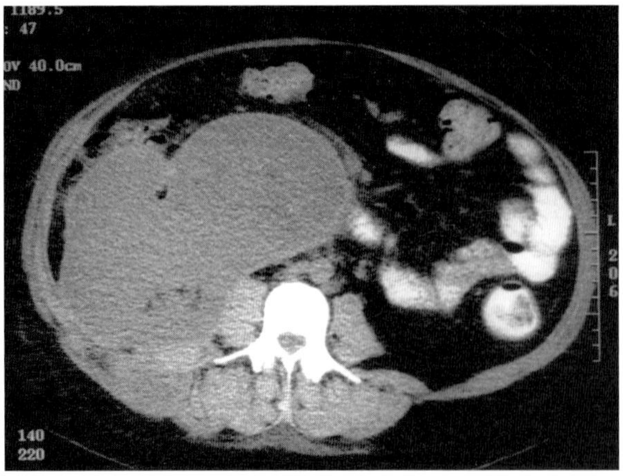

Fig. 52.1. CT scan of a patient with severe pancreatitis and a large peripancreatic collection tracking behind the ascending colon. At operation, the collection contained a mixture of fluid and necrotic tissue

scanning is greatly enhanced by intravenous injection of contrast. In certain situations there may be hesitancy to use intravenous contrast, but the information gained usually justifies its use. The contrast-enhanced CT scan delineates normal homogeneously perfused pancreatic tissue from under-perfused or nonviable pancreatic tissue. In addition, extension of inflammation, fluid and necrosis beyond the pancreas into retroperitoneal tissue planes can be appreciated with CT scanning. It is often not possible to distinguish peripancreatic fluid from necrosis and most often there is a combination of both (Fig. 52.1).

Several investigators have developed scoring systems to characterize the CT findings of acute pancreatitis [73]. Balthazar and colleagues have reported a grading system which correlates well with clinical course and has predictive value similar to Ranson's criteria for assessing the risk of infection [74].

Definitive diagnosis of pancreatic infection requires percutaneous CT-guided aspiration or direct operative sampling of tissue or fluid. Blood cultures are often negative or may reflect alternate sites of infection such as pulmonary or central venous lines. Percutaneous CT-guided aspiration of suspicious fluid collections has been found to be safe and accurate for diagnosis but probably not 100% reliable in excluding pancreatic infection [75, 76].

The role of percutaneous CT-guided aspiration in clinical management of pancreatitis continues to be debated. The appearance of peripancreatic fluid collections or necrosis in a patient who is exhibiting recovery from acute pancreatitis does not mandate immediate intervention. Thus, percutaneous aspiration is less useful in this situation. At the other extreme, patients who are failing medical management in association with peripancreatic fluid collections and/or necrosis should probably undergo operation anyway. It is the patient in between the two extremes, with an unresolved illness and positive findings on CT scan, who may benefit from CT-guided aspiration. A positive aspirate mandates surgical intervention while a negative aspirate permits continued close observation. It is important to remember that patients should be re-aspirated if fluid collections or inflammatory masses persist and illness continues.

Gerzof and colleagues have reviewed the role of CT-guided aspiration in diagnosis and management of pancreatic inflammatory masses [77]. They evaluated the outcome of 92 aspirations in the setting of acute pancreatitis. Fifty of these aspirates were sterile. All of these were judged to be true negatives on the basis of cultures obtained at the time or surgery or by resolution of the pancreatic mass or fluid collection without surgery. Forty-two aspirates were judged to have been positive and all of these were confirmed by surgery or catheter drainage. Of these 42, six were initially negative but positive on reaspiration. There were no significant complications related to the procedure. The authors emphasized that CT appearance together with clinical findings cannot distinguish sterile vs. infected inflammatory masses. They also demonstrated that pancreatic infection occurs earlier than previously suspected, with 55% of infections occurring within 14 days of the onset of pancreatitis. Their study and others [78–81] emphasize the useful role of percutaneous aspiration in the evaluation and management of complicated pancreatitis.

52.7.3 Management of Sterile Pancreatic Necrosis

Many patients with sterile pancreatic or peripancreatic necrosis can be managed non-operatively. However, this assumes a negative CT-guided aspirate and a resolving clinical course. Repeated aspirates may be necessary in order to reduce the possibility of false negative results. Several authors have emphasized the need for operative débridement in selected cases of sterile necrosis [82–84]. There is clearly a subset of patients with sterile necrosis and clinical deterioration who probably benefit from an aggressive surgical approach as outlined in the next section on management of pancreatic infection. There is no role for percutaneous catheter drainage in sterile necrosis as this will serve only to provide a route for secondary bacterial infection.

52.7.4 Management of Infected Necrosis

The vast majority of secondary pancreatic infections are associated with pancreatic and peripancreatic necrosis. As a result, these infections are not managed adequately using percutaneous techniques. Surgical treatment requires adequate exposure of the pancreas through a generous incision – either midline or bilateral subcostal. Patients with wide costal angles may be easier to explore through subcostal incisions. The incision should be designed to achieve exposure of the pancreas and both paracolic gutters as directed by CT findings. The anterior surface of the pancreas should be visualized by entering the lesser sac, if possible. Also, the base of the transverse mesocolon should be examined as should the paraduodenal area, tail of the pancreas and the retroperitoneal spaces behind the ascending and descending colon. Resection and débridement should be limited to that which is easily performed by digital dissection, using blunt forceps or by gently pinching away necrotic tissue. Extensive resections with concomitant hemorrhage should be avoided. We believe a series of repeated gentle débridements is better tolerated (and more effective) than one or two major operations with heavy blood loss. At the initial operation, one should make a decision regarding number and frequency of re-explorations. Traditional management has consisted of a single extensive débridement and placement of closed-suction drains [82]. However, in recent years there has been increasing consensus about the merits of repeated laparotomies for management of necrotizing pancreatitis [83–87].

The repeated laparotomy approach involves a less extensive initial débridement but multiple re-operations at 24–48 h apart. There are several advantages of this method. Pancreatitis is a unique inflammatory disease, which may persist over a period of several days or weeks. This is fundamentally different from other abdominal inflammatory disorders such as appendicitis, perforated ulcer or diverticulitis. Tissue damage, necrosis and infection evolve over time and may progress slowly. Thus a more prolonged (or repeated) surgical approach may be better suited for the disease process. We believe it is best to débride necrotic tissue gently. This way, bleeding is minimized but, more importantly, débridement is more complete and infection is better controlled. Repeated operations can be tailored according to the patient's physiological condition and complications such as colonic necrosis or intestinal fistula can be recognized as they occur. One disadvantage of the multiple laparotomy approach may be an increased risk of bowel injury associated with gauze packing. This is especially likely with open packing techniques or when gauze remains in contact with the intestine for longer than 48 h. Our technique at the Medical College of Wisconsin involves repeated gentle débridement with temporary abdominal closure using either a Silastic sheet or a Velcro device, the Wittmann Patch (Starsurgical, Burlington, WI). The latter is especially useful and well suited to the repeated laparotomy concept. Using either technique, it is possible to keep the abdominal contents enclosed and appropriately moist such that iatrogenic fistulas are avoided. We use gauze packing only at the initial débridement or as required for bleeding – but we try not to débride extensively such that bleeding occurs. All débridements are performed in the operating room. The numbers of débridements vary but have ranged from 5 to 26. Using the concepts of multiple, gentle débridements and temporary abdominal closure, we achieved excellent results in a series of renal transplant recipients who developed necrotizing pancreatitis [88].

In an effort to reduce the morbidity of repeated laparotomies, some centers have attempted a single laparotomy with closed continuous lavage [89]. In 2006, Farkas et al. reported their single center results of treating 220 patients with infected pancreatic necrosis [91]. Their surgical approach was to perform a necrosectomy of any devitalized tissue via bilateral subcostal incisions, which was followed by intraoperative lavage using 8–12 l of normal saline. Subsequently, 4–11 large rubber drains were placed in the retroperitoneal space to allow postoperative closed continuous lavage, which lasted an average of 44.5 days with a median of 9.5 l of normal saline used per day. Their overall mortality rate was 7.7%. However, 48 (21.8%) patients required subsequent surgery, 37 of whom developed a late abscess. Five patients developed a colonic fistula that required surgical resection with colectomy. Pancreatic fistulas occurred in 24 patients, all of which closed either spontaneously or with octreotide/TPN therapy. Total hospital stay of surviving patients was a median of 45.5 days.

The overall results for surgical management of infected pancreatic necrosis have improved significantly in recent years [82, 84, 87]. With adherence to the above-mentioned principles, mortality rates have declined into the 10–20% range.

52.7.5 Management of Pancreatic Abscess and Infected Pancreatic Pseudocysts

Occasionally a pure pancreatic abscess (without necrosis) may present. These probably originate as peripancreatic fluid collections which then become secondarily infected. As an isolated fluid collection it may respond to percutaneous catheter drainage. Infected pseudocysts may also be managed effectively with percutaneous drainage. In either case, a pancreatic fistula may ensue if the fluid collection (or pseudocyst) exhibits a connection to the pancreatic ductal system. This can be determined by performing an ERCP either before or after drainage. In the case of a suspected pancreatic abscess, it should be re-emphasized that the majority of these "fluid collections" are in fact found to contain substantial amounts of necrotic tissue (as illustrated in Fig. 52.1). Therefore surgical drainage remains the preferred treatment.

52.8 Summary

The overall risk of pancreatic infection in acute pancreatitis is approximately 5 % but this may rise to 30 – 50 % in cases of severe pancreatitis. The natural history of pancreatic infection is that it arises most commonly from enteric bacteria. There is sufficient evidence for a beneficial effect of prophylactic antibiotics in severe pancreatitis such that patients who meet appropriate criteria, early in the course of severe pancreatitis, should receive a course of antibiotic therapy such as imipenem or meropenem until clinical recovery occurs. The presence of pancreatic or peripancreatic necrosis itself does not mandate surgical intervention, but should prompt consideration of a diagnostic percutaneous aspirate to detect early infection. Patients with negative aspirates should undergo repeated aspirates as dictated by clinical progress or surgical intervention if deterioration occurs. Patients with positive aspirates should undergo prompt surgical intervention, as there is no role for medical or percutaneous management of infection in the presence of pancreatic or peripancreatic necrosis. Patients who are admitted to a medical service for management of acute pancreatitis should be seen in consultation by surgeons experienced in the management of pancreatic infection.

References

1. Lillemoe KD, Yeo CJ (1998) Management of complications of pancreatitis. Curr Probl Surg 35:1 – 98
2. Trivedi CD, Pitchumoni CS (2005) Drug-induced pancreatitis: an update. J Clin Gastroenterol 39:709 – 716
3. Farion AM, Ricci GL, Sianesi M, et al. (1987) Physiopathologic role of microlithiasis in gallstone pancreatitis. Surg Gynecol Obstet 164:252 – 6
4. Klar E, Warshaw AL (1995) Infections of the pancreas. In: Howard RJ, Simmons RL (eds) Surgical infectious diseases. Appleton & Lange, Norwalk, CT, pp 1059 – 67
5. Ranson JHC, Rifkind DM, Roses DF, et al. (1974) Prognostic signs and the role of operative management in acute pancreatitis. Surg Gynecol Obstet 139:69 – 81
6. Blamey SL, Imrie CW, O'Neill J, Gilmour WH, Carter DC (1984) Prognostic factors in acute pancreatitis. Gut 25:1340 – 6
7. Knaus WA, Draper EA, Wagner DP, et al. (1985) APACHE II: a severity of disease classification system. Crit Care Med 13:818 – 29
8. Bradley EL (1993) A clinically based classification system for acute pancreatitis. Summary of the International Symposium on Acute Pancreatitis, Atlanta, GA, 1992. Arch Surg 128:586 – 90
9. Heath DI, Cruickshank A, Gudgeon M, Jehanli A, Shenkin A, Imrie CW (1993) Role of interleukin-6 in mediating the acute phase protein response and potential as an early means of severity assessment in acute pancreatitis. Gut 34:41 – 5
10. Kellum JM, Demeester TR, Elkins RC, et al. (1972) Respiratory insufficiency secondary to acute pancreatitis. Ann Surg 175:657 – 62
11. Kimura T, Toung JK, Margolis S, et al. (1979) Respiratory failure in acute pancreatitis: a possible role for triglycerides. Ann Surg 189:509 – 14
12. Maciver AG, Metcalfe IL, Possmayer F, et al. (1977) Altercation of surfactant chemistry in experimental acute pancreatitis. J Surg Res 23:311 – 4
13. Ranson JHC, Turner JW, Roses DF (1974) Respiratory complications in acute pancreatitis. Ann Surg 179:557 – 66
14. Jacobs ML, Daggett WM, Cirett JM, et al. (1977) Acute pancreatitis: analysis of factors influencing survival. Ann Surg 186:43 – 51
15. Powell JJ, Miles R, Siriwardena AK (1998) Antibiotic prophylaxis in the initial management of severe acute pancreatitis. Br J Surg 85:582 – 587
16. Takase K, Takeyama Y, Nishikawa J, Ueda T, Hori Y, Yamamoto M, Kuroda Y (1999) Apoptotic cell death of renal tubules in experimental severe acute pancreatitis. Surgery 125:411 – 20
17. Ho HS, Frey CF (1997) The role of antibiotic prophylaxis in severe acute pancreatitis. Arch Surg 132:487 – 493
18. Widdison AL, Karanija ND, Reber HA (1994) Routes of spread of pathogens into the pancreas in a feline model of acute pancreatitis. Gut 35:1306 – 10
19. Lange JF, van Gool J, Tytgat GN (1987) The protective effect of a reduction in intestinal flora on mortality of acute haemorrhagic pancreatitis in the rat. Hepatogastroenterology 34:28 – 30
20. Webster MW, Pasculle AW, Myerowitz RL, et al. (1979) Postinduction bacteremia in experimental acute pancreatitis. Am J Surg 138:419 – 20
21. Tarpila E, Nystrom PO, Franzen L, et al. (1993) Bacterial translocation during acute pancreatitis in rats. Eur J Surg 159:109 – 13
22. Runkel NS, Moody FG, Smith GS, et al. (1991) The role of the gut in the development of sepsis in acute pancreatitis. J Surg Res 51:18 – 23
23. Medich DS, Lee TK, Melhem MF, et al. (1993) Pathogenesis of pancreatic sepsis. Am J Surg 165:46 – 50
24. Arendt T, Wendt M, Olszewski M, et al. (1997) Cerulein-induced acute pancreatitis in rats: does bacterial translocation occur via a transperitoneal pathway? Pancreas 15: 291 – 6
25. Luiten EJ, Hop WC, Endtz HP, et al. (1998) Prognostic importance of Gram-negative intestinal colonization preceding pancreatic infection in severe acute pancreatitis. Results of a controlled clinical trial of selective decontamination. Intensive Care Med 24:438 – 45
26. Beger HG, Bittner R, Block S, et al. (1986) Bacterial contamination of pancreatic necrosis. A prospective clinical study. Gastroenterology 91:433 – 8
27. Gerzof SG, Banks PA, Robbins AH, et al. (1987) Early diagnosis of pancreatic infection by computed tomography-guided aspiration. Gastroenterology 93:1315 – 20
28. Bassi C, Falconi M, Girelli R, et al. (1989) Microbiological findings in severe acute pancreatitis. Surg Res Commun 5:1 – 4
29. Banks PA (1991) Infected necrosis: morbidity and therapeutic consequences. Hepatogastroenterology 38:116 – 19
30. Uhl W, Buchler M, Malfertheiner P, et al. (1991) PMN-elastase in comparison with CRP, antiproteases, and LDH as indicators of necrosis in human acute pancreatitis. Pancreas 6:253 – 9
31. Schmid SW, Uhl W, Steinle A, et al. (1996) Human pancreas-specific protein. A diagnostic and prognostic marker in acute pancreatitis and pancreas transplantation. Int J Pancreatol 19:165 – 70
32. Klar E, Herfarth C, Messmer K (1990) Therapeutic effect of isovolumic hemodilution with dextran 60 on the impair-

ment of pancreatic microcirculation in acute biliary pancreatitis. Ann Surg 211:346–53

33. Choi TK, Mok, F, Zahn WH, et al. (1989) Somatostatin in the treatment of acute pancreatitis: a prospective randomized controlled trial. Gut 30:223–7
34. D'Amico D, Favia G, Biasiato R, et al. (1990) The use of somatostatin in acute pancreatitis – results of a multicenter trial. Hepatogastroenterology 37:92–8
35. Buchler M, Malfertheiner P, Uhl W, et al. (1993) Gabexate mesilate in human acute pancreatitis. Gastroenterology 104:1165–70
36. Valderrama R, Perez-Mateo M, Navarro S (1992) Multicenter double-blind trial of gabexate mesilate (FOY) in unselected patients with acute pancreatitis. Digestion 51:65–70
37. Targarona MJ, Barreda CL, Arroyo BC, Orellana VA, Portanova RM (2005) Total enteral nutrition as prophylactic therapy for pancreatic necrosis infection in severe acute pancreatitis. Pancreatology 6:58–64
38. Kaushik N, Pietraszewski M, Holst JJ, O'Keefe SJD (2005) Enteral feeding without pancreatic stimulation. Pancreas 31:353–359
39. Olah A, Belagyi T, Issekutz A, Gamal ME, Bengmark A (2002) Randomized clinical trial of specific lactobacillus and fibre supplement to early enteral nutrition in patients with acute pancreatitis. Br J Surg 89:1103–7
40. Schmid SW, Uhl W, Friess H (1999) The role of infection in acute pancreatitis. Gut 45:311–316
41. Farkas G, Marton J, Mandi Y, Szederkenyi E (1996) Surgical strategy and management of infected pancreatic necrosis. Br J Surg 83:930–933
42. Foitzik T, Fernandez-del Castillo C, Ferraro MG, et al. (1995) Pathogenesis and prevention of early pancreatic infection in experimental acute necrotizing pancreatitis. Ann Surg 222:179–85
43. Bradley EL III (1993) A fifteen-year experience with open drainage for infected pancreatic necrosis. Surg Gynecol Obstet 177:215–222
44. Luiten EJ, Hop WC, Lange JF, et al. (1997) Differential prognosis of Gram-negative versus Gram-positive infected and sterile pancreatic necrosis; results of a randomized trial in patients with severe acute pancreatitis treated with adjuvant selective decontamination. Clin Infect Dis 25: 811–16
45. Finegold SM (1995) Anaerobic bacteria. In: Howard RJ, Simmons RL (eds) Surgical infectious disease. Appleton & Lange, Norwalk, CT, pp 6–81
46. Foizik TF, Fernandez-del Castillo C, Ferraro MJ, Mithofer K, Rattner DW, Warshaw AL (1995) Pathogenesis and prevention of early pancreatic infection in experimental acute necrotizing pancreatitis. Ann Surg 222:179–85
47. Mithofer K, Fernandez-del Castillo C, Ferraro MG, Lewandrowski K, Rattner DW, Warshaw AL (1996) Antibiotic treatment improves survival in experimental acute necrotizing pancreatitis. Gastroenterology 110:232–40
48. Widdison A, Karanjia ND, Reber HA (1994) Antimicrobial treatment of pancreatic infection in cats. Br J Surg 81: 886–89
49. Trudel JL, Wittnich C, Brown RA (1994) Antibiotics bioavailability in acute experimental pancreatitis. J Am Coll Surg 178:475–9
50. Roberts EA, Williams RJ (1979) Ampicillin concentrations in pancreatic fluid bile obtained at endoscopic retrograde cholangiopancreatography (ECRP). Scand J Gastroenterol 14:669–72
51. Buchler M, Malfertheiner P, Friess H, Isenmann R, Vanek E, Grimm H, et al. (1992) Human pancreatic tissue concentration of bactericidal antibiotics. Gastroenterology 103: 1902–8
52. Foitzik T, Hotz HG, Kinzig M, Sorgel F, Buhr HJ (1997) Influence of changes in pancreatic tissue morphology and capillary blood flow on antibiotic tissue concentrations in the pancreas during the progression of acute pancreatitis. Gut 40:526–30
53. Drewelow B, Koch K, Otto C, Franke A, Reithling AK (1992) Penetration of ceftazidime into human pancreas. Infection 21:229–34
54. Bassi C, Pederzoli P, Vesentini S, Falconi M, Bonora A, Abbas H, et al. (1994) Behavior of antibiotics during human necrotizing pancreatitis. Antimicrob Agents Chemother 38:830–6
55. Pederzoli P, Bassi C, Vesentini S, Campedelli A (1993) A randomized multicentre clinical trial of antibiotic prophylaxis of septic complications in acute pancreatitis with imipenem. Surg Gynecol Obstet 176:480–3
56. Sainio V, Kemppainen E, Puolakkainen P, Taavitsainen M, Kivisaari L, Valtonen V, et al. (1995) Early antibiotic treatment in acute necrotizing pancreatitis. Lancet 346:663–7
57. Schwartz M, Isenmann R, Meyer H, Beger HG (1997) Antibiotic use in necrotizing pancreatitis. Results of a controlled study. Dtsch Med Wochenschr 122:356–61
58. Golub R, Siddiqi F, Pohl D (1998) Role of antibiotics in acute pancreatitis: A meta-analysis. J Gastrointestinal Surg 2:496–503
59. Nordback I, Sand F, Saaristo R, Paajanen H (2001) Early treatment with antibiotics reduces the need for surgery in acute necrotizing pancreatitis – a single-center randomized study. J Gastrointest Surg 5:113–20
60. Maravi-Poma E, Gener J, Alvarez-Lerma F, Olaechea P, Blanco A, Dominguez-Munoz JE (2003) Early antibiotic treatment (prophylaxis) of septic complications in severe acute necrotizing pancreatitis: a prospective, randomized, multicenter study comparing two regimens with imipenem-cilastatin. Intensive Care Med 29:1974–80
61. Manes G, Rabitti PG, Menchise A, Riccio E, Balzano A, Uomo G (2003) Prophylaxis with meropenem of septic complications in acute pancreatitis: a randomized, controlled trial versus imipenem. Pancreas 27:e79–e83
62. Isenmann R, Runzi M, Kron M, Kahl S, Kraus D, Jung N, Maier L, Malfertheiner P, Goebell H, Beger HG (2004) Prophylactic antibiotic treatment in patients with predicted severe acute pancreatitis: a placebo-controlled doubleblind trial. Gastroenterology 126:997–1004
63. Heinrich S, Schafer M, Rousson V, Clavien P (2006) Evidence-based treatment of acute pancreatitis: a look at established paradigms. Ann Surg 243:154–68
64. Howard TJ, Temple MB (2002) Prophylactic antibiotics alter the bacteriology of infected necrosis in severe acute pancreatitis. J Am Coll Surg 195:759–67
65. Warshaw AL, Jin G (1985) Improved survival in 45 patients with pancreatic abscess. Ann Surg 202:408–17
66. Fedorak IJ, Ko TC, Kjuricin G, et al. (1992) Secondary pancreatic infections: are they distinct clinical entities? Surgery 112:824
67. Wilson C, Heads A, Shenkin A, Imrie CW (1989) C-reactive protein, antiproteases and complement factors as objective markers of severity in acute pancreatitis. Br J Surg 76:177–81
68. Buchler M, Malfertheiner P, Schoetensack C, et al. (1986) Sensitivity of antiproteases, complement factors and C-reactive protein in detecting pancreatic necrosis. Results of a prospective clinical study. Int J Pancreatol 1:227–35
69. Mayer AD, McMahon MJ, Bowen M, Cooper EH (1984) C reactive protein: an aid to assessment and monitoring of acute pancreatitis. J Clin Pathol 37:207–11
70. Puolakkainen P, Valtonen V, Paananen A, Schroder T (1987) C-reactive protein (CRP) and serum phospholipase

A2 in the assessment of the acute pancreatitis. Gut 28: 764–71
71. Schmidt J, Fernandez-del Castillo C, Rattner DW, et al. (1992) Trypsinogen activation peptides in experimental pancreatitis in the rat. Prognostic implications and histopathologic correlates. Gastroenterology 103:1009–16
72. Gudgeon AM, Heath DI, Hurley P, et al. (1990) Trypsinogen activation peptides assay in the early prediction of severity of acute pancreatitis. Lancet 335:4–8
73. Balthazar EJ, Robinson DL, Megibow AJ, Ranson JHC (1990) Acute pancreatitis: value of CT in establishing prognosis. Radiology 174:331–336
74. Balthazar EJ, Ranson JHC, Naidich DP, et al. (1985) Acute pancreatitis: prognostic value of CT. Radiology 156:767–772
75. Fink AS, Hiatt JR, Pitt HA, et al. (1988) Indolent presentation of pancreatic abscess: experience with 100 cases. Arch Surg 123:1067–72
76. Rattner DW, Legemate DA, Lee MJ, Mueller PR, Warshaw AL (1992) Early surgical debridement of pancreatic necrosis is beneficial irrespective of infection. Am J Surg 163: 105–9
77. Gerzof S, Banks P, Robbins AH, Johnson WC, Spechler SJ, Wetzner SM, Snider JM, Langevin RE, Jay ME (1987) Early diagnosis of pancreatic infection by computed tomography-guided aspiration. Gastroenterology 93:1315–20
78. Karlson KB, Martin EC, Fankuchen EI, Mattern RF, Schultz RW, Casarella WJ (1982) Percutaneous drainage of pancreatic pseudocysts and abscesses. Radiology 142:619–24
79. Gerzof SG, Johnson WC, Robbins AH, Spechler SJ, Nabseth DC (1984) Percutaneous drainage of infected pancreatic pseudocysts. Arch Surg 119:888–93
80. Barkin JS, Pereiras R, Hill M, Levi J, Isikoff M, Rogers AI (1982) Diagnosis of pancreatic abscess via percutaneous aspiration. Dig Dis Sci 27:1011–4
81. Hill MC, Dach JL, Barkin J, Isikoff MB, Morse B (1983) The role of percutaneous aspiration in the diagnosis of pancreatic abscess. AJR 141:1035–8
82. Warshaw AL, Gongliang J (1985) Improved survival in 45 patients with pancreatic abscess. Ann Surg 202:408–417
83. Stanten R, Frey CF (1990) Comprehensive management of acute necrotizing pancreatitis and pancreatic abscess. Arch Surg 125:1269–75
84. Bradley EL (1993) A fifteen year experience with open drainage for infected pancreatic necrosis. Sur Gynecol Obstet 177:215–22
85. Malangoni MA, Richardson JD, Shallcross JC, Seiler JG, Polk HC (1986) Factors contributing to fatal outcome after treatment of pancreatic abscess. Ann Surg 6:605–613
86. Pemberton JH, Nagorney DM, Becker JM, Ilstrup D, Dozois RR, Remine WH (1986) Controlled open lesser sac drainage for pancreatic abscess. Ann Surg 203:600–4
87. Orlando R, Welch JP, Akbari CM, Bloom GB, Macaulay WP (1993) Techniques and complications of open packing of infected pancreatic necrosis. Surg Gynecol Obstet 177: 65–71
88. Slakey DP, Johnson CP, Cziperle DJ, Roza AM, Wittman DH, Gray DWR, Roake JA, Britton J, Morris PJ, Adams MB (1997) Management of severe pancreatitis in renal transplant recipients. Ann Surg 225:217–22
89. Werner J, Hartwig W, Hackert T, Buchler MW (2005) Surgery in the treatment of acute pancreatitis – open pancreatic necrosectomy. Scand J Surg 94:130–4
90. Farkas G, Marton F, Mandi Y, Leindler L (2006) Surgical management and complex treatment of infected pancreatic necrosis: 18-year experience at a single center. J Gastrointest Surg 10:278–85

Chapter 53

Urinary Tract Infections

53

D. McRackan, C. Carson

Infection of the urinary tract (UTIs) represents one of the most commonly encountered disease processes in medicine. The spectrum of the illness severity is as wide as that of the patient population affected. In the US alone, urinary tract infections account for over seven million physician visits and require over 100,000 hospitalizations annually [1]. The financial burden of this is over 2 billion dollars per year, 500 million dollars of which is required to contend with nosocomial infections [1]. Of hospitalized patients, 3% develop an infection of the urinary tract, representing 40% of the 2 million nosocomial infections in the US annually [2]. Eighty percent of these infections occur in the setting of an indwelling urethral catheter, and in intensive care units (ICUs) up to 95% may be due to urinary catheterization [3–5]. Device-related infection rates (number of catheter-related UTIs per 1,000 catheter days) range from 9% to 18% in various ICUs worldwide [6–10]. Although the incidence of UTIs in the critically ill has been shown to vary based on the type of ICU, the impact in every unit is significant [6]. UTIs are the most common nosocomial infection in American medical ICUs, where the disease accounts for 31% of hospital acquired infections [5]. In European ICUs the incidence of nosocomial UTI is second only to respiratory infections [7]. The importance of urinary tract infections in the critically ill cannot be overstated. A recent study found that in 16% of ICU patients in septic shock, the source could be traced to the urinary tract [11]. Catheterized ICU patients who develop UTIs have a threefold increase in mortality [12].

For the purposes of evaluation, treatment and prognosis, urinary tract infections are divided into complicated and uncomplicated categories. Complicated UTIs are defined as infections that are associated with conditions that elevate the risk of therapeutic failure [3]. They involve patients with anatomical or functional defects of the urinary tract, or patients with altered defense mechanisms [14, 15]. Subjects include the critically ill or catheterized and as such will be the focus of this chapter.

53.1 Risk Factors

Several factors may predispose the critically ill patient to infection of the urinary tract, the most important of which is catheterization (Table 53.1). Urethral catheterization is the most common identifiable cause of nosocomial UTI and the incidence of infection is directly proportional to the duration of catheterization [3, 16]. The risk of infection with a single catheterization is 1–2% [17]. One study has concluded that insertion of urethral catheters outside of the operating room carries an increased rate of infection in ICU patients [18].

The incidence of UTI has been shown to increase with length of ICU stay [2, 16]. Females, obese, diabetic and elderly patients have higher rates of infection [2, 16]. Patients with serum creatinine greater than 2.0 mg/dl have been shown to have a greater incidence of catheter-related infections as well [19].

Another significant risk factor for urinary infection in any patient is urinary stasis [20]. Stagnancy may occur at any level in the urinary tract from an isolated calyx to the distal urethra. Frequent causes in the critically ill include bladder dysfunction from neurologic injury or from anesthetic. Dysfunctional urethral catheters may lead to stasis of urine. With obstruction there is an increase in bacterial binding to urothelium and stretch injury causes breakdown of the mucosal barrier, allowing invasion [13]. A patient with an infected, obstructed urinary tract represents a urologic emergency.

Table 53.1. Risk factors for UTI in the critically ill

Risk factors
Urethral catheterization
Prolonged ICU stay
Female sex
Obesity
Diabetes mellitus
Advanced age
Renal failure
Urinary stasis

53.2 Etiology

While the majority of uncomplicated community acquired UTIs have *Escherichia coli* as the solitary pathogen, complicated urinary infections involve a broader spectrum of organisms [21, 22]. Patients who are critically ill and/or have indwelling urethral catheters more frequently have polymicrobial infections, often involving atypical species [21, 23]. Although most uropathogens in the critically ill stem from endogenous flora, the sources of exogenous contamination in ICUs are vast. Only the largest studies regarding the etiology of nosocomial UTIs are discussed here, and results are summarized with comparison to uncomplicated UTI in Table 53.2.

The SENTRY study, the largest surveillance series to date, is an ongoing multicenter longitudinal surveillance program encompassing thousands of hospitalized patients from a variety of departments [24, 25]. Urinary tract isolates from North American, European, Latin American and Asian inpatients with nosocomial UTIs have been recorded and compared in terms of species prevalence and antibiotic resistance. In western centers, seven uropathogens accounted for over 90% of isolates. In order of decreasing prevalence, they were *E. coli* (47.3%), *Enterococcus* spp. (12.6%), *Klebsiella* spp. (11.0%), *Pseudomonas* spp. (7.6%), *Proteus* spp. (5.2%), *Enterobacter* spp. (3.5%), and *Citrobacter* spp. (2.8%). The Asia-Western Pacific arm of the study has reported similar rates; however, *Pseudomonas* spp. have been more commonly reported [25]. Of note, *Enterococcus* spp. have very rarely been found in Latin America.

The ESGNI-003 study was a one day prevalence study of multiple departments in over 220 European hospitals in 29 countries [26]. Nosocomial uropathogens from non-catheterized patients were similar in prevalence to the SENTRY study. However, in catheterized patients *Candida* spp. accounted for over 16% of isolates and *Pseudomonas* spp. were significantly more common.

A recent study from the UK focused on catheter-associated UTIs over a 5-year period from one university hospital [27]. *E. coli* and *Enterococcus* spp. were still the most frequently isolated pathogens, but *Proteus* spp. and *Pseudomonas* spp. were more commonly identified. Similar studies, performed in Italian and French centers, showed *Pseudomonas* spp. to be second only to *E. coli* in causing infection in patients with indwelling catheters (24% and 22% respectively) [28a, 29]. Indeed, *Pseudomonas* spp. have repeatedly been shown to plague patients with structural abnormalities of the urinary tract [29]. Atypical infections in patients with indwelling catheters include a large variety of organisms, including *Serratia*, *Stenotrophomonas* and *Providencia* spp. [23, 30, 31].

Duration of catheterization is significant when considering the possible etiology of UTI. In the first 4 days after catheterization, bacteriuria is usually not yet polymicrobial. In these first days, *E. coli* is the most common pathogen [23]. In the weeks following, the organism is more difficult to predict. In the intensive care setting many organisms become more likely to cause UTI over time, including *Enterococcus*, *Klebsiella* and *Candida* species [21, 32].

Fungal UTIs are a particular concern with catheterized and critically ill patients. *Candida* spp. have been found to be the uropathogen implicated in up to 20% of the UTIs in Western ICUs and it has been reported that up to 40% of patients with chronic indwelling catheters develop fungal UTIs [2, 32]. *Candida albicans* and *Candida glabrata* are by far the most common isolates [33].

Because of the vast array of organisms capable of causing urinary infection in the critically ill, one should base treatment on specific culture results and not attempt to predict etiology. Broad spectrum antibiotics administered at the outset of infection should be geared toward the coverage of all likely pathogens.

Table 53.2. The isolation frequency of major uropathogens in nosocomial UTIs found in the SENTRY study, ESGNI study and by Wazait et al. compared to data from the ECO-SENS Project (a European international multicenter survey of uncomplicated cystitis) [28]

Pathogen	SENTRY [24] North America, European Union, Latin America, (nosocomial UTI)	SENTRY [25] Asia-Pacific region (nosocomial UTI)	ESGNI [26] (nosocomial UTI)	Wazait [27] (catheter-associated nosocomial UTI)	ECO-SENS Project [28] (uncomplicated community UTI)
E. coli	47.3%	37.8%	35.3%	30.9%	53.3%
Enterococci	12.6%	10.8%	15.2%	17.2%	–
Klebsiella spp.	11.0%	12.3%	9.8%	–	2.2%
P. aeruginosa	7.6%	11.1%	5.4%	11.2%	2.7%
P. miribilis	5.2%	4.0%	6.7%	15.6%	4.4%
Enterobacter spp.	3.5%	4.5%	4.5%	–	–
Citrobacter spp.	2.8%	2.4%	2.7%	–	–
S. aureus	2.5%	3.7%	3.1%	9.5%	–

53.3 Pathogenesis

The outcome of the host-pathogen interplay depends on several factors. Uropathogens must first establish an anatomic pathway of invasion. Once the organism gains access to the urinary tract, infection may occur if bacterial virulence outweighs host defenses. In critically ill patients, immunocompromise may allow multiple organisms with minimal virulence to flourish. In fact, patients with diabetes mellitus, renal disease and chronic indwelling urethral catheters are often infected with organisms that lack typical virulence factors seen in community acquired UTIs [34, 35].

53.3.1 Conduits of Infection

53.3.1.1 Ascending Infection

By far, the most common route of urinary infection is ascent from the perineum to the bladder via the urethra. Bacteria originate from the fecal or vaginal flora [20]. Risk of infection via this route is increased in patients with urethral catheters or fecal soiling, both of which are common in the critically ill [36]. In patients with cystitis, bacteria may extend to the upper urinary system in half of the cases; pyelonephritis is most commonly established by this mechanism [20]. Although baseline vesicoureteral reflux may intensify the colonization of the upper tracts, it is not required. Ureteric peristalsis has been shown to be hindered by gram negative endotoxins and anatomic obstruction to urinary flow, thus propagating ascending infection [37].

As stated, urethral catheterization is a major risk factor for bacterial ascent and subsequent infection. Organisms colonizing the urethral meatus or distal urethra may easily be carried into the bladder by catheterization [3]. Once in place, bacteria may ascend along the luminal surface of the catheter (intraluminal ascent) or along the outside surface (extraluminal ascent) [38]. Several authors have suggested that in female patients, the extraluminal route is more common, as bacteria of the fecal or vaginal flora climb periurethrally [36, 39]. These authors state that male patients are more often infected via intraluminal pathways as a consequence of nonsterile equipment or disruption of drainage systems. Other authors have found that extraluminal invasion is more common in both sexes [38]. Gram positive organisms and yeasts are most likely to ascend by the extraluminal route [38].

Within the catheterized bladder, there exist two potential sources of infectious organisms. *Planktonic* organisms are those that grow in suspension, floating in urine [40]. Other bacteria may establish and thrive in organic layers that coat the catheter surface, called *biofilms* [41]. These layers, which are similar to those found on indwelling vascular catheters, are formed by secreted bacterial polysaccharides with host proteins and salts from normal urine [42]. Biofilms are thought to provide a barrier to antibiotics and host defenses and may traumatize urothelium with crystal formation [41].

53.3.1.2 Hematogenous Spread

Hematogenous seeding of the urinary tract is a much less frequent cause of UTI than ascending infection. However, bacteremia can be an important cause of suppurative infections of the kidney including renal and perinephric abscesses [43]. Hematogenous spread may also be implicated in infection of the kidneys by *Candida* spp., which may spread from central venous catheters [20]. There is evidence that urinary tract obstruction may increase risk of infection by hematogenous spread as organisms from the blood stream are prevented from being cleared in the urine [44].

53.3.1.3 Lymphatic Spread

Although rarely seen, renal or peri-renal infection via lymphatic seeding may occur in the setting of a severe retroperitoneal infectious process, including bowel perforation [45].

53.3.2 Host Defenses

Within the urinary tract, there exist multiple impediments to bacterial colonization and multiplication. Many of these defense mechanisms are evoked during acute infection while others are active in the normal urinary tract. In addition, some of these defenses are gender-specific.

Arguably the most important host characteristic in avoidance of bacterial invasion is unimpeded urinary flow. The normal voiding mechanism serves to rid the urinary tract of microorganisms that may have gained access via the urethra or blood stream [44, 46]. Stagnancy at any level may allow bacterial multiplication and urothelial binding. Overdistension from obstruction also interferes with local mucosal defenses [13]. This circumstance is frequently seen in the outpatient setting in patients who fail to completely empty their bladder due to neurologic disease or benign prostatic hypertrophy. Recurrent UTIs frequently complicate the urologic care in these groups. In the intensive care setting, urinary impedance may be caused by neurologic bladder dysfunction, catheter malfunction, or mass effect on the upper urinary tract from retroperitoneal processes.

The composition of urine is a major factor in the prevention of infection. Dilute urine in the well-hydrated patient inhibits bacterial growth and may promote cell lysis via low osmolality [47]. The baseline acidity of urine has been shown to decrease bacterial multiplication and when pH drifts upward, bacterial growth is enhanced [48]. Urea, a main component of urine, has significant antibacterial action [49].

Several proteins found in normal urine have been shown to provide a barrier to infection. Tamm-Horsfall protein (uromodulin), which is secreted by the distal tubule, is abundant in human urine. It has been shown to bind fimbriae of multiple uropathogens and facilitate removal by polymorphonuclear leukocytes [50, 51]. Lactoferrin, the known iron scavenger, exists in urine as well. By binding all available iron it exerts a significant antibacterial effect [52]. Other urinary proteins, such as urokinase-type plasminogen activator, are suspected to have antibacterial activity but are still under investigation [53]. The lining of the lower urinary tract plays an important role in maintaining a sterile environment. In both human and murine models, growth of normal bladder urothelium is slow, often taking weeks to months to fully regenerate [54]. However, when infection occurs, this turnover rate increases sharply causing the urothelium to slough [55]. The shed epithelium is then removed by the urine, thereby cleansing the bladder of existing bacteria.

If the previously described host defenses should fail and uropathogens begin to penetrate the urothelium, an immune response will be elicited. When the integrity of the urothelium is violated, polymorphonuclear leukocytes are recruited to the sight of injury by several cytokines, most importantly IL-1, IL-6 and IL-8 [56–58]. This begins an elaborate cascade leading to bacterial degradation. Within days the humoral immune response is initiated as antibodies are formed to components of the bacterial cell wall, most notably O and K lipopolysaccharides [59]. The humoral response has been shown to be much more profound when the upper urinary tracts are involved in the infection. Patients without a fully competent immune system (e.g., transplant recipients, poorly controlled diabetics, or patients with AIDS) have long been known to have increased rates of UTI [60].

Both sexes have developed unique measures to guard against UTI. As stated, in females, the vaginal flora is an important source for ascending infection [20]. A proper estrogen balance helps create a healthier environment in two ways. First, estrogen stimulates the regeneration and sloughing of vaginal mucosa which allows removal of adherent bacteria [61]. It also creates a more hospitable environment for the proliferation of lactobacilli. These species create and maintain an acidic vaginal fluid which inhibits the proliferation of gram negative bacteria [62]. Bacterial adherence to vaginal mucosa has been found to be reduced in women expressing a variety of cell surface antigens. The best studied is the expression of Lewis blood group antigens A and B, which decrease the likelihood of UTI by making bacterial binding sites less available [63].

In males, the most important preventive factor is urethral length, which is a significant anatomic obstacle to ascending infection [64]. Secondarily, there are many protective proteins in prostatic secretions including prostatic antibacterial factor which likely play a role in defense once invasion has occurred [65, 66].

53.3.3 Bacterial Virulence Factors

Uropathogens have developed a multitude of mechanisms by which to establish infection and evade host defenses. Nearly 30 separate virulence factors have been discovered for *E. coli* alone [67]. The type and number of these factors present in a given pathogen often determine the severity of infection. Many virulence genes are easily exchanged between organisms by horizontal gene transfer [68].

Once bacteria have ascended into the urinary tract, the extent to which they adhere to the urothelium is a critical event in the establishment of infection [69]. The most important and thoroughly studied virulence factors in *E. coli* are adhesins, surface glycoproteins usually protruding from pilli with the capability to tightly bind to urothelial cell surfaces [13]. The most abundant and significant adhesin in uropathogenic *E. coli* is the type 1 pillus [70]. Type 1 pilli allow *E. coli* to attach to epithelium and avoid being flushed out in the urine. These attachments are vital in strains causing cystitis but not pyelonephritis [71]. Recently, studies have shown that type 1 pilli are important for additional reasons. First, these adhesins promote invasion of individual urothelial cells. This allows uropathogenic *E. coli* to evade extracellular defenses while multiplying within host cells [55]. Additionally, type 1 pilli have been shown to promote biofilm formation [72]. Several other adhesins, e.g., S, P, and Dr pilli, have been shown to be important in adherence and internalization in various areas of the urinary tract [55, 73, 74]. P fimbriae in particular are associated with acute uncomplicated pyelonephritis via interaction with renal cell membranes [75]. Studies have shown that *E. coli* can exhibit a phenomenon called phase variation, wherein they switch from a piliated to non-piliated form to avoid neutrophilic targeting of these structures [76, 77].

Uropathogenic *E. coli* very frequently secrete toxins that are thought to aid in tissue invasion. Hemolysin is produced by the majority of *E. coli* responsible for acute urinary infection [78]. This toxin causes urothelial disruption and allows tissue penetration [79]. Investigation is underway on several potentially significant *E.*

coli toxins including cytotoxic necrotizing factor type 1, which has been shown to promote apoptosis in human urothelial cells [80].

A large percentage of *E. coli* strains with the propensity to cause pyelonephritis contain surface polysaccharides called K antigens [81]. These structures provide increased pathogenic potential by preventing complement activation on the bacterial cell wall [79]. Both the presence and number of K antigen structures on the bacterial surface correlate with virulence [82].

Because other species less commonly cause urinary infection, their pathogenic mechanisms are less extensively studied than *E. coli*. However, this is an area of active research. Recently a virulence gene was found in *S. aureus* that enables the bacteria to resist degradation within the urinary tract by neutrophils. This may be a mechanism shared by *Enterococcus* spp. and *Pseudomonas aeruginosa* as related genes exist in these species [83].

53.4 Diagnosis

How to define and properly diagnose UTI in the critically ill is often challenging. The chance of a catheterized patient having bacterial colonization of their urinary tract is 3–10% per day of indwelling catheterization [84]. Using modern closed collecting systems, one-half of patients will exhibit bacteriuria by 2 weeks [3]. Colonization is frequently difficult to differentiate clinically from infection since the majority of catheterized patients with UTIs are asymptomatic [85]. Bacteriuria alone requires no treatment [86].

The diagnosis of a UTI in the catheterized ICU patient generally requires pyuria (the presence of white blood cells in the urine) and significant bacterial growth in the urine. The Center for Disease Control's recommendations for the diagnosis of UTI with and without an indwelling catheter are listed in Tables 53.3 and 53.4, respectively [87]. However, there is some debate as to the validity of the recommendations.

Several authors have argued that using a cutoff of 10^5 microorganisms/ml of urine may lead to underdiagnosis. Bacterial doubling time in urine is relatively slow and bladder emptying is immediate in a properly working catheter. In a non-catheterized patient, UTI leads to frequent voiding. These facts have led to the idea that significant infection may not immediately reach 10^5 organisms/ml and that, with a symptomatic patient, 10^2 organisms/ml may be sufficient for the diagnosis [88]. It has been shown that nearly 40% of patients with less than 10^5 bacteria/ml will exceed the 10^5 cutoff within 3 days if untreated [89]. Lowering the criteria for the density of uropathogen required for the diagnosis of UTI would increase the number of UTIs diagnosed and would therefore have significant economic impact. There is currently not enough information available for definite recommendations in this regard.

Table 53.3. CDC criteria for the diagnosis of uncomplicated UTI

At least one of the following signs and symptoms without any other recognized cause:
Fever > 38.4 °C
Urgency
Frequency
Dysuria
Suprapubic tenderness
PLUS
A positive urine culture with > 10^5 microorganisms/ml and/or urinalysis > 10^3 WBC/mm^3

Table 53.4. CDC criteria for the diagnosis of catheter-associated UTI

Presence of Foley catheter
PLUS one of the following signs and symptoms without any other recognized cause:
Fever > 38.4 °C
Urgency
Frequency
Dysuria
Suprapubic tenderness
PLUS
A positive urine culture with > 10^5 microorganisms/ml and/or urinalysis > 10^3 WBC/mm^3

It is vital that when a urine specimen is taken from a catheterized patient with a suspected UTI, it is done so in a way that minimizes contamination. In patients with recently placed catheters, the best way is to draw urine from a catheter port. If no port is available, catheter puncture with a sterile needle is acceptable [90]. In chronically catheterized patients, the best urine specimen is one taken immediately after placement of a new catheter as this will be a true representation of planktonic organisms [91]. Specimens should never be taken from collection bags, as they are frequently colonized with organisms not actually present in the urine [86].

53.5 Radiographic Evaluation

In the majority of adults with acute urinary infection, imaging is unnecessary. However, there exist two subsets of patients in which a radiographic workup is fully warranted to exclude sources of bacteria that are not amenable to eradication by antibiotics alone. The goal of imaging in these patients is to find surgical causes of infection.

The first group includes patients with febrile UTIs that remain symptomatic 48–72 h after the initiation of appropriate antibiotic treatment [92, 93]. In this population, it is prudent to rule out perinephric or renal abscesses which develop as a consequence of acute pyelonephritis and often require formal drainage procedures. Diabetic patients may develop emphysematous pyelonephritis (see below), which rarely responds to medical treatment and carries a high mortality rate [94].

The second group of patients that should undergo imaging for a febrile UTI are those patients with preexisting risk factors for infection that may require surgical treatment [95]. This includes patients with:

1. A history of urinary calculi in whom a large infectious stone may contain an overwhelming bacterial burden or in whom there may exist ureteric obstruction.
2. Sickle cell disease, who are predisposed to renal papillary necrosis and subsequent ureteric obstruction.
3. A history of genitourinary manipulation or surgery that may predispose to obstruction.
4. Neurologic bladder dysfunction, in whom there is an increased risk of urinary calculi and renal scarring.
5. Poorly controlled diabetes mellitus, in whom there is an increased risk of abscess formation or emphysematous pyelonephritis.
6. End stage renal disease, in whom there is an increased risk of emphysematous pyelonephritis.

In patients with UTI that warrant imaging, the diagnostic test of choice is computed tomography (CT), which most accurately displays the severity of renal disease and detects the presence and cause of urinary obstruction [95]. If the patient is unable to be transported to the CT scanner, bedside ultrasound may be used. This modality can accurately detect pelvicalyceal dilation (indicating possible obstruction), pus in the collecting system (pyonephrosis), and large abscesses [93, 96, 97]. However, it has its limitations, including the inability to differentiate between air and calculi in the collecting system [93]. Ultrasound is also less sensitive than CT in detecting focal abscesses [92]. Magnetic resonance imaging (MRI) use is generally reserved for hemodynamically stable patients with compromised renal function, who require contrasted imaging. Although MRI may accurately delineate renal infection and obstruction, it is inferior to CT in visualizing renal calculi [98].

The findings of acute pyelonephritis on CT include focal or generalized renal enlargement with wedge-shaped areas of focal attenuation after contrast administration [99]. Usually, there are no abnormal findings on ultrasound and MRI shows global renal enlargement with mild perinephric fluid [98, 100, 101]. These descriptions must be contrasted with those of emphysematous pyelonephritis and perirenal or renal abscesses, all of which are discussed below.

53.6 Treatment

When considering treatment for a urinary infection in the critically ill patient, several factors must be considered. The most immediate goals of the physician are to rapidly and definitively eradicate the specific uropathogen and reduce morbidity and mortality. However, as in other nosocomial infections, minimizing the emergence and spread of resistant microorganisms is critical.

The specific choice of antibiotic for a critically ill patient with a UTI is made difficult by a dearth of clinical trials in this area. Therefore, the decision must be based on the following factors:

- Published data on susceptibility of common nosocomial uropathogens
- Resistance rates within a given hospital or intensive care unit
- Patient factors including allergies and renal function
- Need for intravenous versus oral treatment
- Cost

53.6.1 The Decision to Treat

As stated above, differentiating the truly infected patient from one with asymptomatic bacteriuria can be troublesome. However, this distinction is vital to prevent the over-treatment of UTIs and the emergence of bacterial resistance. There is no clinical benefit in treating catheterized patients with asymptomatic colonization of the urinary tract [102]. In fact, treatment leads to rapid reinfection by more resistant species, thereby complicating medical care [103, 104]. Similarly, there is no benefit to treating asymptomatic funguria in the catheterized patient, as this does not lessen the risk of *Candida* UTI [105]. The only patients who warrant treatment of asymptomatic bacteriuria are pregnant females [106].

When a high index of clinical suspicion exists for UTI, a urine culture should be sent prior to initiating treatment. Whenever possible, therapy should be delayed until culture results are available [107].

53.6.2 Empiric Treatment

A large percentage of critically ill patients require antibiotic treatment immediately after cultures are sent. This includes patients who are moderately to severely symptomatic and those with impending hemodynamic instability as a result of infection [86]. Many require IV treatment to prevent sepsis or because of impaired gastrointestinal absorption [106]. Initial therapy should adequately cover gram negative pathogens and *Enterococcus* spp. [86]. For several years, aminoglycosides (typically gentamicin) have been widely used as empiric treatment for gram negative uropathogens and are frequently used in combination with ampicillin for *Enterococcus* coverage [21]. These drugs are available by IV formulation and are cost-effective. However, aminoglycosides carry significant risk of nephrotoxicity and ototoxicity and serum levels must be closely monitored [21]. Other initial parenteral options are the fluoroquinolones, second or third generation cephalosporins, or carbapenems [108]. Many authors have advocated the use of antipseudomonal treatment as the initial empiric therapy for any patient in the intensive care setting or who exhibits signs of hemodynamic instability [21, 107, 108]. *Pseudomonas* spp. are known to be highly resistant in the hospital setting and any patient who fails to respond to several days of treatment with one of the aforementioned antibiotic classes should certainly be placed on antipseudomonal therapy because of sepsis risk [108]. Recommended therapy for empiric coverage of *Pseudomonas* spp. includes an acylaminopenicillin with beta-lactamase inhibitor (piperacillin/tazobactam), a third generation cephalosporin such as ceftazidime or a carbapenem such as imipenem [108]. The fluoroquinolones are an appropriate choice for pseudomonal coverage, but reports suggest that resistance is on the rise and this class must be used with caution [109].

Once culture results are available, patients should be immediately switched from empiric to specific antibiosis. Maintaining broad-spectrum antibiotics in this setting risks the development of resistance to a relatively limited armament of effective therapy.

Whenever the diagnosis of UTI is suspected in a catheterized patient, the catheter should be replaced prior to beginning antibiotic treatment. This removes the existing biofilm and decreases rate of relapse [86]. Replacement of the catheter prior to treatment has been shown to improve clinical outcomes [110]. Urine cultures should be sent from the new catheter to be certain that growth reflects planktonic organisms and not those from the biofilm.

53.6.3 Duration of Treatment

The duration of antimicrobial treatment for UTI in the critically ill patient is not well established. Most authors recommend 7–14 days of treatment if there is an appropriate clinical response (resolution of fever by 48 h) [21, 86]. Once defervescence has occurred, patients may be switched to oral antibiotics if they have a functional gastrointestinal tract.

53.7 Antibiotic Resistance

Critically ill and hospitalized patients are highly prone to infection by multi-drug resistant uropathogens due to selection pressures from widespread antibiotic usage [21]. While resistance varies widely by time and location, it is helpful to recognize broad patterns that may direct empiric therapy. Susceptibility of the most common uropathogens is reviewed here and their susceptibilities, as listed in the SENTRY study, are summarized in Table 53.5 [24, 25].

53.7.1 *Escherichia coli*

Escherichia coli resistance patterns in nosocomial UTIs have been thoroughly investigated by the SENTRY study [24, 25]. In western centers, *E. coli* susceptibility to amoxicillin/clavulanate and cefuroxime is very high (>95%). Resistance to trimethoprim/sulfamethoxazole is over 30% in Western centers, with the highest resistance rates found in Latin America. *E. coli* resistance to trimethoprim/sulfamethoxazole has doubled since 1990 in the US [111]. Uropathogenic *E. coli* remains sensitive to fluoroquinolones worldwide, but in Latin America and Asia Pacific regions resistance rates are up to 18%. *E. coli* is predictably very sensitive to broad spectrum antibiotics such as piperacillin/tazobactam, imipenem and amikacin.

53.7.2 *Pseudomonas aeruginosa*

Pseudomonas spp. have high resistance rates worldwide to a multitude of antibiotics. In Western centers, fluoroquinolone resistance exceeds 37% and in Latin America over half of isolates exhibit resistance. The ESGNI study found that less than 50% of species were sensitive to fluoroquinolones and non-amikacin aminoglycosides [26]. Karlowski et al. recently published *Pseudo-*

Table 53.5. SENTRY study all-region resistance rates (percentages) for the most common urinary tract isolates [24]

Antimicrobial	*E. coli*	*Klebsiella* spp.	*P. aeruginosa*	Enterococci
Ampicillin	45	76	100	12
Amoxicillin/clavulanate	5	10	99	12
Cefuroxime	4	17	100	–
Ciprofloxacin	11	10	37	47
Garenoxacin	11	8	44	–
Nitrofurantoin	3	16	100	1
Trimethoprim/sulfamethoxazole	31	23	99	35
Vancomycin	–	–	–	5

monas resistance rates from American ICUs. In this study, isolates displayed over 20% resistance to both ciprofloxacin and levafloxacin and resistance rates were found to increase over the 5-year study [112]. These reported sensitivity rates were lower than similar studies performed only 2 years prior [113]. In American ICUs, *Pseudomonas* spp. remain highly sensitive to amikacin (>93%) and piperacillin/tazobactam (>91%), which is similar to rates reported in Asian centers [24, 112]. Isolates from Western centers show virtually no sensitivity to ampicillin, amoxicillin/clavulanate, cefuroxime and trimethoprim/sulfamethoxazole [24].

53.7.3 *Enterococcus* spp.

The prevalence and resistance patterns of *Enterococcus* show a large amount of variation by region. In Western centers, susceptibility to ampicillin remains high (>88%), and no resistance is found in Latin America, where *Enterococcus* infection of the urinary tract is less common. Asian centers have slightly higher rates of resistance to ampicillin at 18%. Sensitivity of *Enterococcus* spp. to fluoroquinolones varies widely by formulation: in Western centers, sensitivity to garenfloxacin is over 85% while that of ciprofloxacin is only 44%. *Enterococcus* has been shown to have high resistance to ciprofloxacin in other recent studies [114]. Vancomycin-resistant *Enterococcus* spp. have only been detected in significant quantities in North America, where resistance is approximately 7%.

53.7.4 *Klebsiella* spp.

Considerable regional variation in susceptibility patterns has been reported for *Klebsiella* spp., but in Western centers, fluoroquinolone sensitivity remains very high. Cefuroxime is the least active antibiotic in these locations. Asian centers report over 94% sensitivity to both cefepime and imipenem. Worldwide, resistance of *Klebsiella* spp. to amoxicillin/clavulanate remains low.

53.8 Prevention

For decades, investigators have evaluated a variety of modalities to prevent the establishment of UTI in hospitalized patients with indwelling catheters. The most significant development to date has been the widespread use of closed sterile urinary catheter drainage systems, which have dramatically decreased the rate of UTI [115]. Several trials have involved the use of silver-coated catheters and results have been variable [116–119]. A meta-analysis of these studies showed that the use of silver alloy, but not silver oxide-coated, catheters reduced UTI [120]. However, there is currently not enough information in terms of efficacy and cost for recommendations to be made in this regard. A few studies have investigated regular meatal cleansing in preventing catheter associated UTI, but no benefit has been observed [115, 121]. Attempts have been made to reduce UTIs by periodically irrigating the bladder with antibiotic solutions. However, no benefit has been found and investigators noted that bacterial resistance expanded during the study [122].

To date, there have been very few studies on the prevention of UTI specifically in the critically ill, and therefore concrete guidelines do not exist. However, the following recommendations can be made:

1. Only personnel who have been properly educated in aseptic technique should insert urethral catheters.
2. Unobstructed urinary flow should be maintained at all times: kinking of the catheter should be avoided and the drainage system should always be below the level of the bladder.
3. Manipulation of catheters should be minimized and only performed after thorough hand washing.
4. Catheterization should be avoided whenever possible and indwelling catheters should be removed as soon as possible [115, 123].

53.9 Complications

After infection of the urinary tract is established, the disease may follow one of three clinical courses:

1. Infection may resolve as a consequence of appropriate use of antimicrobial therapy
2. Infection may become more widespread and generalized (diffuse pyelonephritis)
3. The infection may coalesce and become isolated in one portion of the kidney (abscess formation)

Serious infections of the urinary tract in the critically ill may have significant acute and chronic consequences. Acute complications, including renal or perinephric abscesses and emphysematous pyelonephritis, are important causes of morbidity and mortality from UTI, and often require immediate surgical intervention to prevent sepsis.

53.9.1 Renal Abscess

Renal abscesses, by definition, are isolated to the renal parenchyma. They are often diagnosed in otherwise healthy individuals; however, several factors increase the risk. These include urinary tract obstruction or ma-

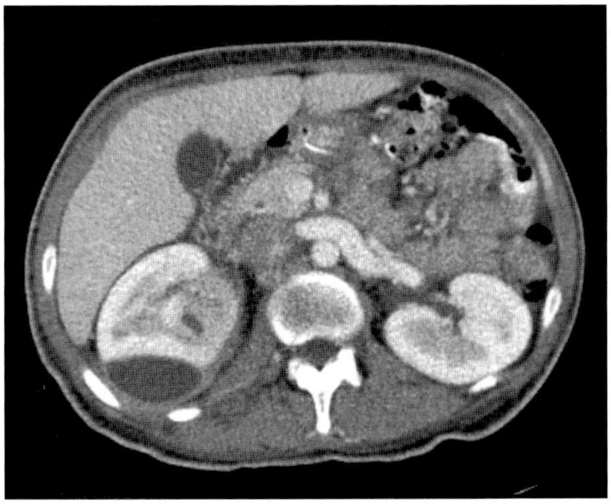

Fig. 53.1. Contrasted CT scan showing a right-sided renal abscess within the renal capsule compressing the adjacent parenchyma

nipulation, polycystic kidney disease, primary infection elsewhere in the body (e.g., intravascular catheters), immune compromise and diabetes mellitus [124–126]. Over half of the renal abscesses in adults are associated with renal calculi or previously damaged kidneys [127]. The majority of renal abscesses are established by ascending infection, and causative uropathogens may include any of those previously discussed. A significant percentage are caused by *S. aureus* hematogenous spread from cutaneous sites. Because the infection is walled off from the collecting system, blood cultures are usually positive with negative urine cultures and pyuria may be absent [128, 129].

The imaging modality of choice for renal abscesses is the contrasted CT scan. Findings include a marginated area of decreased attenuation within the parenchyma without enhancement after the administration of contrast [101] (Fig. 53.1). Up to half will show a peripheral rim of enhancement [92]. If the patient is unsuitable for CT, bedside ultrasound may be performed. Findings on ultrasound may include an intrarenal fluid collection with a thickened wall and contained echoes [130].

Treatment for renal abscesses depends on the size of the abscess as well as the patient's hemodynamic stability and immune function. In a stable immunocompetent patient, abscesses under 3 cm in size may be treated with empiric parenteral antibiotics and closely followed. In a host with evidence of impending hemodynamic compromise or with an impaired immune system, this same abscess should be surgically drained (ideally percutaneously by CT guidance). Renal abscesses over 3 cm in any patient are unlikely to respond to medical therapy alone and require drainage. Again, percutaneous drainage under radiographic guidance is preferred. If this fails or is contraindicated, open surgical drainage may be necessary [131].

53.9.2
Perinephric Abscess

The perinephric abscess is a focal infection between the renal capsule and Gerota's fascia. The majority of perinephric abscesses result from the rupture of a renal abscess into the perinephric space [129]. However, several other mechanisms exist, including hematogenous spread from cutaneous sites and direct extension from other sites of intra-abdominal injury including colon [132]. Risk factors are the same as for renal abscesses, and 25% of patients are diabetic [133]. As in renal abscesses, urine culture usually fails to isolate the responsible uropathogen. Unlike renal abscesses, however, blood cultures also fail to isolate the responsible bacteria more than half the time [134]. Therefore, specific antibiosis should be based only on abscess fluid cultures. Empiric treatment should be similar to that for renal abscesses and serious UTI, as the same uropathogens are involved. Perinephric abscesses are polymicrobial over 25% of the time [127, 134]. Again, CT is the imaging modality of choice due to high sensitivity and anatomic detail [135]. CT can also define extension beyond Gerota's fascia, which may occur with treatment delay.

Unlike renal abscesses, antibiotic treatment alone for perinephric abscesses is rarely curative and primary treatment involves drainage; this is most commonly performed by a radiographically guided percutaneous approach. Open surgical intervention is warranted if percutaneous drainage fails or is contraindicated. With delay in diagnosis or treatment, mortality from perinephric abscesses may approach 50% [129].

53.9.3
Emphysematous Pyelonephritis

Emphysematous pyelonephritis (EPN) is an acute necrotizing parenchymal infection caused by gas-forming uropathogens [136, 137]. The disease process is poorly understood, relatively rare and carries a high mortality rate of 43% [136]. Certain factors have repeatedly been found in association with EPN and are assumed to be essential to pathogenesis. These include high tissue glucose, impaired tissue perfusion, and defective immune response [138]. Up to 90% of patients with EPN are poorly controlled diabetics [139]. The most common causative agents are *E. coli, Klebsiella*, and *Proteus;* urine cultures are almost always positive [140]. Patients usually present with acute pyelonephritis with fever nonresponsive to several days of antibiotics. Almost all patients display fever, vomiting and flank pain [136]. The diagnostic modality of choice is CT because of the ability to differentiate intraparenchymal gas (the hallmark of EPN) from gas within the collecting system (which may only signify an upper UTI) [141]

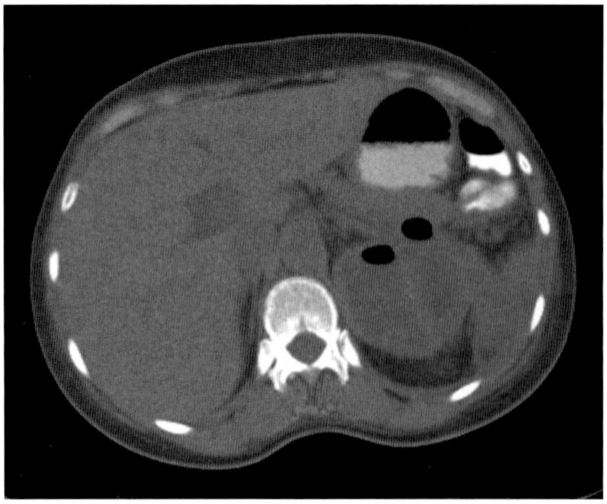

Fig. 53.2. CT performed without intravenous contrast showing left-sided emphysematous pyelonephritis, with two discrete areas of gas within the renal parenchyma

(Fig. 53.2). Ultrasound often fails to make this separation.

Patients with EPN treated with medical therapy alone have much higher mortality rates than those treated surgically [139, 141]. Therefore, the standard of care has classically been open extirpation. However, in many cases patients with EPN are unfit to undergo open surgical drainage or nephrectomy. In some cases, nephrectomy for EPN may make a patient dialysis-dependent. In these instances, percutaneous drainage with empiric broad-spectrum antibiotics may be appropriate [142].

53.10 Conclusions

Urinary infection in critically ill patients is a very common cause of morbidity and mortality. The disease involves a wide spectrum of uropathogens with diverse mechanisms of establishing infection. These microorganisms often cause life-threatening illness which requires immediate medical and often surgical intervention. Urinary catheterization is the most important factor in the development of this infection and should therefore be minimized. It is important for physicians to accurately diagnose and properly treat urinary infection in the ICU setting with the goals of reducing infectious complications and slowing the development of antibiotic resistance.

References

1. Foxman B, Brown P (2003) Epidemiology of urinary tract infections: transmission and risk factors, incidence, and costs. Infect Dis Clin North Am 17(2):227–41
2. Laupland KB, Zygun DA, Davies HD, Church DL, Louie TJ, Doig CJ (2002) Incidence and risk factors for acquiring nosocomial urinary tract infection in the critically ill. J Crit Care 17(1):50–7
3. Sedor J, Mulholland SG (1999) Hospital-acquired urinary tract infections associated with the indwelling catheter. Urol Clin North Am 26(4):821–8
4. Merle V, Germain JM, Bugel H, Nouvellon M, Lemeland JF, Czernichow P, Grise P (2002) Nosocomial urinary tract infections in urologic patients: assessment of a prospective surveillance program including 10,000 patients. Eur Urol 41(5):483–9
5. Richards MJ, Edwards JR, Culver DH, Gaynes RP (1999) Nosocomial infections in medical intensive care units in the United States. National Nosocomial Infections Surveillance System. Crit Care Med 27(5):887–92
6. Emori TG, Banerjee SN, Culver DH, Gaynes RP, Horan TC, Edwards JR, Jarvis WR, Tolson JS (1991) Nosocomial infections in elderly patients in the United States, 1986–1990. National Nosocomial Infections Surveillance System. Am J Med 91(3B):289S–293S
7. Vincent JL, Bihari DJ, Suter PM, Bruining HA, White J, Nicolas-Chanoin MH, Wolff M, Spencer RC, Hemmer M (1995) The prevalence of nosocomial infection in intensive care units in Europe. Results of the European Prevalence of Infection in Intensive Care (EPIC) Study. EPIC International Advisory Committee. JAMA 274(8):639–44
8. Zolldann D, Spitzer C, Hafner H, Waitschies B, Klein W, Sohr D, Block F, Lutticken R, Lemmen SW (2005) Surveillance of nosocomial infections in a neurologic intensive care unit. Infect Control Hosp Epidemiol 26(8):726–31
9. Rosenthal VD, Guzman S, Crnich C (2004) Device-associated nosocomial infection rates in intensive care units of Argentina. Infect Control Hosp Epidemiol 25(3):251–5
10. Trilla A (1994) Epidemiology of nosocomial infections in adult intensive care units. Intensive Care Med 20 Suppl 3:S1–4
11. Rosser CJ, Bare RL, Meredith JW (1999) Urinary tract infections in the critically ill patient with a urinary catheter. Am J Surg 177(4):287–90
12. Platt R, Polk BF, Murdock B, Rosner B (1982) Mortality associated with nosocomial urinary-tract infection. N Engl J Med 307(11):637–42
13. Hooton TM (2000) Pathogenesis of urinary tract infections: an update [review]. J Antimicrob Chemother 46 Suppl 1:1–7; discussion 63–5
14. Ronald AR, Harding GK (1997) Complicated urinary tract infections. Infect Dis Clin North Am 11(3):583–92
15. Melekos MD, Naber KG (2000) Complicated urinary tract infections [review]. Int J Antimicrob Agents 15(4):247–56
16. Leone M, Albanese J, Garnier F, Sapin C, Barrau K, Bimar MC, Martin C (2003) Risk factors of nosocomial catheter-associated urinary tract infection in a polyvalent intensive care unit. Intensive Care Med 29(7):1077–80
17. Turck M, Goffe B (1962) The urethral catheter and urinary tract infection. J Urol 88:834–7
18. Shapiro M, Simchen E, Izraeli S, Sacks TG (1984) A multivariate analysis of risk factors for acquiring bacteriuria in patients with indwelling urinary catheters for longer than 24 hours. Infect Control 5(11):525–32
19. Saint S, Lipsky BA (1999) Preventing catheter-related bacteriuria: should we? Can we? How? [Review] Arch Intern Med 159(8):800–8

20. Sobel JD (1997) Pathogenesis of urinary tract infection. Role of host defenses. Infect Dis Clin North Am 11(3): 531–49
21. Carson C, Naber KG (2004) Role of fluoroquinolones in the treatment of serious bacterial urinary tract infections. Drugs 64(12):1359–73
22. Kahlmeter G; ECO.SENS (2003) An international survey of the antimicrobial susceptibility of pathogens from uncomplicated urinary tract infections: the ECO.SENS Project. J Antimicrob Chemother 51(1):69–76
23. Warren JW (2001) Catheter-associated urinary tract infections. Int J Antimicrob Agents 17(4):299–303
24. Gordon KA, Jones RN; SENTRY Participant Groups (Europe, Latin America, North America) (2003) Susceptibility patterns of orally administered antimicrobials among urinary tract infection pathogens from hospitalized patients in North America: comparison report to Europe and Latin America. Results from the SENTRY Antimicrobial Surveillance Program (2000). Diagn Microbiol Infect Dis 45(4): 295–301
25. Turnidge J, Bell J, Biedenbach DJ, Jones R (2002) Pathogen occurrence and antimicrobial resistance trends among urinary tract infection isolates in the Asia-Western Pacific Region: report from the SENTRY Antimicrobial Surveillance Program, 1998–1999. Int J Antimicrob Agents 20(1): 10–7
26. Bouza E, San Juan R, Munoz P, Voss A, Kluytmans J (2001) A European perspective on nosocomial urinary tract infections II. Report on incidence, clinical characteristics and outcome (ESGNI-004 study). European Study Group on Nosocomial Infection. Clin Microbiol Infect 7(10):532–42
27. Wazait HD, Patel HR, Veer V, Kelsey M, Van Der Meulen JH, Miller RA, Emberton M (2003) Catheter-associated urinary tract infections: prevalence of uropathogens and pattern of antimicrobial resistance in a UK hospital (1996–2001). BJU Int 91(9):806–9
28. Kahlmeter G (2003) Prevalence and antimicrobial susceptibility of pathogens in uncomplicated cystitis in Europe. The ECO.SENS study. Int J Antimicrob Agents 22 Suppl 2:49–52
28a. Bochicchio GV, Joshi M, Shih D, Bochicchio K, Tracy K, Scalea TM (2003) Reclassification of urinary tract infections in critically ill trauma patients: a time-dependent analysis. Surg Infect (Larchmt) 4(4):379–85
29. Coker C, Poore CA, Li X, Mobley HL (2000) Pathogenesis of *Proteus mirabilis* urinary tract infection. Microbes Infect 2(12):1497–505
30. Maki DG, Hennekens CG, Phillips CW, Shaw WV, Bennett JV (1973) Nosocomial urinary tract infection with *Serratia marcescens:* an epidemiologic study. J Infect Dis 128(5): 579–87
31. VanCouwenberghe CJ, Farver TB, Cohen SH (1997) Risk factors associated with isolation of *Stenotrophomonas (Xanthomonas) maltophilia* in clinical specimens. Infect Control Hosp Epidemiol 18(5):316–21
32. Zolldann D, Spitzer C, Hafner H, Waitschies B, Klein W, Sohr D, Block F, Lutticken R, Lemmen SW (2005) Surveillance of nosocomial infections in a neurologic intensive care unit. Infect Control Hosp Epidemiol 26(8):726–31
33. Leone M, Albanese J, Antonini F, Michel-Nguyen A, Blanc-Bimar MC, Martin C (2003) Long-term epidemiological survey of *Candida* species: comparison of isolates found in an intensive care unit and in conventional wards. J Hosp Infect 55(3):169–74
34. Brauner A, Katouli M, Ostenson CG (1995) P-fimbriation and haemolysin production are the most important virulence factors in diabetic patients with *Escherichia coli* bacteraemia: a multivariate statistical analysis of seven bacterial virulence factors. J Infect 31(1):27–31
35. Karkkainen UM, Ikaheimo R, Katila ML, Sivonen A, Siitonen A (2000) Low virulence of *Escherichia coli* strains causing urinary tract infection in renal disease patients. Eur J Clin Microbiol Infect Dis 19(4):254–9
36. Hooton TM, Johnson C, Winter C, Kuwamura L, Rogers ME, Roberts PL, Stamm WE (1991) Single-dose and three-day regimens of ofloxacin versus trimethoprim-sulfamethoxazole for acute cystitis in women. Antimicrob Agents Chemother 35(7):1479–83
37. Thulesius O, Araj G (1987) The effect of uropathogenic bacteria on ureteral motility. Urol Res 15(5):273–6
38. Tambyah PA, Halvorson KT, Maki DG (1999) A prospective study of pathogenesis of catheter-associated urinary tract infections. Mayo Clin Proc 74(2):131–6
39. Daifuku R, Stamm WE (1984) Association of rectal and urethral colonization with urinary tract infection in patients with indwelling catheters. JAMA 252(15):2028–30
40. Stamm WE, Hooton TM, Johnson JR, Johnson C, Stapleton A, Roberts PL, Moseley SL, Fihn SD (1989) Urinary tract infections: from pathogenesis to treatment. J Infect Dis 159(3):400–6
41. Matsukawa M, Kunishima Y, Takahashi S, Takeyama K, Tsukamoto T (2005) Bacterial colonization on intraluminal surface of urethral catheter. Urology 65(3):440–4
42. Watnick P, Kolter R (2000) Biofilm, city of microbes. J Bacteriol 182(10):2675–9
43. Brook I (2004) Urinary tract and genito-urinary suppurative infections due to anaerobic bacteria. Int J Urol 11(3):133–41
44. Measley RE Jr, Levison ME (1991) Host defense mechanisms in the pathogenesis of urinary tract infection. Med Clin North Am 75(2):275–86
45. Bechtold RE, Dyer RB, Zagoria RJ, Chen MY (1996) The perirenal space: relationship of pathologic processes to normal retroperitoneal anatomy. Radiographics 16(4): 841–54
46. Hinman F Jr, Cox CE (1966) The voiding vesical defense mechanism: the mathematical effect of residual urine, voiding interval and volume on bacteriuria. J Urol 96(4):491–8
47. Kaye D (1968) Antibacterial activity of human urine. J Clin Invest 47(10):2374–9
48. Patterson JE, Andriole VT (1997) Bacterial urinary tract infections in diabetes. Infect Dis Clin North Am 11(3): 735–50
49. Mulholland SG (1979) Lower urinary tract antibacterial defense mechanisms. Invest Urol 17(2):93–7
50. Toma G, Bates JM Jr, Kumar S (1994) Uromodulin (Tamm-Horsfall protein) is a leukocyte adhesion molecule. Biochem Biophys Res Commun 200(1):275–82
51. Orskov I, Ferencz A, Orskov F (1980) Tamm-Horsfall protein or uromucoid is the normal urinary slime that traps type 1 fimbriated *Escherichia coli.* Lancet 1(8173):887
52. Abrink M, Larsson E, Gobl A, Hellman L (2000) Expression of lactoferrin in the kidney: implications for innate immunity and iron metabolism. Kidney Int 57(5):2004–10
53. Jin T, Bokarewa M, Tarkowski A (2005) The role of urokinase in innate immunity against *Staphylococcus aureus.* Microbes Infect 7(9–10):1170–5
54. Jost SP, Gosling JA, Dixon JS (1989) The morphology of normal human bladder urothelium. J Anat 167:103–15
55. Bower JM, Eto DS, Mulvey MA (2005) Covert operations of uropathogenic *Escherichia coli* within the urinary tract. Traffic 6(1):18–31
56. Benson M, Jodal U, Agace W, Hellstrom M, Marild S, Rosberg S, Sjostrom M, Wettergren B, Jonsson S, Svanborg C

(1996) Interleukin (IL)-6 and IL-8 in children with febrile urinary tract infection and asymptomatic bacteriuria. J Infect Dis 174(5):1080–4
57. Lin SJ, Huang JL (1998) Circulating interleukin (IL)-1 beta, IL-6 and tumor necrosis factor-alpha in children with febrile infection – a comparison with C-reactive protein. Asian Pac J Allergy Immunol 16(2–3):105–9
58. Otto G, Braconier J, Andreasson A, Svanborg C (1999) Interleukin-6 and disease severity in patients with bacteremic and nonbacteremic febrile urinary tract infection. J Infect Dis 179(1):172–9
59. Mattsby-Baltzer I, Claesson I, Hanson LA, Jodal U, Kaijser B, Lindberg U, Peterson H (1981) Antibodies to lipid A during urinary tract infection. J Infect Dis 144(4):319–28
60. Tolkoff-Rubin NE, Rubin RH (1997) Urinary tract infection in the immunocompromised host. Lessons from kidney transplantation and the AIDS epidemic. Infect Dis Clin North Am 11(3):707–17
61. Raz R, Stamm WE (1993) A controlled trial of intravaginal estriol in postmenopausal women with recurrent urinary tract infections. N Engl J Med 329(11):753–6
62. Hooton TM, Scholes D, Hughes JP, Winter C, Roberts PL, Stapleton AE, Stergachis A, Stamm WE (1996) A prospective study of risk factors for symptomatic urinary tract infection in young women. N Engl J Med 335(7):468–74
63. Gaffney RA, Schaeffer AJ, Anderson BE, Duncan JL (1994) Effect of Lewis blood group antigen expression on bacterial adherence to COS-1 cells. Infect Immun 62(7):3022–6
64. Hinman F Jr, Cox CE (1967) Residual urine volume in normal male subjects. J Urol 97(4):641–5
65. Fair WR, Parrish RF (1981) Antibacterial substances in prostatic fluid. Prog Clin Biol Res 75A:247–64
66. Lipsky BA (1989) Urinary tract infections in men. Epidemiology, pathophysiology, diagnosis, and treatment. Ann Intern Med 110(2):138–50
67. Johnson JR, Kuskowski MA, Gajewski A, Sahm DF, Karlowsky JA (2004) Virulence characteristics and phylogenetic background of multidrug-resistant and antimicrobial-susceptible clinical isolates of *Escherichia coli* from across the United States, 2000–2001. J Infect Dis 190(10):1739–44
68. Johnson JR, Lockman HA, Owens K, Jelacic S, Tarr PI (2003) High-frequency secondary mutations after suicide-driven allelic exchange mutagenesis in extraintestinal pathogenic *Escherichia coli*. J Bacteriol 185(17):5301–5. Erratum in: J Bacteriol 2003 185(22):6746
69. Ofek I, Beachey EH (1980) Bacterial adherence. Adv Intern Med 25:503–32
70. Le Bouguenec C (2005) Adhesins and invasins of pathogenic *Escherichia coli*. Int J Med Microbiol 295(6–7):471–8
71. Gunther NW 4th, Lockatell V, Johnson DE, Mobley HL (2001) In vivo dynamics of type 1 fimbria regulation in uropathogenic *Escherichia coli* during experimental urinary tract infection. Infect Immun 69(5):2838–46
72. Schembri MA, Klemm P (2001) Biofilm formation in a hydrodynamic environment by novel fimh variants and ramifications for virulence. Infect Immun 69(3):1322–8
73. Foxman B, Zhang L, Tallman P, Palin K, Rode C, Bloch C, Gillespie B, Marrs CF (1995) Virulence characteristics of *Escherichia coli* causing first urinary tract infection predict risk of second infection. J Infect Dis 172(6):1536–41
74. Guignot J, Bernet-Camard MF, Pous C, Plancon L, Le Bouguenec C, Servin AL (2001) Polarized entry of uropathogenic Afa/Dr diffusely adhering *Escherichia coli* strain IH11128 into human epithelial cells: evidence for alpha5beta1 integrin recognition and subsequent internalization through a pathway involving caveolae and dynamic unstable microtubules. Infect Immun 69(3):1856–68
75. Johnson JR (1991) Virulence factors in *Escherichia coli* urinary tract infection. Clin Microbiol Rev 4(1):80–128
76. Hultgren SJ, Schwan WR, Schaeffer AJ, Duncan JL (1986) Regulation of production of type 1 pili among urinary tract isolates of *Escherichia coli*. Infect Immun 54(3):613–20
77. Eisenstein BI (1981) Phase variation of type 1 fimbriae in *Escherichia coli* is under transcriptional control. Science 214(4518):337–9
78. Funfstuck R, Tschape H, Stein G, Vollandt R, Schneider S (1989) Virulence of *Escherichia coli* strains in relation to their hemolysin formation, mannose-resistant hemagglutination, hydroxamate production, K 1-antigen and the plasmid profile in patients with chronic pyelonephritis. Clin Nephrol 32(4):178–84
79. Funfstuck R, Stein G (1997) Pathogenetic aspects of urinary tract infection. Wien Med Wochenschr 147(19–20):465–9
80. Mills M, Meysick KC, O'Brien AD (2000) Cytotoxic necrotizing factor type 1 of uropathogenic *Escherichia coli* kills cultured human uroepithelial 5637 cells by an apoptotic mechanism. Infect Immun 68(10):5869–80
81. Loftus JC, Smith JW, Ginsberg MH (1994) Integrin-mediated cell adhesion: the extracellular face. J Biol Chem 269(41):25235–8
82. Kaijser B, Ahlstedt S (1977) Protective capacity of antibodies against *Escherichia coli* and K antigens. Infect Immun 17(2):286–9
83. Peschel A, Jack RW, Otto M, Collins LV, Staubitz P, Nicholson G, Kalbacher H, Nieuwenhuizen WF, Jung G, Tarkowski A, van Kessel KP, van Strijp JA (2001) *Staphylococcus aureus* resistance to human defensins and evasion of neutrophil killing via the novel virulence factor MprF is based on modification of membrane lipids with l-lysine. J Exp Med 193(9):1067–76
84. Haley RW, Hooton TM, Culver DH, Stanley RC, Emori TG, Hardison CD, Quade D, Shachtman RH, Schaberg DR, Shah BV, Schatz GD (1981) Nosocomial infections in U.S. hospitals 1975–1976: estimated frequency by selected characteristics of patients. Am J Med 70(4):947–59
85. Tambyah PA, Maki DG (2000) Catheter-associated urinary tract infection is rarely symptomatic: a prospective study of 1,497 catheterized patients. Arch Intern Med 160(5):678–82
86. Nicolle LE (2005 Catheter-related urinary tract infection. Drugs Aging 22(8):627–39
87. National Nosocomial Infections Surveillance (NNIS) (1998) System report, data summary from October 1986-April 1998, issued June 1998. Am J Infect Control 26(5):522–33
88. Stamm WE, Hooton TM (1993) Management of urinary tract infections in adults. N Engl J Med 329(18):1328–34
89. Stark RP, Maki DG (1984) Bacteriuria in the catheterized patient. What quantitative level of bacteriuria is relevant? N Engl J Med 311(9):560–4
90. Grahn D, Norman DC, White ML, Cantrell M, Yoshikawa TT (1985) Validity of urinary catheter specimen for diagnosis of urinary tract infection in the elderly. Arch Intern Med 145(10):1858–60
91. Tenney JH, Warren JW (1988) Bacteriuria in women with long-term catheters: paired comparison of indwelling and replacement catheters. J Infect Dis 157(1):199–202
92. Soulen MC, Fishman EK, Goldman SM, Gatewood OM (1989) Bacterial renal infection: role of CT. Radiology 171(3):703–7
93. Webb JA (1997) The role of imaging in adult acute urinary tract infection. Eur Radiol 7(6):837–43
94. Lautin EM, Gordon PM, Friedman AC, Dourmashkin L,

Fromowitz F (1979) Emphysematous pyelonephritis: optimal diagnosis and treatment. Urol Radiol 1(2):93–6
95. Baumgarten DA, Baumgartner BR (1997) Imaging and radiologic management of upper urinary tract infections. Urol Clin North Am 24(3):545–69
96. Ellenbogen PH, Scheible FW, Talner LB, Leopold GR (1978) Sensitivity of gray scale ultrasound in detecting urinary tract obstruction. AJR Am J Roentgenol 130(4): 731–3
97. Lee JK, Baron RL, Melson GL, McClennan BL, Weyman PJ (1981) Can real-time ultrasonography replace static B-scanning in the diagnosis of renal obstruction? Radiology 139(1):161–5
98. Rusinek H, Kaur M, Lee VS (2004) Renal magnetic resonance imaging. Curr Opin Nephrol Hypertens 13(6):667–73
99. Gold RP, McClennan BL, Rottenberg RR (1983) CT appearance of acute inflammatory disease of the renal interstitium. AJR Am J Roentgenol 141(2):343–9
100. Kass EJ, Silver TM, Konnak JW, Thornbury JR, Wolfman MG (1976) The urographic findings in acute pyelonephritis: non-obstructive hydronephrosis. J Urol 116(5):544–6
101. Talner LB, Davidson AJ, Lebowitz RL, Dalla Palma L, Goldman SM (1994) Acute pyelonephritis: can we agree on terminology? Radiology 192(2):297–305
102. Garibaldi RA, Burke JP, Dickman ML, Smith CB (1974) Factors predisposing to bacteriuria during indwelling urethral catheterization. N Engl J Med 291(5):215–9
103. Warren JW, Tenney JH, Hoopes JM, Muncie HL, Anthony WC (1982) A prospective microbiologic study of bacteriuria in patients with chronic indwelling urethral catheters. J Infect Dis 146(6):719–23
104. Alling B, Brandberg A, Seeberg S, Svanborg A (1975) Effect of consecutive antibacterial therapy on bacteriuria in hospitalized geriatric patients. Scand J Infect Dis 7(3):201–7
105. Kauffman CA, Vazquez JA, Sobel JD, Gallis HA, McKinsey DS, Karchmer AW, Sugar AM, Sharkey PK, Wise GJ, Mangi R, Mosher A, Lee JY, Dismukes WE (2000) Prospective multicenter surveillance study of funguria in hospitalized patients. The National Institute for Allergy and Infectious Diseases (NIAID) Mycoses Study Group. Clin Infect Dis 30(1):14–8
106. Nicolle LE (2001) A practical guide to antimicrobial management of complicated urinary tract infection. Drugs Aging 18(4):243–5
107. Wagenlehner FM, Weidner W, Naber KG (2005) Emergence of antibiotic resistance amongst hospital-acquired urinary tract infections and pharmacokinetic/pharmacodynamic considerations. J Hosp Infect 60(3):191–200
108. Naber KG, Bergman B, Bishop MC, Bjerklund-Johansen TE, Botto H, Lobel B, Jinenez Cruz F, Selvaggi FP; Urinary Tract Infection (UTI) Working Group of the Health Care Office (HCO) of the European Association of Urology (EAU) (2001) EAU guidelines for the management of urinary and male genital tract infections. Urinary Tract Infection (UTI) Working Group of the Health Care Office (HCO) of the European Association of Urology (EAU). Eur Urol 40(5):576–88
109. Jones RN, Beach ML, Pfaller MA (2001) Spectrum and activity of three contemporary fluoroquinolones tested against *Pseudomonas aeruginosa* isolates from urinary tract infections in the SENTRY Antimicrobial Surveillance Program (Europe and the Americas; 2000): more alike than different! Diagn Microbiol Infect Dis 41(3):161–3
110. Raz R, Schiller D, Nicolle LE (2000) Chronic indwelling catheter replacement before antimicrobial therapy for symptomatic urinary tract infection. J Urol 164(4): 1254–8
111. Gupta K, Hooton TM, Stamm WE (2001) Increasing antimicrobial resistance and the management of uncomplicated community-acquired urinary tract infections. Ann Intern Med 135(1):41–50
112. Karlowsky JA, Draghi DC, Jones ME, Thornsberry C, Friedland IR, Sahm DF (2003) Surveillance for antimicrobial susceptibility among clinical isolates of *Pseudomonas aeruginosa* and *Acinetobacter baumannii* from hospitalized patients in the United States, 1998 to 2001. Antimicrob Agents Chemother 47(5):1681–8
113. Pfaller MA, Jones RN, Doern GV, Kugler K (1998) Bacterial pathogens isolated from patients with bloodstream infection: frequencies of occurrence and antimicrobial susceptibility patterns from the SENTRY antimicrobial surveillance program (United States and Canada, 1997). Antimicrob Agents Chemother 42(7):1762–70
114. Fung-Tomc JC, Gradelski E, Valera L, Kolek B, Bonner DP (2000) Comparative killing rates of fluoroquinolones and cell wall-active agents. Antimicrob Agents Chemother 44(5):1377–80
115. Leone M, Garnier F, Avidan M, Martin C (2004) Catheter-associated urinary tract infections in intensive care units. Microbes Infect 6(11):1026–32
116. Johnson JR, Roberts PL, Olsen RJ, Moyer KA, Stamm WE (1990) Prevention of catheter-associated urinary tract infection with a silver oxide-coated urinary catheter: clinical and microbiologic correlates. J Infect Dis 162(5):1145–50
117. Riley DK, Classen DC, Stevens LE, Burke JP (1995) A large randomized clinical trial of a silver-impregnated urinary catheter: lack of efficacy and staphylococcal superinfection. Am J Med 98(4):349–56
118. Schaeffer AJ, Story KO, Johnson SM (1988) Effect of silver oxide/trichloroisocyanuric acid antimicrobial urinary drainage system on catheter-associated bacteriuria. J Urol 139(1):69–73
119. Liedberg H, Lundeberg T (1990) Silver alloy coated catheters reduce catheter-associated bacteriuria. Br J Urol 65(4):379–81
120. Elmore JG, Sullivan SD, Emerson SS, Koepsell TD (1998) The efficacy of silver alloy-coated urinary catheters in preventing urinary tract infection: a meta-analysis. Am J Med 105(3):236–41
121. Huth TS, Burke JP, Larsen RA, Classen DC, Stevens LE (1992) Randomized trial of meatal care with silver sulfadiazine cream for the prevention of catheter-associated bacteriuria. J Infect Dis 165(1):14–8
122. Warren JW, Platt R, Thomas RJ, Rosner B, Kass EH (1978) Antibiotic irrigation and catheter-associated urinary-tract infections. N Engl J Med 299(11):570–3
123. Saint S, Lipsky BA (1999) Preventing catheter-related bacteriuria: should we? Can we? How? Arch Intern Med 1999 159(8):800–8
124. Yen DH, Hu SC, Tsai J, Kao WF, Chern CH, Wang LM, Lee CH (1999) Renal abscess: early diagnosis and treatment. Am J Emerg Med 17(2):192–7
125. Segura JW, Kelalis PP (1973) Localized renal parenchymal infections in children. J Urol 109(6):1029–32
126. Klein DL, Filpi RG (1977) Acute renal carbuncle. J Urol 118(6):912–5
127. Salvatierra O Jr, Bucklew WB, Morrow JW (1967) Perinephric abscess: a report of 71 cases. J Urol 98(3):296–302
128. Schiff M Jr, Glickman M, Weiss RM, Ahern MJ, Touloukian RJ, Lytton B, Andriole VT (1977) Antibiotic treatment of renal carbuncle. Ann Intern Med 87(3):305–8
129. Dembry LM, Andriole VT (1997) Renal and perirenal abscesses. Infect Dis Clin North Am 11(3):663–80

130. Hoddick W, Jeffrey RB, Goldberg HI, Federle MP, Laing FC (1983) CT and sonography of severe renal and perirenal infections. AJR Am J Roentgenol 140(3):517–20
131. Siegel JF, Smith A, Moldwin R (1996) Minimally invasive treatment of renal abscess. J Urol 155(1):52–5
132. Saiki J, Vaziri ND, Barton C (1982) Perinephric and intranephric abscesses: a review of the literature. West J Med 136(2):95–102
133. Thorley JD, Jones SR, Sanford JP (1974) Perinephric abscess. Medicine (Baltimore) 53(6):441–51
134. Edelstein H, McCabe RE (1988) Perinephric abscess. Modern diagnosis and treatment in 47 cases. Medicine (Baltimore) 67(2):118–31
135. Hoddick W, Jeffrey RB, Goldberg HI, Federle MP, Laing FC (1983) CT and sonography of severe renal and perirenal infections. AJR Am J Roentgenol 140(3):517–20
136. Michaeli J, Mogle P, Perlberg S, Heiman S, Caine M (1984) Emphysematous pyelonephritis. J Urol 131(2):203–8
137. Evanoff GV, Thompson CS, Foley R, Weinman EJ (1987) Spectrum of gas within the kidney. Emphysematous pyelonephritis and emphysematous pyelitis. Am J Med 83(1):149–54
138. Huang JJ, Chen KW, Ruaan MK, Tsai HM (1994) Recurrent emphysematous pyelonephritis. A case report. Int Urol Nephrol 26(4):389–93
139. Cook DJ, Achong MR, Dobranowski J (1989) Emphysematous pyelonephritis. Complicated urinary tract infection in diabetes. Diabetes Care 12(3):229–32
140. Flores G, Nellen H, Magana F, Calleja J (2002) Acute bilateral emphysematous pyelonephritis successfully managed by medical therapy alone: a case report and review of the literature. BMC Nephrol 3:4
141. Stein JP, Spitz A, Elmajian DA, Esrig D, Freeman JA, Grossfeld GD, Ginsberg DA, Skinner DG (1996) Bilateral emphysematous pyelonephritis: a case report and review of the literature. Urology 47(1):129–34
142. Hall JR, Choa RG, Wells IP (1988) Percutaneous drainage in emphysematous pyelonephritis – an alternative to major surgery. Clin Radiol 39(6):622–4

Chapter 54

Neurosurgical Infections in Intensive Care Unit Patients

54

E.M. Brown

54.1 Introduction

At any point in time a high proportion of the beds on the general intensive care units (ICUs) of hospitals with neurosurgical services will be occupied by neurosurgical patients; indeed, on occasions, most of the beds may be occupied by such patients. The majority of neurosurgical patients requiring ICU admission will comprise those who have sustained head injuries, subarachnoid haemorrhages or complications of neurosurgical procedures. Only a minority will be admitted with serious intracranial or spinal infections, while others will develop neurosurgical infections while they are on the ICU. This chapter is devoted to common primary and secondary neurosurgical infections in the ICU population. Although all such infections are encountered relatively infrequently they are nonetheless important causes of morbidity and mortality. They may also delay a patient's discharge from hospital, necessitate further surgery and increase the overall cost of hospital care. Prompt diagnosis and combined medical and surgical interventions, therefore, remain the cornerstone of efforts to minimize the incidences of adverse outcomes. The reader should be aware however that current practice in, and recommendations for, the treatment of infections in neurosurgical patients owe little to evidence-based medicine. This situation exists not because there have been too few clinical trials that have been undertaken in an attempt to address these issues, but, rather, because the published literature is dominated by studies that suffer from flaws in their design and/or execution. The recommendations contained herein are therefore based on a less than robust published literature, working party reports, which are predominantly consensus statements, and personal experience.

54.2 Primary Infections

54.2.1 Brain Abscess

54.2.1.1 Epidemiology

Brain abscess is a focal (or, less frequently, multifocal) process that develops within the brain parenchyma. It is the second most common infection of the central nervous system (CNS) after bacterial meningitis and is the most common space-occupying infection of the CNS. Nonetheless, it is a relatively rare disease, with a reported incidence that varies from 0.32 to 1.1 hospital admissions per 100,000; therefore, between four and ten cases will present annually to a neurosurgical department. The incidence of brain abscess is higher in immunocompromised patients, and those hospitals to which large numbers of patients with the acquired immunodeficiency syndrome (AIDS) are admitted can expect higher incidences. The mean age of patients is 35–40 years, with a peak incidence in the second and third decades; approximately 25% of all brain abscesses occur in children (peak incidence 4–7 years of age). There is a male preponderance, with a male:female ratio of 2–3:1.

54.2.1.2 Pathogenesis

Brain abscesses develop as consequences of implantation in the brain substance of bacteria or bacterial emboli from either local or distant septic foci. While certain pre-existing brain diseases, such as intracerebral haematoma, neoplasms and strokes, may serve as foci for abscess formation, predisposing lesions are rarely identified. In the majority of cases, organisms gain access by direct spread from contiguous infected foci, e.g., acute or chronic otitis media (with or without mastoiditis), sinusitis, dental infections and meningitis (albeit rarely). Middle ear and sinugenic infections together account for 40–70% of brain abscesses, although the widespread administration of antibiotic therapy to patients with otitis media has led to a decrease in the incidence attributable to the former in most developed countries. The incidence of odontogenic abscess is approximately 10 %. Metastatic or haematogenous spread from a distant focus accounts for 20 – 25 % of brain abscesses. The most common sources are chronic pyogenic lung diseases, such as empyema, bronchiectasis and lung abscesses, which are now uncommon in developed countries. Others include osteomyelitis, intra-abdominal infections, pelvic infections, skin and soft tissue infections, septicaemias and infective endocarditis. Cyanotic congenital cardiac disease in patients with right-to-left shunts, particularly Fallot's tetralogy, is associated with 5 – 10 % of cases overall, but up to 25 % of all brain abscesses in children. Brain abscesses complicate cavernous sinus thrombosis secondary to septic thrombophlebitis of the anterior facial vein or malignant tumours involving the cranial bones. Organisms may also gain access to the brain following implantation through a penetrating wound of the head which may be traumatic or iatrogenic, i.e., following neurosurgery or in association with an intracranial pressure monitor; this route accounts for 5 – 10 % of brain abscesses. In infants and children, congenital malformations, especially meningomyelocele, encephalocele and sinuses connecting the exterior to the spinal or cerebral meninges, represent frequent pathways for infection. Finally, 10 – 30 % of cases are cryptogenic.

Most abscesses (75 – 90 %) are solitary, occurring, in descending order of frequency, in the frontal, temporal, frontoparietal, parietal, cerebellar and occipital lobes; the locations in the brain reflect the site of predisposing, and usually adjacent, foci of infection. For example, frontal lobe abscesses are characteristically secondary to frontal or ethmoidal sinusitis or dental sepsis, while temporal lobe abscesses and cerebellar abscesses are secondary to infections in the middle ear/mastoid cavity or sphenoidal sinuses. Brainstem and thalamic abscesses are characteristically the result of haematogenous spread from a distant focus. Multiple lesions, on the other hand, account for 5 – 25 % of abscesses. They are almost always metastatic, spreading via the bloodstream from distant foci of infection, and are most frequently located in the area of the brain supplied by the middle cerebral artery (parietal, anterior temporal and posterior frontal lobes).

54.2.1.3 *Pathology*

Irrespective of the origin of the infection, brain abscesses are thought to develop in areas of pre-existing necrosis, this being a principal requirement for their initiation. The first stage in the development of an abscess is an acute cerebritis which normally lasts about 3 days. This is followed by a late cerebritis of 4 – 9 days' duration, culminating in a necrotic central focus. The formation of a collagen capsule around the developing abscess starts after 10 days and is usually complete by 14 days. The capsule, which limits the spread of infection within the brain, tends to be thinner on the medial aspect, thereby accounting for the tendency of abscesses, on rare occasions, to rupture into the ventricles. Metastatic abscesses are characteristically less well encapsulated and this may account for their tendency to spread. The oedema surrounding an abscess often occupies a greater volume than the abscess itself and therefore makes an important contribution to raised intracranial pressure.

54.2.1.4 *Aetiology*

As many as 50 % of brain abscesses are monomicrobial and a similar percentage are polymicrobial. Between 20 % and 25 % are culture-negative, either because the patient has already received antibiotic treatment or because laboratory diagnostic techniques have been less than optimal. The range of pathogens reflects the broad spectrum of primary sources of infection. Aerobic bacteria have been isolated from between 50 % and 75 % of lesions and anaerobes from 25 – 50 %. Streptococci, predominantly microaerophilic and anaerobic species, are the most commonly recovered organisms (40 – 70 %), regardless of the source. Abscesses that are secondary to penetrating trauma have, in the past, been caused by *Staphylococcus aureus*, but Enterobacteriaceae and *Pseudomonas aeruginosa* are increasing in frequency. Aerobic Gram-negative bacilli (AGNB), particularly *Proteus* spp. and *P. aeruginosa*, are also common pathogens in patients with otogenic brain abscesses. A very broad range of other bacterial species are occasionally isolated. Finally, in immunocompromised patients, a wide variety of uncommon bacteria are being identified with increasing frequency; these include mycobacteria, *Listeria monocytogenes*, *Actinomyces* spp. and *Nocardia* spp.

54.2.1.5 *Clinical Manifestations*

The clinical spectrum of patients with brain abscesses ranges from fulminating to indolent and can vary in duration from hours to weeks. Other contributing factors include the size and location of the abscess, the virulence of the pathogen(s) and the presence of co-morbidities. Headache is the most common symptom (occurring in ≥ 75 % of patients). If it is the only complaint there is a high likelihood of misdiagnosis and if accompanied by a discharging ear there is a risk that it will be attributed to otitis media. Nausea and vomiting, presumably secondary to raised intracranial pressure, are common, affecting approximately 50 % of patients.

Other prominent features are fever (40–60%), dizziness, impaired consciousness and papilloedema (40–60%). Focal neurological signs (in 50% of patients) vary according to the location of the abscess, but may include hemiparesis, focal seizures and visual and speech disturbances. Diffuse neurological dysfunction is usually associated with abscesses in the occipital or temporal lobe and is characterized by coma, generalized seizures, behavioural disturbances and confusion. Meningism, which is a feature in approximately 25% of cases, is also characteristic of abscesses in the occipital or temporal lobe and may be secondary to concomitant meningitis or rupture of the abscess into a ventricle or the subarachnoid space. Other clinical features may reflect the extracranial underlying disease, e.g., ear or nasal discharge. Multiple microabscesses usually present as a diffuse encephalopathy.

The differential diagnosis in patients with brain abscesses includes a myriad of other diseases, the most common being herpes simplex encephalitis, subdural empyema, cerebral metastasis, bacterial meningitis, primary brain tumour, vascular lesions, tuberculosis and toxoplasmosis.

54.2.1.6 Diagnosis

The principal diagnostic procedures are radiological. A plain skull X-ray is often normal in patients with brain abscesses, but may show a mid-line shift (in >50% of patients), gas in the abscess cavity (rare) or evidence of sinusitis or mastoiditis. A contrast-enhanced computed tomography (CT) scan is the single most useful investigation and is more sensitive than radionuclide brain scans once the abscess has progressed beyond the cerebritis stage. It usually shows a ring-enhancing lesion surrounded by oedema or, less commonly, either nodular enhancement or areas of low attenuation without enhancement. Displacement of the ventricles by the adjacent abscess is often evident and signs of sinusitis or middle ear disease/mastoiditis should also be sought. The CT scan lacks specificity, however, and it may be difficult to distinguish brain abscesses from other mass lesions, especially neoplasms. Magnetic resonance imaging (MRI) is at least as specific and sensitive as CT and may be superior, especially in the early (cerebritis) stage of the disease and in terms of detecting multiple small abscesses. However, in common with the CT scan, it suffers from not being able to reliably differentiate between an abscess and a neoplasm. Demonstration of a hypo-intense rim on T_2-weighted MRI images, which is unusual in this lesion, but occasionally seen, can be very helpful in facilitating the diagnosis. Radionuclide scanning is sometimes helpful, particularly when used in conjunction with ^{99m}Tc-HMPAO. It is very rarely needed when MRI is available and is most likely to be of value following surgery. Finally, a white cell scan, a ^{99m}Tc-HMPAO scan, magnetic resonance spectroscopy and positron emission tomography (PET) have been shown to be effective diagnostic tools, particularly in terms of differentiating brain abscesses from neoplasms.

Lumbar puncture is generally unhelpful, the findings on microscopy tending to be highly variable and non-specific; organisms are isolated from <10% of CSF samples, principally in patients with concurrent meningitis or ventriculitis. It may also be a dangerous procedure, leading to brainstem herniation in up to one-third of patients. It should be performed, therefore, only if meningitis is suspected, when the benefits outweigh the risks and when a CT scan confirms that it is safe to do so. Electroencephalography (EEG) is usually abnormal in patients with brain abscesses, but the findings are non-specific. For this reason, it is considered a non-essential investigation. The peripheral white blood cell (WBC) count is raised in 30–60% of patients and the serum CRP concentration will be markedly elevated in many cases; however, normal values of these parameters should not rule out the diagnosis. Blood cultures are positive in 10–20% of patients and are essential investigations if a systemic focus is suspected. They may be particularly helpful in patients who are not managed surgically. When present, samples of sputum or nasal or ear discharge should also be cultured.

54.2.1.7 Surgical Management

Most patients with brain abscesses undergo surgery as part of their management. Surgery is associated with a number of advantages, including confirmation of the diagnosis, removal of infected and necrotic material, relief of raised intracranial pressure, accurate identification of the aetiological agent(s) (thereby facilitating optimal antimicrobial therapy) and enhancement of the activities of antibiotics.

Removal of pus is achieved by craniotomy and drainage or excision of the abscess or by aspiration through a burr hole, preferably with CT- or MRI-guided stereotaxy. The type of procedure is dictated by the depth, size and location of the abscess, the number of abscesses, the stage of development, the clinical status of the patient and the risk of post-operative complications. The superiority of one or the other of these techniques remains controversial. Some neurosurgeons claim that there are more frequent sequelae (mainly epilepsy), greater morbidity from trauma and a higher incidence of mortality with excision. Others have suggested that excision is associated with a lower incidence of mortality and offers immediate decompression, a lower recurrence rate, a shorter period of hospitalization and a shorter course of antibiotics. The overall consensus is that there is probably no difference between the two options, but that aspiration is appropriate for patients who are too ill to undergo a more extensive surgical procedure, who have multiple abscesses or whose abscesses are poorly encapsulated or in deep, critical or less accessible areas of the brain, while excision should be undertaken in the presence of foreign material, in patients with superficial, solitary or multiloculated abscesses and for abscesses that fail to resolve following aspiration. If patients have shown favourable clinical responses to antibiotic treatment, further aspirations of the abscess cavity are unnecessary.

Conservative (non-surgical) management should be restricted to highly selected groups of patients who are neurologically intact and who fulfil the following criteria: small abscesses (< 3 cm in diameter); poor medical condition which precludes surgery; high density lesion (cerebritis); no predisposing factors; multiple abscesses; and inaccessible abscesses or those in deep or eloquent brain locations. The best results are obtained when bacteria are identified in blood cultures. A number of reports have confirmed that patients can be managed successfully without surgery, but the strategy relies on CT monitoring in order to detect exacerbations as early as possible.

54.2.1.8
Antimicrobial Chemotherapy

Several antibiotics, including benzylpenicillin, ampicillin, cefuroxime, chloramphenicol, co-trimoxazole, ceftazidime and metronidazole, have been detected in brain abscess pus in therapeutic concentrations, but this is not necessarily predictive of therapeutic efficacy; there is little information currently available regarding the penetration of newer agents.

The complexity of the physiological, surgical, pharmacological and bacteriological parameters that influence the outcome of treatment of patients with brain abscesses, together with a lack of data from prospective, randomized clinical trials, have undermined efforts to make recommendations for optimal empirical therapy. For many years, a combination of penicillin and chloramphenicol was the most widely used regimen and, indeed, most patients responded favourably to it. More recently, however, extended-spectrum β-lactams, particularly third-generation cephalosporins, in combination with metronidazole, have become increasingly popular.

The initial choice of empirical antibiotic therapy can be facilitated by a number of considerations, including the location of the abscess, the precipitating source of infection (e.g., middle ear infection, a history of sinusitis or trauma, etc.), the odour of the pus (which suggests the presence of anaerobes) and a Gram's stain of the pus. Treatment should be initiated as soon as the diagnosis is confirmed. The recommendations summarized in Table 54.1 constitute appropriate first-line empirical therapy. Treatment should be modified, if necessary, in the light of the results obtained from culturing aspirated pus. Initially, all antibiotics should be administered by the intravenous route. The efficacy of instilling antibiotics directly into the abscess cavity is unconfirmed. Moreover, antibiotics administered by this

Table 54.1. Sites, predominant pathogens and initial empirical antibiotic therapy of patients with brain abscesses

Source	Site	Predominant pathogens	Antimicrobial regimens[a]
Paranasal sinuses	Frontal lobe	Streptococci (particularly those belonging to the milleri group), anaerobes, *Haemophilus* spp.	Cefuroxime 1.5 g tds, cefotaxime 2 g qds or ceftriaxone 3–4 g od and metronidazole 500 mg tds
Teeth	Frontal lobe	Streptococci, anaerobes, *Haemophilus* spp.	Cefuroxime 1.5 g tds and metronidazole 500 mg tds
Middle ear (less often, sphenoidal sinuses)	Temporal lobe	Enterobacteriaceae, *P. aeruginosa*, anaerobes, streptococci	Flucloxacillin 3–4 g qds and metronidazole 500 mg tds plus either ceftazidime 2 g tds or gentamicin 5 mg/kg od[b]
Middle ear (less often, sphenoidal sinuses)	Cerebellum	Enterobacteriaceae, *P. aeruginosa*, anaerobes, streptococci	Flucloxacillin 3–4 g qds and metronidazole 500 mg tds plus either ceftazidime 2 g tds or gentamicin 5 mg/kg od[b]
Penetrating trauma/ post-operative	According to site of wound	*S. aureus*, Enterobacteriaceae	Flucloxacillin 2–3 g qds or cefuroxime 1.5 g tds, cefotaxime 2 g qds or ceftriaxone 3–4 g od
Metastatic and cryptogenic	Multiple lesions (usually in area supplied by middle cerebral artery)	Streptococci, *S. aureus*, anaerobes, Enterobacteriaceae, *P. aeruginosa*	Depends on source: benzylpenicillin 1.8–2.4 g 6-hourly if infective endocarditis or cyanotic congenital heart disease; alternatively, cefuroxime 1.5 g tds or cefotaxime 2 g qds or ceftriaxone 3–4 g od with or without metronidazole 500 mg tds

[a] Adult dosages, [b] Serum concentrations must be monitored

route may diffuse rapidly into the surrounding tissues and precipitate seizures. Current evidence does not support the routine instillation of antimicrobial agents into brain abscess cavities.

The optimal duration of treatment of patients with brain abscesses remains a controversial issue, current practice owing more to tradition than to scientific evidence. Recommendations have ranged from 4–8 weeks of parenteral therapy, followed by prolonged courses of oral therapy (assuming suitable agents are available), if the abscess has been excised or aspirated, and even longer (up to 12 weeks of parenteral therapy) when management has been conservative. The lack of uniformity of opinion regarding an optimal duration is due both to a failure to attempt to resolve this question by prospective clinical trials and to the absence of reliable criteria for monitoring patients' responses to therapy. Serial CT and MRI scans cannot be used to provide an objective endpoint for discontinuing antibiotics because scan appearances may suggest ongoing infection for up to 10 weeks after the successful completion of therapy. The antibiotics can be discontinued once the serum CRP concentration falls to within the normal range, provided that patients have undergone either drainage or excision of their abscesses, that the abscesses are solitary, that there is improvement in the clinical condition and that the fever has resolved. In most cases this will be within 2 weeks of starting appropriate therapy. In a minority of patients the CRP concentrations will be within the normal range, or only slightly elevated, at the time of presentation. The most likely explanation for this observation is that the abscess has been completely walled off and the infection no longer exposed to the physiological processes that drive the inflammatory response – analogous to sequestra in patients with chronic osteomyelitis. Although, in these patients, the CRP cannot be used to monitor response to therapy, it may still not be necessary to administer antibiotics for more than 2 weeks, so long as the abscess has been excised or drained. A further complication is that, while the CRP is a very sensitive criterion for monitoring response to therapy, it is not specific. Therefore, if there is an intercurrent infection or other inflammatory process, such as a deep vein thrombosis or pulmonary embolism, the CRP concentration may remain elevated. Finally, if there is an absence of systemic signs of infection, at least 1 week of oral therapy has been completed, the serum CRP concentration has fallen markedly below 100 mg/l, the patient is able to tolerate antibiotics by mouth and appropriate agents are available, treatment can be switched from the parenteral route to the oral route.

54.2.1.9 Adjunctive Therapy

Steroids are commonly used to reduce oedema, but are of no proven benefit in terms of reducing the incidences of morbidity or neurological sequelae or the duration of hospital stay. The consensus is that they should be avoided unless there is marked oedema with raised intracranial pressure and rapid neurological deterioration; even then, they should be used for short periods only. Anticonvulsants may be appropriate in patients with seizures and are often started empirically as prophylaxis.

54.2.1.10 Prognosis and Complications

In the past, the incidence of mortality has ranged from 20–50%. More recently, however, incidences of 5–20% have been reported. This improved outcome has been attributed to more sensitive and specific radiological techniques (which allow earlier diagnosis and better localization), superior surgical techniques (in particular, the introduction of stereotactic brain biopsy and aspiration), more reliable microbiological methods and more effective antibiotic therapy. Outcome does not appear to be influenced by the location of the abscess, the number of abscesses, predisposing factors, the nature of the pathogen(s) or the type of surgery. A poor prognosis is, however, related to the initial clinical status of the patient, particularly the level of consciousness (which is indirectly related to a delay in diagnosis), and is associated with rapidly progressing neurological impairment, multiple, deep or multiloculated abscesses and rupture of the abscess into a ventricle.

Complications include cortical thrombophlebitis (leading to focal epilepsy or hemiparesis), rupture into a ventricle or subarachnoid space (leading to meningitis and/or ventriculitis, coma and death), tension pneumocephalus and non-communicating hydrocephalus. Neurological sequelae (25–50%) include hemiparesis, cranial nerve palsies, epilepsy, memory deficits, behavioural disorders, ataxia, blindness and hemianopia.

Intraventricular rupture is a particularly serious complication and is associated with a mortality rate exceeding 80%. As well as the administration of appropriate antibiotics systemically, management should comprise open craniotomy with aggressive debridement of the abscess cavity and lavage of the ventricular system with normal saline containing one or more appropriate antibiotics suitable for intraventricular instillation, i.e., vancomycin and gentamicin, each at a concentration of 10 mg/l.

54.2.2 Subdural Empyema

54.2.2.1 Epidemiology

Infection of the subdural space may occasionally be localized by adhesions forming an abscess, but the wide extent of this potential space and the relative avascularity of its walls are such that pus, once formed, normally spreads too rapidly for effective adhesions to develop. It is then no longer an abscess but a subdural empyema. Subdural empyema occurs less commonly than brain abscess, but still accounts for approximately 20 % of all intracranial infections; a typical neurosurgical department will therefore see between two and three cases per year. While all ages are affected, 76 % of cases occur in the second and third decades. There is a male preponderance, the male : female ratio being 4 : 1.

54.2.2.2 Pathogenesis

In 50 – 70 % of patients infection spreads to the dura, either directly or, more often, indirectly via venous drainage, from the paranasal sinuses (particularly the frontal and ethmoid sinuses). Frontal sinusitis may cause thrombophlebitis of the anterior part of the superior sagittal sinus, with infection then spreading to the subdural space bilaterally. The circular and petrosal sinuses may be infected from the sphenoid air sinuses and both middle cranial fossae may then be involved. A further 10 – 20 % of subdural empyemas originate in the middle ear or mastoid cavity; infection spreads directly into the subdural space via erosion of the tegmen tympani or bone adjacent to the air cells and dura mater or, indirectly, by way of a progressive thrombophlebitis of the perforating veins. Otogenic subdural empyema is initially localized posteriorly or on the tentorium. In 5 % of cases spread is from a distant focus, usually the lungs, via the bloodstream. Subdural empyema may also develop following trauma or neurosurgery or in association with dental infection, facial infection, brain abscess, meningitis (the principal predisposing disease in infants), cranial osteomyelitis or infected subdural haematoma; in 15 % of cases the source is unknown.

54.2.2.3 Pathology

Large collections of pus may develop, not only on the surfaces of the cerebral hemispheres, but also in the interhemispheric fissure, at the base of the brain and between the inferior surfaces of the cerebral hemispheres and the tentorium; the posterior fossa is rarely involved and fewer than 10 % of infections are infratentorial. The empyema may be loculated. Eventually, pus may accumulate focally to form multiple abscesses. Oedema of the brain parenchyma develops rapidly and contributes to the mass effect. Focal osteomyelitis and extradural abscess co-exist in up to 50 % of patients.

54.2.2.4 Aetiology

The organisms associated with subdural empyema closely resemble those causing brain abscesses although, unlike brain abscess, most infections are monomicrobial. Streptococci (aerobic, anaerobic and microaerophilic) are the predominant pathogens, being isolated from 50 – 75 % of patients. Anaerobes account for 5 – 10 % of pathogens, and *S. aureus* (15 – 25 %) and Enterobacteriaceae and *P. aeruginosa* (together accounting for 5 – 10 % of infections) are usually associated with head trauma or neurosurgery. A miscellany of other organisms, including *Haemophilus influenzae*, *Streptococcus pneumoniae*, *Neisseria meningitidis* and Group B β-haemolytic streptococci, has also been isolated. The aetiological agents in infants are the same as those causing leptomeningitis. In approximately one-third of cases no pathogens are isolated, either because patients were receiving antibiotics when the specimens were obtained or because of suboptimal culture techniques.

54.2.2.5 Clinical Manifestations

The signs and symptoms of subdural empyema are the consequences of the combined effects of raised intracranial pressure, focal pressure, meningitis, systemic effects and the underlying infection. Acute subdural empyema has been described as the most imperative surgical emergency. Patients present with a history of short duration, and the course of the disease is rapid and fulminating. The most common clinical features are headache, fever, meningism, nausea and/or vomiting, impaired consciousness, focal neurological deficits (including hemiparesis, hemiplegia and dysphasia) and focal or generalized seizures. Because of the rapid course of the disease process papilloedema develops in fewer than 50 % of patients. Concurrent sinusitis or otitis media has been reported in 60 – 90 % of cases. In the absence of appropriate treatment the neurological signs become exaggerated and the intracranial pressure increases, with transtentorial and tonsillar herniation.

In patients with subacute subdural empyemas the history is longer (usually weeks) and infection is usually secondary to trauma or surgery. Patients complain of chronic localized headache, and tenderness and erythema are present over the craniotomy incision or the site of the trauma.

In infancy the clinical features are similar to those in adults, i.e., high fever, seizures, vomiting, lethargy, irritability, a bulging fontanelle, neck stiffness and coma.

The clinical features of subdural empyema are non-specific and the following conditions must be included in the differential diagnosis: brain abscess; extradural abscess; cortical thrombophlebitis; meningitis; thrombosis of the cavernous or lateral sinus; sphenoid sinus empyema; tuberculous meningitis; encephalitis; septic infarct secondary to endocarditis; and exacerbation of otitis media or sinusitis.

54.2.2.6 Diagnosis

A high clinical suspicion and prompt diagnosis are essential to a successful outcome. Plain skull films are rarely helpful, although they may demonstrate concurrent sinusitis or otitis media and/or pineal shift. An unenhanced CT scan is often normal. Contrast enhancement, which is mandatory, frequently demonstrates very subtle changes with only slight displacement of the enhancing capsule away from the vault. However, these changes are non-specific and not invariably present, especially in the early stages of the disease. Because of its greater sensitivity and specificity MRI with gadolinium enhancement has become the diagnostic procedure of choice.

Peripheral WBC counts are usually high ($20-30\times10^9$/l). EEG often reveals non-specific abnormalities and is therefore not particularly helpful. Similarly, the findings in the CSF are non-specific and are usually consistent with the presence of a parameningeal focus; however, the WBC count is not invariably elevated. On the grounds that a lumbar puncture rarely provides valuable diagnostic information and may cause brainstem herniation this procedure is justified in only the most exceptional circumstances.

54.2.2.7 Surgical Management

In most cases the rapid progression of a subdural empyema necessitates early surgical intervention, although small numbers of patients have been treated conservatively. Surgical drainage relieves intracranial pressure and facilitates both optimal antibiotic therapy and the activities of the antibiotics administered. Drainage can be achieved either by multiple burr holes with irrigation of the subdural space or by craniotomy, but neurosurgeons are at variance regarding the superior approach. Advocates of craniotomy claim that it is associated with a higher incidence of survivors, better decompression and lower rates of complications and reaccumulation. It is the surgery of choice for patients with posterior fossa empyema if the pus is too tenacious to be removed through a burr hole or if there is reaccumulation of pus. On the other hand, if infection of the cranial bone flap complicates craniotomy, replacement of the flap may not be possible until the infection has resolved, thereby leaving a defect. Recurrences, which may be multiple, are common, necessitating further surgery in up to 50% of patients. Serial serum CRP concentrations should be used to monitor patients' responses. Failure of the CRP concentration to fall or a rise following an initial decline in a patient who is receiving appropriate antibiotic therapy in adequate dosages is probably the earliest indication of reaccumulation.

54.2.2.8 Antimicrobial Chemotherapy

Although treatment is almost invariably empirical the choice of agents can be guided by knowledge of the predominant pathogens, the presumed source and the odour and a Gram's stain of the pus. A second- or third-generation cephalosporin, such as cefuroxime 1.5 g qds, cefotaxime 2–3 g qds or ceftriaxone 3–4 g od or 2 g bd, in combination with metronidazole 500 mg tds, would be appropriate empirical therapy of most patients with subdural empyema. Neonates, in whom subdural empyemas are often secondary to meningitis, can be given the same regimen, but without the metronidazole. Patients who develop subdural empyemas following neurosurgery should receive a combination of flucloxacillin 2–3 g qds and ceftazidime 2 g tds. Therapy should be modified, if necessary, in the light of culture and susceptibility test results. Initially, all antibiotics should be administered by the intravenous route. Instillation of antibiotics into the subdural space is a common practice, but there is no evidence that it is beneficial and β-lactam antibiotics may be epileptogenic. There is no consensus regarding the optimal duration of therapy and no clinical trials have been conducted with the aim of resolving this issue. Most patients have been treated for between 3 and 4 weeks, although, in common with patients with brain abscesses, antibiotics can be discontinued once the serum CRP concentration returns to normal. This will usually be 2 weeks after starting appropriate therapy.

Therapeutic adjuncts include prophylactic anticonvulsants and mannitol and steroids to reduce intracranial pressure.

54.2.2.9 Prognosis and Complications

Without prompt diagnosis and the initiation of effective treatment subdural empyema is rapidly fatal. In the past, mortality rates have ranged from 25–40% but, more recently, with the introduction of better diagnostic and therapeutic measures, rates have fallen to between 10% and 20%; if the patient is alert at the time of presentation, mortality rates are usually less than 10%, but may be up to 75% if the patient is comatose.

When therapeutic intervention is timely there is a high likelihood of complete recovery in survivors. Reaccumulation of pus, which is almost invariably sterile, occurs in up to 50% of patients on as many as three occasions, thereby necessitating further surgery. Other complications include focal or generalized seizures, hemiparesis, aphasia, septic venous thrombosis, corticothrombophlebitis, intracranial abscess, epidural abscess and osteomyelitis.

54.2.3 Spinal Extradural (Epidural) Abscess

54.2.3.1 Epidemiology

Spinal extradural abscess is a localized suppurative infection of the space between the outermost layer of the meninges, the dura mater, and the vertebral column. It is an uncommon disease and even large neurosurgical centres can expect no more than 5 cases per year. While all ages are affected, the mean age is between 50 and 60 years; the disease is rare in infants and young children. The male:female ratio has been reported as varying from 1–2:1.

54.2.3.2 Pathogenesis

Spinal extradural abscesses almost always originate from foci of infection elsewhere in the body, with spread to the extradural space either via the bloodstream or the lymphatic system, or directly from a contiguous focus of infection. Skin and soft tissue infections are the most common sources of bacteraemias leading to extradural infections, but other foci include infective endocarditis, pharyngitis, mastoiditis, pneumonia, urinary tract infections, periodontal infections, intra-abdominal infections and infected vascular catheters. Abscesses may also occur following direct spread from vertebral osteomyelitis (present in more than 50% of chronic abscesses, but in only 15% of acute abscesses), perinephric, retropharyngeal or psoas abscesses, decubitus ulcers or persistent/congenital dermal sinus tracts. Infections have been reported, albeit rarely, following penetrating injuries, lumbar punctures, spinal surgery, epidural anaesthesia and CT-guided needle biopsy and in association with the use of temporary epidural catheters. A history of prior back trauma has been noted in 10–35% of patients, leading to suggestions that haematomas or damaged tissues may predispose to haematogenous seeding. Other predisposing conditions include diabetes, intravenous drug abuse, degenerative joint disease and renal or liver failure.

54.2.3.3 Pathology

Owing to the lack of resistance to the longitudinal spread of infection through the extradural space, several (on average, between three and six) vertebral segments are affected, although there have been reports of the entire length of the spinal cord being involved. Involvement of the thoracic spine occurs in 50–80% of cases, the lumbar spine in 17–38% and the cervical spine in 10–25%; in children, infection usually affects the cervical and lumbar regions. Abscesses are located posterior to the cord in more than 70% of patients, but they may also be anterior or circumferential. Acute abscesses consist of granulation tissue containing loculated pus, while chronic abscesses consist of both granulation and fibrous tissues. As the abscess enlarges it may compress the spinal cord, cause vascular occlusion secondary to septic thrombophlebitis or extend into the subdural or subarachnoid space.

54.2.3.4 Aetiology

Pathogens are isolated either from blood cultures or intraoperative specimens or both. *S. aureus* is the predominant aetiological agent, accounting for 60–90% of infections. Other common organisms include streptococci (approximately 20%), AGNB (approximately 15%) and anaerobes (up to 7%); a very broad range of bacterial and fungal species have been reported less frequently and multiple organisms have been isolated from 5–10% of patients.

54.2.3.5 Clinical Manifestations

Spinal extradural abscesses may develop acutely or chronically. Acute cases are more likely to exhibit the classical features of infection, i.e., high fevers, rigors and raised peripheral WBC counts, consistent with spread by the haematogenous route, while chronic cases are more likely to be secondary to slowly developing contiguous foci of infection, particularly vertebral osteomyelitis. Meningism is a not-uncommon presentation and usually results from the proximity of the abscess to the meninges, i.e., a parameningeal focus, as opposed to infection in the CSF compartment. Classically, the disease progresses through four phases: phase I, focal vertebral pain at the affected level of the spine, with localized tenderness and fever; phase II, nerve root pain, with radiculopathy and/or paraesthesiae; phase III, weakness, with motor and sensory deficits and/or bladder or bowel dysfunction; and phase IV, paralysis. The first three phases progress at rates varying from days in acute cases to weeks or months in chronic cases. However, the weakness phase (III) can progress to the paralysis phase (IV) within hours, irrespective of whether the course of the disease is acute or chronic.

Back pain, with or without neurological deficits, may be attributed to an enormous range of disease processes. This, and the relative rarity of spinal extradural abscess, have led to a high percentage of patients with this disease being initially misdiagnosed, although the presence of systemic signs of infection may help to narrow the spectrum. Included in the differential diagnosis of spinal extradural abscess are the following: musculoskeletal pain secondary to strain or trauma; vertebral or intervertebral disc space disease (degenerative or inflammatory); vertebral osteomyelitis; tuberculous osteomyelitis; transverse myelitis (associated with bacterial, viral or parasitic infection, vaccination or autoimmune disease); meningitis; intradural or extradural neoplasms (primary or metastatic); Guillain-Barré syndrome; vascular lesions; spinal subdural abscess; epidural lipomatosis; epidural sarcoidosis; intraspinal infection; and spinal cord haematoma.

54.2.3.6 Diagnosis

Spinal extradural abscess should be considered in any patient with back pain and one or both of radicular symptoms and meningism, especially in the presence of the signs of infection. Prompt diagnosis is essential if permanent neurological sequelae are to be avoided.

Plain X-ray films of the spine are normal in many patients, but they may show signs of vertebral osteomyelitis or other findings suggestive of infection in the spinal canal. CT, with contrast enhancement, is useful in diagnosing vertebral osteomyelitis and distinguishing between extradural and subdural infections. However, as it is a relatively insensitive technique for diagnosing extradural abscesses and as it may fail to define the longitudinal extent of the infection, it is rarely used. Gadolinium-enhanced MRI is superior to CT and is currently the diagnostic procedure of choice in the initial evaluation of patients with suspected extradural abscesses. It usually shows an heterogeneously enhancing extradural mass with compression of the adjacent neural structures. MRI accurately identifies both extradural abscess and osteomyelitis, differentiates between extradural abscess and other spinal cord lesions with which it can be confused and precisely delineates the longitudinal extent of the infection and loculations of inflammatory tissue.

A raised peripheral WBC count and ESR are common findings, especially in patients with acute disease, but are non-specific and therefore unreliable. Samples of blood for culture should always be taken and yield a pathogen in up to 70% of cases. A lumbar puncture should not be performed routinely because of the risk of spreading infection to the subdural or subarachnoid space. Examination of CSF typically shows ranges characteristic of a parameningeal focus of inflammation, with a raised WBC count of usually no more than 150 cells/mm^3 (much less if the abscess is chronic) and comprising a mixture of polymorphonuclear leucocytes and lymphocytes or predominantly polymorphonuclear leucocytes; the protein concentration is raised (markedly in the presence of a complete block) and the glucose concentration is normal, unless there is coincidental meningitis. A Gram's stain is usually negative and the CSF is sterile in up to 80% of cases. Material obtained from the abscess should always be submitted for Gram's stain and culture.

54.2.3.7 Surgical Management

Surgical drainage with decompression laminectomy, as soon as the diagnosis is made in order to optimize neurological recovery and to reduce the potential for rapid progression to complete and permanent paralysis, is considered to be the cornerstone of surgical management. The extent of the procedure will depend on the extent of the abscess, as demonstrated by radiological imaging. In children, a limited laminectomy may be undertaken to minimize the risk of subsequent spinal deformity. Occasionally, anterior spinal decompression is necessary, particularly when the cervical spine is involved and pus is present in the ventral extradural space. Immediate stabilization with graft, and even plates and screws, has recently been used successfully in the acute stage. It has been recommended that a wound drain be inserted at the time of primary drainage as a means of preventing recurrence of the extradural collection. Primary closure of the wound reduces both the amount of discomfort experienced by the patient and the duration of hospital stay. CT-guided percutaneous needle aspiration has been used as an alternative to laminectomy in selected patients, but this approach has not been validated by clinical trials and it should not normally be used in place of surgery. Antibiotic therapy alone may be considered if a patient's general condition precludes surgery or if the patient has no or only minimal neurological deficit on presentation. The latter group should be monitored closely with regular neurological examinations and MRI studies, and surgical intervention should be implemented immediately in the event of sudden neurological deterioration.

54.2.3.8
Antimicrobial Chemotherapy

The initial empirical regimen, the choice of which can be facilitated by a Gram's stain of any pus that is obtained at surgery, should provide cover against the predominant pathogen, *S. aureus*. Flucloxacillin 2–3 g qds is therefore the drug of choice, with a first-generation cephalosporin, such as cefradine 2–3 g qds, for patients who are allergic to penicillins and a glycopeptide (vancomycin or teicoplanin) for those with infections likely to be caused by methicillin-resistant *S. aureus* (MRSA). If there is any reason to suspect AGNB, a second- or third-generation cephalosporin (cefuroxime 1.5 g tds, cefotaxime 2–3 g qds or ceftriaxone 3–4 g od or 2 g bd) or a fluoroquinolone (ciprofloxacin 400–600 mg bd) would be appropriate, unless *P. aeruginosa* is a possibility, in which case ceftazidime 2 g tds (together with flucloxacillin) should be administered. An anti-anaerobic agent, such as metronidazole 500 mg tds, should be added to the empirical regimen if anaerobes are suspected on the basis of the original focus of infection and/or foul-smelling pus. Treatment should be modified, if necessary, in the light of the results of culture and susceptibility testing. Initially, all antibiotics should be administered by the intravenous route. While the optimal duration of therapy has not been determined, most patients have received antibiotics for 3–4 weeks, although shorter courses may be equally effective. The response to treatment should be monitored by serial measurements of the serum CRP concentration. If there is concurrent osteomyelitis the drugs should be given for a total of 6 weeks. The role of steroids in the management of patients with spinal extradural abscess is controversial. They have not been shown convincingly to improve outcome and, with prompt diagnosis, early surgical decompression and effective antibiotic therapy, are probably unnecessary.

54.2.3.9
Prognosis and Complications

The likelihood of complete recovery is high if intervention is begun before or during the second (root pain) phase of the disease, i.e., before there is significant neurological deficit. The prognosis worsens rapidly when there is a delay in making the diagnosis and once weakness develops. There is little likelihood of full recovery if surgery is delayed by more than 24 h after the onset of paralysis and no chance if the delay is more than 48 h. The overall incidence of mortality is reported to be 13 %, but 5 % in patients treated surgically.

54.3
Secondary Infections

54.3.1
External Ventricular Drain-Associated Ventriculitis

54.3.1.1
Epidemiology

External ventricular drains (EVDs) are essential monitoring devices in neurosurgery and direct portals for the removal of CSF (as temporary means of controlling raised intracranial pressure) or the injection of therapeutic agents. Their benefits must be balanced against the complications associated with their use. The most important of these complications is infection (ventriculitis) which, after operative site/wound infection, is the commonest secondary infection in neurosurgical patients. The risk of developing ventriculitis is lowest during the first 4 days that the drain is in situ, rises over the first 10 days and falls off markedly thereafter. The incidence has been reported to be as high as 40 %, but more commonly between 4 % and 11 %, and is directly related to the effectiveness of the aseptic techniques employed in inserting and maintaining the drain. Although some investigators have described an association between infection and intraventricular haemorrhage [5, 7], those involved in a recently published, large, prospective study found no such association [4]; this latter group did however identify length of EVD placement and CSF fluid leakage about the drain as independent risk factors. It has been proposed that the infection rate could be lowered by prophylactically exchanging EVDs at 5-day intervals [5]. However, it was subsequently demonstrated that the infection rate in patients in whom EVDs were replaced after < 5 days was not lower than that in patients in whom the drains were exchanged at intervals of > 5 days [3]. The investigators therefore recommended that drains should be removed from non-infected patients as early as is practicable, but that they should not be exchanged routinely. In other centres, an antibiotic with predominantly Gram-positive activity is given as a single dose by the parenteral route before EVD insertion and is continued while the EVD remains in situ [4]. Not surprisingly, most (82 %) of the pathogens identified at that institution are Gram-negative bacteria which are associated with mortality rates of up to 58 %, markedly higher than those associated with Gram-positive bacteria. In addition, two retrospective studies of the efficacy of antibiotic prophylaxis in patients with external CSF drainage devices [1, 6] failed to demonstrate reduced incidences of ventriculitis, but showed that this intervention is associated with increased healthcare costs. In view of the absence of any discernible benefit and the risk of selecting for multidrug-resistant AGNB, prophylactic antibiotics should not be routinely administered to patients with EVDs.

54.3.1.2
Aetiology

In common with intravascular line-related infections, the predominant aetiological agents are coagulase-negative staphylococci (CoNS), followed by *S. aureus* (including MRSA). The remainder comprises a wide range of other Gram-positive bacteria, including α-haemolytic streptococci, and, with increasing frequency, especially among patients who have received prolonged and/or multiple courses of antibiotics, AGNB. Yeasts are recognized, albeit rare, pathogens.

54.3.1.3
Clinical Manifestations

The clinical features of EVD-associated ventriculitis typically bear little resemblance to those of bacterial meningitis, either because many of the aetiological agents exhibit only low-grade virulence (and, hence, do not elicit brisk inflammatory responses in the CSF compartment) or because the patients are sedated and/or paralyzed. The signs and symptoms may therefore be subtle, or even inapparent. Pyrexia is an almost invariable finding and may be the only sign in patients who are unresponsive. On the other hand, fever is a common finding in neurosurgical patients and is not pathognomonic of infection. Headache, nausea and/or vomiting and, less frequently, altered mental status may be observed in responsive patients, but signs of raised intracranial pressure are uncommon owing to the presence of the EVD.

54.3.1.4
Diagnosis

Microscopic examination of CSF may reveal a marked pleiocytosis. More commonly, however, few, or even no, WBCs may be seen because many of the causes of EVD-associated ventriculitis cause minimal inflammatory responses. Bacteria may be detected on a Gram's stain, but the definitive diagnostic criterion is the isolation of a presumptive pathogen on direct, as opposed to enrichment, culture of the CSF. However, the incidence of contamination is high in this setting and the diagnosis should therefore be confirmed by identifying the same bacterium in a second specimen.

54.3.1.5
Antimicrobial Chemotherapy

In most cases antibiotic therapy can be administered by the intraventricular route. If the pathogen is a CoNS the patient should be treated by instilling vancomycin (5–20 mg, depending on the volume of distribution, i.e., 5 mg for patients with volumes of distribution which are less than normal, 10 mg for those with normal volumes, 15 mg for those with volumes which are moderately greater than normal and 20 mg for those with volumes which are markedly greater than normal) directly into the ventricles via the EVD and then clamping the drain for approximately 15 min. The dosing frequency will depend on the volume of CSF drained during the 24 h since the previous dose and must be reviewed daily. If there is no, or minimal, drainage (<50 ml/day) doses need to be repeated on only every third day. If the amount of drainage is between 50 ml and 100 ml dosing should be on alternate days. If the volume is between 100 ml and 150 ml a daily dose should be administered. For patients whose output exceeds 150 ml in a 24-h period the baseline dosage should be increased by 5 mg for each 50 ml. A 5–7 day course is usually adequate. Patients with ventriculitis caused by *S. aureus* (regardless of whether the isolate is methicillin-susceptible or -resistant) should receive the same regimen as those with infections caused by CoNS, but the duration of therapy should be 2 weeks; systemic rifampicin (600 mg bd) can be administered as a therapeutic adjunct, particularly in cases of severe infection. Those with infections caused by AGNB should receive a third-generation cephalosporin (cefotaxime, ceftriaxone or ceftazidime) or meropenem, depending on the susceptibility of the pathogen. In addition, gentamicin, in dosages ranging from 2–5 mg, according to the patient's volume of distribution, should be administered intraventricularly via the EVD. The dosing frequency is based on the volume of CSF that has drained over the 24 h since the preceding dose and is the same as that described above for vancomycin (but increasing the baseline dosage by 1 mg for each 50 ml of CSF in excess of 150 ml); the frequency must be assessed daily. Colistin (50,000–200,000 IU, depending on the volume of distribution) can be substituted for gentamicin in the event of resistance to the latter drug, again with the same dosing frequency as for vancomycin (but increasing the baseline dosage by 25,000 IU for each 50 ml in excess of 150 ml) and with daily assessment. The duration of therapy should be 2–3 weeks. The dosing regimens are summarized in Table 54.2. It must be pointed out that the product licenses of the antibiotics recommended herein for intraventricular use do not cover this route of administration. However, many hundreds of patients have received drugs by this route and, to date, no adverse effects have been reported when formulations suitable for administration into the CSF compartment have been employed. Moreover, intraventricular administration is highly effective, ensures maximum concentrations at the site of infection, avoids systemic toxicity, exerts negligible pressures in terms of selecting resistant strains and, when used as the only therapeutic intervention, is markedly less expensive than parenteral treatment. Finally, if the EVD is no lon-

Table 54.2. Antibiotic treatment regimens for patients with EVD-associated ventriculitis

Antibiotic	Dosage according to CSF VD[a]				Dosing frequency (per 24 h since previous dose)			
	<Normal	Normal	Moderately >normal	Markedly >normal	<50 ml	50–100 ml	100–150 ml	>150 ml
Vancomycin	5 mg	10 mg	15 mg	20 mg	Every third day	Alternate days	Daily	Daily + 5 mg for each 50 ml, or part thereof, >150 ml
Gentamicin	2 mg	3 mg	4 mg	5 mg	Every third day	Alternate days	Daily	Daily + 1 mg for each 50 ml, or part thereof, >150 ml
Colistin	50,000 IU	100,000 IU	150,000 IU	200,000 IU	Every third day	Alternate days	Daily	Daily + 25,000 IU for each 50 ml, or part thereof, >150 ml

[a] Volume of distribution

ger required, it should be removed immediately after administration of the last dose of antibiotic in order to avoid relapse or reinfection; otherwise, it should be replaced for the same reason.

54.3.2 Post-neurosurgical Bacterial Meningitis

54.3.2.1 Epidemiology

In a study of 151 adult patients with nosocomial bacterial meningitis [2] 68 (45%) had recently undergone neurosurgery. Nonetheless, the incidence of bacterial meningitis complicating neurosurgical procedures (excluding patients with CSF shunts or external CSF drainage devices) is low, varying from 0.5% in patients who have undergone clean procedures with antibiotic prophylaxis to 6% in those who have undergone clean-contaminated procedures (those that traverse an area colonized by bacteria, e.g., an air-filled sinus) without prophylactic cover. Craniotomy following trauma or for the resection of tumour is the procedure most frequently associated with post-operative meningitis. Close proximity to the heavily colonized scalp, or the need to enter the frontal, sphenoidal or mastoid air sinuses, allows direct contamination of the operative field and secondary CSF leakage facilitates the entry of potential pathogens into the subarachnoid space.

54.3.2.2 Aetiology

AGNB, including *Escherichia coli, Klebsiella pneumoniae, Enterobacter* spp., *P. aeruginosa* and, increasingly, *Acinetobacter* spp., which together account for 60–70% of cases, followed by *S. aureus*, are the most common aetiological agents. In patients with defects of the dura and CSF leaks (rhinorrhoea or otorrhoea) who have not received prophylactic antibiotics, *S. pneumoniae* and, less frequently, other constituents of the upper respiratory tract flora are the principal pathogens, whereas in those who have received antibiotics as prophylaxis or for other reasons AGNB predominate.

54.3.2.3 Clinical Manifestations

The clinical features of post-neurosurgical meningitis, which usually presents within the first 7–10 days following surgery, are indistinguishable from those of community-acquired meningitis, i.e., headache, fever, neck stiffness, nausea and vomiting and, occasionally, an altered level of consciousness. However, the onset is sometimes insidious and it may be difficult to differentiate bacterial meningitis from the neurological symptoms and signs that are common in the early post-operative period or that are associated with the underlying disease. Another cause of the 'meningeal syndrome' that also presents approximately 7–10 days into the post-neurosurgical period is chemical or aseptic meningitis. This condition occurs more than twice as frequently as bacterial meningitis and is thought to be the result of chemical irritation of the meninges, caused either by blood or blood degradation products which are introduced into the subarachnoid space during surgery or by factors released by dural substitutes. The course and symptoms are identical to those in patients with bacterial meningitis, but patients normally respond favourably to high dosages of corticosteroids.

54.3.2.4 Diagnosis

In the acute stages of bacterial meningitis meningeal enhancement may be seen, although this is not particularly helpful and its absence does not exclude meningitis. Examination of the CSF is the definitive diagnostic procedure, but a CT scan is frequently performed first in order to determine that a lumbar puncture is safe. When a lumbar puncture is unsafe it may be necessary to carry out a ventricular puncture (although ventricular and lumbar CSF samples in patients with obstructive hydrocephalus may differ markedly in terms of the cell counts and biochemical profiles) or to treat empirically. The CSF protein concentration and WBC count (with a predominance of polymorphonuclear leucocytes) are almost always elevated. However, if the sample has been obtained within 12 h of the onset of symptoms the cell count may be low or even within the normal range; a repeat CSF examination (where practical) 24 h later usually demonstrates a marked pleiocytosis. The glucose concentration is normally depressed in the presence of infection, but a Gram's stain may be negative in up to 70% of patients with culture-positive infections. In common with the clinical presentation, CSF parameters (both cellular and biochemical) may be altered in the post-operative period as a result of either the surgery itself or aseptic meningitis. Indeed, the ranges of values of CSF variables found in infected patients overlap significantly with those found in non-infected post-operative patients, thereby confounding efforts to confirm the diagnosis. The desirability of avoiding the needless administration of antibiotics to patients with aseptic meningitis and the potentially devastating consequences associated with giving steroids to patients with bacterial meningitis have prompted a search for alternative diagnostic tests that both reliably and rapidly distinguish between the two disease processes. Currently, however, no validated single test or combination of tests has been shown to have sufficient specificity and sensitivity for it to be used to discriminate, with the 100% accuracy that is required, between bacterial and aseptic meningitis at the time of presentation. Until this problem has been resolved, isolation of a pathogen from the CSF of post-operative neurosurgical patients must remain the definitive diagnostic criterion, although this means that the diagnosis can be made only retrospectively.

54.3.2.5 Antimicrobial Chemotherapy

Owing to the difficulties of accurately identifying patients with bacterial meningitis prospectively and the morbidity and mortality resulting from delays in initiating therapy, all patients who present with the clinical and laboratory features of post-operative meningitis should receive empirical antibiotic therapy. If the CSF is subsequently found to be sterile (usually after 2–3 days), antibiotic treatment can be discontinued, providing that antibiotics had not been given during the 24–48 h before the lumbar puncture was performed.

A third-generation cephalosporin, such as cefotaxime 2–3 g qds or ceftriaxone 3–4 g od or 2 g bd, should be administered as initial empirical therapy, unless the patient has already received broad-spectrum antibiotics, in which case ceftazidime 2 g tds should be prescribed in order to provide cover against *P. aeruginosa*. Where high rates of resistance to third-generation cephalosporins are observed meropenem 2 g tds should be prescribed. Meropenem is also the drug of choice for patients with infections caused by *Acinetobacter* spp., which tend to be resistant to multiple antibiotics. (The incidence of seizures in neurosurgical patients receiving meropenem is low, i.e., <1%, compared with up to 7% in patients given imipenem-cilastatin.) The only other therapeutic option for patients with infections caused by multidrug-resistant AGNB is trimethoprim-sulfamethoxazole, although, owing to increasing rates of resistance to this agent, it should not be administered unless the pathogen is confirmed to be susceptible. In the absence of robust evidence of efficacy, fluoroquinolones, such as ciprofloxacin, should not be used as therapy of patients with meningitis caused by AGNB. Those with infections caused by methicillin-susceptible strains of *S. aureus* should be treated with flucloxacillin 2–3 g qds, with or without rifampicin 600 mg bd. Either vancomycin 1 g bd or teicoplanin 12 mg/kg body weight od (after three loading doses given at 12-h intervals) is the drug of choice for the treatment of patients with meningitis caused by strains of MRSA and should be administered in combination with rifampicin 600 mg bd. However, glycopeptides penetrate poorly into the CSF compartment and, if the patient has failed to respond to systemic therapy, it may be necessary to implant a ventricular access device, such as an Ommaya reservoir, and to instil vancomycin (10 mg every third day) directly into the ventricles. Treatment should be modified, if necessary, once the results of culture and susceptibility testing are available. Because AGNB can develop resistance to β-lactams during courses of therapy, ideally, CSF should be obtained for culture at regular intervals (every 4–5 days) in order to ensure that sterilization has been achieved. If a patient with infection caused by an AGNB

Table 54.3. Systemic[a] antibiotic therapy of neurosurgical patients with post-operative bacterial meningitis

Clinical setting/pathogen	Regimen
First-line empirical therapy	Cefotaxime 2–3 g qds or ceftriaxone 3–4 g od or 2 g bd
Patient has recently received a broad-spectrum antibiotic or confirmed *P. aeruginosa*	Ceftazidime 2 g tds
Suspected or confirmed ESBL-producing Enterobacteriaceae or *Acinetobacter* sp.	Meropenem 2 g tds
Methicillin-susceptible *S. aureus*	Flucloxacillin 2–3 g qds with or without rifampicin 600 mg bd
Methicillin-resistant *S. aureus*	Vancomycin 1 g bd[b] or teicoplanin 12 mg/kg body weight od (after three loading doses) plus rifampicin 600 mg bd

[a] If intraventricular instillation is indicated, the following regimens, administered every third day, are appropriate: vancomycin 10 mg; gentamicin 3–4 mg; colistin 50,000–200,000 IU
[b] Serum concentrations must be monitored

is severely ill, the response to therapy is delayed or the pathogen is not eradicated by systemic treatment alone, gentamicin (3–4 mg, assuming a normal adult CSF volume of distribution) or, in the event of resistance to gentamicin, colistin (between 50,000 IU and 200,000 IU, assuming a normal adult CSF volume of distribution) should be given intraventricularly every third day; the threshold for doing so should be low. The total duration of therapy should be 2 weeks if the pathogen is *S. aureus* and up to 3 weeks if it is an AGNB. The various dosing regimens are summarized in Table 54.3.

References

1. Alleyne CH Jr, Hassan M, Zabramski JM (2000) The efficacy and cost of prophylactic and periprocedural antibiotics in patients with external ventricular drains. Neurosurgery 47:1124–1129
2. Durand ML, Calderwood SB, Weber DJ, et al. (1993) Acute bacterial meningitis in adults. A review of 493 episodes. N Engl J Med 328:21–28
3. Holloway KL, Barnes T, Choi S, et al. (1996) Ventriculostomy infections: the effect of monitoring duration and catheter exchange in 584 patients. J Neurosurg 85:419–424
4. Lyke KE, Obasanjo OO, Williams MA, et al. (2001) Ventriculitis complicating use of intraventricular catheters in adult neurosurgical patients. Clin Infect Dis 33:2028–2033
5. Mayhall CG, Archer NH, Lamb VA, et al. (1984) Ventriculostomy-related infections. A prospective epidemiologic study. N Engl J Med 310:553–559
6. Rebuck JA, Murry KR, Rhoney DH, et al. (2000) Infection related to intracranial pressure monitors in adults: analysis of risk factors and antibiotic prophylaxis. J Neurol Neurosurg Psychiatry 69:381–384
7. Stenager E, Gerner-Smidt P, Kock-Jensen C (1986) Ventriculostomy-related infections – an epidemiological study. Acta Neurochir (Wien) 83:20–23

Further Reading

Infection in Neurosurgery Working Party of the British Society for Antimicrobial Chemotherapy (2000) The management of neurosurgical patients with postoperative bacterial or aseptic meningitis or external ventricular drain-associated ventriculitis. Br J Neurosurg 14:7–12

Infection in Neurosurgery Working Party of the British Society for Antimicrobial Chemotherapy (2000) The rational use of antibiotics in the treatment of brain abscess. Br J Neurosurg 14:525–530

Chapter 55

Biliary Tract Infections

55

D. Holena, S.R. Eachempati, P.S. Barie

Infections of the biliary tree are similar to those found elsewhere in the body in that therapy consists of antibiotics directed at the causative pathogens and source control, typically in the form of drainage. Prior to the development of antibiotics, biliary tract infections carried a dismal prognosis and open surgical drainage was the only treatment modality available. The morbidity and mortality has decreased with the judicious use of potent antibiotics and the development of newer, less invasive modalities for drainage, but biliary tract infections remain an important cause and occasional complication of critical illness. Unless diagnosed and treated aggressively, multiple organ dysfunction syndrome (MODS) and death may ensue rapidly. Hepatobiliary infections can be subdivided into those that involve primarily the hepatic parenchyma (e.g., pyogenic liver abscess, amebic abscess, echinoccocal disease) and those that arise from the biliary tree (e.g., cholangitis, biloma), but all infections involve both systems to some degree. Signs and symptoms of hepatobiliary infection commonly include abdominal pain, fever, nausea, and vomiting; clinical presentation may range in severity from the appearance of a chronic disease state to overt septic shock. Leukocytosis is common to all, but whereas patterns of liver enzyme abnormalities are observed for different entities, the degree of overlap is such that it may be difficult to make a definitive diagnosis based on history, physical examination, and laboratory values alone. Furthermore, in the critically ill patient, it may be difficult to distinguish liver dysfunction caused by primary infection from that caused by MODS. Imaging of the biliary tree is often of paramount importance in the diagnosis and treatment of biliary tract infections, but ultimately a thorough working knowledge of the differential diagnosis and treatment of biliary tract infections is the key to successful management.

55.1 Cholangitis

Cholangitis is an acute infection of the biliary tree. The pathogenesis of cholangitis requires both obstruction and bacterial superinfection. The etiology of biliary obstruction can be divided conceptually into intrinsic and extrinsic causes. The most common cause of intrinsic obstruction in the Western world is choledocholithiasis as a consequence of gallbladder calculi [1]. Stones may form primarily in the common bile duct as well, although this is less common in Western countries and more frequent among Asian populations. Primary cancers of the biliary tree, benign strictures caused by trauma or ischemia, and disease processes such as primary sclerosing cholangitis or Caroli's disease (a congenital disorder characterized by multifocal, segmental dilatation of intrahepatic bile ducts) may also lead to intrinsic obstruction. Both primary and metastatic malignant disease of the abdominal viscera may cause extrinsic obstruction, as more rarely can benign processes such as Mirizzi's syndrome, in which an impacted stone in the gallbladder compresses the common bile duct. The nature of the obstruction contributes to the disease process, with obstruction from stones being more likely to cause cholangitis than malignant obstruction [2].

Bile is sterile in the normal biliary tree, owing to several factors. Bile itself has bacteriostatic properties, and forward flow of bile from the hepatic ducts into the duodenum serves as a flushing mechanism. In addition, the sphincter of Oddi serves as an anatomic barrier between the gut and the biliary tree, preventing reflux of enteric flora. Bile salts excreted by the liver influence the microbiology of the small bowel and serve to absorb intraluminal endotoxins. Bile salts may also exhibit a trophic effect on small bowel mucosa, thus helping to prevent bacterial and endotoxin translocation. In the absence of biliary flow, normal bacterial ecology is perturbed, leading to bacterial overgrowth as well as degradation of mucosal defenses. The hepatic reticuloendothelial system serves to filter translocated bacteria and endotoxin and is impaired when the biliary tree is obstructed, increasing further the risk of infection [3, 4]. Bacteria may gain access to the biliary tree either via the portal vein or by ascending directly from the duodenum; support exists for both mechanisms in animal models [5, 6]. In addition, pathogens may be introduced iatrogenically during surgical, endoscopic, or percutaneous biliary interventions

Charcot's triad of fever, right upper quadrant pain, and jaundice is seen in 50 – 70 % of patients upon presentation of cholangitis, with fever being the most consistent clinical feature (90 %) [7]. With the addition of hypotension and altered mental status (i.e., severe sepsis or septic shock), Reynolds' pentad is said to be present. Laboratory studies in cholangitis typically reveal leukocytosis, and direct hyperbilirubinemia is seen in 88 – 100 % of patients. Alkaline phosphatase is elevated in the majority (78 %) as well [8]. Transaminitis is usually mild but may be marked in cases of acute obstruction.

Bile cultures obtained in cholangitis are positive 80 – 100 % of the time, with positive blood cultures found in up to two-thirds of patients. The concordance rate between bile and blood cultures ranges between 33 % and 84 %, with bile cultures demonstrating greater than one organism in roughly half of all cases. The typical flora are enteric in origin with *Klebsiella* spp., *E. coli, Enterococcus* spp., and *Enterobacter* spp. being most common. Cutaneous flora, oral flora, and pseudomonads may be found more frequently in cholangitis than occurs in the postoperative and post-interventional setting [9].

Radiologic imaging of patients with cholangitis can be accomplished using ultrasound (US), computed tomography (CT) scan, or magnetic resonance imaging (MRI). Ultrasound reliably detects cholelithiasis as well as intrahepatic and extrahepatic ductal dilation, but is only 50 % sensitive for detecting choledocholithiasis. Computed tomography detects ductal dilation with 98 % accuracy and is superior to ultrasound in defining the level of obstruction, but may fail to visualize stones as only 10 – 15 % of stones are calcified and therefore radiopaque. Because stones can be visualized on MRI, magnetic resonance cholangiopancreatography (MRCP) provides the most complete noninvasive imaging information as to the etiology of biliary obstruction. Whereas MRCP can be most elucidating, it is expensive, time-consuming, and not universally available. In addition, it does not allow for therapeutic intervention. By contrast, endoscopic retrograde cholangiopancreatography (ERCP) and percutaneous transhepatic cholangiopancreatography (PTC) are both 90 – 100 % sensitive for defining the site and nature of biliary obstruction [4]. Either can be used not only diagnostically but also therapeutically to decompress the biliary tree, obtain tissue specimens, and place biliary stents. Both ERCP and PTC have a small incidence of complications that may precipitate ICU admission. In the stable patient with suspected cholangitis, ultrasound should be considered the investigation of first choice, followed by further imaging as needed with CT or MRCP. Because of the potential for intervention, ERCP should be considered strongly in unstable patients and in other cases where intervention is likely to be necessary (Fig. 55.1). Hemodynamic instability in the setting of suspected or confirmed bacterial cholangitis is a true emergency that requires immediate biliary decompression.

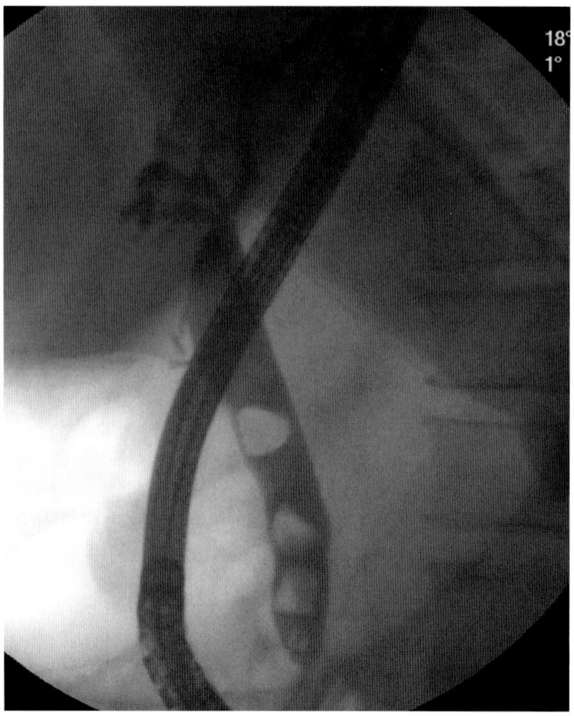

Fig. 55.1. ERCP demonstrating choledocholithiasis with dilatation of the biliary tree

Treatment of cholangitis consists of immediate fluid resuscitation and broad-spectrum antibiotics followed by urgent or emergent biliary decompression. Numerous antibiotic regimens have been demonstrated to be successful, including a single broad-spectrum agent such as a ureidopenicillin [10] (e.g., piperacillin/tazobactam); a ureidopenicillin plus metronidazole; mono- or combination therapy with fluoroquinolones; or combination therapy with an extended-spectrum cephalosporin, ampicillin, and metronidazole [11 – 13]. Selection of antibiotics must take into consideration local bacterial resistance patterns and cost. The majority of patients will respond to initial medical therapy followed by biliary decompression, but 10 – 15 % will undergo clinical decompensation requiring emergent decompression [14, 15].

In the past, surgical drainage by cholecystectomy and common bile duct decompression was the only method of decompression available; in the emergency setting the mortality was as high as 40 % [7]. Currently, the less invasive techniques of ERCP and PTC have technical success rates that exceed 90 %. There are class I data to demonstrate ERCP is the safest and most efficacious treatment for acute cholangitis. The success rate is greater than 90 %, and the mortality rate of 10 % is considerably lower than that of surgery [16].

Through ERCP a sphincterotomy can be performed to facilitate drainage and removal of calculi. Alternatively, a temporizing stent or nasobiliary tube may be placed. Complications of ERCP include pancreatitis, perforation, hemorrhage, aspiration, systemic sepsis, and failure to clear the duct.

Percutaneous transhepatic biliary drainage can be used to treat cholangitis in over 90 % of cases, but it carries 30 % morbidity from complications such as hemorrhage, pneumothorax, subphrenic abscess, and bile peritonitis. The mortality for PTC is estimated to be between 5 % and 10 %, similar to that of ERCP [1, 17]. Although the morbidity is higher, PTC may be used preferentially in situations such as intrahepatic choledocholithiasis, intrasegmental cholangitis from proximal bile duct stricture or neoplasm, or when ERCP is not feasible secondary to surgically altered upper gastrointestinal tract anatomy (e.g., after Roux-en-Y reconstruction) or challenging native anatomic variations (such as when the ampulla of Vater is located within a duodenal diverticulum).

Surgery is now used infrequently in the primary management of acute cholangitis. In situations that require surgery to address an underlying problem, as in the case of cholangitis caused by a resectable malignant obstruction, patients may often be temporized by ERCP or PTC. This converts an emergency operation with its attendant mortality into an elective procedure, which can be performed at lower risk after the patient has been stabilized. Surgery is indicated in patients who fail less invasive treatment methods, and standard surgical therapy consists of a cholecystectomy, choledochotomy, biliary drainage, and T-tube placement. Techniques to perform this technique laparoscopically have been developed, but are not in every surgeon's armamentarium.

In a case of mild cholangitis as a result of choledocholithiasis, the patient should undergo elective cholecystectomy (either after ERCP or intraoperative common bile duct exploration) upon recovery to prevent further episodes. In the event that the patient is not a candidate for such a procedure, the patient should be monitored expectantly.

55.2 Liver Abscess

The underlying etiology and treatment of pyogenic liver abscesses has shifted dramatically in the past century. At the turn of the twentieth century, hepatic abscesses were typically the result of intra-abdominal bacterial infections, most commonly appendicitis; in the pre-antibiotic era, cure depended upon prompt surgical drainage. With the advent of antimicrobial agents, primary infection seeding the liver via the portal vein has greatly diminished as a cause of hepatic abscess. The most common cause of liver abscesses is now ascending biliary tract infection [18] (e.g., cholangitis, direct extension of acute suppurative cholecystitis).

The incidence of hepatic abscess ranges from 8 to 20 cases per 100,000 hospital admissions [19]. The average age of presentation is in the 6th decade of life. Most published series suggest that hepatic abscesses occur fairly uniformly across gender, geographic, and ethnic lines. Hepatic abscesses can be categorized by site of route of invasion into the liver; 30 – 60 % arise from the infection of the biliary tree. Seeding from the portal vein accounts for 10 – 25 % of abscesses and is typically a result of intra-abdominal sources of infection such as diverticulitis. Systemic seeding via the hepatic artery occurs in 1 – 10 % of cases from processes such as bacterial endocarditis, dental abscesses, or interventions such as hepatic artery chemoembolization, intraoperative cryoablation, or radiofrequency ablation [18]. These techniques directed at unresectable malignant liver neoplasms result in necrosis of tumor and hepatic parenchyma; secondary superinfection leading to abscess formation may occur. Direct extension from adjacent organ infection (e.g., cholecystitis or pyelonephritis) causes 2 – 10 % of cases, whereas rarer causes include blunt and penetrating trauma to the liver (<1 %). Liver abscess complicates fewer than 1 % of blunt liver injuries managed non-operatively and is more common in patients requiring damage-control laparotomy and perihepatic packing to control hemorrhage [20]. Liver abscess may be cryptogenic in 25 – 50 % of cases [21], but further investigation of the biliary tree may reveal a biliary source in more than half of these patients [22].

The most common presenting symptoms in patients with pyogenic hepatic abscess are fever and chills, abdominal pain, and weight loss. A history of non-specific abdominal complaints and constitutional symptoms is common, and presentation can range from the appearance of a chronic disease state to overt septic shock. The laboratory workup demonstrates leukocytosis in most patients, with liver enzymes being moderately abnormal as well. Alanine aminotransferase (ALT), aspartate aminotransferase (AST), and serum bilirubin concentration may demonstrate only mild elevations except in patients with underlying liver disease, who may have more pronounced abnormalities. Of the liver enzymes, alkaline phosphatase is most sensitive, being elevated out of proportion to ALT and AST in approximately two-thirds of patients [21].

Due to the protean manifestations of liver abscess and the number of disease processes that may share a similar presentation, radiographic imaging is crucial in confirming the diagnosis. Ultrasound and CT are the two most frequently employed modalities of investigation, both having greater than 95 % sensitivity. One-

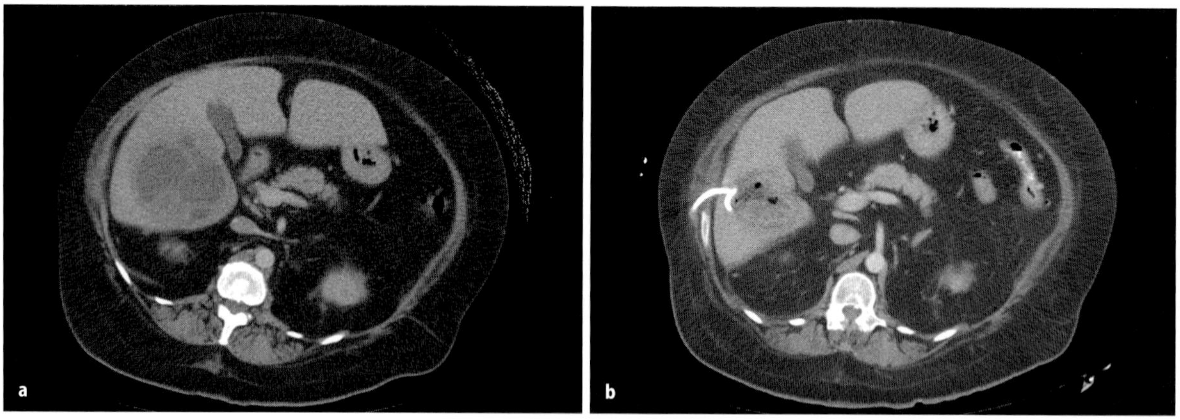

Fig. 55.2. a CT findings of multiloculated pyogenic abscess of the right lobe of the liver. **b** Successful CT-guided drainage of multiloculated pyogenic abscess of the right lobe of the liver

half of patients will present with more than one abscess, and approximately 75% of all liver abscesses will be found in the right lobe of the liver [23]. Both CT (Fig. 55.2A, B) and ultrasound can be used to perform guided drainage, but ultrasonic drainage is advantageous in that it can be used at the bedside of the critically ill patient. Magnetic resonance imaging is more costly and time-consuming than either US or CT, but may be more sensitive in discriminating between pyogenic liver abscesses and primary or secondary malignant liver tumors.

Pyogenic liver abscesses are equally likely to be polymicrobial as monomicrobial, and approximately 5–27% show no growth in culture. In many cases, failure to speciate bacteria in culture may reflect that the patients have been treated with antibiotics prior to specimen collection. The bacteriologic flora found in liver abscesses seems to reflect the underlying source of the infection, but overall the most common gram-negative aerobes found in pyogenic liver abscesses are *E. coli* and *Klebsiella* spp., while the most common gram positive aerobes found are *Enterococcus* spp., *S. viridans*, and *S. aureus*. Among cultured anaerobes, *Bacteroides* species predominate [19].

Options for treatment range from antibiotics alone to open surgical drainage. Historically, medical management of pyogenic liver abscess carries a mortality of 60–100% [24]. However, several recent case series demonstrate success rates of up to 80% when multiple (miliary) abscesses, too small or too numerous for percutaneous drainage, are treated with antibiotics alone; for carefully selected cases this may be a reasonable starting approach [23]. Although antibiotics are a necessary adjunct to the treatment of hepatic abscesses, most authorities agree that this approach is not sufficient except in the case of very small abscesses or in patients in whom intervention poses a prohibitive risk. The preferred method of treatment is broad-spectrum antibiotics in conjunction with drainage of all abscesses. For most of the twentieth century, open surgery was the only method available for drainage; today most hepatic abscesses can be treated successfully by image-guided percutaneous techniques. Computed tomography and ultrasound-guided drainage catheter placement both carry a success rate of 70–93%. Image-guided needle aspiration may also be employed in the treatment of small hepatic abscesses. Success rates between the two techniques are equivalent, but 50% of all patients undergoing needle aspiration will require more than one aspiration [25].

Surgical drainage is indicated in patients who fail percutaneous management, require surgical management of the underlying problem, or have abscesses that are not amenable to minimally invasive techniques because of their location. Surgical options include simple drainage and formal resection. Prior to the era of percutaneous drainage the optimum surgical approach was much debated; for anterior abscesses, a standard right subcostal incision is used. Posterior abscesses may be accessed through the bed of the 12th rib, whereas abscesses in the dome of the liver may be drained trans-diaphragmatically, albeit with an increased risk of empyema. Liver resection should be considered in those patients with extensive tissue loss or with intrahepatic stones, which may serve as a nidus for recurrent infection.

In the early 1900s the mortality associated with hepatic abscess was reported to approach 80%; today, most series quote a mortality rate of between 6% and 31% [18]. Factors associated with worse prognosis include an underlying diagnosis of malignant disease, multiple abscesses, and a high presenting Acute Physiology and Chronic Health Evaluation (APACHE) II score [26].

55.3 Amebic Liver Abscess

Amebic liver abscess is the most common extraintestinal sequela of *E. histolytica* infection, but occurs in only 1% of afflicted patients. Uncommon in North America, *E. histolytica* is endemic in parts of Central and South America, sub-Saharan Africa, India, and Indonesia. The typical patient is a male in the third to fourth decade of life who resides in or has recently traveled to an endemic area. Liver abscess may occur as early as 4 days after exposure but typically takes 2–4 weeks to develop [27]. Risk factors for development of amebic liver abscess include immunodeficiency states such as human immunodeficiency virus infection, underlying malignant disease, poor nutrition, corticosteroid use, and after splenectomy [27].

As in patients with pyogenic liver abscess, those with amebic liver abscess most commonly present with fever and chills, abdominal pain, and weight loss. Jaundice occurs less commonly than in pyogenic liver abscesses, being found in only 10% of patients [28]. Whereas patients with amebic liver abscess may have a history of dysenteric symptoms, most will not have concurrent symptoms upon presentation.

The most common laboratory abnormality is leukocytosis. Alkaline phosphatase is elevated in 80% of patients with chronic presentations, but may not be elevated in the acute setting. Aspartate aminotransferase (AST) is elevated in only 25% of patients, and hyperbilirubinemia is rare. Suspicion of amebic liver abscess should prompt measurement of amebic serology as measured by the indirect hemagglutination test, which is positive in 90–100% of cases. If the test is negative and clinical suspicion remains high, serology should be rechecked in 7–10 days [27]. This test may be less useful in endemic areas, as serology may remain positive for up to 20 years in the case of a previous infection. Amebae will be detected by stool antigen in less than one-half of those presenting with amebic liver abscess [29].

Amebic abscess may be imaged with CT, US, or MRI, all of which are very sensitive but poorly specific for this entity. Computed tomography and MRI demonstrate round, well-demarcated lesions that are located in the right lobe in 75% of cases. Up to 50% of patients will have an elevated right hemidiaphragm on chest radiography [30].

In contradistinction to pyogenic liver abscesses, the mainstay of treatment for amebic liver abscess is antimicrobial therapy. The recommended treatment consists of metronidazole 750 mg orally or intravenously three times daily for 7–10 days, which carries a cure rate of greater than 90%. All patients who are treated for extraintestinal manifestations of amebiasis must also be treated with a luminal decontaminant such as paromomycin (30 mg/kg orally per day in three divided doses, for 10 days) to eradicate intestinal *E. histolytica* [29].

In the case where it is unclear whether a liver abscess is pyogenic, amebic, or amebic with pyogenic superinfection, needle aspiration or catheter drainage may be used to help make the diagnosis. Aspirate of amebic abscess consists primarily of necrotic hepatocytes and has a characteristic „anchovy paste" appearance. Upon microscopy the amebae will be seen less than 20% of the time. Percutaneous drainage may also be indicated when patients fail to respond to metronidazole within 96 h. Other relative indications for percutaneous drainage include a lesion size greater than 5 cm or for abscesses in the left lobe of the liver, which are believed to have a higher risk of rupture than abscesses in other portions of the liver [30].

Complications of amebic liver abscess include rupture of the abscess into the pleura, pericardium, or peritoneum. These events happen rarely but may be catastrophic when they occur. Uncomplicated amebic liver abscess has an excellent prognosis, with a mortality of less than 1% for uncomplicated disease. Mortality may be higher in complicated cases and has been shown to be associated with hyperbilirubinemia, hypoalbuminemia, large abscess cavity volume, and multiple abscesses [31].

55.4 Echinoccoccal Liver Disease

Cystic hydatid disease must be considered in patients presenting with cholangitis associated with cavitary lesions of the liver. This clinical entity is rare in developed countries but remains a problem in South and Central America, the Middle East, some sub-Saharan countries, and parts of Asia and the former Soviet Union. Both *Echinococcus granulosus* and *E. multilocularis* may cause cystic hydatid disease in humans, but *E. granulosus* accounts for roughly 95% of cases.

The definitive hosts of the tapeworm *E. granulosus* are dogs, wolves, and foxes. The adult form of the parasite lives and lays eggs in the small intestine of its host; these eggs contain embryos (known as oncospheres) that are then shed in the stool, only to be ingested by the sheep or other species (e.g., human beings), which serve as intermediate hosts. Once in the gastrointestinal tract of the intermediate host, the eggs hatch, releasing the oncospheres. These embryos penetrate the intestinal mucosa of the host and migrate to distant organs via the bloodstream or lymphatics. Once in the viscera, the oncospheres develop into multilayered cystic cavities that eventually give rise to the adult forms of the parasite. These cysts may occur anywhere throughout the body, but the vast majority occur in the liver

(68%), lung (17%), kidney (3.7%) and spleen (2.8%) [32, 33].

Most human beings infected with *E. granulosus* are asymptomatic. In the initial phase of the disease, the hydatid cyst is dormant and does not cause major pathology. The cyst may remain in this asymptomatic state for the life of the host, or complications of infection may occur as growth occurs. The presenting signs and symptoms of hydatid cyst disease will vary based on the underlying behavior of the cyst; if the cyst expands and exerts a mass effect on adjacent structures, patients may present with jaundice, hepatomegaly, or ascites from portal vein compression. The cyst may also rupture into the biliary tree, resulting in the clinical picture of obstructive jaundice, cholangitis, or liver abscess as detritus from the cyst obstructs the biliary tree.

Liver enzymes in patients with hydatid disease of the liver may be normal or demonstrate elevations in AST, ALT, and serum bilirubin concentration. When rupture occurs, these elevations may be marked and associated with eosinophilia and hyperamylasemia [32]. Serologic diagnosis of *E. granulosus* infection can be made using enzyme-linked immunosorbent assay (ELISA) with a sensitivity of 84–94% [14, 34]; similar tests for *E. multilocularis* are slightly more specific (95–100%) [2].

Computed tomography, US, and MRI may all be used to image the liver in echinococcal disease. The sensitivity of CT for detecting hydatid cyst disease in the liver ranges between 61% and 96% [35, 36], whereas the sensitivity of ultrasound is 90–95%. The major advantage of CT over US is in imaging the number and size of hepatic cysts, as well as the presence of extrahepatic disease [37, 38]. In addition, CT may be more useful than US in imaging suspected rupture of echinococcal cysts. Magnetic resonance imaging is more time-consuming and costly than CT, but may be more sensitive in demonstrating communication between a cyst and the biliary tree.

When the diagnosis is uncertain despite thorough radiologic and serologic investigation, ERCP is the next test of choice. Endoscopic retrograde cholangiopancreatography may reveal communication between cysts and the biliary tree or intraductal filling defects. In patients with obstructive symptoms or cholangitis, a sphincterotomy may be performed and the common bile duct swept clean of debris as a temporizing measure prior to definitive treatment.

Medical therapy for echinococcal cyst disease consists oral benzimidazoles, with albendazole being the agent of choice because of its superior gastrointestinal absorption. Whereas antihelminthic therapy plays an important adjunctive role in the treatment of hydatid cyst disease, medical therapy alone is ineffective in 70% of cases [39]. Definitive treatment typically consists of drainage of the cyst cavity and sterilization of its contents with a scolicidal agent. Options for cyst evacuation and sterilization include open surgical technique, laparoscopic surgery, and percutaneous intervention. All techniques are similar in that the cyst is first cannulated and aspirated, at which point a scolicidal agent (most often hypertonic saline or ethanol) is instilled for a set period of time. Scolicidal agents should be used with great care in cases where the cyst has been demonstrated to communicate with the biliary tree because the bile ducts will also be exposed. For this reason, formalin should never be used for this purpose as it has been associated with the development of bile duct sclerosis [40]. Open surgery allows for more controlled evacuation of cyst contents than do either laparoscopic or percutaneous approaches; morbidity is increased and hospitalization is prolonged stay but cysts can be drained that are located in regions of the liver which are not amenable to laparoscopic or percutaneous approaches. Techniques described range from simple drainage, to resection of the cyst without violation of the cyst wall (pericystectomy), to formal hepatic resection.

55.5 Calculous Cholecystitis

Calculous cholecystitis occurs when gallstones migrate from the gallbladder into the cystic duct, causing outflow obstruction. This obstruction causes inflammation and edema of the gallbladder wall, which is initially sterile but may be followed by bacterial superinfection; bile cultures at the time of cholecystectomy for acute cholecystitis are positive in only 15–30% of cases [41]. Acute calculous cholecystitis presents with fever, right upper quadrant pain, nausea, and vomiting. Physical examination may range from arrest of inspiration due to tenderness on palpation in the right upper quadrant (Murphy sign) to guarding with rebound tenderness in advanced cases marked by peritonitis. Concomitant jaundice may occur and suggests the presence of choledocholithiasis. Leukocytosis is common, whereas liver enzymes are typically elevated in uncomplicated cases of acute cholecystitis. Ultrasound is a highly sensitive and specific test (95% and 97%, respectively) for acute cholecystitis and is the initial test of choice. Diagnostic findings include the presence of stones in the gallbladder, thickening of the gallbladder wall (>3.5 mm), pericholecystic fluid, and tenderness with application of the US probe (sonographic Murphy sign) [42].

Computed tomography is less sensitive in the diagnosis of acute calculous cholecystitis than US, but may also demonstrate thickening of the gallbladder wall, pericholecystic fluid, and gallstones. It is important to note that the majority of gallbladder calculi are not radiopaque and thus may not be visualized on CT. Nuclear scintigraphy may also be used to demonstrate nonfilling of the gallbladder, suggesting obstruction of the cystic duct; this study is less useful in patients with serum bilirubin >3 mg/dl, as this test is based upon hepatic excretion of the scintigraphic agent. When biliary cultures are positive in cases of acute calculous cholecystitis, typical pathogens include *Enterococcus* spp., *Klebsiella* spp., and Enterobacteriaceae [19].

Most cases of acute calculous cholecystitis resolve with bowel rest, fluid resuscitation, and intravenous antibiotics, and are ultimately treated by surgical removal of the gallbladder. If the patient initially responds to medical therapy, cholecystectomy can either be performed 24–48 h after admission or 6 weeks later as an elective procedure. Approximately 80% of patients will respond initially to medical therapy; the remainder progress rapidly to gangrene and perforation of the gallbladder with subsequent development of subhepatic abscess or peritonitis. These patients clearly warrant admission to the intensive care unit for resuscitation prior to definitive treatment. Gangrene of the gallbladder is associated with a 30% mortality rate and unfortunately tends to occur in older, sicker patients [43]. Emphysematous cholecystitis is a severe manifestation of acute cholecystitis that occurs with a predilection for elderly and diabetic patients. It is defined by the presence of gas in the gallbladder wall as visualized on US or CT and is characterized polymicrobial infection including *Clostridium* spp., *E. coli*, *Klebsiella* spp., and *Streptococcus* spp. Roughly one-half of all cases of emphysematous cholecystitis are acalculous; the reported mortality ranges from 15% to 25% [44, 45].

Gallstone pancreatitis may coexist in up to 5% of patients presenting with acute calculous cholecystitis; whereas most common duct stones will pass spontaneously; ERCP to clear the common bile duct and ampulla is mandatory in the presence of persistent obstruction. Cholecystectomy should be performed on the same hospital admission after resolution of pancreatitis. Rarely, gallstones may fistulize to the bowel and present as obstruction (gallstone ileus). Treatment is by surgical exploration, enterotomy, and removal of the offending stone; whether or not cholecystectomy and fistula excision should be performed at the same operation is a matter of some debate in surgical circles and depends upon the clinical status of the patient and the findings at laparotomy.

55.6 Acalculous Cholecystitis

The diagnosis of acalculous cholecystitis must always be entertained in the patient with sepsis for whom no clear source of infection can be determined. Defined as cholecystitis in the absence of cholelithiasis, cases of acalculous cholecystitis have been reported in age groups ranging from pediatric to geriatric but most often occur in the setting of severe illness or injury. It may also occur in the postoperative setting, particularly in men after emergency surgery complicated by large-volume blood loss. One review of 31,710 cases of cardiac surgery found a 0.05% incidence of acalculous cholecystitis [46]; in open abdominal aortic aneurysm repair, the incidence has been reported to be between 0.7% and 0.9% [47, 48]. Acalculous cholecystitis has also been described in the adult outpatient population, particularly in elderly men with atherosclerotic disease [49, 50].

The etiology of acalculous cholecystitis has yet to be elucidated fully, but it is most likely to be a manifestation of splanchnic ischemia-reperfusion injury. Alternatively, biliary stasis associated with critical illness may lead to distention of the gallbladder, which in combination with hypoperfusion may cause ischemia and ultimately necrosis. Factors such as mechanical ventilation, total parenteral nutrition use, cytokine activation, and endotoxemia have also been implicated [51].

Acute acalculous cholecystitis is more likely to be complicated than calculous disease; necrosis of the gallbladder is found in over 50% of cases, whereas perforation occurs in 20% of cases. A grave condition in patients who are often already critically ill, the mortality for acute acalculous cholecystitis approaches 30% [52].

The diagnosis of acalculous cholecystitis can be difficult to make. Patients who are able to communicate may report abdominal pain localizing to the right upper quadrant or diffuse pain in the case of peritonitis. Fever is usually present. Physical examination may reveal signs ranging from localized tenderness in the right upper quadrant to frank peritonitis. A right upper quadrant mass consisting of the gallbladder or a phlegmon may be palpable. All too often, however, the al-

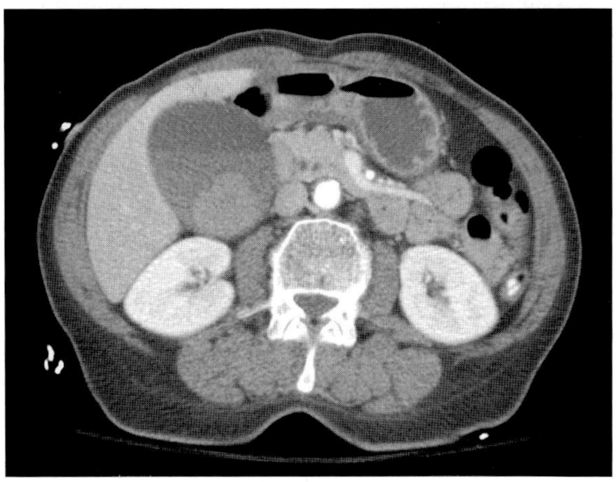

Fig. 55.3. Hemorrhagic acalculous cholecystitis imaged by CT scan. Clot (solid matter) and unclotted blood (fluid density within the bile) is visible within the lumen of a markedly distended gallbladder

tered mental status that accompanies critical illness may obscure any useful information that might be obtained from the history and physical examination. Laboratory values are non-specific but usually include leukocytosis and elevated liver enzymes, particularly of bilirubin, transaminases, and alkaline phosphatase. Hyperbilirubinemia, perhaps representative of the cholestasis of sepsis, is typical and occurs more often than in calculous cholecystitis.

Ultrasound is perhaps the ideal radiologic study to investigate the diagnosis of acalculous cholecystitis [53]. Ultrasound may reveal hydrops of the gallbladder, pericholecystic fluid, or gallbladder wall thickening. When a cut-off of 3.5 mm is used for wall thickness, US has a sensitivity of 98.5 % and a specificity of 80 % [54]. Ultrasound is also convenient in that it can be done at the bedside of patients too ill to be transported to the radiology suite and followed immediately by percutaneous drainage. Computed tomography is equally accurate in the diagnosis of acalculous cholecystitis [55] (Fig. 55.3), but requires that the patient be stable enough to be transported. The primary advantage of CT scan over US is the ability to evaluate other potential sources of intra-abdominal infection. Whereas a radionucleotide biliary scan is an excellent diagnostic modality for patients with community-onset acute cholecystitis, interpretation in critically ill patients can be confounded by false-positive scans due to fasting, liver disease, or parenteral nutrition, which are sufficiently common to diminish the utility of radionucleotide imaging in this population.

Upon making the diagnosis of acalculous cholecystitis, a decision about the method of source control must be made and empiric antibiotic therapy must be started. Even though up to one-half of cases of acute acalculous cholecystitis are associated with culture-negative bile (at least initially, considering that ischemia-reperfusion is paramount and superinfection is a secondary phenomenon), empiric antibiotics are needed because distinguishing sterile from infected cases can be clinically impossible owing to the massive inflammatory response. The organisms most frequently cultured from the bile in acalculous cholecystitis are *E. coli*, *Klebsiella* spp., and *E. faecalis* [51]. In the setting of critical illness, consideration for patterns of antimicrobial resistance amongst local bacterial flora must be considered when instituting empiric intravenous antibiotic therapy.

The treatment of cholecystitis, whether calculous or acalculous, has traditionally been by cholecystectomy. However, patients with acalculous cholecystitis are often critically ill at the time of diagnosis and may be poor surgical candidates. In the past decade, other methods of source control have been investigated. Percutaneous cholecystostomy tube placement is a minimally invasive alternative to surgical removal of the gallbladder that is increasingly favored over cholecystectomy [56, 57]. It can be performed with <10 % morbidity and has a mortality rate of 20–36 % [58], similar to that seen in open surgery and reflective of the serious nature of this complication for the critically ill patient. In this technique, the gallbladder is punctured through an anterior transhepatic approach under US guidance and a drainage catheter is placed using the Seldinger technique. A tube study may be performed at the time of catheter placement to confirm that the gallbladder communicates with the biliary tree (i.e., the cystic duct is patent). If it does not and concomitant cholangitis is suspected, further drainage of the biliary tree must be performed with ERCP or PTC. Complications of percutaneous cholecystostomy include hemorrhage, biliary peritonitis, and tube dislodgement. Hypotension may occur at the time of tube placement and is presumed to be caused by procedure-related bacteremia. Patients with uncomplicated acalculous cholecystitis should improve rapidly after gallbladder decompression; failure to improve should raise suspicions of an incorrect diagnosis or inadequate source control. Under such conditions, open exploration is mandated.

Upon resolution of acalculous cholecystitis, patients treated with percutaneous cholecystostomy may safely have their tubes removed once a normal tube study has been completed (e.g., the cystic duct is demonstrated to be patent). Percutaneous cholecystostomy is definitive treatment in this group.

55.7 Postoperative Biliary Tract Infections

Perihepatic infections may occur as a result of commonly performed hepatobiliary surgical procedures. Postoperative bile leaks may occur after any operation

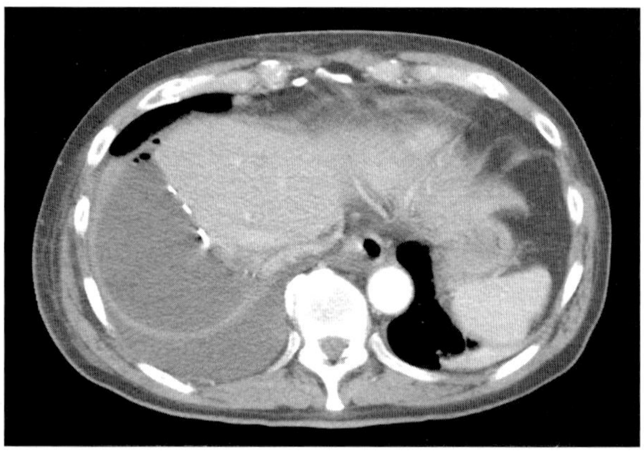

Fig. 55.4. A CT of the abdomen demonstrating a biloma after right hepatectomy for hepatocellular carcinoma. An abscess within the larger biloma (surrounded by the contrast-enhanced rim of tissue) is evident

in which a portion of the biliary tree is transected [such as hepatectomy (Fig. 55.4), hepatico-enterostomy, orthotopic liver transplantation, or cholecystectomy]. This fluid may then become infected secondarily by microbial flora introduced at the time of operation, bacteria present in the biliary tree from preoperative instrumentation, or by translocation from the gut, leading to an infected intrahepatic or perihepatic collection known as a biloma.

Laparoscopic cholecystectomy is one of the most frequently performed operations in the world and is generally safe and well tolerated. Bile leaks, however, occur in up to 1% of patients undergoing laparoscopic cholecystectomy. Removal of the gallbladder may lead to bile leakage from the transected cystic duct, the hepatic bed of the gallbladder, or from incidental injury to other portions of the biliary tree during dissection. Patients with postoperative bile collections may present with right upper quadrant pain, fever, nausea, vomiting or jaundice, but the presence of bile in the abdomen even when no infection is present may cause a sterile peritonitis. Discrimination between sterile bile peritonitis and infection may be difficult without culture of the collection. Postoperative fluid collections may be imaged with a variety of studies including US, CT, and MRI. Diagnosis of bile leakage can be made either by image-guided aspiration of the collection or nuclear scintigraphy. Whereas nuclear scintigraphy is an excellent study for making the diagnosis of bile leak, it is not useful in determining the origin of the leak. For this reason ERCP is used to determine the anatomy of the biliary leak, with some leaks being amenable to concomitant endoscopic therapy.

Treatment of postoperative bile leakage hinges first upon drainage and then definitive treatment targeted at addressing the underlying problem. If the leak originates from the bed of the gallbladder, percutaneous drainage alone is indicated. Extravasation of bile from the cystic duct is best managed endoscopically by stent placement with or without sphincterotomy to allow bile to drain preferentially through the ampulla rather than via the cystic duct [59]. Major duct injuries discovered at ERCP generally require surgical management.

Although the mortality of liver resection has decreased in the last several decades, morbidity rates still approach 50% in some large series. Perihepatic and intra-abdominal abscess complicates 8–30% of major liver resections and is associated with preoperative biliary stenting, hepaticoenterostomy, increased operative time, greater extent of resection, and the need for blood transfusion [20, 60]. Preoperative hyperbilirubinemia as a result of biliary obstruction occurs frequently in patients with biliary tract malignancies (e.g., cholangiocarcinoma, hepatocellular carcinoma) and current literature suggests that such patients are at increased risk for complications of surgical resection [61]. For this reason, preoperative biliary stenting has been investigated as a means to reduce postoperative morbidity. Recent data demonstrate clearly that preoperative stent placement to alleviate biliary obstruction leads to increased rates of bactibilia and postoperative infectious complications [62, 63].

Resection of hepatic parenchyma leaves dead space in the abdomen that collects bile and blood and is in proximity to ischemic tissue at the resection line. Bacterial superinfection may occur, leading to the formation of a perihepatic or intrahepatic abscess. Infected bilomas are heralded by fever, right upper quadrant pain, leukocytosis, and elevated liver enzymes. Imaging modalities for post-hepatectomy abscesses include CT (Fig. 55.4), US and MRI as discussed in the prior section on pyogenic hepatic abscess. Cultures reveal that 50–75% of postoperative perihepatic abscesses are polymicrobial, with bacteria of enteric origin (e.g., *E. coli, Enterococcus* spp.) predominating [3]. Image-guided percutaneous drainage is the treatment of choice where feasible, with re-operation reserved for those patients in whom percutaneous drainage is not possible or unsuccessful.

Liver transplantation is the only long-term treatment modality available for patients with end-stage liver disease. Despite recent advances in surgical technique and perioperative management, transplantation is plagued by complication rates ranging from 24% to 64%. The incidence of biliary leak after orthotopic liver transplantation is between 10% and 40%, with these leaks most commonly arising from hepatic resection lines, T-tube sites and biliary anastomoses [64]. Patients may have symptoms and laboratory values as described above and may present up to 6 months after transplantation. Computed tomography is used to image the collection, which may be intrahepatic in up to two-thirds of cases. Endoscopic retrograde cholangiopancreaticography, PTC, or cholangiogram through a pre-existing T-tube may be used to delineate the origin of the leak. Most collections may be drained percutaneously, and in the event of direct communication with the biliary tree ERCP can be used to re-establish preferential enteric drainage. Because the blood supply to the biliary tree is derived from the hepatic artery, anastomotic leaks in the transplant setting may occur as a result of ischemia from hepatic artery thrombosis. For this reason assessment of the patency of the graft hepatic artery must be determined. Whereas some cases of biloma associated with hepatic artery thrombosis may respond to more conservative measures, up to two-thirds will require re-transplantation [65].

Cholangitis may also occur in the postoperative setting, particularly when an anastomosis has been created directly between the biliary tree and intestine. Such a construction allows for reflux of enteric bacteria into the biliary tree and may be exacerbated by stenosis at the anastomotic site. Because of surgically altered anatomy, the anastomotic site may not be amenable to ERCP, in which case PTC may be performed. Recurrent cholangitis that fails less invasive intervention may ultimately require surgical revision or retransplantation [65].

55.8 Cholestasis of Sepsis

Sepsis has been described as a cause of jaundice in the critically ill patient for well over 150 years, but only in the past several decades have strides have been made in revealing the underlying pathogenesis. Endotoxemia as a result of systemic infection leads to intrahepatic cholestasis, resulting in clinical jaundice [66]. Investigation on the molecular level has elucidated the relevant mechanisms. Animal models demonstrate that endotoemia has a plethora of effects on both hepatocytes and bile duct epithelial cells. Portal vein perfusion with endotoxin leads to a significant decrease in basal bile flow and bile acid secretion [67]. This reduction in flow can be ameliorated by pre-treatment with dexamethasone, which blocks endotoxin-mediated release of cytokines such as tumor necrosis factor (TNF)-α and interleukin (IL)-1 [68]. Endotoxin-mediated reduction in bile flow is prevented by administration of anti-TNF antibodies [69]. Current evidence suggests that endotoxin and cytokines act on hepatocytes at the cellular level by causing down-regulation and redistribution of cell membrane transport proteins responsible for bile-acid dependent bile flow at the canicular membrane. Consistent with this mechanism is the finding of direct hyperbilirubinemia in the cholestasis of sepsis in the presence of otherwise normal or only mildly deranged liver function tests [62]. Elevated bilirubin reflecting endotoxemia may precede other clinical signs of infection and may be more pronounced in patients with pre-existing liver disease [63]. In the septic patient with hyperbilirubinemia, imaging studies are indicated to investigate the possibility of primary pathology of the liver or biliary tree. Once this has been ruled out therapeutic efforts are directed at identifying and eradicating the underlying source of infection.

References

1. Kadakia SC (1993) Biliary tract emergencies: acute cholecystitis, acute cholangitis, and acute pancreatitis. Med Clin North Am 77:1015
2. Lanier AP, Trujillo DE, Schantz PM, et al. (1987) Comparison of serologic tests for the diagnosis and follow-up of alveolar hydatid disease. Am J Trop Med Hyg 37:609
3. Krige JEJ, Bornman PC (2002) Infections in hepatic, biliary and pancreatic surgery. In: Blumgart L, Fong Y (eds) Surgery of the liver and biliary tract. Elsevier, London, p 151
4. Yusoff IF (2003) Diagnosis and management of cholecystitis and cholangitis. Gastroenterol Clin North Am 32:1145
5. Sung JY, Leung JWC, Shaffer EA, et al. (1992) Ascending infection of the biliary tract after surgical sphincterotomy and biliary stenting. J Gastroenterol Hepatol 7:240
6. Sung JY, Shaffer EA, Olson ME, et al. (1991) Bacterial invasion of the biliary system by way of the portal-venous system. Hepatology 14:313
7. Boey JH, Way LW (1980) Acute cholangitis. Ann Surg 191: 264
8. Pessa ME, Hawkins IF, Vogel SB (1987) The treatment of acute cholangitis: Percutaneous transhepatic biliary drainage before definitive therapy. Ann Surg 205:389
9. Shimada K, Noro T, Inamatsu T, et al. (1981) Bacteriology of acute obstructive suppurative cholangitis of the aged. J Clin Microbiol 14:522
10. Thompson JE, Jr, Pitt HA, Doty JE, et al. (1990) Broad spectrum penicillin as an adequate therapy for acute cholangitis. Surg Gynecol Obstet 171:275
11. Leung JW, Ling TK, Chan RC, et al. (1994) Antibiotics, biliary sepsis, and bile duct stones. Gastrointest Endosc 40: 716
12. Sung JJ, Lyon DJ, Suen R, et al. (1995) Intravenous ciprofloxacin as treatment for patients with acute suppurative cholangitis: a randomized, controlled clinical trial. J Antimicrob Chemother 35:855
13. Thompson J, Bennion RS, Pitt HA (1994) An analysis of infectious failures in acute cholangitis. HPB Surg 8:139
14. Hanau LH, Stiegbigel NH (2000) Acute (ascending) cholangitis. Infect Dis Clin North Am 14:521
15. Saik RP, Greenburg AG, Farris JM (1975) Spectrum of cholangitis. Am J Surg 130:143
16. Sugiyama M, Atomi Y (1998) The benefits of endoscopic nasobiliary drainage without sphincterotomy for acute cholangitis. Am J Gastroenterol 93:2065
17. Joseph PK, Bizer LS, Sprayregen SS, et al. (1986) Percutaneous transhepatic biliary drainage: results and complications in 81 patients. JAMA 255:2763
18. Huang C, Pitt HA, Lipsett PA, et al. (1996) Pyogenic hepatic abscess. Changing trends over 42 years. Ann Surg 223:600
19. Johannsen EC (2000) Pyogenic liver abscesses. Infect Dis Clin North Am 14:547
20. Garwood RA, Sawyer RG, Thompson L, et al. (2004) Infectious complications after hepatic resection. Am Surg 70: 787
21. Kaplan GG, Gregson DB, Laupland KB (2004) Population-based study of the epidemiology of and the risk factors for pyogenic liver abscess. Clin Gastroenterol Hepatol 2:1032
22. Wong WM, Wong BCYM, Hui CK, et al. (2002) Pyogenic liver abscesses: retrospective analysis of 80 cases over a 10-year period. J Gastoenterol Hepatol 17:1001
23. Rahimian J, Wilson T, Oram V, et al. (2004) Pyogenic liver abscess: Recent trends in etiology and mortality. Clin Infect Dis 39:1654
24. Chu K, Fan S, Lai ECS, et al. (1996) Pyogenic liver abscess. An audit of experience over the last decade. Arch Surg 131:148
25. Yu SC, Ho SS, Lau WY, et al. (2004) Treatment of pyogenic liver abscess: prospective randomized comparison of catheter drainage and needle aspiration. Hepatology 39:932
26. Perez JAA, Gonzalez JJ, Baldonedo RF, et al. (2001) Clinical course, treatment, and multivariate analysis of risk factors for pyogenic liver abscess. Am J Surg 181:177
27. Seeto RK, Rockey DC (1999) Amebic liver abscess: Epidemiology, clinical features, and outcome. West J Med 170:104
28. Maltz G, Knauer CM (1991) Amebic liver abscess: A 15-year experience. Am J Gastroenterol 86:704

29. Haque R, Huston CD, Hughes M, et al. (2003) Amebiasis. N Engl J Med 348:1565
30. Stanley SL, Jr (2003) Amoebiasis. Lancet 361:1025
31. Sharma MP, Dasarathy, S, Verma, N, et al. (1996) Prognostic markers in amebic liver abscess: a prospective study. Am J Gastroenterol 91:2584
32. Aucott JN, Ravdin JI (1993) Amebiasis and „nonpathogenic" intestinal protozoa. Infect Dis Clin North Am 7:467
33. Grove DI, Warren KS, Mahmoud AAF (1976) Algorithms in the diagnosis and management of exotic diseases: Echinococcosis. J Infect Dis 133:354
34. Zarzosa MP, Orduna Domingo A, Gutierrez P, et al. (1999) Evaluation of six serological tests in diagnosis and postoperative control of pulmonary hydatid disease patients. Diagn Microbiol Infect Dis 35:255
35. Di Palma A, Ettorre GC, Scapati C (1991) The role of computerized tomography in the diagnosis of hydatid disease. Radiol Med 82:430
36. Miguet JP, Bresson-Hadni S, Vuitton D (1989) Echinococcosis of the liver. In: McIntyre N, Benhamou JP, Bircher J, et al. (eds) Oxford textbook of clinical hepatology. Oxford University Press, Oxford, p 721
37. Dhar P, Chaudhary A, Desai R, et al. (1996) Current trends in the diagnosis and management of cystic hydatid disease of the liver. J Commun Dis 28:221
38. Safioleas M, Misiakos E, Manti C, et al. (1994) Diagnostic evaluation and surgical management of hydatid disease of the liver. World J Surg 18:859
39. Balik AA, Basoglu M, Çelebi F, et al. (1999) Surgical treatment of hydatid disease of the liver: review of 304 cases. Arch Surg 134:166
40. Ammann RW, Eckert J (1996) Cestodes. Echinococcus. Gastroenterol Clin North Am 25:655
41. Den-Hoed PT, Boelhouwer RU, Veen HF, et al. (1998) Infections and bacteriological data after laparoscopic and open gallbladder surgery J Hosp Infect 39:27
42. Shea A, Berlin JA, Escarce JJ, et al. (1994) Revised estimates of diagnostic test sensitivity and specificity in suspected biliary tract disease. Arch Intern Med 154:2573
43. Stefanidis D, Sirinek KR, Bingener J (2006) Gallbladder perforation: risk factors and outcome. J Surg Res 131:204
44. Garcia-Sancho Tellez L, Rodriguez-Montes JA, Fernandez de Lis S, et al. (1999) Acute emphysematous cholecystitis; report of twenty cases. Hepatogastroenterology 46:2144
45. Mentzer RM, Golden GT, Chandler JG, et al. (1975) A comparative appraisal of emphysematous cholecystitis. Am J Surg 129:10
46. Barie PS (1993) Acalculous and postoperative cholecystitis. In: Barie PS, Shires GT (eds) Surgical intensive care. Little, Brown, Boston, p 837
47. Hagino RT (1997) Acalculous cholecystitis after aortic reconstruction. J Am Coll Surg 184:245
48. Ouriel K, Green RM, Ricotta JJ, et al. (1984) Acute acalculous cholecystitis complicating abdominal aortic aneurysm resection. J Vasc Surg 1:646
49. Savoca PE, Longo WE, Zucker KA, et al. (1990) The increasing prevalence of acalculous cholecystitis in outpatients. Results of a 7-year study. Ann Surg 211:433
50. Ryu JK, Ryu KH, Kim KH (2003) Clinical features of acute acalculous cholecystitis. J Clin Gastroenterol 36:166
51. Barie PS, Eachempati SR (2003) Acute acalculous cholecystitis. Curr Gastroenterol Rep 5:302
52. Wang AJ, Wang TE, Lin CC, et al. (2003) Clinical predictors of severe gallbladder complications in acute acalculous cholecystitis. World J Gastroenterol 9:2821
53. Shuman WP (1984) Low sensitivity of sonography and cholescintigraphy in acalculous cholecystitis. AJR Am J Roentgenol 142:531
54. Deitch EA (1981) Acute acalculous cholecystitis: Ultrasonic diagnosis. Am J Surg 142:290
55. Mirvis SE (1987) CT diagnosis of acalculous cholecystitis. J Comput Assist Tomogr 11:83
56. Akhan O, Akinci D, Ozmen MN (2002) Percutaneous cholecystostomy. Eur J Radiol 43:229
57. Davis CA, Landercasper J, Gundersen LH, Lambert PJ (1999) Effective use of percutaneous cholecystostomy in high-risk surgical patients: Techniques, tube management, and results. Arch Surg 134:727
58. Byrne MF, Suhocki P, Mitchell RM, et al. (2003) Percutaneous cholecystostomy in patients with acute cholecystitis: experience of 45 patients at a US referral center. J Am Coll Surg 197:206
59. Cuschieri A (2002) Cholecystitis. In: Blumgart LH, Fong Y (eds) Surgery of the liver and biliary tract. WB Saunders, London, p 665
60. Jarnagin WR, Gonen M, Fong Y, et al. (2002) Improvement in perioperative outcome after hepatic resection. Ann Surg 236:397
61. Cherqui D, Benoist S, Benoit M, et al. (2000) Major liver resection for carcinoma in jaundiced patients without preoperative biliary drainage. Arch Surg 135:302
62. Hochwald SN, Burke EC, Jarnagin WR, et al. (1999) Association of preoperative biliary stenting with increased postoperative infectious complications in proximal cholangiocarcinoma. Arch Surg 134:261
63. Faust TW, Reddy KR (2004) Postoperative jaundice. Clin Liver Dis 8:151
64. Federle MP, Kapoor V (2003) Complications of liver transplantation imaging and intervention. Radiol Clin North Am 41:1289
65. Said A, Safdar N, Lucey MR, et al. (2004) Infected bilomas in liver transplant recipients, incidence, risk factors, and implications for prevention Am J Transplant 23:574
66. Hosotsubo K, Nishimura M, Nishimura S (2000) Hyperbilirubinaemia after major thoracic surgery: comparison between open-heart surgery and oesophagectomy. Crit Care 4:180
67. Roelofsen H, Shoemaker B, Bakker C, et al. (1995) Impaired hepatocanalicular organic anion transport in endotoxemic rats. Am J Physiol 269:427
68. Roelofsen H, Van Der Veere CN, Ottenhoff R, et al. (1994) Decreased bilirubin transport in the perfused liver of endotoxemic rats. Gastroenterology 107:1075
69. Whiting JF, Green RM, Rosenbluth AB, et al. (1995) Tumor necrosis factor-alpha decreases hepatocyte bile salt uptake and mediates endotoxin induced cholestasis. Hepatology 22:1273

Subject Index